2006

Nursing Spectrum DRUG Handbook

www.nursesdrughandbook.com

Common abbreviations

The abbreviations below are commonly used by nurses. Not all of them, however, are acceptable. Those in red marked with a Clinical Alert logo 🔊 were identified as contributing to medication errors in the 2004 National Patient Safety Goals of the Joint Commission on Accreditation of Healthcare Organizations (JCAHO) and by the Institute for Safe Medication Practices. To avoid mistakes and to ensure JCAHO compliancy, spell out the entire term.

Abbreviation	Term
ABG	arterial blood gas
a.c.	before meals
ACE	angiotensin-converting enzyme
ACLS	advanced cardiac life support
ACTH	adrenocorticotropic hormone
🔊 AD	right ear
ADH	antidiuretic hormone
ADLs	activities of daily living
AICD	automatic implantable cardiac defibrillator
AIDS	acquired immunodeficiency syndrome
ALP	alkaline phosphatase
ALT	alanine aminotransferase
APTT	activated partial thromboplastin time
🔊 AS	left ear
AST	aspartate aminotransferase
🔊 AU	each ear
AV	atrioventricular
B_1	beta$_1$
B_2	beta$_2$
BCLS	basic cardiac life support
b.i.d.	twice daily
BP	blood pressure
BSA	body surface area
🔊 B.T.	bedtime
BUN	blood urea nitrogen
$\bar{c}$	with
C	Celsius
cAMP	cyclic 3', 5' adenosine monophosphate
CBC	complete blood count
🔊 cc	cubic centimeter
CI	cardiac index
CK	creatine kinase
cm	centimeter
CMV	cytomegalovirus
CNS	central nervous system
COPD	chronic obstructive pulmonary disease
CR	controlled release
CV	cardiovascular
CVA	cerebrovascular accident
CYP	cytochrome
D_5W	dextrose 5% in water
DIC	disseminated intravascular coagulation
🔊 D/C	discharge, discontinue
dl	deciliter
DNA	deoxyribonucleic acid
ECG	electrocardiogram
EEG	electroencephalogram
EENT	eyes, ears, nose, and throat
F	Fahrenheit
FDA	Food and Drug Administration
g	gram
G	gauge
GABA	gamma-aminobutyric acid
GFR	glomerular filtration rate
GGT	gamma-glutamyltransferase
GI	gastrointestinal
GnRH	gonadotropin-releasing hormone
gr	grain
gtt	drops
G6PD	glucose-6-phosphate dehydrogenase
GU	genitourinary
H_1	histamine$_1$
H_2	histamine$_2$
HCL	hydrochloride

🔊 Clinical alert. **Do not use.**

HCT	hematocrit
HDL	high-density lipoprotein
Hg	mercury
Hgb	hemoglobin
HIV	human immunodeficiency virus
HMG-CoA	3-hydroxy-3-methylglutaryl coenzyme A
HR	heart rate
🔊 h.s.	at bedtime
🔊 H.S.	half-strength
🔊 I.J.	injection
I.M.	intramuscular
🔊 I.N.	intranasal
INR	International Normalized Ratio
IPPB	intermittent positive-pressure breathing
🔊 IU	international unit
I.V.	intravenous
K	potassium
kg	kilogram
KVO	keep vein open
L	liter
lb	pound
LD	lactate dehydrogenase
LDL	low-density lipoprotein
m	meter
m^2	square meters
🔊 µg	microgram
MAO	monoamine oxidase
mcg	microgram
MDI	metered-dose inhaler
mEq	milliequivalent
mg	milligram
🔊 $MgSO_4$	magnesium sulfate
ml	milliliter
mm	millimeter
mm^3	cubic millimeters
mm Hg	millimeters of mercury
mmol	millimole
🔊 MS	morphine sulfate
🔊 MSO_4	morphine sulfate
Na	sodium
NA	not applicable
NaCl	sodium chloride
ng	nanogram
NG	nasogastric
N.P.O.	nothing by mouth
NSAID	nonsteroidal anti-inflammatory drug
🔊 O.D.	right eye
🔊 O.S.	left eye
OTC	over the counter
🔊 O.U.	each eye
oz	ounce
p.c.	after meals
PCA	patient-controlled analgesia
per	through, by
P.O.	by mouth
P.R.	by rectum
p.r.n.	as needed
PT	prothrombin time
PTT	partial thromboplastin time
PVC	premature ventricular contraction
q	every
🔊 Q.D.	every day
🔊 q.h.s.	at bedtime
q.i.d.	four times daily
🔊 Q.O.D.	every other day
RBC	red blood cell
RDA	recommended dietary allowance
RNA	ribonucleic acid
RSV	respiratory syncytial virus
SA	sinoatrial
🔊 S.C.	subcutaneous
SI	International System of Units
SIADH	syndrome of inappropriate antidiuretic hormone secretion
S.L.	sublingual
🔊 S.Q.	subcutaneous
SSRI	selective serotonin reuptake inhibitor
T_3	triiodothyronine
T_4	thyroxine
TCA	tricyclic antidepressant
t.i.d.	three times daily
🔊 T.I.W.	three times a week
tRNA	transfer ribonucleic acid
tsp	teaspoon
🔊 U	unit
USP	United States Pharmacopeia
VMA	vanillylmandelic acid
WBC	white blood cell

🔊 Clinical alert. **Do not use.**

2006

Nursing Spectrum DRUG Handbook

2006 Nursing Spectrum DRUG Handbook

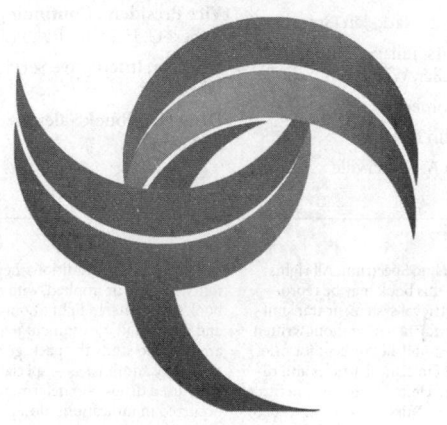

Patricia Dwyer Schull, RN, MSN

www.nursesdrughandbook.com

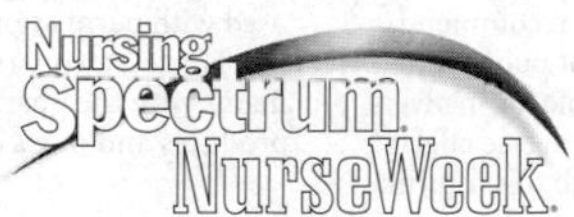

This book was developed by MedVantage Publishing, LLC, and published by Nursing Spectrum.

MedVantage Publishing Staff

Director: Patricia Dwyer Schull, RN, MSN

Clinical Manager: Minnie Bowen Rose, BSN, MEd

Editorial Manager: Kathy E. Goldberg

Design Manager: Stephanie Peters

Website Development Manager: Don Saul

Research Coordinator and Analyst: Lois Piano, RN, MSN, EdD

Clinical Editors: Julie M. Gerhart, MS, RPh; Cheryl A. Grandinetti, PharmD; Sandy Keefe, RN, MSN; Cynthia Saver, RN, MS; Jeannette Wick, RPh

Editors: Karen Comerford, Jessica Baskin Taylor, Doris Weinstock

Designers: Joseph J. Clark, Jan Greenberg

Editorial Assistants: Julia S. Knipe (supervisor), Judy A. Muller, William M. Schull

Indexer: Karen Comerford

Cover Design: John Hubbard

Illustrator: Kevin A. Somerville

Nursing Spectrum Staff

President and Publisher: Patti McCook Rager, RN, MSN, MBA

Executive Vice President, Professional Services: Fred J. DiCostanzo, RN, MA

Senior Vice President, Editorial Services/ Editor in Chief: Judith Mitiguy, RN, MS

Senior Vice President, Marketing and Research: John F. Leggett

Executive Vice President, Advertising, Marketing, and Interactive Services: Steven H. Hauber

Executive Vice President, Circulation, Production, and Systems: Melyni Serpa

Executive Vice President, Finance: Jim Filiaggi

Vice President, Continuing Education: Robert G. Hess, Jr., RN, PhD

Director, Interactive Services: Doug Jankowski

Drug Handbook Sales Associate: Lesley McGerald

 Printed in the United States of America. For information, write Nursing Spectrum, 2655 Villa Creek Dr., Suite 250, Dallas, TX 75234, or visit www.nursesdrughandbook.com.

ISSN: 1550-0543
ISBN-13: 978-1-930745-02-5
ISBN-10: 1-930745-02-8

A note from the publisher

Welcome to *2006 Nursing Spectrum Drug Handbook,* the second edition of our drug reference for nurses. We are so gratified with the response of practicing nurses, nursing students, and faculty members to our premier edition. Many busy professional nurses have taken the time to e-mail or write to us at Nursing Spectrum, thanking us for helping them stay current on drug administration. You have told us you love the depth of drug content, the safe drug administration insert, and the additional safety features integrated throughout the book. You have described the book as reliable, practical, concise, and clear, and have compared it favorably to other nursing drug handbooks. In addition, you've told us that the book's companion website, nursesdrughandbook.com, is user friendly, easy to navigate, and brimming with useful patient teaching materials and drug updates.

I am sure you'll be equally pleased with the enhancements you'll find in *2006 Nursing Spectrum Drug Handbook.* In an effort to make the second edition even better than the first, we asked dozens of nurses to evaluate the premier edition. Based on this feedback, the second edition—which you now hold in your hands—reflects key changes that will help you give medications more safely. Drug monographs have been updated, with new indications and Clinical Alerts included as appropriate. Brand new monographs have been added for newly approved drugs, and coverage of herbs and supplements has been expanded.

What's more, the book's safety theme is even more prominent. The full-color safe drug administration insert (a personal favorite of mine) has doubled in length to 32 pages and now includes several new treatment algorithms. Also, dark borders have been added so you can find the insert more easily. Many of the appendices have been updated or expanded, and new appendices have been added on such topics as life-threatening adverse reactions, anesthetic drugs, and infusion rates for commonly infused drugs. The book's companion website, nursesdrughandbook.com, now offers free PDA monograph downloads to give you quick access to information on many commonly prescribed drugs.

On a personal note, I'd like to express my gratitude to every nurse who purchased the premier edition of *Nursing Spectrum Drug Handbook.* Your enthusiastic reception of the book tells us that it's right on target with Nursing Spectrum's mission of educating, recognizing, and supporting nurses. I am pleased that we had the opportunity to add this important book to our portfolio of publications, programs, and services. Please consider this second edition proof of our continuing commitment to serving nurses.

Patti Rager, RN, MSN, MBA
President & Publisher
Nursing Spectrum

Contents

Part 3
Appendices

Foreword

Adverse drug events are the business of all health professionals, but they are of greatest importance to nurses. The Institute of Medicine put these errors on the national agenda in 1999 when its report *To Err is Human: Building a Safer Health System* identified adverse drug events (ADEs) as the cause of roughly 7,000 deaths annually.

Statistics published since then are equally alarming: In 2001, researchers estimated that ADEs injure or kill more than 770,000 hospital patients annually. A 2002 study published in the *New England Journal of Medicine* found that one in four patients suffered observable ADEs that year.

Because of these published statistics, a great deal of attention has been paid to error-reducing protocols and strategies by the nursing profession to ensure patient safety in drug administration. Guidelines have been established to create a safe working environment and to promote teamwork and better communication among colleagues.

In the battle against ADEs, nurses stand at the front lines, collectively administering drugs to millions of patients each day. The nurse carries out the final step in the administration process. She also performs patient assessment, which can reveal unique signs and symptoms of ADEs. In fact, nurses are the only health care team members who regularly detect and document ADE indicators visible at the bedside. A recent study found that nurses and RN case managers reported 84% of the serious ADEs documented in a healthcare facility's system.

To promptly and accurately detect ADEs, you must possess an adequate knowledge base—and an easily accessible source of accurate and up-to-date drug information. That's where *Nursing Spectrum Drug Handbook* comes in. Since the first edition was published a year ago, this book has become the trusted bedside drug reference of many thousands of nurses.

The reasons for this trust are obvious. Nurses find the book easy to use and easy to read. Most importantly, they value it because it helps them keep patients safe. The emphasis on safety comes through loud and clear, from the eye-catching Clinical Alerts in each monograph to the unique safe drug administration insert and the well-chosen appendix topics.

With all of this and more, *2006 Nursing Spectrum Drug Handbook* is indispensable for any nurse. I am confident it will quickly become the drug reference you turn to most often.

Harriet R. Feldman, RN, PhD, FAAN
Dean and Professor
Lienhard School of Nursing
Chair, Institutional Review Board
Pace University
Pleasantville and New York City, New York

Advisors

Vicki L. Buchda, RN, MS
Director of Nursing
Mayo Clinic in Scottsdale
Scottsdale, Ariz.

Pamela R. Dellinger, RN, PhD, CHCR
Recruitment Specialist
Lincoln Medical Center
Lincolnton, N.C.

Gloria F. Donnelly, RN, PhD, FAAN
Dean and Professor
College of Nursing and Health Professions
Drexel University
Philadelphia, Pa.

Harriet R. Feldman, RN, PhD, FAAN
Dean and Professor
Lienhard School of Nursing
Chair, Institutional Review Board
Pace University
Pleasantville and New York City, N.Y.

Linda Groah, RN, MS, CNOR, CNAA, FAAN
Director of Hospital Operations
Kaiser Permanente Medical Center
San Francisco, Calif.

David Hawkins, PharmD
Professor and Senior Associate Dean of Pharmacy
Southern School of Pharmacy
Mercer University
Atlanta, Ga.

Peggy Kalowes, RN, MSN, CNRN, PhD
Assistant Professor
Department of Nursing
California State University
Long Beach, Calif.

Terris E. Kennedy, RN, PhD
Chief Nursing Officer
Vice President for Patient Care Services
Shore Memorial Hospital
Nassawadox, Va.

James A. Koestner, BS, PharmD
Critical Care Pharmacist
Vanderbilt University Medical Center
Nashville, Tenn.

Ann Barrow McKenzie, RN, MSN
Coordinator of College Relations
College of Nursing
Villanova University
Villanova, Pa.

Claire M. Young, RN, MBA
Chief Nursing Officer
Chair, Division of Nursing
The Cleveland Clinic Foundation
Cleveland, Ohio

Contributors and reviewers

Sue Apple, RN, DNSc
Assistant Professor
School of Nursing and Health Studies
Georgetown University
Washington, D.C.

Nancy Balkon, PhD, ANP-C, APRN
Clinical Associate Professor
School of Nursing
Stony Brook University
Stony Brook, N.Y.

Cathy L. Bartels, PharmD, FAAIM
Associate Professor
Creighton University Medical Center
Omaha, Neb.

Barbara Barzoloski-O'Connor, RN, MSN
Infection Control Manager
Howard County General Hospital
Columbia, Md.

Melanie Boock, RN, BSN
Nursing Supervisor
Emergency Room Staff Nurse
Vail Valley Medical Center
Vail, Colo.

Vicky Borders-Hemphill, PharmD
Medical Writer
Clinton, Md.

Terry M. Bottomley, RN
Charge Nurse
Emergency Department
Wooster Community Hospital
Wooster, Ohio

Cheryl A. Bozman, RRT, RN, BSN
Clinical Educator
Oakwood Hospital and Medical Center
Dearborn, Mich.

Susan C. Braun, RN, MS
Clinical Instructor
University of Illinois
Chicago, Ill.

Jason D. Buckway, RN, BSN
Intermediate Care Nurse Manager
McKay-Dee Hospital Center
Intermountain Health Care
Ogden, Utah

Joseph T. Catalano, RN, PhD
Professor and Chairman
Department of Nursing
East Central University
Ada, Okla.

Linda C. Copel, RN, CS, PhD, CFLE, DAPA
Associate Professor
College of Nursing
Villanova University
Villanova, Pa.

Justin G. Dalton, RN, BSN
Clinical Nurse Educator
McKay-Dee Hospital Center
Intermountain Health Care
Ogden, Utah

Teresa Dowdell, BS, RPh
Associate Professor
College of Nursing
University of South Florida
Tampa, Fla.

Julie M. Gerhart, MS, RPh
Pharmacy Affairs Manager
Merck & Co., Inc.
West Point, Pa.

Cheryl A. Grandinetti, PharmD
Senior Clinical Research Pharmacist
Pharmaceutical Management Branch
Cancer Therapy Evaluation Program
Division of Cancer Treatment and Diagnosis
National Cancer Institute
Clarksburg, Md.

Franklin R. Grollman, PharmD, BCOP
Clinical Pharmacist
National Naval Medical Center
Bethesda, Md.

Helena M. Hardin, RN
Assistant Clinical Manager
Cardiac and Medical Intensive Care Unit
Oakwood Hospital and Medical Center
Dearborn, Mich.

Nancy Hargis, RN, BSN
Nurse Manager
Emergency Department
Shore Memorial Hospital
Nassawadox, Va.

Monica Holmberg, PharmD
Phoenix Indian Medical Center
Phoenix, Ariz.

Sandy Keefe, RN, MSN
Freelance Nurse Writer
El Dorado Hills, Calif.

Frank J. Krivanek, PharmD
Clinical Coordinator
Director of Pharmacy Practice Residency Program
Mount Carmel West
Columbus, Ohio

Nancy L. Laplante, RN, BSN
Instructor
Nursing Department
Neumann College
Aston, Pa.

Travis W. Linneman, PharmD
Pharmacy Practice Resident
Barnes-Jewish Hospital at Washington University School of Medicine
Saint Louis, Mo.

Mary Jane J. McDevitt, RN, BS
Home Care Nurse
Delaware County Memorial Hospital
Drexel Hill, Pa.

Miranda L. Moyer, RN, BSN
Staff Nurse
Nursing Care Services
Colmar, Pa.

Keith M. Olsen, PharmD, FCCP, FCCM
Professor of Pharmacy
College of Pharmacy
University of Nebraska Medical Center
Omaha, Neb.

Lois A. Piano, RN, MSN, EdD
Senior Research Associate
Curtis Analytic Partners
Philadelphia, Pa.

Christine Price, PharmD
Primary Clinical Coordinator
Morton Plant Mease Health Care
Clearwater, Fla.

Barbara Putrycus, RN, MSN, CCRN
Director
Operating Room Services
Oakwood Hospital and Medical Center
Dearborn, Mich.

Michelle Renaud, RN, PhD
Assistant Professor
Pacific Lutheran University
Tacoma, Wash.

Cynthia Saver, RN, MS
President
CLS Development, Inc.
Columbia, Md.

Melinda K. Schott, RPh, PharmD
Staff Pharmacist
Stop & Shop Pharmacy
Wallingford, Conn.

Ann Schlaffer, RN, PNP
Pediatric Nurse Practitioner
Eastern Shore Rural Health
Atlantic, Va.

AnnMarie Smith, RN, BSN, MA
Clinical Instructor
The Cleveland Clinic Foundation
Cleveland, Ohio

Mary E. Stassi, RN, C
Health Occupations Coordinator
St. Charles Community College
St. Peters, Mo.

Barbara Tassone, RN, CNP
Nurse Practitioner
Greater Baltimore Medical Center
Baltimore, Md.

Tracey R. Troop, RN
Nurse
Intensive Care Unit
Abington Memorial Hospital
Abington, Pa.

Vera Usinowicz, RN, MS, CCRN
Clinical Nurse Specialist
Critical Care Unit
The Valley Hospital
Ridgewood, N.J.

Jeannette Yeznach Wick, RPh, MBA, FASCP
Senior Clinical Research Pharmacist
National Cancer Institute
Bethesda, Md.

Preface and user's guide

Achieving clinical excellence in administering and monitoring drugs has never been more crucial—or more challenging—for the nurse. Medication errors and harmful side effects make the headlines often these days. In the past year alone, several top-selling drugs have been taken off the market and others have new "black box" warnings on their labels. Labels on some antidepressants now warn of a link to suicidal behavior; those for many nonsteroidal anti-inflammatory drugs (including ibuprofen and naproxen) caution of an increased risk for heart attacks, strokes, and GI bleeding. Other drugs also have been withdrawn—for instance, Lotronex in 2000 (but subsequently reintroduced) and Vioxx in 2004 (also expected to return to the market).

At the same time, newly approved drugs are being marketed directly to consumers. In the past, use of a new drug increased gradually. If unexpected adverse effects emerged, relatively few patients had been exposed to the risk. But these days, new drugs may skyrocket into widespread use before some side effects are known.

Undoubtedly, the intensified emphasis on adverse drug events (ADEs) makes the nurse's job more formidable. Public opinion polls consistently portray nursing as one of the most trusted professions, and patients look to us for guidance about their medicines.

Studies show we're doing a good job in protecting them. A recent analysis of 334 medication errors associated with 264 ADEs over a 6-month period discovered that nurses were the healthcare professionals most likely to detect and intercept errors in medication ordering, transcription, or dispensing. Nearly half of the errors examined were intercepted before they caused adverse events—and 87% of these were intercepted by nurses.

For our patients' sake, we can't let down our guard. We must demand that our managers and employers promote a culture of safety that maximizes error prevention and mitigation, promotes blame-free error reporting, and takes a systems approach to reducing medication errors. Major nursing organizations and the Joint Commission on Accreditation of Healthcare Organizations (JCAHO) have taken the lead by regulating certain practice areas and creating guidelines to help prevent ADEs (such as those stemming from ambiguous abbreviations or use of high-risk drugs).

On an individual level, each nurse must learn as much as possible about the drugs she administers. *2006 Nursing Spectrum Drug Handbook* has been developed with this in mind. By helping you gain a thorough understanding of drugs and stay abreast of emerging drug data, we will serve as your advocate, helping you keep your patients safe from medication errors and untoward drug effects.

Targeting excellence

The quality, relevance, and success of any book for nurses hinges on whether it meets the needs of its target audience. For the premier edition of *Nursing Spectrum Drug Handbook*, we based the book's format, theme, features, and design on the feedback I received when I met with nurses around the country.

To help determine how to refine and update the book for this second edition, we took the same approach, asking more than 60 practicing nurses, student nurses, nursing school deans, and nursing executives to review the premier edition. Their overwhelmingly positive response to the book was heartening, and their comments on specific aspects and features were enlightening. We also took into account the many comments we've received from nurses who purchased the first edition.

New for this edition

Based on reviewers' and readers' feedback and our own analysis of the premier edition, we have made several key changes for this edition. We have:

- added 40 new monographs, including newly approved drugs
- updated preexisting monographs with the latest information on new indications, new dosages, new off-label uses, and new safety warnings
- included more Clinical Alerts—especially for high-alert drugs
- expanded our coverage of herbs and nutritional supplements
- added a 14-page chart on anesthetic drugs (complete with administration and patient teaching guidelines), as well as a chart to help you identify life-threatening adverse reactions
- included more laboratory values to help you monitor blood drug levels and detect adverse reactions
- doubled the size of the full-color insert on safe drug administration, which now includes additional sanctioned treatment guidelines for life-threatening emergencies
- introduced new appendix topics
- provided access to free PDA-downloadable monographs of commonly used drugs on our companion website, www.nursesdrughandbook.com.

Continuing outstanding features

Individual drug monographs are the core of any drug handbook. Like the premier edition, *2006 Nursing Spectrum Drug Handbook* presents alphabetically arranged monographs for approximately 1,000 generic drugs and 3,000 trade drugs.

To help ensure that this information is accurate and current, new material was reviewed and updated by more than 60 practicing nurses and pharmacists, and then edited by our highly experienced team of clinical and editorial experts. Our advisory board of well-known nurse-leaders and pharmacists also contributed valuable guidance during the development phase.

Other continuing features of this book include:

- red Clinical Alert logos, which highlight critical administration and safety considerations
- scored tablet icons to denote each "Indications and dosages" section so you can find this crucial data instantly
- detailed administration guidelines for every drug, with specific instructions on oral, I.M., I.V., subcutaneous, and other routes when applicable
- life-threatening adverse reactions shown in **boldface**
- interactions with other drugs, diagnostic tests, foods, herbs and nutritional supplements, and behaviors
- photogallery of common tablets and capsules
- comprehensive index that allows you to look up a drug by its generic name, trade name, or indications
- patient monitoring guidelines, including ongoing assessment, follow-up laboratory test results that suggest adverse reactions, and warning signs of an untoward event.

General drug administration guidelines

From the time a prescriber orders a drug to the time the patient receives it, the process of drug administration may involve up to 200 individual steps. Missteps can happen at any point in this process—but you can help prevent some of these errors long before the dose is prepared.

During the initial patient evaluation, for instance, review the patient's current drug regimen, obtain drug allergy information, measure height and weight, and check the diagnosis and other baseline data to help determine the patient's risk for an adverse reaction. Also, make sure you're familiar with the drug's action, expected benefits, adverse reactions, and interaction potential in light of such patient factors as diagnosis and medical condition.

The "five rights" of drug administration

Nurses are legally responsible for applying and ensuring the "five rights" of drug administration. To help achieve these goals, use the following strategies:

- **Right patient.** Always confirm the patient's identity before administering a drug. Check his ID bracelet and ask him to state his name; then confirm his name, age, and allergies. JCAHO requires the use of two identifiers, such as the patient number, his telephone number, or his Social Security number. Ideally, match the ordered treatment to the patient using his name bracelet and ID number, comparing it to the drug order transcribed in the medication administration record (MAR). Be especially cautious if your patient is confused, because he may answer to the wrong name.
- **Right drug.** Giving the wrong drug is the most common type of medication error. It typically results from such factors as look-alike and sound-alike drug names, similar drug labels and packaging, and poor communication. Never try to decipher an illegible drug order, and never give a drug if you're not sure why it was prescribed.

To make sure you give the right drug, match the drug label against the order in the MAR *three times*—once when you remove the container from the patient's drug drawer, again before you remove the dose from the container, and finally, before you return the container to the drawer or discard it. Never give a drug from a container that is unlabeled or has an unreadable label, and never borrow a drug from another patient.

In an effort to reduce "wrong-drug" and other medication errors, many hospitals are adopting new technologies, such as bar-code point-of-care medication administration systems. Keep in mind, though, that after such a system is implemented, it must be monitored closely for problems, and staff members must receive adequate training in its use.

- **Right dosage.** Check the dosage against the order in the MAR. Determine if it's appropriate based on the patient's age, size, vital signs, and condition. If the dose needs to be measured, use appropriate equipment—for instance, an oral syringe rather than a parenteral syringe to measure an oral liquid drug. Be on the look-out for misinterpretation of orders, incorrect calculation of volumes and infusion rates, misreading of decimal points, and labeling errors.

When administering a drug that can cause serious harm if given incorrectly (such as I.V. insulin or heparin) or when giving an infusion to a pediatric patient, always double-check the dosage and pump settings; then verify these with a colleague.

- **Right time.** Incorrect timing of drug administration accounted for 43% of medication errors reported in a 2002 study published in the *Archives of Internal Medicine*. Although most medications are not time-sensitive, dose timing can be critical if the patient must maintain a specific blood drug level, or to ensure accurate laboratory test values or avoid interactions with other drugs.

Usually, a dose should be given within 30 minutes before or after the time specified in the order, in accordance with your facility's established protocols (for example, at 9 A.M., 1 P.M., and 6 P.M. or at 10 A.M., 2 P.M., and 7 P.M.). Always administer a dose as it's prepared.

To maximize the drug's therapeutic efficacy, determine whether it should be given with or without food and whether it could interact with or impede the absorption of concurrently administered drugs. If the patient's scheduled for diagnostic testing, determine whether to withhold the dose until after the test.

• **Right route.** Many drugs can be given by multiple routes. The prescriber chooses the route based on such factors as the patient's condition and the desired onset of action. In turn, the prescribed dosage is based on the administration route. Generally, oral dosages of a given drug are greater than injected dosages, so a serious overdose may occur if a dose intended for oral administration is given by injection instead.

Also, keep in mind that most serious error outcomes occur when the I.V. route is used. (Only a few high-risk drugs, such as warfarin, some chemotherapy drugs, and a few sedatives, are given orally.) Also be aware that I.M. drugs should not be given I.V. because of the potential for adverse effects.

Finally, be aware that some drugs or drug forms (for instance, sustained-release tablets or capsules) should never be crushed. Crushing can alter the dosage delivered, causing the patient to receive a bolus of a drug that's meant to be released slowly over several hours.

Additional nursing responsibilities

Of course, the nurse's responsibilities don't stop with these five rights. Documentation, monitoring, and patient teaching are also crucial.

After giving the drug, always document that it was administered. Document the dose as soon as it is given—never before. When documenting, use only accepted abbreviations and avoid those that are used rarely or that could be misread or misinterpreted. (See *Avoiding dangerous abbreviations.*)

If the patient refuses a medication, report this to the prescriber immediately. Then record his refusal on both the MAR and the patient's record; include your initials, full name, and credentials on both records.

During the course of drug therapy, monitor the patient to determine drug efficacy and detect signs and symptoms of an adverse reaction or interaction. Teach the patient the name of the prescribed drug, its dosage, administration route, dosing frequency and times, and duration of therapy. Make sure he knows how to recognize the drug's therapeutic effects, adverse reactions, and interactions with other drugs, foods, herbs, and behaviors.

User's guide to *2006 Nursing Spectrum Drug Handbook*

This book is organized in three main parts.

Part 1: A to Z drug monographs

Part 1 presents individual drug monographs in alphabetical order by generic name. Each monograph starts with basic information, including dosages and administration guidelines. Next come adverse reactions, interactions, nursing care to provide during drug therapy, and teaching points to review with the patient. Within each monograph, information is presented in the following order.

Generic name. A drug's generic name is the nonproprietary name, typically assigned by the manufacturer. When more than one therapeutic form of the drug is available, generic names of

Avoiding dangerous abbreviations

To help reduce medication errors, all healthcare team members must use abbreviations correctly. The Joint Commission on the Accreditation of Healthcare Organizations (JCAHO) mandates that healthcare organizations standardize a list of abbreviations, acronyms, and symbols that should not be used. Organizations must approve a minimum required list of prohibited abbreviations, which includes the first five items shown below. JCAHO also advises organizations to consider adding the remaining items to their "Do not use" list.

Abbreviation	Potential problem	Solution
U (for "unit")	Mistaken as "0," "4," or "cc"	Write "unit."
IU (for "international unit")	Mistaken as "IV" ("intravenous") or 10 ("ten")	Write "international unit."
Q.D., Q.O.D. (for "once daily," "every other day")	Mistaken for each other. Period after "Q" may be mistaken for "I"; "O" may be mistaken for "I."	Write "daily" or "every other day."
Trailing zero (X.0 mg) (prohibited only for drug-related notations); lack of leading zero (.X mg)	Decimal point is missed.	Never write a zero by itself after decimal point (X mg); always use a zero before decimal point (0.X mg).
MS MSO_4 $MgSO_4$	Confused for one another. May mean "morphine sulfate" or "magnesium sulfate."	Write "morphine sulfate" or "magnesium sulfate."
μg (for "microgram")	Mistaken for "mg" (milligrams), resulting in 1,000-fold overdose	Write "mcg."
H.S. (for "half-strength" or "at bedtime")	Mistaken for "half-strength" or "hour of sleep" ("at bedtime")	Write "half-strength" or "at bedtime."
q.H.S. (for "at bedtime")	Mistaken for "every hour"	Write "at bedtime."
T.I.W. (for "3 times a week")	Mistaken for "3 times a day" or "twice weekly"	Write "3 times weekly" or "three times weekly."
S.C. or S.Q. (for "subcutaneous")	Mistaken for "S.L." (sublingual) or "5 every"	Write "Sub-Q," "subQ," or "subcutaneously."
D/C (for "discharge")	Misinterpreted as "discontinue"	Write "discharge."
cc (for "cubic centimeters")	Mistaken for "U" (units) if poorly written	Write "ml" for milliliters.
AS, AD, AU (for "left ear," "right ear," "both ears")	Mistaken for OS, OD, or OU	Write "left ear," "right ear," or "both ears."

Understanding pregnancy risk categories

Whenever possible, pregnant women should avoid drug therapy. The risks of taking drugs during pregnancy range from relatively minor fetal defects (such as ear tags or extra digits) to fetal death.

When drug therapy is considered, the drug's benefits to the mother must be weighed against the risk to the fetus. Ideally, the drug should provide clear benefits to the mother without harming the fetus. To help prescribers and pregnant patients assess a drug's risk-to-benefit ratio, the Food and Drug Administration assigns one of five pregnancy risk categories to each drug. In addition, certain drugs are not rated.

Category A: No evidence of risk exists. Adequate, well-controlled studies in pregnant women don't show an increased risk of fetal abnormalities during any trimester.

Category B: The risk of fetal harm is possible but remote. Animal studies show no fetal risk; however, controlled studies haven't been done in humans. Or animal studies do show a risk to the fetus, but adequate studies in pregnant women haven't shown such a risk.

Category C: Fetal risk can't be ruled out. Although animal studies show risks, adequate, well-controlled human studies are lacking. Despite the potential fetal risks, use of the drug may be acceptable because of benefits to the mother.

Category D: Positive evidence of fetal risk exists. Nevertheless, potential benefits from the drug may outweigh the risk. For example, the drug may be acceptable in a life-threatening situation or serious disease if safer drugs can't be used or are ineffective.

Category X: Contraindicated during pregnancy. Studies in animals or humans or reports of adverse reactions show evidence of fetal risk that clearly outweighs any possible benefit to the patient.

Category NR: Not rated.

these forms are listed alphabetically.

Trade names. A drug's common trade, or brand, name is the proprietary, trademarked name under which it's marketed. Trade-name and generic drugs are therapeutically equivalent in strength, quality, performance, and use; when interchanged, they have the same effects and no differences. However, they may vary in preservatives, color, shape, labeling, and, possibly, scoring. In the monographs, trade-name drugs available only in Canada are marked with a maple leaf for easy identification.

Pharmacologic and therapeutic classes. This section specifies the drug's pharmacologic class (based on its pharmacologic properties and action—for example, sulfonamide or corticosteroid) and therapeutic class (based on approved therapeutic uses of the drug—for instance, antineoplastic or antihypertensive). Many drugs fall into multiple therapeutic classes.

Pregnancy risk category. This section lists the category assigned by the Food and Drug Administration (FDA) to indicate the drug's potential danger to the fetus when taken during pregnancy. (See *Understanding pregnancy risk categories*.)

Controlled substance schedule. Narcotics, stimulants, and certain other drugs fall under the Controlled Substances Act. The Drug Enforcement Agency assigns each of these drugs a category, or schedule, based on its abuse potential and other factors. (See *Schedules of controlled substances*.) This section, when applicable, provides the drug's assigned schedule.

Action. This section summarizes how the drug achieves its therapeutic effect—the action that takes place when it reaches its target site and combines with cellular drug receptors to cause certain physiologic responses. When a drug's action isn't known or when researchers have proposed theories for the action but haven't clarified it definitively, we state this fact.

Availability. This section lists the physical forms in which the drug is produced and dispensed, plus available strengths (the amount of active ingredient present) for each form.

Indications and dosages. Marked with a red scored tablet icon for quick identification, this section details the drug's FDA-approved indications for adults, children, infants, and neonates (when appropriate), along with the recommended dosages, administration routes, and dosing frequency for each indication. The indications and dosages shown reflect current clinical trends, not unequivocal standards, and must be considered in light of the patient's condition and diagnosis. (Although we've made every effort to ensure the accuracy of all dosages, we urge you to become familiar with the official package insert for each drug you administer.)

Dosage adjustment. This section tells which patient groups (such as children or elderly patients), diseases, or disorders (such as renal or hepatic dysfunction) may necessitate dosage adjustment.

Off-label uses. Here you'll find a list of off-label (unlabeled or unapproved) uses of the drug, when applicable. Off-label drug use has become increasingly common as clinical research moves ahead of the FDA's approval process. In some cases, off-label use has become the standard of care.

Contraindications. This section lists conditions that contraindicate use of the drug, such as preexisting diseases. As a rule, never give a drug to a patient who has a history of hypersensitivity to that drug.

Drugs commonly implicated in hypersensitivity reactions include antibiotics, histamines, iodides, phenothia-

Schedules of controlled substances

The Controlled Substances Act of 1970 regulates the production and distribution of stimulants, narcotics, depressants, hallucinogens, and anabolic steroids. Drugs regulated by this law fall into five categories, or schedules, based on their abuse potential, medicinal value, and harmfulness. Schedule I drugs are the most hazardous; schedule V drugs, the least hazardous.

Schedule I: High potential for abuse; no currently accepted medical use in the United States. Using the drug even under medical supervision is thought to be unsafe.

Schedule II: High potential for abuse; currently accepted medical use in the United States (or currently accepted medical use with severe restrictions). Abuse may lead to severe psychological or physical dependence. Emergency telephone orders for limited quantities may be authorized, but the prescriber must provide a written, signed prescription order.

Schedule III: Lower abuse potential than schedule I and II drugs; currently accepted medical use in the United States. Abuse may lead to a moderate or low degree of physical dependence or high psychological dependence. Telephone orders are permitted.

Schedule IV: Lower abuse potential than schedule I, II, or III drugs; currently accepted medical use in the United States. Abuse may lead to limited physical dependence or psychological dependence. Telephone orders are permitted.

Schedule V: Low abuse potential compared to drugs in other schedules; currently accepted medical use in the United States. Abuse may lead to limited physical dependence or to psychological dependence. Some schedule V drugs may be available in limited quantities without a prescription (if state law permits).

High-alert drugs

SAFETY GUIDELINES

Certain drugs expose patients to an increased risk of significant harm when used in error. The Institute for Safe Medication Practices (ISMP) has created a list of high-alert drugs based on voluntary medication error reports, harmful medication errors described in the literature, practitioner feedback, and expert reviews. The ISMP has identified both high-alert drug classes (or categories) and specific high-alert drugs.

High-alert drug classes and categories

- adrenergic agonists, I.V.
- adrenergic antagonists, I.V.
- cardioplegic solutions
- chemotherapeutic agents
- dextrose (20% or greater)
- dialysis solutions
- epidural and intrathecal drugs
- general anesthetics
- glycoprotein IIb/IIIa inhibitors
- hypoglycemics, oral
- inotropic drugs, I.V.
- liposomal drug forms
- moderate sedation agents, I.V. (or oral agents for children)
- narcotics and opioids
- neuromuscular blocking agents
- thrombolytics and fibrinolytics, I.V.
- total parenteral nutrition solutions

Specific high-alert drugs

- amiodarone, I.V.
- colchicine, injection
- heparin, low molecular weight
- heparin, unfractionated, I.V.
- insulin, subcutaneous and I.V.
- lidocaine, I.V.
- magnesium sulfate injection
- methotrexate, oral nononcologic use
- nesiritide
- potassium chloride for injection
- potassium phosphates injection
- sodium chloride injection
- sodium nitroprusside for injection
- warfarin

zines, tranquilizers, anesthetics, diagnostic agents (such as iodinated contrast media), and biologic agents (such as insulin, vaccines, and antitoxins).

Precautions. For some patients, a specific drug may pose an increased risk of untoward effects—yet the doctor prescribes it because, in his judgment, the potential benefits outweigh the risks. For instance, many drugs can be dangerous for elderly patients, pregnant or breastfeeding women, young children, and patients with renal or hepatic dysfunction. This section tells you which patients to whom you must administer the drug cautiously. Precautions can be especially important if you're administering a high-alert drug. (See *High-alert drugs.*)

Administration. Here you'll find information to help you prepare the drug and administer it correctly and safely, regardless of the route—including whether to give it with or without food, how to mix it for I.V. or I.M. use, and what flow rate to use.

Route, onset, peak, and duration. Presented in table form, this section provides a pharmacokinetic profile—onset of action, peak blood level, and duration of action—for each route by which the drug is administered.

Adverse reactions. Occurring in roughly 30% of hospital patients, adverse reactions are undesirable and unintended drug effects, which can range from mild to life-threatening. They may arise immediately and suddenly, or may take weeks or even months to develop.

Adverse reactions can be especially dangerous if a medication error occurs in a patient who's receiving a high-alert drug. The sickest patients—those in the intensive care unit—typically receive anywhere from 20 to 40 different drugs. These patients are the most vulnerable to adverse reactions, drug interactions, and life-threatening consequences of a medication error. In this section, we list the most commonly reported adverse reactions by body system. Life-threatening reactions appear in **boldface.**

Interactions. With Americans taking more prescription and nonprescription drugs than ever, you're likely to encounter patients experiencing the effects of drug interactions. Many people also take herbs and nutritional supplements that can interact with drugs to cause dangerous effects or to impede a drug's intended effect. This section presents documented and clinically significant interactions that may occur if the drug is used concurrently with other drugs, specific foods, and certain herbs or supplements, or if it's combined with certain behaviors (for instance, smoking or alcohol use). It also describes the drug's effects on diagnostic test results, which can be especially important for hospital patients.

Patient monitoring. Close patient monitoring is essential during drug therapy (and in some cases, even after therapy ends) to help gauge whether the drug is effective and to detect untoward reactions or interactions. Early detection of troublesome side effects or drug inefficacy allows timely adjustments in therapy and may prevent patient injury or avoid a treatment delay.

To monitor your patient effectively, not only must you be familiar with the drug you're administering and its intended outcome. You must also consider how this drug might interact with other drugs that your patient is receiving, and determine whether his medical condition, vital signs, or recent laboratory findings make him more vulnerable to interactions or adverse effects. This section discusses important nursing assessments and interventions, such as monitoring blood drug levels to help determine the correct dosage and to prevent toxicity.

Patient teaching. The nurse's responsibility for teaching patients about their care has never been greater. What's more, patients are now demanding more information about their treatment. This section describes key teaching points you should cover with a patient who's receiving the drug, including essential information needed to create a patient teaching plan and protect your patient even after discharge. Topics include how and when the patient should take the drug, which symptoms he should report immediately, and which drugs, foods, herbs, or behaviors he should avoid during drug therapy.

Part 2: Drug classes, vitamins and minerals, herbs and supplements

Part 2 presents collective monographs on therapeutic drug classes and abbreviated monographs on vitamins, minerals, herbs, and nutritional supplements. Monographs on therapeutic drug classes familiarize you with the overall attributes of an entire drug class. These monographs also give you an idea of which drug the prescriber may order if a particular drug in the same class is unsuitable for your patient.

The use of herbal remedies and supplements is soaring—yet many users and health care practitioners are in the dark about these products' adverse effects and potential interactions with prescription and over-the-counter drugs. This section gives basic information that may help your patient use herbs more safely.

Part 3: Appendices, selected references, and index

Appendices serve as handy references on important drug topics and related issues—everything from normal laboratory values for monitoring and detecting drug levels to annual costs of commonly used drugs. New to this edition are a table on commonly used anesthetic drugs and a chart that describes life-threatening adverse reactions—information that can help you detect these reactions quickly.

Website and other bonuses

Our website, www.nursesdrughandbook.com, gives you 24-hour access to hundreds of drug monographs, online versions of the book's safe drug administration insert, drug news (including new approvals and indications), continuing education modules that focus on drug administration, and patient teaching aids on common drugs (which you can customize and give to patients). Also, in 2006, this website will provide access to monographs of many commonly used drugs, which you can download free to your personal digital assistant. We'll keep adding more features, so visit often.

I'm certain *2006 Nursing Spectrum Drug Handbook* will enhance your practice and help you make drug therapy safer and more effective for your patients. No matter how complex the drug or the drug regimen, this book will serve as a reliable resource that will help you master the demands of drug administration.

Acknowledgments

Completing a project of this scope and intensity takes considerable effort and hard work by a dedicated team. I consider myself extremely fortunate in that respect, because many generous and accomplished people have helped me immensely. I can't thank them enough—but I will try.

I owe a special debt of gratitude to the thoughtful, tireless, patient, and incredibly knowledgeable MedVantage team—Minnie Rose (clinical manager), Kathy Goldberg (editorial manager), Stephanie Peters (design manager), Julia Knipe (administration manager), and the clinical editors, text editors, copy editors, and designers whose diligence plays a large role in helping this project meet high standards of quality.

Thanks also to the entire Nursing Spectrum team, including the marketing and sales staff, website team, and especially Patti Rager, Steve Hauber, John Leggett, Cindy Poe, Lesley McGerald, Lisa Marie Edelman, Penny Schneider, and John Petry. I value their wisdom, guidance, ongoing support, and enthusiasm for this project.

I'd like to thank our advisors, contributors, and reviewers for generously sharing their time and clinical expertise. Their assistance and advice have been invaluable.

All my thanks to my wonderful husband, children, grandchildren, extended family, and friends. Their unflagging love and support are ongoing sources of strength to me.

Finally, thanks to all of the nurses everywhere who work conscientiously to help ensure that patients receive the best possible care. I'm especially grateful to those of you who've written or e-mailed me with kind words for *Nursing Spectrum Drug Handbook*. Know that I appreciate your enthusiastic support and will continue to work hard to bring you the tools you need to safeguard your patients.

Patricia Dwyer Schull, RN, MSN
Author

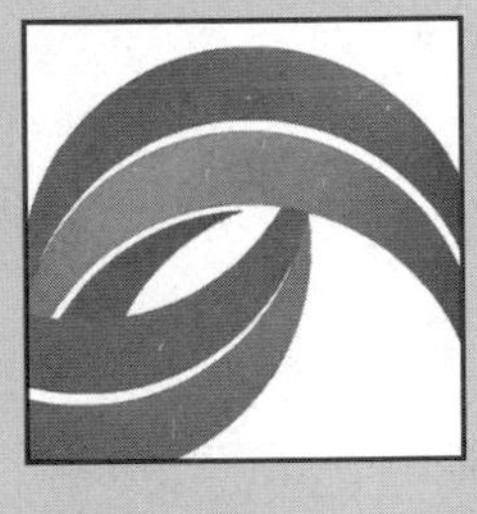

Part 1

Drugs A to Z

Safe drug administration

Photogallery of common tablets and capsules

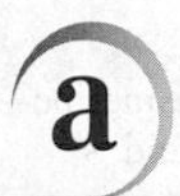

abacavir sulfate

Ziagen

Pharmacologic class: Carbocyclic nucleoside reverse transcriptase
Therapeutic class: Antiretroviral
Pregnancy risk category C

Action

Converts via intracellular enzymes to active metabolite carbovir triphosphate, which inhibits activity of human immunodeficiency virus-1 (HIV-1) reverse transcriptase. Inhibits viral reproduction by interfering with DNA and RNA synthesis

Availability

Oral solution: 20 mg/ml
Tablets: 300 mg

Indications and dosages

➢ HIV-1 infection
Adults: 300 mg P.O. b.i.d.
Children ages 3 months to 16 years: 8 mg/kg P.O. b.i.d., to a maximum dosage of 300 mg b.i.d.

Contraindications

- Hypersensitivity to drug
- Hepatic disease, lactic acidosis
- Breastfeeding
- Children younger than age 3 months

Precautions

Use cautiously in:

- impaired renal function, bone marrow suppression
- risk factors for hepatic disease
- elderly patients
- pregnant patients.

Administration

- Always give in combination with other antiretrovirals.

🔊 Be aware that drug may cause fatal hypersensitivity reactions.

- Give with food if GI upset occurs.

Route	Onset	Peak	Duration
P.O.	Unknown	0.5-1.7 hr	Unknown

Adverse reactions

CNS: headache, weakness, insomnia
GI: nausea, vomiting, diarrhea, poor appetite, pancreatitis
Hematologic: neutropenia, severe anemia
Hepatic: hepatic failure
Metabolic: mild hyperglycemia, **lactic acidosis**
Skin: rash, **erythema multiforme, toxic epidermal necrolysis**
Other: body fat redistribution, **Stevens-Johnson syndrome, fatal hypersensitivity reaction**

Interactions

Drug-drug. *Methadone:* Increased oral methadone clearance
Drug-diagnostic tests. *Alanine aminotransferase, aspartate aminotransferase, creatine phosphokinase, gamma-glutamyltransferase, glucose, triglycerides:* increased levels
Drug-herbs. *St. John's wort:* decreased drug blood level and reduced drug effect
Drug-behaviors. *Alcohol use:* increased drug half-life and concentration

Patient monitoring

🔊 Assess for severe lactic acidosis, especially in women and obese patients.

🔊 Evaluate closely for signs and symptoms of hypersensitivity reaction, which can be fatal. These include fever, rash, fatigue, nausea, vomiting, diarrhea, abdominal pain, dyspnea, cough, and pharyngitis.

◀ Never restart therapy if patient has experienced a previous hypersensitivity reaction to this drug.
- Check for liver enlargement.
- Monitor CBC, serum electrolytes, and liver and kidney function test results.

Patient teaching

- Advise patient to take drug with food to minimize GI upset.
- Instruct patient to refrigerate drug but not to freeze it.

◀ Teach patient how to recognize hypersensitivity reaction. Instruct him to stop taking drug and contact prescriber immediately if signs or symptoms of such a reaction occur.

◀ Tell patient to contact prescriber if he develops a rash (possible sign of Stevens-Johnson syndrome).

- Inform patient that drug doesn't cure HIV but lowers viral count.
- Instruct patient to obtain medication guide and warning card with each refill.
- Tell patient he'll undergo frequent blood and urine testing during therapy.
- Advise patient to consult prescriber before drinking alcohol or using herbs.
- As appropriate, review all other significant and life-threatening adverse reactions and interactions, especially those related to the drugs, tests, herbs, and behaviors mentioned above.

abacavir sulfate and lamivudine

Epzicom

Pharmacologic class: Nucleoside analogue
Therapeutic class: Antiretroviral agent
Pregnancy risk category C

Action

Abacavir converts to its active metabolite (carbovir triphosphate), and lamivudine is phosphorylated to its active metabolite (lamivudine triphosphate) by intracellular enzymes. These metabolites inhibit activity of human immunodeficiency virus-1 (HIV-1) reverse transcriptase. Drug interferes with DNA and RNA synthesis, thereby inhibiting viral reproduction.

Availability

Tablets: 600 mg abacavir/300 mg lamivudine

Indications and dosages

➢ HIV-1 infection
Adults: 1 tablet P.O. daily

Contraindications

- Hypersensitivity to abacavir, lamivudine, or other product components
- Hepatic impairment

Precautions

Use cautiously in:

- treatment-experienced patients (cross-resistance may occur)
- concurrent hepatitis B infection
- renal impairment
- elderly patients
- pregnant or breastfeeding patients
- children (safety and efficacy not established).

Administration

◀ Before administering, ask patient if he's allergic to abacavir or lamivudine.

- Always give in combination with other antiretrovirals.
- Administer with plenty of water, with or without food.
- Know that drug isn't recommended for patients who would require dosage adjustment, because tablet shouldn't be broken.

Route	Onset	Peak	Duration
P.O.	Unknown	Unknown	Unknown

a

Adverse reactions

CNS: paresthesia, peripheral neuropathy, insomnia, depression or depressed mood, migraine, fatigue, malaise, weakness, dizziness, vertigo, anxiety, abnormal dreams, **seizures**
GI: nausea, diarrhea, abdominal pain, gastritis, stomatitis, pancreatitis
Hematologic: lymphadenopathy, splenomegaly, **anemia (including pure red-cell aplasia and severe anemias progressing with therapy), aplastic anemia**
Hepatic: posttreatment exacerbation of hepatitis B, hepatic steatosis
Metabolic: hyperglycemia, **lactic acidosis**
Musculoskeletal: muscle weakness, **rhabdomyolysis**
Respiratory: abnormal breath sounds, wheezing
Skin: alopecia, toxic epidermal necrolysis, **erythema multiforme, Stevens-Johnson syndrome**
Other: body fat redistribution, fever, allergic reactions including urticaria and **anaphylaxis**

Interactions

Drug-drug. *Nelfinavir, sulfamethoxazole/trimethoprim:* increased lamivudine blood level
Drug-diagnostic tests. *Amylase, bilirubin, creatine kinase, glucose, lipase, triglycerides:* elevated levels
Liver function tests: abnormal results
Platelet count: decreased
Drug-behaviors. *Alcohol use:* increased abacavir blood level

Patient monitoring

- Monitor patients (especially women and overweight patients) for signs and symptoms of lactic acidosis.
- Monitor hepatic function closely during therapy and for at least several months afterward.

Patient teaching

[Clinical alert] Advise patient not to use drug if he is allergic to abacavir or lamivudine.

- Instruct patient to take drug exactly as prescribed.
- Tell patient to take drug with plenty of water, with or without food.

[Clinical alert] Instruct patient to stop taking drug and get immediate medical attention if he experiences such allergic symptoms as fatigue, general ill feeling, achiness, rash, fever, difficulty breathing, cough, throat inflammation, or severe nausea, vomiting, diarrhea, or abdominal pain.

[Clinical alert] Caution patient never to take drug again if he experiences an allergic reaction.

[Clinical alert] Tell patient to make sure he receives medication guide and warning card issued with each new prescription and refill. Teach him to carry card at all times and to read it each time he refills prescription, to ensure he has the most current drug information.

[Clinical alert] Advise patient to contact prescriber right away if he develops symptoms of liver impairment (unusual tiredness, weakness, nausea, itching, yellowing of eyes or skin, tenderness on upper right side of abdomen, or flulike symptoms).

[Clinical alert] Tell patient not to stop taking drug without consulting prescriber. If he stops taking it for any reason other than allergic reaction, he must consult prescriber before restarting, because serious or life-threatening reactions may occur.

- Emphasize that drug doesn't cure HIV infection.
- Tell HIV-infected women not to breastfeed infants, to avoid risk of transmitting HIV infection.
- Inform patient that he'll have regular blood tests during drug therapy.
- As appropriate, review all other significant and life-threatening adverse

reactions and interactions, especially those related to the drugs, tests, and behaviors mentioned above.

abciximab

ReoPro✤

Pharmacologic class: Platelet aggregation inhibitor

Therapeutic class: Antithrombotic, antiplatelet drug

Pregnancy risk category C

Action

Inhibits fibrinogen binding and platelet-platelet interaction by impeding fibrinogen binding to platelet receptor sites, thereby prolonging bleeding time

Availability

Injection: 2 mg/ml (5-ml vials containing 10 mg)

Indications and dosages

➢ Adjunct to aspirin and heparin to prevent acute cardiac ischemic complications in patients undergoing percutaneous coronary intervention (PCI)

Adults: 0.25 mg/kg I.V. bolus given 10 to 60 minutes before start of PCI, followed by infusion of 0.125 mcg/kg/minute for 12 hours. Maximum dosage is 10 mcg/minute.

➢ Adjunct to aspirin and heparin in patients with unstable angina who haven't responded to conventional medical therapy and will undergo PCI within 24 hours

Adults: 0.25 mg/kg I.V. bolus, followed by 18- to 24-hour infusion of 10 mcg/minute, ending 1 hour after PCI

Contraindications

- Hypersensitivity to drug or murine proteins
- Active internal bleeding
- Bleeding diathesis
- Severe, uncontrolled hypertension
- Thrombocytopenia (< 100,000 cells/mm^3)
- Neutropenia
- Aneurysm
- Arteriovenous malformation
- History of cerebrovascular accident
- Oral anticoagulant therapy within past 7 days (unless prothrombin time is < 1.2 times control)

Precautions

Use cautiously in:

- patients receiving drugs that affect hemostasis (such as thrombolytics, anticoagulants, or antiplatelet drugs)
- pregnant or breastfeeding patients.

Administration

- Give through separate I.V. line with no other drugs.
- Avoid noncompressible I.V. sites, such as subclavian or jugular vein.

🔊 Stop continuous infusion after failed PCI.

- Restrict patient to bed rest for 6 to 8 hours after drug withdrawal or 4 hours after heparin withdrawal (whichever occurs first).
- After catheter removal, apply pressure to femoral artery for at least 30 minutes.

Route	Onset	Peak	Duration
I.V.	Rapid	30 min	48 hr

Adverse reactions

CNS: dizziness, anxiety, agitation, abnormal thinking, hypoesthesia, difficulty speaking, confusion, weakness, **cerebral ischemia, coma**

CV: pseudoaneurysm, palpitations, vascular disorders, arteriovenous fistula, hypotension, peripheral edema, weak pulse, intermittent claudication, bradycardia, **ventricular or supraventricular tachycardia, atrial fibrillation or flutter, atrioventricular block,**

nodal arrhythmias, pericardial effusion, embolism, thrombophlebitis
EENT: abnormal or double vision
GI: nausea, vomiting, diarrhea, constipation, dyspepsia, ileus, gastroesophageal reflux, enlarged abdomen, dry mouth
GU: urinary tract infection, urine retention or urinary incontinence, painful or frequent urination, abnormal renal function, cystalgia, prostatitis
Hematologic: anemia, **leukocytosis, thrombocytopenia, bleeding**
Metabolic: diabetes mellitus, **hyperkalemia**
Musculoskeletal: myopathy, myalgia, increased muscle tension, reduced muscle stretching ability
Respiratory: pneumonia, crackles, rhonchi, bronchitis, pleurisy, **pleural effusion, bronchospasm, pulmonary edema, pulmonary embolism**
Skin: pallor, cellulitis, petechiae, pruritus, bullous eruptions, diaphoresis
Other: abscess, peripheral coldness, development of human antichimeric antibodies

Interactions

Drug-drug. *Drugs that affect hemostasis (such as aspirin, dextran, dipyridamole, heparin, nonsteroidal anti-inflammatory drugs, oral anticoagulants, thrombolytics, and ticlopidine):* increased bleeding risk
Drug-diagnostic tests. *Activated partial thromboplastin time (APTT), clotting time, prothrombin time (PT):* increased values
Platelets: decreased count

Patient monitoring

- Assess platelet count before, during, and after therapy.

🔊 Monitor catheter insertion site frequently for bleeding.

🔊 During catheter insertion and for 6 hours after catheter removal, frequently monitor digital pulse in leg where catheter was inserted.

- Monitor CBC, PT, APTT, and International Normalized Ratio.
- Minimize arterial or venous punctures, automatic blood pressure cuff use, I.M. injections, nasotracheal or nasogastric intubation, and urinary catheterization.
- Use indwelling venipuncture device, such as heparin lock, to draw blood.

Patient teaching

- Tell patient what to expect during and after drug administration.
- Advise patient to minimize GI upset by eating small, frequent servings of food and drinking plenty of fluids.

🔊 Instruct patient to immediately report unusual bleeding or bruising.

- Caution patient to avoid activities that may cause injury. Advise him to use soft toothbrush and electric razor to avoid gum and skin injury.
- Inform patient that he'll undergo regular blood testing during therapy.

acamprosate calcium

Campral

Pharmacologic class: Gamma-aminobutyric acid (GABA) analogue
Therapeutic class: Detoxification agent
Pregnancy risk category C

Action

Unclear. May interact with glutamate and GABA neurotransmitter systems centrally, restoring balance between neuronal excitation and inhibition (which is altered by chronic alcoholism).

Availability

Tablets (enteric-coated): 333 mg

Indications and dosages

➤ To maintain abstinence from alcohol in patients with alcohol dependence who are abstinent when treatment begins
Adults: 2 tablets P.O. t.i.d.

Dosage adjustment

- Moderate renal impairment

Contraindications

- Hypersensitivity to drug
- Severe renal impairment

Precautions

Use cautiously in:
- mild to moderate renal impairment
- suicidal ideation or behavior
- elderly patients
- breastfeeding patients
- children.

Administration

- Give without regard to meals.
- Don't crush or break enteric-coated tablet.
- Know that drug helps maintain alcohol abstinence only when used as part of treatment program that includes counseling and support.

Route	Onset	Peak	Duration
P.O.	Unknown	3-8 hr	Unknown

Adverse reactions

CNS: apathy, confusion, agitation, neurosis, malaise, somnolence, abnormal thinking, vertigo, asthenia, anxiety, depression, dizziness, insomnia, paresthesia, tremor, withdrawal syndrome headache, migraine, abnormal dreams, hallucinations, **seizures, suicidal ideation or suicide attempt**
CV: chest pain, palpitations, syncope, hypotension, angina pectoris, varicose veins, phlebitis, peripheral edema, orthostatic hypotension, vasodilation, tachycardia, hypertension, **myocardial infarction**
EENT: abnormal vision, amblyopia, hearing loss, tinnitus, rhinitis, pharyngitis
GI: nausea, vomiting, diarrhea, constipation, abdominal pain, dyspepsia, flatulence, belching, gastroenteritis, gastritis, esophagitis, hematemesis, dry mouth, anorexia, pancreatitis, **rectal hemorrhage, GI hemorrhage**
GU: urinary frequency, urinary tract infection, urinary incontinence, erectile dysfunction, increased or decreased libido, metrorrhagia, vaginitis
Hematologic: anemia, ecchymosis, eosinophilia, lymphocytosis, **thrombocytopenia**
Hepatic: hepatic cirrhosis
Metabolic: hyperglycemia, diabetes mellitus, hyperuricemia, gout, avitaminosis
Musculoskeletal: joint, muscle, neck, or back pain
Respiratory: cough, dyspnea, bronchitis, epistaxis, pneumonia, **asthma**
Skin: pruritus, sweating
Other: abnormal taste, increased thirst, increased appetite, weight gain or loss, pain, infection, flulike symptoms, chills, abscess, hernia, allergic reaction, accidental or intentional injury, **intentional overdose**

Interactions

Drug-drug. *Naltrexone:* increased acamprosate blood level
Drug-diagnostic tests. *Bilirubin, eosinophils, lymphocytes:* increased levels
Liver function tests: abnormal results
Red blood cells: decreased count

Patient monitoring

Monitor patient for depression or expressed suicidal ideation.
- Monitor creatinine clearance during therapy.

Patient teaching

- Instruct patient to swallow tablet whole, with or without food.

a

• Advise patient to keep taking drug exactly as prescribed, even if he has a relapse. Encourage him to discuss any renewed alcohol consumption with prescriber.
Instruct patient to contact prescriber immediately if he experiences seizure, chest pain, suicidal thoughts, or symptoms of liver problems (such as unusual tiredness or yellowing of skin or eyes).
• Caution patient to move slowly to a sitting or standing position, to avoid dizziness or light-headedness from a sudden blood pressure decrease.
• Advise patient to avoid driving and other hazardous activities until he knows how drug affects concentration, alertness, vision, coordination, and physical dexterity.
• Instruct female patient to notify prescriber if she becomes or intends to become pregnant or to breastfeed during therapy.
• Inform patient that drug helps maintain abstinence from alcohol only when used as part of treatment program that includes counseling and support.
• Emphasize that drug doesn't eliminate or diminish alcohol withdrawal symptoms.
• As appropriate, review all other significant and life-threatening adverse reactions and interactions, especially those related to the drugs and tests mentioned above.

acarbose

Prandase*, Precose

Pharmacologic class: Alpha-glucosidase inhibitor
Therapeutic class: Hypoglycemic
Pregnancy risk category B

Action

Improves blood glucose control by slowing carbohydrate digestion in intestine and prolonging conversion of carbohydrates to glucose

Availability

Tablets: 25 mg, 50 mg, 100 mg

Indications and dosages

➢ Treatment of type 2 (non-insulin-dependent) diabetes mellitus when diet alone doesn't control blood glucose
Adults: Initially, 25 mg P.O. t.i.d. Increase q 4 to 8 weeks as needed until maintenance dosage is reached. Maximum dosage is 100 mg P.O. t.i.d. for adults weighing more than 60 kg (132 lb); 50 mg P.O. t.i.d. for adults weighing 60 kg or less.

Contraindications

• Hypersensitivity to drug
• Renal dysfunction
• Type 1 diabetes mellitus, diabetic ketoacidosis
• GI disease
• Cirrhosis
• Colonic ulcers
• Inflammatory bowel disease
• Intestinal obstruction
• Pregnancy or breastfeeding

Precautions

Use cautiously in:
• patients receiving concurrent hypoglycemic drugs
• children.

Administration

• Give with first bite of patient's three main meals.
• Know that drug prevents breakdown of table sugar (sucrose). Thus, mild hypoglycemia must be corrected with oral glucose (such as D-glucose or dextrose), and severe hypoglycemia may warrant I.V. glucose or glucagon injection.

• Be aware that drug may be used alone or in combination with insulin, metformin, or sulfonylureas (such as glipizide, glyburide, or glimepiride).

Route	Onset	Peak	Duration
P.O.	Rapid	1 hr	Unknown

Adverse reactions

GI: diarrhea, abdominal pain, flatulence
Metabolic: hypoglycemia (when used with insulin or sulfonylureas)
Other: edema, hypersensitivity reaction (rash)

Interactions

Drug-drug. *Activated charcoal, calcium channel blockers, corticosteroids, digestive enzymes, diuretics, estrogen, hormonal contraceptives, isoniazid, nicotinic acid, phenothiazines, phenytoin, sympathomimetics, thyroid products:* decreased therapeutic effect of acarbose
Digoxin: decreased digoxin blood level and reduced therapeutic effect
Insulin, sulfonylureas: hypoglycemia
Drug-diagnostic tests. *Alanine aminotransferase, aspartate aminotransferase:* increased levels
Calcium, vitamin B_6*:* decreased levels
Hematocrit: decreased

Patient monitoring

• Monitor patient for hypoglycemia if he's taking drug concurrently with insulin or sulfonylureas.
• Stay alert for hyperglycemia during periods of increased stress.
• Assess GI signs and symptoms to differentiate drug effects from those caused by paralytic ileus.
• Check 1-hour postprandial glucose level to gauge drug's efficacy.
• Monitor liver function test results. Report abnormalities so that dosage adjustments may be made as needed.

Patient teaching

• Inform patient that drug may cause serious interactions with many common medications, so he should tell all prescribers he's taking it.
• Teach patient about other ways to control blood glucose level, such as recommendations regarding diet, exercise, weight reduction, and stress management.
• Stress importance of testing urine and blood glucose regularly.
• Teach patient about signs and symptoms of hypoglycemia. Tell him that although this drug doesn't cause hypoglycemia when used alone, hypoglycemic symptoms may arise if he takes it with other hypoglycemics.
• Urge patient to keep oral glucose on hand to correct mild hypoglycemia; inform him that sugar in candy won't correct hypoglycemia.
• Inform patient that GI symptoms such as flatulence may result from delayed carbohydrate digestion in intestine.
• Advise patient to obtain medical alert identification and to carry or wear it at all times.
• As appropriate, review all other significant and life-threatening adverse reactions and interactions, especially those related to the drugs and tests mentioned above.

acebutolol hydrochloride

Monitan✱, Rhotral✱, Sectral

Pharmacologic class: Beta-adrenergic blocker (selective)

Therapeutic class: Antihypertensive, antiarrhythmic (class II)

Pregnancy risk category B

Action

At low doses, selectively inhibits response to adrenergic stimulation by blocking cardiac $beta_1$-adrenergic receptors (with little effect on $beta_2$-adrenergic receptors of bronchial and vascular smooth muscle). At high doses, inhibits both $beta_1$- and $beta_2$-adrenergic receptors, causing airway resistance.

Availability

Capsules: 200 mg, 400 mg
Tablets: 100 mg, 200 mg, 400 mg

Indications and dosages

➢ Hypertension
Adults: Initially, 400 mg P.O. daily or 200 mg b.i.d.; optimal response usually occurs at 400 to 800 mg daily. For severe hypertension, increase dosage gradually to a maximum of 1,200 mg daily in two divided doses.
➢ Premature ventricular arrhythmias
Adults: Initially, 200 mg P.O. b.i.d. Increase dosage gradually until optimum response occurs, usually at 600 to 1,200 mg daily.

Dosage adjustment

- Renal impairment
- Elderly patients

Off-label uses

- Acute phase of myocardial infarction (MI)
- Stable angina

Contraindications

- Hypersensitivity to drug
- Heart failure or cardiogenic shock
- Second- or third-degree heart block
- Severe bradycardia
- Obstructive airway disease
- Breastfeeding

Precautions

Use cautiously in:
- renal or hepatic impairment, inadequate cardiac function, peripheral or mesenteric vascular disease, hyperthyroidism, diabetes mellitus
- elderly patients
- pregnant patients
- children.

Administration

Withhold drug and notify prescriber if patient's apical pulse is below 60 beats/minute.
- Before surgery, notify anesthesiologist that patient is receiving drug.
- Avoid dosages above 800 mg daily in elderly patients.

Route	Onset	Peak	Duration
P.O. (blood pressure effect)	1-1.5 hr	2-8 hr	12-24 hr
P.O. (antiarrhythmic effect)	1 hr	4-6 hr	Up to 10 hr

Adverse reactions

CNS: fatigue, lethargy, insomnia, dizziness, depression, short-term memory loss, emotional lability, anxiety, confusion, headache, partial sensation loss, hemiparesis
CV: hypotension, chest pain, palpitations, peripheral vascular insufficiency, peripheral vasodilation, worsening arterial insufficiency, claudication, **bradycardia, heart failure, intensified atrioventricular nodal block**
EENT: dry burning eyes, abnormal or blurred vision, eye irritation and pain, conjunctivitis, tinnitus, pharyngitis
GI: nausea, vomiting, diarrhea, constipation, dyspepsia, abdominal pain, dry mouth, anorexia, **mesenteric arterial thrombosis, ischemic colitis**
GU: frequent or difficult urination, nocturia, diminished libido, impotence, Peyronie's disease
Hematologic: agranulocytosis, nonthrombocytopenic purpura
Metabolic: type 2 diabetes mellitus, hypoglycemia in nondiabetic patients, increased hypoglycemic response to insulin
Musculoskeletal: joint, back, or muscle pain
Respiratory: dyspnea, wheezing, cough, shortness of breath, **bronchospasm, bronchoconstriction**
Skin: rash, pruritus, diaphoresis

Other: fever, thirst, edema, pneumonitis, pleurisy, lupus erythematosus–like illness, hypersensitivity reaction, **pulmonary granuloma, pleuropulmonary fibrosis**

Interactions

Drug-drug. *Alpha agonists (such as nasal decongestants and other beta-adrenergic blockers):* increased risk of severe hypertension
Aluminum or calcium salts, barbiturates, cholestyramine, colestipol, indomethacin, nonsteroidal anti-inflammatory drugs, penicillin, rifampin, salicylates, sulfinpyrazone: decreased antihypertensive effect
Anticholinergics, hydralazine, methyldopa, prazosin: increased risk of bradycardia and hypotension
Beta$_2$-agonists (such as theophylline): decreased beta$_2$-agonist effect, possibly leading to bronchoconstriction
Calcium channel blockers (nondihydropyridine): synergistic effects
Cardiac glycosides: additive negative effect on sinoatrial (SA) or atrioventricular node conduction, slowing or completely suppressing SA node activity
Catecholamine-depleting drugs: marked bradycardia, hypertension, vertigo, syncope, and orthostatic blood pressure changes
Diuretics: increased hypotensive effect
Epinephrine: increased risk of blocked sympathomimetic effects
Ergot alkaloids: increased risk of peripheral ischemia and gangrene
Glyburide in patients with type 2 diabetes: decreased hypoglycemic effect
Lidocaine: increased lidocaine blood level and possible toxicity
Drug-diagnostic tests. *Alkaline phosphatase, antinuclear antibody titers, bilirubin, blood urea nitrogen, lactate dehydrogenase, low-density lipoproteins, transaminases:* increased levels
Glucose tolerance test: altered tolerance
Drug-herbs. *Aloe, buckthorn bark or berry, cascara bark, rhubarb root, senna leaf or fruit:* increased acebutolol effect
Ephedra (ma huang): arrhythmias

Patient monitoring

- Carefully monitor blood pressure during initial dosage titration. Notify prescriber of significant or abrupt blood pressure decrease.
- Observe for orthostatic hypotension, especially when giving drug with other antihypertensives.
- Watch closely for marked bradycardia or hypotension if giving drug with reserpine or other catecholamine-depleting agents.
- Be aware that drug may mask signs and symptoms of hypoglycemia in patients with diabetes mellitus or hyperthyroidism.

🔊 Taper dosage gradually over 2 weeks when discontinuing. Abrupt withdrawal may exacerbate angina or trigger MI, especially in patients with coronary artery disease.

Patient teaching

- Teach patient how to take his pulse. Tell him to notify prescriber if pulse rate is below 60 beats/minute.
- Caution patient to avoid driving and other hazardous activities until he knows how drug affects concentration, alertness, and vision.
- Tell patient to watch for and report hypoglycemia signs and symptoms.
- Instruct patient with bronchospastic disease to keep bronchodilator on hand at all times.
- Instruct patient to store drug in tight container at room temperature, protected from light.
- As appropriate, review all other significant and life-threatening adverse reactions and interactions, especially those related to the drugs, tests, and herbs mentioned above.

a

acetaminophen

Abenol✱, Acephen, Aceta, Acetaminophen, Actimol, Aminofen, Apacet, Apo-Acetaminophen✱, Arthritis Foundation Pain Reliever, Aspirin Free, Aspirin Free Anacin, Aspirin Free Pain Relief, Atasol✱, Banesin, Children's Pain Reliever, Children's Tylenol Soft Chews, Dapa, Dolono, Datril, Dynafed✱, Dynafed E.X., Exdol✱, Feverall, Genapap, Genebs, Halenol, Halenol Children's, Infant's Pain Reliever, Liquiprin, Mapap, Maranox, Neopap, Oraphen-PD, Panadol, Redutemp, Ridenol, Robigesic✱, Silapap, St. Joseph Aspirin-Free Drops, Tapanol, Tempra, Tylenol, Tylenol Arthritis, Uni-Ace

Pharmacologic class: Synthetic nonopioid *p*-aminophenol derivative

Therapeutic class: Analgesic, antipyretic

Pregnancy risk category B

Action

Unclear. Pain relief may result from inhibition of prostaglandin synthesis in CNS, with subsequent blockage of pain impulses. Fever reduction may result from vasodilation and increased peripheral blood flow in hypothalamus, which dissipates heat and lowers body temperature.

Availability

Caplets, capsules: 160 mg, 500 mg, 650 mg (extended-release)
Drops: 100 mg/ml
Elixir: 80 mg/2.5 ml, 80 mg/5 ml, 120 mg/5 ml, 160 mg/5 ml
Gelcaps: 500 mg
Liquid: 160 mg/5 ml, 500 mg/15 ml
Solution: 80 mg/1.66 ml, 100 mg/1 ml, 120 mg/2.5 ml, 160 mg/5 ml, 167 mg/5 ml
Suppositories: 80 mg, 120 mg, 125 mg, 300 mg, 325 mg, 650 mg
Suspension: 32 mg/ml, 160 mg/5 ml
Syrup: 160 mg/5 ml
Tablets (chewable): 80 mg, 160 mg
Tablets (extended-release): 160 mg, 325 mg, 500 mg, 650 mg
Tablets (film-coated): 160 mg, 325 mg, 500 mg

Indications and dosages

➢ Mild to moderate pain caused by headache, muscle ache, backache, minor arthritis, common cold, toothache, or menstrual cramps; fever
Adults: 325 to 650 mg P.O. q 4 to 6 hours, or 1,000 mg three or four times daily. Or two extended-release caplets or tablets P.O. q 8 hours, to a maximum dosage of 4,000 mg/day. Or 650 mg P.R. q 4 to 6 hours, to a maximum dosage of 4,000 mg/day.
Children: 10 to 15 mg/kg, or as indicated below:

Oral use

Age	Usual dosage	Maximum dosage
11-12 years	480 mg q 4 hr	5 doses in 24 hr
9-10 years	400 mg q 4 hr	5 doses in 24 hr
6-8 years	320 mg q 4 hr	5 doses in 24 hr
4-5 years	240 mg q 4 hr	5 doses in 24 hr
2-3 years	160 mg q 4 hr	5 doses in 24 hr
1 year	120 mg q 4 hr	5 doses in 24 hr
4-11 months	80 mg q 4 hr	5 doses in 24 hr
0-3 months	40 mg q 4 hr	5 doses in 24 hr

Rectal use

Age	Usual dosage	Maximum dosage
12 years and older	325-650 mg q 4 hr	4,000 mg/day
11-12 years	320-480 mg q 4 hr	2,880 mg/day

(continued)

Rectal use *(continued)*

Age	Usual dosage	Maximum dosage
6-11 years	325 mg q 4 hr	2,600 mg/day
3-6 years	120-125 mg q 6 hr	720 mg/day
1-3 years	80 mg q 4 hr	
3-11 months	80 mg q 6 hr	

Dosage adjustment
- Renal or hepatic impairment

Contraindications
- Hypersensitivity to drug

Precautions
Use cautiously in:
- anemia, hepatic or renal disease
- elderly patients
- pregnant or breastfeeding patients
- children younger than age 2.

Administration
- Be aware that although most patients tolerate drug well, toxicity can occur with a single dose.
- Know that acetylcysteine may be ordered to treat acetaminophen toxicity, depending on patient's blood drug level. Activated charcoal is used to treat acute, recent acetaminophen overdose (within 1 hour of ingestion).
- Determine overdose severity by measuring acetaminophen blood level no sooner than 4 hours after overdose ingestion (to ensure that peak concentration has been reached).

Route	Onset	Peak	Duration
P.O.	0.5-1 hr	10-60 min	3-8 hr (dose dependent)
P.R.	0.5-1 hr	10-60 min	3-4 hr

Adverse reactions
Hematologic: thrombocytopenia, hemolytic anemia, neutropenia, leukopenia, pancytopenia
Hepatic: jaundice, **hepatotoxicity**
Metabolic: hypoglycemic coma
Skin: rash, urticaria
Other: hypersensitivity reactions (such as fever)

Interactions
Drug-drug. *Activated charcoal, cholestyramine, colestipol:* decreased acetaminophen absorption
Barbiturates, carbamazepine, diflunisal, hydantoins, isoniazid, rifabutin, rifampin, sulfinpyrazone: increased risk of hepatotoxicity
Hormonal contraceptives: decreased acetaminophen efficacy
Oral anticoagulants: increased anticoagulant effect
Phenothiazines (such as chlorpromazine, fluphenazine, thioridazine): severe hypothermia
Zidovudine: increased risk of granulocytopenia
Drug-diagnostic tests. *Home glucose measurement systems:* altered results
Urine 5-hydroxyindole acetic acid: false-positive result
Drug-behaviors. *Alcohol use:* increased risk of hepatotoxicity

Patient monitoring
🔊 Observe for acute toxicity and overdose. Signs and symptoms of acute toxicity are as follows—*Phase 1:* Nausea, vomiting, anorexia, malaise, diaphoresis. *Phase 2:* Right upper quadrant pain or tenderness, liver enlargement, elevated bilirubin and hepatic enzyme levels, prolonged prothrombin time, oliguria (occasional). *Phase 3:* Recurrent anorexia, nausea, vomiting, and malaise; jaundice; hypoglycemia; coagulopathy; encephalopathy; possible renal failure and cardiomyopathy. *Phase 4*: Either recovery or progression to fatal complete hepatic failure.

Patient teaching
- Caution parents or other caregivers not to give acetaminophen to children

younger than age 2 without consulting prescriber first.
- Tell patient, parents, or other caregivers not to use drug concurrently with other acetaminophen-containing products.
- Advise patient, parents, or other caregivers to contact prescriber if fever or other symptoms persist despite taking recommended amount of drug.
- Inform patients with chronic alcoholism that drug may increase risk of severe liver damage.
- As appropriate, review all other significant and life-threatening adverse reactions and interactions, especially those related to the drugs, tests, and behaviors mentioned above.

acetazolamide

Acetazolam✦, AK-Zol, Apo-Acetazolamide✦, Dazamide, Diamox, Diamox Sequels, Storzolamide

Pharmacologic class: Carbonic anhydrase inhibitor
Therapeutic class: Diuretic, antiglaucoma drug, anticonvulsant, altitude agent, urinary alkalinizer
Pregnancy risk category C

Action

Inhibits carbonic anhydrase in kidney, decreasing water reabsorption and increasing excretion of sodium, potassium, and bicarbonate. Lowers intraocular pressure by decreasing aqueous humor production. May raise seizure threshold by reducing carbonic anhydrase in CNS, thereby decreasing neuronal conduction.

Availability

Capsules (sustained-release): 500 mg
Injection: 500 mg/vial
Tablets: 125 mg, 250 mg

Indications and dosages

➤ Open-angle (chronic simple) glaucoma (given with miotics)
Adults: 250 mg P.O. one to four times daily, or 500-mg sustained-release capsule P.O. once or twice daily. Don't exceed total daily dosage of 1 g.

➤ Preoperative treatment of closed-angle (secondary) glaucoma
Adults: 250 mg P.O. q 4 hours or 250 mg P.O. b.i.d.; in acute cases only, 500 mg P.O. followed by 125 to 250 mg P.O. q 4 hours. For rapid relief of increased intraocular pressure, 500 mg I.V., repeated in 2 to 4 hours; then 125 to 250 mg P.O. q 4 to 6 hours.
Children: 10 to 15 mg/kg/day P.O. in divided doses q 6 to 8 hours, or 5 to 10 mg/kg I.V. q 6 hours

➤ Seizure disorder (given with other anticonvulsants)
Adults and children: 250 mg P.O. daily when given with another anticonvulsant, or 8 to 30 mg/kg daily P.O. in one to four divided doses. Usual dosage range is 375 mg to 1 g daily.

➤ Drug-induced edema or edema secondary to heart failure
Adults: Initially, 250 to 375 mg P.O. daily. If diuresis fails, give dose on alternate days, or give for 2 days alternating with day of rest.
Children: 5 mg/kg P.O. daily, or 150 mg/m^2 P.O. or I.V. once daily in morning

➤ Acute high-altitude (mountain) sickness
Adults: 500 mg to 1 g P.O. daily in divided doses, or sustained-release capsule q 12 to 24 hours. Dosing should begin 24 to 48 hours before ascent and continue during ascent and for 48 hours after reaching desired altitude. For rapid ascent, 1-g P.O. dose is recommended.

Dosage adjustment

- Mild renal failure

Off-label uses

- Acute pancreatitis
- Alkalosis after open-heart surgery
- Hereditary ataxia
- Peptic ulcer
- Periodic paralysis
- Renal calculi
- Phenobarbital or lithium overdose
- Hydrocephalus in infants

Contraindications

- Hypersensitivity to drug or sulfonamides
- Adrenocortical insufficiency
- Closed-angle glaucoma
- Severe pulmonary obstruction
- Severe renal disease, hypokalemia, hyponatremia
- Hepatic disease

Precautions

Use cautiously in:

- respiratory, renal, or hepatic disease; diabetes mellitus, hypercalcemia, gout, adrenocortical insufficiency
- pregnant or breastfeeding patients.

Administration

Before giving, ask if patient is pregnant. Drug may cause fetal toxicity.

- Direct I.V. administration is preferred. When giving by direct I.V. route, reconstitute 500-mg vial with more than 5 ml of sterile water for injection; administer over 1 minute.
- When giving drug intermittently, further dilute with normal saline solution or dextrose solution and infuse over 4 to 8 hours.
- Be aware that I.M. administration is painful because solution is alkaline.
- If necessary, crush tablets and mix in nonsweet, nonalcoholic syrup or nonglycerin solution.

Route	Onset	Peak	Duration
P.O.	1 hr	2-4 hr	8-12 hr
P.O. (sustained)	2 hr	8-12 hr	18-24
I.V., I.M.	1-2 min	15-18 min	4-5 hr

Adverse reactions

CNS: weakness, nervousness, irritability, drowsiness, confusion, dizziness, depression, tremor, headache, paresthesia, flaccid paralysis, **seizures**
EENT: transient myopia, tinnitus, hearing dysfunction, sensation of lump in throat
GI: nausea, vomiting, diarrhea, constipation, melena, abdominal distention, dry mouth, anorexia
GU: dysuria, hematuria, glycosuria, polyuria, crystalluria, renal colic, renal calculi, **uremia, sulfonamide-like renal lesions, renal failure**
Hematologic: thrombocytopenia, leukopenia, agranulocytosis, hemolytic anemia, thrombocytopenic purpura, pancytopenia, bone marrow depression with aplastic anemia
Hepatic: hepatic insufficiency
Metabolic: hypokalemia, hyperglycemia and glycosuria, hyperuricemia and gout, **metabolic acidosis, hyperchloremic acidosis**
Respiratory: hyperpnea
Skin: rash, pruritus, urticaria, photosensitivity, hirsutism, cyanosis
Other: altered taste and smell, weight loss, fever, excessive thirst, pain at I.M. injection site, hypersensitivity reaction, **Stevens-Johnson syndrome**

Interactions

Drug-drug. *Amphetamines, procainamide, quinidine, tricyclic antidepressants:* decreased excretion and enhanced or prolonged effect of these drugs, leading to toxicity
Amphotericin B, corticosteroids, corticotrophin, other diuretics: increased risk of hypokalemia
Lithium, phenobarbital, salicylates: increased excretion of these drugs, possibly reducing their efficacy
Methenamine compounds: inactivation of these drugs
Phenytoin, primidone: severe osteomalacia

Salicylates: increased risk of salicylate toxicity
Drug-diagnostic tests. *Ammonia, bilirubin, calcium, chloride, glucose, uric acid:* increased levels
Thyroid iodine uptake: decreased in patients with hyperthyroidism or normal thyroid function
Urinary protein (with some reagents): false-positive result
Drug-behaviors. *Sun exposure:* increased risk of photosensitivity

Patient monitoring

Evaluate for signs and symptoms of sulfonamide sensitivity; drug can cause fatal hypersensitivity.
Monitor laboratory test results for hematologic changes; blood glucose, potassium, bicarbonate, and chloride levels; and liver and kidney function changes.
• Observe for signs and symptoms of bleeding tendency.
• Monitor fluid intake and output.

Patient teaching

• Advise patient to take drug with food if GI upset occurs.
• Caution patient to avoid driving and other hazardous activities until he knows how drug affects concentration and alertness.
• Tell patient to eat potassium-rich foods (such as seafood, bananas, and oranges) if taking drug long term or receiving other potassium-depleting drugs.
• Advise patient to avoid activities that can cause injury. Advise him to use soft toothbrush and electric razor to avoid gum and skin injury.
• Tell patient to report significant numbness or tingling.
• Inform patient that he'll undergo regular blood testing during therapy.
• As appropriate, review all other significant and life-threatening adverse reactions and interactions, especially those related to the drugs, tests, and behaviors mentioned above.

acetylcysteine (*N*-acetylcysteine)

Acetadote, Mucomyst✱, Mucomyst 10, Mucosil-10, Mucosil-20, Parvolex✱

Pharmacologic class: *N*-acetyl derivative of naturally occurring amino acid (L-cysteine)

Therapeutic class: Mucolytic, acetaminophen antidote

Pregnancy risk category B

Action

Decreases viscosity of secretions, promoting secretion removal through coughing, postural drainage, and mechanical means. In acetaminophen overdose, maintains and restores hepatic glutathione, needed to inactivate toxic metabolites.

Availability

Injection: 200 mg/ml
Solution: 10%, 20%

Indications and dosages

➢ Mucolytic agent in adjunctive treatment of acute and chronic bronchopulmonary disease (bronchitis, bronchiectasis, chronic asthmatic bronchitis, emphysema, pneumonia, primary amyloidism of lungs, tuberculosis, tracheobronchitis), pulmonary complications of cystic fibrosis, atelectasis, or pulmonary complications related to surgery, posttraumatic chest conditions, tracheostomy care, or use during anesthesia
Adults and children: *Nebulization (face mask, mouthpiece, tracheostomy)*— 6 to 10 ml of 10% solution or

3 to 5 ml of 20% solution three or four times daily. Dosage range is 2 to 20 ml of 10% solution or 1 to 10 ml of 20% solution q 2 to 6 hours.
Nebulization (tent or croupette)—Volume of 10% or 20% solution that will maintain heavy mist for desired period
Instillation (direct)—1 to 2 ml of 10% to 20% solution q 1 hour p.r.n.
Instillation via syringe attached to percutaneous intratracheal catheter—2 to 4 ml of 10% solution or 1 to 2 ml of 20% solution q 1 to 4 hours
➢ Diagnostic bronchial studies
Adults and children: Two to three doses of 2 to 4 ml of 10% solution or 1 to 2 ml of 20% solution by nebulization or intratracheal instillation before procedure
➢ Acetaminophen overdose
Adults, elderly patients, children: Give immediately if 24 hours or less have elapsed since acetaminophen ingestion. Use the following protocol: Empty stomach by lavage or emesis induction, and then have patient drink copious amounts of water. If activated charcoal has been given, perform lavage before giving acetylcysteine. Draw blood for acetaminophen plasma assay and baseline aspartate aminotransferase (AST), alanine aminotransferase (ALT), prothrombin time, bilirubin, blood glucose, blood urea nitrogen, electrolyte, and creatinine clearance levels. If ingested acetaminophen dose is in toxic range, give acetylcysteine 140 mg/kg P.O. as loading dose from 20% solution. Administer 17 maintenance doses of 70 mg/kg P.O. q 4 hours, starting 4 hours after loading dose. Repeat procedure until acetaminophen blood level is safe. If patient vomits loading dose or any maintenance dose within 1 hour of administration, repeat that dose.

Off-label uses
- Unstable angina

Contraindications
- Hypersensitivity to drug (except with antidotal use)
- Status asthmaticus (except with antidotal use)

Precautions
Use cautiously in:
- renal or hepatic disease, Addison's disease, alcoholism, brain tumor, bronchial asthma, seizure disorder, hypothyroidism, respiratory insufficiency, psychosis
- elderly patients
- pregnant or breastfeeding patients.

Administration
- Separate administration times of this drug and antibiotics.
- Use plastic, glass, or stainless steel container when giving by nebulizer, because solution discolors on contact with rubber and some metals.
- Once solution is exposed to air, use within 96 hours.
- Dilute solution before administering for acetaminophen overdose, to reduce risk of vomiting and reduce drug's unpleasant odor and irritating or sclerosing properties.
- Chill solution and have patient sip through straw, or, if necessary, give by nasogastric tube when administering for acetaminophen overdose.

Route	Onset	Peak	Duration
P.O.	30-60 min	1-2 hr	Unknown
Instillation, inhalation	1 min	5-10 min	2-3 hr

Adverse reactions
CNS: dizziness, drowsiness, headache
CV: hypotension, hypertension, tachycardia
EENT: severe rhinorrhea

GI: nausea, vomiting, stomatitis, constipation, anorexia
Hepatic: hepatotoxicity
Respiratory: hemoptysis, tracheal and bronchial irritation, increased secretions, wheezing, chest tightness, **bronchospasm**
Skin: urticaria, rash, clamminess, angioedema
Other: tooth damage, chills, fever

Interactions

Drug-drug. *Activated charcoal:* increased absorption and decreased efficacy of acetylcysteine
Nitroglycerin: increased nitroglycerin effects, causing hypotension and headache
Drug-diagnostic tests. *Liver function tests:* abnormal results

Patient monitoring

- Monitor respirations, cough, and character of secretions.

Patient teaching

- Instruct patient to report worsening cough and other respiratory symptoms.
- Advise patient to mix oral form with juice or cola to mask bad taste and odor.
- As appropriate, review all other significant and life-threatening adverse reactions and interactions, especially those related to the drugs and tests mentioned above.

acetylsalicylic acid (aspirin)

Acuprin, Apo-Asa✤, Apo–ASEN✤, Arthrinol✤, Arthrisin✤, Arthritis Foundation Pain Reliever, Artria S.R.✤, ASA, Aspergum, Aspirin✤, Aspir-Low, Aspirtab, Astrin✤, Bayer, Coryphen✤, Easprin, Ecotrin, Empirin, Entrophen✤, Genprin, Halfprin, Headache Tablet✤, Healthprin, Heartline, Norwich, Novasen✤, PMS-ASA✤, Sal-Adult✤, Sal-Infant✤, Sloprin, St. Joseph, Supasa✤, Sureprin, ZORprin

Pharmacologic class: Nonsteroidal anti-inflammatory drug (NSAID)
Therapeutic class: Nonopioid analgesic, antipyretic, antiplatelet drug
Pregnancy risk category C (with full dose in third trimester: ***D***)

Action

Reduces pain and inflammation by inhibiting prostaglandin production. Fever reduction mechanism unknown; may be linked to decrease in endogenous pyrogens in hypothalamus resulting from prostaglandin inhibition. Exerts antiplatelet effect by inhibiting synthesis of prostacyclin and thromboxane A_2.

Availability

Gum (chewable): 227 mg
Suppositories: 60 mg, 120 mg, 200 mg, 300 mg, 325 mg, 600 mg, 650 mg
Tablets: 81 mg, 325 mg, 500 mg
Tablets (chewable): 81 mg
Tablets (enteric-coated, delayed-release): 81 mg, 162 mg, 325 mg, 500 mg, 650 mg, 975 mg
Tablets (extended-release): 650 mg, 800 mg
Tablets (film-coated): 325 mg, 500 mg

Indications and dosages

➢ Mild pain or fever

Adults: 325 to 500 mg P.O. q 3 hours, or 325 to 650 mg P.O. q 4 hours, or 650 to 1,000 mg P.O. q 6 hours, to a maximum dosage of 4,000 mg/day. *Extended-release tablets*—650 mg to 1,300 mg q 8 hours, not to exceed 3,900 mg/day; or 800 mg q 12 hours.

Children: 10 to 15 mg/kg P.O. or P.R. q 4 hours, not to exceed total daily dosage of 3.6 g, or up to 60 to 80 mg/kg/day. See chart below.

Age (years)	Dosage (q 4 hr)
12-14	648 mg
11-12	486 mg
9-10	405 mg
6-8	324 mg
4-5	243 mg
2-3	162 mg

➢ Mild to moderate pain caused by inflammation (as in rheumatoid arthritis or osteoarthritis)

Adults: Initially, 2,400 to 3,600 mg P.O. daily in divided doses. Dosage may be increased by 325 to 1,200 mg daily at intervals of at least 1 week. Usual maintenance dosage is 3.6 to 5.4 g/day P.O. in divided doses, to a maximum dosage of 6 g/day.

➢ Juvenile rheumatoid arthritis

Children: 60 to 130 mg/kg/day P.O. in children weighing 25 kg (55 lb) or less, or 2,400 to 3,600 mg P.O. daily in children weighing more than 25 kg P.O.; give in divided doses q 6 to 8 hours.

➢ Acute rheumatic fever

Adults: 5 to 8 g/day P.O. in divided doses

Children: Initially, 100 mg/kg/day P.O. in individual doses for first 2 weeks; then maintenance dosage of 75 mg/kg/day P.O. in divided doses for next 4 to 6 weeks

➢ To reduce the risk of transient ischemic attacks (TIAs) or cerebrovascular accident in men with a history of TIAs caused by emboli

Adults: 650 mg P.O. b.i.d or 325 mg P.O. q.i.d.

➢ To reduce the risk of myocardial infarction (MI) in patients with a history of MI or unstable angina

Adults: 75 to 325 mg/day P.O.

➢ Kawasaki disease

Children: Initially during acute febrile period, 80 to 180 mg/kg/day P.O. in four divided doses. Maintenance dosage is 3 to 10 mg/kg/day given as a single dose for up to 8 weeks or until platelet count and erythrocyte sedimentation rate return to normal.

➢ Thromboembolic disorders

Adults: 325 to 650 mg P.O. once or twice daily

Contraindications

- Hypersensitivity to salicylates, other NSAIDs, or tartrazine
- Renal impairment
- Severe hepatic impairment
- Hemorrhagic states or blood coagulation defects
- Vitamin K deficiency caused by dehydration
- Concurrent anticoagulant use
- Pregnancy (third trimester) or breastfeeding

Precautions

Use with extreme caution, if at all, in:

- hepatic disorders, anemia, asthma, gastritis, Hodgkin's disease
- heart failure or other conditions in which high sodium content is harmful (buffered aspirin)
- patients receiving other salicylates or NSAIDs concurrently
- elderly patients
- children and adolescents.

Administration

Never administer to child or adolescent who has signs or symptoms of chickenpox or flulike illness.

Don't give within 6 weeks after administration of live varicella virus vaccine, because of risk of Reye's syndrome.
• Give with food or large amounts of water or milk to minimize GI irritation.
• Know that extended-release and enteric-coated forms are best for long-term therapy.
• Be aware that aspirin should be discontinued at least 1 week before surgery because it may inhibit platelet aggregation.

Route	Onset	Peak	Duration
P.O. (tablets)	15-30 min	1-2 hr	4-6 hr
P.O. (chewable)	Rapid	Unknown	1-4 hr
P.O. (enteric-coated)	5-30 min	2-4 hr	8-12 hr
P.O. (extended)	5-30 min	1-4 hr	3-6 hr
P.R.	5-30 min	3-4 hr	1-4 hr

Adverse reactions

EENT: hearing loss, tinnitus, ototoxicity
GI: nausea, vomiting, abdominal pain, dyspepsia, epigastric distress, heartburn, anorexia, **GI bleeding**
Hematologic: thrombocytopenia, hemolytic anemia, leukopenia, agranulocytosis, shortened red blood cell life span
Hepatic: hepatotoxicity
Metabolic: hyponatremia, hypokalemia, **hypoglycemia**
Respiratory: wheezing, hyperpnea, **pulmonary edema with toxicity**
Skin: rash, urticaria, bruising, angioedema
Other: hypersensitivity reactions, **salicylism or acute toxicity**

Interactions

Drug-drug. *Acidifying drugs (such as ammonium chloride):* increased salicylate blood level
Activated charcoal: decreased salicylate absorption
Alkalinizing drugs (such as antacids): decreased salicylate blood level
Angiotensin-converting enzyme (ACE) inhibitors: decreased antihypertensive effect
Anticoagulants, NSAIDs, thrombolytics: increased bleeding risk
Carbonic anhydrase inhibitors (such as acetazolamide): salicylism
Corticosteroids: increased salicylate excretion and decreased blood level
Furosemide: increased diuretic effect
Live varicella virus vaccine: increased risk of Reye's syndrome
Methotrexate: decreased methotrexate excretion and increased blood level, causing greater risk of toxicity
Nizatidine: increased salicylate blood level
Spironolactone: decreased spironolactone effect
Sulfonylureas (such as chlorpropamide, tolbutamide): enhanced sulfonylurea effects
Tetracycline (oral): decreased absorption of tetracycline (with buffered aspirin)
Drug-diagnostic tests. *Alanine aminotransferase, alkaline phosphatase, amylase, aspartate aminotransferase, coagulation studies, $Paco_2$, uric acid:* increased values
Cholesterol, glucose, potassium, protein-bound iodine, sodium, thyroxine, triiodothyronine: decreased levels
Pregnancy test, protirelin-induced thyroid stimulating hormone, radionuclide thyroid imaging, serum theophylline (Schack and Waxler method), urine catecholamines, urine glucose, urine hydroxyindoleacetic acid, urine ketones (ferric chloride method), urine vanillylmandelic acid: test interference
Tests using phenosulfonphthalein as diagnostic agent: decreased urinary excretion of phenosulfonphthalein
Urine protein: increased level
Drug-food. *Urine-acidifying foods:* increased salicylate blood level

Drug-herbs. *Anise, arnica, cayenne, chamomile, clove, fenugreek, feverfew, garlic, ginger, ginkgo biloba, ginseng, horse chestnut, kelpware, licorice:* increased bleeding risk
Drug-behaviors. *Alcohol use:* increased bleeding risk

Patient monitoring

- Watch for signs and symptoms of hypersensitivity and other adverse reactions, especially bleeding tendency.
- Stay alert for signs and symptoms of acute toxicity, such as diplopia, ECG abnormalities, generalized seizures, hallucinations, hyperthermia, oliguria, acute renal failure, incoherent speech, irritability, restlessness, tremor, vertigo, confusion, disorientation, mania, lethargy, laryngeal edema, anaphylaxis, and coma.
- Monitor elderly patients carefully because they're at greater risk for salicylate toxicity.
- With prolonged therapy, frequently assess hemoglobin, hematocrit, International Normalized Ratio, and kidney function test results.
- Check salicylate blood levels frequently.
- Evaluate patient for signs and symptoms of ototoxicity (hearing loss, tinnitus, ataxia, and vertigo).

Patient teaching

- Tell patient to report ototoxicity symptoms, unusual bleeding, and bruising.
- Caution patient to avoid activities that may cause injury. Advise him to use soft toothbrush and electric razor to avoid gum and skin injury.
- Instruct patient to tell all prescribers he's taking drug, because it may cause serious interactions with many common medications.
- Tell patient not to take other over-the-counter preparations containing aspirin.
- Inform patient that he may need to undergo regular blood testing during therapy.
- As appropriate, review all other significant and life-threatening adverse reactions and interactions, especially those related to the drugs, tests, foods, herbs, and behaviors mentioned above.

acitretin
Soriatane

Pharmacologic class: Second-generation retinoid
Therapeutic class: Antipsoriatic
Pregnancy risk category X

Action
Unclear. Promotes normal growth cycle of skin cells, possibly by targeting retinoid receptors in these cells and adjusting factors that affect epidermal proliferation and synthesis of RNA and DNA.

Availability
Capsules: 10 mg, 25 mg

Indications and dosages
➤ Severe psoriasis, including erythrodermic and generalized pustule types
Adults and elderly patients: Initially, 25 to 50 mg/day P.O. as a single dose with main meal. If initial response is satisfactory, give maintenance dosage of 25 to 50 mg/day P.O.

Off-label uses
- Darier's disease (keratosis follicularis)
- Lamellar ichthyosis (in children)
- Lichen planus
- Nonbullous and bullous ichthyosiform erythroderma
- Palmoplantar pustulosis
- Sjögren-Larsson syndrome

Contraindications

- Hypersensitivity to drug or paraben (used as preservative in gelatin capsule)
- Pregnancy or anticipated pregnancy within 3 years after drug discontinuation (drug has teratogenic and embryotoxic effects)
- Women of childbearing age who may not use reliable contraception during therapy and for at least 3 years after drug discontinuation
- Breastfeeding

Precautions

Use cautiously in:

- hepatic or renal impairment, diabetes mellitus, obesity
- elevated cholesterol or triglyceride levels
- elderly patients.

Administration

Verify that patient isn't pregnant before giving drug.

- Give as a single dose with main meal.

Route	Onset	Peak	Duration
P.O.	Unknown	Unknown	Unknown

Adverse reactions

CNS: headache, depression, insomnia, drowsiness, fatigue, migraine, rigors, abnormal gait, nerve inflammation, hyperesthesia, paresthesia, **pseudotumor cerebri**
EENT: abnormal or blurred vision, dry eyes, eye irritation, eyebrow and eyelash loss, eyelid inflammation, cataract, conjunctivitis, corneal epithelial abnormality, reduced night vision, photophobia, recurrent styes, earache, tinnitus, hearing loss, epistaxis, rhinitis, sinusitis, **papilledema**
GI: nausea, vomiting, diarrhea, constipation, abdominal pain, gastritis, stomatitis, esophagitis, melena, painful straining at stool, pancreatitis, lip inflammation and cracking, dry mouth, anorexia
GU: abnormal urine, dysuria, atrophic vaginitis, leukorrhea
Hepatic: abnormal hepatic function, jaundice, **hepatitis**
Metabolic: poor blood glucose control
Musculoskeletal: joint, muscle, back, and bone pain; arthritis; bone disorders; spinal bone overgrowth; increased muscle tone or rigidity; tendinitis
Respiratory: coughing, increased sputum, laryngitis
Skin: dry skin, pruritus, skin atrophy, skin peeling, abnormal skin odor, sticky skin, seborrhea, dermatitis, diaphoresis, cold clammy skin, skin infection, rash, pyrogenic granuloma, skin ulcers, skin fissures, sunburn, flushing, purpura, nail disorder, inflammation of tissue surrounding nails, abnormal hair texture, alopecia
Other: abnormal taste, glossitis, tongue ulcers, gingival bleeding, gingivitis, edema, thirst, hot flashes

Interactions

Drug-drug. *Glyburide:* increased blood glucose clearance
Methotrexate: increased risk of hepatotoxicity
Oral contraceptives ("minipill"): decreased contraceptive efficacy
Drug-diagnostic tests. *Alanine aminotransferase, aspartate aminotransferase, triglycerides:* increased levels
Low-density lipoproteins: decreased level
Drug-behaviors. *Alcohol use:* interference with acitretin elimination, possible drug toxicity

Patient monitoring

- Monitor patient who has early signs or symptoms of pseudotumor cerebri, such as headache, nausea, vomiting, and visual disturbances. Discontinue drug immediately if papilledema occurs.

• Check blood lipid levels before therapy begins and every 1 to 2 weeks during therapy.
• Monitor blood glucose levels and kidney and liver function test results.
• If drug causes open skin lesions resulting from dermatitis or blisters, watch for signs and symptoms of infection.
• Assess for pain, stinging, and itching. Apply cool compresses as needed for relief.
Be aware that women taking this drug must avoid alcohol-containing foods, beverages, medications, and over-the-counter products during therapy and for 2 months afterward.

Patient teaching

• Instruct patient to take drug with main meal to minimize GI upset.
• Tell patient to avoid driving and other hazardous activities until he knows how drug affects concentration, alertness, and vision.
• Caution patient not to drink alcohol during therapy.
Advise females to use effective contraception for at least 1 month before starting drug, throughout entire course of therapy, and for 3 years after discontinuing drug.
• Explain that disease may seem to worsen at start of therapy.
• Tell contact lens wearers that lens intolerance may develop.
• As appropriate, review all other significant and life-threatening adverse reactions and interactions, especially those related to the drugs, tests, and behaviors mentioned above.

activated charcoal

Actidose, Actidose-Aqua, CharcoAid, CharcoAid 2000, Charco Caps, Liqui-Char

Pharmacologic class: Carbon residue
Therapeutic class: Antiflatulent, antidote
Pregnancy risk category C

Action

Binds to poisons, toxins, irritants, and drugs, forming a barrier between particulate material and GI mucosa that inhibits absorption of this material in GI tract. As an antiflatulent, reduces intestinal gas volume and relieves related discomfort.

Availability

Capsules: 260 mg
Granules: 15 g/120 ml
Liquid: 15 g/120 ml, 50 g/240 ml, 208 mg/1 ml
Oral suspension: 12.5 g/60 ml, 15 g/75 ml, 25 g/120 ml, 30 g/120 ml, 50 g/240 ml
Powder: 15, 30, 40, 130, 240 g/container

Indications and dosages

➢ Poisoning
Adults: 25 to 100 g P.O. (or 1 g/kg, or about 10 times the amount of poison ingested) as a suspension in 120 to 240 ml (4 to 8 oz) of water
Children: Initially, 1 to 2 g/kg P.O. (or 10 times the amount of poison ingested) as a suspension in 120 to 240 ml (4 to 8 oz) of water
➢ Flatulence
Adults: 600 mg to 5 g P.O. as a single dose, or 975 mg to 3.9 g in divided doses

Off-label uses

• Diarrhea

a

- GI distress
- Hypercholesterolemia

Contraindications
None

Precautions
Use cautiously in:
- patients who have aspirated corrosives or hydrocarbons and are vomiting.

Administration
🔊 Don't try to give activated charcoal to semiconscious patient.
🔊 If signs of aspiration occur, stop giving drug immediately to avoid fatal airway obstruction or infection.
- Administer by large-bore nasogastric tube after gastric lavage, as needed.
- Give within 30 minutes of poison ingestion when possible.
- Mix powder with tap water to form thick syrup. Add fruit juice or flavoring to improve taste.
- Be aware that drug inactivates ipecac syrup.
- Know that drug is ineffective in poisoning from ethanol, methanol, and iron salts.
- Don't give children more than one dose of drug product containing sorbitol (sweetener).
- When used for indications other than as antidote, give drug at least 2 hours before or 1 hour after other drugs.

Route	Onset	Peak	Duration
P.O.	Immediate	Unknown	Unknown

Adverse reactions
GI: nausea, vomiting, diarrhea, constipation, black stools, **intestinal obstruction**

Interactions
Drug-drug. *Acetaminophen, barbiturates, carbamazepine, digitoxin, digoxin, furosemide, glutethimide, hydantoins, methotrexate, nizatidine, phenothiazines, phenylbutazones, propoxyphene, salicylates, sulfonamides, sulfonylurea, tetracycline, theophyllines, tricyclic antidepressants, valproic acid:* decreased absorption of these drugs
Ipecac syrup: ipecac absorption and inactivation
Drug-food. *Milk, ice cream, sherbet:* decreased absorptive activity of drug

Patient monitoring
- Monitor patient for constipation.
- If patient vomits soon after receiving dose, ask prescriber if dose should be repeated.

Patient teaching
- Instruct patient to drink six to eight glasses of fluid daily to prevent constipation.
- Tell patient that stools will be black as charcoal is excreted from body.
- As appropriate, review all other significant and life-threatening adverse reactions and interactions, especially those related to the drugs and foods mentioned above.

acyclovir
acyclovir sodium
Alti-Acyclovir✦, Avirax✦, Zovirax

Pharmacologic class: Acyclic purine nucleoside analogue
Therapeutic class: Antiviral
Pregnancy risk category B

Action
Inhibits viral DNA polymerase, thereby inhibiting replication of viral DNA. Specific for herpes simplex types 1 (HSV-1) and 2 (HSV-2), varicella-zoster virus, Epstein-Barr virus, and cytomegalovirus (CMV).

Availability

Capsules: 200 mg
Cream: 5% in 2-g tube
Injection: 50 mg/ml
Ointment: 5% in 15-g tube
Powder for injection: 500 mg/vial, 1,000 mg/vial
Suspension: 200 mg/5 ml
Tablets: 400 mg, 800 mg

Indications and dosages

➢ Acute treatment of herpes zoster (shingles)
Adults: 800 mg P.O. q 4 hours while awake (five times/day) for 7 to 10 days
➢ Initial episode of genital herpes
Adults: 200 mg P.O. q 4 hours while awake (1,000 mg/day) for 10 days
➢ Chronic suppressive therapy for recurrent genital herpes episodes
Adults: 400 mg P.O. b.i.d., or 200 mg P.O. three to five times daily for up to 12 months
➢ Intermittent therapy for recurrent genital herpes episodes
Adults: 200 mg P.O. q 4 hours while awake (five times/day) for 5 days, initiated at first sign or symptom of recurrence
➢ Management of initial episodes of genital herpes and limited, non-life-threatening mucocutaneous herpes simplex virus infections in immunocompromised patients
Adults: Apply approximately ½" ribbon of ointment per 4 square inches of surface area to sufficiently cover all lesions q 3 hours, six times daily for 7 days.
➢ Treatment of recurrent herpes labialis (cold sores)
Adults and adolescents ages 12 and older: Apply cream to infected area five times daily for 4 days.
➢ Varicella (chickenpox)
Adults and children weighing more than 40 kg (88 lb): 800 mg P.O. q.i.d. for 5 days
Children older than age 2: 20 mg/kg P.O. q.i.d. for 5 days
➢ Mucosal and cutaneous HSV-1 and HSV-2 in immunocompromised patients
Adults and children older than age 12: 5 mg/kg I.V. infusion over 1 hour given q 8 hours for 7 days
Children younger than age 12: 10 mg/kg I.V. infusion over 1 hour given q 8 hours for 7 days
➢ Herpes simplex encephalitis
Adults and children older than age 12: 10 mg/kg I.V. over 1 hour given q 8 hours for 10 days
Children ages 3 months to 12 years: 20 mg/kg I.V. over 1 hour given q 8 hours for 10 days
Children from birth to 3 months: 10 mg/kg I.V. over 1 hour given q 8 hours for 10 days
➢ Varicella zoster infections in immunocompromised patients
Adults and adolescents older than age 12: 10 mg/kg I.V. over 1 hour given q 8 hours for 7 days
Children younger than age 12: 20 mg/kg I.V. over 1 hour given q 8 hours for 7 days

Dosage adjustment

- Renal impairment
- Obesity (adult dosage based on ideal weight)
- Elderly patients

Off-label uses

- Herpes zoster encephalitis
- CMV and HSV infection after bone marrow or kidney transplantation
- Infectious mononucleosis
- Varicella pneumonia

Contraindications

- Hypersensitivity to drug or valacyclovir

Precautions

Use cautiously in:
- preexisting serious neurologic, hepatic, pulmonary, or fluid or electrolyte abnormalities

- renal impairment
- obesity
- pregnant or breastfeeding patients.

Administration

- Make sure patient is adequately hydrated before starting therapy.
- Give I.V. infusion over at least 1 hour to minimize renal damage.
- Don't give by I.V. bolus or by I.M. or subcutaneous route.
- Be aware that absorption of topical acyclovir is minimal.

Route	Onset	Peak	Duration
P.O.	Variable	1.5-2 hr	4 hr
I.V.	Immediate	1 hr	8 hr
Topical	Unknown	Unknown	Unknown

Adverse reactions

CNS: aggressive behavior, dizziness, malaise, weakness, paresthesia, headache; with I.V. use—**encephalopathic changes** (lethargy, tremors, obtundation, confusion, hallucinations, agitation, seizures, coma)
CV: peripheral edema
EENT: vision abnormalities
GI: nausea, vomiting, diarrhea
GU: proteinuria, hematuria, crystalluria, vaginitis, candidiasis, changes in menses, vulvitis, oliguria, **renal failure, glomerulonephritis**
Hematologic: anemia, lymphadenopathy, **thrombocytopenia, thrombotic thrombocytopenic purpura/hemolytic uremic syndrome** (in immunocompromised patients), **disseminated intravascular coagulation, hemolysis, leukopenia, leukoclastic vasculitis**
Hepatic: jaundice, **hepatitis**
Musculoskeletal: myalgia
Skin: photosensitivity rash, pruritus, angioedema, alopecia, urticaria, severe local inflammatory reactions (with I.V. extravasation), **toxic epidermal necrolysis, erythema multiforme**
Other: gingival hyperplasia, fever, excessive thirst, pain at injection site, **anaphylaxis, Stevens-Johnson syndrome**

Interactions

Drug-drug. *Interferon:* additive effect
Nephrotoxic drugs: increased risk of nephrotoxicity
Probenecid: increased acyclovir blood level
Zidovudine: increased CNS effects, especially drowsiness
Drug-diagnostic tests. *Alanine aminotransferase, aspartate aminotransferase, bilirubin, blood urea nitrogen:* increased levels

Patient monitoring

- Monitor fluid intake and output.
- Assess for signs and symptoms of encephalopathy.
- Evaluate patient frequently for adverse reactions, especially bleeding tendency.
- Monitor CBC with white cell differential and kidney function test results.

Patient teaching

- Instruct patient to keep taking drug exactly as prescribed, even after symptoms improve.
- Advise patient to drink enough fluids to ensure adequate urinary output.
- Tell patient to monitor urine output and report significant changes.
- Instruct patient to immediately report unusual bleeding or bruising. (Clinical alert)
- Caution patient to avoid driving and other hazardous activities until he knows how drug affects concentration and alertness.
- Advise patient to minimize GI upset by eating small, frequent servings of food and drinking plenty of fluids.
- Tell patient to use soft toothbrush and electric razor to avoid injury to gums and skin.
- Advise patient to avoid sexual intercourse when visible herpes lesions are present.

• Inform patient that he may need to undergo regular blood testing during therapy.
• As appropriate, review all other significant and life-threatening adverse reactions and interactions, especially those related to the drugs and tests mentioned above.

adalimumab

Humira

Pharmacologic class: Biological modifier

Therapeutic class: Antirheumatic (disease-modifying), immunomodulator

Pregnancy risk category B

Action

Human immunoglobulin (Ig) G1 monoclonal antibody that binds to human tumor necrosis factor (TNF), which plays a role in inflammation and immune responses. Also modulates biological responses induced or modulated by TNF.

Availability

Injection (preservative-free): 40 mg/0.8 ml

Indications and dosages

➢ To reduce signs and symptoms of moderately to severely active rheumatoid arthritis and slow disease progression in patients ages 18 and older who don't respond adequately to disease-modifying antirheumatics

Adults: 40 mg subcutaneously every other week

Contraindications

• Hypersensitivity to drug
• Active infection, including chronic or localized infection

Precautions

Use cautiously in:
• preexisting or recent onset of demyelinating disorders, immunosuppression, or lymphoma
• elderly patients
• pregnant or breastfeeding patients
• children.

Administration

• Give subcutaneously; rotate injection sites.
• Be aware that patients not receiving methotrexate concurrently may benefit from dosage increase to 40 mg weekly.
• Store in refrigerator and protect from light.

Route	Onset	Peak	Duration
Subcut.	Slow	75-187 hr	Unknown

Adverse reactions

CNS: headache, **demyelinating disease**
CV: hypertension, **arrhythmias**
EENT: sinusitis
GI: nausea, vomiting, abdominal pain
GU: urinary tract infection, hematuria
Metabolic: hyperlipidemia, hypercholesterolemia
Musculoskeletal: back pain
Respiratory: upper respiratory tract infection
Skin: rash
Other: accidental injury, pain and swelling at injection site, flulike symptoms, lupuslike syndrome, fungal infection, allergic reactions, **tuberculosis reactivation, malignancies**

Interactions

Drug-drug. *Immunosuppressants (including corticosteroids):* serious infection
Live-virus vaccines: serious illness
Drug-diagnostic tests. *Alkaline phosphatase:* elevated level

Patient monitoring

[Clinical alert] Monitor for signs and symptoms of infection if patient is receiving con-

a

current corticosteroids or other immunosuppressants (because of risk that infection may progress).
• Monitor CBC.

Patient teaching

• Teach patient how to recognize and report signs and symptoms of allergic response and other adverse reactions.
• Inform patient that drug lowers resistance to infection. Instruct him to immediately report fever, cough, breathing problems, and other infection symptoms.
• Instruct patient to minimize GI upset by eating small, frequent servings of healthy food and drinking plenty of fluids.
• As appropriate, review all other significant and life-threatening adverse reactions and interactions, especially those related to the drugs and tests mentioned above.

adefovir dipivoxil

Hepsera

Pharmacologic class: Nucleotide reverse transcriptase inhibitor
Therapeutic class: Antiviral
Pregnancy risk category C

Action

Inhibits hepatitis B virus (HBV) DNA polymerase and suppresses HBV replication

Availability

Tablets: 10 mg

Indications and dosages

➤ Chronic HBV with active viral replication plus persistent elevations in alanine aminotransferase (ALT) or aspartate aminotransferase (AST) or histologically active disease
Adults: 10 mg P.O. daily

Dosage adjustment

• Renal impairment

Contraindications

• Hypersensitivity to drug

Precautions

Use cautiously in:
• lactic acidosis, renal or hepatic impairment
• elderly patients
• pregnant or breastfeeding patients
• children.

Administration

• Offer human immunodeficiency virus (HIV) testing before starting therapy. (Drug may increase resistance to antiretrovirals in HIV patients.)
• Give with or without food.

Route	Onset	Peak	Duration
P.O.	Rapid	0.6-4 hr	Unknown

Adverse reactions

CNS: headache
GI: nausea, vomiting, diarrhea, abdominal pain, flatulence, dyspepsia, anorexia, pancreatitis
GU: renal dysfunction
Hepatic: severe hepatomegaly with steatosis, hepatitis exacerbation (if therapy is withdrawn)
Metabolic: lactic acidosis
Respiratory: pneumonia
Other: fever, infection, pain, antiretroviral resistance in patients with unrecognized HIV

Interactions

Drug-drug. *Acetaminophen, aspirin, indomethacin:* granulocytopenia
Acyclovir, adriamycin, amphotericin B, benzodiazepines, cimetidine, dapsone, doxorubicin, experimental nucleotide analogue, fluconazole, flucytosine, ganciclovir, indomethacin, interferon, morphine, phenytoin, probenecid, sulfonamide, trimethoprim, vinblastine,

vincristine: increased risk of nephrotoxicity
Drug-diagnostic tests. *Amylase, blood glucose, blood urea nitrogen, creatine kinase, hepatic enzymes, lipase:* elevated levels

Patient monitoring

- Monitor fluid intake and output.
- Watch for hematuria.
- Assess for signs and symptoms of lactic acidosis, especially in women and overweight patients.
- Check for liver enlargement.
- Monitor liver and kidney function test results.
- After therapy ends, monitor patient for evidence of serious hepatitis exacerbation.

Patient teaching

- Advise patient to take drug with or without food.
- Instruct patient to drink plenty of fluids to ensure adequate urine output.
- Advise patient to monitor urine output and color and to report significant changes.
- Tell patient that drug may cause weakness. Discuss appropriate lifestyle adjustments.
- Caution patient not to take over-the-counter analgesics without prescriber's approval.
- Inform patient that he'll undergo regular blood testing during therapy.
- As appropriate, review all other significant and life-threatening adverse reactions and interactions, especially those related to the drugs and tests mentioned above.

adenosine

Adenocard, Adenoscan

Pharmacologic class: Endogenous nucleoside
Therapeutic class: Antiarrhythmic
Pregnancy risk category C

Action

Converts paroxysmal supraventricular tachycardia (PSVT) to normal sinus rhythm by slowing conduction through atrioventricular (AV) node and interrupting reentry pathway. Also used as a diagnostic agent in thallium scanning.

Availability

Injection: 3 mg/ml

Indications and dosages

Adenocard—

➢ PSVT, including that associated with Wolff-Parkinson-White syndrome (after attempting vagal maneuvers, when appropriate)
Adults and children weighing more than 50 kg (110 lb): Initially, 6 mg by rapid I.V. bolus over 1 to 2 seconds. If desired effect isn't achieved within 1 to 2 minutes, give 12 mg by rapid I.V. bolus; may repeat 12-mg I.V. bolus dose as needed. Maximum single dosage is 12 mg.
Children weighing less than 50 kg (110 lb): 0.05 to 0.1 mg/kg by rapid I.V. bolus. If this dosage proves ineffective, increase in 1 to 2 minutes by 0.05 mg/kg q 2 minutes, to a maximum single dosage of 0.3 mg/kg. Maximum single dosage is 12 mg.

Adenoscan—

➢ Diagnosis of coronary artery disease in conjunction with thallium-201 myocardial perfusion scintigraphy in

patients unable to exercise adequately during testing
Adults: 140 mcg/kg/minute by I.V. infusion over 6 minutes, for a total dosage of 0.84 mg/kg. Required dose of thallium-201 is injected at midpoint (after first 3 minutes) of Adenoscan infusion.

Off-label uses

- Diagnosis of supraventricular arrhythmias
- Pulmonary hypertension

Contraindications

- Hypersensitivity to drug
- Second- or third-degree AV block
- Sinus node disease
- Bronchoconstrictive lung disease

Precautions

Use cautiously in:

- asthma, angina
- elderly patients
- pregnant patients
- children.

Administration

- Administer I.V. injection as a rapid bolus directly into vein whenever possible during cardiac monitoring.
- Flush I.V. line immediately with normal saline solution to drive drug into bloodstream.
- Don't give more than 12 mg as a single dose.
- Don't administer through central line (may cause prolonged asystole).

Route	Onset	Peak	Duration
I.V.	Immediate	10 sec	20-30 sec

Adverse reactions

CNS: light-headedness, dizziness, apprehension, headache, tingling in arms, numbness
CV: chest pain, palpitations, hypotension, ST-segment depression, **first- or second-degree AV block, atrial tachyarrhythmias, other arrhythmias**
EENT: blurred vision, tightness in throat
GI: nausea, pressure in groin
Musculoskeletal: discomfort in neck, jaw, and arms
Respiratory: chest pressure, dyspnea and urge to breathe deeply, hyperventilation
Skin: burning sensation, facial flushing, sweating
Other: metallic taste

Interactions

Drug-drug. *Carbamazepine:* worsening of progressive heart block
Digoxin, verapamil: increased risk of ventricular fibrillation
Dipyridamole: increased adenosine effect
Theophylline: decreased adenosine effect
Drug-food. *Caffeine:* decreased adenosine effect
Drug-herbs. *Aloe, buckthorn bark or berry, cascara sagrada, rhubarb root, senna leaf or fruits:* increased adenosine effect
Guarana: decreased adenosine effect
Drug-behaviors. *Smoking:* increased risk of tachycardia

Patient monitoring

- Monitor heart rhythm for new arrhythmias after administering dose.
- Check vital signs. Assess for chest pain or pressure, dyspnea, and sweating.

[Clinical alert] Watch for bronchoconstriction in patients with asthma, emphysema, or bronchitis.

- Ask patient if he has recently used aloe, buckthorn, cascara sagrada, guarana, rhubarb root, or senna. If response is positive, notify prescriber.

Patient teaching

- Advise patient to report problems at infusion site.
- Tell patient he may experience 1 to 2 minutes of flushing, chest pain and

pressure, and breathing difficulty during administration. Assure him that these effects will subside quickly.

- Advise patient to minimize GI upset by eating small, frequent servings of healthy food and drinking plenty of fluids.
- As appropriate, review all other significant and life-threatening adverse reactions and interactions, especially those related to the drugs, foods, herbs, and behaviors mentioned above.

agalsidase beta

Fabrazyme, Fibrazyme

Pharmacologic class: Homodimeric glycoprotein
Therapeutic class: Recombinant human alpha-galactosidase enzyme
Pregnancy risk category B

Action

Provides exogenous source of alpha-galactosidase A (which is deficient in Fabry disease) and reduces deposits of globotriaosylceramide in kidney and other body tissues

Availability

Powder for reconstitution: 37 mg (5 mg/ml)

Indications and dosages

➣ Fabry disease

Adults: 1 mg/kg I.V. q 2 weeks. Infuse no faster than 0.25 mg/minute; if tolerated, increase rate by 0.05 to 0.08 mg/minute in subsequent infusions.

Contraindications

None

Precautions

Use cautiously in:

- cardiac dysfunction
- pregnant or breastfeeding patients
- children.

Administration

- Premedicate with antipyretics, as prescribed.
- To reconstitute, slowly inject 7.2 ml of sterile water for injection into vial; then roll and tilt vial gently to mix drug.
- Don't shake drug, and don't use filter needles.
- Dilute reconstituted solution with normal saline injection to a final volume of 500 ml.
- Infuse through separate I.V. line; don't mix with other drugs.

Route	Onset	Peak	Duration
I.V.	End of infusion	90 min	Up to 5 hr

Adverse reactions

CNS: anxiety, depression, dizziness, paresthesias
CV: dependent edema, chest pain, **cardiomegaly**
EENT: rhinitis, sinusitis, laryngitis, pharyngitis
GI: nausea, dyspepsia
GU: testicular pain
Musculoskeletal: arthrosis, bone pain
Respiratory: bronchitis, **bronchospasm**
Skin: pallor
Other: pain, allergic reactions, **infusion reactions** (hypertension, chest tightness, dyspnea, fever, rigors, hypotension, abdominal pain, pruritus, myalgia, headache, urticaria)

Interactions

Drug-drug. *Amiodarone, chloroquine, gentamicin, monobenzone:* inhibition of intracellular agalsidase activity

Patient monitoring

- Watch closely for signs and symptoms of allergic or infusion reaction.

a

• Monitor vital signs and fluid intake and output. Stay alert for dependent edema, blood pressure changes, and chest pain.
• Measure temperature. Watch for signs and symptoms of infection (particularly EENT and respiratory infections).
• Evaluate patient's mood. Report significant anxiety or depression.

Patient teaching

Clinical alert: Teach patient to recognize and immediately report signs and symptoms of allergic or infusion reaction.
• Caution patient to avoid driving and other hazardous activities until he knows how drug affects mood, balance, and blood pressure.
• Advise patient to report signs and symptoms of infection (particularly EENT and respiratory infections).
• Inform patient that drug can cause depression and anxiety. Instruct him to notify prescriber if these effects occur.
• As appropriate, review all other significant and life-threatening adverse reactions and interactions, especially those related to the drugs mentioned above.

albumin (human normal serum)

5%: Albumarc, Albuminar-5, Albunex, Albutein 5%, Buminate 5%, Plasbumin-5
25%: Albumarc, Albuminar-25, Albutein 25%, Buminate 25%, Plasbumin-25

Pharmacologic class: Blood product, colloid
Therapeutic class: Volume expander
Pregnancy risk category C

Action

Provides colloidal oncotic pressure, increases circulating plasma volume, regulates fluid balance, and helps maintain normal blood volume. Also acts as carrier for intermediate metabolites in transport.

Availability

Albumin 5% injection: 50-ml, 250-ml, 500-ml, and 1,000-ml vials
Albumin 25% injection: 20-ml, 50-ml, and 100-ml vials

Indications and dosages

➢ Hypovolemia with shock
Adults: Initially, 500 ml of 5% solution by rapid I.V. infusion, repeated in 30 minutes if desired effect isn't achieved
Children: 50 ml of 5% solution by I.V. infusion, repeated in 15 to 30 minutes if desired effect isn't achieved, or 2.5 to 5 ml of 25% solution/kg by I.V. infusion, repeated after 10 to 30 minutes. Total dosage shouldn't exceed 20 ml/kg.
Neonates and infants: 10 to 20 ml/kg by I.V. infusion based on response, delivered at 25% to 50% of adult rate. Total dosage shouldn't exceed 20 ml/kg.
➢ Severe burns
Adults: For initial therapy, give large volumes of crystalloids and lesser amounts of 5% solution I.V. to maintain plasma volume. After 24 hours, may increase 5% albumin I.V. to maintain plasma albumin level of about 2.5 g +/- 0.5 g/100 ml, or total serum protein level of about 5.2 g/100 ml.
➢ Acute hypoproteinemia
Adults: 50 to 70 g/day (200 to 280 ml) of 25% solution by I.V. infusion (if edema is present or considerable albumin has been lost); not to exceed 2 ml/minute
Children: 25 g/day (100 ml) of 25% solution by I.V. infusion (if edema is present or considerable albumin has been lost); not to exceed 2 ml/minute

➢ Erythrocyte resuspension
Adults: Usual dosage is 25 g of albumin I.V. per liter of erythrocytes.
➢ Hyperbilirubinemia/erythroblastosis fetalis
Infants: 1 g/kg (4 ml/kg of 25% solution) I.V. within 1 to 2 hours before exchange transfusion
➢ Acute nephrosis
Adults: Initially, 100 ml of 25% solution I.V., repeated daily for 7 days if needed (given concurrently with loop diuretic)

Contraindications
• Hypersensitivity to drug
• Cardiac failure, hypervolemia, or pulmonary edema
• Severe anemia

Precautions
Use cautiously in:
• dehydration, renal failure, hepatic disease, hypertension, low cardiac reserve, pulmonary disease
• pregnant patients.

Administration
• Be sure patient is well hydrated before giving drug.
• Adhere to prescribed infusion rate, which varies with patient's age, clinical condition, and diagnosis. Don't administer too rapidly.
• Deliver by I.V. infusion with no further dilution. If slower administration is desired, mix 200 ml of 25% albumin with 300 ml of 10% glucose solution, and give by continuous drip at a rate of 100 ml/hour.
• Know that for erythrocyte resuspension, albumin 25% is added to isotonic suspension of washed red cells immediately before transfusion.
• Withhold angiotensin-converting enzyme (ACE) inhibitors 24 hours before giving albumin, if possible.

Route	Onset	Peak	Duration
I.V.	Immediate	End of infusion	Several hr

Adverse reactions
CNS: headache, light-headedness, dizziness
CV: tachycardia, hypotension, **fluid overload**
EENT: blurred vision, tightness in throat
GI: nausea, vomiting, increased salivation
Musculoskeletal: back pain
Respiratory: respiratory changes, hyperventilation, dyspnea, chest pressure, **pulmonary edema**
Skin: rash, urticaria, flushing
Other: metallic taste, chills, fever, groin pressure

Interactions
Drug-drug. *ACE inhibitors:* increased risk of atypical reactions
Drug-diagnostic tests. *Alkaline phosphatase:* false increase

Patient monitoring
• Check vital signs and assess fluid intake and output frequently.
🔊 Monitor for hemorrhage and shock after injury or surgery. Rapid postinfusion blood pressure increase may cause bleeding from severed vessels.
🔊 Monitor for signs and symptoms of heart failure and pulmonary edema.
• Monitor hemoglobin, hematocrit, protein, and electrolyte levels.

Patient teaching
• Inform patient that he'll undergo regular blood testing during therapy.
• As appropriate, review all other significant and life-threatening adverse reactions and interactions, especially those related to the drugs and tests mentioned above.

albuterol (salbutamol)
Proventil, Ventolin

albuterol sulfate (salbutamol sulfate)
AccuNeb, Airet, Asmol♣, Gen-Salbutamol♣, Novo-Salmol♣, Proventil HFA, Proventil Repetabs, Ventolin HFA, Volmax

Pharmacologic class: Sympathomimetic ($beta_2$-adrenergic agonist)
Therapeutic class: Bronchodilator, antiasthmatic
Pregnancy risk category C

Action
Relaxes smooth muscles by stimulating $beta_2$-receptors, thereby causing bronchodilation and vasodilation

Availability
Aerosol: 90 mcg/actuation
Oral solution: 2 mg/5 ml
Solution for inhalation: 0.083% (3 ml), 0.5% (0.5 and 20 ml), 0.63 mg/3 ml, 1.25 mg/3 ml
Syrup: 2 mg/5 ml
Tablets: 2 mg, 4 mg
Tablets (extended-release): 4 mg, 8 mg

Indications and dosages
➢ To prevent and relieve bronchospasm in patients with reversible obstructive airway disease
Adults and children ages 12 and older: *Tablets*—2 to 4 mg P.O. three or four times daily, not to exceed 32 mg daily. *Extended-release tablets*—4 to 8 mg P.O. q 12 hours, not to exceed 32 mg daily in divided doses. *Syrup*—2 to 4 mg (1 to 2 tsp or 5 to 10 ml) three or four times daily, not to exceed 8 mg q.i.d. *Aerosol*—one to two inhalations q 4 to 6 hours to relieve bronchospasm; two inhalations q.i.d. to prevent bronchospasm. *Solution for inhalation*—2.5 mg three to four times daily by nebulization, delivered over 5 to 15 minutes.
Children ages 6 to 12: *Tablets*—2 mg P.O. three or four times daily; maximum daily dosage is 24 mg, given in divided doses. *Extended-release tablets*—4 mg q 12 hours; maximum daily dosage is 24 mg/kg given in divided doses. *Syrup*—2 mg (1 tsp or 5 ml) three or four times daily, not to exceed 24 mg.
Children ages 2 to 12 weighing more than 15 kg (33 lb): *Solution for inhalation*—2.5 mg three to four times/day by nebulization
Children ages 2 to 6: *Syrup*—Initially, 0.1 mg/kg P.O. t.i.d., not to exceed 2 mg (1 tsp) t.i.d. Maximum dosage is 4 mg (2 tsp) t.i.d.
➢ To prevent exercise-induced bronchospasm
Adults and children older than age 4 (older than age 12 with Proventil): Two inhalations 15 minutes before exercise

Dosage adjustment
- Sensitivity to beta-adrenergic stimulants
- Elderly patients

Off-label uses
- Chronic obstructive pulmonary disease
- Hyperkalemia with renal failure
- Preterm labor management

Contraindications
- Hypersensitivity to drug

Precautions
Use cautiously in:
- cardiac disease, hypertension, diabetes mellitus, glaucoma, seizure disorder, hyperthyroidism, exercise-induced bronchospasm, prostatic hypertrophy
- elderly patients

• pregnant or breastfeeding patients
• children.

Administration

• Give extended-release tablets whole; don't crush or mix with food.
• Administer solution for inhalation by nebulization over 5 to 15 minutes, after diluting 0.5 ml of 0.5% solution with 2.5 ml of sterile normal saline solution.
• Know that children weighing less than 15 kg (33 lb) who require less than 2.5 mg/dose should receive 0.5% inhalation solution.

Route	Onset	Peak	Duration
P.O.	15-30 min	2-3 hr	6-12 hr
P.O. (extended)	30 min	2-3 hr	12 hr

Adverse reactions

CNS: dizziness, excitement, headache, hyperactivity, insomnia
CV: hypertension, palpitations, tachycardia, chest pain
EENT: conjunctivitis, dry and irritated throat, pharyngitis
GI: nausea, vomiting, anorexia, heartburn, GI distress, dry mouth
Metabolic: hypokalemia
Musculoskeletal: muscle cramps
Respiratory: cough, dyspnea, wheezing, **paradoxical bronchospasm**
Skin: pallor, urticaria, rash, angioedema, flushing, sweating
Other: tooth discoloration, increased appetite, **hypersensitivity reaction**

Interactions

Drug-drug. *Beta-adrenergic blockers:* inhibited albuterol action, possibly causing severe bronchospasm in asthmatic patients
Digoxin: decreased digoxin blood level
MAO inhibitors: increased cardiovascular adverse effects
Oxytoxics: severe hypotension
Potassium-wasting diuretics: ECG changes, hypokalemia
Theophylline: increased risk of theophylline toxicity
Drug-food. *Caffeine-containing foods and beverages (such as coffee, tea, chocolate):* increased stimulant effect
Drug-herbs. *Cola nut, ephedra (ma huang), guarana, yerba maté:* increased stimulant effect

Patient monitoring

🔊 Stay alert for hypersensitivity reactions and paradoxical bronchospasm. Stop drug immediately if these occur.
• Monitor serum electrolyte levels.

Patient teaching

• Tell patient to swallow extended-release tablets whole and not to mix them with food.
🔊 Teach patient signs and symptoms of hypersensitivity reaction and paradoxical bronchospasm. Tell him to stop taking drug immediately and contact prescriber if these occur.
🔊 Instruct patient to notify prescriber immediately if prescribed dosage fails to provide usual relief, because this may indicate seriously worsening asthma.
• Advise patient to limit intake of caffeine-containing foods and beverages and to avoid herbs unless prescriber approves.
• Caution patient to avoid driving and other hazardous activities until he knows how drug affects concentration and alertness.
• Advise patient to establish effective bedtime routine and to take drug well before bedtime to minimize insomnia.
• As appropriate, review all other significant and life-threatening adverse reactions and interactions, especially those related to the drugs, foods, and herbs mentioned above.

a

aldesleukin (interleukin-2, IL-2)

Proleukin

Pharmacologic class: Interleukin-2 (IL-2), human recombinant (cytokine)
Therapeutic class: Antineoplastic (miscellaneous)
Pregnancy risk category C

Action

Activates cellular immunity and inhibits tumor growth by increasing lymphocytes and cytokines, which lyse tumor cells

Availability

Injection: 22 million international units/vial

Indications and dosages

➢ Metastatic renal cell carcinoma and metastatic melanoma

Adults older than age 18: 600,000 international units/kg I.V. given over 15 minutes q 8 hours for a maximum of 14 doses, followed by 9 days of rest. Repeat for another 14 doses, for a maximum of 28 doses per course.

Off-label uses

- Colorectal cancer
- Kaposi's sarcoma
- Non-Hodgkin's lymphoma

Contraindications

- Hypersensitivity to drug
- Arrhythmias, cardiac tamponade, seizures, severe GI bleeding, coma or toxic psychosis lasting more than 48 hours
- Organ allograft
- Abnormal thallium stress test or pulmonary function test results

Precautions

Use cautiously in:

- anemia, bacterial infections, heart disease, CNS metastases, hepatic disease, pulmonary disease, renal disease, thrombocytopenia
- pregnant or breastfeeding patients
- children.

Administration

- Make sure patient's thallium stress test and pulmonary function test results are normal before giving.

Clinical alert: Don't give if patient is drowsy or severely lethargic; contact prescriber immediately.

- Reconstitute drug according to label directions with 1.2 ml of sterile water for injection by injecting diluent against side of vial (to prevent excessive foaming).
- Further dilute reconstituted dose with 50 ml of 5% dextrose injection.
- Administer I.V. infusion over 15 minutes.
- Don't use in-line filter.

Route	Onset	Peak	Duration
I.V.	5 min	13 min	3-4 hr

Adverse reactions

CNS: dizziness, mental status changes, syncope, sensory or motor dysfunction, headache, fatigue, rigors, weakness, malaise, poor memory, depression, sleep disturbances, hallucinations
CV: bradycardia, sinus tachycardia, premature atrial complexes, premature ventricular contractions, **arrhythmias, myocardial ischemia, cardiac arrest, capillary leak syndrome and severe hypotension, myocardial infarction**
EENT: reversible vision changes, conjunctivitis
GI: nausea, vomiting, diarrhea, constipation, dyspepsia, abdominal pain, stomatitis, anorexia, **intestinal perforation, ileus, GI bleeding**
GU: hematuria, proteinuria, dysuria, **renal failure, oliguria or anuria**

Hematologic: anemia, purpura, eosinophilia, **thrombocytopenia, coagulation disorders, leukopenia, leukocytosis**
Hepatic: jaundice, ascites
Metabolic: hyperglycemia, **hypoglycemia, acidosis, alkalosis**
Musculoskeletal: joint and back pain, myalgia
Respiratory: cough, chest pain, tachypnea, wheezing, dyspnea, pulmonary congestion, **pulmonary edema, respiratory failure, apnea, pleural effusion**
Skin: erythema, pruritus, rash, dry skin, petechiae, urticaria, exfoliative dermatitis
Other: weight gain or loss, fever, chills, edema, infection, pain or reaction at injection site, hypersensitivity reaction

Interactions

Drug-drug. *Aminoglycosides, asparaginase, cytotoxic chemotherapy agents, doxorubicin, indomethacin, methotrexate:* increased toxicity
Antihypertensives: increased hypotensive effect
Glucocorticoids: reduced antitumor effects
Drug-diagnostic tests. *Alkaline phosphatase, bilirubin, glucose, blood urea nitrogen, creatinine, potassium, transaminases:* increased levels
Calcium, glucose, magnesium, phosphorus, potassium, protein sodium, uric acid: decreased levels

Patient monitoring

- Monitor heart rate and rhythm, vital signs, and fluid intake and output.
- Assess for signs and symptoms of hypersensitivity reaction and infection.
- Monitor for adverse CNS effects. Report these immediately.
- Evaluate chest X-rays.
- Monitor CBC, electrolyte levels, and liver and kidney function test results.

Patient teaching

[Clinical alert] Tell patient that drug lowers resistance to infections. Advise him to immediately report fever, cough, breathing problems, and other signs or symptoms of infection.

[Clinical alert] Advise patient to immediately report chest pain, irregular or fast heart beats, easy bruising or bleeding, or abdominal pain.

- Instruct patient to minimize GI upset by eating small, frequent servings of food and drinking plenty of fluids.
- Provide dietary counseling. Refer patient to dietitian if adverse GI effects significantly limit food intake.
- Notify patient that he'll undergo blood testing and have chest X-rays taken during therapy.
- As appropriate, review all other significant and life-threatening adverse reactions and interactions, especially those related to the drugs and tests mentioned above.

alemtuzumab

Campath

Pharmacologic class: Monoclonal antibody
Therapeutic class: Antineoplastic
Pregnancy risk category C

Action

Binds to CD52 antigen on surface of B- and T-lymphocytes, monocytes, macrophages, "natural killer" cells, and granulocytes. Lyses leukemic cells and reduces tumor size.

Availability

Solution for injection: 30 mg/3 ml

a

Indications and dosages

➢ Chronic lymphocytic (B-cell) leukemia when fludarabine therapy fails

Adults: Initially, 3 mg/day I.V. given over 2 hours; if tolerated, increase to 10 mg/day, to a maximum single dose of 30 mg/day. Then give a maintenance dose of 30 mg three times weekly on nonconsecutive days (such as Monday, Wednesday, Friday) for up to 12 weeks.

Dosage adjustment

- Hematologic toxicity

Contraindications

- Type I hypersensitivity or anaphylactic reaction to drug or its components
- Active systemic infection
- Immunodeficiency (as in human immunodeficiency virus infection)

Precautions

Use cautiously in:

- pregnant or breastfeeding patients
- children.

Administration

Clinical alert: Withhold drug and contact prescriber if patient has signs or symptoms of systemic infection at time of scheduled infusion.

Clinical alert: Don't give by I.V. push or bolus.

- Withdraw dose from ampule and filter with sterile, low-protein-binding, 5-micron filter.
- Dilute with 100 ml of normal saline solution or dextrose 5% in water.
- Infuse over 2 hours.
- Protect I.V. solution from light.

Route	Onset	Peak	Duration
I.V.	Unknown	Unknown	Unknown

Adverse reactions

CNS: tremor, malaise, dizziness, depression, insomnia, drowsiness, weakness, headache, abnormal sensations, fatigue

CV: peripheral edema, chest pain, hypotension, hypertension, tachycardia, **supraventricular tachycardia**

EENT: rhinitis, pharyngitis, epistaxis

GI: nausea, vomiting, constipation, diarrhea, dyspepsia, abdominal pain, stomatitis, anorexia

Hematologic: anemia, **thrombocytopenia, pancytopenia, bone marrow hypoplasia, neutropenia, bone marrow depression**

Metabolic: hypokalemia, hypomagnesemia

Musculoskeletal: myalgia, bone or back pain

Respiratory: cough, bronchitis, dyspnea, pneumonitis, **bronchospasm**

Skin: herpes simplex infection, urticaria, pruritus, diaphoresis

Other: edema, fever, candidiasis, infection, **infusion-related reactions, sepsis**

Interactions

Drug-drug. *Live-virus vaccines:* decreased drug efficacy and increased adverse effects

Drug-diagnostic tests. *CD4+ T lymphocytes, hematocrit, hemoglobin, lymphocytes, neutrophils, platelets, red blood cells, white blood cells:* decreased values

Patient monitoring

- Assess for hypotension during infusion.
- Monitor vital signs frequently throughout entire course of therapy.
- Monitor CBC, CD4+ level, electrolyte levels, and platelet count.

Patient teaching

Clinical alert: Inform patient that drug lowers resistance to infection. Instruct him to immediately report fever, cough, breathing problems, sore throat, and other signs or symptoms.

Clinical alert: Tell patient to immediately report irregular or fast heart beats or easy bruising or bleeding.

- Caution patient to avoid driving and other hazardous activities until he

knows how drug affects concentration and alertness.

- Advise patient to minimize GI upset by eating small, frequent servings of food and drinking plenty of fluids.
- Instruct patient to follow regular bedtime routine and avoid bedtime stimulants.
- Encourage patient to discuss activity recommendations and pain management with prescriber.
- Inform patient that he'll undergo regular blood testing during therapy.
- As appropriate, review all other significant and life-threatening adverse reactions and interactions, especially those related to the drugs and tests mentioned above.

alendronate sodium

Fosamax

Pharmacologic class: Bisphosphonate
Therapeutic class: Bone-resorption inhibitor
Pregnancy risk category C

Action

Impedes bone resorption by inhibiting osteoclast activity, absorbing calcium phosphate crystal in bone, and directly blocking dissolution of hydroxyapatite crystal of bone

Availability

Tablets: 5 mg, 10 mg, 35 mg, 40 mg, 70 mg

Indications and dosages

➢ Paget's disease of bone
Adults: 40 mg P.O. daily for 6 months
➢ Prevention of osteoporosis in postmenopausal women
Adults: 5 mg P.O. daily or 35 mg P.O. once weekly
➢ Glucocorticoid-induced osteoporosis in adults with low bone mineral density who are receiving daily glucocorticoid doses equivalent to 7.5 mg or more of prednisone
Adults: 5 mg P.O. daily. For postmenopausal women not receiving estrogen, recommended dosage is 10 mg P.O. once daily.
➢ Osteoporosis in postmenopausal women; to increase bone mass in men with osteoporosis
Adults: 10 mg P.O. daily or 70 mg P.O. once weekly

Contraindications

- Hypersensitivity to bisphosphonates
- Hypocalcemia
- Renal insufficiency
- Esophageal abnormalities

Precautions

Use cautiously in:

- renal insufficiency, esophageal disease, GI ulcers, gastritis
- pregnant or breastfeeding patients
- children.

Administration

- Give with 6 to 8 oz of water before first food, beverage, or medication of day.
- Don't give food, other beverages, or oral drugs for at least 30 minutes after giving dose.
- Keep patient upright for at least 30 minutes after giving dose to avoid serious esophageal irritation.
- Be aware that aspirin and nonsteroidal anti-inflammatory drugs (NSAIDs) may worsen GI upset. Discuss alternative analgesics with prescriber.

Route	Onset	Peak	Duration
P.O.	1 mo	3-6 mo	3 wk-7 mo

Adverse reactions

CNS: headache
CV: hypertension
GI: nausea, vomiting, diarrhea, constipation, abdominal pain, acid regurgita-

tion, esophageal ulcer, flatulence, dyspepsia, abdominal distention, dysphagia
GU: urinary tract infection
Hematologic: anemia
Metabolic: hypomagnesemia, hypophosphatemia, hypokalemia, **fluid overload**
Musculoskeletal: bone or muscle pain
Skin: rash, redness, photosensitivity
Other: abnormal taste

Interactions

Drug-drug. *Antacids, calcium supplements:* decreased alendronate absorption
NSAIDs, salicylates: increased risk of GI upset
Ranitidine: increased alendronate effect
Drug-diagnostic tests. *Calcium, phosphate:* decreased levels
Drug-food. *Any food, caffeine (as in coffee, tea, cocoa), mineral water, orange juice:* decreased drug absorption

Patient monitoring

- Monitor for signs and symptoms of GI irritation, including ulcers.
- Monitor blood pressure.
- Evaluate blood calcium and phosphate levels.

Patient teaching

Tell patient to immediately report serious vomiting, severe chest or abdominal pain, difficulty swallowing, or abdominal swelling.
- Instruct patient to take drug first thing in the morning on an empty stomach, with 6 to 8 oz of water only.
- Tell patient not to lie down, eat, drink, or take other oral medications for 30 minutes after taking dose.
- Advise patient to take only those pain relievers suggested by prescriber. Inform him that some over-the-counter pain medications (such as aspirin and NSAIDs) may worsen drug's adverse effects.
- As appropriate, review all other significant and life-threatening adverse reactions and interactions, especially those related to the drugs, tests, and foods mentioned above.

alfuzosin

Uroxatral, Xatral✱

Pharmacologic class: Alpha$_1$-adrenergic receptor blocker
Therapeutic class: Benign prostatic hyperplasia agent
Pregnancy risk category B

Action

Selectively inhibits alpha$_1$-adrenergic receptors in lower urinary tract, relaxing smooth muscle in bladder neck and prostate

Availability

Tablets (extended-release): 10 mg

Indications and dosages

➤ Signs and symptoms of benign prostatic hyperplasia
Adults: 10 mg P.O. once daily with food, given at same meal each day

Contraindications

- Hypersensitivity to drug or its components
- Moderate or severe hepatic impairment
- Concomitant use of potent CYP-4503A4 inhibitors (such as itraconazole, ketoconazole, or ritonavir)

Precautions

Use cautiously until prostate cancer is ruled out. Also use cautiously in:
- coronary, hepatic, or renal insufficiency
- congenital or acquired QT prolongation.

Administration
- Administer with food.
- Don't crush or break tablet.

Route	Onset	Peak	Duration
P.O.	Unknown	8 hr	Unknown

Adverse reactions
CNS: dizziness, headache, fatigue
EENT: sinusitis, pharyngitis
GI: nausea, constipation abdominal pain, dyspepsia
Respiratory: upper respiratory tract infection, bronchitis
Other: pain

Interactions
Drug-drug. *Atenolol, cimetidine, diltiazem, itraconazole, ketoconazole, ritonavir:* increased alfuzosin blood level
Drug-food. *Any food:* increased alfuzosin absorption

Patient monitoring
- Monitor patient for adverse reactions, such as dizziness.

Patient teaching
- Instruct patient to take drug with food at same time each day.
- Tell patient not to break, chew, or crush tablet.
- Caution patient to avoid driving and other hazardous activities until he knows if drug makes him dizzy.
- As appropriate, review all other significant adverse reactions and interactions, especially those related to the drugs and foods mentioned above.

alitretinoin
Panretin

Pharmacologic class: Second-generation retinoid
Therapeutic class: Topical antineoplastic
Pregnancy risk category D

Action
Binds to and activates intracellular retinoid receptor subtypes, regulating expression of genes that control cellular differentiation and proliferation

Availability
Topical gel: 0.1%

Indications and dosages
➢ Treatment of cutaneous lesions in patients with AIDS-related Kaposi's sarcoma
Adults: Apply to lesions b.i.d., gradually increasing to t.i.d. or q.i.d. according to individual lesion tolerance

Contraindications
- Hypersensitivity to retinoids or other drug components

Precautions
Use cautiously in:
- photosensitivity
- concomitant use of insecticides containing diethyltoluamide (DEET)
- elderly patients
- pregnant or breastfeeding patients
- children.

Administration
- Apply generous amount of gel to affected area. Let dry for 3 to 5 minutes before covering with clothing.

Route	Onset	Peak	Duration
Topical	Unknown	Unknown	Unknown

Adverse reactions
CNS: paresthesia
Skin: rash, pruritus, exfoliative dermatitis, skin disorder at application site (such as abrasion, burning, blisters, excoriation, scab, cracking, crusting, drainage, eschar, fissure, oozing, peeling, redness, or swelling), edema
Other: pain, increased sensitivity to sunlight or sun lamps

Interactions
Drug-behaviors. *DEET-containing insect repellents:* increased adverse reactions to DEET

Patient monitoring
- Monitor patient for serious adverse effects, especially burns caused by exposure to sunlight or sun lamps.

Patient teaching
- Instruct patient to apply generous amount of gel to affected skin area and let dry for 3 to 5 minutes before covering area with clothing.
- Caution patient to avoid applying gel to mucous membranes or to normal skin surrounding lesions.

Clinical alert: Inform patient that drug increases sensitivity to sunlight and that exposure to sunlight or sun lamps (even through window glass or on a cloudy day) may cause serious burn of treated areas. Caution him to avoid such exposure.
- Tell patient to avoid insect repellents containing DEET during therapy.
- Emphasize importance of keeping all medical appointments so prescriber can check progress and monitor for unwanted drug effects.
- As appropriate, review all other significant adverse reactions and interactions, especially those related to the behaviors mentioned above.

a

allopurinol
Apo-Allopurinol✤, Lopurin, Zyloprim

allopurinol sodium
Aloprim

Pharmacologic class: Xanthine oxidase inhibitor
Therapeutic class: Antigout drug
Pregnancy risk category C

Action
Inhibits conversion of xanthine to uric acid and increases reutilization of hypoxanthine and xanthine for nucleic acid synthesis, thereby decreasing uric acid levels in both serum and urine

Availability
Injection: 500 mg/30-ml vial
Tablets: 100 mg, 300 mg

Indications and dosages
➢ Gout in patients with frequent disabling attacks; gout resulting from hyperuricemia, acute or chronic leukemia, psoriasis, or multiple myeloma
Adults: 200 to 300 mg P.O. daily in mild cases or 400 to 600 mg P.O. daily in severe cases, to a maximum dosage of 800 mg/day; or 200 to 400 mg/m²/day I.V. as a single infusion or in equally divided doses q 6, 8, or 12 hours
Children ages 6 to 10: 300 mg P.O. daily
Children younger than age 6: 150 mg P.O. daily
➢ To prevent acute gout attacks
Adults: 100 mg P.O. daily; increase by 100 mg at weekly intervals without exceeding maximum dosage of 800 mg, until uric acid level falls to 6 mg/dl or less
➢ Recurrent calcium oxalate calculi
Adults: 200 to 300 mg P.O. daily in single dose or divided doses

➢ To prevent uric acid nephropathy during cancer chemotherapy
Adults: 600 to 800 mg P.O. daily for 2 to 3 days, accompanied by high fluid intake

Dosage adjustment
- Renal impairment

Off-label uses
- Hematemesis caused by gastritis induced by nonsteroidal anti-inflammatory drugs
- Pain from acute pancreatitis
- Seizures refractory to standard therapy

Contraindications
- Hypersensitivity to drug
- Idiopathic hemochromatosis

Precautions
Use cautiously in:
- acute gout attack, renal insufficiency, dehydration
- pregnant or breastfeeding women.

Administration
- Don't mix I.V. form with other drugs or give through same I.V. port as drugs that may be incompatible.
- Give I.V. solution within 10 hours of reconstitution.
- Divide doses larger than 300 mg.
- Don't refrigerate reconstituted I.V. solution.
- Give oral form with or right after meals.
- Don't give oral form with mineral water, orange juice, or caffeinated beverages.

Route	Onset	Peak	Duration
P.O.	2-3 days	0.5-2 hr	1-2 wk
I.V.	Unknown	0.5 hr	Unknown

Adverse reactions
CNS: drowsiness, dizziness, headache, peripheral neuropathy, neuritis, paresthesia
CV: hypersensitivity vasculitis, **necrotizing vasculitis**
EENT: retinopathy, cataract, epistaxis
GI: nausea, vomiting, diarrhea, abdominal pain, dyspepsia, gastritis
GU: exacerbation of gout and renal calculi, **uremia, renal failure**
Hematologic: eosinophilia, anemia, **thrombocytopenia, bone marrow depression, agranulocytosis, leukocytosis, aplastic anemia, leukopenia**
Hepatic: cholestatic jaundice, **hepatomegaly, hepatitis, hepatic necrosis**
Musculoskeletal: myopathy, joint pain
Skin: rash; alopecia; maculopapular, urticarial, or purpuric lesions; severe furunculosis of nose; ichthyosis; bruising; **scaly or exfoliative erythema multiforme; toxic epidermal necrolysis**
Other: abnormal taste, loss of taste, fever, chills

Interactions
Drug-drug. *Amoxicillin, ampicillin, bacampicillin:* increased risk of rash
Anticoagulants (except warfarin): increased anticoagulant effect
Antineoplastics: increased risk of myelosuppression
Azathioprine, mercaptopurine: inhibition of allopurinol metabolism
Chlorpropamide: increased hypoglycemic effects
Diazoxide, diuretics, mecamylamine, pyrazinamide: increased uric acid levels
Ethacrynic acid, thiazide diuretics: increased risk of allopurinol toxicity
Uricosurics: increased uric acid excretion
Urine-acidifying drugs (ammonium chloride, ascorbic acid, potassium or sodium phosphate): increased risk of renal calculi
Xanthines: increased theophylline levels

Drug-diagnostic tests. *Alanine aminotransferase, alanine phosphatase, aspartate aminotransferase, bilirubin, eosinophils:* increased levels
Granulocytes, hemoglobin, platelets, white blood cells: decreased levels
Drug-food. *Caffeine-containing beverages and foods, mineral water, orange juice:* decreased drug absorption, increased uric acid level
Drug-behaviors. *Alcohol use:* increased uric acid level

Patient monitoring

- Assess fluid intake and output. Intake should be sufficient to yield daily output of at least 2 L of slightly alkaline urine.
- Monitor uric acid level to help evaluate drug efficacy.

Patient teaching

Clinical alert: Instruct patient to promptly report painful urination, bloody urine, rash, eye irritation, or swelling of lips and mouth.
- Tell patient to take drug with food or milk, exactly as prescribed.
- Explain that gout attacks may not ease significantly until 2 to 6 weeks of therapy.
- Caution patient to avoid driving and other hazardous tasks until he knows how drug affects concentration and alertness.
- Advise patient to avoid alcohol, caffeine-containing beverages and foods, mineral water, and orange juice during therapy.
- As appropriate, review all other significant and life-threatening adverse reactions and interactions, especially those related to the drugs, tests, foods, and behaviors mentioned above.

a

almotriptan malate

Axert

Pharmacologic class: Serotonin (5-hydroxytryptamine [5-HT]) receptor agonist
Therapeutic class: Vascular headache suppressant, antimigraine drug
Pregnancy risk category C

Action

Promotes vascular constriction and relieves migraine by stimulating specific 5-HT receptors in intracranial blood vessels and sensory trigeminal nerves

Availability

Tablets: 6.25 mg, 12.5 mg

Indications and dosages

➢ Acute migraine
Adults: Single dose of 6.25 to 12.5 mg P.O. at first sign or symptom of migraine; may repeat if symptoms reappear within 2 hours. Don't exceed two doses in a 24-hour period.

Contraindications

- Hypersensitivity to drug
- Ischemic heart disease, myocardial infarction (MI), cerebrovascular accident, uncontrolled hypertension
- Ischemic bowel disease
- Basilar or hemiplegic migraine
- MAO inhibitor use in past 14 days
- Use of other 5-HT agonists or ergotamine-containing or ergot-type drugs within past 24 hours

Precautions

Use cautiously in:
- impaired renal or hepatic function
- cardiovascular risk factors
- pregnant or breastfeeding patients
- children younger than age 18 (use not recommended).

Administration

• Give with or without food.
• Wait at least 2 hours after initial dose before giving repeat dose.
• Don't exceed two doses in 24 hours.
Don't give within 14 days of MAO inhibitors or within 24 hours of other 5-HT agonists or ergotamine-containing or ergot-type drugs.

Route	Onset	Peak	Duration
P.O.	Variable	1-3 hr	Unknown

Adverse reactions

CNS: headache, anxiety, dizziness, fatigue, malaise, weakness, cold or hot sensations, sedation, numbness, burning or tingling sensations
CV: blood pressure changes, palpitations, tachycardia, **coronary artery vasospasm, MI, ventricular fibrillation, ventricular tachycardia**
EENT: vision changes; nasal, throat, and mouth discomfort
GI: nausea, abdominal distress, dysphagia, dry mouth
Musculoskeletal: weakness, stiff neck, muscle pain
Respiratory: chest tightness or pressure
Skin: sweating, flushing

Interactions

Drug-drug. *CYP2D6 inhibitors (erythromycin, itraconazole, ritonavir):* increased almotriptan effect
Ergot derivatives, other 5-HT agonists: prolonged vasoactive action
Ketoconazole and other CYP3A inhibitors: increased almotriptan blood level, leading to toxicity
MAO inhibitors: decreased almotriptan absorption
Selective serotonin reuptake inhibitors: weakness, hyperreflexia, poor coordination

Patient monitoring

• Assess patient's cardiovascular status, noting chest tightness or pressure.
• Monitor vital signs.

Patient teaching

Tell patient to immediately report chest tightness or pressure.
• Inform patient that he may take drug with or without food.
• If second dose is needed, tell patient to take it at least 2 hours after first.
• Caution patient not to take more than two doses in 24 hours.
• Instruct patient to avoid driving and other hazardous activities until he knows how drug affects concentration and alertness.
• As appropriate, review all other significant and life-threatening adverse reactions and interactions, especially those related to the drugs mentioned above.

alosetron hydrochloride

Lotronex

Pharmacologic class: Serotonin receptor antagonist
Therapeutic class: Agent for irritable bowel syndrome
Pregnancy risk category B

Action

Inhibits activation of nonselective cation channels, resulting in modulation of enteric nervous system

Availability

Tablets: 0.5 mg, 1 mg

Indications and dosages

➢ Women with severe, diarrhea-predominant irritable bowel syndrome (IBS) unresponsive to conventional therapy
Adult women: Initially, 1 mg P.O. daily. After 4 weeks, may increase to 1 mg P.O. b.i.d.

a

Contraindications
• Hypersensitivity to drug or its components
• Current constipation or history of chronic or severe constipation
• History of complications related to constipation
• History of intestinal obstruction, stricture, toxic megacolon, GI perforation, or adhesion
• History of ischemic colitis, impaired intestinal circulation, thrombophlebitis, or hypercoagulable state
• Current Crohn's disease or ulcerative colitis, active diverticulitis, or history of these disorders
• Inability to understand or comply with patient-physician agreement for drug

Precautions
Use cautiously in:
• hepatic insufficiency
• elderly patients
• pregnant or breastfeeding patients
• children.

Administration
🔊 Before administering, know that drug is approved with the following marketing restrictions: Ensure that patient understands that drug has serious risks, patient reads and signs patient-physician agreement, and patient follows directions in accompanying medication guide.
• Know that anatomical and biochemical abnormalities of GI tract should be ruled out before drug therapy starts.
• Give with or without food.
🔊 Don't administer drug if patient is constipated.
🔊 Stop therapy immediately if patient develops constipation or signs or symptoms of ischemic colitis.

Route	Onset	Peak	Duration
P.O.	Rapid	1 hr	Unknown

Adverse reactions
CNS: anxiety, malaise
CV: increased blood pressure, extrasystoles, tachyarrhythmias, **arrhythmias**
GI: nausea; constipation; GI pain, discomfort, or spasms; abdominal distention; regurgitation or gastroesophageal reflux; hemorrhoids; decreased salivation; dyspepsia; **ischemic colitis; GI perforation; small-bowel mesenteric ischemia**
GU: urinary frequency
Hematologic: hemorrhage
Respiratory: breathing disorders
Skin: sweating, urticaria
Other: fatigue, cramps, disturbed temperature regulation

Interactions
Drug-drug. *Hydralazine, isoniazid, procainamide:* altered blood levels of these drugs
Drug-diagnostic tests. *Blood glucose, calcium, phosphate:* increased or decreased level

Patient monitoring
🔊 Monitor patient closely for adverse reactions, especially such GI reactions as constipation and signs or symptoms of ischemic colitis.

Patient teaching
🔊 Make sure patient knows about drug's marketing restrictions, which stipulate that she understands drug has serious risks, that she reads and signs patient-physician agreement, and that she follows directions in accompanying medication guide.
• Tell patient to take drug exactly as prescribed, with or without food.
🔊 Instruct patient to contact prescriber immediately if she develops constipation or symptoms of insufficient blood flow to bowel (such as new or worsening pain in bowels or bloody bowel movements).
• As appropriate, review all other significant and life-threatening adverse

reactions and interactions, especially those related to the drugs and tests mentioned above.

alprazolam

Apo-Alpraz✤, Novo-Alprazol✤, Nu-Alpraz✤, Xanax, Xanax TS✤, Xanax XR

Pharmacologic class: Benzodiazepine
Therapeutic class: Anxiolytic
Controlled substance schedule IV
Pregnancy risk category D

Action

Unclear. Thought to act at limbic, thalamic, and hypothalamic levels of CNS to produce sedative, anxiolytic, skeletal muscle relaxant, and anticonvulsant effects.

Availability

Solution: 1 mg/ml
Tablets (extended-release): 0.5 mg, 1 mg, 2 mg, 3 mg
Tablets (immediate-release): 0.25 mg, 0.5 mg, 1 mg, 2 mg

Indications and dosages

➢ Anxiety disorders

Adults: Initially, 0.25 to 0.5 mg P.O. t.i.d. Maximum dosage is 4 mg daily in divided doses.

Elderly patients: Initially, 0.25 mg P.O. two or three times daily. Maximum dosage is 4 mg daily in divided doses.

➢ Panic disorders

Adults: *Immediate-release tablets*—Initially, 0.5 mg P.O. t.i.d. Increase by a maximum of 1 mg at intervals of 3 to 4 days, with a maximum dosage of 10 mg daily in divided doses. *Extended-release tablets*—Initially, 0.5 to 1 mg P.O. daily. Usual dosage is 3 to 6 mg daily, with a maximum dosage of 10 mg daily.

Dosage adjustment

- Hepatic impairment

Off-label uses

- Agoraphobia
- Depression
- Premenstrual syndrome

Contraindications

- Hypersensitivity to benzodiazepines
- Narrow-angle glaucoma
- Psychosis
- Shock
- Coma
- Labor and delivery
- Pregnancy or breastfeeding

Precautions

Use cautiously in:
- hepatic dysfunction
- history of attempted suicide or drug dependence
- elderly patients.

Administration

- Don't give with grapefruit juice.
- Make sure patient swallows extended-release tablets whole without chewing or crushing.

Clinical alert: Don't withdraw drug suddenly. Seizures and other withdrawal symptoms may occur unless dosage is tapered carefully.

Route	Onset	Peak	Duration
P.O.	30 min	1-2 hr	4-6 hr

Adverse reactions

CNS: dizziness, drowsiness, depression, fatigue, light-headedness, disorientation, anger, hostility, euphoria, hypomanic episodes, restlessness, confusion, crying, delirium, headache, stupor, rigidity, tremor, paresthesia, vivid dreams, extrapyramidal symptoms
CV: bradycardia, tachycardia, hypertension, hypotension, palpitations, **CV collapse**
EENT: blurred or double vision, nystagmus, nasal congestion

GI: gastric disorders, dysphagia, anorexia, increased salivation, dry mouth
GU: menstrual irregularities, urinary retention, urinary incontinence, libido changes, gynecomastia
Hematologic: blood dyscrasias such as eosinophilia, **agranulocytosis, leukopenia, and thrombocytopenia**
Hepatic: hepatic dysfunction (including **hepatitis**)
Musculoskeletal: muscle rigidity, joint pain
Skin: dermatitis, rash, pruritus, urticaria, increased sweating
Other: weight loss or gain, hiccups, fever, edema, psychological drug dependence, drug tolerance

Interactions

Drug-drug. *Antidepressants, antihistamines, opioids, other benzodiazepines:* increased CNS depression
Barbiturates, rifampin: increased metabolism and decreased efficacy of alprazolam
Cimetidine, disulfiram, erythromycin, fluoxetine, hormonal contraceptives, isoniazid, ketoconazole, metoprolol, propoxyphene, propranolol, valproic acid: decreased metabolism and increased action of alprazolam
Digoxin: increased risk of digoxin toxicity
Levodopa: decreased antiparkinsonian effect
Theophylline: increased sedative effect
Tricyclic antidepressants (TCAs): increased TCA blood levels
Drug-diagnostic tests. *Alanine aminotransferase, alkaline phosphatase, aspartate aminotransferase, lactate dehydrogenase:* elevated levels
Drug-food. *Grapefruit juice:* decreased drug metabolism and increased blood level
Drug-herbs. *Chamomile, hops, kava, skullcap, valerian:* increased CNS depression
Drug-behaviors. *Alcohol use:* increased CNS depression
Smoking: decreased alprazolam efficacy

Patient monitoring

- Watch for excessive CNS depression if patient is concurrently taking antidepressants, other benzodiazepines, antihistamines, or opioids.
- If patient is taking TCAs concurrently, watch for increase in adverse TCA effects.
- Monitor CBC and liver and kidney function test results.
- Monitor vital signs and weight.
- Report signs of drug abuse, including frequent requests for early refills.

Patient teaching

- Instruct patient to swallow extended-release tablets whole without crushing or chewing.

(Clinical alert) Tell patient that drug may make him more depressed, angry, or hostile. Urge him to contact prescriber immediately if he thinks he's dangerous to himself or others.

- Inform patient that drug may cause tremors, muscle rigidity, and other movement problems. Advise him to report these effects to prescriber.

(Clinical alert) Caution patient not to stop taking drug suddenly. Withdrawal symptoms, including seizures, may occur unless drug is tapered carefully.

- Advise patient to avoid driving and other hazardous activities until he knows how drug affects concentration and alertness.
- As appropriate, review all other significant and life-threatening adverse reactions and interactions, especially those related to the drugs, tests, foods, herbs, and behaviors mentioned above.

alprostadil

Caverject, Edex, Muse, Prostin VR Pediatric

Pharmacologic class: Prostaglandin E_1
Therapeutic class: Impotence agent, ductus arteriosus patency adjunct
Pregnancy risk category NR

Action

Produces vasodilation, inhibits platelet aggregation, and stimulates intestinal and uterine smooth muscles. In ductus arteriosus patency, relaxes smooth muscle of ductus arteriosus. In erectile dysfunction, promotes erection by relaxing trabecular smooth muscle and dilating cavernosal arteries.

Availability

Injection: 5 mcg/ml, 10 mcg/ml, 20 mcg/ml, 40 mcg/ml, 500 mcg/ml
Pellets: 125 mcg, 250 mcg, 500 mcg, 1,000 mcg
Powder for injection: 5 mcg/ml, 10 mcg/ml, 20 mcg/ml

Indications and dosages

➤ Palliative therapy for infants to temporarily maintain patency of ductus arteriosus

Infants: 0.05 to 0.1 mcg/kg/minute I.V. (Prostin VR Pediatric). Once therapeutic response occurs, reduce infusion to lowest dosage required to maintain response. Maximum dosage is 0.4 mcg/kg/minute.

➤ Erectile dysfunction of vasculogenic, psychogenic, or mixed etiology

Adults: *Intracavernosal*—Initial dosage in medical setting is 2.5 mcg (Caverject, Edex). If partial response occurs, give second 2.5-mcg dose after 1 hour; then increase in increments of 5 to 10 mcg until patient achieves suitable erection lasting no more than 1 hour. If no response to initial 2.5-mcg dose occurs, may increase second dose to 7.5 mcg within 1 hour; then increase in 5- to 10-mcg increments at intervals of at least 24 hours until patient achieves suitable erection. No more than two doses should be repeated for at least 24 hours. Patient should self-administer alprostadil no more often than three times weekly, waiting at least 1 day between doses.
Intraurethral—Initial dosage in medical setting is 125 mcg or 250 mcg (Muse pellet), titrated to lowest possible dosage. If no response occurs, subsequent doses may be increased to 500 or 1,000 mcg as needed. No more than two urethral pellets should be used within a 24-hour period.

➤ Erectile dysfunction of pure neurogenic cause

Adults: *Intracavernosal*—Initial dosage in medical setting is 1.25 mcg. If no response occurs, a second 1.25-mcg dose may be given after 1 hour; no more than two doses should be administered in a 24-hour period. If additional dose titration is required, 5 mcg may be given over next 24 hours, followed by increases in 5-mcg increments until optimal response occurs.

Off-label uses

- Angiography of penile vasculature
- Atherosclerosis
- Gangrene and pain due to vascular disease

Contraindications

- Hypersensitivity to drug
- Penile deformity or implant
- Conditions that predispose patient to priapism
- Respiratory distress syndrome
- Men who engage in sexual intercourse with pregnant women (unless condoms are used)
- Children (intracavernous use)
- Urethral stricture, balanitis, severe hypospadias, acute or chronic urethri-

tis, thrombocythemia, polycythemia (all with intraurethral use)

Precautions

Use cautiously in:
- bleeding tendencies
- neonates.

Administration

- Reconstitute powder for injection with 1 ml of diluent supplied or bacteriostatic water for injection with benzyl alcohol.
- Be aware that each brand of powder for injection contains varying amounts of alprostadil before reconstitution, but all brands deliver same amount when administered.
- Inject concentrate into diluent in infusion chamber. Don't let concentrate touch plastic side of chamber.
- Infuse at 0.05 to 0.1 mcg/kg/minute. When therapeutic response occurs, reduce to lowest dosage that maintains response.
- Don't give faster than 0.4 mcg/kg/minute.
- Don't give by direct injection or intermittent infusion. Use infusion pump for continuous infusion.
- In infants, use large peripheral vein or central vein or give through umbilical artery catheter at ductus level.

Route	Onset	Peak	Duration
I.V.	20 min	1-2 hr	Length of infusion
Intra-cavernous	5-20 min	5-20 min	1-6 hr

Adverse reactions

Except where otherwise noted, reactions below pertain to Prostin VR Pediatric.
CNS: dizziness, headache (intracavernous use); **seizures**
CV: hypertension (intracavernous use); tachycardia, edema, hypotension, **bradycardia, cardiac arrest**
EENT: nasal congestion (intracavernous use)
GI: diarrhea
GU: penile, urethral, or testicular pain; urethral burning; trauma; prolonged erection; priapism; penile fibrosis; penile edema; penile disorders; prostate enlargement, hypertrophy, or pain (all with intracavernous use)
Hematologic: disseminated intravascular coagulation (DIC), inhibited platelet aggregation
Metabolic: hypokalemia
Musculoskeletal: cortical proliferation of long bones (long-term infusions), back pain (intracavernous use)
Respiratory: respiratory tract infection, cough (intracavernous use); **apnea**
Skin: flushing; hematoma or bruising at injection site; penile rash (intracavernous use)
Other: flulike symptoms (intracavernous use); fever; **sepsis**

Interactions

Drug-drug. *Anticoagulants:* increased risk of bleeding
Cyclosporine: decreased cyclosporine blood level
Vasoactive agents: safety and efficacy not established
Drug-diagnostic tests. *Potassium:* decreased level

Patient monitoring

- [Clinical alert] Monitor infant's cardiopulmonary status. Be prepared to provide respiratory support for apnea (most likely to occur during first hour of infusion).
- [Clinical alert] Evaluate infant for adverse cardiovascular effects (especially bradycardia) and adverse CNS reactions (especially seizures), which are more common in smaller infants and after 48 hours of infusion.
- [Clinical alert] Monitor infant's arterial pressure with umbilical artery catheter, auscultation, or Doppler transducer.
- [Clinical alert] Assess infant for signs of sepsis and for bleeding caused by DIC.

• Monitor blood oxygenation, systemic blood pressure, and blood pH to evaluate drug efficacy.
• Monitor infant's clotting studies and serum electrolyte levels.
• With intracavernous use, monitor patient for hypotension.

Patient teaching

• Explain reason for drug use to parents. Provide updates on drug efficacy.
• Tell parents about adverse effects and subsequent nursing interventions, as appropriate.
• If patient is using drug to treat erectile dysfunction, review administration guidelines (after initial treatment) to ensure proper use.
• Tell patient with erectile dysfunction to report signs and symptoms of infection (such as foul penile discharge), other adverse reactions, and prolonged erection (more than 6 hours).
• Advise patient with erectile dysfunction not to have sexual intercourse with a pregnant woman without using a condom.
• As appropriate, review all other significant and life-threatening adverse reactions and interactions, especially those related to the drugs and tests mentioned above.

alteplase (tissue plasminogen activator, recombinant)

Activase, Activase rt-PA✱, Cathflo Activase, Lysatec rt-PA✱

Pharmacologic class: Plasminogen activator
Therapeutic class: Thrombolytic
Pregnancy risk category C

Action

Converts plasminogen to plasmin, which in turn breaks down fibrin and fibrinogen, thereby dissolving thrombus

Availability

Injection: 2-mg single-patient vials; 50-mg, 100-mg vials

Indications and dosages

➢ Lysis of thrombi obstructing coronary arteries in acute myocardial infarction (MI)
3-hour infusion—
Adults: 100 mg I.V. over 3 hours as follows: 60 mg over first hour (give 6 to 10 mg as bolus over first 1 to 2 minutes), then 20 mg I.V. over second hour, then 20 mg I.V. over third hour
Adults weighing less than 65 kg (143 lb): 1.25 mg/kg I.V. in divided doses over 3 hours, not to exceed 100 mg
Accelerated infusion—
Adults weighing more than 67 kg (147 lb): Give total dosage of 100 mg as follows: 15 mg I.V. bolus over 1 to 2 minutes, then 50 mg I.V. over next 30 minutes, then 35 mg I.V. over next 60 minutes.
Adults weighing 67 kg (147 lb) or less: 15 mg I.V. bolus over 1 to 2 minutes, followed by 0.75 mg/kg I.V. over next 30 minutes (not to exceed 50 mg), followed by 0.5 mg/kg I.V. over next hour, not to exceed 35 mg
➢ Acute ischemic cerebrovascular accident (CVA)
Adults: 0.9 mg/kg I.V. over 1 hour, to a maximum dosage of 90 mg, with 10% of total dosage given as I.V. bolus within first minute
➢ Acute massive pulmonary embolism
Adults: 100 mg I.V. over 2 hours, followed by heparin

Off-label uses

• Blocked venous catheter (2-mg bolus injected into catheter for adults and children ages 2 years and older)

a

• Small-vessel occlusion by microthrombi
• Peripheral arterial thromboembolism

Contraindications

• Active MI or pulmonary embolism in patients with increased bleeding risk
• Previous CVA, history of intracranial hemorrhage, uncontrolled hypertension, seizures, or active internal bleeding

Precautions

Use cautiously in:
• hypersensitivity to anistreplase or streptokinase
• GI or genitourinary bleeding, ophthalmic hemorrhage, organ biopsy, severe hepatic or renal disease
• elderly patients
• pregnant or breastfeeding patients
• children.

Administration

🔈 Be aware that intracranial hemorrhage must be ruled out before therapy begins.
• Give I.V. only, using controlled-infusion device.
🔈 To treat acute ischemic CVA, give within 3 hours of initial signs or symptoms.
🔈 If uncontrolled bleeding occurs, stop infusion and notify prescriber immediately.
• Reconstitute with unpreserved sterile water for injection, using large-bore needle to shoot diluent stream directly into powder. Wait a few minutes for foam to settle, and then draw up dose and administer right away.

Route	Onset	Peak	Duration
I.V.	Unknown	Unknown	Unknown

Adverse reactions

CNS: cerebral hemorrhage, cerebral edema, CVA (with accelerated infusion)
CV: hypotension, bradycardia, recurrent ischemia, **pericardial effusion, pericarditis, mitral regurgitation, electromechanical dissociation, arrhythmias, cardiogenic shock, heart failure, cardiac arrest, cardiac tamponade, myocardial rupture, embolization, venous thrombosis**
GI: nausea, vomiting, **GI bleeding**
GU: GU tract bleeding
Hematologic: spontaneous bleeding, bone marrow depression
Musculoskeletal: musculoskeletal pain
Respiratory: pulmonary edema
Skin: bruising, flushing
Other: fever, edema, phlebitis or bleeding at I.V. site, hypersensitivity reaction (including rash, **anaphylactic reaction, laryngeal edema**), **sepsis**

Interactions

Drug-drug. *Aspirin, drugs affecting platelet activity (such as abciximab, heparin, dipyridamole, oral anticoagulants, vitamin K antagonists):* increased risk of bleeding
Drug-diagnostic tests. *Blood urea nitrogen:* elevated level

Patient monitoring

• Monitor vital signs, ECG, and neurologic status.
• Maintain strict bed rest.
• Watch for signs and symptoms of bleeding tendency and hemorrhage.
• Monitor patient on Cathflo Activase for GI bleeding, venous thrombosis, and sepsis.
• Evaluate results of clotting studies.

Patient teaching

🔈 Instruct patient to immediately report adverse reactions, especially unusual bleeding or bruising.
• Stress importance of strict bed rest.
• Tell patient to avoid activities that can cause injury. Advise him to use soft toothbrush and electric razor to avoid gum and skin injury.

• Advise patient that he'll undergo regular blood testing during therapy.
• As appropriate, review all other significant and life-threatening adverse reactions and interactions, especially those related to the drugs and tests mentioned above.

aluminum hydroxide

AlternaGEL, Alu-Cap, Alugel✦, Alu-Tab, Amphojel, Dialume

Pharmacologic class: Inorganic salt
Therapeutic class: Antacid
Pregnancy risk category NR

Action

Dissolves in acidic gastric secretions, releasing anions that partially neutralize gastric hydrochloric acid. Also elevates gastric pH, inhibiting the action of pepsin (an effect important in peptic ulcer disease).

Availability

Capsules: 400 mg, 475 mg, 500 mg
Oral suspension: 320 mg/5 ml, 450 mg/5 ml, 600 mg/5 ml, 675 mg/5 ml
Tablets: 300 mg, 500 mg, 600 mg

Indications and dosages

➢ Hyperacidity
Adults: 500 to 1,500 mg (tablet or capsule) P.O. 1 hour after meals and at bedtime; or 5 to 30 ml (oral suspension) between meals and at bedtime, as needed or directed

Off-label uses

• Bleeding from stress ulcers
• Gastroesophageal reflux disease

Contraindications

• Signs or symptoms of appendicitis or inflamed bowel

Precautions

Use cautiously in:
• gastric outlet obstruction, hypercalcemia, hypophosphatemia, massive upper GI hemorrhage
• patients using other aluminum products concurrently
• patients on dialysis
• pregnant or breastfeeding patients.

Administration

• Administer with water or fruit juice.
• Give 1 hour after meals and at bedtime.
• In reflux esophagitis, administer 20 to 40 minutes after meals and at bedtime.
• Don't give within 1 to 2 hours of antibiotics, histamine$_2$ (H_2) blockers, iron preparations, corticosteroids, or enteric-coated drugs.
• Provide care as appropriate if patient becomes constipated.

Route	Onset	Peak	Duration
P.O.	15-30 min	30 min	30 min-3 hr

Adverse reactions

CNS: malaise (with prolonged use), **neurotoxicity, encephalopathy**
GI: constipation, anorexia (with prolonged use), **intestinal obstruction**
Metabolic: hypophosphatemia (with prolonged use)
Musculoskeletal: osteomalacia and chronic phosphate deficiency with bone pain, malaise, muscle weakness (with prolonged use)
Other: aluminum toxicity

Interactions

Drug-drug. *Allopurinol, anti-infectives (including quinolones, tetracyclines), corticosteroids, diflunisal, digoxin, ethambutol, H_2 blockers, hydantoins, iron salts, isoniazid, penicillamine, phenothiazines, salicylates, thyroid hormone, ticlopidine:* decreased effects of these drugs

Enteric-coated drugs: premature release of these drugs in stomach
Drug-diagnostic tests. *Gastrin:* increased level
Phosphate: decreased level
Some imaging studies: test interference
Drug-food. *Milk, other foods high in vitamin D:* milk-alkali syndrome (nausea, vomiting, distaste for food, headache, confusion, hypercalcemia, hypercalciuria)

Patient monitoring

- Monitor long-term use of high doses if patient is on sodium-restricted diet. (Drug contains sodium.)
- Assess for GI bleeding.
- Watch for constipation.
- With long-term use, monitor blood phosphate level and assess for signs and symptoms of hypophosphatemia (anorexia, malaise, muscle weakness). Also monitor bone density.

Patient teaching

- Tell patient to take drug 1 hour after meals and at bedtime.
- Caution patient not to take drug within 1 to 2 hours of anti-infectives, H_2 blockers, iron, corticosteroids, or enteric-coated drugs.
- Advise patient to take drug with water or fruit juice.
- Instruct patient to report signs and symptoms of GI bleeding and hypophosphatemia (appetite loss, malaise, muscle weakness).
- Recommend increased fiber and fluid intake and regular physical activity to help ease constipation.
- Inform patient that drug contains sodium, so he should discuss drug therapy with health care providers if he's later told to consume a low-sodium diet.
- Advise patient that he'll need to undergo periodic blood testing and bone mineral density tests if he's receiving long-term therapy.
- As appropriate, review all other significant and life-threatening adverse reactions and interactions, especially those related to the drugs, tests, and foods mentioned above.

amantadine hydrochloride

Symmetrel

Pharmacologic class: Anticholinergic-like agent
Therapeutic class: Antiviral, antiparkinsonian
Pregnancy risk category C

Action

Antiviral action unclear; may prevent penetration of influenza A virus into host cell. Antiparkinsonian action unknown; may ease parkinsonian symptoms by increasing dopamine release, preventing dopamine reuptake into presynaptic neurons, stimulating dopamine receptors, or enhancing dopamine sensitivity.

Availability

Capsules (liquid-filled): 100 mg
Syrup: 50 mg/5 ml
Tablets: 100 mg

Indications and dosages

➢ Symptomatic treatment or prophylaxis of influenza type A virus in patients with respiratory conditions
Adults older than age 65 with normal renal function: 100 mg P.O. once daily
Adults to age 64 with normal renal function: 200 mg (tablets) or 4 tsp of syrup P.O. daily in a single dose, or 100 mg tablet or 2 tsp of syrup P.O. b.i.d.
Children ages 9 to 12: 100 mg P.O. q 12 hours
Children ages 1 to 9 or weighing less than 45 kg (99 lb): 4.4 to 8.8 mg/kg/day of syrup P.O. q 12 hours, not to exceed 150 mg daily

➢ Parkinson's disease
Adults: Initially, 100 mg P.O. daily, increased to 100 mg b.i.d. if needed. If patient doesn't respond adequately, give 200 mg b.i.d., up to 400 mg/day.
➢ Drug-induced extrapyramidal reactions
Adults: 100 mg to 300 mg P.O. daily in divided doses

Dosage adjustment
- Renal impairment

Contraindications
- Hypersensitivity to drug
- Untreated closed-angle glaucoma

Precautions
Use cautiously in:
- cardiac disease, hepatic disease, renal impairment, seizure disorder, psychiatric problems
- elderly patients
- pregnant or breastfeeding patients.

Administration
- For antiviral use, start therapy within 24 to 48 hours of symptom onset and continue for 24 to 48 hours after symptoms resolve.
- When giving as prophylactic antiviral, start therapy as soon as possible and continue for at least 10 days after exposure to virus.
- When giving with influenza vaccine, continue drug for 2 to 3 weeks while patient develops antibody response to vaccine.

Route	Onset	Peak	Duration
P.O.	48 hr	2 wk	Unknown

Adverse reactions
CNS: depression, dizziness, drowsiness, insomnia, light-headedness, anxiety, irritability, hallucinations, confusion, ataxia, headache, nervousness, abnormal dreams, agitation, fatigue, delusions, aggressive behavior, manic reaction, psychosis, slurred speech, euphoria, abnormal thinking, amnesia, increased or decreased motor activity, paresthesia, tremor, abnormal gait, delirium, stupor, **coma**
CV: orthostatic hypotension, tachycardia, peripheral edema, **heart failure, cardiac arrest, arrhythmias**
EENT: blurred vision, mydriasis, keratitis, photosensitivity, optic nerve palsy, nasal congestion
GI: nausea, vomiting, diarrhea, constipation, dry mouth, dysphagia, anorexia
GU: urine retention, decreased libido
Hematologic: leukocytosis
Musculoskeletal: involuntary muscle contractions
Respiratory: tachypnea, **acute respiratory failure, pulmonary edema**
Skin: purplish skin discoloration, rash, pruritus, diaphoresis
Other: edema, fever, allergic reactions including **anaphylaxis**

Interactions
Drug-drug. *Anticholinergics, antihistamines, phenothiazines, quinidine, tricyclic antidepressants:* increased atropine-like adverse effects
CNS stimulants: increased CNS stimulation
Hydrochlorothiazide, triamterene: increased amantadine effects
Drug-diagnostic tests. *Alanine aminotransferase, alkaline phosphatase, aspartate aminotransferase, bilirubin, blood urea nitrogen, creatine kinase, creatinine, gamma-glutamyltransferase, lactate dehydrogenase:* increased levels
Drug-herbs. *Angel's trumpet, jimsonweed, scopolia:* increased cardiac and anticholinergic-like effects
Drug-behaviors. *Alcohol use:* increased CNS adverse reactions

Patient monitoring
🔊 Monitor patient for depression and suicidal ideation.
- Watch for mental status changes, especially in elderly patients.

a

• Stay alert for worsening of psychiatric problems if patient has a history of such problems or substance abuse.
• Monitor for orthostatic hypotension.
• Evaluate for signs and symptoms of fluid overload.
• Monitor kidney and liver function test results.

Patient teaching

Caution patient that taking more than prescribed dosage may lead to serious adverse reactions or even death.
• Advise patient to establish effective bedtime routine and to take drug several hours before bedtime to minimize insomnia.
• Caution patient to avoid driving and other hazardous activities until he knows how drug affects concentration and alertness.
• Advise patient to minimize GI upset by eating small, frequent servings of foods and drinking plenty of fluids.
• Instruct patient to contact prescriber if he develops signs or symptoms of depression.
• As appropriate, review all other significant and life-threatening adverse reactions and interactions, especially those related to the drugs, tests, herbs, and behaviors mentioned above.

amifostine

Ethyol

Pharmacologic class: Organic thiophosphate cytoprotective drug
Therapeutic class: Antineoplastic
Pregnancy risk category C

Action

Undergoes conversion to free thiol, an active metabolite that reduces toxic effects of cisplatin on renal tissue

Availability

Powder for injection: 500-mg anhydrous base and 500 mg mannitol in 10-ml vials

Indications and dosages

➤ To reduce cumulative renal toxicity of cisplatin therapy in patients with ovarian cancer or non-small-cell lung cancer
Adults: 910 mg/m² I.V. daily as a 15-minute infusion, starting 30 minutes before chemotherapy
➤ To reduce moderate to severe xerostomia in patients undergoing postoperative radiation treatment for head or neck cancer
Adults: 200 mg/m² I.V. daily as a 3-minute infusion, starting 15 to 30 minutes before standard fraction radiation therapy

Off-label uses

• Protection of lung fibroblasts from damaging effects of paclitaxel

Contraindications

• Hypersensitivity to drug
• Hypotension
• Concurrent antihypertensive therapy that can't be discontinued for 24 hours before amifostine treatment
• Definitive radiotherapy

Precautions

Use cautiously in:
• arrhythmias, heart failure, ischemic heart disease, renal impairment, hearing impairment, hypocalcemia, myasthenia gravis, nausea, vomiting, hypotension, obesity
• history of cerebrovascular accident or transient ischemic attacks
• elderly patients
• pregnant patients (safety and efficacy not established)
• breastfeeding patients
• children (safety and efficacy not established).

Administration

• Ensure that patient is adequately hydrated before starting drug.
• Give antiemetics before and during therapy.
• Reconstitute single-dose vial with 9.7 ml of sterile normal saline injection.
• Don't mix with other drugs or solutions.
• Know that drug also can be prepared in polyvinyl chloride bags.
• Don't infuse longer than 15 minutes; doing so increases risk of adverse reactions.
Clinical alert: Keep patient supine during administration.

Route	Onset	Peak	Duration
I.V.	5-8 min	Unknown	Unknown

Adverse reactions

CNS: dizziness, drowsiness, rigors
CV: hypotension
GI: nausea, vomiting
Metabolic: hypocalcemia
Respiratory: dyspnea, sneezing
Skin: flushing, rash, urticaria, **erythema multiforme**
Other: chills, warm sensation, hiccups, allergic reactions

Interactions

Drug-drug. *Antihypertensives:* increased risk of hypotension
Drug-diagnostic tests. *Calcium:* decreased level

Patient monitoring

• Monitor blood pressure.
• Assess for severe nausea and vomiting.
• Monitor fluid intake and output.
• Monitor blood calcium level. Give calcium supplements as ordered.

Patient teaching

• Emphasize importance of remaining supine during drug administration to prevent hypotension.
• Caution patient to avoid driving and other hazardous activities until he knows how drug affects concentration and alertness.
• Advise patient to minimize GI upset by eating small, frequent servings of food and drinking plenty of fluids.
• Provide dietary counseling. Refer patient to dietitian if adverse GI effects significantly limit food intake.
• Inform patient that sneezing is a normal effect of drug.
• As appropriate, review all other significant and life-threatening adverse reactions and interactions, especially those related to the drugs and tests mentioned above.

amikacin sulfate

Amikin

Pharmacologic class: Aminoglycoside
Therapeutic class: Anti-infective
Pregnancy risk category D

Action

Interferes with protein synthesis in bacterial cells by binding to 30S ribosomal subunit, leading to bacterial cell death

Availability

Injection: 50 mg/ml, 250 mg/ml

Indications and dosages

➢ Severe systemic infections caused by sensitive strains of *Pseudomonas aeruginosa, Escherichia coli,* or *Proteus, Klebsiella, Serratia, Enterobacter, Actinobacter, Providencia, Citrobacter,* or *Staphylococcus* species
Adults, children, and older infants: 15 mg/kg/day I.V. or I.M. in two to three divided doses q 8 to 12 hours in 100 to 200 ml of dextrose 5% in water (D_5W) over 30 to 60 minutes. Maximum dosage is 1.5 g/day.

a

Neonates: Initially, 10 mg/kg I.M., then 7.5 mg/kg I.M. q 12 hours

➢ Uncomplicated urinary tract infections caused by susceptible organisms

Adults, children, and older infants: 250 mg I.M. or I.V. twice daily

Dosage adjustment

- Renal impairment (adults)
- Patients undergoing hemodialysis

Off-label uses

- *Mycobacterium avium-intracellulare* infection

Contraindications

- Hypersensitivity to aminoglycosides
- Renal or hepatic disease
- Myasthenia gravis
- Parkinsonism
- Breastfeeding

Precautions

Use cautiously in:

- decreased renal function, neuromuscular disorders
- elderly patients
- pregnant patients.

Administration

- Don't physically mix amikacin with other drugs. Administer separately.
- For I.V. use, dilute in 100 to 200 ml of normal saline solution or D_5W and give over 30 to 60 minutes.
- Ensure adequate fluid intake to avoid dehydration.
- Draw peak blood level 1 hour after I.M. infusion or 30 to 60 minutes after I.V. infusion.
- Draw trough blood level just before next dose.

Route	Onset	Peak	Duration
I.V.	Immediate	30 min	8-12 hr
I.M.	Variable	1 hr	8-12 hr

Adverse reactions

CNS: dizziness, vertigo, tremor, numbness, depression, confusion, lethargy, headache, paresthesia, ataxia, **neuromuscular blockade, seizures, neurotoxicity**

CV: hypotension, hypertension, palpitations

EENT: nystagmus and other visual disturbances, ototoxicity, hearing loss, tinnitus

GI: nausea, vomiting, splenomegaly, stomatitis, increased salivation, anorexia

GU: azotemia, increased urinary excretion of casts, polyuria, painful urination, impotence, **nephrotoxicity**

Hematologic: purpura, eosinophilia, **leukemoid reaction, aplastic anemia, neutropenia, agranulocytosis, leukopenia, thrombocytopenia, pancytopenia, hemolytic anemia**

Hepatic: hepatomegaly, hepatic necrosis, hepatotoxicity

Musculoskeletal: joint pain, muscle twitching

Respiratory: apnea

Skin: rash, alopecia, urticaria, itching, exfoliative dermatitis

Other: weight loss, superinfection, pain and irritation at I.M. site

Interactions

Drug-drug. *Acyclovir, amphotericin B, cephalosporin, cisplatin, diuretics, vancomycin:* increased risk of ototoxicity and nephrotoxicity

Depolarizing and nondepolarizing neuromuscular junction blockers, general anesthetics: increased amikacin effect, possibly leading to respiratory depression

Dimenhydrinate: masking of ototoxicity signs and symptoms

Indomethacin: increased trough and peak amikacin levels

Parenteral penicillin: amikacin inactivation

Drug-diagnostic tests. *Alanine aminotransferase, alkaline phosphatase, aspar-*

tate aminotransferase, bilirubin, blood urea nitrogen, creatinine, lactate dehydrogenase, nonprotein nitrogen, nitrogen compounds (such as urea): increased levels
Calcium, potassium, magnesium, sodium: decreased levels
Reticulocytes: increased or decreased count

Patient monitoring

- Monitor kidney function test results and urine cultures, output, protein, and specific gravity.
- Monitor results of peak and trough drug blood levels.
- Evaluate for signs and symptoms of ototoxicity (hearing loss, tinnitus, ataxia, and vertigo).
- Assess for secondary superinfections, particularly upper respiratory tract infections.

Patient teaching

Clinical alert: Inform patient that drug may cause hearing loss, seizures, and other neurologic problems. Tell him to report these symptoms immediately.

- Instruct patient to immediately report fever, cough, breathing problems, sore throat, and other signs and symptoms of infection.
- Caution patient to avoid driving and other hazardous activities until he knows how drug affects concentration and alertness.
- Instruct patient to notify prescriber if he's urinating much more or much less than normal.
- Advise patient to minimize GI upset by eating small, frequent servings of food and drinking plenty of fluids.
- Inform patient that he'll undergo regular blood and urine testing during therapy.
- As appropriate, review all other significant and life-threatening adverse reactions and interactions, especially those related to the drugs and tests mentioned above.

amiloride hydrochloride

Midamor

Pharmacologic class: Pyrazine-carbonyl-guanidine
Therapeutic class: Potassium-sparing diuretic
Pregnancy risk category B

Action

Inhibits sodium reabsorption at distal convoluted renal tubule, cortical collecting tubule, and collecting duct, thereby causing sodium and fluid loss and potassium retention

Availability

Tablets: 5 mg

Indications and dosages

➤ Adjunctive therapy (with thiazide or other potassium-wasting diuretics) to help restore a normal serum potassium level; to prevent hypokalemia in patients at risk (such as those receiving cardiac glycosides)
Adults: 5 mg P.O. daily as adjunct to usual antihypertensive or diuretic; may increase to 20 mg daily with careful electrolyte monitoring
➤ Monotherapy in patients with heart failure or hypertension
Adults: Initially, 5 mg P.O. daily; if needed, increase to 10 mg P.O. daily. In persistent hypokalemia, may increase to 15 to 20 mg P.O. daily with careful electrolyte monitoring.

Contraindications

- Hypersensitivity to drug
- Impaired renal function
- Concurrent use or ingestion of potassium supplements or other potassium-sparing diuretics
- Serum potassium level > 5.5 mEq/L
- Children

a

Precautions

Use cautiously in:
- hepatic insufficiency, cardiopulmonary disease, diabetes mellitus, renal disease
- elderly patients
- pregnant patients.

Administration

- Administer with meals.

Never give to patient concurrently receiving potassium supplements or other potassium-sparing diuretics.

Route	Onset	Peak	Duration
P.O.	2 hr	6-10 hr	24 hr

Adverse reactions

CNS: headache, weakness, fatigue, dizziness, paresthesia, **encephalopathy**
GI: nausea, vomiting, constipation, abdominal pain, flatulence
GU: polyuria, erectile dysfunction
Metabolic: electrolyte imbalances (when used with other diuretics), **hyperkalemia**
Musculoskeletal: muscle cramps
Respiratory: cough, dyspnea
Skin: rash
Other: appetite changes

Interactions

Drug-drug. *Angiotensin-converting enzyme (ACE) inhibitors, cyclosporine, potassium supplements, other potassium-sparing diuretics, tacrolimus:* increased risk of severe hyperkalemia
Digoxin: decreased digoxin efficacy
Lithium: reduced lithium clearance and increased risk of lithium toxicity
Nonsteroidal anti-inflammatory drugs (NSAIDs): reduced diuretic and antihypertensive effects of amiloride
Drug-diagnostic tests. *Blood urea nitrogen, potassium:* increased levels
Chloride, hemoglobin, magnesium, neutrophils, sodium: decreased levels
Liver function tests: decreased values
Drug-food. *Foods high in potassium, salt substitutes containing potassium:* hyperkalemia
Drug-herbs. *Licorice:* increased risk of hypokalemia

Patient monitoring

- Monitor blood chemistry and liver and kidney function test results, CBC, and electrolyte levels (especially potassium).
- Assess for signs and symptoms of hyperkalemia, especially in patients also taking ACE inhibitors or indomethacin.
- Evaluate patient for orthostatic hypertension.

Patient teaching

Instruct patient to immediately report signs and symptoms of hyperkalemia (tingling, fatigue, muscle weakness or paralysis).
- Tell patient to avoid high-potassium salt substitutes and foods.
- Advise patient to minimize GI upset by taking drug with meals; eating small, frequent servings of healthy food; and drinking plenty of fluids.
- Encourage patient to discuss activity recommendations and pain management with prescriber. Advise him to avoid NSAIDs, which interfere with drug's action.
- Caution patient to avoid driving and other hazardous activities until he knows how the drug affects concentration and alertness.
- Inform patient that he'll undergo regular blood testing during therapy.
- As appropriate, review all other significant and life-threatening adverse reactions and interactions, especially those related to the drugs, tests, foods, and herbs mentioned above.

amino acids

amino acid injection
FreAmine, HepatAmine, Primene✦, Vamin N✦

crystalline amino acid infusions
Aminosyn, FreAmine III, Novamine, Travasol, TrophAmine

crystalline amino acid infusions with dextrose
Aminosyn (various strengths), Travasol (various strengths)

crystalline amino acid infusions with electrolytes
Aminosyn (various strengths), FreAmine (various strengths), ProcalAmine, Travasol (various strengths)

crystalline amino acid infusions with electrolytes in dextrose
Aminosyn (various strengths)

hepatic failure or hepatic encephalopathy formulations
HepatAmine

high metabolic stress formulations
Aminosyn-HBC, BranchAmin 4%, FreAmine-HBC

renal failure formulations
Aminess 5.2%, Aminosyn-RF 5.2%, 5.4% NephrAmine, RenAmin

Pharmacologic class: Protein substrate
Therapeutic class: Caloric drug, nitrogen product
Pregnancy risk category C

Action
Provide substrate for protein synthesis (anabolism) or help conserve existing body protein (protein-sparing effect)

Availability
Injection: Many strengths and concentrations are available. Specific formulation to use depends on patient's status, underlying disease or disorder, and duration of therapy.

Indications and dosages
Indications and dosages given below are limited to those used in common nutritional therapies.

➤ Total parenteral nutrition (TPN) supplement for patients with negative nitrogen balance secondary to inability of GI tract to absorb protein, patients unable to receive adequate nutrition through tube feedings, and patients requiring bowel rest
Adults: 1 to 1.7 g/kg/day I.V. (by peripheral vein) with low concentration of dextrose solution as required, or 500 ml amino acids I.V. injection (by central vein), mixed with 500 ml of concentrated dextrose injection, electrolytes, and vitamins, given over 8 hours
Children: Follow manufacturer's directions and use with caution.

➤ Nutritional supplement for patients with high metabolic stress
Adults: With adequate calories, 1.5 g/kg/day I.V. May be mixed with other solutions, as directed, and given by peripheral vein if amino acid solution

contains minimal calories and central route isn't indicated.

➢ Nutritional supplement for patients with renal failure

Adults: 250 to 600 ml of Aminosyn I.V. daily, depending on formulation. If needed, mix formulations with other solutions before infusing.

Children: Initially, start with low dosage, following manufacturer's directions. Increase to maximum daily dosage of 0.5 to 1g/kg I.V. If needed, mix formulations with other solutions before infusing.

➢ Nutritional supplement in patients with hepatic failure or hepatic encephalopathy

Adults: 80 to 120 g of amino acids (12 to 18 g of nitrogen) I.V. daily, mixed with other solutions as required. May be given by peripheral vein if central route isn't indicated.

Contraindications

- Hypersensitivity to amino acids
- Intracranial or intraspinal hemorrhage
- Severe renal or hepatic disease
- Metabolic disorders

Precautions

Use cautiously in:

- heart failure, hypertension, diabetes mellitus, hepatic or renal impairment
- elderly patients
- pregnant patients
- children.

Administration

- Don't give by I.V. push or bolus.
- Don't give hypertonic solutions via peripheral vein.

◀ Begin I.V. infusion slowly. Control infusion rate carefully with infusion pump; monitor infusion rate closely.

- For subclavian administration, infuse into midsuperior vena cava.
- Use strict aseptic technique when mixing and preparing solution. Replace all I.V. equipment every 24 hours.
- Check infusion site often for infection, phlebitis, and tissue damage.
- Change I.V. sets every 24 hours.
- Don't stop therapy abruptly, because rebound hypoglycemia may occur.

Route	Onset	Peak	Duration
I.V.	Immediate	Immediate	Unknown

Adverse reactions

CNS: headache, dizziness, confusion, **loss of consciousness**

CV: hypertension, tachycardia, **heart failure, venous thrombosis, circulatory overload**

GI: nausea, vomiting, abdominal pain

GU: osmotic diuresis, glycosuria

Hepatic: jaundice, **fatty liver, hepatic impairment**

Metabolic: rebound hypoglycemia (with abrupt cessation of long-term infusion), hyperglycemia, fatty acid deficiency, electrolyte imbalances, hyperammonemia, hypophosphatemia, hypocalcemia, dehydration, **metabolic acidosis and alkalosis, uremia, hyperosmolar hyperglycemic nonketotic syndrome**

Musculoskeletal: osteoporosis

Respiratory: pulmonary edema

Skin: rash, generalized flushing, warm sensation, papular eruptions, urticaria, extravasation necrosis, phlebitis or tissue sloughing at injection site

Other: fever, chills, pain, hypersensitivity reaction, **catheter sepsis**

Interactions

Drug-drug. *Tetracycline:* reduced protein-sparing effects of amino acids

Drug-diagnostic tests. *Blood urea nitrogen (BUN):* increased

Patient monitoring

- When initiating therapy, monitor blood glucose level frequently until stabilized. Then monitor daily.
- Monitor serum electrolyte levels. Report unusual electrolyte losses (for in-

stance, from nasogastric tube, vomiting, drainage, or diarrhea).
• Watch for circulatory overload in patients with cardiac insufficiency.
• Monitor BUN.
• Evaluate fractional urine regularly for glycosuria, which may signal glucose intolerance and sepsis onset.
🔊 Assess for sepsis continually; check temperature every 4 hours.
• Evaluate patient's nutritional status regularly.

Patient teaching

🔊 Tell patient that TPN infusion may increase risk of infection. Advise him to immediately report fever, chills, and other signs and symptoms.
• Instruct patient to report unusual pain, redness, swelling, and other changes at infusion site.
• Advise patient to notify prescriber of vomiting or diarrhea.
• Caution patient to avoid driving and other hazardous activities until he knows how drug affects concentration and alertness.
• As appropriate, review all other significant and life-threatening adverse reactions and interactions, especially those related to the drugs mentioned above.

aminocaproic acid

Amicar, EACA

Pharmacologic class: Carboxylic acid derivative

Therapeutic class: Antihemorrhagic, antifibrinolytic

Pregnancy risk category C

Action

Interferes with plasminogen activator substances and blocks action of fibrinolysin (plasmin)

Availability

Injection: 250 mg/ml
Syrup: 250 mg/ml
Tablets: 500 mg

Indications and dosages

➤ Excessive bleeding caused by fibrinolysis
Adults: 5 g P.O. during first hour; then 1 to 1.25 g/hour until drug blood level of 0.13 mg/ml is reached and sustained and bleeding is controlled. Or 4 to 5 g in 250 ml of compatible diluent I.V. over 1 hour, followed by continuous infusion of 1 g/hour in 50 ml of diluent. Continue for 8 hours or until bleeding stops. Maximum daily dosage is 30 g.

Off-label uses

• Dental extractions
• Hemorrhage

Contraindications

• Hypersensitivity to drug
• Upper urinary tract bleeding
• Disseminated intravascular coagulation
• Neonates (injectable form)

Precautions

Use cautiously in:
• heart, hepatic, or renal failure.

Administration

• Dilute I.V. form in sterile water for injection, normal saline solution, dextrose 5% in water, or Ringer's solution for injection. Give at prescribed rate.
• Know that oral and I.V. doses are the same.

Route	Onset	Peak	Duration
P.O.	1 hr	2 hr	Unknown
I.V.	1 hr	Unknown	3 hr

Adverse reactions

CNS: dizziness, malaise, headache, delirium, hallucinations, weakness, **seizures**

CV: hypotension, ischemia, **thrombophlebitis, cardiomyopathy, bradycardia, arrhythmias**
EENT: conjunctival suffusion, tinnitus, nasal congestion
GI: nausea, vomiting, diarrhea, abdominal pain, dyspepsia
GU: intrarenal obstruction, renal failure
Hematologic: bleeding tendency, generalized thrombosis, agranulocytosis, leukopenia, thrombocytopenia
Musculoskeletal: myopathy, **rhabdomyolysis**
Respiratory: dyspnea, **pulmonary embolism**
Skin: rash, pruritus

Interactions

Drug-drug. *Estrogens, hormonal contraceptives:* increased risk of hypercoagulation
Activated prothrombin, prothrombin complex concentrates: increased signs of active intravascular clotting
Drug-diagnostic tests. *Alanine aminotransferase, aldolase, aspartate aminotransferase, blood urea nitrogen, creatinine, creatine kinase, potassium:* increased levels
Drug-herbs. *Alfalfa, anise, arnica, astragalus, bilberry, black currant seed oil, capsaicin, cat's claw, celery, chaparral, clove oil, dandelion, dong quai, evening primrose oil, feverfew, garlic, ginger, ginkgo, papaya extract rhubarb, safflower oil, skullcap:* increased anticoagulant effect
Coenzyme Q10, St. John's wort: reduced anticoagulant effect

Patient monitoring

• Monitor vital signs, fluid intake and output, and ECG.
◀ Assess for signs and symptoms of thrombophlebitis and pulmonary embolism.
◀ Monitor neurologic status, especially for signs of impending seizure.
• Monitor kidney and liver function test results, serum electrolyte levels, and CBC with white cell differential.
• Evaluate for blood dyscrasias, particularly bleeding tendencies.

Patient teaching

• Tell patient that drug may significantly affect many body systems. Assure him that he'll be monitored closely.
◀ Instruct patient to immediately report signs and symptoms of thrombophlebitis, pulmonary embolism, or unusual bleeding.
• Tell patient he'll undergo frequent blood testing during therapy.
• As appropriate, review all other significant and life-threatening adverse reactions and interactions, especially those related to the drugs, tests, and herbs mentioned above.

aminophylline (theophylline, ethylenediamine)

Truphylline

Pharmacologic class: Xanthine
Therapeutic class: Bronchodilator
Pregnancy risk category C

Action

Unclear. Thought to directly relax smooth muscle of bronchial airways and increase pulmonary blood flow by inhibiting phosphodiesterase.

Availability

Injection: 250 mg/10 ml
Oral liquid: 105 mg/5 ml
Suppositories: 250 mg, 500 mg
Tablets: 100 mg, 200 mg

Indications and dosages

➢ Symptomatic relief of bronchospasm in patients with acute symptoms who require rapid theophyllinization

Adults (nonsmokers): 0.7 mg/kg/hour I.V. for first 12 hours. Maintenance dosage is 0.5 mg/kg/hour I.V.

Children ages 9 to 16: 1 mg/kg/hour I.V. for first 12 hours. Maintenance dosage is 0.8 mg/kg/hour I.V.

Children ages 6 months to 9 years: 1.2 mg/kg/hour I.V. for first 12 hours. Maintenance dosage is 1 mg/kg/hour I.V.

➢ Chronic bronchial asthma

Adults and children: Dosage is highly individualized. Common initial dosage is 16 mg/kg/24 hours I.V. or 400 mg/ 24 hours I.V. in divided doses at 6- or 8-hour intervals. If needed, dosage may be increased 25% at 3-day intervals.

Dosage adjustment

- Heart failure
- Hepatic disease
- Elderly patients
- Smokers

Off-label uses

- Dyspnea in patients with chronic obstructive pulmonary disease (COPD)

Contraindications

- Hypersensitivity to xanthine compounds or ethylenediamine
- GI disease
- Seizure disorders

Precautions

Use cautiously in:

- COPD, diabetes mellitus, glaucoma, renal or hepatic disease, heart failure or other cardiac or circulatory impairment, hypertension, hyperthyroidism, peptic ulcer, severe hypoxemia
- elderly patients
- neonates, infants, and young children.

Administration

- For I.V. use, dilute according to label directions and infuse at a rate no faster than 25 mg/minute.
- Don't give in I.V. solutions containing invert sugar, fructose, or fat emulsions.
- Give oral form at meals with 8 oz of water.

Route	Onset	Peak	Duration
P.O. (extended)	Variable	Variable	Variable
P.O. (liquid)	15-60 min	1-7 hr	Variable
I.V.	Immediate	Immediate	6-8 hr
P.R.	Unknown	Unknown	Unknown

Adverse reactions

CNS: irritability, dizziness, nervousness, restlessness, headache, insomnia, stammering speech, abnormal behavior, mutism, unresponsiveness alternating with hyperactivity, **seizures**

CV: palpitations, sinus tachycardia, extrasystoles, **marked hypotension, arrhythmias, circulatory failure**

GI: nausea, vomiting, diarrhea, epigastric pain, hematemesis, gastroesophageal reflux, anorexia

GU: urine retention (in men with enlarged prostate), diuresis, increased excretion of renal tubular cells and red blood cells, proteinuria

Metabolic: hyperglycemia

Musculoskeletal: muscle twitching

Respiratory: tachypnea, **respiratory arrest**

Skin: flushing

Other: fever, hypersensitivity reactions (including exfoliative dermatitis and urticaria)

Interactions

Drug-drug. *Adenosine:* decreased antiarrhythmic effect of adenosine

Barbiturates, nicotine, phenytoin, rifampin: decreased aminophylline blood level

Beta-adrenergic blockers: antagonism of aminophylline effects

Calcium channel blockers, cimetidine, ciprofloxacin, disulfiram, erythromycin,

hormonal contraceptives, influenza vaccine, interferon, methotrexate: elevated aminophylline blood level
Carbamazepine, isoniazid, loop diuretics (such as furosemide): increased or decreased aminophylline blood level
Ephedrine, other sympathomimetics: toxicity, arrhythmias
Lithium: increased lithium excretion
Drug-diagnostic tests. *Aspartate aminotransferase, glucose:* increased levels
Drug-herbs. *Cayenne:* increased risk of aminophylline toxicity
Drug-behaviors. *Smoking:* increased aminophylline elimination

Patient monitoring

Monitor aminophylline blood level. Adjust dosage if patient has signs or symptoms of toxicity (tachycardia, headache, anorexia, nausea, vomiting, diarrhea, restlessness, and irritability).
- Assess for arrhythmias, especially after giving loading dose.
- Check vital signs and fluid intake and output.
- Monitor patient's response to drug, and assess pulmonary function test results.

Patient teaching

- Advise patient to take oral doses at meals with 8 oz of water.
- Caution patient to avoid driving and other hazardous activities until he knows how drug affects concentration and alertness.
- Tell patient to minimize GI upset by eating small, frequent servings of food and drinking plenty of fluids.
- Advise patient to establish effective bedtime routine to minimize insomnia.
- Caution patient not to change aminophylline brands.
- If patient smokes, tell him to notify prescriber if he stops smoking; dosage may need to be adjusted.
- As appropriate, review all other significant and life-threatening adverse reactions and interactions, especially those related to the drugs, tests, herbs, and behaviors mentioned above.

amiodarone hydrochloride

Cordarone, Pacerone

Pharmacologic class: Adrenergic blocker
Therapeutic class: Antiarrhythmic (class III)
Pregnancy risk category D

Action

Prolongs duration and refractory period of action potential. Slows electrical conduction, electrical impulse generation from sinoatrial node, and conduction through accessory pathways. Also dilates blood vessels.

Availability

Injection: 50 mg/ml in 3-ml ampules
Tablets: 200 mg, 400 mg

Indications and dosages

➢ Life-threatening ventricular arrhythmias

Adults: 150 mg in 100 ml of dextrose 5% in water (D_5W) by rapid I.V. infusion over 10 minutes; then dilute 900 mg in 500 ml of D_5W and administer 360 mg by slow I.V. infusion over next 6 hours; then 540-mg I.V. maintenance infusion over next 18 hours. Or 800 to 1,600 mg P.O. daily in one to two doses for 1 to 3 weeks; then 600 to 800 mg P.O. daily in one to two doses for 1 month; then 400-mg P.O. daily as maintenance dosage.

Off-label uses

- Atrioventricular (AV) nodal reentry tachycardia (with parenteral use)

• Conversion of atrial fibrillation to normal sinus rhythm

Contraindications

• Hypersensitivity to drug
• Cardiogenic shock
• Second- or third-degree AV block
• Marked sinus bradycardia
• Breastfeeding
• Neonates

Precautions

Use cautiously in:
• electrolyte imbalances, severe pulmonary or hepatic disease, thyroid disorders
• history of heart failure
• elderly patients
• pregnant patients
• children.

Administration

🔈 Know that I.V. amiodarone is a high-alert drug.
🔈 Give loading dose only in hospital setting with continuous ECG monitoring.
• Administer oral loading dose in two equal doses with meals. Give maintenance dose daily or in two divided doses to minimize GI upset.
• Don't give I.V. unless patient is on continuous ECG monitoring.
• Dilute I.V. drug with dextrose 5% in water and use in-line filter. Drug isn't compatible with normal saline solution.
• Use central venous catheter when giving repeated doses. If possible, use dedicated catheter for drug.

Route	Onset	Peak	Duration
P.O.	Variable	3-7 hr	Wks-mos
I.V.	Hrs	Unknown	Variable

Adverse reactions

CNS: dizziness, fatigue, headache, insomnia, paresthesia, peripheral neuropathy, poor coordination, involuntary movements, tremor, sleep disturbances
CV: hypotension, **heart failure, worsening arrhythmia, AV block, sinoatrial node dysfunction, bradycardia, asystole, cardiac arrest, cardiogenic shock, electromechanical dissociation, ventricular tachycardia**
EENT: corneal microdeposits, corneal or macular degeneration, visual disturbances, dry eyes, eye discomfort, optic neuritis or neuropathy, scotoma, lens opacities, photophobia, visual halos, **papilledema**
GI: nausea, vomiting, constipation, abdominal pain, abnormal salivation, anorexia
GU: decreased libido
Hematologic: coagulation abnormalities, thrombocytopenia
Hepatic: nonspecific hepatic disorders, **hepatic dysfunction**
Metabolic: hypothyroidism, hyperthyroidism
Respiratory: cough, **adult respiratory distress syndrome, pulmonary inflammation or fibrosis, pulmonary edema**
Skin: flushing, photosensitivity, toxic epidermal necrolysis
Other: abnormal taste and smell, edema, fever, **Stevens-Johnson syndrome**

Interactions

Drug-drug. *Anticoagulants:* increased prothrombin time (PT)
Beta-adrenergic blockers: increased risk of bradycardia and hypotension
Calcium channel blockers: increased risk of AV block (with verapamil, diltiazem) or hypotension (with any calcium channel blocker)
Cholestyramine: decreased amiodarone blood level
Cimetidine, ritonavir: increased amiodarone blood level
Class I antiarrhythmics (disopyramide, flecainide, lidocaine, mexiletine, procainamide, quinidine): increased blood levels of these drugs, leading to toxicity

Cyclosporine: elevated cyclosporine and creatinine blood levels
Dextromethorphan: impaired dextromethorphan metabolism (with amiodarone therapy of 2 weeks or longer)
Digoxin: increased digoxin blood level, leading to toxicity
Fentanyl: increased bradycardia, hypotension
Fluoroquinolones: increased risk of life-threatening arrhythmias
Methotrexate: impaired methotrexate metabolism, possibly causing toxicity (with amiodarone use longer than 2 weeks)
Phenytoin: decreased amiodarone blood level or increased phenytoin blood level (with amiodarone use longer than 2 weeks)
Theophylline: increased theophylline blood level (with amiodarone use longer than 1 week)
Drug-diagnostic tests. *Kidney function tests:* abnormal results

Patient monitoring

Monitor patient closely. Drug may cause serious or life-threatening adverse reactions.
Watch for slow onset of life-threatening arrhythmias, especially after giving loading dose.
Monitor ECG continuously during loading dose and when dosage is changed.
- Check patient's blood pressure, pulse, and heart rhythm regularly.
- Assess for signs and symptoms of lung inflammation.
- Monitor baseline and subsequent chest X-rays, as well as pulmonary, liver, and thyroid function test results.
- Closely monitor patient who's receiving other drugs concurrently because amiodarone can interact with many drugs. Check digoxin blood level if patient is receiving digoxin; monitor PT or International Normalized Ratio if patient is receiving anticoagulants.

Patient teaching

Inform patient that drug may cause serious adverse reactions. Instruct him to report these immediately.
- Tell patient to take oral doses with meals. Advise him to divide daily dose into two doses if drug causes GI upset.
- Tell patient that adverse reactions are most common with high doses and may become more frequent after 6 months of therapy.
- Inform patient that he'll undergo regular blood testing, chest X-rays, and pulmonary function tests during therapy.
- As appropriate, review all other significant and life-threatening adverse reactions and interactions, especially those related to the drugs and tests mentioned above.

amitriptyline hydrochloride

Apo-Amitriptyline, Levate✤, Novotriptyn✤

Pharmacologic class: Tricyclic compound
Therapeutic class: Antidepressant
Pregnancy risk category D

Action

Unclear. Inhibits norepinephrine and serotonin reuptake at presynaptic neuron, increasing levels of these neurotransmitters in brain. Also has sedative, anticholinergic, and mild peripheral vasodilating effects.

Availability

Injection: 10 mg/ml
Syrup: 10 mg/5 ml
Tablets: 10 mg, 25 mg, 50 mg, 75 mg, 100 mg, 150 mg

Indications and dosages

➢ Depression

Adults: 75 mg P.O. daily in divided doses; may increase gradually to 150 mg/day. Or start with 50 to 100 mg P.O. at bedtime and increase by 25 to 50 mg as needed, to a total dosage of 150 mg. Hospitalized patients initially may receive 100 mg P.O. daily, with gradual increases as needed to a total dosage of 300 mg P.O. With I.M. use, give 20 to 30 mg q.i.d.

Dosage adjustment

- Elderly patients
- Adolescents
- Outpatients

Off-label uses

- Analgesic adjunct for phantom limb pain or chronic pain

Contraindications

- Hypersensitivity to drug or other tricyclic antidepressants (TCAs)
- MAO inhibitor use within past 14 days
- Children younger than age 12

Precautions

Use cautiously in:

- seizures, cardiovascular disease, renal or hepatic impairment, urinary retention, hyperthyroidism, increased intraocular pressure, closed-angle glaucoma, prostatic hypertrophy, bipolar disorder, schizophrenia, paranoia
- elderly patients
- pregnant or breastfeeding patients.

Administration

- Administer full dose at bedtime to minimize orthostatic hypotension.
- Give injectable form by I.M. route only.
- Don't withdraw drug suddenly. Instead, taper dosage gradually.
- If patient is scheduled for surgery, discuss dosage tapering with prescriber.
- Be aware that drug is often used in conjunction with psychotherapy.

Route	Onset	Peak	Duration
P.O.	2-4 wk	2-6 wk	Unknown
I.M.	2-3 wk	2-6 wk	Unknown

Adverse reactions

CNS: headache, fatigue, agitation, numbness, paresthesia, peripheral neuropathy, weakness, restlessness, panic, anxiety, dizziness, drowsiness, difficulty speaking, excitement, hypomania, psychosis exacerbation, extrapyramidal effects, poor coordination, hallucinations, insomnia, nightmares, **seizures, coma, suicidal behavior or ideation (especially in children and adolescents)**

CV: ECG changes, tachycardia, hypertension, orthostatic hypotension, **arrhythmias, heart block, myocardial infarction**

EENT: blurred vision, dry eyes, mydriasis, abnormal visual accommodation, increased intraocular pressure, tinnitus

GI: nausea, vomiting, constipation, dry mouth, epigastric pain, anorexia, **paralytic ileus**

GU: urinary retention, delayed voiding, urinary tract dilation, gynecomastia

Hematologic: agranulocytosis, thrombocytopenia, thrombocytopenic purpura, leukopenia

Metabolic: changes in blood glucose level

Skin: photosensitivity rash, urticaria, flushing, diaphoresis

Other: increased appetite, weight gain, high fever, edema, hypersensitivity reaction

Interactions

Drug-drug. *Activated charcoal:* decreased amitriptyline absorption

Adrenergics, anticholinergics, anticholinergic-like drugs: increased anticholinergic effects
Amiodarone, cimetidine, quinidine, ritonavir: increased amitriptyline effects
Barbiturates: decreased amitriptyline blood level, increased CNS and respiratory effects
Clonidine: hypertensive crisis
CNS depressants (including antihistamines, opioids, sedative-hypnotics): increased CNS depression
Drugs metabolized by CYP-4502D6 (such as other antidepressants, phenothiazines, carbamazepine, class 1C antiarrhythmics): decreased amitriptyline clearance, possibly causing toxicity
Guanethidine: antagonism of antihypertensive action
Levodopa: delayed or decreased levodopa absorption, hypertension
MAO inhibitors: hypotension, tachycardia, potentially fatal reactions
Rifabutin, rifampin, rifapentine: decreased amitriptyline blood level and effects
Selective serotonin reuptake inhibitors: increased risk of toxicity
Sympathomimetics: increased pressor effect of direct-acting sympathomimetics (epinephrine, norepinephrine), possibly causing arrhythmias; decreased pressor effect of indirect-acting sympathomimetics (ephedrine, metaraminol)
Drug-diagnostic tests. *Eosinophils, liver function tests:* increased values
Glucose, granulocytes, platelets, white blood cells: increased or decreased levels
Drug-herbs. *Angel's trumpet, jimsonweed, scopolia:* increased anticholinergic effects
Chamomile, hops, kava, skullcap, valerian: increased CNS depression
St. John's wort: decreased drug blood level and reduced efficacy
Drug-behaviors. *Alcohol use:* increased CNS sedation
Smoking: increased drug metabolism and altered effects
Sun exposure: increased risk of photosensitivity reaction

Patient monitoring

- Evaluate for signs and symptoms of psychosis. If present, discuss possible dosage change with prescriber.
- Assess for changes in patient's mood or mental status.

[Clinical alert] Monitor for signs and symptoms of depression and assess for suicidal ideation (especially in child or adolescent).

- Check blood pressure for orthostatic hypertension.
- Monitor CBC with white cell differential, glucose levels, and liver function test results.

Patient teaching

[Clinical alert] Instruct patient, parent, or caregiver to contact prescriber if severe mood changes or suicidal thoughts occur (especially if patient is child or adolescent).

- Tell patient that drug may cause temporary blood pressure decrease if he stands up suddenly. Advise him to rise slowly and carefully.
- Caution patient to avoid driving and other hazardous activities until he knows how drug affects concentration and alertness.
- Advise patient to minimize GI upset by eating small, frequent servings of food and drinking plenty of fluids.
- Inform patient that he'll undergo frequent blood testing during therapy.
- As appropriate, review all other significant and life-threatening adverse reactions and interactions, especially those related to the drugs, tests, herbs, and behaviors mentioned above.

amlodipine besylate

Norvasc L

Pharmacologic class: Calcium channel blocker

Therapeutic class: Antihypertensive

Pregnancy risk category C

Action

Inhibits influx of extracellular calcium ions, thereby decreasing myocardial contractility, relaxing coronary and vascular muscles, and decreasing peripheral resistance

Availability

Tablets: 2.5 mg, 5 mg, 10 mg

Indications and dosages

➢ Essential hypertension, chronic stable angina pectoris, and vasospastic angina (Prinzmetal's angina)

Adults: 5 to 10 mg P.O. once daily

Dosage adjustment

- Hepatic impairment
- Elderly patients

Off-label uses

- Pulmonary hypertension
- Raynaud's disease

Contraindications

- Hypersensitivity to drug

Precautions

Use cautiously in:

- aortic stenosis, severe hepatic impairment, heart failure
- elderly patients
- pregnant or breastfeeding patients.
- children.

Administration

- Be aware that this drug may be given alone or with other drugs to relieve hypertension or angina.

Route	Onset	Peak	Duration
P.O.	Unknown	6-9 hr	24 hr

Adverse reactions

CNS: headache, dizziness, drowsiness, light-headedness, fatigue, weakness, lethargy

CV: peripheral edema, angina, bradycardia, hypotension, palpitations

GI: nausea, abdominal discomfort

Musculoskeletal: muscle cramps, muscle pain or inflammation

Respiratory: shortness of breath, dyspnea, wheezing

Skin: rash, pruritus, urticaria, flushing

Interactions

Drug-drug. *Beta-adrenergic blockers:* increased risk of adverse effects

Fentanyl, nitrates, other antihypertensives, quinidine: additive hypotension

Drug-behaviors. *Acute alcohol ingestion:* additive hypotension

Patient monitoring

🔈 Monitor patient for worsening angina.

- Monitor heart rate and rhythm and blood pressure, especially at start of therapy.

🔈 Assess for heart failure; report signs and symptoms (peripheral edema, dyspnea) to prescriber promptly.

🔈 Give sublingual nitroglycerin, as prescribed, if patient has signs or symptoms of acute myocardial infarction (especially when dosage is increased).

Patient teaching

- If patient also uses sublingual nitroglycerin, tell him he can take nitroglycerin as needed for acute angina.
- Caution patient to avoid driving and other hazardous activities until he

knows how drug affects concentration and alertness.
• As appropriate, review all other significant adverse reactions, especially those related to the drugs and behaviors mentioned above.

amoxapine

Asendin

Pharmacologic class: Tricyclic compound
Therapeutic class: Antidepressant
Pregnancy risk category C

Action

Unclear. Inhibits reuptake of norepinephrine or serotonin at presynaptic neuron, thereby increasing levels of these neurotransmitters in brain. Also has sedative, anticholinergic, and mild peripheral vasodilatory properties.

Availability

Tablets: 25 mg, 50 mg, 100 mg, 150 mg

Indications and dosages

➢ Depression accompanied by anxiety or agitation
Adults: Initially, 50 mg P.O. two or three times daily, increased to 100 mg two or three times daily by end of first week. If starting dosage (up to 300 mg/day) is tolerated but ineffective for at least 2 weeks, dosage may be increased. For outpatients, maximum suggested dosage is 400 mg/day; for hospitalized patients, 600 mg/day.

Dosage adjustment

• Elderly patients

Off-label uses

• Analgesic adjunct for phantom limb pain or chronic pain

Contraindications

• Hypersensitivity to drug or other tricyclic antidepressants (TCAs)
• MAO inhibitor use within past 14 days
• Patients younger than age 16

Precautions

Use cautiously in:
• renal or hepatic impairment, prostatic hypertrophy, hyperthyroidism, angle-closure glaucoma, bipolar disorder, schizophrenia
• elderly patients
• pregnant or breastfeeding patients.

Administration

🔊 Don't give drug if patient has taken MAO inhibitors within past 14 days.
• If desired, give daily dose up to 300 mg at bedtime.
• If patient is scheduled for surgery, discuss need for dosage tapering with prescriber.

Route	Onset	Peak	Duration
P.O.	Unknown	2-4 hr	2-4 wk

Adverse reactions

CNS: agitation, restlessness, fatigue, panic, anxiety, dizziness, drowsiness, difficulty articulating words, excitement, hypomania, psychosis exacerbation, extrapyramidal effects, tardive dyskinesia, poor coordination, hallucinations, headache, insomnia, nightmares, numbness, paresthesia, peripheral neuropathy, weakness, **neuroleptic malignant syndrome, seizures, coma, suicidal behavior or ideation** (especially **in children and adolescents**)
CV: ECG changes, hypertension, orthostatic hypotension, **arrhythmias, heart block, myocardial infarction, tachycardia**
EENT: blurred vision, dry eyes, mydriasis, abnormal visual accommodation, increased intraocular pressure, tinnitus

GI: nausea, vomiting, constipation, anorexia, epigastric pain, dry mouth, **paralytic ileus**
GU: urine retention, delayed voiding, urinary tract dilation, gynecomastia
Hematologic: agranulocytosis, thrombocytopenia, thrombocytopenic purpura, leukopenia
Metabolic: changes in blood glucose level
Skin: photosensitivity rash, urticaria, flushing, diaphoresis
Other: increased appetite, weight gain, high fever, edema, hypersensitivity reactions

Interactions

Drug-drug. *Adrenergics, anticholinergics, anticholinergic-like drugs:* increased anticholinergic effects
Amiodarone, cimetidine, quinidine, ritonavir: increased amoxapine effects
Barbiturates: reduced amoxapine blood level, increased CNS and respiratory effects
Clonidine: hypertensive crisis
CNS depressants (including antihistamines, opioids, sedative-hypnotics): increased CNS depression
Drugs metabolized by CYP450 2D6 (such as other antidepressants, carbamazepine, class IC antiarrhythmics, phenothiazines): decreased amoxapine clearance, possible toxicity
Guanethidine: antagonism of antihypertensive action
Levodopa: delayed or decreased levodopa absorption, hypertension
MAO inhibitors: hypotension, tachycardia, extreme excitation, fever, hyperpyrexia, seizures
Rifabutin, rifampin, rifapentine: decreased amoxapine blood level and effects
Selective serotonin reuptake inhibitors: increased toxicity
Sympathomimetics: increased pressor effects of direct-acting sympathomimetics (epinephrine, norepinephrine), possibly causing arrhythmias; decreased pressor effects of indirect-acting sympathomimetics (ephedrine, metaraminol)
Valproic acid: increased valproic acid blood level, greater risk of adverse reactions
Drug-diagnostic tests. *Eosinophils, liver function tests:* increased values
Glucose, granulocytes, platelets, white blood cells: increased or decreased values
Drug-herbs. *Evening primrose:* lower seizure threshold, increased risk of seizures
Drug-behaviors. *Alcohol use:* increased CNS sedation
Smoking: increased metabolism and altered drug effects
Sun exposure: increased risk of photosensitivity reactions

Patient monitoring

🔊 Watch for signs and symptoms of neuroleptic malignant syndrome (high fever, rapid pulse and breathing, profuse sweating).
• Monitor patient for signs and symptoms of psychosis. If these occur, consult prescriber.
• Evaluate patient for development of tardive dyskinesia (involuntary movements of face, arms, legs, and trunk).
• Assess for changes in mood and mental status.
• Check blood pressure for orthostatic hypertension.
🔊 Watch for signs and symptoms of depression, and assess for suicidal ideation.
• Monitor CBC with white cell differential, glucose level, and kidney and liver function test results.

Patient teaching

🔊 Tell patient to contact prescriber immediately if he develops high fever, rapid pulse and breathing, profuse sweating, changes in mental status, or involuntary movements.

a

Instruct patient to promptly report severe mood changes or suicidal thoughts.
- Caution patient to avoid driving and other hazardous activities until he knows how drug affects concentration and alertness.
- Tell patient that stopping drug suddenly can cause withdrawal symptoms.
- Advise patient to rise slowly and carefully to avoid dizziness.
- Caution patient that drug may cause serious interactions with many common drugs. Instruct him to tell all prescribers that he's taking this drug.
- Advise patient to minimize GI upset by eating small, frequent servings of food and drinking plenty of fluids.
- Tell patient he'll undergo frequent blood testing during therapy.
- As appropriate, review all other significant and life-threatening adverse reactions and interactions, especially those related to the drugs, tests, herbs, and behaviors mentioned above.

amoxicillin

amoxicillin trihydrate

Amoxil, Amoxil Pediatric Drops, Apo-Amoxil*, Dispermox, Novamoxin*, Nu-Amoxil*, Trimox, Trimox Pediatric Drops

Pharmacologic class: Aminopenicillin
Therapeutic class: Anti-infective
Pregnancy risk category B

Action

Inhibits cell-wall synthesis during bacterial multiplication, leading to cell death. Shows enhanced activity toward gram-negative bacteria compared to natural and penicillinase-resistant penicillins.

Availability

Capsules: 250 mg, 500 mg
Powder for oral suspension: 50 mg/ml and 125 mg/5 ml (pediatric), 200 mg/5 ml, 250 mg/5 ml, 400 mg/5 ml
Tablets: 500 mg, 875 mg
Tablets for oral suspension: 200 mg, 400 mg
Tablets (chewable): 125 mg, 200 mg, 250 mg, 400 mg

Indications and dosages

➢ Uncomplicated gonorrhea
Adults and children weighing at least 40 kg (88 lb): 3 g P.O. as a single dose
Children ages 2 and older weighing less than 40 kg (88 lb): 50 mg/kg P.O. given with probenecid 25 mg/kg P.O. as a single dose

➢ Bacterial endocarditis prophylaxis for dental, GI, and GU procedures
Adults: 2 g P.O. 1 hour before procedure
Children: 50 mg/kg P.O. 1 hour before procedure

➢ Lower respiratory tract infections caused by streptococci, pneumococci, non-penicillinase-producing staphylococci, and *Haemophilus influenzae*
Adults and children weighing more than 20 kg (44 lb): 875 mg P.O. q 12 hours or 500 mg P.O. q 8 hours
Children weighing less than 20 kg (44 lb): 45 mg/kg/day P.O. in divided doses q 12 hours or 40 mg/kg/day P.O. in divided doses q 8 hours

➢ Ear, nose, and throat infections caused by streptococci, pneumococci, non-penicillinase-producing staphylococci, and *H. influenzae;* GU infections caused by *Escherichia coli, Proteus mirabilis,* and *Streptococcus faecalis;* skin and soft-tissue infections caused by streptococci, susceptible staphylococci, and *E. coli*
Adults and children weighing more than 20 kg (44 lb): 500 mg P.O. q 12 hours or 250 mg P.O. q 8 hours

Children weighing less than 20 kg (44 lb): 45 mg/kg/day P.O. in divided doses q 12 hours or 20 to 40 mg/kg P.O. in divided doses q 8 hours

➢ Postexposure anthrax prophylaxis

Adults: 500 mg P.O. t.i.d. for 60 days

Children: 80 mg/kg/day P.O. t.i.d. for 60 days

Dosage adjustment

- Renal impairment
- Hemodialysis
- Infants ages 3 months and younger

Off-label uses

- *Chlamydia trachomatis* infection in pregnant patients

Contraindications

- Hypersensitivity to drug or any penicillin

Precautions

Use cautiously in:

- severe renal insufficiency, infectious mononucleosis, hepatic dysfunction
- pregnant patients.

Administration

Ask about history of penicillin allergy before giving.

- Give with or without food.
- Store liquid form in refrigerator when possible.
- Know that maximum dosage for infants ages 3 months and younger is 30 mg/kg/day divided q 12 hours.

Route	Onset	Peak	Duration
P.O.	30 min	1-2 hr	8-12 hr

Adverse reactions

CNS: lethargy, hallucinations, anxiety, confusion, agitation, depression, dizziness, fatigue, hyperactivity, insomnia, behavioral changes, **seizures** (with high doses)

GI: nausea, vomiting, diarrhea, bloody diarrhea, abdominal pain, gastritis, stomatitis, glossitis, black "hairy" tongue, furry tongue, enterocolitis, **pseudomembranous colitis**

GU: vaginitis, nephropathy, **interstitial nephritis**

Hematologic: eosinophilia, anemia, **thrombocytopenia, thrombocytopenic purpura, leukopenia, hemolytic anemia, agranulocytosis, bone marrow depression**

Hepatic: cholestatic jaundice, hepatic cholestasis, **cholestatic hepatitis, nonspecific hepatitis**

Respiratory: wheezing

Skin: rash

Other: superinfections (oral and rectal candidiasis), fever, **anaphylaxis**

Interactions

Drug-drug. *Allopurinol:* increased risk of rash

Chloramphenicol, macrolides, sulfonamides, tetracycline: decreased amoxicillin efficacy

Hormonal contraceptives: decreased contraceptive efficacy

Probenecid: decreased renal excretion

Drug-diagnostic tests. *Alanine aminotransferase, alkaline phosphatase, eosinophils, lactate dehydrogenase:* increased levels

Granulocytes, hemoglobin, platelets, white blood cells: decreased values

Direct Coombs' test, urine glucose, urine protein: false-positive results

Drug-food. *Any food:* delayed or reduced drug absorption

Drug-herbs. *Khat:* decreased antimicrobial efficacy

Patient monitoring

- Monitor for signs and symptoms of hypersensitivity reaction.

Evaluate for seizures when giving high doses.

- Monitor patient's temperature and watch for other signs and symptoms of superinfection (especially oral or rectal candidiasis).

a

Patient teaching

Instruct patient to immediately report signs and symptoms of hypersensitivity reactions, such as rash, fever, or chills.

- Tell patient he may take drug with or without food.
- Tell patient not to chew or swallow tablets for suspension, because they're not meant to be dissolved in mouth.
- Advise patient to minimize GI upset by eating small, frequent servings of food and drinking plenty of fluids.
- Tell patient taking hormonal contraceptives that drug may reduce contraceptive efficacy. Suggest she use alternative birth control method.
- Inform patient that drug lowers resistance to other types of infections. Instruct him to report new signs and symptoms of infection, especially in mouth or rectum.
- Tell parents they may give liquid form of drug directly to child or may mix it with foods or beverages.
- As appropriate, review all other significant and life-threatening adverse reactions and interactions, especially those related to the drugs, tests, foods, and herbs mentioned above.

amoxicillin and clavulanate potassium

Augmentin, Augmentin ES-600, Augmentin XR, Clavulin♣

Pharmacologic class: Aminopenicillin
Therapeutic class: Anti-infective
Pregnancy risk category B

Action

Amoxicillin inhibits transpeptidase, preventing cross-linking of bacterial cell wall and leading to cell death. Addition of clavulanate (a beta-lactam) increases drug's resistance to beta-lactamase (an enzyme produced by bacteria that may inactivate amoxicillin).

Availability

Oral suspension: 125 mg amoxicillin with 31.25 mg clavulanic acid/5 ml, 200 mg amoxicillin with 28.5 mg clavulanic acid/5 ml, 250 mg amoxicillin with 62.5 mg clavulanic acid/5 ml, 400 mg amoxicillin with 57 mg clavulanic acid/5 ml, 600 mg amoxicillin with 42.9 mg clavulanic acid/5 ml
Tablets (chewable): 125 mg amoxicillin with 31.25 mg clavulanate, 200 mg amoxicillin with 28.5 mg clavulanate, 250 mg amoxicillin with 62.5 mg clavulanate, 400 mg amoxicillin with 57 mg clavulanate
Tablets (extended-release): 1,000 mg amoxicillin with 62.5 mg clavulanate
Tablets (film-coated): 250 mg amoxicillin with 125 mg clavulanate, 500 mg amoxicillin with 125 mg clavulanate, 875 mg amoxicillin with 125 mg clavulanate

Indications and dosages

➤ Lower respiratory tract infections, otitis media, sinusitis, skin and skin-structure infections, and urinary tract infections (UTIs) caused by susceptible strains of gram-negative and gram-positive organisms

Adults and children weighing more than 40 kg (88 lb): 500 mg q 12 hours or 250 mg P.O. q 8 hours (based on amoxicillin component). For severe infections, 875 mg P.O. q 12 hours or 500 mg P.O. q 8 hours.

➤ Serious infections and community-acquired pneumonia

Adults and children weighing more than 40 kg (88 lb): 875 mg P.O. q 12 hours or 500 mg P.O. q 8 hours

Infants and children ages 3 months and older weighing less than 40 kg (88 lb): 20 to 45 mg/kg/day P.O. in divided doses q 12 hour or 20 to 40 mg/kg/day in divided doses q 8 hours,

based on severity of infection and amoxicillin component (125 mg/5 ml or 250 mg/5 ml suspension)
Infants younger than 3 months: 30 mg/kg/day P.O. (based on amoxicillin component) divided q 12 hours. (125 mg/5 ml oral suspension is recommended.)
➢ Recurrent or persistent acute otitis media caused by *Streptococcus pneumoniae, Haemophilus influenzae,* or *Moraxella catarrhalis* in children ages 2 and younger and in children who have received antibiotic therapy within last 3 months
Children ages 3 months to 12 years: 90 mg/kg/day of Augmentin ES-600 P.O. q 12 hours for 10 days

Dosage adjustment
- Renal impairment
- Hemodialysis
- Infants ages 3 months and younger

Contraindications
- Hypersensitivity to drug or any penicillin
- Phenylketonuria (some products)
- History of cholestatic jaundice or hepatic dysfunction associated with this drug

Precautions
Use cautiously in:
- severe renal insufficiency, infectious mononucleosis
- pregnant patients.

Administration
Clinical alert: Ask about history of penicillin allergy before giving.
- Give with or without food.
- Know that maximum dosage for infants ages 3 months and younger is 30 mg/kg/day divided q 12 hours.
- Be aware that 12-hour dosing is recommended to reduce diarrhea.
- Refrigerate oral suspension when possible, or store at room temperature for up to 7 days.

Route	Onset	Peak	Duration
P.O.	Unknown	1-2.5 hr	6-8 hr
P.O. (extended)	Unknown	1-4 hr	Unknown

Adverse reactions
CNS: lethargy, hallucinations, anxiety, confusion, agitation, depression, dizziness, fatigue, hyperactivity, insomnia, behavioral changes, **seizures** (with high doses)
GI: nausea, vomiting, diarrhea, abdominal pain, stomatitis, glossitis, gastritis, black "hairy" tongue, furry tongue, enterocolitis, **pseudomembranous colitis**
GU: vaginitis, nephropathy, **interstitial nephritis**
Hematologic: anemia, **thrombocytopenia, thrombocytopenic purpura, leukopenia, hemolytic anemia, agranulocytosis, bone narrow depression, eosinophilia**
Hepatic: cholestatic hepatitis
Respiratory: wheezing
Skin: rash
Other: superinfections (oral and rectal candidiasis), fever, **anaphylaxis**

Interactions
Drug-drug. *Allopurinol:* increased risk of rash
Chloramphenicol, macrolides, sulfonamides, tetracycline: decreased amoxicillin efficacy
Hormonal contraceptives: decreased contraceptive efficacy
Probenecid: decreased renal excretion and increased blood level of amoxicillin
Drug-food. *Any food:* delayed or reduced drug absorption
Drug-herbs. *Khat:* decreased antimicrobial effect

Patient monitoring

- Monitor patient carefully for signs and symptoms of hypersensitivity reaction.

🔊 Monitor for seizures when giving high doses.

- Check patient's temperature and watch for other signs and symptoms of superinfection, especially oral or rectal candidiasis.

Patient teaching

🔊 Instruct patient to immediately report signs or symptoms of hypersensitivity reaction, such as rash, fever, or chills.

- Tell patient he may take drug with or without food.
- Inform patient that drug lowers resistance to some types of infections. Instruct him to report new signs or symptoms of infection (especially of mouth or rectum).
- Advise patient to minimize GI upset by eating small, frequent servings of food and drinking plenty of fluids.
- Tell patient taking hormonal contraceptives that drug may reduce contraceptive efficacy. Suggest she use alternative birth control method.
- Inform parents that they may give liquid form of drug directly to child or may mix it with foods or beverages.
- As appropriate, review all other significant and life-threatening adverse reactions and interactions, especially those related to the drugs, foods, and herbs mentioned above.

amphotericin B cholesteryl sulfate

Amphotec

amphotericin B desoxycholate

Amphocin, Fungizone Intravenous

amphotericin B lipid complex

Abelcet

amphotericin B liposome

AmBisome

Pharmacologic class: Systemic polyene antifungal

Therapeutic class: Antifungal

Pregnancy risk category B

Action

Binds to sterols in fungal cell membrane, increasing permeability. This allows potassium to exit the cell, causing fungal impairment or death.

Availability

Amphotericin B cholesteryl sulfate—
Injection: 50 mg, 100 mg
Amphotericin B desoxycholate—
Injection: 50-mg vial
Oral suspension: 100 mg/ml in 24-ml bottles
Amphotericin B lipid complex—
Suspension for injection: 100 mg/20-ml vials
Amphotericin B liposome—
Injection: 50 mg

Indications and dosages

➤ Invasive aspergillosis

Adults: *Amphotericin B desoxycholate*—For patients with good cardio renal function who tolerate test dose, give 0.25 to 0.3 mg/kg daily by slow I.V.

infusion (0.1 mg/ml over 2 to 6 hours). Gradually increase to 0.5 to 0.6 mg/kg daily. Patients with neutropenia or rapidly progressing, potentially fatal infections may require higher dosages (1 to 1.5 mg/kg daily).
Adults and children ages 1 month and older: *Amphotericin B liposome*—3 to 5 mg/kg I.V. daily
➢ Invasive aspergillosis in patients with renal impairment or unacceptable toxicity who can't tolerate or don't respond to amphotericin B desoxycholate in effective doses
Adults and children: *Amphotericin B cholesteryl sulfate*—3 to 4 mg/kg daily I.V. Dilute in dextrose 5% in water (D_5W) and give by continuous infusion at 1 mg/kg/hour. *Amphotericin B lipid complex*—5 mg/kg daily I.V. prepared as 1-mg/ml infusion and delivered at a rate of 2.5 mg/kg/hour.
➢ Systemic histoplasmosis
Adults: *Amphotericin B desoxycholate*—If patient tolerates test dose, gradually increase from initial recommended dosage of 0.25 to 0.3 mg/kg daily by slow I.V. infusion (0.1 mg/ml over 2 to 6 hours) to usual dosage of 0.5 to 0.6 mg/kg daily I.V. for 4 to 8 weeks; higher dosages (0.7 to 1 mg) may be necessary for rapidly progressing, potentially fatal infections.
➢ Systemic coccidioidomycosis and blastomycosis
Adults: *Amphotericin B desoxycholate*—If patient tolerates test dose, gradually increase from initial recommended dosage of 0.25 to 0.3 mg/kg daily by slow I.V. infusion (0.1 mg/ml over 2 to 6 hours) to usual dosage of 0.5 to 1 mg/kg daily I.V. for 4 to 12 weeks.
➢ Systemic cryptococcosis
Adults: *Amphotericin B desoxycholate*—If patient tolerates test dose, gradually increase from initial recommended dosage of 0.25 to 0.3 mg/kg daily by slow I.V. infusion (0.1 mg/ml over 2 to 6 hours) to usual dosage of 0.3 to 1 mg/kg daily I.V. (with or without flucytosine) for 2 weeks to several months. For patients with human immunodeficiency virus (HIV) infection, usual dosage is 0.7 mg/kg daily I.V. for 4 weeks, followed by 0.7 mg/kg I.V. given on alternate days for 4 additional weeks. If patient can't tolerate or doesn't respond to amphotericin B desoxycholate, give amphotericin B cholesteryl sulfate at a dosage of 3 to 6 mg/kg daily I.V.
Adults and children ages 1 month and older: *Amphotericin B liposome*—3 to 5 mg/kg daily I.V.
➢ Cryptococcal meningitis in HIV-infected patients
Adults: *Amphotericin B desoxycholate*—If patient tolerates test dose, gradually increase from initial recommended dosage of 0.25 to 0.3 mg/kg daily by slow I.V. infusion (0.1 mg/ml over 2 to 6 hours) to usual dosage of 0.3 to 1 mg/kg daily I.V. (with or without flucytosine) for 2 weeks to several months. *Amphotericin B lipid complex*—5 mg/kg I.V. infusion daily for 6 weeks, followed by 12 weeks of oral fluconazole therapy. *Amphotericin B liposome*—6 mg/kg I.V. infusion daily.
➢ Disseminated candidiasis
Adults: *Amphotericin B desoxycholate*—If patient tolerates test dose, gradually increase from initial recommended dosage of 0.25 to 0.3 mg/kg daily by slow I.V. infusion (0.1 mg/ml over 2 to 6 hours) to usual dosage of 0.4 to 0.6 mg/kg daily by slow I.V. infusion for 7 to 14 days (low-risk patients) or for 6 weeks (high-risk patients). For hepatosplenic candidiasis, 1 mg/kg daily I.V. given with oral flucytosine; for severe or refractory esophageal candidiasis in HIV-infected patients, 0.3 mg/kg daily I.V. for at least 5 to 7 days; for candiduria, 0.3 mg/kg daily I.V. for 3 to 5 days.
Adults and children ages 1 month and older: *Amphotericin B liposome*—3 to 5 mg/kg/day I.V. for 5 to 7 days

➢ Systemic zygomycosis, including mucormycosis
Adults: *Amphotericin B desoxycholate*—If patient tolerates test dose, gradually increase from initial recommended dosage of 0.25 to 0.3 mg/kg daily by slow I.V. infusion (0.1 mg/ml over 2 to 6 hours) to usual dosage of 1 to 1.5 mg/kg daily I.V. for 2 to 3 months. For rhinocerebral phycomycosis form, total dosage is 3 g I.V.
➢ Systemic disseminated sporotrichosis
Adults: *Amphotericin B desoxycholate*—If patient tolerates test dose, gradually increase from initial recommended dosage of 0.25 to 0.3 mg/kg daily by slow I.V. infusion (0.1 mg/ml over 2 to 6 hours) to usual dosage of 0.4 to 0.5 mg/kg daily I.V. for 2 to 3 months.
➢ Cutaneous leishmaniasis
Adults and children: *Amphotericin B desoxycholate*—If patient tolerates test dose, gradually increase from initial recommended dosage of 0.25 to 0.5 mg/kg/day given by slow I.V. infusion (0.1 mg/ml over 2 to 6 hours) until 0.5 to 1 mg/kg/day is reached; then give every other day. Usual duration is 3 to 12 weeks.
➢ Visceral leishmaniasis in immunocompetent patients
Adults and children ages 1 month and older: *Amphotericin B liposome*—3 mg/kg given I.V. over 2 hours on days 1 through 5, 14, and 21. Repeat course if initial treatment fails to clear parasites.
➢ Visceral leishmaniasis in immunocompromised patients
Adults and children ages 1 month and older: *Amphotericin B liposome*—4 mg/kg given I.V. over 2 hours on days 1 through 5, 10, 17, 24, 31, and 38
➢ Empiric therapy for presumed fungal infection in febrile, neutropenic patients
Adults: *Amphotericin B desoxycholate*—If patient tolerates test dose, gradually increase from initial recommended dosage of 0.25 to 0.3 mg/kg daily by slow I.V. infusion (0.1 mg/ml over 2 to 6 hours) to usual dosage of 0.25 to 1 mg/kg daily I.V. *Amphotericin B liposome*—3 mg/kg daily given I.V. over 120 minutes for 2 weeks

Off-label uses

- Chemoprophylaxis in immunocompromised patients
- Coccidioidal arthritis
- Prophylaxis of fungal infections in bone-marrow transplant recipients, patients with primary amoebic meningoencephalitis caused by *Naegleria fowleri*, and patients with ocular aspergillosis

Contraindications

- Hypersensitivity to drug and its components
- Severe respiratory distress

Precautions

Use cautiously in:
- renal impairment, electrolyte abnormalities
- pregnant or breastfeeding patients
- children.

Administration

- Know that amphotericin B should be given only by health care professionals thoroughly familiar with drug, its administration, and adverse reactions.

🔊 Before giving first dose of conventional amphotericin B (desoxycholate form), test dose may be ordered (due to widely varying tolerance and clinical status) as follows: 1 mg in 20 ml of D_5W over 20 to 30 minutes; monitor vital signs every 30 minutes for next 2 hours.

- Know that if desoxycholate form is discontinued for 1 week or longer, drug should be restarted at 0.25 mg/kg daily, with dosage then increased gradually.

• Pretreat with antihistamines, antipyretics, or corticosteroids, as prescribed.
• Give through separate I.V. line, using infusion pump and in-line filter with pores larger than 1 micron.
• Choose distal vein for I.V. site. Alternate sites regularly.
• Mix with 10 ml of sterile water to reconstitute. Don't mix with sodium chloride, other electrolytes, or bacteriostatic products.
• Flush I.V. line with 5% dextrose injection before and after infusion.
• Keep dry form of drug away from light. Once mixed with fluid, solution can be kept in light for up to 8 hours.
Know that total daily dosage of amphotericin B desoxycholate form should never exceed 1.5 mg/kg.

Route	Onset	Peak	Duration
P.O.	Unknown	Unknown	Unknown
I.V.	Rapid	End of infusion	24 hr

Adverse reactions

CNS: anxiety, confusion, headache, insomnia, weakness, depression, dizziness, drowsiness, hallucinations, speech difficulty, ataxia, vertigo, stupor, psychosis, **seizures**
CV: hypotension, hypertension, tachycardia, phlebitis, chest pain, orthostatic hypotension, vasodilation, **asystole, atrial fibrillation, bradycardia, cardiac arrest, shock, supraventricular tachycardia**
EENT: double or blurred vision, amblyopia, eye hemorrhage, hearing loss, tinnitus, epistaxis, rhinitis, sinusitis, pharyngitis
GI: nausea, vomiting, diarrhea, melena, abdominal pain, abdominal distention, dry mouth, oral inflammation, oral candidiasis, anorexia, **GI hemorrhage**
GU: painful urination, hematuria, albuminuria, glycosuria, excessive urea buildup, urine of low specific gravity, nephrocalcinosis, **renal failure, renal tubular acidosis, oliguria, anuria**
Hematologic: eosinophilia; normochromic, normocytic, or hypochromic anemia; **leukocytosis; thrombocytopenia; leukopenia; agranulocytosis; coagulation disorders**
Hepatic: jaundice, **acute hepatic failure, hepatitis**
Metabolic: hypomagnesemia, hypokalemia, hypocalcemia, hypernatremia, hyperglycemia, dehydration, hypoproteinemia, hypervolemia, hyperlipidemia, **acidosis**
Musculoskeletal: muscle, joint, neck, or back pain
Respiratory: increased cough, hypoxia, lung disorders, hyperventilation, wheezing, dyspnea, hemoptysis, tachypnea, **asthma, bronchospasm, respiratory failure, pulmonary edema, pleural effusion**
Skin: discoloration, bruising, flushing, pruritus, urticaria, acne, rash, sweating, nodules, skin ulcers, alopecia, maculopapular rash
Other: gingivitis, fever, infection, peripheral or facial edema, weight changes, pain or reaction at injection site, tissue damage with extravasation, hypersensitivity reactions including **anaphylaxis**

Interactions

Drug-drug. *Antineoplastics (such as mechlorethamine):* renal toxicity, bronchospasm, hypotension
Cardiac glycosides: increased risk of digitalis toxicity (in potassium-depleted patients)
Corticosteroids: increased potassium depletion
Cyclosporine, tacrolimus: increased creatinine levels
Flucytosine: increased flucytosine toxicity
Imidazoles (clotrimazole, fluconazole, ketoconazole, miconazole): antagonism of amphotericin B effects

a

Leukocyte transfusion: pulmonary reactions
Nephrotoxic drugs (such as antibiotics, pentamidine): increased risk of renal toxicity
Thiazides: increased electrolyte depletion
Skeletal muscle relaxants: increased skeletal muscle relaxation
Zidovudine: increased myelotoxicity and nephrotoxicity
Drug-diagnostic tests. *Alanine aminotransferase, alkaline phosphatase, aspartate aminotransferase, bilirubin, blood urea nitrogen, creatinine, gamma-glutamyltransferase, lactate dehydrogenase, nitrogenous compounds (urea), uric acid:* increased levels
Calcium, hemoglobin, magnesium, platelets, potassium, protein: decreased levels
Eosinophils, glucose, white blood cells: increased or decreased levels
Liver function tests: abnormal results
Prothrombin time: prolonged
Drug-herbs. *Gossypol:* increased risk of renal toxicity

Patient monitoring

Clinical alert: Monitor for infusion-related reactions (fever, chills, hypotension, GI symptoms, breathing difficulties, and headache). Stop infusion and notify prescriber immediately if reaction occurs.

Clinical alert: After giving test dose, monitor vital signs and temperature every 30 minutes for 2 to 4 hours, as ordered.

- Assess fluid intake and output.
- Monitor kidney and liver function test results and serum electrolyte levels.
- Assess for signs and symptoms of ototoxicity (hearing loss, tinnitus, ataxia, and vertigo).

Patient teaching

Clinical alert: Advise patient to contact prescriber immediately if he has fever, chills, headache, vomiting, diarrhea, cough, or breathing problems.

- Instruct patient to report hearing loss, dizziness, or unsteady gait.
- Caution patient to avoid driving and other hazardous activities until he knows how drug affects concentration, alertness, and vision.
- Instruct patient to drink plenty of fluids.
- Tell patient to monitor urine output and report significant changes.
- Advise patient to minimize GI upset by eating small, frequent servings of food and drinking plenty of fluids.
- As appropriate, review all other significant and life-threatening adverse reactions and interactions, especially those related to the drugs, tests, and herbs mentioned above.

ampicillin sodium

Ampicin✤, Apo-Ampi✤, Marcillin, Novo-Ampicillin✤, Nu-Ampi✤, Penbritin✤, Polycillin, Principen

Pharmacologic class: Aminopenicillin
Therapeutic class: Anti-infective
Pregnancy risk category B

Action

Destroys bacteria by inhibiting bacterial cell-wall synthesis during microbial multiplication

Availability

Capsules: 250 mg, 500 mg
Oral suspension: 125 mg/5 ml, 250 mg/5 ml
Powder for injection: 125 mg, 250 mg, 500 mg, 1 g, 2 g, 10 g

Indications and dosages

➢ Respiratory tract, skin, and soft-tissue infections caused by *Haemophilus influenzae*, staphylococci, and streptococci

Adults and children weighing 40 kg (88 lb) or more: 250 to 500 mg I.V. or I.M. q 6 hours
Adults and children weighing less than 40 kg (88 lb): 25 to 50 mg/kg/day I.M. or I.V. in divided doses q 6 to 8 hours
Adults and children weighing more than 20 kg (44 lb): 250 mg P.O. q 6 hours
Children weighing 20 kg (44 lb) or less: 50 mg/kg/day P.O. in divided doses q 6 to 8 hours
➢ Bacterial meningitis caused by *Neisseria meningitidis, Escherichia coli,* group B streptococci, or *Listeria monocytogenes*; septicemia caused by *Streptococcus* species, penicillin G–susceptible staphylococci, enterococci, *E. coli, Proteus mirabilis,* or *Salmonella* species
Adults: 150 to 200 mg/kg/day by continuous I.V. infusion or I.M. injection in equally divided doses q 3 to 4 hours, to a maximum dosage of 14 g
Children: 100 to 200 mg/kg/day I.V. in divided doses q 3 to 4 hours
➢ GI or urinary tract infections, including *Neisseria gonorrhoeae* infection in women
Adults and children weighing more than 40 kg (88 lb): 500 mg I.M. or I.V. q 6 hours
Adults and children weighing 40 kg (88 lb) or less: 50 to 100 mg/kg/day I.M. or I.V. in equally divided doses q 6 to 8 hours
➢ Endocarditis prophylaxis for dental, oral, or upper respiratory tract procedures
Adults: 2 g I.M. or I.V. within 30 minutes before procedure
Children: 50 mg/kg I.V. or I.M. within 30 minutes before procedure
➢ Prevention of bacterial endocarditis before GI or GU surgery or instrumentation
High-risk adults: 2 g I.M. or I.V. with gentamicin 1.5 mg/kg I.M. or I.V. within 30 minutes before procedure. Six hours later, give ampicillin 1 g I.M. or I.V., or amoxicillin 1 g P.O.
High-risk children: 50 mg/kg I.M. or I.V. with 1.5 mg/kg of gentamicin I.M. or I.V. within 30 minutes before procedure; 6 hours later, give ampicillin 25 mg/kg I.M. or I.V. or ampicillin 25 mg/kg P.O.
Moderate-risk adults: 2 g I.M. or I.V. within 30 minutes before procedure
Moderate-risk children: 50 mg/kg I.M. or I.V. within 30 minutes before procedure
➢ Prophylaxis for neonatal group B streptococcal disease
Adult women: During labor, loading dose of 2 g I.V.; then 1 g I.V. q 4 hours until delivery
➢ *N. gonorrhoeae* infections
Adults: Single dose of 3.5 g P.O. given with 1 g probenecid
Children weighing 40 kg (88 lb) or more: 500 mg I.M. or I.V. q 6 hours
Children weighing less than 40 kg (88 lb): 50 mg/kg/day in divided doses q 6 to 8 hours
➢ Urethritis caused by *N. gonorrhoeae* (in males)
Adults and children weighing 40 kg (88 lb) or more: 500 mg I.V. or I.M., repeated 8 to 12 hours later
➢ Prophylaxis against sexually transmitted diseases in adult rape victims
Adults: 3.5 g P.O. with 1 g probenecid as a single dose

Dosage adjustment

• Renal impairment

Contraindications

• Hypersensitivity to penicillins, cephalosporins, imipenem, or other beta-lactamase inhibitors

Precautions

Use cautiously in:
• severe renal insufficiency, infectious mononucleosis
• pregnant or breastfeeding patients.

a

Administration
- Ask patient about history of penicillin allergy before giving.
- For I.V. use, mix powder with bacteriostatic water for injection in amount listed on label.
- For direct I.V. injection, give over 10 to 15 minutes. Don't exceed 100 mg/minute.
- For intermittent I.V. infusion, mix with 50 to 100 ml of normal saline solution and give over 15 to 30 minutes.
- Change I.V. site every 48 hours.
- Give oral doses 1 hour before or 2 hours after meals.

Route	Onset	Peak	Duration
P.O.	30 min	2 hr	6-8 hr
I.V.	Immediate	5 min	6-8 hr
I.M.	15 min	1 hr	6-8 hr

Adverse reactions
CNS: lethargy, hallucinations, anxiety, confusion, agitation, depression, fatigue, dizziness, **seizures**
CV: vein irritation, **thrombophlebitis, heart failure**
EENT: blurred vision, itchy eyes
GI: nausea, vomiting, diarrhea, abdominal pain, enterocolitis, gastritis, stomatitis, glossitis, black "hairy" tongue, furry tongue, oral or rectal candidiasis, **pseudomembranous colitis**
GU: vaginitis, nephropathy, **interstitial nephritis**
Hematologic: anemia, eosinophilia, **agranulocytosis, hemolytic anemia, leukopenia, thrombocytopenic purpura, thrombocytopenia, neutropenia**
Hepatic: nonspecific hepatitis
Musculoskeletal: arthritis exacerbation
Respiratory: wheezing, dyspnea, hypoxia, **apnea**
Skin: rash, urticaria, fever, diaphoresis
Other: pain at injection site, superinfections, hyperthermia, hypersensitivity reaction, **anaphylaxis, serum sickness**

Interactions
Drug-drug. *Allopurinol:* increased risk of rash
Chloramphenicol: synergistic or antagonistic effects
Hormonal contraceptives: decreased contraceptive effect, increased risk of breakthrough bleeding
Probenecid: decreased renal excretion of ampicillin, increased ampicillin blood level
Tetracyclines: reduced bactericidal effect
Drug-diagnostic tests. *Conjugated estrone, estradiol, estriol-glucuronide, total conjugated estriols:* increased levels in pregnant patients
Granulocytes, hemoglobin, platelets, white blood cells: decreased levels
Coombs' test, urine glucose: false-positive results
Eosinophils: increased count
Drug-food. *Any food:* reduced ampicillin efficacy

Patient monitoring
- Watch for signs and symptoms of hypersensitivity reaction.

Monitor for seizures when giving high doses.
- Frequently measure patient's temperature and check for signs and symptoms of superinfection, especially oral or rectal candidiasis.
- Monitor for bleeding tendency or hemorrhage.

Patient teaching
- Tell patient to take oral dose with 8 oz of water 1 hour before or 2 hours after a meal.

Instruct patient to immediately report signs and symptoms of hypersensitivity reaction, such as rash, fever, or chills.
- Inform patient that drug lowers resistance to certain other infections. Tell him to report new signs or symptoms of infection, especially in mouth or rectum.

• Advise patient to minimize GI upset by eating small, frequent servings of food and drinking plenty of fluids.
Instruct patient to promptly report unusual bleeding or bruising.
• Tell patient to avoid activities that can cause injury. Advise him to use soft toothbrush and electric razor to avoid gum and skin injury.
• Inform patient taking hormonal contraceptives that drug may reduce contraceptive efficacy. Advise her to use alternative birth control method.
• As appropriate, review all other significant and life-threatening adverse reactions and interactions, especially those related to the drugs, tests, and foods mentioned above.

ampicillin sodium and sulbactam sodium

Unasyn

Pharmacologic class: Aminopenicillin/beta-lactamase inhibitor
Therapeutic class: Anti-infective
Pregnancy risk category B

Action

Destroys bacteria by inhibiting bacterial cell-wall synthesis during microbial multiplication. Addition of sulbactam enhances drug's resistance to beta-lactamase, an enzyme that can inactivate ampicillin.

Availability

Injection: Vials; piggyback vials containing 1.5 g (1 g ampicillin sodium and 0.5 g sulbactam sodium), 3 g (2 g ampicillin sodium and 1 g sulbactam sodium), and 15 g (10 g ampicillin sodium and 5 g sulbactam sodium)

Indications and dosages

➤ Intra-abdominal, gynecologic, and skin-structure infections caused by susceptible beta-lactamase-producing strains

Adults and children weighing 40 kg (88 lb) or more: 1.5 to 3 g (1 g ampicillin and 0.5 g sulbactam to 2 g ampicillin and 1 g sulbactam) I.M. or I.V. q 6 hours. Maximum dosage is 4 g sulbactam daily.

Children ages 1 year and older: 75 mg (50 mg ampicillin and 25 mg sulbactam)/kg I.V. q 6 hours

Dosage adjustment

• Renal impairment

Contraindications

• Hypersensitivity to penicillins, cephalosporins, imipenem, or other beta-lactamase inhibitors

Precautions

Use cautiously in:
• severe renal insufficiency, infectious mononucleosis
• pregnant or breastfeeding patients.

Administration

• Ask patient about history of penicillin allergy before giving.
• Let vial stand several minutes until foam has evaporated before administering drug.
• Don't mix I.V. form with other I.V. drugs.
• Give direct I.V. dose over 10 to 15 minutes.
• Give intermittent infusion in 50 to 100 ml of compatible solution over 15 to 30 minutes.
• Change I.V. site every 48 hours.
• Don't give I.M. to children.

Route	Onset	Peak	Duration
I.V.	Immediate	End of infusion	6-8 hr
I.M.	Rapid	1 hr	6-8 hr

Adverse reactions

CNS: lethargy, hallucinations, anxiety, confusion, agitation, depression, fatigue, dizziness, **seizures**
CV: vein irritation, **thrombophlebitis, heart failure**
EENT: blurred vision, itchy eyes
GI: nausea, vomiting, diarrhea, abdominal pain, enterocolitis, gastritis, stomatitis, glossitis, black "hairy" tongue, furry tongue, oral and rectal candidiasis, **pseudomembranous colitis**
GU: hematuria, hyaline casts in urine, vaginitis, nephropathy, **interstitial nephritis**
Hematologic: anemia, eosinophilia, **agranulocytosis, hemolytic anemia, leukopenia, thrombocytopenic purpura, thrombocytopenia, neutropenia**
Hepatic: nonspecific hepatitis
Musculoskeletal: arthritis exacerbation
Respiratory: wheezing, dyspnea, hypoxia, **apnea**
Skin: rash, urticaria, diaphoresis
Other: pain at injection site, fever, hyperthermia, superinfections, hypersensitivity reactions, **anaphylaxis, serum sickness**

Interactions

Drug-drug. *Allopurinol:* increased risk of rash
Chloramphenicol: synergistic or antagonistic effects
Hormonal contraceptives: decreased contraceptive efficacy, increased risk of breakthrough bleeding
Probenecid: decreased renal excretion and increased blood level of ampicillin
Tetracyclines: reduced bactericidal effect
Drug-diagnostic tests. *Alanine aminotransferase, alkaline phosphatase, aspartate aminotransferase, bilirubin, blood urea nitrogen, creatine kinase, creatinine, gamma-glutamyltransferase, eosinophils, lactate dehydrogenase:* increased levels
Estradiol, estriol-glucuronide, granulocytes, hemoglobin, lymphocytes, neutrophils, platelets, white blood cells: decreased levels
Coombs' test: false-positive result
Urinalysis: red blood cells, hyaline casts

Patient monitoring

- Monitor for signs and symptoms of hypersensitivity reaction.
- Check for signs and symptoms of infection at injection site.

Clinical alert: Monitor for seizures when giving high doses.

- Watch for bleeding tendency and hemorrhage.
- Check patient's temperature and watch for other signs and symptoms of superinfection, especially oral or rectal candidiasis.
- Monitor CBC and liver function test results.

Patient teaching

Clinical alert: Instruct patient to immediately report signs and symptoms of hypersensitivity reaction, such as rash, fever, or chills.

- Tell patient to report signs and symptoms of infection or other problems at injection site.
- Advise patient to minimize GI upset by eating small, frequent servings of food and drinking plenty of fluids.
- Inform patient that drug lowers resistance to certain infections. Instruct him to report new signs or symptoms of infection, especially in mouth or rectum.

Clinical alert: Tell patient to promptly report unusual bleeding or bruising.

- Inform patient taking hormonal contraceptives that drug may reduce contraceptive efficacy. Advise her to use alternative birth control method.
- Instruct patient to avoid activities that can cause injury. Advise him to use soft toothbrush and electric razor to avoid gum and skin injury.

• Inform patient that he may need to undergo regular blood testing during therapy.
• As appropriate, review all other significant and life-threatening adverse reactions and interactions, especially those related to the drugs and tests mentioned above.

amprenavir

Agenerase

Pharmacologic class: Protease inhibitor
Therapeutic class: Antiretroviral
Pregnancy risk category C

Action

Inhibits replication of human immunodeficiency virus-1 (HIV-1) by interfering with HIV-1 protease, thereby blocking viral maturation and causing formation of noninfectious virions

Availability

Capsules: 50 mg, 150 mg
Oral solution: 15 mg/ml

Indications and dosages

➢ Treatment of HIV-1 infection
Adults and children ages 13 to 16 weighing more than 50 kg (110 lb): *Capsules*—1,200 mg P.O. b.i.d. *Oral solution*—1,400 mg P.O. b.i.d.
Children ages 4 to 12, and children ages 13 to 16 weighing less than 50 kg (110 lb): *Capsules*—20 mg/kg P.O. b.i.d. or 15 mg/kg P.O. t.i.d., to a maximum dosage of 2,400 mg/day, given with other antiretrovirals. *Oral solution*—22.5 mg/kg P.O. b.i.d. or 17 mg/kg P.O. t.i.d., to a maximum dosage of 2,800 mg/day, given with other antiretrovirals

Dosage adjustment

• Renal or hepatic impairment

Contraindications

• Hypersensitivity to drug
• Renal or hepatic failure
• Concomitant metronidazole or disulfiram use
• Pregnancy
• Children younger than age 4

Precautions

Use cautiously in:
• hepatic or renal impairment, diabetes mellitus, hemophilia
• patients receiving concurrent amiodarone, parenteral lidocaine, tricyclic antidepressants, or quinidine.

Administration

Stop drug if patient develops signs or symptoms of Stevens-Johnson syndrome.
• Don't give with meals or grapefruit juice or within 1 hour of antacids.
• Be aware that capsules and oral solution aren't interchangeable on a milligram-to-milligram basis.

Route	Onset	Peak	Duration
P.O.	Rapid	1-2 hr	8-12 hr

Adverse reactions

CNS: depression, dizziness, mood disorders, headache, anxiety, peripheral paresthesia, oral and perioral paresthesia, mood disorders
GI: nausea, vomiting, diarrhea, abdominal pain
Hematologic: acute hemolytic anemia, spontaneous bleeding (in patients with hemophilia A or B)
Metabolic: hyperglycemia, hypertriglyceridemia, hypercholesterolemia, cushingoid appearance (moon face, buffalo hump)
Skin: rash, pruritus
Other: abnormal taste, abnormal fat redistribution, peripheral wasting, breast enlargement, **Stevens-Johnson syndrome**

a

Interactions

Drug-drug. *Abacavir, cimetidine, pimozide, ritonavir:* increased amprenavir blood level
Amiodarone, benzodiazepines, calcium channel blockers, cisapride, ergot alkaloids, lidocaine (systemic), quinidine, tricyclic antidepressants: competitive interference, resulting in life-threatening reactions
Antacids: interference with amprenavir absorption
Anticonvulsants: decreased amprenavir blood level; increased carbamazepine blood level (with carbamazepine)
Antihistamines, dapsone, lovastatin, simvastatin: increased levels of these drugs, possibly leading to toxicity
Azole antifungals (itraconazole, ketoconazole): changes in blood level of either drug
Clozapine, sildenafil: increased blood levels of these drugs
Erythromycin: increased blood levels of both drugs
Hormonal contraceptives: reduced contraceptive efficacy
Indinavir: increased amprenavir blood level, decreased indinavir blood level
Rifampin, saquinavir: decreased amprenavir blood level, increased rifampin or saquinavir blood level
Warfarin: inhibition of warfarin metabolism, possibly resulting in life-threatening effects
Zidovudine: increased levels of both drugs
Drug-diagnostic tests. *Cholesterol, glucose, triglycerides:* increased levels
Drug-food. *Fatty foods, grapefruit juice:* interference with drug absorption
Drug-herbs. *St. John's wort:* more than 50% reduction in amprenavir blood level

Patient monitoring

🔊 Watch for signs and symptoms of depression; assess for suicidal ideation.
- Monitor blood glucose, triglyceride, and cholesterol levels.
- Monitor clotting functions in patients with hemophilia.
- Evaluate body fat distribution throughout course of therapy.
- Assess dental hygiene and monitor oral health in patients with oral or perioral paresthesia.

Patient teaching

🔊 Tell patient to contact prescriber if rash or signs or symptoms of depression occur.
- Instruct patient not to take drug with fatty foods, grapefruit juice, or antacids, because they impede drug absorption.
- Caution patient to avoid driving and other hazardous activities until he knows how drug affects concentration and alertness.
- Advise patient to minimize GI upset by eating small, frequent servings of foods and drinking plenty of fluids.
- Inform patient that drug may interfere with hormonal contraceptive use. Suggest she use alternative birth control measure.
- Advise patient that he'll undergo regular blood testing during therapy.
- As appropriate, review all other significant and life-threatening adverse reactions and interactions, especially those related to the drugs, tests, foods, and herbs mentioned above.

amyl nitrite

Amyl Nitrite, Aspirols, Vaporole

Pharmacologic class: Coronary vasodilator
Therapeutic class: Antianginal
Pregnancy risk category C

Action

Relaxes vascular smooth muscle, thereby dilating large coronary vessels, decreasing systemic vascular resistance, reducing afterload, decreasing cardiac output, and relieving angina

Availability

Ampules: 0.3 ml

Indications and dosages

➢ Acute angina attack
Adults: 0.18 to 0.3 ml by inhalation, repeated in 3 to 5 minutes if needed
➢ Antidote for cyanide poisoning
Adults and children: 0.3 ml by inhalation for 15 to 60 seconds q 5 minutes until sodium nitrite infusion is available

Contraindications

- Hypersensitivity to drug

Precautions

Use cautiously in:
- glaucoma, hypotension, hyperthyroidism, severe anemia, early myocardial infarction
- elderly patients
- pregnant or breastfeeding patients.

Administration

- Crush ampule and wave under patient's nose one to six times. If needed, repeat in 3 to 5 minutes.

Route	Onset	Peak	Duration
Inhalation	30 sec	Unknown	3-5 min

Adverse reactions

CNS: headache, dizziness, weakness, syncope, restlessness
CV: orthostatic hypotension, flushing, palpitations, **tachycardia**
EENT: increased intraocular pressure
GI: nausea, vomiting, fecal incontinence
GU: urinary incontinence
Hematologic: hemolytic anemia, methemoglobinemia
Skin: cutaneous vasodilation, rash, pallor, facial and neck flushing

Interactions

Drug-drug. *Aspirin:* increased amyl nitrite blood level and action
Calcium channel blockers: increased risk of symptomatic orthostatic hypotension
Sildenafil: increased risk of hypotension
Sympathomimetics: decreased antianginal effects, hypotension, tachycardia
Drug-behaviors. *Alcohol use:* severe hypotension, cardiovascular collapse

Patient monitoring

- Monitor vital signs. Stay alert for tachycardia and orthostatic hypotension.
- Assess for bowel and bladder incontinence.
- Monitor neurologic response. Watch closely for dizziness and syncope.
- Assess level of headache pain.
- In long-term therapy, monitor CBC.

Patient teaching

- Teach patient to crush capsule and wave it under his nose until angina is relieved (usually after one to six inhalations).
- Tell patient that drug often causes dizziness, orthostatic hypotension, and syncope. Advise him to sit or lie down until these effects subside.
- Inform patient that drug often causes headache. Instruct him to follow prescriber's recommendations for pain relief.
- Tell patient that drug may cause fecal or urinary incontinence. Encourage him to use bathroom frequently to avoid accidents.
- As appropriate, review all other significant and life-threatening adverse reactions and interactions, especially those related to the drugs and behaviors mentioned above.

anagrelide hydrochloride

Agrylin

Pharmacologic class: Hematologic drug

Therapeutic class: Antiplatelet drug

Pregnancy risk category C

Action

Unclear. May reduce platelet production by decreasing megakaryocytic hypermaturation, thereby decreasing platelet count and inhibiting platelet aggregation (at higher doses).

Availability

Capsules: 0.5 mg, 1 mg

Indications and dosages

➢ Essential thrombocythemia

Adults: 0.5 mg P.O. q.i.d. or 1 mg P.O. b.i.d. for 1 week. Adjust as needed to lowest effective dosage that maintains platelet count below 600,000/mm^3. Maximum dosage is 10 mg daily or 2.5 mg as a single dose.

Dosage adjustment

- Hepatic or renal disease

Contraindications

- Prolonged exposure to sunlight
- Women who are or may become pregnant

Precautions

Use cautiously in:

- renal, hepatic, or cardiac dysfunction
- pregnant or breastfeeding patients
- children younger than age 16.

Administration

- Give 1 hour before or 2 hours after meals.

Route	Onset	Peak	Duration
P.O.	Immediate	1 hr	48 hr

Adverse reactions

CNS: amnesia, confusion, depression, dizziness, drowsiness, weakness, headache, syncope, insomnia, migraine, nervousness, pain, paresthesia, malaise, **seizures, cerebrovascular accident**

CV: angina, chest pain, hypertension, palpitations, orthostatic hypotension, peripheral edema, vasodilation, **arrhythmias, tachycardia, heart failure, hemorrhage, myocardial infarction, cardiomyopathy, cardiomegaly, atrial fibrillation, complete heart block, pericarditis**

EENT: amblyopia, abnormal or double vision, visual field abnormalities, tinnitus, epistaxis, rhinitis, sinusitis

GI: nausea, vomiting, diarrhea, constipation, abdominal pain, melena, gastric or duodenal ulcers, dyspepsia, aphthous stomatitis, anorexia, flatulence, gastritis, pancreatitis, **GI hemorrhage**

GU: painful urination, hematuria

Hematologic: lymphadenoma, **bleeding tendency, anemia, thrombocytopenia**

Metabolic: dehydration

Musculoskeletal: leg cramps; joint, back, muscle, neck pain

Respiratory: bronchitis, dyspnea, pneumonia, respiratory disease, **asthma, pulmonary infiltrates, pulmonary fibrosis, pulmonary hypertension**

Skin: bruising, pruritus, rash, alopecia, urticaria, skin disease, photosensitivity reaction

Other: chills, fever, flulike symptoms, edema

Interactions

Drug-drug. *Sucralfate:* interference with anagrelide absorption

Drug-diagnostic tests. *Hemoglobin, platelets:* decreased values

Hepatic enzymes: elevated values

Drug-food. *Any food:* decreased drug bioavailability

Drug-herbs. *Evening primrose oil, feverfew, garlic, ginger, ginkgo biloba, ginseng, grapeseed:* increased antiplatelet effect

Patient monitoring

🔊 Watch for signs and symptoms of vasodilation, heart failure, and arrhythmias in patients with cardiovascular disease.
- For first 2 weeks, monitor CBC and liver and kidney function test results.
- Monitor platelet count regularly until maintenance dosage is established.
- Check regularly for adverse reactions, especially bleeding tendency.
- Monitor blood pressure for orthostatic hypertension.

Patient teaching

- Instruct patient to take drug 1 hour before or 2 hours after meals.
- Tell patient that drug may cause a temporary blood pressure decrease if he sits or stands up suddenly. Tell him to rise slowly and carefully.

🔊 Instruct patient to report unusual bleeding or bruising or difficulty breathing.

🔊 Tell patient to avoid prolonged exposure to sunlight.
- Caution patient to avoid driving and other hazardous activities until he knows how drug affects concentration, alertness, and vision.
- Inform patient using hormonal contraceptives that drug may interfere with contraceptive efficacy. Advise her to use alternative birth control method.
- Tell patient to avoid activities that may cause injury. Tell him to use soft toothbrush and electric razor to avoid gum and skin injury.
- Advise patient to minimize GI upset by eating small, frequent servings of food and drinking plenty of fluids.
- Notify patient that he'll undergo regular blood testing during therapy.
- As appropriate, review all other significant and life-threatening adverse reactions and interactions, especially those related to the drugs, tests, foods, and herbs mentioned above.

anakinra

Kineret

Pharmacologic class: Interleukin-1 (IL-1) blocker

Therapeutic class: Immunomodulator, antirheumatic

Pregnancy risk category B

Action

Inhibits binding of IL-1 with IL type I receptors, thereby mediating immunologic, inflammatory, and other physiologic responses

Availability

Prefilled glass syringes: 100 mg/0.67 ml

Indications and dosages

➢ Moderately to severely active rheumatoid arthritis in patients ages 18 and older who don't respond to disease-modifying antirheumatics alone

Adults: 100 mg/day subcutaneously, given at same time each day

Contraindications

- Hypersensitivity to drug or *Escherichia coli*–derived protein
- Serious infections

Precautions

Use cautiously in:
- immunosuppression, active infection, chronic illness, renal impairment
- elderly patients
- pregnant or breastfeeding patients
- children.

a

Administration

Withhold drug and notify prescriber if patient shows signs or symptoms of active infection.

Use extreme caution if patient is concurrently receiving drugs that block tumor necrosis factor (TNF), because of increased risk of serious infection.

- Give entire dose from prefilled syringe.
- Don't freeze or shake syringe.

Route	Onset	Peak	Duration
Subcut.	Slow	3-7 hr	Unknown

Adverse reactions

CNS: headache
EENT: sinusitis
GI: nausea, diarrhea, abdominal pain
Hematologic: thrombocytopenia, neutropenia
Respiratory: upper respiratory tract infection
Skin: rash, pruritus, injection site reaction or bruising, rash, erythema, inflammation
Other: flulike symptoms, infections

Interactions

Drug-drug. *Etanercept, infliximab, other drugs that block TNF:* increased risk of serious infection
Live-virus vaccines: vaccine inefficacy
Drug-diagnostic tests. *Neutrophils:* decreased count

Patient monitoring

- Monitor CBC with white cell differential.
- Assess injection site for reactions.

Patient teaching

Tell patient to immediately report signs or symptoms of infection.

- Advise patient to report signs and symptoms of allergic response.
- Instruct patient to take drug at same time each day for best response.
- Teach patient about proper drug disposal (in puncture-resistant container). Also caution him against reusing needles, syringes, and drug product.
- Tell patient not to freeze or shake drug.
- As appropriate, review all other significant and life-threatening adverse reactions and interactions, especially those related to the drugs and tests mentioned above.

anastrozole

Arimidex

Pharmacologic class: Nonsteroidal aromatase inhibitor
Therapeutic class: Antineoplastic
Pregnancy risk category D

Action

Reduces serum estradiol levels with no significant effect on adrenocorticoid or aldosterone level; decreases stimulating effect of estrogen on tumor growth

Availability

Tablets: 1 mg

Indications and dosages

➤ Postmenopausal women with hormone receptor-unknown or hormone receptor-positive advanced breast cancer or with advanced breast cancer after tamoxifen therapy; adjuvant treatment for hormone receptor-positive breast cancer
Adults: 1 mg P.O. daily

Contraindications

- Pregnancy
- Children

Precautions

Use cautiously in:

- women of childbearing age
- breastfeeding patients.

Administration

• Verify that patient isn't pregnant before giving drug.

Route	Onset	Peak	Duration
P.O.	>24 hr	Unknown	<6 days

Adverse reactions

CNS: headache, weakness, dizziness, depression, paresthesia, lethargy
CV: chest pain, peripheral edema, vasodilation, hypertension, **thromboembolic disease**
EENT: pharyngitis
GI: nausea, vomiting, diarrhea, constipation, abdominal pain, anorexia, dry mouth
GU: vaginal bleeding, leukorrhea, vaginal dryness, pelvic pain
Musculoskeletal: bone or back pain, muscle weakness
Respiratory: dyspnea, cough
Skin: rash
Other: food distaste, weight gain, swelling, hot flashes, flulike symptoms, tumor flare

Interactions

Drug-diagnostic tests. *Hepatic enzymes, low-density lipoproteins, total cholesterol:* increased levels

Patient monitoring

Check regularly for signs and symptoms of thromboembolic disease, especially dyspnea and chest pain.
• Monitor for circulatory overload (suggested by peripheral edema, cough, and dyspnea).
• Assess for signs and symptoms of depression. Evaluate patient for suicidal ideation.
• Monitor liver function test results.

Patient teaching

Advise patient to immediately report signs and symptoms of thromboembolic disease and circulatory overload.
Emphasize importance of preventing pregnancy during therapy.
• Tell patient to contact prescriber if she develops signs or symptoms of depression.
• Caution patient to avoid driving and other hazardous activities until she knows how drug affects concentration and alertness.
• Advise patient to minimize GI upset by eating small, frequent servings of food and drinking plenty of fluids.
• Inform patient that she'll undergo regular blood testing during therapy.
• As appropriate, review all other significant and life-threatening adverse reactions and interactions, especially those related to the tests mentioned above.

anistreplase (anisoylated plasminogen streptokinase activator complex, APSAC)

Eminase

Pharmacologic class: Plasminogen activator
Therapeutic class: Thrombolytic enzyme
Pregnancy risk category C

Action

Combines with plasminogen to form activated complex, which converts plasminogen to plasmin and causes lysis of thrombi in arteries

Availability

Powder for injection: 30 units/vial

Indications and dosages

➢ Management of acute myocardial infarction (MI), including lysis of thrombi obstructing coronary arteries, reduction of infarct size, improvement

of ventricular function, and prevention of death
Adults: 30 units by direct I.V. injection given over 2 to 5 minutes, starting as soon as possible after onset of acute MI symptoms

Contraindications
• Hypersensitivity to anistreplase or streptokinase
• Active or recent internal bleeding
• Cerebrovascular accident within past 2 months
• Aneurysm
• Uncontrolled hypertension
• Severe hepatic disease
• Breastfeeding

Precautions
Use cautiously in:
• hemorrhagic conditions, hepatic or renal disease
• patients receiving warfarin concurrently
• elderly patients
• pregnant patients
• children.

Administration
• Don't further dilute reconstituted solution before giving drug or adding to infusion fluids.
• Don't add other drugs to vial or syringe.
• Gently roll vial to mix. To minimize foaming, don't shake.

Route	Onset	Peak	Duration
I.V.	Immediate	45 min	4-6 hr

Adverse reactions
CNS: dizziness, fever, headache, **intracranial hemorrhage**
CV: conduction disorders, hypotension, **arrhythmias**
EENT: epistaxis
GI: nausea, vomiting, abdominal pain, constipation, **GI hemorrhage**
GU: hematuria, proteinuria, vaginal bleeding
Hematologic: eosinophilia, **bleeding tendency**
Musculoskeletal: joint pain or stiffness, myalgia, back or bone pain
Respiratory: hemoptysis, dyspnea, **bronchospasm**
Skin: hematoma, urticaria, pruritus, flushing, angioedema, delayed purpuric rash
Other: bleeding at puncture site, ankle edema, chills, fever, gum or mouth hemorrhages, **shock, anaphylaxis**

Interactions
Drug-drug. *Drugs that alter platelet function (such as aspirin, dipyridamole, heparin, oral anticoagulants):* increased bleeding risk
Drug-diagnostic tests. *Alpha$_2$-antiplasmin, factor V, factor VIII, fibrinogen and plasminogen activity, hematocrit, hemoglobin:* decreased values
Eosinophils, International Normalized Ratio, partial thromboplastin time, prothrombin time: increased values

Patient monitoring
🔊 Monitor patient for signs and symptoms of anaphylaxis.
🔊 Watch for bleeding tendency and hemorrhaging.
• Assess neurologic status and vital signs regularly.
• Evaluate patient for arrhythmias, conduction disorders, and hypotension.
• Monitor CBC and blood coagulation studies.

Patient teaching
• Tell patient to report signs and symptoms of allergic reaction.
• Instruct patient to report unusual bleeding or bruising.
• Caution patient to avoid activities that can cause injury. Advise him to use soft toothbrush and electric razor to avoid gum and skin injury.

- Explain to patient that he will be on bed rest during entire course of treatment and will be monitored closely.
- Advise patient to minimize GI upset by eating small, frequent servings of food and drinking plenty of fluids.
- Caution patient not to use aspirin during therapy.
- Inform patient that he'll undergo regular blood testing during therapy.
- As appropriate, review all other significant and life-threatening adverse reactions and interactions, especially those related to the drugs and tests mentioned above.

antihemophilic factor (AHF, factor VIII)

Alphanate, Bioclate, HelixateFS, Hemofil M, Humate-P, Hyate:C, Koate-DVI, Kogenate FS, Monarc-M, Monoclate-P, Recombinate, ReFacto

Pharmacologic class: Hemostatic
Therapeutic class: Antihemophilic
Pregnancy risk category C

Action

Promotes conversion of prothrombin to thrombin (necessary for hemostasis and blood clotting). Also replaces missing or deficient clotting factors, thereby controlling or preventing bleeding.

Availability

I.V. injection: 250, 500, 1,000, or 1,500 international units/vial in numerous preparations

Indications and dosages

➢ Spontaneous hemorrhage in patients with hemophilia A (factor VIII deficiency)
Adults and children: Dosage is highly individualized, calculated as follows: AHF required (international units) equals weight (kg) multiplied by desired factor VIII increase (% of normal) multiplied by 0.5.

To control bleeding, desired factor VIII level is 20% to 40% of normal for minor hemorrhage; 30% to 60% of normal for moderate hemorrhage; or 60% to 100% of normal for severe hemorrhage. To prevent spontaneous hemorrhage, desired factor VIII level is 5% of normal.

Contraindications

- Hypersensitivity to drug or to mouse, hamster, or bovine protein

Precautions

Use cautiously in:
- hepatic disease
- blood types A, B, and AB
- patients receiving factor VIII inhibitors
- pregnant patients
- neonates and infants.

Administration

- Before giving, verify that patient has no history of hypersensitivity to drug or to mouse, hamster, or bovine protein.
- Follow prescriber's instructions regarding hepatitis B prophylaxis before starting therapy.
- Refrigerate concentrate until ready to reconstitute drug.
- Warm bottles of concentrate and diluent to room temperature before mixing.
- Roll bottle gently between hands until drug is well-mixed.
- After drug is reconstituted, don't refrigerate, shake, or store near heat.
- Don't mix with other I.V. solutions.
- Use plastic (not glass) syringe and filter.

Route	Onset	Peak	Duration
I.V.	Immediate	1-2 hr	Unknown

a

Adverse reactions

CNS: headache; lethargy; fatigue; dizziness; jitteriness; drowsiness; depersonalization; tingling in arms, ears, and face
CV: chest tightness, angina pectoris, tachycardia, slight hypotension, **thrombosis**
EENT: blurred or abnormal vision, eye disorder, otitis media, epistaxis, rhinitis, sore throat
GI: nausea, vomiting, diarrhea, constipation, stomachache, abdominal pain, gastroenteritis, anorexia,
Hematologic: forehead bruises, **increased bleeding tendency, thrombocytopenia, hemolytic anemia, intravascular hemolysis, hyperfibrinogenemia**
Hepatic: hepatitis B transmission
Musculoskeletal: myalgia, muscle weakness, bone pain, finger pain
Respiratory: dyspnea, coughing, wheezing, **bronchospasm**
Skin: rash, acne, flushing, diaphoresis, urticaria
Other: taste changes, allergic reaction, fever, chills, cold feet, cold sensations, infected hematoma, stinging at injection site, **anaphylaxis, human immunodeficiency virus transmission**

Interactions

Drug-diagnostic tests. *Bilirubin, creatine kinase:* increased levels
Hemoglobin, platelets: decreased values

Patient monitoring

🔈 Monitor for signs and symptoms of anaphylaxis and hemolysis.
🔈 Watch for bleeding tendency and hemorrhaging.
- Check vital signs regularly.
- Monitor CBC and coagulation studies.

🔈 Assess for severe headache (may indicate intracranial hemorrhage).

Patient teaching

🔈 Tell patient to immediately report signs and symptoms of allergic response or bleeding tendency.
- Caution patient not to use aspirin during therapy.
- Instruct patient to contact prescriber if drug becomes less effective.
- Tell patient to report signs or symptoms of hepatitis B.
- Caution patient to avoid driving and other hazardous activities until he knows how drug affects concentration, alertness, and vision.
- Advise patient to minimize GI upset by eating small, frequent servings of food and drinking plenty of fluids.
- Notify patient that he'll undergo regular blood testing during therapy.
- As appropriate, review all other significant and life-threatening adverse reactions and interactions, especially those related to the tests mentioned above.

antithrombin III, human (AT-III, heparin cofactor 1)

Thrombate III

Pharmacologic class: Blood derivative, coagulation inhibitor
Therapeutic class: Antithrombin
Pregnancy risk category B

Action

Inactivates thrombin and activated forms of factors IXa, Xa, XIa, and XIIa, thereby inhibiting coagulation and thromboembolism formation

Availability

Injection: 500 international units, 1,000 international units

Indications and dosages

➢ Thromboembolism related to AT-III deficiency

Adults: Initial dosage is individualized to amount required to increase AT-III activity to 120% of normal (determined 20 minutes after administration). Usual infusion rate is 50 to a maximum of 100 international units/minute I.V. Dosage calculation is based on anticipated 1.4% increase in plasma AT-III activity produced by 1 international unit/kg of body weight.

Use this formula to calculate dosage: Required dosage (international units) equals desired activity (%) minus baseline AT-III activity (%) multiplied by weight (kg) divided by 1.4 (international units/kg).

Maintenance dosage is individualized to amount required to maintain AT-III activity at 80% of normal.

Contraindications

None

Precautions

Use cautiously in:

- pregnant or breastfeeding patients
- children (safety and efficacy not established).

Administration

- Mix powder with 10 ml of sterile water, normal saline solution, or dextrose 5% in water.
- Use filter needle provided by manufacturer to draw up solution.
- Don't shake vial.
- Know that drug may be diluted further in same solution if desired.
- Don't mix with other solutions.
- Infuse over 10 to 20 minutes.
- Administer within 3 hours of reconstitution.

🔊 If adverse reactions occur, decrease infusion rate or, if indicated, stop infusion until symptoms disappear.

Route	Onset	Peak	Duration
I.V.	Immediate	Unknown	4 days

Adverse reactions

CNS: dizziness, light-headedness, headache
CV: vasodilation, reduced blood pressure, chest pain
EENT: perception of "film" over eyes
GI: nausea, sensation of intestinal fullness
GU: diuresis
Musculoskeletal: muscle cramps
Respiratory: dyspnea, shortness of breath
Skin: urticaria, oozing lesions, hives, hematoma
Other: foul taste, chills, fever

Interactions

Drug-drug. *Heparin:* increased anticoagulant effect

Patient monitoring

- Monitor AT-III activity levels regularly.

🔊 Watch for signs and symptoms of too-rapid infusion, such as dyspnea and hypertension.

- Monitor vital signs and temperature.
- Assess fluid intake and output to detect dehydration.

Patient teaching

🔊 Instruct patient to immediately report chest tightness, dizziness, and fever.

- Caution patient to avoid driving and other hazardous activities until he knows how drug affects concentration and alertness.
- Advise patient to minimize GI upset and unpleasant taste by eating small, frequent servings of healthy food and drinking plenty of fluids.
- Tell patient that he'll undergo regular blood testing during therapy.
- As appropriate, review all other significant adverse reactions and interac-

tions, especially those related to the drugs mentioned above.

aprepitant

Emend

Pharmacologic class: Substance P and neurokinin-1 antagonist

Therapeutic class: Adjunctive antiemetic

Pregnancy risk category B

Action

Augments antiemetic activity of ondansetron (a 5-hydroxytryptamine$_3$-receptor antagonist) and dexamethasone. Also inhibits cisplatin-induced emesis.

Availability

Capsules: 80 mg, 125 mg

Indications and dosages

➤ To prevent acute and delayed nausea and vomiting caused by highly emetogenic cancer chemotherapy

Adults: 125 mg P.O. 1 hour before chemotherapy on day 1; then 80 mg P.O. once daily in morning on days 2 and 3. Give with 12 mg dexamethasone P.O. and 32 mg ondansetron I.V. on day 1, and with 8 mg dexamethasone P.O. on days 2 to 4.

Contraindications

- Hypersensitivity to drug
- Concurrent pimozide, terfenadine, astemizole, or cisapride therapy
- Breastfeeding

Precautions

Use cautiously in:

- patients receiving concurrent warfarin or CYP3A4 inhibitors
- pregnant patients.

Administration

- Give 1 hour before chemotherapy on day 1, together with other antiemetics as prescribed.
- Give on mornings of days 2 and 3.

Route	Onset	Peak	Duration
P.O.	Unknown	Unknown	Unknown

Adverse reactions

CNS: dizziness, neuropathy, headache, insomnia, asthenia, fatigue
EENT: tinnitus
GI: nausea, vomiting, constipation, diarrhea, epigastric discomfort, gastritis, heartburn, abdominal pain, anorexia
Hematologic: neutropenia
Other: fever, dehydration, hiccups

Interactions

Drug-drug. *CYP3A4 inducers (carbamazepine, phenytoin, rifampin):* decreased aprepitant blood level
CYP3A4 inhibitors (azole antifungals, clarithromycin, nefazodone, ritonavir): increased aprepitant blood level
Dexamethasone, methylprednisolone: increased steroid exposure
Docetaxel, etoposide, ifosfamide, imatinib, irinotecan, paclitaxel, vinblastine, vincristine, vinorelbine: increased blood levels of these drugs
Hormonal contraceptives: decreased contraceptive efficacy
Paroxetine: decreased efficacy of either drug
Pimozide: increased blood level and toxic effects of aprepitant
Tolbutamide, warfarin: CYP2C9 induction, decreased efficacy of these drugs

Patient monitoring

- Monitor neurologic status. Institute measures to prevent injury as needed.
- Assess nutritional and hydration status.
- Monitor CBC.

Patient teaching

- Tell patient that drug may cause CNS effects. Explain that he'll be monitored to ensure his safety.
- Advise patient to minimize GI upset by eating small, frequent servings of foods and drinking plenty of fluids.
- Caution patient to avoid driving and other hazardous activities until he knows how drug affects concentration, hearing, strength, balance, and alertness.
- As appropriate, review all other significant and life-threatening adverse reactions and interactions, especially those related to the drugs mentioned above.

argatroban

Acova

Pharmacologic class: L-arginine–derived thrombin inhibitor
Therapeutic class: Anticoagulant
Pregnancy risk category B

Action

Binds rapidly to site of thrombi, neutralizing conversion of fibrinogen to fibrin, activation of coagulation factors, and platelet aggregation (processes required for thrombus formation)

Availability

Injection: 100 mg/ml in 2.5-ml vials

Indications and dosages

➢ Treatment or prophylaxis of thrombosis in patients with heparin-induced thrombocytopenia
Adults: 2 mcg/kg/minute as a continuous I.V. infusion, to a maximum dosage of 10 mcg/kg/minute. Adjust dosage as needed to maintain activated partial thromboplastin time (APTT) at 1.5 to 3 times initial baseline value (not to exceed 100 seconds).

➢ Anticoagulation during percutaneous coronary intervention in patients who have or are at risk for heparin-induced thrombocytopenia
Adults: Start continuous I.V. infusion at 25 mcg/kg/minute and give loading dose of 350 mcg/kg by I.V. bolus over 3 to 5 minutes. Check activated clotting time (ACT) 5 to 10 minutes after bolus dose is given; adjust dosage until ACT is between 300 and 450 seconds. If ACT is below 300 seconds, give additional I.V. bolus dose of 150 mcg/kg; then increase infusion rate to 30 mcg/kg/minute, and check ACT after 5 to 10 minutes. If ACT exceeds 450 seconds, decrease infusion rate to 15 mcg/kg/minute, and check ACT after 5 to 10 minutes. Maintain adjusted infusion dosage once therapeutic ACT has been reached.

Dosage adjustment

- Hepatic impairment

Contraindications

- Hypersensitivity to drug
- Overt major bleeding

Precautions

Use cautiously in:

- hepatic impairment or disease, intracranial bleeding
- pregnant or breastfeeding patients
- children younger than age 18.

Administration

- Stop all parenteral anticoagulants before starting argatroban.
- Dilute in normal saline solution, dextrose 5% in water, or lactated Ringer's solution to a concentration of 1 mg/ml.
- Inject contents of 2.5-ml vial into 250-ml bag of diluent.
- Protect solution from direct sunlight.

Route	Onset	Peak	Duration
I.V.	Rapid	1-3 hr	Duration of infusion

a

Adverse reactions

CNS: headache
CV: hypotension, unstable angina, **atrial fibrillation, cardiac arrest, ventricular tachycardia, cerebrovascular disorders**
GI: nausea, vomiting, diarrhea, abdominal pain, anorexia, **GI bleeding**
GU: urinary tract infection, minor GU tract bleeding and hematuria, **renal dysfunction**
Hematologic: groin bleeding, brachial bleeding, **hypoprothrombinemia, thrombocytopenia, bleeding or hemorrhage**
Respiratory: cough, dyspnea, pneumonia, hemoptysis
Skin: rash, bleeding at puncture site
Other: allergic reaction, pain, infection, fever, **sepsis, anaphylaxis**

Interactions

Drug-drug. *Oral anticoagulants:* prolonged prothrombin time, increased International Normalized Ratio, increased risk of bleeding
Thrombolytics: increased risk of intracranial bleeding
Drug-diagnostic tests. *Hematocrit, hemoglobin:* decreased values

Patient monitoring

- Monitor patient for signs and symptoms of anaphylaxis.
- Evaluate patient for bleeding tendency and hemorrhage.
- Assess neurologic status and vital signs frequently.
- Monitor CBC and coagulation studies, especially partial thromboplastin time.
- Check for signs and symptoms of serious arrhythmias and hypotension.

Patient teaching

- Instruct patient to immediately report allergic reaction and unusual bleeding or bruising.
- Tell patient to avoid activities that can cause injury. Advise him to use a soft toothbrush and electric razor to avoid gum and skin injury.
- Advise patient to minimize GI upset by eating small, frequent servings of food and drinking plenty of fluids.
- Tell patient that he'll undergo regular blood testing during therapy.
- As appropriate, review all other significant and life-threatening adverse reactions and interactions, especially those related to the drugs and tests mentioned above.

aripiprazole

Abilify

Pharmacologic class: Quinolone-derived atypical antipsychotic agent
Therapeutic class: Antipsychotic, neuroleptic
Pregnancy risk category C

Action

Unclear. Thought to exert partial agonist activity at central dopamine D_2 and type 1A serotonin (5-HT_{1A}) receptors and antagonistic activity at serotonin 5-HT_{2A} receptors. Also has alpha-adrenergic and histamine$_1$-blocking properties.

Availability

Tablets: 10 mg, 15 mg, 20 mg, 30 mg

Indications and dosages

➤ Schizophrenia
Adults: 10 to 15 mg P.O. daily. If needed, increase to 30 mg daily after 2 weeks.
➤ To maintain stability in schizophrenic patients
Adults: 15 mg P.O. daily. Therapy may continue for up to 26 weeks with periodic evaluations.
➤ Acute manic and mixed episodes associated with bipolar disorder
Adults: 30 mg P.O. daily for up to 3 weeks

Dosage adjustment

• Concurrent use of potent CYP3A4 inhibitors (such as ketoconazole), CYP2D6 inhibitors (such as fluoxetine, paroxetine, quinidine), or CYP3A4 inducers (such as carbamazepine)

Contraindications

• Hypersensitivity to drug

Precautions

Use cautiously in:
• cerebrovascular disease, hypotension, seizure disorder, suicidal ideation
• high risk for aspiration pneumonia
• pregnant or breastfeeding patients
• children and adolescents (safety and efficacy not established).

Administration

• Give with or without food.
• Don't administer with grapefruit juice.

Route	Onset	Peak	Duration
P.O.	Slow	3-5 hr	Unknown

Adverse reactions

CNS: drowsiness, insomnia, akathisia, agitation, anxiety, headache, lightheadedness, drowsiness, tremor, tardive dyskinesia, **seizures, neuroleptic malignant syndrome, increased suicide risk**
CV: orthostatic hypotension, hypertension, peripheral edema, chest pain, **bradycardia, tachycardia**
EENT: rhinitis
GI: nausea, vomiting, diarrhea, constipation, jaundice, abdominal pain, esophageal motility disorders
GU: urinary incontinence
Respiratory: cough
Skin: rash
Other: fever

Interactions

Drug-drug. *CNS depressants:* increased sedation
Drugs that induce CYP3A4: decreased aripiprazole effect
Drugs that inhibit CYP3A4 or CYP2D6: serious toxic effects
Other antipsychotic agents: increased extrapyramidal effects
Drug-herbs. *Kava:* increased CNS depression
Drug-behaviors. *Alcohol use:* increased sedation

Patient monitoring

🔊 Watch for signs and symptoms of depression, and evaluate patient for suicidal ideation.
• Monitor neurologic status closely. Watch for tardive dyskinesia.
🔊 Evaluate patient for neuroleptic malignant syndrome (fever, altered mental status, rigid muscles, arrhythmia, tachycardia, sweating). Stop drug and notify prescriber if these signs and symptoms occur.
• Monitor blood pressure, pulse, and weight.

Patient teaching

🔊 Instruct patient to contact prescriber if he experiences depression or has suicidal thoughts.
• Advise patient to establish effective bedtime routine to minimize insomnia.
• Inform patient that symptoms will subside slowly over several weeks.
• Tell patient he may take drug with or without food.
• Caution patient to avoid driving and other hazardous activities until he knows how drug affects concentration and alertness.
• Tell patient that drug may cause urinary incontinence.
• Advise patient to minimize GI upset by eating small, frequent servings of food and drinking plenty of fluids.
• Caution patient to avoid strenuous exercise and hot environments whenever possible.

• As appropriate, review all other significant and life-threatening adverse reactions and interactions, especially those related to the drugs, herbs, and behaviors mentioned above.

arsenic trioxide

Trisenox

Pharmacologic class: Nonmetallic element, white arsenic
Therapeutic class: Antineoplastic
Pregnancy risk category D

Action

Unclear. May cause morphologic changes and DNA fragmentation in promyelocytic leukemia cells, causing cell death and degradation of or damage to PML/RAR alpha (a fusion protein).

Availability

Injection: 1 mg/ml

Indications and dosages

➢ Acute promyelocytic leukemia (APL) in patients who have relapsed or are refractory to retinoid and anthracycline chemotherapy

Adults and children ages 5 and older: *Induction phase*—0.15 mg/kg I.V. daily until bone marrow remission occurs, to a maximum of 60 doses. *Consolidation phase*—0.15 mg/kg I.V. daily for 25 doses over 5 weeks, starting 3 to 6 weeks after completion of induction phase.

Contraindications

- Hypersensitivity to drug
- Pregnancy

Precautions

Use cautiously in:

- renal impairment, cardiac abnormalities
- elderly patients
- breastfeeding patients
- children.

Administration

Know that drug is carcinogenic. Follow facility policy for preparing and handling antineoplastics.

- Dilute in 100 to 250 ml of dextrose 5% in water or normal saline solution.
- Don't mix with other drugs.
- Infuse over 1 to 2 hours (may infuse over 4 hours if patient has vasomotor reaction).

Route	Onset	Peak	Duration
I.V.	Unknown	Unknown	Unknown

Adverse reactions

CNS: headache, insomnia, paresthesia, dizziness, tremor, drowsiness, anxiety, confusion, agitation, rigors, weakness, **seizures, coma**

CV: ECG abnormalities, palpitations, chest pain, hypotension, hypertension, tachycardia, **prolonged QT interval, torsades de pointes**

EENT: blurred vision, painful red eye, dry eyes, eye irritation, swollen eyelids, tinnitus, earache, nasopharyngitis, postnasal drip, epistaxis, sinusitis, sore throat

GI: nausea, vomiting, constipation, diarrhea, abdominal pain, fecal incontinence, dyspepsia, dry mouth, mouth blisters, oral candidiasis, anorexia, **GI hemorrhage**

GU: urinary incontinence, intermenstrual bleeding, renal impairment, **oliguria, renal failure, vaginal hemorrhage**

Hematologic: anemia, lymphadenopathy, **leukocytosis, thrombocytopenia, neutropenia, disseminated intravascular coagulation, hemorrhage**

Metabolic: hypokalemia, hypomagnesemia, hyperglycemia, acidosis, **hypoglycemia, hyperkalemia**

Musculoskeletal: joint, muscle, bone, back, neck, or limb pain

Respiratory: dyspnea, cough, hypoxia, wheezing, crackles, tachypnea, decreased breath sounds, crepitation, hemoptysis, rhonchi, upper respiratory tract infection, **pleural effusion**
Skin: flushing, erythema, pallor, bruising, petechiae, pruritus, dermatitis, dry skin, hyperpigmentation, urticaria, skin lesions, herpes simplex infection, local exfoliation, diaphoresis, night sweats
Other: fever, facial edema, weight gain or loss, bacterial infection, pain and edema at injection site, **hypersensitivity reaction, sepsis**

Interactions

Drug-drug. *Drugs that can cause electrolyte abnormalities (such as amphotericin B, diuretics):* increased risk of electrolyte abnormalities
Drugs that can prolong QT interval (antiarrhythmics, thioridazines, some quinolones): increased QT-interval prolongation
Drug-diagnostic tests. *Alanine aminotransferase, aspartate aminotransferase, calcium, magnesium, white blood cells:* increased levels
Glucose, potassium: altered levels
Hemoglobin, neutrophils, platelets: decreased values

Patient monitoring

[Clinical alert] Watch for signs and symptoms of APL differentiation syndrome (fever, dyspnea, weight gain, pulmonary infiltrates, and pleural or pericardial effusions).
• Evaluate vital signs and neurologic status.
[Clinical alert] Obtain baseline ECG; monitor ECG at least weekly.
• Assess for arrhythmias and conduction disorders.
[Clinical alert] Discontinue drug and notify prescriber if patient develops syncope, tachycardia, or arrhythmias.
• Monitor serum electrolyte levels, CBC, and coagulation studies.
• Assess for hypoglycemia and hyperglycemia if patient is diabetic.

Patient teaching

[Clinical alert] Instruct patient to immediately report signs and symptoms of allergic responses, fever, breathing problems, and seizures.
• Tell patient that drug increases risk of serious infection. Instruct him to report signs or symptoms of infection.
[Clinical alert] Emphasize importance of avoiding pregnancy during therapy.
• Caution patient to avoid driving and other hazardous activities until he knows how drug affects concentration and alertness.
• Tell patient to minimize GI upset by eating small, frequent servings of food and drinking plenty of fluids.
• Advise patient to establish effective bedtime routine to minimize insomnia.
• Notify patient that he'll undergo regular blood testing during therapy.
• As appropriate, review all other significant and life-threatening adverse reactions and interactions, especially those related to the drugs and tests mentioned above.

asparaginase

Elspar, Kidrolase*

Pharmacologic class: Enzyme
Therapeutic class: Antineoplastic (miscellaneous)
Pregnancy risk category C

Action

Hydrolyzes asparagine (an amino acid needed for malignant cell growth in acute lymphocytic leukemia), resulting in leukemic cell death

Availability

Injection: 10,000 international units/vial (with mannitol)

Safe drug administration

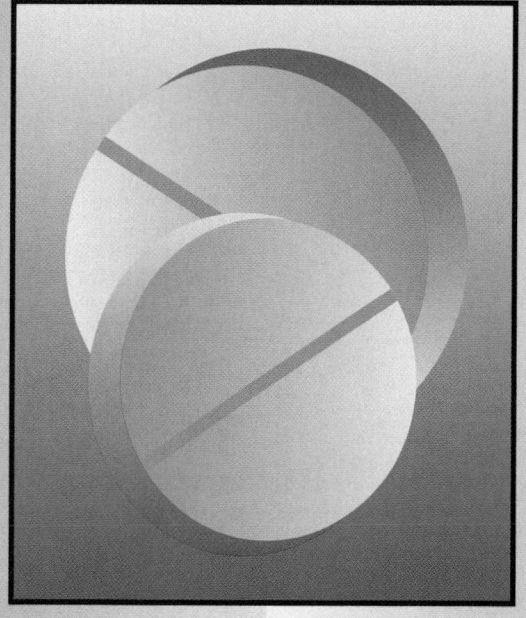

The following guidelines on preparing, administering, and monitoring drug therapy will help you ensure patient safety and drug effectiveness.

Drug compatibilities

Use the table below to determine if you can safely mix two drugs together in the same syringe or administer them together through the same I.V. line.

KEY
C: compatible
I: incompatible
✳: conflicting data exist
Blank space: no data available

	acyclovir sodium	amikacin	amiodarone	amphotericin B	aztreonam	calcium chloride	calcium gluconate	cefazolin	cefepime	ceftazidime	clindamycin	cyclosporine	dexamethasone	digoxin	diltiazem	diphenhydramine	dobutamine	dopamine	enalaprilat
acyclovir sodium															I		I	I	
amikacin			C	I	C	C	C	C	C	I	C	C	C	C	C	C			C
amiodarone		C		C		C	C	I		I	C			I			C	C	
amphotericin B		I	C		I										C	✳		I	I
aztreonam		C		I		C	C			C	C		C		C	C	C	C	C
calcium chloride		C	C														✳	C	
calcium gluconate		C	C		C			I			I		C			C	✳		C
cefazolin		C	I		C		I				✳	C	C		C				C
cefepime		C									C								
ceftazidime		I	I		C						C				C				C
clindamycin		C	C		C		I	✳	C	C		C							C
cyclosporine		C						C			C							✳	
dexamethasone		C			C		C	C								✳			
digoxin			I														I		
diltiazem	I	C		C	C			C			C						C	C	
diphenhydramine		C		✳	C		C						✳						
dobutamine	I		C		C	✳	✳							I	C			C	C
dopamine	I		C	I	C	C						✳			C		C		C
enalaprilat		C		I	C		C	C		C	C						C	C	
epinephrine		C	C			✳	✳										C		
esmolol		C	C			C		C		C	C			C			C	C	C
famotidine	C		C	C			C	C		C			C	C		C	C	C	C
fluconazole		C		C				C		C	C	C							
furosemide		✳	✳												I	I	I		

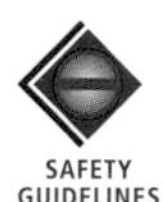

epinephrine		C	C			*	*										C					C		C
esmolol		C	C			C		C		C	C			C	C		C	C	C			C		I
famotidine	C		C	C			C	C		C			C	C		C	C	C	C	C	C		C	*
fluconazole		C	C				C			C	C											C		
furosemide		*	*													I	I			C	I	*		
heparin		I		I	C		C	*	C	*	C		C	C	*	*	*	C	C	C	C	C		C
hydrocortisone		C		I	C	C	C				C		C		*			C	C	C	C	C	C	C
hydromorphone hydrochloride																								
imipenem and cilastatin sodium					C										C							C		
insulin			C		C			C						I	*		*	I			C	C		
labetalol		C	C				C	C		C	C						C	C	C		C	C		I
levofloxacin		C									C		C				C	C		C				I
lorazepam		C	C		I								*		C	I						C		C
magnesium		C	*	*	C	I	*	C			I	*					*		C		C	C		
methylprednisolone			C	C	C		C	C			C					I		C	C			C		
metoprolol																								
metronidazole		C	C		I			*	C	C	C	C						*	C		C		C	
midazolam		C	C				C	C		I	C		*	C			*	C			C	C		I
milrinone		C	C			C	C	C			C		C	C			C	C		C				I
morphine		C	C		C	C		C		C	C		C	C		C	C	C	C		C	C	C	I
nitroglycerin			C														C	C			C	C		C
nitroprusside			*			C											C	C	C	C	C	C		C
norepinephrine															C		C	C				C		
ondansetron		C		I	C			C		C	C	*	*			C		C				C		I
phenylephrine			C				C									C	C					C		
potassium chloride		C	C				C	C	C	C			C	C		*	*	C	C	C	C	C	C	I
propofol		I		I	C	I	C	C		C	C	C	C	C		C	C	C	C	C	C	C		C
sodium bicarbonate		C	I	I	C	I	I			I							I	I						C
tobramycin			C		C		C	C	I	*	*	C							C		C			*
vancomycin		C	C		*		C	*	C	*		C	I			C			C		C	C		
vecuronium			C					C									C	C		C	C			

Drug compatibilities (continued)

KEY
C: compatible
I: incompatible
*: conflicting data exist
Blank space: no data available

	acyclovir sodium	amikacin	amiodarone	amphotericin B	aztreonam	calcium chloride	calcium gluconate	cefazolin	cefepime	ceftazidime	clindamycin	cyclosporine	dexamethasone	digoxin	diltiazem	diphenhydramine	dobutamine	dopamine	enalaprilat
heparin		I		I	C		C	*	C	*	C		C	C	*	*	*	C	C
hydrocortisone		C		I	C	C	C				C		C		*	C		C	C
hydromorphone hydrochloride																			
imipenem and cilastatin sodium			I		C										C				
insulin			C		C			C						I	*		*	I	
labetalol		C	C				C	C		C	C						C	C	C
levofloxacin		C									C		C				C	C	
lorazepam		C	C		I								C		C	I			
magnesium		C	*	*	C	I	*	C			I	C					*		C
methylprednisolone			C	C	C		C				C				*	I		C	C
metoprolol																			
metronidazole		C	C		I			*	C	C	C	C						*	C
midazolam		C	C				C	C		I	C		*	C			*	C	
milrinone		C	C			C	C	C		C	C		C	C	C		C	C	
morphine		C	C		C	C		C		C	C		C	C		C	C	C	C
nitroglycerin			C												C		C	C	
nitroprusside			*			C											C	C	C
norepinephrine			C												C		C	C	
ondansetron		C		I	C			C		C	C	*	*			C		C	
phenylephrine			C				C									C	C		
potassium chloride		C	C		C		C	C	C	C				C	C		*	*	C
propofol		I		I	C	I	C	C		C	C	C	C	C		C	C	C	C
sodium bicarbonate		C	I		C	I	I			I					*		I	I	
tobramycin			C		C		C	C	I	*	*	C			C				C
vancomycin		C	C		*		C	*	C	*			I		C	C			C
vecuronium			C					C									C	C	

	epinephrine	esmolol	famotidine	fluconazole	furosemide	heparin	hydrocortisone	hydromorphone hydrochloride	imipenem and cilastatin sodium	insulin	labetalol	levofloxacin	lorazepam	magnesium	methylprednisolone	metoprolol	metronidazole	midazolam	milrinone	morphine	nitroglycerin	nitroprusside	norepinephrine	ondansetron	phenylephrine	potassium chloride	propofol	sodium bicarbonate	tobramycin	vancomycin	vecuronium
	C	C	C	C	C		*		C	I	*	I	C	C	*		C	C	C	I	*	C		C	C	C	C	C	I	*	C
	C	C	C		C	*				C			C	*			C	I		C				C			C	C			C
						C							C					C						C		C		I			
			C			C				C			I					I	I					C							
		C	C			I	C		C		I	I		C				C	C	C	C	C	I			C	C	*	C	C	
		C	C		I	*				I				C			C	C		C	C	C	C			C	C	*	C	C	
	C				I	I				I			C							C	I	I			C			C		C	
			C		C	C	C	C	I			C					C		C					*		C	C			C	C
		C	C			C	*			C	C						C		C	C		C		C		C	C	I	C	C	
			C			*											C	*	C	C				*		I	I				
																				C											
		C		C		C	C				C		C	C	C			C	C	C									C		
		C	C		I	C	I	C	I	C	C				*		C		C	C	C	C	C	C		C	*	I	C	C	C
	C				I	C			I	C			C	C	C		C	C		C	C	C	C			C	C	C	C	C	C
		C	C	C	I	I	C			C	C	C		C	C	C	C	C	C			C	C	C		C	C	I	C	C	C
		C	C		C	*				C	C	I						C	C			C					C				C
	C	C	C		C	C				C	C	I		C				C	C	C	C		C			C					C
			C							I	C							C	C	C		C					C				
			C		I	C	C	C	C				*		*			C		C						C	C	I		C	
			C			C						C															I			C	
	C	C	C	C	I	C		C	C		C	C		C	C				C	C	C		C		C		C	C			
	C	C	C		C	C	C			C	C		C	C	C			*	C	C	C		C	C	I			C	I	C	C
					C	C	C	I		*	*	C		I				I	C	I				I		C	C			I	
		C			*	I			C	C			C			C	C	C	C							I					
		C	C			*	I			C	C	C	C	C				C	C	C				C	C		C	I			C
		C				C	C						C					C	C	C	C	C					C			C	

Conversions and calculations

Accurate conversions and calculations are crucial to ensuring safe drug administration. Use the tables below when you need to convert one unit to another, find equivalent measures, convert temperatures between Celsius and Fahrenheit, or calculate dosages or administration rates.

Metric measures

Solids

1 milligram (mg) = 1,000 micrograms (mcg)
1 gram (g) = 1,000 mg
1 kilogram (kg) = 1,000 g

Liquids

1 milliliter (ml) = 1 cubic centimeter (cc)
1 ml = 1,000 microliters (mcl)
1 cc = 1,000 mcl
1 liter (L) = 1,000 ml
1 L = 1,000 cc

Household to metric equivalents

1 teaspoon (tsp) = 5 ml
1 tablespoon (tbs) = 15 ml
1 ounce (oz) = 30 ml
2 tbs = 30 ml
1 oz = 30 g
1 pound (lb) = 454 g
2.2 lb = 1 kg
1 inch = 2.54 centimeters (cm)

Temperature conversions

To convert Celsius (°C) to Fahrenheit (°F)

Use the following equation:
(°C × 1.8) + 32 = °F
Example: 38 °C times 1.8 is 68.4; 68.4 plus 32 equals 100.4 °F.

To convert °F to °C

(°F– 32) × 1.8 = °C
Example: 98.6 °F minus 32 is 66.8.; 66.8 times 1.8 equals 37 °C.

Calculating dosages and administration rates

$$\text{Concentration of solution in mg/ml} = \frac{\text{mg of drug}}{\text{ml of solution}}$$

$$\text{Infusion rate in mg/minute} = \frac{\text{mg of drug}}{\text{ml of solution}} \times \text{flow rate (ml/hour)} \div 60 \text{ minutes}$$

$$\text{Concentration of solution in mcg/ml} = \frac{\text{mg of drug} \times 1{,}000}{\text{ml of solution}}$$

Infusion rate in mcg/minute =

$$\frac{\text{mg of drug} \times 1{,}000}{\text{ml of solution}} \times \text{flow rate (ml/hour)} \div 60 \text{ minutes}$$

Infusion rate in mcg/kg/minute =

$$\frac{\text{mg of drug} \times 1{,}000}{\text{ml of solution}} \times \text{flow rate (ml/hour)} \div 60 \text{ minutes} \div \text{weight in kg}$$

Infusion rate in ml/hour = ml of solution ÷ 60 minutes

$$\text{Infusion rate in gtt/minutes} = \frac{\text{ml of solution}}{\text{time in minutes}} \times \text{drip factor (gtt/ml)}$$

Drug names that look or sound alike

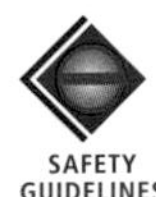

The drug names below can easily be confused, either verbally or in writing, because they either sound alike or have similar spellings. Generic names of these drugs appear in regular type; trade names are capitalized and in **boldface**.

Accupril, Accutane
Accutane, Anturane
acetazolamide, acetohexamide
acetylcholine, acetylcysteine
Aciphex, Aricept
Adderall, Inderal
albuterol, atenolol
Aldactazide, Aldactone
Aldomet, Aldoril
Aldoril, Elavil
alfentanil, fentanyl, **Sufenta, sufentanil**
Allegra, Viagra
alprazolam, diazepam, lorazepam, midazolam
Altace, alteplase
Alupent, Atrovent
amantadine, rimantadine
Ambien, Amen
Amicar, Amikin
amiloride, amiodarone, amlodipine
amitriptyline, nortriptyline
amoxicillin, **Augmentin**
Anafranil, enalapril
Apresazide, Apresoline
Asacol, Os-Cal, Oxytrol
Atarax, Ativan
atenolol, timolol
Avinza, Invanz
azithromycin, erythromycin
baclofen, **Bactroban**
Benadryl, Bentyl, Benylin, Betalin
bepridil, **Prepidil**
Betagan, BetaGen
Bumex, Buprenex
bupivacaine, ropivacaine
bupropion, buspirone
Calan, Colace
calcifediol, calcitriol
Capitrol, captopril
Cardene, Cardizem
Cardene, codeine
cefazolin, cefprozil
cefotaxime, ceftizoxime
cefuroximine, deferoxamine
Cefzil, Kefzol
Celebrex, Celexa
Celebrex, Cerebyx
chlorpromazine, chlorpropamide, promethazine
Ciloxan, Cytoxan
ciprofloxacin, ofloxacin
Clinoril, Clozaril
clofazimine, clonidine, clozapine
clomiphene, clomipramine
clonazepam, clorazepate
clonidine, quinidine
clotrimazole, co-trimoxazole
codeine, **Lodine**
Coreg, Zomig
Cozaar, Zocor
cyclobenzaprine, cyproheptadine
cycloserine, cyclosporine
dacarbazine, procarbazine
dactinomycin, daunorubicin
danazol, **Dantrium**
dapsone, **Diprosone**
Darvon, Diovan
daunorubicin, idarubicin
Decadron, Percodan
desipramine, imipramine
Desogen, desonide
desoximetasone, dexamethasone
Desoxyn, digitoxin, digoxin
diazepam, **Ditropan**
diazoxide, **Dyazide**
dimenhydrinate, diphenhydramine
Diprivan, Ditropan

(continued)

Drug names that look or sound alike (continued)

dipyridamole, disopyramide
dobutamine, dopamine
doxapram, doxazosin, doxepin, doxycycline
Doxil, Paxil, Plavix
dronabinol, droperidol
dyclonine, dicyclomine
Dynacin, DynaCirc
Echogen, Epogen
Elavil, Equanil, Mellaril
Eldepryl, enalapril
Elmiron, Imuran
eloxatin, **Exelon**
enalapril, ramipril
Entex, Tenex, Xanax
ephedrine, epinephrine
esmolol, **Osmitrol**
Estraderm, Estratab, Estratest
Estraderm, Testoderm
ethosuximide, methsuximide
etidronate, etretinate
Eurax, Urex
Evista, E-vista
Femara, FemHRT
fenoprofen, flurbiprofen
Fioricet, Fiorinal
Flaxedil, Flexeril
Flomax, Fosamax
flunisolide, fluocinonide
fluoxetine, fluvastatin, fluvoxamine, paroxetine
flurazepam, temazepam
folic acid, folinic acid
Foradil, Toradol
fosinopril, lisinopril, **Risperdal**
fosphenytoin, phenytoin
furosemide, torsemide
glimepiride, glipizide, glyburide
Granulex, Regranex
guaifenesin, guanfacine
Haldol, Stadol
heparin, **Hepsera, Hespan**
Hycodan, Vicodin
hydralazine, hydroxyzine
hydromorphone, morphine
Hyperstat, Nitrostat
imipenem, **Omnipen**
imipramine, **Norpramin**
Inderal, Inderide, Isordil
Intropin, Isoptin
Lamasil, Lomotil
Lamictal, Lamisil
lamivudine, lamotrigine
Lanoxin, Lasix, Lonox
Levatol, Lipitor
Levbid, Lithobid
Levitra, Raptiva
Librax, Librium
Loniten, Lotensin, lovastatin
Lorabid, Slo-bid
losartan, valsartan
Mandol, nadolol
Maxidex, Maxzide
Mazicon, Mevacor, Mivacron
mebendazole, methimazole
meclizine, memantine
melphalan, **Mephyton**
meperidine, meprobamate
Mesantoin, Mestinon
metaproterenol, metoprolol
methicillin, mezlocillin
methotrexate, metolazone
metoprolol, misoprostol
minoxidil, **Monopril**
mithramycin, mitomycin
naloxone, naltrexone
Naprelan, Naprosyn
Navane, Nubain
nelfinavir, nevirapine
Neurontin, Noroxin
niacinamide, nicardipine
nicardipine, nifedipine, nimodipine
Norpace, Norpramin
Ocufen, Ocuflox
olanzapine, olsalazine
Orinase, Ornade
oxaprozin, oxazepam
oxycodone, **OxyContin**

paclitaxel, paroxetine
Panadol, pindolol, **Plendil**
pancuronium, pipecuronium
Parlodel, pindolol
paroxetine, pralidoxime, pyridoxine
Pelamine, pemoline
pentobarbital, phenobarbital
pentosan, pentostatin
Percocet, Percodan, Procet
Phenaphen, Phenergan
phenelzine, **Phenylzin**
phentermine, phentolamine
pioglitazone, rosiglitazone
Pitocin, Pitressin
Pravachol, Prevacid
Pravachol, propranolol
prednisolone, prednisone, primidone
Premarin, Primaxin
Prilosec, Prinivil, Proventil
Prilosec, Prozac
ProAmatine, protamine
probenecid, **Procanbid**
promazine, promethazine
Proscar, Provera, Prozac
protamine, **Protopam, Protropin**
Quarzan, Questran
quinidine, quinine
ranitidine, rimantadine
Relpax, Revex, Revia
Reminyl, Robinul
reserpine, **Risperdal**
Restoril, Vistaril
Retrovir, ritonavir
ribavirin, riboflavin
rifabutin, rifampin
Rifadin, Rifamate, Rifater
Rifadin, Ritalin, ritodrine
Roxanol, Roxicet
Salbutamol, salmeterol
saquinavir, **Sinequan**
selegiline, **Stelazine**
Septa, Septra
Serentil, Serevent
Seroquel, Serzone
Solu-Cortef, Solu-Medrol
somatropin, sumatriptan
Spiriva, Stalevo
Sufenta, Survanta
sulfadiazine, sulfasalazine, sulfisoxazole
sumatriptan, zolmitriptan
Tambocor, tamoxifen
tegaserod, **Tegretol, Toradol**
Tequin, Ticlid
terbinafine, terbutaline, terfenadine
terbutaline, tolbutamide
terconazole, tioconazole
testolactone, testosterone
thiamine, **Thorazine**
tiagabine, tizanidine
Ticar, Tigan
Timoptic, Viroptic
Tobradex, Tobrex
tolazamide, tolbutamide
tolnaftate, **Tornalate**
Trandate, Tridate
Trendar, Trental
tretinoin, trientine
triamcinolone, **Triaminicin, Triaminicol**
triaminic, **Triaminicin**
triamterene, trimipramine
trifluoperazine, triflupromazine
Ultracef, Ultracet
Urised, Urispas
valacyclovir, valganciclovir
Vancenase, Vanceril
Vanceril, Vansil
VePesid, Versed
verapamil, **Verelan**
Verelan, Virilon
vinblastine, vincristine, vindesine, vinorelbine
Wellbutrin, Wellcovorin, Wellferon
Xanax, Zantac
Zantac, Zyrtec
Zestril, Zostrix
Zocor, Zoloft
Zofran, Zosyn
Zymar, Zyprexa, Zyrtec

Tablets and capsules *not* to crush

Crushing extended-release or other long-acting oral drug forms can cause the ingredients to be released all at once instead of gradually. Similarly, crushing can break the coating of enteric-coated drugs, leading to GI irritation. Other drugs may taste bad or have carcinogenic or teratogenic potential when crushed. Never crush the trade-name drugs listed below.

Accutane
Aciphex
Adalat CC
Aerolate
Aggrenox
Allegra D
Artane Sequels
Arthrotec
Asacol
Bayer EC
Bellergal-S
Biaxin XL
Boniva
Calan SR
Carbatrol
Carbiset-TR
Cardene SR
Cardizem CD, LA, SR
Carter's Little Pills
Cartia XT
Ceclor CD
CellCept
Choledyl SA
Claritin-D
Colace
Colestid
Compazine Spansules
Concerta
Cotazym-S
Covera-HS
Creon
Cytovene
Cytoxan
Deconamine SR
Depakene
Depakote
Desoxyn Gradumets
Dexedrine Spansule
Diamox Sequels
Dilacor XR
Dilatrate-SR
Disobrom
Ditropan XL
Donnatal Extentabs
Donnazyme
Drixoral
Dulcolax
DynaCirc CR
Easprin
Ecotrin
Effexor XR
Entex LA
Erythromycin Base
Eskalith CR
Factive
Feocyte
Feosol
Ferro-Sequel
Feratab
Flomax
Glucotrol XL
Guaifed
Ilotycin
Imdur
Inderal LA
Inderide LA
Indocin SR
Isoptin SR
Isordil Sublingual, Tembids
Isosorbide Dinitrate Sublingual
Kadian
Kaon-Cl
K-Dur
Klor-Con
Klotrix
K-Tab
Levbid
Levsinex Timecaps
Lexxel
Lithobid

Lodine XL
Lodrane LD
Macrobid
Mestinon Timespans
Methylin ER
Micro-K Extencaps
Monafed
MS Contin
Naldecon
Naprelan
Nexium
Nia-Bid
Niaspan
Nicotinic Acid
Nitro-Bid
Nitroglyn
Nitrong
Nitrostat
Norflex
Norpace CR
Novafed A
Oramorph SR
OxyContin
Pancrease MT
PCE
Pentasa
Perdiem
Phazyme
Phyllocontin
Plendil
Pneumomist
Prelu-2
Prevacid
Prilosec
Pro-Banthine
Procainamide HCL SR
Procardia
Proscar
Protonix
Proventil Repetabs
Prozac
Quibron-T/SR
Quinaglute Dura-Tabs
Quinidex Extentabs
Respaire SR
Respbid
Reyataz
Ritalin-SR
Roxanol SR
Ru-Tuss
Sinemet CR
Slo-bid Gyrocaps
Slo-Niacin
Slo-Phyllin GG, Gyrocaps
Slow FE
Slow-K
Slow-Mag
Sorbitrate SA
Striant
Sudafed 12 Hour
Sular
Sustaire
Tavist-D
Tegretol-XR
Teldrin
Ten-K
Tenuate Dospan
Tessalon Perles
Theobid Duracaps
Theochron
Theoclear LA
Theo-Dur
Theolair-SR
Theo-Sav
Theospan-SR
Theo-24
Theovent
Theo-X
Thorazine Spansules
Tiazac
Toprol XL
T-Phyl
Tranxene-SD
Trental
Triaminic
Trilafon Repetabs
Trinalin Repetabs
Tuss-Ornade Spansules
Tylenol Extended Relief
Ultrase MT
Uniphyl
Verelan
Volmax
Voltaren, XR
Wellbutrin SR, XL
Xanax-XR
ZORprin
Zyban
Zymase

Identifying injection sites

Injection sites vary with administration route. The instructions below describe proper identification sites for I.M., subcutaneous, and I.V. drugs.

To begin, wash your hands, put on gloves, and locate the appropriate site. Clean the site with an alcohol pad, and administer the injection as described here.

I.M. injections

You can administer an I.M. injection into the muscles shown below. In these illustrations, specific injection sites are shaded.

Deltoid site

- Locate the lower edge of the acromial process.
- Insert the needle 1" to 2" below the acromial process at a 90-degree angle.

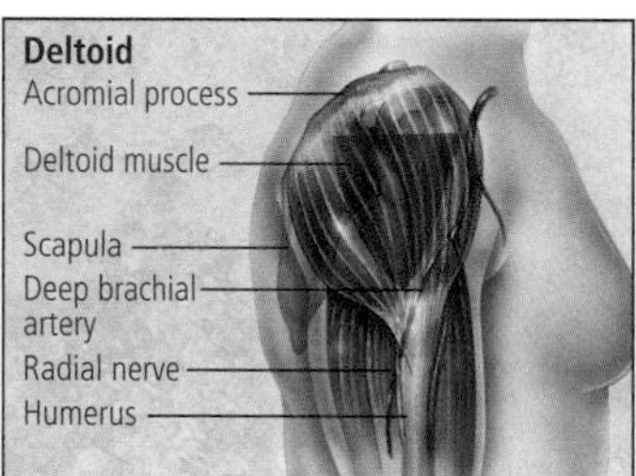

Dorsogluteal site

- Draw an imaginary line from the posterior superior iliac spine to the greater trochanter.
- Insert the needle at a 90-degree angle above and outside the drawn line.
- You can administer a Z-track injection through this site. After drawing up the drug, change the needle, displace the skin lateral to the injection site, withdraw the needle, and then release the skin.

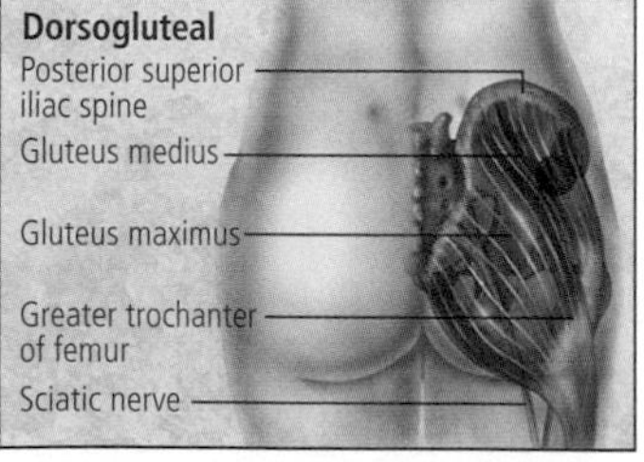

Ventrogluteal site

- With the palm of your hand, locate the greater trochanter of the femur.
- Spread your index and middle fingers posteriorly from the anterior superior iliac spine to the furthest area possible. This is the correct injection site.
- Remove your fingers and insert the needle at a 90-degree angle.

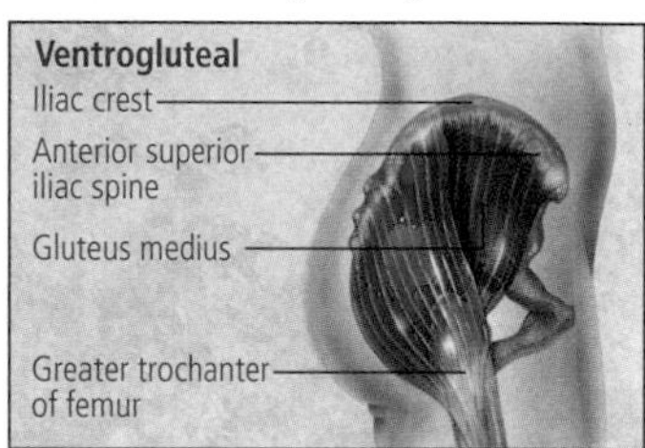

Vastus lateralis and rectus femoris sites

- Find the lateral quadriceps muscle for the vastus lateralis, or the anterior thigh for the rectus femoris.
- Insert the needle at a 90-degree angle into the middle third of the muscle, parallel to the skin surface.

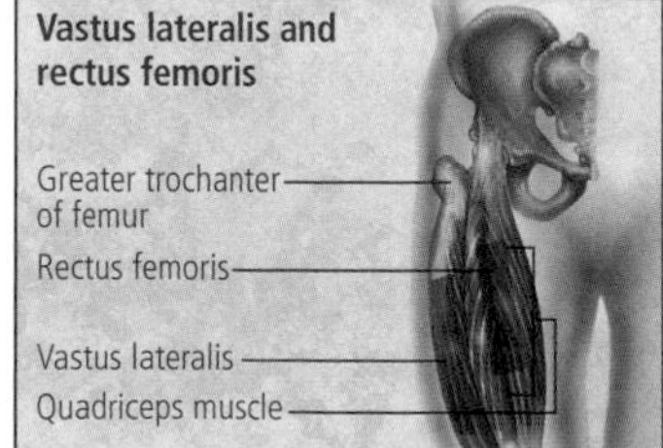

Subcutaneous injections

Subcutaneous drugs can be injected into the fat pads on the abdomen, buttocks, upper back, and lateral upper arms and thighs (shaded in the illustrations below). If your patient requires frequent subcutaneous injections, make sure to rotate injection sites.

- Gently gather and elevate or spread subcutaneous tissue.
- Insert the needle at a 45- or 90-degree angle, depending on the drug or the amount of subcutaneous tissue at the site.

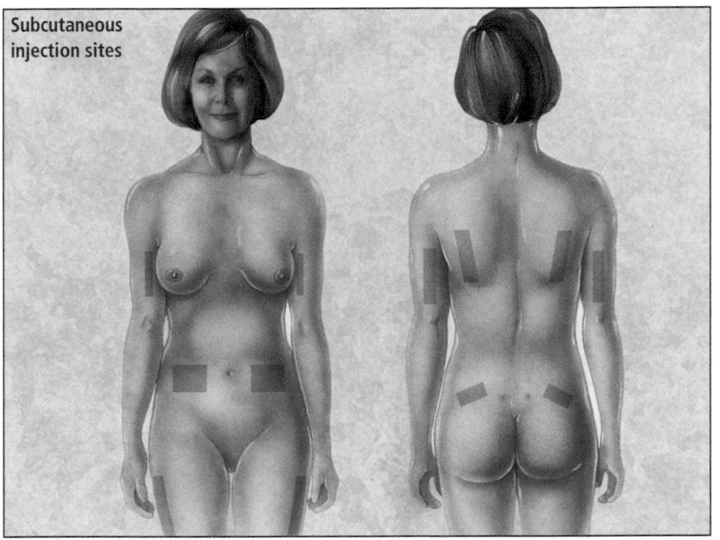

I.V. injections

I.V. drugs can be injected into the veins of the arms and hands. The illustration at right shows commonly used sites.

- Locate the vein using a tourniquet.
- Insert the catheter at a slight angle (about 10 degrees).
- Release the tourniquet when blood appears in the syringe or tubing.
- Slowly inject the drug into the vein.

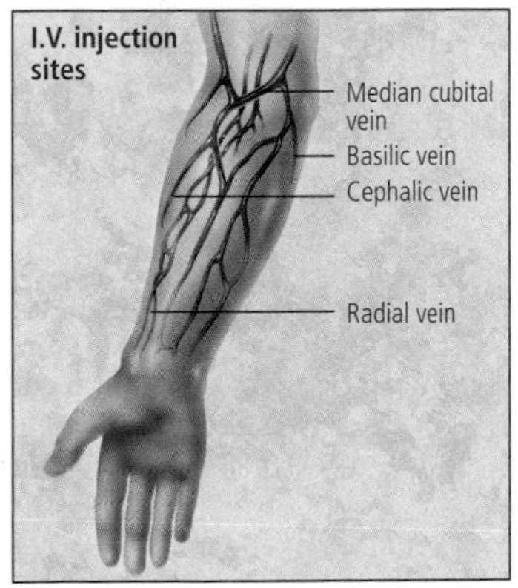

Monitoring blood levels

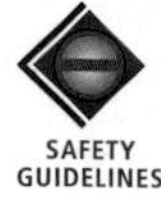

The table below shows therapeutic and toxic blood levels for selected drugs. Keep in mind that such levels may vary slightly among laboratories.

Drug	Therapeutic blood level	Toxic blood level
acetaminophen	10 to 20 mcg/ml	> 150 mcg/ml
alprazolam	0.025 to 0.102 mcg/ml	Not defined
amikacin	Peak: 25 to 35 mcg/ml	> 35 mcg/ml
	Trough: 5 to 10 mcg/ml	> 10 mcg/ml
aminophylline	10 to 20 mcg/ml	> 20 mcg/ml
amiodarone	1 to 2.5 mcg/ml	> 2.5 mcg/ml
amitriptyline	120 to 250 ng/ml	> 500 ng/ml
amobarbital	1 to 5 mcg/ml	> 10 mcg/ml
atenolol	0.2 to 0.7 mcg/ml	35 mcg/ml
bepridil	1 to 2 ng/ml	> 2 ng/ml
calcium	9 to 10.5 mg/dl	> 12 mg/dl
carbamazepine	4 to 14 mcg/ml	> 15 mcg/ml
clonazepam	10 to 80 ng/ml	> 100 ng/ml
creatinine	0.6 to 1.2 mg/dl	> 4 mg/dl
cyclosporine	50 to 300 ng/ml	> 400 ng/ml
desipramine	115 to 300 ng/ml	> 400 ng/ml
diazepam	0.5 to 2 mcg/ml	> 3 mcg/ml
digoxin	0.8 to 2 ng/ml	Adults: > 2.5 ng/ml
	Trough (> 12 hours after dose):	Children: > 3 ng/ml
	Heart failure: 0.8 to 1.5 ng/ml	
	Arrhythmias: 1.5 to 2 ng/ml	
diltiazem	0.05 to .40 mcg/ml	3.7 to 6.1 mcg/ml
diphenylhydantoin	10 to 20 mcg/ml	20 to 50 mcg/ml
disopyramide	2 to 8 mcg/ml	> 8 mcg/ml
ethchlorvynol	2 to 8 mcg/ml	> 20 mcg/ml
ethosuximide	40 to 100 mcg/ml	> 100 mcg/ml
flecainide	0.2 to 1 mcg/ml	> 1 mcg/ml
fluconazole	5 to 15 mcg/ml	Not defined
fluoxetine	0.09 to 0.40 mcg/ml	Not defined
gentamicin	Peak: 4 to 12 mcg/ml	> 12 mcg/ml
	Trough: 1 to 2 mcg/ml	> 2 mcg/ml
glucose	70 to 110 mg/dl	> 300 mg/dl
glutethimide	2 to 6 mcg/ml	> 5 mcg/ml
haloperidol	5 to 20 ng/ml	> 20 ng/ml
hydromorphone	0.008 to 0.049 mcg/ml	Not defined

Drug	Therapeutic blood level	Toxic blood level
imipramine	225 to 300 ng/ml	> 500 ng/ml
kanamycin	Peak: 25 to 35 mcg/ml	> 35 to 40 mcg/ml
	Trough (mild to moderate infection): 1 to 4 mcg/ml	> 10 to 15 mcg/ml
	Trough (severe infection): 4 to 8 mcg/ml	> 10 to 15 mcg/ml
lidocaine	1.5 to 6 mcg/ml	> 6 mcg/ml
lithium	0.6 to 1.2 mEq/L	> 1.5 mEq/L
lorazepam	50 to 240 ng/ml	300 to 600 ng/ml
magnesium	12 to 32 mcg/ml	80 to 120 mcg/ml
meperidine	100 to 550 ng/ml	> 1,000 ng/ml
meprobamate	6 to 12 mcg/ml	> 60 mcg/ml
methsuximide	10 to 40 mcg/ml	> 44 mcg/ml
metoprolol	0.03 to 0.27 mcg/ml	Not defined
mezlocillin	35 to 45 mcg/ml	> 45 mcg/ml
milrinone	150 to 250 ng/ml	> 250 ng/ml
nifedipine	0.025 to 0.1 mcg/ml	> 0.1 mcg/ml
nortriptyline	50 to 140 ng/ml	> 300 ng/ml
oxazepam	0.2 to 1.4 mcg/ml	> 2 mcg/ml
paroxetine	0.031 to 0.062 mcg/ml	Not defined
phenobarbital	10 to 40 mcg/ml	> 40 mcg/ml
phenytoin	10 to 20 mcg/ml	> 20 mcg/ml
potassium	3.5 to 5.0 mEq/L	> 6 mEq/L
primidone	4 to 12 mcg/ml	> 12 mcg/ml
procainamide	4 to 8 mcg/ml	> 10 mcg/ml
propofol	2 to 16 mcg/ml	Not defined
propranolol	50 to 200 ng/ml	> 200 ng/ml
quinidine	2 to 5 mcg/ml	> 5 mcg/ml
salicylates	100 to 300 mcg/ml	> 300 mcg/ml
sertraline	0.055 to 0.25 mcg/ml	Not defined
sodium	135 to 145 mEq/L	> 160 mEq/L
streptomycin	25 mcg/ml	> 25 mcg/ml
theophylline	10 to 20 mcg/ml	> 20 mcg/ml
tobramycin	Peak: 4 to 12 mcg/ml	> 12 mcg/ml
	Trough: 1 to 2 mcg/ml	> 2 mcg/ml
tocainide	4 to 10 mcg/ml	Not defined
valproic acid	50 to 100 mcg/ml	> 100 mcg/ml
vancomycin	Peak: 20 to 40 mcg/ml	> 40 mcg/ml
	Trough: 5 to 15 mcg/ml	> 15 mcg/ml
verapamil	0.08 to 0.3 mcg/ml	Not defined
zolpidem	0.003 to 0.018 mcg/ml	Not defined

Effects of dialysis on drug therapy

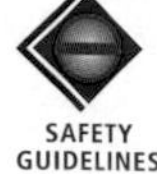

A patient receiving a drug that's removed by hemodialysis (HD) or peritoneal dialysis (PD) will need supplemental doses of that drug. The chart below shows which drugs are removed by dialysis and therefore will necessitate supplemental dosing during or after dialysis. Drugs listed as "unlikely" haven't been studied; however, because of their chemical properties, dialysis is unlikely to remove them.

Generic drug	Removed by HD	Removed by PD
acetaminophen	Yes	No
acyclovir	Yes	No
adenosine	Unlikely	Unlikely
albumin	Unlikely	Unlikely
alendronate	No	No data
allopurinol	Yes	No data
alprazolam	No	Unlikely
amikacin	Yes	Yes
amiodarone	No	No
amitriptyline	No	No
amlodipine	No	No
amoxicillin	Yes	No
amphotericin B	No	No
ampicillin	Yes	No
ascorbic acid	Yes	Yes
aspirin	Yes	Yes
atenolol	Yes	No
atorvastatin	No	Unlikely
aztreonam	Yes	No
bleomycin	No	No
bumetanide	No	Unlikely
bupropion	No	No
buspirone	No	No data
candesartan	No	No data
captopril	Yes	No
carbamazepine	No	No
carbenicillin	Yes	No
carboplatin	Yes	No data
carisoprodol	Yes	Yes
carmustine	No	No data
cefaclor	Yes	Yes
cefadroxil	Yes	No
cefazolin	Yes	No
cefepime	Yes	Yes
cefmetazole	Yes	No
cefonicid	No	No
cefoperazone	No	No
cefotaxime	Yes	No
cefotetan	Yes	Yes
cefoxitin	Yes	No
cefpodoxime	Yes	No
ceftazidime	Yes	Yes
ceftriaxone	No	No
cefuroxime	Yes	No
cephalexin	Yes	No
chloramphenicol	Yes	No
chlorpheniramine	Yes	No
cimetidine	No	No
ciprofloxacin	No	No
citalopram	No	Unlikely
clindamycin	No	No
clofibrate	No	No
clonazepam	No	Unlikely
clonidine	No	No
codeine	No	Unlikely
colchicine	No	No
cyclophosphamide	Yes	No data
cyclosporine	No	No
dapsone	Yes	No data
desipramine	No	No
dexamethasone	No	No
diazepam	No	Unlikely
diazoxide	Yes	Yes
dicloxacillin	No	No
digoxin	No	No
diltiazem	No	No
diphenhydramine	Unlikely	Unlikely
divalproex	No	No
dobutamine	No	No
dopamine	No	Unlikely
doxazosin	No	No

Generic drug	Removed by HD	Removed by PD
doxepin	No	No
doxycycline	No	No
drotrecogin alfa	Unlikely	Unlikely
edetate calcium	Yes	Yes
enalapril	Yes	Yes
exoxaparin	No	Unlikely
epinephrine	No data	No data
epoetin alfa	No	No
ertapenem	Yes	No data
erythromycin	No	No
esmolol	Yes	Yes
estradiol	No	No data
ethacrynic acid	No	Unlikely
etoposide	No	No
famciclovir	Yes	No data
famotidine	No	No
felodipine	No	Unlikely
fenofibrate	No	Unlikely
filgrastim	No	Unlikely
flecainide	No	Unlikely
fluconazole	Yes	Yes
flucytosine	Yes	Yes
fluoxetine	No	No
folic acid	Yes	No data
foscarnet	Yes	No data
furosemide	No	Unlikely
gabapentin	Yes	No data
ganciclovir	Yes	No data
gemfibrozil	No	No
gentamicin	Yes	Yes
glyburide	No	Unlikely
haloperidol	No	No
heparin	No	No
hydralazine	No	No
hydrochlorothiazide	No	Unlikely
hydrocodone	No data	No data
hydromorphone	No data	No data
hydroxyzine	No	No
ibuprofen	No	Unlikely
ibutilide	No data	No data
imipenem	Yes	Yes
imipramine	No	No
indomethacin	No	Unlikely
insulin	No	No
irbesartan	No	No data

Generic drug	Removed by HD	Removed by PD
isoniazid	No	No
isosorbide dinitrate	No	No
isosorbide mononitrate	Yes	No
isradipine	No	No
ketoconazole	No	No
ketoprofen	Unlikely	Unlikely
labetalol	No	No
lansoprazole	No	Unlikely
levetiracetam	Yes	No data
levofloxacin	Unlikely	Unlikely
lidocaine	No	Unlikely
linezolid	Yes	No data
lisinopril	Yes	No data
lithium	Yes	Yes
loracarbef	Yes	No data
loratadine	No	No
lorazepam	No	Unlikely
losartan	No	No
lovastatin	Unlikely	Unlikely
loxapine	No data	No data
mannitol	Yes	Yes
maprotiline	No	Unlikely
melphalan	No	No data
meperidine	No	Unlikely
mercaptopurine	Yes	No data
meropenem	Yes	No data
mesalamine	Yes	Unlikely
mesna	No data	No data
metformin	Yes	No data
methadone	No	No
methicillin	No	No
methotrexate	Yes	No
methyldopa	Yes	Yes
methylprednisolone	Yes	No data
metoclopramide	No	No
metoprolol	Yes	No data
metronidazole	Yes	No
mexiletine	Yes	No
mezlocillin	Yes	No
miconazole	No	No
midazolam	No	Unlikely
minoxidil	Yes	Yes
morphine	No data	No

(continued)

Generic drug	Removed by HD	Removed by PD
nadolol	Yes	No data
nafcillin	No	No
nalbuphine	No data	No data
naloxone	No data	No data
naltrexone	No data	No data
naproxen	No	Unlikely
neomycin	Yes	yes
nicardipine	No	Unlikely
nifedipine	No	No
nilutamide	No data	No data
nimodipine	No	No
nitrofurantoin	Yes	No data
nitroglycerin	No	No
nitroprusside	Yes	Yes
nortriptyline	No	No
octreotide	Yes	No data
ofloxacin	Yes	No
olanzapine	No	No
omeprazole	Unlikely	Unlikely
ondansetron	Unlikely	Unlikely
oxazepam	No	Unlikely
oxycodone	No data	No data
paclitaxel	No	Unlikely
pancuronium	No data	No data
pantoprazole	No	No data
paroxetine	No	Unlikely
penicillin	Yes	No
phenobarbital	Yes	Yes
phenytoin	No	No
piperacillin	Yes	No
pravastatin	No	No data
prazepam	No	Unlikely
prazosin	No	No
prednisone	No	No
primidone	Yes	No data
procainamide	Yes	No
promethazine	No	No data
propafenone	No	No
propofol	Unlikely	Unlikely
propoxyphene	No	No
propranolol	No	No
propylthiouracil	No	No data
pseudoephedrine	No	Unlikely
quinapril	No	No
quinidine	No; removed by hemoperfusion	No

Generic drug	Removed by HD	Removed by PD
quinine	No	No
ramipril	No	No data
ranitidine	No	No
reserpine	No	No
reteplase	No data	No data
rifampin	No	No
risperidone	No data	No data
ritodrine	Yes	Yes
ritonavir	Unlikely	No
rosiglitazone	No	Unlikely
rosuvastatin	No	No data
salsalate	Yes	No
sertraline	No	Unlikely
simvastatin	Unlikely	Unlikely
sotalol	Yes	No data
stavudine	Yes	No data
streptomycin	Yes	Yes
sulbactam	Yes	No
sulfamethoxazole	Yes	No
sulfisoxazole	Yes	Yes
tamoxifen	No data	No data
tazobactam	Yes	No
temazepam	No	Unlikely
terazosin	No	No
tetracycline	No	No
theophylline	Yes	No
thiamine	No	Unlikely
ticarcillin	Yes	No
timolol	No	No
tirofiban	Yes	No data
tobramycin	Yes	Yes
torsemide	No	Unlikely
tramadol	No	No data
trimethoprim	Yes	No
valacyclovir	Yes	No
valproic acid	No	No
valsartan	No	Unlikely
vancomycin	No	No
venlafaxine	No	Unlikely
verapamil	No	No
warfarin	No	No
zalcitabine	No data	No data
ziprasidone	No	Unlikely
zolpidem	No	Unlikely

Anaphylaxis: Treatment guidelines

A hypersensitivity reaction may occur when a patient comes in contact with a certain agent, such as a drug, food, or other foreign protein. In some patients, this reaction progresses to life-threatening anaphylaxis, marked by sudden development of urticaria and respiratory distress. If this reaction continues, it may precipitate vascular collapse, leading to shock and, occasionally, death.

Hypersensitivity reaction

↓

Adults: Epinephrine 0.2 to 0.5 ml of 1:1,000 solution subcutaneously; repeat q 10 to 15 minutes to maximum dosage of 1 mg.
Children: Epinephrine 10 mcg/kg of 1:1,000 solution subcutaneously, to maximum of 500 mcg/dose; may repeat q 15 minutes for 2 doses, then q 4 hours p.r.n.

↓

Adults or children: Diphenhydramine 1 to 2 mg/kg I.V.

↓

Adults: Hydrocortisone 100 mg I.V. initially; then administer as indicated.
Children: Hydrocortisone 0.16 to 1 mg/kg I.V. given once or twice daily

↓

If poor response, use anaphylaxis algorithm.

Anaphylaxis

↓

Administer CPR if patient loses circulation or breathing; follow Advanced Cardiac Life Support guidelines.

↓

If hypotension occurs, give vasopressors (such as dopamine, norepinephrine, or neosynephrine). Provide fluid resuscitation with large volumes of normal saline or lactated Ringer's solution.

↓

Adults and children: If bronchospasm occurs, give 1 to 2 inhalations of inhaled bronchodilator and consider loading dose of 6 mg/kg theophylline I.V., followed by maintenance dose as indicated.

↓

Adults: Epinephrine 0.2 to 0.5 ml of 1:1,000 solution subcutaneously; repeat q 10 to 15 minutes to maximum dosage of 1 mg.
Children: Epinephrine 10 mcg/kg of 1:1,000 solution subcutaneously, to maximum of 500 mcg/dose; may repeat dose q 15 minutes for 2 doses, then q 4 hours as needed

↓

If patient doesn't respond to subcutaneous epinephrine, dilute epinephrine to yield 1:10,000 solution. For adults, infuse at 1 mcg/minute; may titrate to 2 to 10 mcg/minute. For children, infuse at 0.1 mcg/kg/minute.

KEY:
CPR: cardiopulmonary resuscitation

Adult cardiac arrest: Treatment guidelines

If you suspect your patient is in cardiac arrest, take appropriate steps, as described below.

↓

Assess responsiveness.

↓

Unresponsive
Begin primary survey.
Activate emergency response system.
Call for defibrillator.
Assess breathing (open airway; look, listen, and feel for breathing).

↓

Not breathing
Give two slow breaths.
Assess pulse; if pulseless, start chest compressions.
Attach monitor or defibrillator (if available).

↓

No pulse
Continue CPR.
Assess heart rhythm.

↓ (left branch)

VF or VT on monitor
Attempt defibrillation (up to three shocks if VF/VT persists).

↓

Administer CPR for 1 minute. (→ return to *No pulse*; ↓ Conduct secondary ABCD survey)

↓ (right branch)

Asystole or PEA on monitor

↓

Administer CPR for up to 3 minutes. (→ return to *No pulse*; ↓ Conduct secondary ABCD survey)

Conduct secondary ABCD survey

Airway: Attempt to insert airway device.
Breathing: Confirm and secure airway device; provide ventilation and oxygenation.
Circulation: Obtain I.V. access; administer adrenergic drug; consider antiarrhythmics, buffer agents, and pacing.
For asystole or PEA, give epinephrine 1 mg I.V.; repeat every 3 to 5 minutes.
For VF/VT, give vasopressin 40 units I.V. for one dose, or give epinephrine 1 mg I.V., repeated every 3 to 5 minutes.
Differential diagnosis: Search for and treat reversible causes.

KEY ABCD: airway, breathing, circulation, differential diagnosis
CPR: cardiopulmonary resuscitation
PEA: pulseless electrical activity
VF: ventricular fibrillation
VT: ventricular tachycardia

Source: American Heart Association

Pediatric cardiac arrest: Treatment guidelines

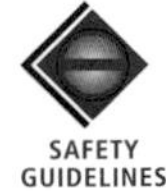

For a pediatric patient in suspected cardiac arrest, take the following steps.

↓

Assess responsiveness.

↓

Unresponsive
Begin primary survey.
Activate emergency response system.
Call for defibrillator.
Assess breathing (open airway; look, listen, and feel for breathing).

↓

Not breathing
Give two slow breaths.
Assess pulse. Start chest compressions if patient is pulseless.

↓

No pulse
Continue CPR.
Assess heart rhythm.

↓

VF or VT on monitor
Attempt defibrillation (up to three shocks if VF/VT persists).
First shock: 2 J/kg; second shock: 2 to 4 J/kg; subsequent shocks: 4 J/kg.
Then repeat sequence of CPR, drugs*, defibrillation, rhythm assessment.

Asystole or PEA on monitor
Give epinephrine 0.01 mg/kg (0.1 ml/kg of 1:10,000 solution) I.V. or I.O.
Continue CPR for 3 minutes; then reassess heart rythm.

↓

Conduct secondary ABCD survey
Airway: Attempt to insert airway device.
Breathing: Confirm and secure airway device; ventilate and oxygenate.
Circulation: Obtain I.V. access; defibrillate and give drugs as appropriate.
*For VF/VT, give epinephrine 0.01 mg/kg (0.1 ml/kg of 1:10,000 solution) I.V. or I.O.; repeat q 3 to 5 minutes; then consider amiodarone or lidocaine.
For asystole, give epinephrine 0.01 mg/kg (0.1 ml/kg of 1:10,000 solution) I.V. or I.O.; repeat q 3 to 5 minutes.
Differential diagnosis: Search for and treat reversible causes, including hypoxemia, hypovolemia, metabolic disorders, and thromboembolism.

KEY
ABDC: airway, breathing, circulation, differential diagnosis
CPR: cardiopulmonary resuscitation
I.O.: intraosseus
J: joules
PEA: pulseless electrical activity
VF: ventricular fibrillation
VT: ventricular tachycardia

Source: American Heart Association

Ischemic chest pain: Treatment guidelines

Chest pain suggestive of ischemia

Immediate assessment (within 10 minutes):
- Measure vital signs and oxygen saturation.
- Obtain I.V. access, 12-lead ECG, and initial serum cardiac marker levels.
- Perform brief history and physical exam; focus on eligibility for fibrinolytic therapy.
- Evaluate initial electrolyte and coagulation studies.
- Request and review portable chest x-ray within 30 minutes.

Assess initial 12-lead ECG.

- ST elevation or new LBBB (strongly suggests injury) • ST-elevation AMI

Start adjunctive treatments (as indicated; no reperfusion delay):
- Beta-adrenergic blockers I.V.
- Nitroglycerin I.V., heparin I.V.
- ACE inhibitors (after 6 hours or when stable)

Time from symptom onset?

> 12 hours

< 12 hours

Choose reperfusion strategy based on local resources.
- Angiography
- PCI (angioplasty +/- stent)
- Cardiothoracic surgery backup

- If signs of cardiogenic shock, PCI is treatment of choice.
- If PCI not available, use fibrinolytics (if no contraindications).

Fibrinolytic therapy chosen:
- front-loaded alteplase or
- streptokinase or
- APSAC or
- reteplase or
- tenecteplase

Goal: Door-to-drug within 30 minutes

Primary PCI chosen:
- Door-to-balloon inflation within 30 minutes to 2 hours
- Experienced operators
- High-volume medical center
- Cardiac surgical capability

KEY
ACE: angiotensin-converting enzyme
AMI: acute myocardial infarction
APSAC: anisoylated plasminogen streptokinase activator complex
LBBB: left bundle-branch block
PCI: percutaneous coronary intervention

Source: American Heart Association

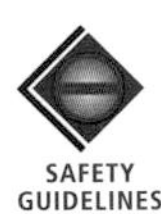

Immediate general treatment:
- Oxygen at 4 L/minute
- Aspirin 160 to 325 mg
- Nitroglycerin S.L. or spray
- Morphine I.V. (if nitroglycerin does not relieve pain)

Use MONA as memory aid: Morphine, Oxygen, Nitroglycerin, Aspirin.

EMS personnel can perform immediate assessment and treatment, including 12-lead ECG and review for fibrinolytic eligibility.

- ST depression or dynamic T-wave inversion (strongly suggests ischemia)
- High-risk unstable angina/non-ST-elevation AMI

- Non-diagnostic ECG: no ST segment or T-wave changes
- Intermediate- or low-risk unstable angina

Meets criteria for unstable or new-onset angina? Or troponin positive?

Yes → **Start adjunctive treatments** (as indicated, no contraindications):
- Heparin
- Aspirin 160 to 325 mg daily
- Glycoprotein IIb/IIIa inhibitors
- Nitroglycerin I.V.
- Beta-adrenergic receptor blockers

No → **Admit to ED (monitored bed).**
- Obtain serial serum markers (including troponin).
- Repeat ECG/continuous ST monitoring .
- Consider imaging study.

Assess clinical status.

High-risk patient, defined by:
- persistent symptoms
- recurrent ischemia
- depressed left ventricular function
- widespread ECG changes
- previous AMI, PCI, or CABG.

Perform cardiac catheterization. Anatomy suitable for revascularization?

Yes → **Revascularization:**
- PCI
- CABG

No → **Admit to critical care unit.**

Clinically stable?

Evidence of ischemia or infarction?

Yes → **Admit to critical care unit.**

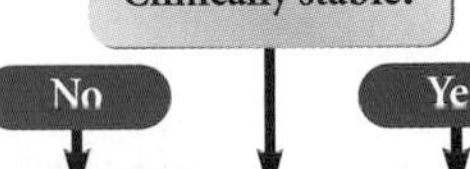

Admit to critical care unit.
- Continue or start treatment.
- Obtain serial cardiac markers and ECG.
- Consider imaging study.

No → Discharge acceptable

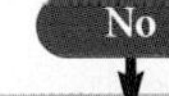

- Arrange follow-up

Stroke: Treatment guidelines

This algorithm for the treatment of cerebrovascular accident (stroke) or suspected stroke is based on the one created by the American Heart Association.

Suspected stroke

Within 10 minutes of arrival at ED:
- Assess ABCs and vital signs.
- Give oxygen.
- Obtain I.V. access; draw blood.
- Check blood glucose level; treat accordingly.
- Obtain 12-lead ECG.
- Perform neurocheck.
- Alert stroke team.

Within 25 minutes of arrival at ED:
- Review patient history.
- Establish symptom onset (< 3 hours required for fibrinolytics).
- Perform physical exam.
- Obtain noncontrast CT scan; read CT scan (< 45 minutes of arrival).
- Obtain lateral C-spine X-ray (if comatose or history of trauma).

CT scan shows intracerebral or subarachnoid hemorrhage (SAH)?

No

Probable ischemic stroke:
- CT scan exclusions?
- Improving neurologic deficits?
- Fibrinolytic exclusions?
- Symptom onset > 3 hours?

No to above

Patient is candidate for fibrinolytic therapy?

Yes

- Obtain informed consent.
- Begin fibrinolytic therapy within 1 hour of arrival at ED.
- Monitor neurologic status; obtain CT scan if condition deteriorates.
- Monitor BP; treat as indicated.
- Admit to CCU.
- Withhold anticoagulants and antiplatelet drugs for 24 hours.

No

Yes

Consult neurosurgery.

Treat for acute hemorrhage:
- Reverse anticoagulants and bleeding disorder.
- Monitor neurologic status.
- Treat hypertension if patient is conscious.

If high suspicion of SAH despite negative CT, perform LP.

Blood on LP

No blood on LP

Initiate supportive care.

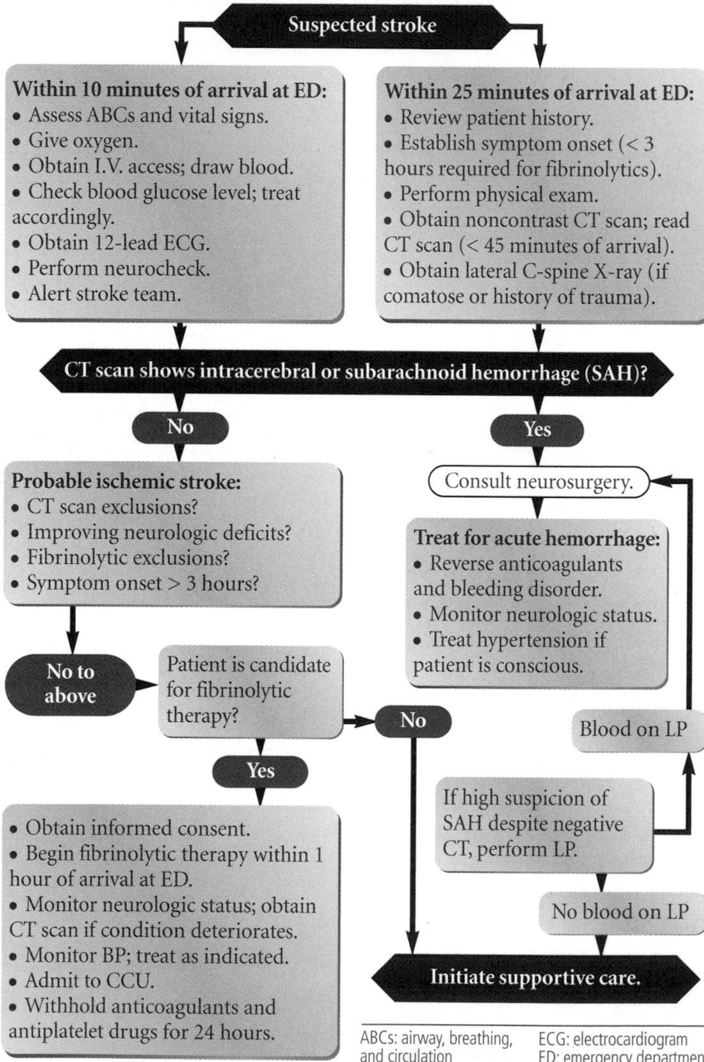

ABCs: airway, breathing, and circulation
BP: blood pressure
CCU: critical care unit
CT: computed tomography
ECG: electrocardiogram
ED: emergency department
LP: lumbar puncture
SAH: subarachnoid hemorrhage

Source: American Heart Association

Hypertensive crisis: Treatment guidelines

Hypertensive crisis is a severe blood pressure rise that can cause irreversible heart, brain, and kidney damage, and even death, unless treated promptly. Suspect this condition if systemic blood pressure is above 240/130 mm Hg without symptoms, or blood pressure is elevated with chest pain, headache, or heart failure.

↓

Immediately reduce blood pressure.
Do not reduce blood pressure by more than 25% of mean arterial pressure over first 2 hours. Consider arterial line insertion for continuous blood pressure monitoring.

↓

Initial drug choices

↓

Systemic blood pressure > 240/130 mm Hg without symptoms, or with headache	**Elevated blood pressure with chest pain or heart failure**	**Elevated blood pressure in pregnant woman with preeclampsia**
Begin nitroprusside I.V. at a rate of 0.1mcg/kg/minute; increase q 3 to 5 minutes to desired effect (maximum: 5 mcg/kg/minute) (drug of choice)	Nitroglycerin I.V. at a rate of 20 to 200 mcg/minute (drug of choice)	Hydralazine 5 to 10 mg I.V. q 20 minutes, to a maximum dosage of 20 mg (drug of choice)
or Fenoldopam I.V. at a rate of 0.05 to 1.6 mcg/kg/minute	**or** Nicardipine I.V. at a rate of 5 to 15 mg/hour	**or** Labetalol 20 mg I.V., followed by 40 mg I.V. 10 minutes later; then 80-mg doses at 10-minute intervals for 2 additional doses, to a maximum cumulative dosage of 220 mg
or Labetalol 20 mg I.V. initially; repeat injection q 10 minutes p.r.n., to maximum dosage of 300 mg	**or** Enalaprilat 1.25 to 5 mg I.V. q 6 hours	

↓

Begin oral antihypertensives when blood pressure decreases to a satisfactory level.

Hyperglycemic crisis: Treatment guidelines

If you suspect your patient has hyperglycemic crisis (also called diabetic ketoacidosis or DKA), complete the initial evaluation. DKA is present if the blood glucose level exceeds 250 mg/dl, arterial pH is below 7.3, bicarbonate level is below 15 mEq/L, and moderate ketonuria is present.

Give I.V. fluid.

Initially, give NSS I.V. at 15 to 20 ml/kg/hour.

When glucose level reaches 250 mg/dl, change to D_5 ½NSS at 150 to 250 ml/hour.

Give insulin.

Give regular insulin 0.15 units/kg as I.V. bolus.

Start infusion of regular insulin at 0.1 unit/kg/hour. If glucose level doesn't fall by 50 to 70 mg/dl in first hour, double the infusion rate q hour until level falls by 50 to 70 mg/dl.

Monitor serum K+ level.

$K^+ < 3.3$ mEq/L: Withhold insulin and give KCl or KPO_4 until level rises to 3.3 mEq/L or higher.

$K^+ \geq 5$ mEq/L: Monitor K^+ level q 2 hours.

$K^+ \geq 3.3$ mEq/L but < 5 mEq/L: Give 20 to 30 mEq KCl in each liter of I.V. fluid to maintain K^+ at 4 to 5 mEq/L.

Assess need for $NaHCO_{3-}$

pH < 6.9: Dilute 100 mmol $NaHCO_{3-}$ in 400 ml SWI; infuse at 200 ml/hour. Repeat dose until pH exceeds 7.0.

pH 6.9 to 7.0: Dilute 50 mmol $NaHCO_{3-}$ in 200 ml SWI; infuse at 200 ml/hour. Repeat $NaHCO_{3-}$ dose until pH exceeds 7.0.

pH > 7.0: Don't give $NaHCO_{3-}$.

Check electrolyte, BUN, creatinine, and glucose levels q 2 to 4 hours until stable. After DKA resolves, continue insulin infusion if patient is NPO status. When oral intake is tolerated, start subcutaneous insulin regimen. Continue I.V. infusion for 1 to 2 hours after subcutaneous insulin therapy begins.

KEY
BUN: blood urea nitrogen
D_5 ½NSS: dextrose 5% in half-normal saline solution
K^+: potassium
KCl: potassium chloride
KPO_4 : potassium phosphate
$NaHCO_{3-}$: sodium bicarbonate
NPO: nothing by mouth
NSS: normal saline solution
SWI: sterile water for injection

Insulin shock: Treatment guidelines

If your patient has signs or symptoms of hypoglycemia, immediately obtain a fingerstick blood glucose level. If the level is 60 mg/dl or lower, have a STAT venous blood glucose level drawn. Then, as appropriate, take the actions described below.

Mild hypoglycemia (fingerstick blood glucose 50 to 60 mg/dl):

Give 4 oz of orange or apple juice, 8 oz of skim milk, or 3 packets of sugar in small amount of water. (Don't give orange juice if serum potassium level is 5 mEq/ml or more or if patient's on dialysis.)

Recheck fingerstick blood glucose level in 15 minutes. If it's 80 mg/dl or lower, repeat treatment.

Observe patient closely for further signs and symptoms of hypoglycemia.

Recheck fingerstick blood glucose level in 1 hour.

Moderate hypoglycemia (fingerstick blood glucose 40 to 50 mg/dl):

Give 4 oz of orange or apple juice, 8 oz of skim milk, or 3 packets of sugar in small amount of water. (Do not give orange juice if serum potassium level is 5 mEq/ml or more or if patient's on dialysis.)

Observe patient closely for further signs and symptoms of hypoglycemia.

Recheck fingerstick blood glucose level in 15 minutes. If glucose remains < 60 mg/dl, consult physician; may give 1 vial dextrose 50% in water (25 g) I.V. over 15 minutes if patient can't take oral carbohydrate.

Severe hypoglycemia (fingerstick blood glucose 40 mg/dl or lower with unconscious or symptomatic patient, or conscious but argumentative patient):

Establish I.V. access; give 1 vial dextrose 50% in water I.V. over 15 minutes.

Monitor fingerstick blood glucose level q 15 minutes until it's 80 mg/dl or higher.

Provide diabetic meal or carbohydrate and protein snack as soon as patient is stable and can eat.

Follow-up care

Stay with the patient if he has moderate or severe hypoglycemia. Monitor blood pressure, heart rate, respiratory rate, and fingerstick blood glucose level every 15 minutes until it reaches 80 mg/dl or higher. Assess level of consciousness and institute safety precautions, as appropriate.

Managing poisonings and overdoses

This chart serves as a quick reference for managing poisonings and drug overdoses. For more detailed instructions, consult your local poison control center. To find your local center, call the American Association of Poison Control Centers at 1-800-222-1222 or visit http://www.aapcc.org/findyour.htm.

Poison or drug	Antidote and dosage
acetaminophen	**acetylcysteine (Acetadote, Mucomyst)** Give P.O. as 5% solution by diluting with carbonated diet beverage. Loading dose: One-time dose of 140 mg/kg. Repeat dose if patient vomits within 1 hour of administration. I.V. dose: 150 mg/kg over 15 minutes. Maintenance dose: 50 mg/kg infused over 4 hours, followed by 100 mg/kg infused over 16 hours.
alpha$_2$-adrenergic agonists opioids	**naloxone (Narcan)** *Adults:* 0.4 to 2 mg I.V., I.M., or subcutaneously; repeat q 2 to 3 minutes, p.r.n. Maximum dosage is 10 mg. *Children > age 5 or ≥ 20 kg:* 2 mg/dose I.V.; repeat q 2 to 3 minutes, p.r.n. *Children < age 5 or < 20 kg:* 0.1 mg/kg I.V.; repeat q 2 to 3 minutes, p.r.n. *Neonates:* Initially, 0.01 mg/kg I.V., repeated q 2 to 3 minutes p.r.n. ***Postoperative opioid-induced respiratory depression*** *Adults:* 0.1 to 0.2 mg I.V. q 2 to 3 minutes, p.r.n. If ordered, give initial adult dose of 0.1 mg I.V. to assess patient's response. Give subsequent doses of 0.4 mg or less (undiluted) by direct injection over 15 seconds, or titrate based on response. As needed, give continuous I.V. infusion, diluting 2 mg of naloxone with 500 ml of normal saline or dextrose 5% in water for a final concentration of 4 mcg/ml; titrate based on patient's response. *Children:* 0.005 to 0.01 mg/kg I.V. q 2 to 3 minutes, p.r.n.. **nalmefene (Revex)** Initially, 0.5 mg/70 kg I.V., followed by a second dose of 1 mg/70 kg I.V. 2 minutes later, if necessary. Doses greater than 1.5 mg/70 kg will likely not improve response and may precipitate withdrawal symptoms.
anticholinergic agents antihistamines atropine	**physostigmine (Antilirium)** *Adults:* 0.5 to 2 mg slow I.V. injection (not to exceed 1 mg/minute). May repeat q 20 minutes until response or adverse effects occur. If initial dose is effective, additional doses of 1 to 4 mg may be given q 30 to 60 minutes as life-threatening signs (arrythmias, seizures, deep coma) recur. *Children:* 0.02 mg/kg I.M. or slow I.V. injection (not to exceed 0.5 mg/minute). May repeat q 5 to 10 minutes until therapeutic response occurs or maximum dosage of 2 mg is given.

Poison or drug	Antidote and dosage
benzodiazepines	**flumazenil (Romazicon)** *Adults:* Initially, 0.2 mg I.V. injected over 30 seconds; follow with 0.3 mg if desired level of consciousness isn't reached. May give further doses of 0.5 mg at 60-second intervals until therapeutic response occurs or cumulative dosage of 3 mg is given. If partial response is achieved at 3 mg, rarely patients may need additional doses up to a total of 5 mg. If sedation recurs, repeat dose at 20-minute intervals. Maximum dosage is 3 mg/hour. *Children:* Initially 0.01 mg/kg (maximum dosage 0.2 mg) with repeat doses of 0.01 mg/kg (maximum dosage 0.2 mg) given q minute to maximum cumulative dosage of 1 mg.
cyanide	Antidote kit contains amyl nitrite, sodium nitrite, sodium thiosulfate. **amyl nitrite** *Adults and children:* Hold amyl nitrite inhalant close to patient's nose or mouth for 30 seconds each minute until I.V. can be established and sodium nitrite infusion started. **sodium nitrite** *Adults:* 300 mg (10 ml) I.V. over 5 minutes *Children:* 0.15 to 0.33 ml/kg, up to 10 ml I.V., over 5 minutes. Methylene blue may be given to adults and children who experience methemoglobinemia from excessive sodium nitrite dosage. Methylene blue dosage is 1 to 2 mg/kg or 25 to 50 mg/mm^2 I.V. infused very slowly over several minutes. If needed, a second dose may be given after 1 hour. Or, 100 to 300 mg P.O. daily. **sodium thiosulfate** Follow sodium nitrite infusion with sodium thiosulfate. *Adults and adolescents:* 12.5 g (50 ml) I.V. at a rate of 2.5 to 5 ml/minute. *Children:* 412.5 mg/kg or 7 g/mm^2 I.V. at a rate of 2.5 to 5 ml/minute.
digoxin	**digoxin immune Fab (Digibind, DigiFab)** Calculate dosage as number of 38-mg vials, using this formula: Digoxin level (in ng) × patient's weight (in kg) divided by 100. Usual dosage range is four to six vials. If ingested amount of digoxin is unknown, give 10 to 20 vials (380 to 800 mg) I.V. over 30 minutes through a 0.22-micron filter. May give bolus dose if cardiac arrest is imminent.
ethylene glycol	**fomepizole (Antizol)** Loading dose: 15 mg/kg I.V. over 30 minutes, followed by 10 mg/kg I.V. over 30 minutes q 12 hours for four doses Maintenance dose: 15 mg/kg I.V. over 30 minutes q 12 hours until ethylene glycol level falls below 20 mg/dl
heparin	**protamine sulfate** Dosage is based on partial thromboplastin time; usually, 1 mg for each 100 units of heparin. Give I.V. over 10 minutes (maximum rate of 5 mg/minute) in doses not exceeding 50 mg. Patients allergic to fish, vasectomized or infertile men, and patients taking protamine-insulin products are at increased risk for protamine hypersensitivity.

(continued)

Managing poisonings and overdoses (continued)

Poison or drug	Antidote and dosage
hypercalcemic emergency	**edetate disodium (Endrate)** *Adults:* 50 mg/kg/day by slow I.V. infusion over at least 3 hours, up to a maximum of 3 g/day. *Children:* 40 mg/kg/day by slow I.V. infusion over at least 3 hours, up to a maximum of 70 mg/kg/day. Dilute with normal saline solution or dextrose 5% in water; don't infuse rapidly. Keep patient in bed for 15 minutes after infusion to avoid orthostatic hypotension. Keep I.V. calcium readily available, because drug may cause profound hypocalcemia, leading to tetany, seizures, arrhythmias, and respiratory arrest. Alternate I.V. sites daily to decrease risk of thrombophlebitis. **Alert:** Do not confuse drug with edetate calcium disodium, used as lead poisoning antidote.
iron	**deferoxamine (Desferal)** ***Acute iron intoxication:*** Initially, 1 g I.M., followed by 500 mg q 4 hours for two doses depending on clinical response, and then 500 mg q 4 to 12 hours, up to 6 g/day. May give I.V. infusion of 10 to 15 mg/kg/hour for first 1 g. Subsequent doses shouldn't exceed 125 mg/hour. Maximum dosage is 6 g in 24 hours. *Chronic iron intoxication:* In adults, 1 to 2 g/day subcutaneously. In children, maximum dosage of 2 g/day subcutaneously.
lead	**edetate calcium disodium (Calcium Disodium Versenate)** ***Acute lead encephalopathy*** *Adults and children:* 1 to 1.5 g/m²/day I.V. or I.M. (preferred) in divided doses at 8- to 12-hour intervals for 5 days. A second course may be given after at least two drug-free days. ***Lead poisoning without encephalopathy*** *Children:* 1 g/m²/day I.V. or I.M. in divided doses for 5 days Dilute I.V. dose with 250 to 500 ml of normal saline solution or dextrose 5% in water. Rapid infusion may be lethal; infuse at rate suggested by manufacturer. Discontinue drug at first sign of renal toxicity. For I.M. injections only, may add procaine hydrochloride to minimize pain at injection site. **Alert:** Do not confuse drug with edetate disodium, used to treat hypercalcemia. **succimer (Chemet)** *Adults:* 10 mg/kg/dose P.O. q 8 hours for 5 days; then 10 mg/kg/dose q 12 hours for 14 days. ***Lead poisoning in children with blood lead levels above 45 mcg/dl*** *Children:* 10 mg/kg P.O. or 350 mg/m² P.O. q 8 hours for 5 days; then decrease to 10 mg/kg P.O. or 350 mg/m² P.O. q 12 hours for 14 days. Treatment lasts 19 days; repeated courses should follow 2-week rest period. Monitor CBC with white cell differential. Stop drug and contact prescriber if neutrophil count drops below 1,200/mm³.

Poison or drug	Antidote and dosage
opioid overdose and dependence	**naloxone hydrochloride (Narcan)** ***Opioid overdose*** *Adults:* 0.4 to 2 mg I.V., I.M., or subcutaneously; repeat q 2 to 3 minutes, p.r.n., up to 10 mg If ordered, give initial adult dose of 0.1 mg I.V. to assess patient's response. Give subsequent doses of 0.4 mg or less (undiluted) by direct injection over 15 seconds, or titrate based on response. As needed, give continuous I.V. infusion, diluting 2 mg of naloxone with 500 ml of normal saline solution or dextrose 5% in water for a final concentration of 4 mcg/ml; titrate based on patient's response. *Children > age 5 or ≥ 20 kg:* 2 mg/dose; repeat q 2 to 3 minutes. *Children < age 5 or < 20 kg:* 0.1 mg/kg; repeat q 2 to 3 minutes. ***Postoperative opioid-induced respiratory depression*** *Adults:* 0.1 to 0.2 mg I.V. q 2 to 3 minutes, p.r.n. *Children:* 0.005 to 0.01 mg/kg q 2 to 3 minutes. ***Opioid dependence*** **naltrexone (Depade, ReVia)** *Adults:* Initially, 25 mg P.O.; give an additional dose of 25 mg if no withdrawal symptoms occur within 1 hour. When patient is receiving 50 mg q 24 hours, a maintenance schedule of 50 to 150 mg/day P.O. may be used. Don't initiate therapy until patient has been opiate-free for 7 to 10 days; do not begin for opioid dependence until a naloxone challenge test has been given. **Alert:** Do not confuse naltrexone with naloxone.
organophosphate insecticides	**pralidoxime (Protopam)** *Adults:* 1 to 2 g I.V. in 100 ml of normal saline solution infused over 15 to 30 minutes. If pulmonary edema occurs, may give as 5% solution I.V. over 5 minutes. May repeat dose in 1 hour if muscle weakness persists; may give additional doses at 10- to 12-hour intervals cautiously if muscle weakness continues. *Children:* 20 to 50 mg/kg (up to 1 g) in 250 ml normal saline solution I.V. over 30 minutes
warfarin	**phytonadione (Vitamin K)** *Adults:* 2.5 to 10 mg subcutaneously. based on prothrombin time/ International Normalized Ratio; may repeat in 6 to 8 hours as needed. In emergency, 2.5 to 25 mg slow I.V. (no faster than 1 mg/minute); may repeat 6 to 8 hours after first dose.
miscellaneous drug overdose	**activated charcoal** *Adults:* 1 to 2 g/kg with at least a 10:1 ratio of activated charcoal to intoxicant (usual dose is 25 to 100 g charcoal in water or sorbitol) and administered P.O. or by nasogastric tube. Do not give doses greater than 100 g. *Children:* 1 to 2 g/kg or 25 to 50 g charcoal. The use of repeated oral charcoal with sorbitol doses is not recommended.

Preventing and treating extravasation

Extravasation—escape of a vesicant drug into surrounding tissues—can result from a damaged vein or from leakage around a venipuncture site. Vesicant drugs (such as daunorubicin and vincristine) can cause severe tissue damage if extravasation occurs.

To help prevent extravasation, make sure the existing I.V. line is patent before you administer a drug by the I.V. route. Check patency by:

- inspecting the site for edema or pain
- flushing the I.V. line with 0.9% sodium chloride solution
- gently aspirating blood from the catheter.

Alternatively, you may insert a new I.V. catheter to ensure correct catheter placement. For vesicant drugs, consider using a central venous catheter.

If extravasation occurs, stop the infusion at once. Aspirate the remaining drug from the catheter and remove the I.V. line (unless you need the catheter to administer an antidote). If the extravasated drug was daunorubicin or doxorubicin, apply a cold compress to the area; if it was vinblastine or vincristine, apply a warm compress. Then instill the appropriate antidote according to facility policy.

Administering antidotes

Antidotes for extravasation typically are either given through the existing I.V. line or injected subcutaneously around the infiltrated site using a 1-ml tuberculin syringe. Be sure to use a new needle for each antidote injection.

Extravasated drug	Antidote and dosage
• aminophylline • calcium solutions • contrast media • dextrose solutions (concentrations of 10% or more) • etoposide • nafcillin • potassium solutions • teniposide • total parenteral nutrition solutions • vinblastine • vincristine • vindesine	**hyaluronidase:** 15 units/ml, as 0.2 ml subcutaneous injection near extravasation site
• dactinomycin	**ascorbic acid injection:** 50 mg
• daunorubicin • doxorubicin	**hydrocortisone sodium succinate:** 100 mg/ml: 50 to 200 mg
• dobutamine • dopamine • epinephrine • metaraminol • norepinephrine	**phentolamine:** 5 to 10 mg diluted in 10 to 15 ml of normal saline solution, administered within 12 hours of extravasation
• mechlorethamine	**sodium thiosulfate 10%:** 10 ml

a

Indications and dosages

➢ Acute lymphocytic leukemia (given with other drugs, such as prednisone or vincristine, as part of antineoplastic regimen)
Children: 1,000 international units/kg I.V. daily for 10 successive days, with asparaginase initiated on day 22 of regimen, or 6,000 international units/m² I.M. on days 4, 7, 10, 13, 16, 19, 22, 25, and 28
➢ Sole agent used to induce remission of acute lymphocytic leukemia
Adults and children: 200 international units/kg I.V. daily for 28 days
➢ Drug desensitization regimen
Adults and children: Initially, 1 international unit I.V. Then double the dosage q 10 minutes until total planned daily dosage has been given.

Contraindications

- Hypersensitivity to drug
- Pancreatitis or history of pancreatitis

Precautions

Use cautiously in:
- bone marrow depression, hepatic or renal disease, CNS depression, clotting abnormalities, infection
- pregnant or breastfeeding patients
- women of childbearing age.

Administration

Administer intradermal skin test as ordered at start of therapy and when drug hasn't been given for 1 week or more.
- Follow prescriber's orders for drug desensitization when indicated (usually before therapy starts and again during retreatment).

Know that drug may be carcinogenic, mutagenic, or teratogenic. Follow appropriate facility policy for handling and preparing.
- Before starting drug, give allopurinol as prescribed to lower risk of neuropathy.
- Add sterile water or normal saline solution (5 ml for I.V. dose, 2 ml for I.M. dose) to powdered drug in vial.
- Filter through 5-micron filter.
- For I.V. use, inject into normal saline solution or dextrose 5% in water and infuse over 30 minutes.
- For I.M. use, give a maximum of 2 ml at any one site.
- Don't use solution unless it's clear.

If drug touches skin or mucous membranes, rinse with copious amounts of water for at least 15 minutes.
- Provide adequate fluid intake to prevent tumor lysis.

Route	Onset	Peak	Duration
I.V.	Immediate	Immediate	23-33 days
I.M.	Immediate	14-24 hr	23-33 days

Adverse reactions

CNS: confusion, drowsiness, depression, hallucinations, fatigue, agitation, headache, lethargy, irritability, **seizures, coma, intracranial hemorrhage and fatal bleeding**
GI: nausea, vomiting, anorexia, abdominal cramps, stomatitis, **hemorrhagic pancreatitis, fulminant pancreatitis**
GU: glycosuria, polyuria, uric acid nephropathy, **uremia, renal failure**
Hematologic: anemia, **leukopenia, hypofibrinogenemia, depression of clotting factor synthesis, bone marrow depression**
Hepatic: fatty liver changes, **hepatotoxicity**
Metabolic: hyperglycemia, hyperuricemia, hypocalcemia, hyperammonemia, **hypoglycemia**
Musculoskeletal: joint pain
Skin: rash, urticaria
Other: chills, fever, weight loss, hypersensitivity reactions, **anaphylaxis, fatal hyperthermia**

Interactions

Drug-drug. *Methotrexate:* decreased methotrexate efficacy
Prednisone: hyperglycemia, increased drug toxicity
Vincristine: hyperglycemia, increased drug toxicity, increased risk of neuropathy
Drug-diagnostic tests. *Alanine aminotransferase, ammonia, aspartate aminotransferase, blood urea nitrogen, glucose, uric acid:* increased levels
Calcium, hemoglobin, white blood cells: decreased levels
Thyroid function tests: interference with test interpretation

Patient monitoring

- Observe for signs and symptoms of anaphylaxis.
- Monitor for bleeding and hemorrhage. Watch closely for signs and symptoms of intracranial hemorrhage.
- Assess vital signs, temperature, and neurologic status.
- Monitor CBC, blood and urine glucose levels, and liver, kidney, and bone marrow function test results.
- Monitor fluid intake and output.

Patient teaching

- Instruct patient to immediately report allergic response, severe abdominal pain, and unusual bleeding or bruising.
- Caution patient to avoid driving and other hazardous activities until he knows how drug affects concentration and alertness.
- Advise patient to drink plenty of fluids to ensure adequate urine output.
- Tell patient to monitor urine output and report significant changes.
- Instruct patient to avoid activities that can cause injury. Tell him to use soft toothbrush and electric razor to avoid injury to gums and skin.
- Advise patient to minimize GI upset by eating small, frequent servings of food and drinking plenty of fluids.
- Tell patient that he'll undergo regular blood testing during therapy.
- As appropriate, review all other significant and life-threatening adverse reactions and interactions, especially those related to the drugs and tests mentioned above.

atenolol

Apo-Atenolol✱, Novo-Atenol✱, Tenormin

Pharmacologic class: Beta-adrenergic blocker (selective)
Therapeutic class: Antianginal, antihypertensive
Pregnancy risk category D

Action

Selectively blocks $beta_1$-adrenergic (myocardial) receptors; decreases cardiac output, peripheral resistance, and myocardial oxygen consumption. Also depresses renin secretion without affecting $beta_2$-adrenergic (pulmonary, vascular, uterine) receptors.

Availability

Injection: 5 mg/10 ml
Tablets: 25 mg, 50 mg, 100 mg

Indications and dosages

➢ Hypertension
Adults: Initially, 50 mg P.O. once daily, increased to 100 mg after 7 to 14 days if needed
➢ Angina pectoris
Adults: Initially, 50 mg P.O. once daily, increased to 100 mg after 7 days if needed. Some patients may require up to 200 mg daily.
➢ Acute myocardial infarction
Adults: Initially, 5 mg I.V. over 5 minutes, followed by 5 mg I.V. 10 minutes later; 10 minutes after last I.V. dose, give 50-mg tablet P.O., then give 50 mg

P.O. in 12 hours. Maintenance dosage is 100 mg P.O. daily or 50 mg b.i.d. for 6 to 9 days.

Dosage adjustment
- Renal impairment
- Elderly patients

Contraindications
- Cardiogenic shock
- Sinus bradycardia
- Greater than first-degree heart block
- Heart failure (unless secondary to tachyarrhythmia treatable with beta-adrenergic blockers)

Precautions
Use cautiously in:
- renal failure, hepatic impairment, pulmonary disease, diabetes mellitus, thyrotoxicosis
- pregnant or breastfeeding patients
- children.

Administration
🔊 If apical pulse is below 60 beats/minute, withhold dose and call prescriber.
- Mix I.V. dose with dextrose or sodium chloride injection solution.
- For I.V. use, administer slowly (no faster than 1 mg/minute).
- Use I.V. solution within 48 hours of mixing.

🔊 Don't discontinue drug suddenly. Instead, taper dosage over 2 weeks.

Route	Onset	Peak	Duration
P.O.	1 hr	2 hr	24 hr
I.V.	5 min	5 min	12 hr

Adverse reactions
CNS: fatigue, lethargy, vertigo, drowsiness, dizziness, depression, disorientation, short-term memory loss
CV: hypertension, intermittent claudication, cold arms and legs, orthostatic hypotension, **bradycardia, arrhythmias, heart failure, cardiogenic shock, myocardial reinfarction**
EENT: blurred vision, dry eyes, eye irritation, conjunctivitis, stuffy nose, rhinitis, pharyngitis, **laryngospasm**
GI: nausea, vomiting, diarrhea, constipation, gastric pain, flatulence, anorexia, **ischemic colitis, retroperitoneal fibrosis, acute pancreatitis, mesenteric arterial thrombosis**
GU: impotence, decreased libido, dysuria, nocturia, Peyronie's disease, **renal failure**
Hematologic: agranulocytosis
Hepatic: hepatomegaly
Metabolic: hypoglycemia
Musculoskeletal: muscle cramps, back and joint pain
Respiratory: dyspnea, wheezing, respiratory distress, **bronchospasm, bronchial obstruction, pulmonary emboli**
Other: decreased exercise tolerance, allergic reaction, fever, development of antinuclear antibodies, hypersensitivity reaction

Interactions
Drug-drug. *Amiodarone, cardiac glycosides, diltiazem, verapamil:* increased myocardial depression, causing excessive bradycardia and heart block
Amphetamines, cocaine, ephedrine, norepinephrine, phenylephrine, pseudoephedrine: excessive hypertension, bradycardia
Ampicillin, calcium salts: decreased antihypertensive and antianginal effects
Aspirin, bismuth subsalicylate, magnesium salicylate, nonsteroidal anti-inflammatory drugs: decreased antihypertensive effect
Clonidine: life-threatening blood pressure increase after clonidine withdrawal or simultaneous withdrawal of both drugs
Dobutamine, dopamine: decrease in beneficial beta-cardiovascular effects
Lidocaine: increased lidocaine levels, greater risk of toxicity
MAO inhibitors: bradycardia

Prazosin: increased risk of orthostatic hypotension
Reserpine: increased hypotension, marked bradycardia
Theophylline: decreased theophylline elimination
Drug-diagnostic tests. *Alanine aminotransferase, alkaline phosphatase, aspartate aminotransferase, antinuclear antibody titer, blood urea nitrogen, creatinine, lactate dehydrogenase, platelets, potassium, uric acid:* increased levels
Glucose: increased or decreased level
Insulin tolerance test: false result
Drug-behaviors. *Alcohol use:* increased hypotension

Patient monitoring

- Watch for signs and symptoms of hypersensitivity reaction.
- Monitor vital signs (especially blood pressure), ECG, and exercise tolerance.
- Check closely for hypotension in hemodialysis patients.
- Monitor blood glucose level regularly if patient is diabetic; drug may mask signs and symptoms of hypoglycemia.

Patient teaching

◀ Instruct patient to immediately report signs and symptoms of allergic response, breathing problems, and chest pain.
- Advise patient to take drug at same time every day.

◀ Inform patient that he may experience serious reactions if he stops taking drug suddenly. Advise him to consult prescriber before discontinuing.
- Caution patient to avoid driving and other hazardous activities until he knows how drug affects concentration and alertness.
- Tell patient that drug may cause a temporary blood pressure decrease if he stands or sits up suddenly. Instruct him to rise slowly and carefully.
- Inform women that drug shouldn't be taken during pregnancy. Urge them to report planned or suspected pregnancy.
- Tell men that drug may cause erectile dysfunction. Advise them to discuss this issue with prescriber.
- As appropriate, review all other significant and life-threatening adverse reactions and interactions, especially those related to the drugs, tests, and behaviors mentioned above.

atomoxetine hydrochloride

Strattera

Pharmacologic class: Selective norepinephrine reuptake inhibitor
Therapeutic class: Antipsychotic agent
Pregnancy risk category C

Action

Unclear. May block norepinephrine reuptake at neuronal synapse.

Availability

Capsules: 10 mg, 18 mg, 25 mg, 40 mg, 60 mg

Indications and dosages

➢ Attention deficit hyperactivity disorder (ADHD)
Adults and children weighing more than 70 kg (154 lb): Initially, 40 mg P.O. daily. After 3 days, may increase to target total daily dosage of 80 mg P.O., given either as a single dose in morning or in evenly divided doses in morning and late afternoon or early evening. If desired response doesn't occur, may increase dosage after 2 to 4 more weeks to a maximum dosage of 100 mg P.O. daily.
Adults and children weighing 70 kg (154 lb) or less: Initially, 0.5 mg/kg/day P.O. Increase after at least 3 days to target daily dosage of 1.2 mg/kg, given either as single daily dose in morning or

as evenly divided doses in morning and late afternoon or early evening.

Dosage adjustment

- Hepatic impairment
- Concurrent use of potent CYP2D6 inhibitors (such as fluoxetine, paroxetine, quinidine) in children weighing less than 70 kg (154 lb)

Contraindications

- Hypersensitivity to drug
- Closed-angle glaucoma
- MAO inhibitor use within past 14 days

Precautions

Use cautiously in:

- hypotension; impaired renal, cardiac, cerebrovascular, hepatic, or endocrine function
- pregnant or breastfeeding patients
- children younger than age 6.

Administration

- Give as a single dose in morning, or give half of total daily dose in morning and other half in late afternoon or early evening.

[Clinical alert] Don't give to patient who has taken MAO inhibitors within past 14 days.

Route	Onset	Peak	Duration
P.O.	Rapid	1-2 hr	Unknown

Adverse reactions

CNS: aggression, insomnia, dizziness, drowsiness, headache, irritability, crying, mood swings, fatigue, rigors
CV: orthostatic hypotension, palpitations, tachycardia
EENT: rhinorrhea, sinusitis
GI: nausea, vomiting, constipation, upper abdominal pain, flatulence, dyspepsia, dry mouth
GU: urinary retention, urinary hesitancy, dysmenorrhea, erectile problems, ejaculation failure, impotence, prostatitis
Musculoskeletal: muscle pain
Respiratory: cough
Skin: dermatitis, sweating
Other: fever, hot flashes, growth retardation (in children), decreased appetite, weight loss

Interactions

Drug-drug. *Albuterol:* increased cardiovascular effects
MAO inhibitors: hyperthermia, myoclonus, rapid changes in vital signs
Potent CYP2D6 inhibitors: increased atomoxetine effects in children weighing less than 70 kg (154 lb)
Vasopressors: hypertensive crisis

Patient monitoring

- Monitor growth in children.
- Assess for weight loss.
- Check blood pressure and pulse, especially after dosage changes.
- Monitor for changes in mood, sleep patterns, and behavior.
- Evaluate for urinary hesitancy or urinary retention and sexual dysfunction.
- Provide dietary counseling. Refer patient to dietitian if adverse GI effects significantly limit food intake.

Patient teaching

- To minimize insomnia, advise patient to establish effective bedtime routine and to take drug in single morning dose or in divided half-doses in morning and late afternoon or early evening.
- Caution patient to avoid driving and other hazardous activities until he knows how drug affects concentration and alertness.
- Advise patient to minimize GI upset by eating small, frequent servings of food and drinking plenty of fluids.
- As appropriate, review all other significant adverse reactions and interactions, especially those related to the drugs mentioned above.

atorvastatin calcium

Lipitor

Pharmacologic class: HMG-CoA reductase inhibitor

Therapeutic class: Lipid-lowering agent

Pregnancy risk category X

Action

Inhibits HMG-CoA reductase, which catalyzes first step in cholesterol synthesis; this action reduces concentrations of serum cholesterol and low-density lipoproteins (LDLs), linked to increased risk of coronary artery disease (CAD). Also moderately increases concentration of high-density lipoproteins (HDLs), associated with decreased risk of CAD.

Availability

Tablets: 10 mg, 20 mg, 40 mg, 80 mg

Indications and dosages

➢ Adjunct to diet for controlling LDL, total cholesterol, apo-lipoprotein B, and triglyceride levels and to increase HDL levels in patients with primary hypercholesterolemia and mixed dyslipidemia; primary dysbetalipoproteinemia in patients unresponsive to diet alone; adjunct to diet to reduce elevated triglyceride levels

Adults: Initially, 10 mg P.O. daily; increase to 80 mg P.O. daily if needed. Adjust dosage according to patient's cholesterol level.

➢ Adjunct to other lipid-lowering treatments in patients with homozygous familial hypercholesterolemia

Adults: 10 to 80 mg P.O. daily

➢ Adjunct to diet to decrease total cholesterol, LDL, and apo-lipoprotein B levels in boys and postmenarchal girls ages 10 to 17 with familial and nonfamilial heterozygous hypercholesterolemia

Boys and girls: Initially, 10 mg P.O. daily; adjust dosage upward or downward based on lipid levels. Maximum dosage is 20 mg daily.

➢ Prevention of cardiovascular disease in patients without clinically evident coronary heart disease (CHD) but with multiple CHD risk factors

Adults: 10 mg P.O. daily

Contraindications

- Hypersensitivity to drug or its components
- Active hepatic disease or unexplained, persistent serum transaminase elevations
- Pregnancy or breastfeeding

Precautions

Use cautiously in:

- renal impairment, hypotension, uncontrolled seizures, myopathy, alcoholism
- severe metabolic, endocrine, or electrolyte disorders
- women of childbearing age
- children younger than age 18.

Administration

- Give with or without food.
- Don't give with grapefruit juice or antacids.

Route	Onset	Peak	Duration
P.O.	Unknown	1-2 hr	Unknown

Adverse reactions

CNS: amnesia, abnormal dreams, emotional lability, headache, hyperactivity, poor coordination, malaise, paresthesia, peripheral neuropathy, drowsiness, syncope, weakness

CV: orthostatic hypotension, palpitations, phlebitis, vasodilation, **arrhythmias**

EENT: amblyopia, altered refraction, glaucoma, eye hemorrhage, dry eyes,

hearing loss, tinnitus, epistaxis, sinusitis, pharyngitis
GI: nausea, vomiting, diarrhea, constipation, abdominal cramps, abdominal or biliary pain, colitis, indigestion, dyspepsia, flatulence, stomach ulcers, gastroenteritis, melena, tenesmus, glossitis, mouth sores, dry mouth, dysphagia, esophagitis, pancreatitis, **rectal hemorrhage**
GU: hematuria, nocturia, dysuria, urinary frequency or urgency, urinary retention, cystitis, nephritis, renal calculi, abnormal ejaculation, decreased libido, erectile dysfunction, epididymitis
Hematologic: anemia, **thrombocytopenia**
Hepatic: jaundice, **hepatic failure, hepatitis**
Metabolic: hyperglycemia, **hypoglycemia**
Musculoskeletal: bursitis, joint pain, back pain, leg cramps, gout, muscle pain or aches, myositis, myasthenia gravis, neck rigidity, torticollis, **rhabdomyolysis**
Respiratory: dyspnea, pneumonia, bronchitis
Skin: alopecia, acne, contact dermatitis, eczema, dry skin, pruritus, rash, urticaria, skin ulcers, seborrhea, photosensitivity, diaphoresis
Other: taste loss, gingival bleeding, fever, facial paralysis, facial or generalized edema, flulike symptoms, infection, appetite changes, weight gain, allergic reaction

Interactions

Drug-drug. *Antacids, colestipol:* decreased atorvastatin blood level
Azole antifungals, cyclosporine, erythromycin, fibric acid derivatives, niacin, other HMG-CoA inhibitors: increased risk of myopathy
Digoxin: increased digoxin level, greater risk of toxicity
Hormonal contraceptives: increased estrogen level
Drug-diagnostic tests. *Alanine aminotransferase, aspartate aminotransferase, creatine kinase:* increased levels
Drug-food. *Grapefruit juice:* increased drug blood level, greater risk of adverse effects
Drug-herbs. *Red yeast rice:* increased risk of adverse effects

Patient monitoring

- Monitor patient for signs and symptoms of allergic response.

[Clinical alert] Evaluate for muscle weakness (a symptom of myositis and possibly rhabdomyolysis).

- Monitor liver function test results and blood lipid levels.

Patient teaching

- Tell patient he may take drug with or without food.

[Clinical alert] Advise patient to immediately report allergic response, irregular heart beats, unusual bruising or bleeding, unusual tiredness, yellowing of skin or eyes, or muscle weakness.

- Instruct patient to avoid grapefruit juice during therapy.
- Caution patient to avoid driving and other hazardous activities until he knows how drug affects concentration, alertness, and vision.
- Advise patient to minimize GI upset by eating small, frequent servings of food and drinking plenty of fluids.
- Inform patient taking hormonal contraceptives that drug increases estrogen levels. Instruct her to tell all prescribers she's taking drug.
- Tell men that drug may cause erectile dysfunction and abnormal ejaculation. Encourage them to discuss these issues with prescriber.
- Tell patient he'll undergo regular blood testing during therapy.
- As appropriate, review all other significant and life-threatening adverse reactions and interactions, especially those related to the drugs, tests, foods, and herbs mentioned above.

atracurium besylate

Tracrium

Pharmacologic class: Nondepolarizing neuromuscular blocker

Therapeutic class: Skeletal muscle relaxant

Pregnancy risk category C

Action

Decreases effects of and response to the neurotransmitter acetylcholine at myoneural junction of skeletal muscles, causing them to relax. Also stimulates histamine release.

Availability

Injection: 10 mg/ml

Indications and dosages

➢ Adjunct to general anesthesia to facilitate endotracheal intubation and relax skeletal muscles during surgery

Adults and children ages 2 and older: Initially, 0.4 to 0.5 mg/kg by I.V. bolus. With prolonged surgery, maintenance dosage of 0.08 to 0.1 mg/kg is given within 20 to 45 minutes; may repeat q 15 to 25 minutes, as needed.

Children ages 1 month to 2 years: 0.3 to 0.4 mg/kg I.V.; repeat if needed.

Off-label uses

- Myasthenia gravis

Contraindications

- Hypersensitivity to drug

Precautions

Use cautiously in:

- elderly patients
- pregnant or breastfeeding patients
- children.

Administration

- Clinical alert: Use only under direct supervision of trained medical staff who can maintain patent airway.
- Clinical alert: Before giving, make sure emergency respiratory equipment is at hand.
- Ensure that patient receives sedative or general anesthetic before giving atracurium.
- Give I.V. only (bolus, intermittent infusion, or continuous infusion). Never give I.M.
- Know that during lengthy procedures, a continuous infusion of 5 to 9 mcg/kg/minute may be given.
- Be aware that patient can hear while drug is in effect. Provide ongoing reassurance.
- Be ready to reverse drug's effects with anticholinesterase drug once spontaneous recovery begins.

Route	Onset	Peak	Duration
I.V.	2 min	3-5 min	35-70 min

Adverse reactions

CNS: inadequate neuromuscular blockade, **prolonged neuromuscular blockade, seizures**

CV: hypotension, **tachycardia, bradycardia**

Respiratory: wheezing, dyspnea, **apnea, bronchospasm, laryngospasm**

Skin: flushing, rash, urticaria, erythema, pruritus

Other: injection site reaction, **anaphylaxis**

Interactions

Drug-drug. *Acetylcholinesterase inhibitors:* inhibition of muscle relaxation and reversal of neuromuscular blockade

Aminoglycosides, enflurane, halothane, isoflurane, lithium, procainamide, trimethaphan, verapamil: increased muscle relaxation

Carbamazepine, phenytoin, theophylline: resistance to or reversal of neuromuscular blockade
Clindamycin, lithium, magnesium salt, opioids, polymyxin antibiotics (colistin, polymyxin B sulfate), procainamide, quinine, thiazide and loop diuretics: enhanced neuromuscular blockade
Corticosteroids: prolonged weakness
Edrophonium, neostigmine, pyridostigmine: atracurium inhibition, reversal of neuromuscular blockade
Succinylcholine: faster atracurium onset, increased depth of muscle relaxation

Patient monitoring

Monitor patient for anaphylaxis and injection site reaction.

- Check vital signs and airway patency until patient recovers completely from drug effects.
- Assess for pain and give analgesics as needed. Be aware that patient may be unable to express pain while drug is in effect.
- Evaluate patient's recovery with muscle strength tests, nerve stimulation, and train-of-four monitoring.
- While drug is in effect, explain events to patient as they occur.

Patient teaching

- Before giving, carefully describe drug effects to patient, explaining that he will be able to hear but won't be able to move.
- As appropriate, review all other significant and life-threatening adverse reactions and interactions, especially those related to the drugs mentioned above.

a

atropine sulfate

AtroPen, Atropine-1

atropine sulfate ophthalmic

Isopto Atropine

Pharmacologic class: Anticholinergic (antimuscarinic)
Therapeutic class: Antiarrhythmic
Pregnancy risk category C

Action

Inhibits acetylcholine at parasympathetic neuroeffector junction of smooth muscle and cardiac muscle, blocking sinoatrial (SA) and atrioventricular (AV) nodes. These actions increase impulse conduction and raise heart rate. In ophthalmic use, blocks cholinergic stimulation to iris and ciliary bodies, causing pupillary dilation and accommodation paralysis.

Availability

Injection: 0.05 mg/ml, 0.1 mg/ml, 0.3 mg/ml, 0.4 mg/ml, 0.5 mg/ml, 0.8 mg/ml, 1 mg/ml
Ophthalmic solution: 0.5%, 1%, 2%
Tablets: 0.4 mg

Indications and dosages

➢ Bradyarrhythmias, symptomatic bradycardia

Adults: 0.5 to 1 mg by I.V. push repeated q 3 to 5 minutes as needed, to a maximum dosage of 2 mg
Children: 0.01 mg/kg I.V. to a maximum dosage of 0.4 mg or 0.3 mg/m^2. May repeat I.V. dose q 4 to 6 hours.

➢ Antidote for anticholinesterase insecticide poisoning

Adults: 2 to 3 mg I.V. repeated q 5 to 10 minutes until symptoms disappear or a toxic level is reached. For severe poisoning, 6 mg q hour.

Children: 0.05 mg/kg I.M. or I.V. repeated q every 10 to 30 minutes until symptoms disappear or a toxic level is reached

➢ Preoperatively to diminish secretions and block cardiac vagal reflexes

Adults and children weighing more than 40.8 kg (90 lb): 0.4 to 0.6 mg I.M., I.V., or subcutaneously 30 to 60 minutes before anesthesia

Children weighing 29.5 to 40.8 kg (65 to 90 lb): 0.4 mg I.M., I.V., or subcutaneously 30 to 60 minutes before anesthesia

Children weighing 18.1 to 29.5 kg (40 to 65 lb): 0.3 mg I.M., I.V., or subcutaneously 30 to 60 minutes before anesthesia

Children weighing 10.9 to18.1 kg (24 to 40 lb): 0.2 mg I.M., I.V., or subcutaneously 30 to 60 minutes before anesthesia

Children weighing 7.3 to10.9 kg (16 to 24 lb): 0.15 mg I.M., I.V., or subcutaneously 30 to 60 minutes before anesthesia

Children weighing 3.2 to7.3 kg (7 to 16 lb): 0.1 mg I.M., I.V., or subcutaneously 30 to 60 minutes before anesthesia

➢ Peptic ulcer disease, functional GI disorders (such as hypersecretory states)

Adults: 0.4 to 0.6 mg P.O. q 4 to 6 hours

Children: 0.01 mg/kg or 0.3/m^2 P.O. q 4 to 6 hours

➢ Parkinsonism

Adults: 0.1 to 0.25 mg P.O. q.i.d.

➢ Antidote for muscarine-induced mushroom toxicity

Adults: 1 to 2 mg/hour I.M. or I.V. until respiratory function improves

➢ Pupillary dilation in acute inflammatory conditions of iris and uveal tract

Adults: Instill one or two drops of 0.5% or 1% solution into eye(s) up to q.i.d.

Children: Instill one or two drops of 0.5% solution into eye(s) up to t.i.d.

➢ To produce mydriasis and cycloplegia for refraction

Adults: Instill one or two drops of 1% solution into eye(s) 1 hour before refraction.

Children: Instill one or two drops of 0.5% solution into eye(s) b.i.d. for 1 to 3 days before examination.

Off-label uses

- Cholinergic-mediated bronchial asthma

Contraindications

- Hypersensitivity to drug or other belladonna alkaloids
- Acute narrow-angle glaucoma
- Adhesions between iris and lens (ophthalmic form)
- Obstructive GI tract disease
- Unstable cardiovascular status
- Asthma
- Myasthenia gravis
- Thyrotoxicosis
- Infants ages 3 months and younger

Precautions

Use cautiously in:

- chronic renal, hepatic, pulmonary, or cardiac disease
- intra-abdominal infection, prostatic hypertrophy
- elderly patients
- pregnant or breastfeeding patients
- children.

Administration

- For I.V. dose, infuse directly into large vein or I.V. tubing over at least 1 minute.
- Be aware that slow I.V. infusion may cause slowing of heart rate.
- Don't administer oral dose within 1 hour of giving antacids.
- Be aware that patients with Down syndrome may be unusually sensitive to drug.

Route	Onset	Peak	Duration
P.O.	0.5-2 hr	1-2 hr	4-6 hr
I.V.	Immediate	2-4 min	4-6 hr
I.M., subcut.	Rapid	15-50 min	4-6 hr

Adverse effects

CNS: headache, restlessness, ataxia, disorientation, delirium, insomnia, dizziness, drowsiness, agitation, nervousness, confusion, excitement
CV: palpitations, **bradycardia, tachycardia**
EENT: photophobia, blurred version, increased intraocular pressure, mydriasis, cycloplegia, nasal congestion
GI: nausea, vomiting, constipation, bloating, dyspepsia, ileus, abdominal distention (in infants), dysphagia, dry mouth
GU: urinary retention, urinary hesitancy, impotence
Skin: decreased sweating, flushing, urticaria, dry skin
Other: thirst, **anaphylaxis**

Interactions

Drug-drug. *Amantadine, antiarrhythmics, anticholinergics, antihistamines, antiparkinsonian drugs, glutethimide, meperidine, muscle relaxants, phenothiazines, tricyclic antidepressants:* increased atropine effects
Antacids, antidiarrheals: decreased atropine absorption
Antimyasthenics: decreased intestinal motility
Cyclopropane: ventricular arrhythmias
Haloperidol: decreased antipsychotic effect
Ketoconazole, levodopa: decreased absorption of these drugs
Metoclopramide: decreased effect of atropine on GI motility
Potassium chloride wax-matrix tablets: increased severity of mucosal lesions
Drug-herbs. *Jaborandi tree, pill-bearing spurge:* decreased drug effect
Jimsonweed: changes in cardiovascular function
Squaw vine: reduced metabolic breakdown of drug
Drug-behaviors. *Sun exposure:* increased risk of photophobia

Patient monitoring

🔊 Watch closely for signs and symptoms of anaphylaxis.
- Monitor heart rate for bradycardia or tachycardia.
- Evaluate fluid intake and output.
- Assess for urine retention or urinary hesitancy.
- Monitor for signs and symptoms of glaucoma.

Patient teaching

🔊 Instruct patient to immediately report allergic response.
🔊 Inform patient that headache, eye pain, and blurred vision may signal glaucoma. Tell him to report these symptoms at once.
- Caution patient to avoid driving and other hazardous activities until he knows how drug affects concentration, alertness, and vision.
- Encourage patient to establish an effective bedtime routine to minimize insomnia.
- Tell patient to apply pressure to inside corner of eye during instillation of ophthalmic solution and for 1 to 2 minutes afterward.
- As appropriate, review all other significant and life-threatening adverse reactions and interactions, especially those related to the drugs, herbs, and behaviors mentioned above.

auranofin
Ridaura

aurothioglucose
Solganal

gold sodium thiomalate
Aurolate

Pharmacologic class: Heavy metal, gold compound
Therapeutic class: Anti-inflammatory
Pregnancy risk category C

Action
Unclear. Exerts anti-inflammatory, antiarthritic, and immunoregulatory actions, including stimulation of cell-mediated immunity, suppression of immunoglobulin synthesis and antibody-dependent cytotoxicity, inhibition of neutrophil release from lysosomal enzymes, selective suppression of macrophage function, inhibition of interleukin secretion by T lymphocytes, and inhibition of neovascularization.

Availability
Capsules (Ridaura): 3 mg
Injection (Aurolate): 50 mg/ml in 2-ml and 10-ml vials for I.M. injection only
Injection (Solganal): 50 mg/ml suspension for I.M. injection (preferably in upper gluteal muscle)

Indications and dosages
➤ Active early rheumatoid arthritis in adults and children when disease isn't adequately controlled by other inflammatory agents or conservative measures
Aurothioglucose—
Adults: Initially, 10 mg I.M. in gluteal muscle once a week; during second and third weeks, 25 mg I.M.; during fourth and subsequent weeks, 50 mg I.M.; then 50 mg I.M. at weekly intervals until patient has received total dosage of 0.8 to 1 g. If patient improves with no signs or symptoms of drug toxicity, give 50 mg I.M. at 3- to 4-week intervals indefinitely.
Children ages 6 to 12: One-fourth of adult dose I.M., depending on body weight, not to exceed 25 mg/dose
Gold sodium thiomalate—
Adults: Initially, 10 mg I.M. in gluteal muscle once a week; during second week, 25 mg I.M.; during third and subsequent weeks, 25 to 50 mg I.M. until major clinical improvement or toxicity occurs or cumulative dose reaches 1 g. Maintenance dosage is 25 to 50 mg I.M. every other week for 2 to 20 weeks. If patient's clinical status remains stable, give maintenance dosage of 25 to 50 mg I.M. q 3 to 4 weeks indefinitely.
Children: Initial test dose of 10 mg I.M.; then 1 mg/kg, not to exceed 50 mg as a single dose. Space doses as described for adult dosage.
➤ Active classic rheumatoid arthritis in patients who don't respond sufficiently to or can't tolerate nonsteroidal anti-inflammatory drugs (NSAIDs)
Auranofin—
Adults: Initially, 6 mg P.O. daily, given in single dose or as 3 mg b.i.d. If response isn't adequate after 6 months, increase to 9 mg P.O. daily, given as 3 mg t.i.d.
Children: Initially, 0.1 mg/kg/day P.O. Maximum dosage is 0.2 mg/kg/day P.O. Maintenance dosage is 0.15 mg/kg/day P.O.

Contraindications
- Hypersensitivity to gold or history of severe gold toxicity
- Systemic lupus erythematosus
- Inflammatory bowel disease
- Pregnancy or breastfeeding

a

Precautions

Use cautiously in:
- renal or hepatic disease, marked hypertension, compromised cardiovascular circulation, Sjögren's syndrome, eczema.

Administration

Give parenteral form by I.M. route only, preferably using gluteal site.
- Administer test dose if prescribed, and monitor patient for reaction.
- Place vial in warm water, and then shake vigorously to mix drug.
- Have patient lie down for 10 to 20 minutes after injection.

Keep dimercaprol readily available to counteract drug toxicity, if needed.

Route	Onset	Peak	Duration
P.O.	Unknown	Unknown	Unknown
I.M.	Slow	4-6 hr	Unknown

Adverse reactions

CNS: dizziness, fainting, malaise
CV: syncope, **bradycardia**
EENT: pharyngitis
GI: nausea, vomiting, diarrhea, dysphagia, abdominal cramps, gastritis, colitis, glossitis, stomatitis, gingivitis, anorexia
GU: vaginitis, **acute tubular necrosis, renal failure, nephrotic syndrome or glomerulitis with proteinuria and hematuria**
Hematologic: eosinophilia, anemia, **leukopenia, thrombocytopenia, granulocytopenia**
Hepatic: jaundice, **hepatitis**
Musculoskeletal: joint pain
Respiratory: cough, shortness of breath, dyspnea, tracheal inflammation, **interstitial pneumonitis, fibrosis, gold bronchitis**
Skin: grayish-blue skin discoloration, erythema, dermatitis, pruritus, flushing, sweating, **exfoliative dermatitis**
Other: metallic taste, **anaphylactic shock**

Interactions

Drug-drug. *Antimalarials, cytotoxic drugs (immunosuppressants other than corticosteroids), penicillamine:* increased risk of adverse hematologic and renal effects
Drug-diagnostic tests. *Hematocrit, hemoglobin, platelets, white blood cells:* decreased levels
Liver function tests: altered results
Urine protein: increased level
Drug-behaviors. *Exposure to sunlight and artificial ultraviolet light*: grayish-blue skin discoloration

Patient monitoring

For 30 minutes after giving dose, monitor patient for signs and symptoms of anaphylaxis.

Stop therapy and consult prescriber if patient complains of itching, rash, or other skin problems.
- Monitor liver and kidney function test results and CBC (especially platelets).

Patient teaching

Instruct patient to stop taking drug and notify prescriber immediately if he develops itching, rash, or other skin problems.
- Explain that drug may take 3 to 4 months to relieve symptoms.

Tell patient to immediately report bleeding tendencies or bruising.
- Tell patient that he may experience more joint pain for 1 to 2 days after each dose, but that pain usually eases.
- Instruct patient to monitor urine output and report significant changes.
- Advise patient to use good oral hygiene. Tell him to report metallic taste.
- Caution patient to avoid driving and other hazardous activities until he knows how drug affects concentration and alertness.

Teach patient about risks of using drug during pregnancy. Advise her to report planned or suspected pregnancy to prescriber.

• Advise patient to minimize GI upset by eating small, frequent servings of foods and drinking plenty of fluids.
• Tell patient that he'll undergo regular blood testing during therapy.
• As appropriate, review all other significant and life-threatening adverse reactions and interactions, especially those related to the drugs, tests, and behaviors mentioned above.

azathioprine
Imuran

azathioprine sodium
Imuran

Pharmacologic class: Purine antagonist
Therapeutic class: Immunosuppressant
Pregnancy risk category D

Action
Prevents proliferation and differentiation of activated B and T cells by interfering with synthesis of purine, DNA, and RNA

Availability
Injection (azathioprine sodium): 100-mg vial
Tablets (azathioprine): 25 mg, 50 mg, 75 mg, 100 mg

Indications and dosages
➢ To prevent rejection of kidney transplant
Adults and children: Initially, 3 to 5 mg/kg/day P.O. or I.V. as a single dose. Give on day of transplantation or 1 to 3 days before day of transplantation; then give 3 to 5 mg/kg/day I.V. after surgery until patient can tolerate P.O. route. Maintenance dosage is 1 to 3 mg/kg/day P.O.

➢ Rheumatoid arthritis
Adults and children: Initially, 1 mg/kg P.O. in one or two daily doses. Increase dosage in steps at 6 to 8 weeks and thereafter at 4-week intervals; use dosage increments of 0.5 mg/kg/day, to a maximum dosage of 2.5 mg/kg/day. Once patient stabilizes, decrease in decrements of 0.5 mg/kg/day to lowest effective dosage.

Dosage adjustment
• Renal disease
• Concurrent allopurinol therapy
• Elderly patients

Off-label uses
• Crohn's disease
• Myasthenia gravis
• Chronic ulcerative colitis

Contraindications
• Hypersensitivity to drug
• Pregnancy or breastfeeding

Precautions
Use cautiously in:
• chickenpox, herpes zoster, impaired hepatic or renal function, decreased bone marrow reserve
• previous therapy with alkylating agents (cyclophosphamide, chlorambucil, melphalan) for rheumatoid arthritis
• elderly patients
• women of childbearing age.

Administration
• For I.V. dose, mix powder with 10 ml of sterile water.
• Use I.V. route only if patient can't tolerate oral dose. Give over 30 to 60 minutes by I.V. push or by infusion in normal saline solution or dextrose 5% in water.
• Give oral doses after meals.

Route	Onset	Peak	Duration
P.O.	6-8 wks	12 wks	Unknown
I.V.	Days-wks	Unknown	Days-wks

a

Adverse reactions

CNS: malaise
EENT: retinopathy
GI: nausea, vomiting, diarrhea, stomatitis, esophagitis, anorexia, mucositis, pancreatitis
Hematologic: anemia, **thrombocytopenia, leukopenia, pancytopenia**
Hepatic: jaundice, **hepatotoxicity**
Musculoskeletal: muscle wasting, joint and muscle pain
Skin: rash, alopecia
Other: chills, fever, **serum sickness, neoplasms, serious infection**

Interactions

Drug-drug. *Allopurinol:* increased therapeutic and adverse effects of azathioprine
Anticoagulants, cyclosporine: decreased actions of these drugs
Atracurium, pancuronium, tubocurarine, vecuronium: reversal of these drugs' actions
Drugs affecting bone marrow and bone marrow cells (such as angiotensin-converting enzyme inhibitors, co-trimoxazole): severe leukopenia
Drug-diagnostic tests. *Alanine aminotransferase, alkaline phosphatase, amylase, aspartate aminotransferase, bilirubin:* increased levels
Albumin, hemoglobin, uric acid: decreased levels
Urine uric acid: decreased level
Drug-herbs. *Astragalus, echinacea, melatonin:* interference with immunosuppressant action

Patient monitoring

- [Clinical alert] Monitor CBC, platelet level, and liver function test results.
- Assess for signs and symptoms of hepatotoxicity (clay-colored stools, pruritus, jaundice, and dark urine).
- Watch for signs and symptoms of infection.
- Monitor for bleeding tendency and hemorrhage.

Patient teaching

- [Clinical alert] Tell patient that drug lowers resistance to infection. Instruct him to immediately report fever, cough, breathing problems, chills, and other symptoms.
- [Clinical alert] Instruct patient to immediately report unusual bleeding or bruising.
- Tell patient that drug effects may not be obvious for up to 8 weeks in immunosuppression and up to 12 weeks for rheumatoid arthritis relief.
- [Clinical alert] Emphasize importance of avoiding pregnancy during therapy and for 4 months afterward.
- Caution patient to avoid activities that may cause injury. Tell him to use soft toothbrush and electric razor to avoid gum and skin injury.
- Advise patient to minimize GI upset by eating small, frequent servings of foods and drinking plenty of fluids.
- Tell patient he'll undergo regular blood testing during therapy.
- As appropriate, review all other significant and life-threatening adverse reactions and interactions, especially those related to the drugs, tests, and herbs mentioned above.

azithromycin, azithromycin dihydrate

Zithromax, Zithromax Tri-Pak, Zithromax Z-Pak

Pharmacologic class: Macrolide
Therapeutic class: Anti-infective
Pregnancy risk category B

Action

Bactericidal and bacteriostatic; inhibits protein synthesis after binding with 50S ribosomal subunit of susceptible organisms. Demonstrates cross-resistance to erythromycin resistant gram-positive strains and resistance to most strains of *Enterococcus faecalis* and methicillin-resistant *Staphylococcus aureus.*

Availability

Capsules: 250 mg, 500 mg
Oral suspension: 100 mg/5 ml in 15-ml bottles; 200 mg/5 ml in 15-ml, 22.5-ml, and 30-ml bottles
Powder for injection: 500 mg in 10-ml vials
Powder for oral suspension: 100 mg/5 ml, 200 mg/5 ml, 1,000 mg/packet
Tablets: 250 mg, 500 mg, 600 mg
Tablets (Tri-Pak): three 500-mg tablets
Tablets (Z-Pak): six 250-mg tablets

Indications and dosages

➢ Mild community-acquired pneumonia, uncomplicated skin and skin-structure infections
Adults: 500 mg P.O. on first day, then 250 mg/day for next 4 days, to a total dosage of 1.5 g
Children ages 6 months and older: 10 mg/kg P.O. (no more than 500 mg/dose) on day 1, then 5 mg/kg (no more than 250 mg/dose) for 4 more days
➢ Community-acquired pneumonia caused by *Chlamydia pneumoniae, Haemophilus influenzae, Mycoplasma pneumoniae, Streptococcus pneumoniae, Legionella pneumophila, Moraxella catarrhalis,* and *S. aureus*
Adults and adolescents ages 16 and older: 500 mg I.V. daily for at least two doses, then 500 mg P.O. daily for a total of 7 to 10 days
Children ages 6 months to 16 years: 10 mg/kg P.O. as a single dose on day 1, then 5 mg/kg P.O. on days 2 through 5
➢ Pharyngitis and tonsillitis
Adults: 500 mg P.O. on day 1, then 250 mg/day for next 4 days, to a total dosage of 1.5 g
Children ages 2 and older: 12 mg/kg P.O. daily for 5 days. Maximum dosage is 500 mg.
➢ Mild to moderate acute exacerbation of chronic obstructive pulmonary disease
Adults: 500 mg/day for 3 days or 500 mg P.O. on day 1, then 250 mg P.O. daily on days 2 through 5
➢ Pelvic inflammatory disease caused by *Chlamydia trachomatis, Neisseria gonorrhoeae,* or *Mycoplasma hominis*
Adults: 500 mg I.V. daily on days 1 and 2, then 250 mg P.O. daily for a total of 7 days. If anaerobes are suspected, give continually with appropriate anti-anaerobic antibiotic, as ordered.
➢ Nongonococcal urethritis or cervicitis caused by *C. trachomatis;* genital ulcers caused by *Haemophilus ducreyi* (chancroid)
Adults: 1g P.O. as a single dose
➢ Urethritis and cervicitis caused by *N. gonorrhoeae*
Adults: 2 g P.O. as a single dose
➢ To prevent disseminated *Mycobacterium avium* complex disease in patients with advanced human immunodeficiency virus
Adults: 1.2 g P.O. once weekly (given alone or with rifabutin)
➢ Acute otitis media
Children ages 6 months and older: 30 mg/kg as a single dose or 10 mg/kg once daily for 3 days; or 10 mg/kg as a single dose on day 1, followed by 5 mg/kg on days 2 through 5

Off-label uses

- Uncomplicated gonococcal infections of cervix, urethra, rectum, and pharynx

Contraindications

- Hypersensitivity to drug, erythromycin, or other macrolide anti-infectives

Precautions

Use cautiously in:
- severe hepatic impairment, severe renal insufficiency, prolonged QT interval
- breastfeeding patients.

Administration

- Obtain specimens for culture and sensitivity testing before starting therapy.
- Administer tablets and single-dose packets with or without food.
- Give oral suspension 1 hour before meals or 2 hours afterward. With 1-g packet, mix entire contents in 2 oz of water.

◀ Don't administer as I.V. bolus or I.M. injection.

- For I.V. use, reconstitute 500-mg vial with 4.8 ml of sterile water for injection.
- As appropriate, dilute solution further using normal or half-normal saline solution, dextrose 5% in water, or lactated Ringer's solution.
- Infuse injection over no less than 60 minutes. Infuse 1 mg/ml over 3 hours or 2 mg/2 ml over 1 hour.
- Know that 1,000-mg packet isn't for pediatric use.

Route	Onset	Peak	Duration
P.O.	Rapid	2.5-3.2 hr	24 hr
I.V.	Rapid	End of infusion	24 hr

Adverse reactions

CNS: dizziness, drowsiness, fatigue, headache, vertigo
CV: chest pain, palpitations
GI: nausea, diarrhea, abdominal pain, cholestatic jaundice, dyspepsia, flatulence, melena, **pseudomembranous colitis**
GU: nephritis, vaginitis, candidiasis
Metabolic: hyperglycemia, **hyperkalemia**
Skin: photosensitivity, rashes, angioedema

Interactions

Drug-drug. *Antacids containing aluminum or magnesium:* decreased peak azithromycin blood level
Carbamazepine, cyclosporine, digoxin, dihydroergotamine, ergotamine, hexobarbital, phenytoin, theophylline, triazolam: increased blood levels of these drugs
Pimozide: prolonged QT interval, ventricular tachycardia
Warfarin: increased International Normalized Ratio
Drug-food. *Any food:* decreased absorption of multidose oral suspension
Drug-behaviors. *Sun exposure:* photosensitivity

Patient monitoring

- Monitor temperature, white blood cell count, and culture and sensitivity results.
- Assess for signs and symptoms of infection.

Patient teaching

- Tell patient he may take tablets with or without food.
- Advise patient to take suspension 1 hour before or 2 hours after meals.
- Remind patient to complete entire course of therapy as ordered, even after symptoms improve.
- As appropriate, review all other significant and life-threatening adverse reactions and interactions, especially those related to the drugs, foods, and behaviors mentioned above.

aztreonam

Azactam

Pharmacologic class: Monobactam
Therapeutic class: Anti-infective
Pregnancy risk category B

Action

Inhibits bacterial cell-wall synthesis during active multiplication by binding with penicillin-binding protein 3, resulting in cell-wall destruction

Availability

Powder for injection: 500-mg vial, 1-g vial, 2-g vial, 1g/50-ml I.V. bag, 2 g/50-ml I.V. bag

Indications and dosages

➢ Infections caused by susceptible gram-negative organisms

Adults: For urinary tract infections, 500 mg or 1 g I.M. or I.V. q 8 or 12 hours; for moderately severe systemic infections, 1 or 2 g I.M. or I.V. q 8 or 12 hours; for severe or life-threatening infections, 2 g I.M. or I.V. q 6 or 8 hours. Maximum dosage is 8 g/day.

Children: For mild to moderate infections, 30 mg/kg I.M. or I.V. q 8 hours; for moderate to severe infections, 30 mg/kg I.M. or I.V. q 6 or 8 hours. Maximum dosage is 120 mg/kg/day.

Dosage adjustment

- Severe renal failure

Contraindications

- Hypersensitivity to drug or its components

Precautions

Use cautiously in:
- renal or hepatic impairment
- elderly patients
- pregnant or breastfeeding patients.

Administration

- Flush I.V. tubing with compatible solution before and after giving drug.
- Compatible solutions include 0.9% sodium chloride injection, 5% or 10% dextrose injection, Ringer's or lactated Ringer's injection, 5% dextrose and 0.9% sodium chloride injection, and 5% dextrose and 0.45% sodium chloride injection.
- After adding diluent to vial or infusion bottle, shake immediately and vigorously.
- For I.V. bolus injection, reconstitute powder for injection by adding 6 to 10 ml of sterile water for injection. Inject prescribed dosage into tubing of compatible I.V. solution slowly over 3 to 5 minutes.
- For intermittent I.V. infusion, reconstitute powder for injection by adding compatible I.V. solution to yield a concentration not exceeding 20 mg/ml. Administer prescribed dosage over 20 to 60 minutes.

🔊 Thaw commercially available frozen drug at room temperature and give by intermittent I.V. infusion only.

- For I.M. injection, reconstitute powder for injection by adding 3 ml of sterile water for injection or 0.9% sodium chloride injection.
- Give I.M. injection deep into large muscle mass.

Route	Onset	Peak	Duration
I.V., I.M.	Organism & dose dependent	1 hr	4-12 hr

Adverse reactions

CV: phlebitis, **thrombophlebitis**

GI: nausea, vomiting, diarrhea (including diarrhea associated with *Clostridium difficile*), **pseudomembranous colitis**

Hematologic: neutropenia

Respiratory: bronchospasm

Skin: rash, toxic epidermal necrolysis

Other: angioedema, **anaphylaxis**

Interactions

Drug-diagnostic tests. *Alanine aminotransferase (ALT), aspartate aminotransferase (AST), creatinine, eosinophils, platelets, prothrombin time (PT), partial thromboplastin time (PTT):* increased values

Coombs' test: positive result

Neutrophils: decreased count

Patient monitoring

🔊 Assess patient closely for signs and symptoms of pseudomembranous colitis.

🔊 Monitor patient carefully for hypersensitivity reaction, especially if he's

allergic to penicillin, carbapenems, or cephalosporins.
• Monitor CBC with differential, AST, ALT, PT, PTT, and serum creatinine values.
• Monitor renal and hepatic function.

Patient teaching

Instruct patient to immediately report severe diarrhea or signs or symptoms of hypersensitivity reaction, such as rash or difficulty breathing.
• Tell female patient to notify prescriber if she is pregnant or breastfeeding.
• As appropriate, review all other significant and life-threatening adverse reactions and interactions, especially those related to the tests mentioned above.

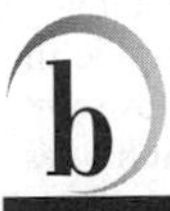

baclofen

Co Baclofen, Kemstro, Lioresal, Lioresal Intrathecal, Liotec✱, Nu-Baclo✱

Pharmacologic class: Skeletal muscle relaxant
Therapeutic class: Antispasmodic
Pregnancy risk category C

Action

Relaxes muscles by acting specifically at spinal end of upper motor neurons

Availability

Intrathecal injection: 10 mg/20 ml (500 mcg/ml), 10 mg/5 ml (2,000 mcg/ml)
Tablets: 10 mg, 20 mg

Indications and dosages

➤ Reversible spasticity associated with multiple sclerosis or spinal cord lesions
Adults: Initially, 5 mg P.O. t.i.d. May increase by 5 mg q 3 days to a maximum dosage of 80 mg/day.
Children ages 4 and older: 25 to 1,200 mcg/day by intrathecal infusion; (average is 275 mcg/day); dosage determined by response during screening phase.
➤ Severe spasticity in patients who don't respond to or can't tolerate oral baclofen
Adults: *Screening phase*—Before pump implantation and intrathecal infusion, give test dose to check responsiveness. Administer 1 ml of 50 mcg/ml dilution over 1 minute by barbotage into intrathecal space. Within 4 to 8 hours, muscle spasms should become less severe or frequent and muscle tone should decrease; if patient's response is inadequate, give second test dose of 75 mcg/1.5 ml 24 hours after first dose. If patient is still unresponsive, may give final test dose of 100 mcg/2 ml 24 hours later. Patients unresponsive to 100-mcg dose aren't candidates for intrathecal baclofen. Following appropriate responsiveness, adjust dosage to twice the screening dose and give over 24 hours. If screening dose efficacy is maintained for 12 hours, don't double the dosage. After 24 hours, increase dosage slowly as needed and tolerated by 10% to 30% daily.
Maintenance therapy—During prolonged maintenance therapy, adjust daily dosage by 10% to 40% as needed and tolerated to maintain adequate control of symptoms. Maintenance dosage ranges from 12 mcg to 2,000 mcg daily.

Dosage adjustment

• Renal impairment
• Seizure disorders
• Elderly patients

Off-label uses
- Cerebral palsy
- Tardive dyskinesia
- Trigeminal neuralgia

Contraindications
- Hypersensitivity to drug
- Rheumatic disorders

Precautions
Use cautiously in:
- epilepsy
- patients who use spasticity to maintain posture and balance
- elderly patients
- pregnant or breastfeeding patients
- children.

Administration
- Give oral doses with food or milk.
- Dilute only with sterile, preservative-free sodium chloride for injection.
- Know that intrathecal infusion should be performed only by personnel who have been trained in the procedure.

Route	Onset	Peak	Duration
P.O.	Unknown	2-3 hr	Unknown
Intrathecal	0.5-1 hr	4 hr	4-8 hr

Adverse reactions
CNS: dizziness, drowsiness, fatigue, confusion, depression, headache, insomnia, hypotonia, difficulty speaking, **seizures**
CV: edema, hypotension, hypertension, palpitations
EENT: blurred vision, tinnitus, nasal congestion
GI: nausea, vomiting, constipation
GU: urinary frequency, dysuria, erectile dysfunction
Metabolic: hyperglycemia
Skin: pruritus, rash, sweating
Other: weight gain, hypersensitivity reactions

Interactions
Drug-drug. *CNS depressants:* increased baclofen effect
MAO inhibitors: increased CNS depression, hypotension
Tricyclic antidepressants: hypotonia
Drug-diagnostic tests. *Alkaline phosphatase, aspartate aminotransferase, glucose:* increased levels
Drug-behaviors. *Alcohol use:* CNS depression

Patient monitoring
- During intrathecal infusion, check pump often for proper functioning and check catheter for patency.
- Monitor patient's response continually to determine appropriate dosage adjustment.

[Clinical alert] Observe closely for signs and symptoms of overdose (drowsiness, light-headedness, dizziness, respiratory depression), especially during initial screening and titration. No specific antidote exists. Immediately remove any solution from pump; if patient has respiratory depression, intubate until drug is eliminated.

Patient teaching
- Advise patient to take oral dose with food or milk.
- Instruct patient to avoid driving and other hazardous activities until he knows how drug affects concentration and alertness.
- Caution patient not to discontinue drug therapy abruptly. Doing so may cause hallucinations and rebound spasticity.
- As appropriate, review all other significant and life-threatening adverse reactions and interactions, especially those related to the drugs, tests, and behaviors mentioned above.

b

balsalazide disodium

Colozal

Pharmacologic class: GI agent
Therapeutic class: Anti-inflammatory
Pregnancy risk category B

Action

Metabolized in colon to mesalamine and then to 5-aminosalicylclic acid, both of which are thought to exert local anti-inflammatory effect by inhibiting prostaglandin and acid metabolites

Availability

Capsules: 750 mg

Indications and dosages

➢ Mild to moderate active ulcerative colitis

Adults: 2.25 g (three 750-mg capsules) P.O. t.i.d. for 8 to 12 weeks

Contraindications

• Hypersensitivity to balsalazide, salicylates, or mesalamine

Precautions

Use cautiously in:
• pyloric stenosis
• breastfeeding patients
• children.

Administration

• Advise patient to swallow capsules whole, either always with or always without food.

Route	Onset	Peak	Duration
P.O.	Unknown	1-2 hr	Unknown

Adverse reactions

CNS: headache, insomnia, dizziness, anxiety, confusion, agitation, **coma**
EENT: blurred vision, eye irritation, tinnitus, earache, epistaxis, sinusitis, sore throat, nasopharyngitis
GI: nausea, vomiting, diarrhea, constipation, abdominal pain, dyspepsia, anorexia, oral blisters, oral candidiasis, **GI hemorrhage**
GU: urinary tract infection
Musculoskeletal: arthralgia; myalgia; bone, back, neck, or limb pain
Respiratory: cough, upper respiratory tract infection
Skin: erythema
Other: generalized pain

Interactions

Drug-drug. *Oral antibiotics:* interference with balsalazide action

Patient monitoring

• Assess character and frequency of stools.
• Monitor CBC and liver and kidney function test results.

Patient teaching

• Instruct patient to take drug only as directed.
• As appropriate, review all other significant and life-threatening adverse reactions and interactions, especially those related to the drugs mentioned above.

basiliximab

Simulect

Pharmacologic class: Monoclonal antibody
Therapeutic class: Immunosuppressant
Pregnancy risk category B

Action

Blocks specific interleukin-2 (IL-2) receptor sites on activated T lymphocytes. Specific binding competitively inhibits IL-2–mediated activation and differentiation of lymphocytes responsible for cell-mediated immunity. Also impairs immunologic response to antigenic challenges.

Availability

Powder for injection: 20 mg in single-use vials

Indications and dosages

➤ Prevention of acute organ rejection in kidney transplantation

Adults and children weighing 35 kg (77 lb) or more: 20 mg I.V. 2 hours before transplantation surgery, then 20 mg I.V. 4 days after surgery. Withhold second dose if complications, hypersensitivity reaction, or graft loss occurs.

Children weighing less than 35 kg (77 lb): 10 mg I.V. 2 hours before transplantation surgery, then 10 mg I.V. 4 days after surgery. Withhold second dose if complications, hypersensitivity reaction, or graft loss occurs.

Contraindications

- Hypersensitivity to drug
- Pregnancy or breastfeeding

Precautions

Use cautiously in:
- elderly patients
- females of childbearing age.

Administration

Give by central or peripheral I.V. route only.
- Reconstitute by adding 5 ml of sterile water for injection to vial for bolus injection, or dilute with normal saline solution or dextrose 5% in water to a volume of 50 ml and infuse over 20 to 30 minutes. Discard any remaining product after preparing each dose.
- Don't infuse other drugs simultaneously through same I.V. line.
- Know that drug should be used only as part of regimen that includes cyclosporine and corticosteroids.

Route	Onset	Peak	Duration
I.V.	2 hr	Unknown	36 days

Adverse reactions

CNS: headache, insomnia, paresthesia, dizziness, drowsiness, tremor, anxiety, confusion, **coma, seizures**
CV: palpitations, edema, chest pain, ECG abnormalities, hypotension, hypertension, **prolonged QT interval**
EENT: blurred vision, eye irritation, tinnitus, earache, epistaxis, nasopharyngitis, sinusitis
GI: nausea, vomiting, diarrhea, constipation, abdominal pain, dyspepsia, anorexia, oral blisters, oral candidiasis, **GI hemorrhage**
GU: urinary incontinence, intermenstrual bleeding, **oliguria, renal failure**
Hematologic: anemia, **disseminated intravascular coagulation, hemorrhage, neutropenia, thrombocytopenia**
Metabolic: hypokalemia, hypomagnesemia, hyperglycemia, **acidosis, hypoglycemia, hyperkalemia**
Musculoskeletal: bone, back, neck, or limb pain
Respiratory: dyspnea, cough, hypoxia, tachypnea, hemoptysis, upper respiratory tract infection, **pleural effusions**
Skin: bruising, pruritus, dermatitis, skin lesions, diaphoresis, night sweats, erythema, hyperpigmentation, urticaria
Other: fever, lymphadenopathy, facial edema, bacterial infection, herpes simplex infection, injection site erythema, hypersensitivity reaction, **sepsis**

Interactions

Drug-drug. *Immunosuppressants:* additive immunosuppression
Drug-diagnostic tests. *Alanine aminotransferase, aspartate aminotransferase, magnesium, calcium, white blood cells:* increased levels
Glucose, potassium: increased or decreased levels

Hemoglobin, neutrophils, platelets: decreased values
Drug-herbs. *Astragalus, echinacea, melatonin:* interference with immunosuppressant action

Patient monitoring

Clinical alert: Watch for signs and symptoms of hypersensitivity reaction. Keep emergency drugs at hand in case these occur.
- Monitor vital signs and observe patient frequently during I.V. infusion.
- Monitor laboratory values and drug blood level.

Patient teaching

- Teach patient about purpose of therapy. Explain that drug decreases the risk of acute organ rejection.
- Tell patient he may be more susceptible to infection because of drug's immunosuppressant effect.
- Inform patient that he'll need lifelong immunosuppressant drug therapy.
- Advise women of childbearing age to use reliable contraception before, during, and for 2 months after therapy.
- As appropriate, review all other significant and life-threatening adverse reactions and interactions, especially those related to the drugs, tests, and herbs mentioned above.

beclomethasone dipropionate

Beclodisk✤, Becloforte✤, Beconase AQ Nasal Spray, QVAR

Pharmacologic class: Corticosteroid
Therapeutic class: Anti-inflammatory agent
Pregnancy risk category C

Action

Unclear. May decrease inflammation by stabilizing leukocytic lysosomal membrane, decreasing number and activity of inflammatory cells, inhibiting bronchoconstriction (leading to direct smooth muscle relaxation), and reducing airway hyperresponsiveness.

Availability

Inhalation aerosol: 40-mcg metered inhalation in 7.3-g canister; 80-mcg metered inhalation in 7.3-g canister
Inhalation capsules: 100 mcg, 200 mcg
Nasal spray: 0.042% (25-g bottle containing 180 metered inhalations)

Indications and dosages

➢ Maintenance treatment of asthma as prophylaxis; asthma patients who require systemic steroids for whom adding an inhaled steroid may reduce or eliminate the need for systemic steroids
Adults and children ages 12 and older: When previous therapy was bronchodilator alone, 40 to 80 mcg by oral inhalation (QVAR) b.i.d.; maximum of 320 mcg b.i.d. When previous therapy was inhaled steroid, 40 to 160 mcg by oral inhalation (QVAR) b.i.d.; maximum of 320 mcg b.i.d.
Children ages 5 to 11: When previous therapy was bronchodilator alone, 40 mcg by oral inhalation (QVAR) b.i.d.; maximum of 80 mcg b.i.d. When previous therapy was inhaled steroid, 40 mcg by oral inhalation (QVAR) b.i.d.; maximum of 80 mcg b.i.d.
➢ Seasonal or perennial rhinitis
Adults and children ages 12 and older: One or two inhalations (42 to 84 mcg Beconase AQ Nasal Spray) in each nostril b.i.d.
Children ages 6 to 12: One inhalation (42 mcg Beconase AQ Nasal Spray) in each nostril b.i.d.

Contraindications

- Hypersensitivity to drug
- Status asthmaticus

Precautions

Use cautiously in:
- active untreated infections, diabetes mellitus, glaucoma, underlying immunosuppression
- patients receiving concurrent systemic corticosteroids
- pregnant or breastfeeding patients
- children younger than age 6.

Administration

- Use spacer device to ensure proper delivery of dose and to help prevent candidiasis and hoarseness.
- After inhalation, tell patient to hold his breath for a few seconds before exhaling.
- For greater efficacy, wait 1 minute between inhalations.
- If patient is also receiving a bronchodilator, administer it at least 15 minutes before beclomethasone.
- Discontinue drug after 3 weeks if symptoms don't improve markedly.

Route	Onset	Peak	Duration
Inhalation (nasal)	5-7 days	3 wk	Unknown
Inhalation (oral)	1-4 wk	Unknown	Unknown

Adverse reactions

CNS: headache
EENT: cataracts, nasal irritation or congestion, epistaxis, perforated nasal septum, nasopharyngeal or oropharyngeal fungal infections, hoarseness, throat irritation
GI: esophageal candidiasis
Metabolic: adrenal suppression
Respiratory: cough, wheezing, **bronchospasm**
Skin: urticaria, **angioedema**
Other: anosmia, Churg-Strauss syndrome, hypersensitivity reactions

Interactions

None significant

Patient monitoring

- Assess patient's mouth daily for signs of fungal infection.
- Observe patient for proper inhaler use.

Patient teaching

- Instruct patient to hold inhaled drug in airway for several seconds before exhaling and to wait 1 minute between inhalations.
- Advise patient to rinse mouth after using inhaler and to wash and dry inhaler thoroughly to help prevent fungal infections and sore throat.
- Encourage patient to document use of drug and his response in a diary.
- If patient is also using a bronchodilator, teach him to use it at least 15 minutes before beclomethasone.
- As appropriate, review all other significant and life-threatening adverse reactions.

benazepril hydrochloride

Lotensin

Pharmacologic class: Angiotensin-converting enzyme (ACE) inhibitor
Therapeutic class: Antihypertensive
Pregnancy risk category C (first trimester), ***D*** (second and third trimesters)

Action

Inhibits conversion of angiotensin I to angiotensin II, a vasoconstrictor that stimulates adrenal glands and promotes aldosterone secretion, thereby reducing sodium and water reabsorption and ultimately decreasing blood pressure. Decreased angiotensin also causes increased potassium level and fluid loss.

Availability
Tablets: 5 mg, 10 mg, 20 mg, 40 mg

Indications and dosages
➢ Hypertension
Adults: Initially, 5 to 10 mg/day P.O. as a single dose. Increase gradually to a maintenance dosage of 20 to 40 mg/day as a single dose or in two divided doses. (Start with 5 mg/day in patients receiving diuretics.)

Dosage adjustment
- Renal impairment

Off-label uses
- Myocardial infarction
- Nephropathy

Contraindications
- Hypersensitivity to drug
- Angioedema (hereditary or idiopathic)
- Pregnancy (particularly in second and third trimesters)

Precautions
Use cautiously in:
- renal or hepatic impairment, hypovolemia, hyponatremia, aortic stenosis, hypertrophic cardiomyopathy, cerebrovascular or cardiac insufficiency
- patients receiving concurrent diuretics
- black patients
- elderly patients
- breastfeeding patients
- children.

Administration
Use extreme caution if patient has family history of angioedema.
- When giving concurrently with diuretics, know that drug may cause excessive hypotension. If possible, stop diuretic therapy 2 to 3 days before starting benazepril.
- Give with or without food.
- Know that drug may be used alone or in conjunction with other antihypertensives.

Route	Onset	Peak	Duration
P.O.	0.5-1 hr	3-4 hr	24 hr

Adverse reactions
CNS: dizziness, drowsiness, fatigue, syncope, light-headedness, headache, insomnia
CV: angina pectoris, hypotension, tachycardia
EENT: sinusitis
GI: diarrhea, nausea, anorexia
GU: proteinuria, erectile dysfunction, decreased libido, **renal failure**
Hematologic: agranulocytosis
Metabolic: hyperkalemia
Respiratory: cough, dyspnea, bronchitis, **asthma, eosinophilic pneumonitis**
Skin: rash, **angioedema**
Other: fever, altered taste

Interactions
Drug-drug. *Allopurinol:* increased risk of hypersensitivity reaction
Antacids: decreased benazepril absorption
Antihypertensives, diuretics, general anesthetics, nitrates, phenothiazines: excessive hypotension
Cyclosporine, indomethacin, potassium-sparing diuretics, potassium supplements: hyperkalemia
Digoxin, lithium: increased lithium blood level, greater risk of lithium toxicity
Nonsteroidal anti-inflammatory drugs: blunting of antihypertensive response
Drug-diagnostic tests. *Alanine aminotransferase, alkaline phosphatase, aspartate aminotransferase, bilirubin, blood urea nitrogen, creatinine, potassium:* increased levels
Antinuclear antibodies: positive result
Sodium: decreased level
Drug-food. *Salt substitutes containing potassium:* hyperkalemia
Drug-herbs. *Capsaicin:* cough

Drug-behaviors. *Acute alcohol ingestion:* increased hypotension

Patient monitoring

- Monitor for signs and symptoms of angioedema, including laryngeal edema and shock.
- Measure blood pressure regularly.
- Monitor CBC, electrolyte levels, kidney and liver function test results, and urinary protein level.

Patient teaching

- Tell patient to immediately report change in urination pattern, difficulty breathing, or swelling of throat or lips.
- Instruct patient to record blood pressure at various intervals daily.
- Tell patient to report dizziness, fainting, or light-headedness during initial therapy.
- Advise patient to increase fluid intake during exercise and in hot weather.
- Caution patient to avoid salt substitutes, which may cause hyperkalemia.
- As appropriate, review all other significant and life-threatening adverse reactions and interactions, especially those related to the drugs, tests, foods, herbs, and behaviors mentioned above.

benztropine mesylate

Apo-Benztropine✤, Cogentin, PMS Benztropine✤

Pharmacologic class: Anticholinergic
Therapeutic class: Antiparkinsonian
Pregnancy risk category C

Action

Inhibits cholinergic excitatory pathways and restores balance of dopamine and acetylcholine in CNS, thereby decreasing excess salivation, rigidity, and tremors (parkinsonian symptoms)

Availability

Injection: 1 mg/ml in 2-ml ampules
Tablets: 0.5 mg, 1 mg, 2 mg

Indications and dosages

➢ Parkinsonism
Adults: Initially, 1 to 2 mg/day P.O. or I.M. at bedtime or in two or four divided doses. Dosage range is 0.5 to 6 mg/day.
➢ Acute dystonic reactions
Adults: Initially, 1 to 2 mg I.M. or I.V., then 1 to 2 mg P.O. b.i.d.
➢ Drug-induced extrapyramidal reactions (except tardive dyskinesia)
Adults: 1 to 4 mg P.O. or I.M. once or twice daily

Dosage adjustment

- Elderly patients

Off-label uses

- Excessive salivation

Contraindications

- Hypersensitivity to drug
- Angle-closure glaucoma
- Tardive dyskinesia
- Children younger than age 3

Precautions

Use cautiously in:

- seizure disorders, arrhythmias, tachycardia, hypertension, hypotension, hepatic or renal dysfunction, alcoholism
- elderly patients
- pregnant or breastfeeding patients.

Administration

- Give after meals to prevent GI upset.
- Crush tablets if patient has difficulty swallowing them.
- Know that I.V. route is seldom used.
- Be aware that entire dose may be given at bedtime. (Drug has long duration of action.)

Route	Onset	Peak	Duration
P.O.	1-2 hr	Unknown	24 hr
I.V., I.M.	15 min	Unknown	24 hr

Adverse reactions

CNS: confusion, depression, dizziness, hallucinations, headache, weakness, memory impairment, nervousness, delusions, euphoria, paresthesia, sensation of heaviness in limbs, **toxic psychosis**
CV: hypotension, palpitations, **tachycardia, arrhythmias**
EENT: blurred vision, diplopia, mydriasis, angle-closure glaucoma
GI: nausea, constipation, dry mouth, **ileus**
GU: urinary hesitancy or retention, dysuria, difficulty maintaining erection
Musculoskeletal: paratonia, muscle weakness and cramps
Skin: rash, urticaria, decreased sweating, dermatoses

Interactions

Drug-drug. *Antacids, antidiarrheals:* decreased benztropine absorption
Antihistamines, bethanechol, disopyramide, phenothiazines, quinidine, tricyclic antidepressants: additive anticholinergic effects
Drug-herbs. *Angel's trumpet, jimsonweed, scopolia:* increased anticholinergic effects
Drug-behaviors. *Alcohol use:* increased sedation

Patient monitoring

- Monitor blood pressure closely, especially in elderly patients.
- Monitor fluid intake and output; check for urinary retention.
- Assess for signs and symptoms of ileus, including constipation and abdominal distention.

Patient teaching

- Advise patient to use caution during activities that require physical or mental alertness, because drug causes sedation.
- Tell patient to avoid increased heat exposure.

◀ Caution patient not to stop therapy abruptly.
- As appropriate, review all other significant and life-threatening adverse reactions and interactions, especially those related to the drugs, herbs, and behaviors mentioned above.

betamethasone
Betnelan✦, Celestone

betamethasone acetate and sodium phosphate
Celestone Soluspan

betamethasone sodium phosphate
Betnesol✦

Pharmacologic class: Glucocorticoid (inhalation)

Therapeutic class: Antiasthmatic, anti-inflammatory (steroidal)

Pregnancy risk category C

Action

Stabilizes lysosomal neutrophils and prevents their degranulation, inhibits synthesis of lipoxygenase products and prostaglandins, activates anti-inflammatory genes, and inhibits various cytokines

Availability

Solution for injection: 4 mg/ml of betamethasone sodium phosphate; 3 mg betamethasone sodium phosphate with 3 mg betamethasone acetate/ml
Suspension for injection (acetate, phosphate): 6 mg (total)/ml
Syrup: 0.6 mg/5 ml
Tablets: 0.6 mg
Tablets (effervescent): 0.5 mg
Tablets (extended-release): 1 mg

Indications and dosages

➢ Inflammatory, allergic, hematologic, neoplastic, autoimmune, and respiratory diseases; prevention of organ rejection after transplantation surgery
Adults: 0.6 to 7.2 mg/day P.O. as a single daily dose or in divided doses; or up to 9 mg I.M. or I.V. of betamethasone sodium phosphate; or 0.5 to 9 mg I.M. of betamethasone sodium phosphate and betamethasone acetate suspension.

➢ Bursitis or tenosynovitis
Adults: 1 ml of suspension intrabursally

➢ Rheumatoid arthritis or osteoarthritis
Adults: 0.5 to 2 ml of suspension intra-articularly

Off-label uses

• Respiratory distress syndrome

Contraindications

• Hypersensitivity to drug
• Breastfeeding

Precautions

Use cautiously in:
• systemic infections, hypertension, osteoporosis, diabetes mellitus, glaucoma, renal disease, hypothyroidism, cirrhosis, diverticulitis, thromboembolic disorders, seizures, myasthenia gravis, heart failure, ocular herpes simplex, emotional instability
• patients receiving systemic corticosteroids
• pregnant patients
• children younger than age 6.

Administration

• Give as a single daily dose before 9:00 A.M.
• Give oral dose with food or milk.
• Administer I.M. injection deep into gluteal muscle (may cause tissue atrophy).
Don't give betamethasone acetate I.V.
• Be aware that typical suspension dosage ranges from one-third to one-half of oral dosage given q 12 hours.
To avoid adrenal insufficiency, taper dosage slowly and under close supervision when discontinuing.
• Know that drug may be given with other immunosuppressants.

Route	Onset	Peak	Duration
P.O.	Unknown	1-2 hr	3-25 days
I.V, I.M. (phosphate)	Rapid	Unknown	Unknown
I.M. (acetate/ phosphate)	1-3 hr	Unknown	1 wk

Adverse reactions

CNS: headache, nervousness, depression, euphoria, psychoses, **increased intracranial pressure**
CV: hypotension, **thrombophlebitis, thromboembolism**
EENT: cataracts, burning and dryness of eyes, rebound nasal congestion, sneezing, epistaxis, nasal septum perforation, difficulty speaking, oropharyngeal or nasopharyngeal fungal infections
GI: nausea, vomiting, anorexia, dry mouth, esophageal candidiasis, peptic ulcers
Metabolic: decreased growth, hyperglycemia, cushingoid appearance, **adrenal insufficiency or suppression**
Musculoskeletal: muscle wasting, muscle pain, osteoporosis, aseptic joint necrosis
Respiratory: cough, wheezing, **bronchospasm**
Skin: facial edema, rash, contact dermatitis, acne, ecchymosis, hirsutism, petechiae, urticaria, **angioedema**
Other: loss of taste, bad taste, weight gain or loss, Churg-Strauss syndrome, increased susceptibility to infection, hypersensitivity reaction

b

Interactions

Drug-drug. *Amphotericin B, loop and thiazide diuretics, ticarcillin:* additive hypokalemia
Barbiturates, phenytoin, rifampin: stimulation of betamethasone metabolism, causing decreased drug effects
Digoxin: increased risk of digoxin toxicity
Fluoroquinolones (such as ciprofloxacin, norfloxacin): increased risk of tendon rupture
Hormonal contraceptives: blockage of betamethasone metabolism
Insulin, oral hypoglycemics: increased betamethasone dosage requirement
Live-virus vaccines: decreased antibody response to vaccine, increased risk of neurologic complications
Nonsteroidal anti-inflammatory drugs: increased risk of adverse GI effects
Drug-diagnostic tests. *Calcium, cholesterol, glucose, potassium:* increased levels
Nitroblue tetrazolium test for bacterial infection: false-negative result
Drug-herbs. *Echinacea:* increased immune-stimulating effects
Ginseng: increased immune-modulating effects
Drug-behaviors. *Alcohol use:* increased risk of gastric irritation and GI ulcers

Patient monitoring

- Monitor weight daily and report sudden increase, which suggests fluid retention.
- Monitor blood glucose level for hyperglycemia.
- Assess serum electrolyte levels for sodium and potassium imbalances.
- Watch for signs and symptoms of infection (which drug may mask).

Patient teaching

- Advise patient to report signs and symptoms of infection.
- Tell patient to report visual disturbances (long-term drug use may cause cataracts).
- Instruct patient to eat low-sodium, high potassium diet.

🔊 Advise patient to carry medical identification describing drug therapy.

- Inform female patients that drug may cause menstrual irregularities.

🔊 Caution patient not to stop taking drug abruptly.

- As appropriate, review all other significant and life-threatening adverse reactions and interactions, especially those related to the drugs, tests, herbs, and behaviors mentioned above.

bethanechol chloride

Duvoid, Myotonachol, PMS-Bethanecol Chloride♣, Urabeth, Urecholine

Pharmacologic class: Cholinergic
Therapeutic class: Urinary and GI tract stimulant
Pregnancy risk category C

Action

Stimulates parasympathetic nervous system and cholinergic receptors, leading to increased muscle tone in bladder and increased frequency of ureteral peristaltic waves. Also stimulates gastric motility, increases gastric tone, and restores rhythmic GI peristalsis.

Availability

Injection: 5 mg/ml
Tablets: 5 mg, 10 mg, 25 mg, 50 mg

Indications and dosages

➤ Postpartal and postoperative nonobstructive urinary retention; urinary retention caused by neurogenic bladder
Adults: 10 to 50 mg P.O. three to four times daily; dosage may be determined by giving 5 or 10 mg q hour until response occurs or a total of 50 mg has

been given. Alternatively, 5 mg subcutaneously three to four times daily; dosage may be determined by giving 2.5 mg subcutaneously q 15 to 30 minutes until response occurs or a total of four doses has been given.

Contraindications

- Hypersensitivity to drug
- GI or GU tract obstruction
- Hyperthyroidism
- Active or latent asthma
- Bradycardia
- Hypotension
- Hypertension
- Atrioventricular conduction defects
- Coronary artery disease
- Seizure disorders
- Parkinsonism
- Peptic ulcer disease

Precautions

Use cautiously in:
- sensitivity to cholinergics or their effects
- pregnant or breastfeeding patients
- children.

Administration

- Give drug on empty stomach 1 hour before or 2 hours after a meal to help prevent nausea and vomiting.

[Clinical alert] Don't give I.M or I.V. Doing so may cause severe symptoms of cholinergic overstimulation, including circulatory collapse and cardiac arrest.

- Keep atropine on hand to counteract severe adverse effects.

Route	Onset	Peak	Duration
P.O.	30-90 min	1 hr	6 hr
Subcut.	5-15 min	15-30 min	2 hr

Adverse reactions

CNS: headache, malaise
CV: bradycardia, hypotension, **heart block, syncope with cardiac arrest**
EENT: excessive lacrimation, miosis
GI: nausea, vomiting, diarrhea, abdominal discomfort, belching
GU: urinary urgency
Respiratory: increased bronchial secretions, **bronchospasm**
Skin: diaphoresis, flushing
Other: hypothermia

Interactions

Drug-drug. *Anticholinergics:* decreased bethanechol efficacy
Cholinesterase inhibitors: additive cholinergic effects
Depolarizing neuromuscular blockers: decreased blood pressure
Ganglionic blockers: severe hypotension
Procainamide, quinidine: antagonism of cholinergic effects
Drug-diagnostic tests. *Amylase, hepatic enzymes, lipase:* increased levels
Drug-herbs. *Angel's trumpet, jimsonweed, scopolia:* antagonism of cholinergic effects

Patient monitoring

- Monitor blood pressure. Be aware that hypertensive patients may experience sudden blood pressure drop.
- Stay alert for orthostatic hypotension, a common adverse effect.
- Monitor vital signs and respiration for 30 to 60 minutes after subcutaneous injection.
- Monitor fluid intake and output and residual urine volume.

Patient teaching

- Tell patient that drug is usually effective within 90 minutes of administration.
- Advise patient to take oral dose on empty stomach 1 hour before or 2 hours after a meal to avoid GI upset.
- Instruct patient to move slowly when sitting up or standing, to avoid dizziness or light-headedness from blood pressure decrease.
- As appropriate, review all other significant and life-threatening adverse

reactions and interactions, especially those related to the drugs, tests, and herbs mentioned above.

bevacizumab

Avastin

Pharmacologic class: Monoclonal antibody
Therapeutic class: Immunologic agent
Pregnancy risk category C

Action

Binds to vascular endothelial growth factor, preventing or reducing microvascular formation and growth and inhibiting metastatic disease progression

Availability

Solution for injection: 25 mg/ml in 4-ml and 16-ml vials

Indications and dosages

➤ First-line treatment of metastatic cancer of colon or rectum (used in combination with 5-fluorouracil-based chemotherapy)
Adults: 5 mg/kg I.V. infusion q 14 days until disease progression occurs

Contraindications

None

Precautions

Use cautiously in:
- hypersensitivity to drug
- cardiovascular disease
- development of immunogenicity
- patients sensitive to infusion reactions
- patients recovering from major surgery
- elderly patients
- pregnant or breastfeeding patients
- children.

Administration

- Withdraw necessary amount for 5 mg/kg dose, and dilute in 100 ml of 0.9% sodium chloride injection.

Don't mix or administer drug with dextrose solutions.

Don't deliver by I.V. push or bolus.

- Initially, infuse drug over 90 minutes. If patient tolerates infusion well, infuse over 60 minutes the second time; if he continues to tolerate it well, infuse each dose over 30 minutes thereafter.

Withhold dose if hypertension occurs.

Stop infusion if patient develops hypertensive crisis, severe bleeding, abdominal pain (may signal intra-abdominal abscess or GI perforation), wound dehiscence, or urinary problems.

- Know that drug is given in combination with 5-fluorouracil-based chemotherapy.
- Be aware that drug shouldn't be given within 28 days after major surgery and that therapy should be suspended several weeks before elective surgery.

Route	Onset	Peak	Duration
I.V.	Unknown	Unknown	Unknown

Adverse reactions

CNS: asthenia, dizziness, headache, confusion, syncope, abnormal gait
CV: hypotension, hypertension, **hypertensive crisis, heart failure, deep-vein thrombosis, intra-abdominal thrombosis, thromboembolism**
EENT: excess lacrimation, **severe epistaxis**
GI: nausea, vomiting, diarrhea, constipation, abdominal pain, stomatitis, dyspepsia, flatulence, colitis, dry mouth, anorexia, **GI perforation, intra-abdominal abscess**
GU: proteinuria, urinary frequency or urgency, **nephrotic syndrome**
Hematologic: leukopenia, neutropenia, hemorrhage
Hepatic: bilirubinemia

Metabolic: hypokalemia
Musculoskeletal: myalgia
Respiratory: upper respiratory tract infection, dyspnea, **massive hemoptysis**
Skin: exfoliative dermatitis, alopecia, dry skin, skin discoloration, skin ulcers, nail disorder, wound-healing complications, **wound dehiscence**
Other: abnormal taste, altered voice, pain, weight loss, **transfusion reaction**

Interactions

Drug-drug. *Irinotecan:* increased concentration of irinotecan metabolite
Drug-diagnostic tests. *Leukocytes, potassium:* decreased levels
Urine protein: increased level

Patient monitoring

🔊 Monitor patient closely for signs and symptoms of thromboembolism and GI perforation (such as abdominal pain, vomiting, and constipation).
🔊 Stay alert for delayed wound healing and wound dehiscence.
- Assess blood pressure frequently.
- Monitor CBC with differential and urine protein and serum electrolyte levels.

Patient teaching

🔊 Tell patient to call prescriber immediately if he experiences dizziness, severe bleeding, stomach pain, or urinary problems or if a wound opens.
- Instruct patient to tell prescriber if he has been exposed to chickenpox or if he has gout, heart disease, viral infection, urinary problems, hepatic disease, or another form of cancer.
- Advise patient to tell prescriber if he has surgery planned; drug may delay wound healing.
- Caution patient not to get immunizations unless prescriber approves.
- Instruct female patient to tell prescriber if she is pregnant, plans to become pregnant, or is breastfeeding.
- As appropriate, review all other significant and life-threatening adverse reactions and interactions, especially those related to the drugs and tests mentioned above.

bicalutamide

Casodex

Pharmacologic class: Nonsteroidal antiandrogen
Therapeutic class: Antineoplastic
Pregnancy risk category X

Action

Antagonizes effects of androgen at cellular level by binding to androgen receptors on target tissues

Availability

Tablets: 50 mg

Indications and dosages

➢ Metastatic prostate cancer
Adults: 50 mg P.O. once daily

Contraindications

- Hypersensitivity to drug

Precautions

Use cautiously in:
- previous hypersensitivity or serious adverse reaction to flutamide or nilutamide
- moderate to severe hepatic impairment
- children.

Administration

- Know that drug is given in combination with luteinizing hormone-releasing hormone (LHRH).
- Administer at same time each day.

Route	Onset	Peak	Duration
P.O.	Unknown	31 hr	Unknown

Adverse reactions

CNS: headache, weakness, dizziness, depression, hypertonia, paresthesia, lethargy
CV: chest pain, peripheral edema, vasodilation, hypertension, **thromboembolic disease**
EENT: pharyngitis
GI: nausea, vomiting, diarrhea, constipation, abdominal pain, anorexia, dry mouth
GU: urinary tract infection
Musculoskeletal: bone and back pain
Respiratory: dyspnea, cough
Skin: rash, alopecia
Other: food distaste, weight gain, edema, pain, hot flashes, flulike symptoms

Interactions

Drug-drug. *Warfarin:* increased bicalutamide effects
Drug-diagnostic tests. *Alanine aminotransferase, alkaline phosphatase, aspartate aminotransferase, bilirubin, cholesterol:* increased levels
Hemoglobin, white blood cells: decreased values

Patient monitoring

- Monitor prostate-significant antigen levels, CBC, and liver and kidney function test results.
- If patient is receiving warfarin concurrently, evaluate prothrombin time and International Normalized Ratio.

Patient teaching

- Instruct patient to take drug at same time each day, along with prescribed LHRH analog.
- Tell patient that any drug-related hair loss should reverse once therapy ends.
- As appropriate, review all other significant and life-threatening adverse reactions and interactions, especially those related to the drugs and tests mentioned above.

biperiden

Akineton

Pharmacologic class: Anticholinergic
Therapeutic class: Antiparkinsonian
Pregnancy risk category C

Action

Inhibits cholinergic excitatory pathways and restores balance of dopamine and acetylcholine in CNS, thereby decreasing such parkinsonian symptoms as excess salivation, rigidity, and tremors

Availability

Injection: 5 mg/ml
Tablets: 2 mg

Indications and dosages

➢ Parkinsonism
Adults: Initially, 2 mg P.O. three to four times daily. Maximum dosage is 16 mg/day.
➢ Extrapyramidal reactions
Adults: 2 mg P.O. one to three times daily; or 2 mg I.M. or I.V., repeated as needed q 30 minutes. Maximum dosage is 8 mg or four doses in 24 hours.

Contraindications

- Hypersensitivity to drug or other anticholinergics
- Angle-closure glaucoma
- Myasthenia gravis
- GI or GU tract obstruction
- Achalasia
- Paralytic ileus or intestinal atony
- Ulcerative colitis
- Prostatic hypertrophy
- Tardive dyskinesia

Precautions

Use cautiously in:
- seizure disorders, arrhythmias, tachy-

cardia, hypotension, hypertension, renal or hepatic dysfunction, chronic illness, alcoholism
• elderly patients
• pregnant or breastfeeding patients.

Administration
• Give before or after meals, depending on patient's response. If dry mouth occurs, give before meals. When giving with meals, allay thirst with water, mints, or chewing gum.
• When giving I.V., inject drug slowly.
• When giving parenterally, have patient rest in prone position for 20 minutes after injection, because drug may cause light-headedness.

Route	Onset	Peak	Duration
P.O.	1 hr	1-1.5 hr	Unknown
I.V.	Immediate	Unknown	1-8 hr
I.M.	15 min	Unknown	Unknown

Adverse reactions
CNS: confusion, incoherence, depression, dizziness, hallucinations, tremor, headache, sedation, weakness, restlessness, delusions, euphoria, memory loss
CV: hypotension, palpitations, tachycardia, **arrhythmias**
EENT: blurred vision, dry eyes, photophobia, mydriasis, increased intraocular pressure, closed-angle glaucoma
GI: nausea, constipation, abdominal distress, difficulty swallowing, dry mouth, **paralytic ileus**
GU: urinary hesitancy or retention
Skin: rash, urticaria, dermatosis, decreased sweating, flushing
Other: increased body temperature, numbness in fingers, cramping, **heat stroke**

Interactions
Drug-drug. *Antacids, antidiarrheals:* decreased biperiden absorption
Antihistamines, disopyramide, phenothiazines, quinidine, tricyclic antidepressants: additive anticholinergic effects
Bethanechol: antagonistic effects
CNS depressants: increased sedative effect
Haloperidol, phenothiazines: masking of extrapyramidal symptoms, tardive dyskinesia, central anticholinergic syndrome
Drug-herbs. *Angel's trumpet, jimsonweed, scopolia:* increased anticholinergic effects
Drug-behaviors. *Alcohol use:* increased CNS depression

Patient monitoring
• Monitor vital signs and cardiac status.
• Watch for urinary retention (more common in males).
• Closely monitor patient with pulmonary disease.

Patient teaching
• Advise patient to take drug with food to minimize GI upset.
• Emphasize importance of avoiding alcohol and other CNS depressants.
• Caution patient against heat exposure and exercising in warm weather, because drug decreases ability to sweat.
• Instruct patient to avoid driving and other hazardous activities until he knows how drug affects concentration and alertness.
• Urge patient to have annual eye examinations because drug increases risk of increased intraocular pressure.
• As appropriate, review all other significant and life-threatening adverse reactions and interactions, especially those related to the drugs, herbs, and behaviors mentioned above.

bisacodyl

Bisac-Evac, Carter's Little Pills, Correctol, Dacodyl, Deficol, Dulcagen, Dulcolax, Feen-a-Mint, Fleet Laxative, Laxit✦, Reliable Gentle Laxative, Theralax, Women's Gentle Laxative

Pharmacologic class: Stimulant laxative

Therapeutic class: Laxative

Pregnancy risk category B

Action

Unclear. Thought to stimulate colonic mucosa, producing parasympathetic reflexes that enhance peristalsis and increase water and electrolyte secretion, thereby causing evacuation of colon.

Availability

Enema: 0.33 mg/ml, 10 mg/ml
Powder for rectal solution: 1.5 mg bisacodyl and 2.5 g tannic acid
Suppositories (rectal): 5 mg, 10 mg
Tablets (enteric-coated): 5 mg

Indications and dosages

➤ Constipation; bowel cleansing for childbirth, surgery, and endoscopic examination

Adults and children ages 12 and older: 5 to 15 mg P.O. Maximum daily dosage is 30 mg/day P.O. or 10 mg P.R.

Children ages 3 to 11: 5 to 10 mg (0.3 mg/kg) P.O. as a single dose or 5 to 10 mg P.R. as a single dose

Children ages 2 and younger: 5 mg P.R. as a single dose

Contraindications

- Hypersensitivity to drug
- Intestinal obstruction
- Gastroenteritis
- Appendicitis

Precautions

Use cautiously in:
- hypersensitivity to tannic acid
- severe cardiovascular disease, anal or rectal fissures
- pregnant or breastfeeding patients.

Administration

- Make sure patient swallows tablets whole without chewing.
- Don't give tablets within 1 hour of dairy products or antacids (may break down enteric coating).
- Know that drug should be used only for short periods.

Route	Onset	Peak	Duration
P.O.	6-12 hr	Variable	Variable
P.R.	15-60 min	Variable	Variable

Adverse reactions

CNS: dizziness, syncope
GI: nausea, vomiting, diarrhea (with high doses), abdominal pain, burning sensation in rectum (with suppositories), laxative dependence, protein-losing enteropathy
Metabolic: hypokalemia, fluid and electrolyte imbalances, **tetany, alkalosis**
Musculoskeletal: muscle weakness (with excessive use)

Interactions

Drug-drug. *Antacids:* gastric irritation, dyspepsia
Drug-diagnostic tests. *Calcium, magnesium, potassium:* decreased levels
Phosphate, sodium: increased levels
Drug-food. *Dairy products:* gastric irritation

Patient monitoring

- Assess stools for frequency and consistency.
- Monitor patient for electrolyte imbalances and dehydration.

Patient teaching

- Instruct patient to swallow (not chew) enteric-coated tablets no sooner than 1 hour before or after ingesting antacids or dairy products. Tell him not to chew tablets.
- Advise patient not to use bisacodyl or other laxatives habitually because this may lead to laxative dependence.
- Suggest other ways to prevent constipation, such as by eating more fruits, vegetables, and whole grains to increase dietary bulk and by drinking 8 to 10 glasses of water daily.
- As appropriate, review all other significant and life-threatening adverse reactions and interactions, especially those related to the drugs, tests, and foods mentioned above.

bismuth subsalicylate

Bismatrol, Bismatrol Extra Strength, Bismed, Pepto-Bismol, Pepto-Bismol Bismuth Maximum Strength, Pink Bismuth, PMS-Bismuth Subsalicylate

Pharmacologic class: Adsorbent
Therapeutic class: Antidiarrheal, antibiotic, antiulcer drug
Pregnancy risk category C

Action

Promotes intestinal adsorption of fluids and electrolytes and decreases synthesis of intestinal prostaglandins. Adsorbent action removes irritants from stomach and soothes irritated bowel lining. Also shows antibacterial activity to eradicate *Helicobacter pylori.*

Availability

Liquid: 130 mg/15 ml, 262 mg/15 ml, 525 mg/15 ml (maximum strength)
Tablets: 262 mg
Tablets (chewable): 262 mg, 300 mg

Indications and dosages

➢ Adjunctive therapy for mild to moderate diarrhea, nausea, abdominal cramping, heartburn, and indigestion accompanying diarrheal illnesses
Adults: Two tablets or 30 ml P.O. (15 ml of maximum strength) q 30 minutes, or two tablets or 60 ml (30 ml of extra/maximum strength) q 60 minutes as needed. Don't exceed 4.2 g in 24 hours.
Children ages 9 to 12: One tablet or 15 ml P.O. (7.5 ml of maximum strength) q 30 to 60 minutes. Don't exceed 2.1 g in 24 hours.
Children ages 6 to 9: 10 ml (5 ml of maximum strength) P.O. q 30 to 60 minutes. Don't exceed 1.4 g in 24 hours.
Children ages 3 to 6: 5 ml (2.5 ml of maximum strength) P.O. q 30 to 60 minutes. Don't exceed 704 mg in 24 hours.
➢ Ulcer disease caused by *H. pylori*
Adults: Two tablets or 30 ml P.O. q.i.d. (15 ml of maximum strength)

Off-label uses

- Chronic infantile diarrhea
- Norwalk virus–induced gastroenteritis

Contraindications

- Hypersensitivity to aspirin
- Elderly patients with fecal impaction
- Children or adolescents during or after recovery from chickenpox or flulike illness

Precautions

Use cautiously in:
- diabetes mellitus, gout
- patients taking concurrent aspirin
- elderly patients
- pregnant or breastfeeding patients
- infants.

Administration
• Know that tablets should be chewed or dissolved in mouth before swallowing.
• Be aware that drug is usually given with antibiotics (such as tetracycline or amoxicillin) when prescribed for ulcer disease.

Route	Onset	Peak	Duration
P.O.	1 hr	Unknown	Unknown

Adverse reactions
EENT: tinnitus, tongue discoloration
GI: nausea, vomiting, diarrhea, constipation, gray-black stools, fecal impaction
Respiratory: tachypnea
Other: salicylate toxicity

Interactions
Drug-drug. *Aspirin, other salicylates:* salicylate toxicity
Corticosteroids, probenecid (large doses), sulfinpyrazone: decreased bismuth efficacy
Enoxacin: decreased enoxacin bioavailability
Methotrexate: increased risk of bismuth toxicity
Tetracycline: decreased tetracycline absorption
Drug-diagnostic tests. *Radiologic GI tract examination:* test interference

Patient monitoring
• Monitor fluid intake and electrolyte levels.
• Monitor stool frequency and appearance.
• Assess infants and debilitated patients for fecal impaction.

Patient teaching
• Instruct patient to chew tablets or dissolve them in mouth before swallowing.
• Inform patient that drug may turn stools gray-black temporarily.
• Tell patient to notify prescriber if he has diarrhea with fever for more than 48 hours.
• As appropriate, review all other significant adverse reactions and interactions, especially those related to the drugs and tests mentioned above.

b

bisoprolol fumarate
Monocor✤, Zebeta

Pharmacologic class: Beta$_1$-adrenergic blocker
Therapeutic class: Antihypertensive
Pregnancy risk category C

Action
Blocks beta$_1$-adrenergic receptors of sympathetic nervous system in heart and kidney, thereby decreasing myocardial excitability, myocardial oxygen consumption, cardiac output, and renin release from kidney. Also lowers blood pressure without affecting beta$_2$-adrenergic (pulmonary, vascular, and uterine) receptor sites.

Availability
Tablets: 5 mg, 10 mg

Indications and dosages
➤ Hypertension
Adults: Initially, 2.5 to 5 mg P.O. daily. Dosages up to 20 mg P.O. daily have been used.

Dosage adjustment
• Renal or hepatic impairment

Contraindications
• Hypersensitivity to drug
• Sinus bradycardia
• Second- or third-degree heart block
• Cardiogenic shock
• Heart failure
• Children (safety and efficacy not established)

Precautions

Use cautiously in:
• renal or hepatic impairment, pulmonary disease, asthma, diabetes mellitus, thyrotoxicosis
• elderly patients
• pregnant or breastfeeding patients.

Administration

• Give with or without food, but be consistent to minimize variations in absorption.
• Check patient's apical pulse before giving. If it's irregular or below 60 beats/minute, withhold dose and notify prescriber.
• Be aware that drug may be given alone or added to diuretic therapy.

Route	Onset	Peak	Duration
P.O.	30-60 min	2 hr	12-15 hr

Adverse reactions

CNS: dizziness, depression, paresthesia, sleep disturbances, hallucinations, memory loss, slurred speech
CV: tachycardia, peripheral vascular insufficiency, claudication, hypotension, sinoatrial or atrioventricular (AV) node block, **second- or third-degree heart block, heart failure, pulmonary edema, cerebrovascular accident, arrhythmias**
EENT: blurred vision, dry eyes, conjunctivitis, tinnitus, rhinitis, pharyngitis
GI: nausea, vomiting, diarrhea, constipation, gastric pain, gastritis, flatulence, anorexia, **ischemic colitis, acute pancreatitis, renal and mesenteric arterial thrombosis**
GU: dysuria, polyuria, nocturia, erectile dysfunction, Peyronie's disease, decreased libido
Hematologic: eosinophilia, **agranulocytosis, thrombocytopenia**
Hepatic: hepatomegaly
Metabolic: hyperglycemia, **hypoglycemia**
Musculoskeletal: arthralgia, muscle cramps
Respiratory: dyspnea, cough, **bronchial obstruction, bronchospasm**
Skin: rash, purpura, pruritus, dry skin, excessive sweating

Interactions

Drug-drug. *Amphetamines, ephedrine, epinephrine, norepinephrine, phenylephrine, pseudoephedrine:* unopposed alpha-adrenergic stimulation
Antihypertensives, aspirin, bismuth subsalicylate, hormonal contraceptives, magnesium salicylate, nitrates, sulfinpyrazone: increased hypotension
Digoxin: additive bradycardia
Dobutamine, dopamine: decrease in beneficial $beta_1$-adrenergic cardiovascular effects
General anesthetics, I.V. phenytoin, verapamil: additive myocardial depression
MAO inhibitors: hypertension (when taken within 14 days of bisoprolol)
Nonsteroidal anti-inflammatory drugs: decreased antihypertensive effect
Thyroid preparations: decreased bisoprolol efficacy
Drug-diagnostic tests. *Alanine aminotransferase, alkaline phosphatase, aspartate aminotransferase, blood urea nitrogen, glucose, low-density lipoproteins, potassium, uric acid:* increased levels
Antinuclear antibodies: increased titers
Insulin tolerance test: test interference
Drug-behaviors. *Acute alcohol ingestion:* additive hypotension
Cocaine use: unopposed alpha-adrenergic stimulation

Patient monitoring

• Closely monitor blood glucose levels in diabetic patients.
• Assess for signs and symptoms of heart failure, including weight gain.
• Stay alert for blood pressure variations. Low blood pressure may indicate overdose.

Patient teaching

- Tell patient to weigh himself daily at same time and to report gain of 3 to 4 lb/day.
- Instruct patient to move slowly when sitting up or standing, to avoid dizziness or light-headedness from blood pressure decrease.
- Caution patient to avoid driving and other hazardous activities until he knows how drug affects concentration and alertness.
- Advise patient to restrict salt intake to help avoid fluid retention.
- Caution patient not to discontinue drug abruptly unless prescriber approves.
- Tell patient to carry medical identification stating that he's taking a beta blocker.
- As appropriate, review all other significant and life-threatening adverse reactions and interactions, especially those related to the drugs, tests, and behaviors mentioned above.

bivalirudin

Angiomax

Pharmacologic class: Thrombin inhibitor

Therapeutic class: Anticoagulant

Pregnancy risk category B

Action

Selectively inhibits thrombin by binding to its receptor sites, causing inactivation of coagulation factors V, VIII, and XII and thus preventing conversion of fibrinogen to fibrin

Availability

Powder for injection: 250 mg/vial

Indications and dosages

➢ Patients with unstable angina who are undergoing percutaneous transluminal angioplasty (PCTA)

Adults: 1 mg/kg I.V. bolus just before PCTA; then start 4-hour I.V. infusion at 2.5 mg/kg/hour. After 4-hour infusion, may give additional I.V. infusion at 0.2 mg/kg/hour for up to 20 hours, along with aspirin as ordered.

Dosage adjustment

- Renal impairment
- Dialysis patients

Off-label uses

- PCTA (regardless of history of unstable angina)
- Anticoagulation during orthopedic surgery

Contraindications

- Hypersensitivity to drug
- Acute coronary syndrome
- Active major bleeding or unstable angina in patients not undergoing PCTA

Precautions

Use cautiously in:

- renal impairment, severe hepatic dysfunction, bacterial endocarditis, cerebrovascular accident, severe hypertension, heparin-induced thrombocytopenia, thrombosis syndrome
- diseases associated with increased risk of bleeding
- concurrent use of other platelet aggregation inhibitors
- pregnant or breastfeeding patients
- children.

Administration

- For I.V. injection and infusion, add 5 ml of sterile water to each 250-mg vial; gently mix until dissolved. Further dilute in 50 ml of dextrose 5% in water or normal saline solution for injection to a final concentration of 5 mg/ml.

- Don't mix with other drugs.
- Don't give by I.M. route.
- Know that drug is intended for use with aspirin.

Route	Onset	Peak	Duration
I.V.	Immediate	Immediate	1-2 hr

Adverse reactions

CNS: headache, anxiety, nervousness, insomnia
CV: hypotension, hypertension, **bradycardia, ventricular fibrillation**
GI: nausea, vomiting, abdominal pain, dyspepsia, **severe spontaneous GI bleeding**
GU: urinary retention, **severe spontaneous GU bleeding**
Hematologic: severe spontaneous bleeding
Musculoskeletal: pelvic or back pain
Other: fever, pain at injection site

Interactions

Drug-drug. *Abciximab, anticoagulants (including heparin, low-molecular-weight heparins, and heparinoids), thrombolytics, ticlopidine:* increased risk of bleeding
Glycoprotein IIb/IIIa inhibitors: safety and efficacy of concomitant use not established
Drug-diagnostic tests. *Activated partial thromboplastin time, prothrombin time:* increased
Drug-herbs. *Ginkgo biloba:* increased risk of bleeding

Patient monitoring

Monitor blood pressure, hemoglobin, and hematocrit. Be aware that decrease in blood pressure or hematocrit may signal hemorrhagic event.
- Monitor venipuncture site closely for bleeding.

Patient teaching

Instruct patient to immediately report bleeding, bruising, or tarry stools.
- Tell patient to avoid activities that can cause injury. Advise him to use soft toothbrush and electric razor to avoid gum and skin injury.
- Advise family members to take classes in cardiopulmonary resuscitation.

bleomycin sulfate

Blenoxane

Pharmacologic class: Antitumor antibiotic
Therapeutic class: Antineoplastic
Pregnancy risk category D

Action

Unclear. Appears to inhibit DNA synthesis and, to a lesser degree, RNA and protein synthesis. Binds to DNA, causing severing of single DNA strands.

Availability

Injection: 15-unit vials, 30-unit vials

Indications and dosages

➢ Hodgkin's lymphoma
Adults: 10 to 20 units/m² I.V., I.M., or subcutaneously once or twice weekly. After 50% response, maintenance dosage is 1 unit/m² I.M. or I.V. daily or 5 units/m² I.M. or I.V. weekly.
➢ Malignant pleural effusion; prevention of recurrent pleural effusions
Adults: 60 units dissolved in 50 to 100 mg of normal saline solution, given through thoracostomy tube
➢ Squamous cell carcinoma of head, neck, skin, penis, cervix, or vulva; non-Hodgkin's lymphoma; testicular carcinoma
Adults and children ages 12 and older: 10 to 20 units/m² I.V., I.M., or subcutaneously once or twice weekly.

Dosage adjustment

- Renal impairment
- Elderly patients

Off-label uses
- Esophageal carcinoma
- Hemangioma
- AIDS-related Kaposi's sarcoma
- Osteosarcoma
- Verrucous carcinoma
- Warts

Contraindications
- Hypersensitivity to drug
- Pregnancy or breastfeeding

Precautions
Use cautiously in:
- renal or pulmonary impairment
- elderly patients
- females of childbearing age.

Administration
- Wash hands before and after preparing drug; wear gloves during handling and preparation.
- For I.M. or subcutaneous use, reconstitute 15-unit vial with 1 to 5 ml and 30-unit vial with 2 to 10 ml of sterile water for injection, normal saline solution for injection, or bacteriostatic water for injection.
- For I.V. infusion, dissolve contents of 15- or 30-unit vial in 5 or 10 ml, respectively, of normal saline solution for injection.
- For intrapleural use, dissolve each 60 units in 50 to 100 ml of normal saline solution for injection, then administer through thoracostomy tube. Clamp tube after instilling drug. During next 4 hours, reposition patient from supine to right and left lateral positions several times. Then unclamp tube and restart suction.
- Premedicate patient with aspirin, as prescribed, to reduce risk of drug fever.

[Clinical alert] Know that cumulative dosages above 400 units should be given with extreme caution because of increased risk of pulmonary toxicity.

Route	Onset	Peak	Duration
I.V.	Immediate	10-20 min	Unknown
I.M., subcut.	15-20 min	30-60 min	Unknown

b

Adverse reactions
CNS: disorientation, weakness, aggressive behavior
CV: hypotension, peripheral vasoconstriction
GI: vomiting, diarrhea, anorexia, stomatitis
Hematologic: anemia, **leukopenia, thrombocytopenia**
Hepatic: hepatotoxicity
Metabolic: hyperuricemia
Respiratory: dyspnea, crackles, **pulmonary fibrosis, pneumonitis**
Skin: alopecia, erythema, rash, urticaria, vesicles, striae, hyperpigmentation, mucocutaneous toxicity
Other: fever, chills, weight loss, **anaphylactic reaction**

Interactions
Drug-drug. *Anesthetics:* increased oxygen requirement
Antineoplastics: increased risk of hematologic and pulmonary toxicity
Cardiac glycosides: decreased cardiac glycoside blood level
Cisplatin: decreased bleomycin elimination, increased risk of toxicity
Fosphenytoin, phenytoin: decreased blood levels of these drugs
Vinblastine: increased risk of Raynaud's syndrome
Drug-diagnostic tests. *Uric acid:* increased level

Patient monitoring
- Assess baseline pulmonary function status before initiating therapy; monitor throughout therapy.
- Monitor chest X-rays and assess breath sounds to detect signs of pulmonary toxicity.
- Assess oral cavity for sores, ulcers, pain, and bleeding.

• Monitor infusion site for irritation, burning, and signs of infection.
• Evaluate closely for signs and symptoms of drug fever.

Patient teaching

• Tell patient to avoid spicy, hot, or rough foods (may cause GI upset).
• Urge patient to use reliable contraceptive method during therapy.
• Tell patient to avoid activities that can cause injury. Advise him to use soft toothbrush and electric razor to avoid gum and skin injury.
• Inform patient that drug may cause hair loss but that hair will grow back after treatment ends.
• As appropriate, review all other significant and life-threatening adverse reactions and interactions, especially those related to the drugs and tests mentioned above.

bortezomib

Velcade

Pharmacologic class: Proteasome inhibitor

Therapeutic class: Antineoplastic

Pregnancy risk category D

Action

Inhibits proteasomes (enzyme complexes that regulate protein homeostasis within cells). Reversibly inhibits chymotrypsin-like activity at 26S proteasome, leading to activation of signaling cascades, cell-cycle arrest, and apoptosis.

Availability

Powder for reconstitution (preservative-free): 3.5 mg (contains 35 mg of mannitol)

Indications and dosages

➢ Multiple myeloma in patients who have undergone at least two previous therapies and demonstrated disease progression during previous therapy

Adults: 1.3 mg/m^2 I.V. twice weekly for 2 weeks (days 1, 4, 8, and 11), followed by 10-day rest period (days 12 to 21). Allow at least 72 hours to elapse between doses. One treatment cycle equals 21 days (3 weeks).

Contraindications

• Hypersensitivity to drug, mannitol, or boron
• Pregnancy

Precautions

Use cautiously in:
• dehydration, hepatic or renal impairment
• history of syncope
• children.

Administration

• Reconstitute drug in vial with 3.5 ml of normal saline for injection.
• Give by I.V. push over 3 to 5 seconds.

Route	Onset	Peak	Duration
I.V.	Unknown	Unknown	Unknown

Adverse reactions

CNS: headache, insomnia, dizziness, anxiety, peripheral neuropathy
CV: tachycardia, hypertension
EENT: throat tightness
GI: nausea, vomiting, diarrhea, abdominal pain, dyspepsia
Hematologic: eosinophilia, anemia, **thrombocytopenia, neutropenia**
Metabolic: dehydration, pyrexia
Respiratory: cough, dyspnea, upper respiratory tract infection
Skin: rash, pruritus, urticaria
Other: altered taste, increased or decreased appetite, fever, chills

Interactions

Drug-drug. *CYP3A4 inducers (including amiodarone, carbamazepine, nevirapine, phenobarbital, phenytoin, and rifampin):* possible decrease in bortezomid serum level and efficacy
CYP3A4 inhibitors (including amiodarone, cimetidine, clarithromycin, delavirdine, diltiazem, disulfiram, erythromycin, fluoxetine, fluvoxamine, nefazodone, nevirapine, propoxyphene, quinupristin, verapamil, zafirlukast, and zileuton): possible increase in bortezomib serum level and efficacy
Drug-food. *Grapefruit juice:* increased bortezomib blood level, greater risk of toxicity

Patient monitoring

- Monitor vital signs and temperature. Especially watch for tachycardia, fever, and hypertension.
- Monitor nutritional and hydration status for changes caused by GI adverse effects.
- Monitor CBC with white cell differential, and watch for signs and symptoms of blood dyscrasias.
- Monitor respiratory status, watching for dyspnea, cough, and other signs and symptoms of upper respiratory tract infection.

Patient teaching

- Inform patient that drug can cause serious blood dyscrasias. Teach him which signs and symptoms to report right away.
- Tell patient drug may cause other significant adverse reactions. Reassure him he will be closely monitored.
- Caution patient to avoid driving and other hazardous activities until he knows how drug affects concentration and alertness.
- Advise patient to minimize adverse GI effects by eating small frequent servings of healthy food and ensuring adequate fluid intake.
- Tell patient to immediately report signs and symptoms of upper respiratory tract infection.
- As appropriate, review all other significant and life-threatening adverse reactions and interactions, especially those related to the drugs and foods mentioned above.

bosentan

Tracleer

Pharmacologic class: Endothelin-receptor antagonist, vasodilator
Therapeutic class: Antihypertensive
Pregnancy risk category X

Action

Binds to and blocks receptor sites for endothelin A and B in endothelium and vascular smooth muscle. This action reduces elevated endothelin levels in patients with pulmonary arterial hypertension, and inhibits vasoconstriction resulting from endothelin-1 (ET-1).

Availability

Tablets: 62.5 mg, 125 mg

Indications and dosages

➤ To improve exercise ability and slow clinical deterioration in patients with pulmonary arterial hypertension who have World Health Organization class III or class IV symptoms
Adults: Initially, 62.5 mg P.O. b.i.d. for 4 weeks; increase to maintenance dosage of 125 mg P.O. b.i.d. In patients older than age 12 who weigh less than 40 kg (88 lb), initial and maintenance dosages are 62.5 mg b.i.d.

Dosage adjustment

- Moderate to severe hepatic dysfunction

• Hepatic injury in patients with alanine aminotransferase or aspartate aminotransferase elevations

Contraindications

• Hypersensitivity to drug
• Severe hepatic impairment
• Patients receiving concurrent cyclosporine or glyburide
• Pregnancy or breastfeeding
• Children younger than age 12 (safety and efficacy not established)

Precautions

Use cautiously in:
• mitral stenosis
• elderly patients.

Administration

• Give tablets in morning and evening, with or without food.

Route	Onset	Peak	Duration
P.O.	Variable	3-5 hr	Unknown

Adverse reactions

CNS: headache, fatigue
CV: edema, hypotension, palpitations
EENT: nasopharyngitis
GI: dyspepsia
Hepatic: hepatic dysfunction, hepatic injury, hepatotoxicity
Skin: pruritus, flushing

Interactions

Drug-drug. *Cyclosporine:* decreased cyclosporine blood level, increased bosentan blood level
Glyburide: decreased blood levels of both drugs, increased risk of hepatic damage
Hormonal contraceptives: decreased bosentan efficacy
Ketoconazole: increased bosentan blood level and effects
Simvastatin and other statins: decreased effects of these drugs
Drug-diagnostic tests. *Hematocrit, hemoglobin:* decreased values
Transaminases: increased values

Patient monitoring

• Assess serum transaminase levels within first 3 days of therapy and then monthly.
• Evaluate hemoglobin level 1 month after therapy and then every 3 months.
• Assess female patient for pregnancy every month during therapy.

Patient teaching

• Tell patient to take drug with or without food in morning and evening.
• Caution female patient to avoid pregnancy, and discuss reliable contraceptive methods. Instruct her to contact prescriber immediately if she thinks she may be pregnant.
• Inform patient that he'll undergo CBC measurement and liver function testing regularly during therapy.
• As appropriate, review all other significant and life-threatening adverse reactions and interactions, especially those related to the drugs and tests mentioned above.

botulinum toxin type A

Botox, Botox Cosmetic

botulinum toxin type B

Myobloc

Pharmacologic class: Neurotoxin
Therapeutic class: Neuromuscular blocker
Pregnancy risk category C

Action

Blocks neuromuscular transmission by binding to receptor sites on motor nerve terminals and inhibiting acetylcholine release, thereby causing localized muscle denervation. As a result, local muscle paralysis occurs, which leads to muscle atrophy and reinnervation due to development of new acetylcholine receptors.

Availability

Toxin type A—
Powder for injection: 100 units/vial
Toxin type B—
Solution for injection: 5,000-units/ml vial

Indications and dosages

Toxin type A

➢ Temporary improvement in appearance of moderate to severe glabellar lines associated with corrugator or procerus muscle activity
Adults ages 65 and younger: *Botox cosmetic only*—Total of 20 units (0.5-ml solution) injected I.M. as divided doses of 0.1 ml into each of five sites: two in each corrugator muscle and one in procerus muscle. Injection usually needs to be repeated q 3 to 4 months to maintain effect.

➢ Blepharospasm
Adults: 1.25 to 2.5 units injected into medial and lateral pretarsal orbicularis oculi of upper eyelid and lateral pretarsal orbicularis oculi of lower eyelid

➢ Strabismus
Adults: 1.25 to 5 units injected into eyelid (dosage varies with strabismus severity). Dose can be repeated in 7 to 14 days if patient has adequate response; with inadequate response, dosage may be doubled.

Toxin types A and B

➢ To relax skeletal muscles and reduce severity of abnormal head position and neck pain associated with cervical dystonia
Adults: *Botox*—Usual dosage is 236 units injected I.M. locally into affected muscles. Dosage ranges from 198 to 300 units. *Myobloc*—2,500 to 5,000 units I.M. injected locally into affected muscles.

Contraindications

- Hypersensitivity to drug
- Active infection at injection site

Precautions

Use cautiously in:
- cardiovascular disease, peripheral neuropathy, neuromuscular disorders
- inflammation at injection site
- pregnant or breastfeeding patients.

Administration

Toxin type A

- Reconstitute toxin type A by slowly injecting preservative-free normal saline solution into drug vial.
- Rotate vial gently to mix drug; then draw up at least 20 units (0.5-ml solution) and expel air bubbles.
- Remove needle used for reconstitution, and attach 30G needle. Then inject drug as divided doses of 0.1 ml into each of five sites (two in each corrugator muscle, one in procerus muscle).
- Prepare eye with several drops of local anesthetic and ocular decongestant, as prescribed, several minutes before injection for blepharospasm or strabismus.
- Be aware that only trained medical personnel should inject this drug.

Toxin type B

- Draw up prescribed dose from preservative-free, 3.5-ml single-use vial.
- Don't shake vial.
- Divide prescribed dose and inject locally into affected muscles.

Route	Onset	Peak	Duration
I.M.	Mins-hrs	Unknown	3-4 mo
I.M. (blepharospasm)	3 days	1-2 wk	3 mo
I.M. (strabismus)	1-2 days	Unknown	1-2 wk

Adverse reactions

CNS: headache, dizziness
CV: hypertension, **arrhythmias, myocardial infarction** (MI)

EENT: blepharoptosis, conjunctivitis, keratitis, eye dryness, double vision, tearing, increased sensitivity to light, sinusitis, pharyngitis
GI: nausea, dyspepsia, difficulty swallowing
Respiratory: pneumonia, bronchitis, upper respiratory tract infection
Skin: skin tightness, ecchymosis
Other: tooth disorder; injection site redness, edema, or pain; flulike symptoms; facial muscle paralysis; infection; **anaphylaxis**

Interactions

Drug-drug. *Aminoglycosides, anticholinesterase compounds, clindamycin, lincomycin, magnesium sulfate, other neuromuscular blockers (such as succinylcholine), polymyxin B, quinidine:* increased risk of adverse effects

Patient monitoring

- Stay alert for signs and symptoms of anaphylaxis, particularly after first dose.
- Monitor vital signs and ECG, watching for evidence of hypertension, arrhythmias, and MI.
- Assess effect of drug on affected muscles; check for paralysis.
- Monitor temperature. Watch for signs and symptoms of respiratory and EENT infections as well as flulike symptoms.

Patient teaching

- Teach patient about desired effect of injection. Advise patient to report paralysis.
- Instruct patient to report signs and symptoms of infection, particularly flulike illness and EENT and respiratory infections.
- Inform patient being treated for blepharospasm (uncontrollable blinking) that he may experience transient eyelid drooping, corneal inflammation, double vision, dry eyes, tearing, and light sensitivity.
- As appropriate, review all other significant and life-threatening adverse reactions and interactions, especially those related to the drugs mentioned above.

bromocriptine mesylate

Alti-Bromocriptine✱, Apo-Bromocriptine✱, Parlodel

Pharmacologic class: Ergot-derivative dopamine agonist
Therapeutic class: Antiparkinsonian
Pregnancy risk category B

Action

Directly stimulates dopamine receptors in hypothalamus, causing release of prolactin-inhibitory factors and thereby relieving akinesia, rigidity, and tremors associated with Parkinson's disease. Also restores testicular or ovarian function and suppresses lactation.

Availability

Capsules: 5 mg
Tablets: 2.5 mg

Indications and dosages

➢ Parkinson's disease
Adults: Initially, 1.25 mg P.O. b.i.d. Increase by 2.5 mg/day q 14 to 28 days depending on therapeutic response. Usual therapeutic dosage is 10 to 40 mg/day.
➢ Acromegaly
Adults: Initially, 1.25 to 2.5 mg/day P.O. for 3 days. Increase up to 1.25 to 2.5 mg/day q 3 to 7 days. Usual therapeutic dosage is 20 to 30 mg/day.
➢ Hyperprolactinemia
Adults: Initially, 1.25 to 2.5 mg/day P.O. Increase gradually q 3 to 7 days up to 2.5 mg two to three times daily.

➢ Neuroleptic malignant syndrome
Adults: Initially, 5 mg P.O. once daily. Increase up to 20 mg/day.
➢ Pituitary tumors
Adults: Initially, 1.25 mg P.O. b.i.d. to t.i.d. Adjust dosage gradually over several weeks to a maintenance dosage of 10 to 20 mg/day given in divided doses.

Contraindications
- Hypersensitivity to drug or other ergot derivatives
- Severe peripheral vascular disease
- Uncontrolled hypertension
- Breastfeeding

Precautions
Use cautiously in:
- impaired hepatic or cardiac function, renal disease, hypertension, pituitary tumor
- psychiatric disorders
- pregnant patients
- children younger than age 15.

Administration
- Give with meals or milk.
- If desired, give at bedtime to minimize dizziness and nausea.

Route	Onset	Peak	Duration
P.O.	2 hr	8 hr	24 hr

Adverse reactions
CNS: confusion, headache, dizziness, fatigue, delusions, nervousness, mania, insomnia, nightmares, **seizures, cerebrovascular accident**
CV: hypotension, palpitations, extrasystoles, **arrhythmias, bradycardia, acute myocardial infarction**
EENT: blurred vision, diplopia, burning sensation in eyes, nasal congestion
GI: nausea, vomiting, diarrhea, constipation, abdominal cramps, anorexia, dry mouth, **GI hemorrhage**
GU: urinary incontinence, polyuria, urinary retention
Musculoskeletal: leg cramps
Skin: urticaria, coolness and pallor of fingers and toes, rash on face and arms, alopecia
Other: metallic taste, digital vasospasm (in acromegaly use only)

Interactions
Drug-drug. *Amitriptyline, estrogens, haloperidol, hormonal contraceptives, imipramine, loxapine, MAO inhibitors, phenothiazines, progestins, reserpine:* interference with bromocriptine effects
Cyclosporine: inhibition of cyclosporine metabolism, leading to cyclosporine toxicity
Erythromycin: increased bromocriptine blood level and greater risk of adverse effects
Levodopa: additive effects of bromocriptine
Risperidone: increased prolactin blood level, interference with bromocriptine effects
Drug-diagnostic tests. *Alanine aminotransferase, alkaline phosphatase, aspartate aminotransferase, blood urea nitrogen, creatine kinase, growth hormone, uric acid:* increased levels
Drug-herbs. *Chaste tree fruit:* decreased bromocriptine effects
Drug-behaviors. *Alcohol use:* disulfiram-like reaction

Patient monitoring
- Monitor blood pressure to detect hypotension.
- When giving drug for hyperprolactinemia, monitor serum prolactin.
- When giving drug for acromegaly, monitor growth hormone levels to help guide dosage adjustment.
- In long-term use, monitor respiratory, hepatic, cardiovascular, and renal function.

Patient teaching
🔈 Caution patient not to drink alcohol because of risk of severe reaction.
- Advise patient to have regular dental exams. Drug causes dry mouth, possi-

bly resulting in caries and periodontal disorders.
• To minimize constipation, instruct patient to exercise regularly, increase dietary fiber intake, and drink plenty of fluids (3,000 ml daily).
• Advise patient who doesn't desire pregnancy to use reliable contraceptive, because drug may restore fertility.
• Caution patient to avoid driving and other hazardous activities until he knows how drug affects concentration and alertness.
• As appropriate, review all other significant and life-threatening adverse reactions and interactions, especially those related to the drugs, tests, herbs, and behaviors mentioned above.

brompheniramine

Bromfenac, Dimetane, Dimetapp Allergy, Nasahist B, ND-Stat

Pharmacologic class: Histamine antagonist
Therapeutic class: Antihistamine
Pregnancy risk category C

Action

Antagonizes effects of histamine at histamine$_1$-receptor sites, but doesn't bind to or inactivate histamine. Also shows anticholinergic, antipruritic, and sedative activity.

Availability

Capsules (liquigels): 4 mg
Elixir: 2 mg/5 ml
Tablets: 4 mg, 8 mg, 12 mg
Tablets (extended-release): 8 mg, 12 mg

Indications and dosages

➢ Symptomatic relief of allergic symptoms caused by histamine release; severe allergic or hypersensitivity reactions

Adults and children ages 12 and older: 4 to 8 mg P.O. three to four times daily, or 8 to 12 mg extended-release tablets P.O. two or three times daily. Maximum dosage is 36 mg/day.
Children ages 6 to 12: 2 mg P.O. q 4 to 6 hours as needed, not to exceed 12 mg/day
Children ages 2 to 6: 1 mg P.O. q 4 to 6 hours p.r.n., not to exceed 6 mg/day

Contraindications

• Hypersensitivity to drug
• Coronary artery disease
• Urinary retention
• Pyloroduodenal obstruction
• Peptic ulcer
• MAO inhibitor use within past 14 days
• Breastfeeding

Precautions

Use cautiously in:
• angle-closure glaucoma, hepatic disease, hyperthyroidism, hypertension, bronchial asthma
• elderly patients
• pregnant patients.

Administration

• Give with food if GI upset occurs.
• Don't break or crush extended-release tablets.

Route	Onset	Peak	Duration
P.O.	15-60 min	2-5 hr	3-24 hr

Adverse reactions

CNS: drowsiness, sedation, dizziness, excitation, irritability, syncope, tremor
CV: hypertension, hypotension, palpitations, tachycardia, extrasystole, **arrhythmias, bradycardia**
EENT: blurred vision, nasal congestion or dryness, dry or sore throat
GI: nausea, vomiting, constipation, dry mouth
GU: urinary retention or hesitancy, dysuria, early menses, decreased libido, impotence

Hematologic: hemolytic anemia, hypoplastic anemia, thrombocytopenia, agranulocytosis, leukopenia, pancytopenia
Respiratory: thickened bronchial secretions, chest tightness, wheezing
Skin: urticaria, rash
Other: increased or decreased appetite, weight gain

Interactions

Drug-drug. *CNS depressants (including opioids and sedative-hypnotics):* additive CNS depression
MAO inhibitors: intensified, prolonged anticholinergic effects
Drug-diagnostic tests. *Allergy tests:* false results
Granulocytes, platelets: decreased counts
Drug-behaviors. *Alcohol use:* increased CNS depression

Patient monitoring

- Monitor respiratory status.
- Stay alert for urinary retention, urinary frequency, and painful or difficult urination. Discontinue drug if these problems occur.
- With long-term use, monitor CBC.
- Monitor elderly patient for dizziness, sedation, and hypotension.
- If patient takes over-the-counter antihistamines, monitor him closely to avoid potential overdose.

Patient teaching

- Advise patient to take drug with meals if GI upset occurs.
- Instruct patient to avoid driving and other hazardous activities until he knows how drug affects concentration and alertness.
- Caution patient to avoid alcohol while taking drug.
- Urge patient to tell all prescribers which drugs and over-the-counter preparations he's taking.
- As appropriate, review all other significant and life-threatening adverse reactions and interactions, especially those related to the drugs, tests, and behaviors mentioned above.

budesonide

Entocort EC, Pulmicort Respules, Pulmicort Turbuhaler, Rhinocort

Pharmacologic class: Corticosteroid (inhalation)
Therapeutic class: Antiasthmatic, steroidal anti-inflammatory
Pregnancy risk category C

Action

Decreases inflammation by inhibiting migration of inflammatory mediators to injury site, where it reverses dilation and increases vessel permeability. Also decreases plasma exudation and mucus secretions within airway.

Availability

Capsules (extended-release): 3 mg
Inhalation powder: 200 mcg/metered inhalation in 200-metered-dose inhaler
Inhalation suspension (Respules): 0.25 mg/2 ml, 0.5 mg/2 ml
Nasal spray: 32 mcg/metered spray (7-g canister)

Indications and dosages

➢ Prophylactic therapy in chronic asthma

Adults previously controlled on bronchodilators alone: One or two inhalations b.i.d. (200 mcg/inhalation)
Adults previously controlled on other inhaled corticosteroids: One or two inhalations b.i.d. Maximum dosage is 800 mcg (four inhalations) b.i.d.
Adults previously controlled on oral corticosteroids: Two to four inhalations b.i.d. Maximum dosage is 800 mcg (four inhalations) b.i.d.

Children ages 6 and older: One inhalation (200 mcg) b.i.d. to a maximum of 400 mcg b.i.d.
Children ages 3 to 6 previously controlled on bronchodilators alone: One or two inhalations b.i.d. (200 mcg/inhalation)
Children ages 3 to 6 previously controlled on other inhaled corticosteroids: One or two inhalations b.i.d.
Children ages 3 to 6 previously controlled on oral corticosteroids: Maximum of two inhalations b.i.d.
Pulmicort Respules—
Children ages 12 months to 8 years previously controlled on bronchodilators alone: 0.25 mg/day as a single dose or in divided doses b.i.d.
Children ages 12 months to 8 years previously controlled on other inhaled corticosteroids: 0.5 mg/day as a single dose or in divided doses of 0.25 mg b.i.d.
Children ages 12 months to 8 years previously controlled on oral corticosteroids: 1 mg/day as a single dose or in divided doses b.i.d. Individualized titration is required.
➢ Seasonal or perennial allergic rhinitis
Adults and children ages 6 and older: Two sprays in each nostril in morning and evening, or four sprays in each nostril in morning. Maintenance dosage is fewest number of sprays needed to control symptoms.
➢ Mild to moderate active Crohn's disease involving ileum, ascending colon, or both
Adults: 9 mg P.O. daily for up to 8 weeks. For recurring episodes of active Crohn's disease, 8-week course can be repeated and tapered to 6 mg P.O. daily for 2 weeks before complete cessation.

Dosage adjustment

- Moderate to severe hepatic disease

Contraindications

- Hypersensitivity to drug
- Status asthmaticus

Precautions

Use cautiously in:

- renal disease, hepatic disease, heart failure, active untreated infections, systemic infections, hypertension, osteoporosis, diabetes mellitus, glaucoma, underlying immunosuppression, hypothyroidism, diverticulitis, nonspecific ulcerative colitis, recent intestinal anastomoses, thromboembolic disorders, seizures, myasthenia gravis, ocular herpes simplex infection
- patients receiving concurrent systemic corticosteroids
- pregnant or breastfeeding patients
- children younger than age 6.

Administration

- If patient also uses a bronchodilator, give that drug at least 15 minutes before budesonide.
- Know that using a spacer reduces risk of candidiasis and hoarseness.
- Make sure patient swallows capsules whole without crushing or chewing them.

Route	Onset	Peak	Duration
P.O.	Unknown	0.5-10 hr	Unknown
Inhalation (nasal)	Immediate	1-2 wk	Unknown

Adverse reactions

CNS: headache, nervousness, depression, euphoria, psychoses, **increased intracranial pressure**
CV: hypotension, Churg-Strauss syndrome, **thrombophlebitis, thromboembolism**
EENT: cataracts, nasal congestion, nasal burning or dryness, epistaxis, perforated nasal septum, hoarseness, nasopharyngeal and oropharyngeal fungal infections

GI: nausea, vomiting, peptic ulcers, anorexia, esophageal candidiasis, dry mouth
Metabolic: hyperglycemia, decreased growth (in children), cushingoid appearance (moon face, buffalo hump), **adrenal suppression or insufficiency**
Musculoskeletal: muscle wasting, muscle pain, osteoporosis, aseptic joint necrosis
Respiratory: cough, wheezing, rebound congestion, **bronchospasm**
Skin: facial edema, rash, petechiae, contact dermatitis, acne, bruising, hirsutism, urticaria
Other: bad taste, anosmia, weight gain or loss, increased susceptibility to infection, **angioedema, hypersensitivity reaction**

Interactions

Drug-drug. *Amphotericin B, mezlocillin, piperacillin, thiazide and loop diuretics, ticarcillin:* additive hypokalemia
Digoxin: increased risk of digoxin toxicity
Erythromycin, indinavir, itraconazole, ketoconazole, ritonavir, saquinavir: increased blood level and effects of budesonide
Fluoroquinolones: increased risk of tendon rupture
Hormonal contraceptives: blockage of budesonide metabolism
Insulin, oral hypoglycemics: increased budesonide requirement
Live-virus vaccines: decreased antibody response to vaccine, increased risk of adverse effects from budesonide
Nonsteroidal anti-inflammatory drugs (including aspirin): increased risk of adverse GI effects
Phenobarbital, phenytoin, rifampin: decreased budesonide efficacy
Somatrem, somatropin: decreased response to budesonide

Drug-food. *Grapefruit, grapefruit juice:* increased blood level and effects of budesonide
High-fat meal: delayed peak budesonide concentration

Patient monitoring

- Monitor respiratory status to evaluate drug efficacy.

🔈 Stay alert for hypersensitivity reactions, especially angioedema.

- Evaluate liver function test results.
- Periodically observe patient for proper inhaler use.
- Assess oral cavity for infection.

Patient teaching

- Teach patient proper use of inhaler.
- Tell patient to swallow capsules whole without crushing or chewing them.

🔈 Instruct patient to contact prescriber immediately if he develops itching, rash, fever, swelling of face and neck, or difficulty breathing.

- Encourage patient to document medication use and his response in diary.
- Advise patient to report signs and symptoms of fungal infections of mouth.
- Tell female patient to inform prescriber if she is pregnant or plans to become pregnant.
- Caution patient to avoid exposure to chickenpox and measles, if possible.
- Emphasize importance of rinsing mouth after each inhaler treatment and washing and drying inhaler thoroughly after each use.
- Instruct patient to avoid high-fat meals, grapefruit, and grapefruit juice.
- As appropriate, review all other significant and life-threatening adverse reactions and interactions, especially those related to the drugs and foods mentioned above.

bumetanide

Bumetanide Injection, Bumex

Pharmacologic class: Loop diuretic
Therapeutic class: Antihypertensive
Pregnancy risk category C

Action

Inhibits reabsorption of sodium and chloride in distal renal tubules and ascending limb of loop of Henle; increases renal excretion of water, sodium, chloride, magnesium, hydrogen, and calcium. Also reduces increased fluid volume caused by renal vasodilation.

Availability

Injection: 0.25 mg/ml
Tablets: 0.5 mg, 1 mg, 2 mg

Indications and dosages

➢ Edema caused by heart failure or hepatic or renal disease; adult nocturia
Adults: 0.5 to 2 mg/day P.O. as a single dose; up to two additional doses may be given q 4 to 5 hours (up to 10 mg/day). Or 0.5 to 1 mg I.V. or I.M., repeated q 2 to 3 hours as needed, up to 10 mg/day.

➢ Hypertension
Adults: 0.5 mg/day P.O. Maximum dosage is 5 mg/day.

Dosage adjustment

- Renal impairment
- Elderly patients

Off-label uses

- Drug-related edema
- Hypercalcemia

Contraindications

- Hypersensitivity to drug or sulfonamides
- Uncorrected electrolyte imbalances
- Hepatic coma
- Anuria and oliguria

Precautions

Use cautiously in:

- severe hepatic disease, electrolyte depletion, diabetes mellitus, worsening azotemia
- elderly patients
- pregnant or breastfeeding patients
- children younger than age 18.

Administration

- Know that oral or I.V. route is preferred, because I.M. administration may cause pain at injection site.
- Be aware that drug may be given alone or with other antihypertensives.
- Dilute with dextrose 5% in water, normal saline solution, or lactated Ringer's injection.
- Give I.V. dose slowly over 2 minutes.
- Give P.O. form with food or milk.

Route	Onset	Peak	Duration
P.O.	30-60 min	1 hr	3-6 hr
I.V.	Within min	15-45 min	3-6 hr
I.M.	40 min	1-2 hr	4-6 hr

Adverse reactions

CNS: dizziness, headache, insomnia, nervousness, vertigo, weakness, paresthesia, confusion, fatigue, hand-flapping tremor, **encephalopathy**
CV: hypotension, ECG changes, chest pain, **thrombophlebitis, arrhythmias**
EENT: blurred vision, nystagmus, hearing loss, tinnitus
GI: nausea, vomiting, diarrhea, constipation, dyspepsia, gastric irritation, dry mouth, anorexia, **acute pancreatitis**
GU: polyuria, nocturia, glycosuria, premature ejaculation, difficulty maintaining erection, **oliguria, renal failure**
Hepatic: jaundice
Metabolic: dehydration, hyperglycemia, hyperuricemia, hypokalemia, hypomagnesemia, **hypochloremic alkalosis**
Musculoskeletal: arthralgia; muscle cramps, aching, or tenderness

Skin: photosensitivity, hives, rash, pruritus, urticaria, diaphoresis
Other: pain, nipple tenderness

Interactions

Drug-drug. *Aminoglycosides, cisplatin:* increased risk of ototoxicity
Amphotericin B, corticosteroids, mezlocillin, other diuretics, piperacillin, stimulant laxatives: additive hypokalemia
Anticoagulants, thrombolytics: increased bumetanide effects
Antihypertensives, nitrates: additive hypotension
Cardiac glycosides: increased risk of digoxin toxicity
Lithium: decreased lithium excretion, possible lithium toxicity
Neuromuscular blockers: prolonged neuromuscular blockade
Nonsteroidal anti-inflammatory drugs, probenecid: inhibition of diuretic response
Drug-diagnostic tests. *Blood urea nitrogen (BUN), cholesterol, creatinine, glucose, nitrogenous compounds:* increased levels
Calcium, magnesium, platelets, potassium, sodium: decreased levels
Drug-herbs. *Dandelion:* interference with diuretic activity
Ginseng: resistance to diuresis
Licorice: rapid potassium loss
Drug-behaviors. *Acute alcohol ingestion:* additive hypotension

Patient monitoring

- Weigh patient at start of therapy, and monitor weight throughout therapy.
- Monitor blood pressure regularly.
- Monitor serum electrolyte, uric acid, urine glucose, and BUN levels.
- Monitor elderly patients for extreme blood pressure changes, orthostatic hypotension, and dehydration.

Patient teaching

- Advise patient to take drug in morning to prevent nocturia, and to take second dose (if required) in late afternoon.
- Instruct patient to move slowly when sitting up or standing, to avoid dizziness or light-headedness from sudden blood pressure drop.
- Caution patient to avoid alcohol because of increased risk of hypotension.
- Advise patient to eat foods high in potassium. Provide other dietary counseling as appropriate to help prevent or minimize electrolyte imbalances.
- Instruct patient to weigh himself often to help detect fluid retention.
- As appropriate, review all other significant and life-threatening adverse reactions and interactions, especially those related to the drugs, tests, herbs, and behaviors mentioned above.

buprenorphine hydrochloride

Buprenex, Subutex

Pharmacologic class: Opioid agonist-antagonist
Therapeutic class: Opioid analgesic
Controlled substance schedule III
Pregnancy risk category C

Action

Unclear. May bind to opiate receptors in CNS, altering perception of and response to painful stimuli while causing generalized CNS depression. Also has partial antagonist properties, which may lead to opioid withdrawal effects in patients with physical drug dependence.

Availability

Injection: 300 mcg (0.3 mg)/ml
Tablets (sublingual): 2 mg, 8 mg

Indications and dosages

➢ Moderate to severe pain

Adults: 0.3 mg I.M. or slow I.V. q 6 hours as needed. Repeat initial dose after 30 to 60 minutes.

Children ages 2 to 12: 2 to 6 mcg (0.002 to 0.006 mg)/kg I.M. or slow I.V. q 4 to 6 hours

➢ Opioid dependence

Adults: 12 to 16 mg/day S.L.

Dosage adjustment

- Elderly patients

Contraindications

- Hypersensitivity to drug
- Elderly patients
- MAO inhibitor use within 14 days

Precautions

Use cautiously in:

- increased intracranial pressure (ICP); respiratory impairment; severe renal, hepatic, or pulmonary disease; hypothyroidism; adrenal insufficiency; undiagnosed abdominal pain; prostatic hypertrophy; systemic lupus erythematosus; gout; kyphoscoliosis; diabetes mellitus; alcoholism
- elderly patients
- pregnant or breastfeeding patients
- children younger than age 13.

Administration

Use extra caution when giving I.V. Drug may cause respiratory depression (especially initial dose).

- Mix with lactated Ringer's injection, dextrose 5% in water, or normal saline solution.
- When giving I.M., rotate injection sites to prevent induration and abscess.
- If patient is immobilized, reposition him frequently and keep head of bed elevated.

Route	Onset	Peak	Duration
I.V.	Immediate	2 min	6 hr
I.M., S.L.	15 min	1 hr	6 hr

Adverse reactions

CNS: confusion, malaise, hallucinations, dizziness, euphoria, headache, unusual dreams, psychosis, slurred speech, paresthesia, depression, tremor, agitation, **seizures, coma, increased ICP**

CV: hypertension, hypotension, palpitations, tachycardia, Wenckebach (Mobitz Type 1) block, **bradycardia**

EENT: blurred vision, diplopia, amblyopia, miosis, conjunctivitis, tinnitus

GI: nausea, vomiting, constipation, flatulence, ileus, dry mouth

GU: urinary retention

Respiratory: hypoventilation, dyspnea, cyanosis, apnea, **respiratory depression**

Skin: diaphoresis, pruritus

Other: physical or psychological drug dependence, drug tolerance

Interactions

Drug-drug. *Antidepressants, antihistamines, sedative-hypnotics:* additive CNS depression

MAO inhibitors: increased CNS and respiratory depression, increased hypotension

Drug-herbs. *Chamomile, hops, kava, skullcap, valerian:* increased CNS depression

Drug-behaviors. *Alcohol use:* increased CNS depression

Patient monitoring

- Monitor respiratory status throughout therapy. Respiratory rate of 12 breaths/minute or less may warrant withholding dose or decreasing dosage.

Patient teaching

- Instruct patient to move slowly when sitting up or standing, to avoid dizziness or light-headedness from sudden blood pressure drop.
- Caution patient to avoid driving and other hazardous activities until he knows how drug affects concentration and alertness.

• Advise patient to increase daily fluid intake to help prevent constipation.
• As appropriate, review all other significant and life-threatening adverse reactions and interactions, especially those related to the drugs, herbs, and behaviors mentioned above.

bupropion hydrochloride

Wellbutrin, Wellbutrin SR, Wellbutrin XL, Zyban

Pharmacologic class: Aminoketone
Therapeutic class: Second-generation antidepressant, smoking-cessation aid
Pregnancy risk category B

Action

Unclear. Thought to decrease neuronal reuptake of dopamine, serotonin, and norepinephrine in CNS. Action as smoking-cessation aid may result from noradrenergic or dopaminergic activity.

Availability

Tablets: 75 mg, 100 mg
Tablets (sustained-release): 100 mg, 150 mg, 200 mg

Indications and dosages

➢ Depression
Adults: Initially, 100 mg P.O. b.i.d. (morning and evening). After 3 days, may increase to 100 mg t.i.d. After 4 weeks, may increase to a maximum dosage of 450 mg/day in divided doses. No single dose should exceed 150 mg. With total daily dosage of 300 mg, wait at least 6 hours between doses; with total daily dosage of 450 mg, wait at least 4 hours between doses. Alternatively, give one 150-mg sustained-release tablet daily; increase to 150-mg sustained-release tablet b.i.d. based on clinical response.

➢ Smoking cessation
Adults: 150-mg sustained-release tablet once daily for 3 days, then 150-mg sustained-release tablet b.i.d. for 7 to 12 weeks. Space doses at least 8 hours apart.

b

Contraindications

• Hypersensitivity to drug
• Seizures
• Anorexia nervosa
• MAO inhibitor use within past 14 days
• Acute alcohol or sedative withdrawal

Precautions

Use cautiously in:
• renal or hepatic impairment, unstable cardiovascular status
• elderly patients
• pregnant or breastfeeding patients
• children.

Administration

• Be aware that sustained-release tablets should be swallowed whole and not crushed or chewed.
• Single dose shouldn't exceed 150 mg for immediate-release tablets or 200 mg for sustained-release tablets.
• Avoid bedtime doses because they may worsen insomnia.
Know that drug shouldn't be withdrawn abruptly.

Route	Onset	Peak	Duration
P.O.	Unknown	2 hr	Unknown
P.O. (sustained)	Unknown	3 hr	Unknown

Adverse reactions

CNS: agitation, headache, insomnia, mania, psychoses, depression, dizziness, drowsiness, tremor, anxiety, nervousness, **seizures**
CV: hypertension, hypotension, tachycardia, palpitations, **complete atrioventricular block**

EENT: blurred vision, amblyopia, auditory disturbances, epistaxis, rhinitis, pharyngitis
GI: nausea, vomiting, dyspepsia, abdominal pain, flatulence, mouth ulcers, dry mouth
GU: urinary frequency, nocturia, vaginal irritation, testicular swelling
Metabolic: hyperglycemia, increased libido, **hypoglycemia, syndrome of inappropriate antidiuretic hormone secretion**
Musculoskeletal: arthralgia, myalgia, leg cramps, twitching, neck pain
Respiratory: bronchitis, increased cough, dyspnea
Skin: photosensitivity, dry skin, pruritus, rash, urticaria, diaphoresis, skin temperature changes
Other: altered taste, increased or decreased appetite, weight gain or loss, hot flashes, fever, allergic reaction, flu-like symptoms

Interactions

Drug-drug. *Benzodiazepine withdrawal, corticosteroids, other antidepressants, over-the-counter stimulants, phenothiazines, theophylline:* increased risk of seizures
Cimetidine: inhibited bupropion metabolism
Levodopa, MAO inhibitors: increased risk of adverse reactions
Ritonavir: increased bupropion blood level
Drug-diagnostic tests. *Glucose:* increased level
Drug-behaviors. *Alcohol use or cessation:* increased risk of seizures
Sun exposure: increased risk of photosensitivity

Patient monitoring

- Monitor blood pressure, ECG, CBC, and renal and hepatic function. Monitor tricyclic antidepressant (TCA) blood level if patient's taking TCAs concurrently.
- Check for oral and dental problems.

Patient teaching

- Instruct patient to swallow sustained-release tablets without crushing or chewing.

Caution patient not to discontinue drug abruptly.

- Emphasize importance of frequent oral hygiene. (Dry mouth increases risk of caries and dental problems.)
- Caution patient to avoid alcohol, because it may increase risk of seizures.
- Advise patient to keep regular appointments for periodic blood tests and hepatic and renal studies.
- As appropriate, review all other significant and life-threatening adverse reactions and interactions, especially those related to the drugs, tests, and behaviors mentioned above.

buspirone hydrochloride

BuSpar

Pharmacologic class: Azaspirodecanedione

Therapeutic class: Anxiolytic

Pregnancy risk category B

Action

Unclear. Thought to bind to serotonin and dopamine receptors in CNS, increasing dopamine metabolism and impulse formation. Also thought to inhibit neuronal firing and reduce serotonin turnover.

Availability

Tablets: 5 mg, 7.5 mg, 10 mg, 15 mg, 30 mg

Indications and dosages

➤ Anxiety disorders; anxiety symptoms

Adults: 5 mg P.O. t.i.d.; increase by 5 mg/day q 2 to 3 days as needed (not to exceed 60 mg/day). Common dosage is 20 to 30 mg/day in divided doses.

Off-label uses
- Parkinsonian syndrome
- Symptomatic relief of depression

Contraindications
- Hypersensitivity to drug
- Severe renal or hepatic impairment
- MAO inhibitor use within past 14 days

Precautions
Use cautiously in:
- patients receiving concurrent anxiolytics or psychotropics
- pregnant or breastfeeding patients
- children.

Administration
- Give with food to minimize GI upset.
- Know that full benefit of drug therapy may take up to 2 weeks.

Route	Onset	Peak	Duration
P.O.	7-10 days	3-4 wk	Unknown

Adverse reactions
CNS: dizziness, drowsiness, nervousness, headache, insomnia, weakness, personality changes, numbness, paresthesia, tremor
CV: chest pain, palpitations, tachycardia, hypertension, hypotension
EENT: blurred vision, conjunctivitis, tinnitus, nasal congestion, sore throat
GI: nausea, vomiting, diarrhea, constipation, abdominal pain, dry mouth
GU: dysuria, urinary frequency or hesitancy, menstrual irregularities, menstrual spotting, libido changes
Musculoskeletal: myalgia
Respiratory: chest congestion, hyperventilation, dyspnea
Skin: rash, alopecia, blisters, pruritus, dry skin, easy bruising, edema, flushing, clammy skin, excessive sweating
Other: altered taste or smell, fever

Interactions
Drug-drug. *Erythromycin, itraconazole:* increased buspirone blood level
MAO inhibitors: hypertension
Trazodone: increased risk of adverse hepatic effects
Drug-food. *Grapefruit juice:* increased buspirone blood level and effects
Drug-herbs. *Hops, kava, skullcap, valerian:* increased CNS depression
Drug-behaviors. *Alcohol use:* increased CNS depression

Patient monitoring
- Monitor mental status closely.
- Assess hepatic and renal function regularly to detect drug toxicity.

Patient teaching
- Instruct patient to take drug with food.
- Advise patient not to use drug to manage everyday stress or tension.
- Instruct patient to avoid driving and other hazardous activities until he knows how drug affects concentration and alertness.
- Caution patient to avoid alcohol because it increases CNS depression.
- Emphasize importance of keeping follow-up appointments to check progress.
- As appropriate, review all other significant adverse reactions and interactions, especially those related to the drugs, foods, herbs, and behaviors mentioned above.

busulfan
Busulfex, Myleran

Pharmacologic class: Alkylating agent
Therapeutic class: Antineoplastic
Pregnancy risk category D

Action
Unclear. Thought to interfere with bacterial cell-wall synthesis by cross-linking strands of DNA and disrupting RNA transcription, which causes cell

to rupture and die. Exhibits minimal immunosuppressant activity.

Availability

Injection: 6 mg/ml in 10-ml ampules
Tablets: 2 mg

Indications and dosages

➢ Chronic myelogenous leukemia
Adults: 4 to 8 mg P.O. daily until white blood cell (WBC) count decreases to 15,000/mm^3; then discontinue drug until WBC count rises to 50,000/mm^3, and then resume as needed.
Children: 0.06 to 0.12 mg/kg/day P.O. or 1.8 to 4.6 mg/m^2/day P.O. Adjust dosage to maintain WBC count at approximately 20,000/mm^3 but not below 10,000/mm^3.
➢ Allogenic hematopoietic stem cell transplantation
Adults: 0.8 mg/kg I.V. q 6 hours for 4 days. Starting 6 hours after 16th dose of busulfan injection, give cyclophosphamide 60 mg/kg/day I.V. over 1 hour for 2 days.

Off-label uses

- Adjunctive therapy in ovarian cancer
- Bone marrow transplantation

Contraindications

- Hypersensitivity to drug
- Patients not definitively diagnosed with chronic myelogenous leukemia
- Pregnancy or breastfeeding

Precautions

Use cautiously in:
- active infections, decreased bone marrow reserve, chronic debilitating disease, depressed neutrophil and platelet counts, seizure disorders, obesity
- patients receiving concurrent myelosuppressive or radiation therapy
- females of childbearing age.

Administration

- Give oral doses on empty stomach.
- When administering I.V., withdraw dose from ampule using 5-micron filter needle. Remove filter needle and use new needle to add busulfan to diluent.
- Dilute for injection using dextrose 5% in water or normal saline solution.
- Follow facility procedures for safe handling, administration, and disposal of chemotherapeutic drugs.

Clinical alert: Be aware that drug is highly toxic and has a narrow therapeutic index.
- Maintain vigorous hydration to reduce risk of renal toxicity.
- Handle patient gently to avoid bruising.

Route	Onset	Peak	Duration
P.O.	1-2 wk	Wks	Up to 1 mo
I.V.	Unknown	Unknown	13 days

Adverse reactions

CNS: anxiety, confusion, depression, dizziness, headache, weakness, **encephalopathy, seizures, cerebral hemorrhage, coma**
CV: chest pain, hypotension, hypertension, tachycardia, ECG changes, **heart block, left-sided heart failure, thrombosis, pericardial effusion, ventricular extrasystole, atrial fibrillation, arrhythmias, cardiac tamponade, cardiomegaly**
EENT: cataracts, ear disorders, epistaxis, pharyngitis
GI: nausea, vomiting, diarrhea, constipation, abdominal pain, dyspepsia, abdominal enlargement, pancreatitis, hematemesis, dry mouth, stomatitis, anorexia
GU: dysuria, hematuria, sterility, gynecomastia, **oliguria**
Hematologic: myelosuppression
Hepatic: hepatitis, hepatomegaly
Metabolic: hypokalemia, hypomagnesemia, hypophosphatemia, hyperuricemia, hyperglycemia

Musculoskeletal: arthralgia, myalgia, back pain
Respiratory: hyperventilation, dyspnea, **pulmonary fibrosis**
Skin: pruritus, rash, acne, alopecia, erythema nodosum, exfoliative dermatitis, hyperpigmentation
Other: allergic reactions, chills, fever, injection site infection or inflammation

Interactions

Drug-drug. *Anticoagulants, aspirin, nonsteroidal anti-inflammatory drugs:* increased risk of bleeding
Live-virus vaccines: decreased antibody response to vaccine, increased risk of adverse reactions
Myelosuppressants: additive bone marrow depression
Nephrotoxic and ototoxic drugs (such as aminoglycosides, loop diuretics): additive nephrotoxicity and ototoxicity
Thioguanine: increased risk of hepatotoxicity
Drug-diagnostic tests. *Alkaline phosphatase, aspartate aminotransferase, bilirubin, nitrogenous compounds (urea):* increased levels
Hemoglobin, WBCs: decreased values

Patient monitoring

- Monitor patient closely for adequate hydration.
- Check for signs and symptoms of local or systemic infections.
- Assess for bleeding and excessive bruising.
- Evaluate oral hygiene regularly.
- Monitor CBC and WBC and platelet counts daily if patient is receiving I.V. busulfan.
- Monitor renal and hepatic function.

🔊 Know that diffuse pulmonary fibrosis ("busulfan lung") is a rare but potentially life-threatening complication, with symptom onset as late as 10 years after therapy.

Patient teaching

- Inform patient that drug doesn't cure leukemia but may induce remission.
- Advise patient to drink plenty of fluids to avoid dehydration.

🔊 Instruct patient to immediately report inability to eat or drink. Prescriber may add another drug to improve appetite.

- Inform patient that he's at increased risk for infection. Advise him to avoid contact with people with known infections and to avoid public transportation, if possible.
- Tell patient he's at increased risk for bleeding and bruising.
- Advise patient to avoid activities that can cause injury and to use soft toothbrush and electric razor to avoid gum and skin injury.
- Inform patient that he'll undergo frequent blood testing to monitor drug effects.
- As appropriate, review all other significant and life-threatening adverse reactions and interactions, especially those related to the drugs and tests mentioned above.

butorphanol tartrate

Stadol, Stadol NS

Pharmacologic class: Opioid agonist-antagonist
Therapeutic class: Opioid analgesic
Controlled substance schedule IV
Pregnancy risk category C

Action

Alters perception of and emotional response to pain by binding with opioid receptors in brain, causing CNS depression. Also exerts antagonistic activity at opioid receptors, which reduces risk of toxicity, drug dependence, and respiratory depression.

Availability

Injection: 1 mg/ml, 2 mg/ml
Nasal spray: 10 mg/ml

Indications and dosages

➢ Moderate to severe pain
Adults: 1 to 4 mg I.M. q 3 to 4 hours as needed, not to exceed 4 mg/dose. Or 0.5 to 2 mg I.V. q 3 to 4 hours as needed. With nasal spray, 1 mg (one spray in one nostril) q 3 to 4 hours, repeated in 60 to 90 minutes if needed.
➢ Labor pains
Adults: 1 to 2 mg I.V. or I.M., repeated after 4 hours as needed
➢ Preoperative anesthesia
Adults: 2 mg I.M. 60 to 90 minutes before surgery
➢ Balanced anesthesia
Adults: 2 mg I.V. shortly before anesthesia induction, or 0.5 to 1 mg I.V. in increments during anesthesia

Dosage adjustment

• Elderly patients

Off-label uses

• Headache
• Symptomatic relief of ureteral colic

Contraindications

• Hypersensitivity to drug

Precautions

Use cautiously in:
• head injury, ventricular dysfunction, coronary insufficiency, respiratory disease, renal or hepatic dysfunction
• history of drug abuse.

Administration

• Make sure solution is clear and free of particulates before giving.
• When using nasal spray, insert tip of the sprayer about ¼" into nostril, point tip backwards, and administer one spray.
• Be aware that I.V. route is preferred for severe pain.
• Know that drug may cause infant respiratory distress in neonate of pregnant patient, especially if given within 2 hours of delivery.

Route	Onset	Peak	Duration
I.V.	2-3 min	30-60 min	3-4 hr
I.M.	10-15 min	30-60 min	3-4 hr
Intranasal	15 min	1-2 hr	4-5 hr

Adverse reactions

CNS: drowsiness, sedation, dizziness, tremor, irritability, syncope, stimulation
CV: hypertension, hypotension, palpitations, bradycardia, tachycardia, extrasystole, **arrhythmias**
EENT: blurred vision, nasal congestion or dryness, dry or sore throat
GI: nausea, vomiting, constipation, epigastric distress, dry mouth, **GI obstruction**
GU: urinary retention or hesitancy, dysuria, early menses, decreased libido, erectile dysfunction
Hematologic: hemolytic anemia, hypoplastic anemia, thrombocytopenia, agranulocytosis, leukopenia, pancytopenia
Respiratory: thickened bronchial secretions, chest tightness, wheezing
Skin: urticaria, rash, diaphoresis
Other: increased or decreased appetite, weight gain, local stinging, **anaphylactic shock, hypersensitivity reaction** (with I.V. use)

Interactions

Drug-drug. *CNS depressants:* additive CNS effects
Drug-behaviors. *Alcohol use:* additive CNS effects

Patient monitoring

• Monitor respiratory status closely, especially after I.V. administration.
• Watch for signs and symptoms of withdrawal in long-term use and in opioid-dependent patients.

• Assess elderly patient closely for sensitivity to drug.

Patient teaching

• Teach patient how to use nasal spray properly.
• Emphasize importance of using drug exactly as prescribed.
• Caution patient that drug may be habit-forming.
• Advise patient to avoid driving and other hazardous activities until he knows how drug affects concentration and alertness.
• As appropriate, review all other significant and life-threatening adverse reactions and interactions, especially those related to the drugs and behaviors mentioned above.

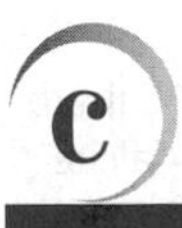

calcitonin (human)

Cibacalcin

calcitonin (salmon)

Calcimar, Caltine, Miacalcin, Miacalcin Nasal Spray, Salmonine

Pharmacologic class: Hormone (calcium-lowering)
Therapeutic class: Hypocalcemic
Pregnancy risk category C

Action

Directly affects bone, kidney, and GI tract. Decreases osteoclastic osteolysis in bone; also reduces mineral release and collagen breakdown in bone and promotes renal excretion of calcium. In pain relief, acts through prostaglandin inhibition, pain threshold modification, or beta-endorphin stimulation.

Availability

Injection: 0.5 mg/ml (human), 1 mg/ml (human), 200 international units/ml in 2-ml vials (salmon)
Nasal spray: 200 international units/actuation in 2-ml bottles (salmon)

Indications and dosages

➢ Postmenopausal osteoporosis
Adults: *Calcitonin (salmon)*—100 international units/day I.M. or subcutaneously, or 200 international units/day intranasally with concurrent supplemental calcium and vitamin D
➢ Paget's disease of bone (osteitis deformans)
Adults: *Calcitonin (salmon)*—Initially, 100 international units/day I.M. or subcutaneously; after titration, maintenance dosage is 50 to 100 international units daily or every other day (three times weekly). *Calcitonin (human)*—0.5 mg I.M. or subcutaneously daily, reduced to 0.25 mg daily.
➢ Hypercalcemia
Adults: *Calcitonin (salmon)*—4 international units/kg I.M. or subcutaneously q 12 hours; after 1 or 2 days, may increase to 8 international units/kg q 12 hours; after 2 more days, may increase further, if needed, to 8 international units q 6 hours.

Contraindications

• Hypersensitivity to drug
• Pregnancy or breastfeeding

Precautions

Use cautiously in:
• renal insufficiency, pernicious anemia
• children.

Administration

Before salmon calcitonin therapy begins, perform skin test, if ordered.
• Bring nasal spray to room temperature before using.
• Give intranasal dose as one spray in one nostril daily; alternate nostrils every day.

• To minimize adverse effects, give at bedtime.
• Rotate injection sites to decrease inflammatory reactions.

Route	Onset	Peak	Duration
I.M., subcut.	15 min	4 hr	8-24 hr
Intranasal	Rapid	0.5 hr	1 hr

Adverse reactions

CNS: headache, weakness, dizziness, paresthesia
CV: chest pain
EENT: epistaxis, nasal irritation, rhinitis
GI: nausea, vomiting, diarrhea, epigastric pain or discomfort
GU: urinary frequency
Musculoskeletal: arthralgia, back pain
Respiratory: dyspnea
Skin: rash
Other: altered taste, allergic reactions including facial flushing, swelling, and **anaphylaxis**

Interactions

Drug-drug. *Previous use of bisphosphonates (alendronate, etidronate, pamidronate, risedronate):* decreased response to calcitonin

Patient monitoring

• Monitor for adverse reactions during first few days of therapy.
• Assess alkaline phosphatase level and 24-hour urinary excretion of hydroxyproline.
• Check urine for casts.

Patient teaching

• Instruct patient to take drug before bedtime to lessen GI upset. Tell him to call prescriber if he can't maintain his usual diet because of GI upset.
• Inform patient using nasal spray that runny nose, sneezing, and nasal irritation may occur during first several days as he adjusts to spray.
• Instruct patient to bring nasal spray to room temperature before using.
• Advise patient to blow nose before using spray, to take intranasal dose as one spray in one nostril daily, and to alternate nostrils with each dose.
• Tell patient to discard unrefrigerated bottles of calcitonin (salmon) nasal spray after 30 days.
• Encourage patient to consume a diet rich in calcium and vitamin D.
• As appropriate, review all other significant adverse reactions and interactions, especially those related to the drugs mentioned above.

calcium acetate

PhosLo, PhosLo Gelcap

calcium carbonate

Alka-Mints, Alkets, Amitone, Calcarb 600, Calci-Chew, Calci-Mix, Calcite 500✤, Calcium 600, Calcium Antacid Extra Strength, Caltrate 600, Chooz, Dicarbosil, Equilet, Florical, Mallamint, Nephro-Calci, Nu-Cal✤, Os-Cal, Os-Cal 500, Oysco, Oyst-Cal 500, Oystercal 500, Rolaids Calcium Rich, Tums, Tums Calcium for Life Bone Health, Tums Calcium for Life PMS, Tums E-X, Tums Ultra

calcium chloride

Calciject✤

calcium citrate

Cal-Citrate-225, Cal-Citrate-250, Citracal, Citracal Liquitabs, Citrus Calcium

calcium glubionate

Calcionate, Calciquid

calcium gluceptate

calcium gluconate

calcium lactate

Cal-Lac

tricalcium phosphate

Posture

Pharmacologic class: Mineral
Therapeutic class: Dietary supplement, electrolyte replacement agent
Pregnancy risk category C (calcium acetate, chloride, glubionate, gluceptate, phosphate), ***NR*** (calcium carbonate, citrate, gluconate, lactate)

Action

Increases serum calcium level through direct effects on bone, kidney, and GI tract. Decreases osteoclastic osteolysis by reducing mineral release and collagen breakdown in bone.

Availability

Calcium acetate—
Gelcaps: 667 mg
Tablets: 667 mg
Calcium carbonate—
Capsules: 1,250 mg
Lozenges: 600 mg
Oral suspension: 1,250 mg
Powder: 6.5 g
Tablets: 650 mg, 1,250 mg, 1,500 mg
Tablets (chewable): 750 mg, 1,000 mg, 1,250 mg
Tablets (gum): 300 mg, 450 mg, 500 mg
Calcium chloride—
Injection: 10% solution
Calcium citrate—
Tablets: 950 mg
Calcium glubionate—
Syrup: 1.8 g/5 ml (contains 115 mg of elemental calcium)
Calcium gluceptate—
Injection: 22% solution
Calcium gluconate—
Injection: 10% solution
Tablets: 500 mg, 650 mg, 975 mg
Calcium lactate—
Tablets: 325 mg, 500 mg, 650 mg
Tricalcium phosphate—
Tablets: 600 mg

Indications and dosages

➢ Hypocalcemic emergency
Adults: 7 to 14 mEq I.V. of 10% calcium gluconate solution, 2% to 10% calcium chloride solution, or 22% calcium gluceptate solution
Children: 1 to 7 mEq calcium gluconate I.V.
Infants: Up to 1 mEq calcium gluconate I.V.

➢ Hypocalcemic tetany
Adults: 4.5 to 16 mEq calcium gluconate I.V., repeated as indicated until tetany is controlled
Children: 0.5 to 0.7 mEq/kg calcium gluconate I.V. three to four times daily as indicated until tetany is controlled
Neonates: 2.4 mEq/kg calcium gluconate I.V. daily in divided doses

➢ Cardiac arrest
Adults: 0.027 to 0.054 mEq/kg calcium chloride I.V., 4.5 to 6.3 mEq calcium gluceptate I.V., or 2.3 to 3.7 mEq calcium gluconate I.V.
Children: 0.27 mEq/kg calcium chloride I.V., repeated in 10 minutes if needed. Check calcium level before giving additional doses.

➢ Magnesium intoxication
Adults: Initially, 7 mEq I.V.; subsequent dosages based on patient response

➢ Exchange transfusions
Adults: 1.35 mEq calcium gluconate I.V. with each 100 ml of citrated blood

➢ Hyperphosphatemia in patients with end-stage renal disease
Adults: Two tablets P.O. daily, given in divided doses t.i.d. with meals. May increase gradually to bring serum phosphate level below 6 mg/dl, provided hypercalcemia doesn't develop.

➢ Dietary supplement
Adults: 500 mg to 2 g P.O. daily

Off-label uses
- Osteoporosis

Contraindications
- Hypersensitivity to drug
- Ventricular fibrillation
- Hypercalcemia and hypophosphatemia
- Cancer
- Renal calculi
- Pregnancy or breastfeeding

Precautions
Use cautiously in:
- renal insufficiency, pernicious anemia, heart disease, sarcoidosis, hyperparathyroidism, hypoparathyroidism
- history of renal calculi
- children.

Administration
Clinical alert: When infusing I.V., don't exceed a rate of 0.5 to 2 ml/minute.
- Keep patient supine for 15 minutes after I.V. administration to prevent orthostatic hypotension.
- Administer P.O. doses 1 to 1½ hours after meals.
- Know that I.M. administration is never recommended.
- Be aware that I.V. route is preferred in children.

Route	Onset	Peak	Duration
P.O.	Unknown	Unknown	Unknown
I.V.	Immediate	Immediate	0.5-2 hr

Adverse reactions
CNS: headache, weakness, dizziness, syncope, paresthesia
CV: mild blood pressure decrease, **bradycardia, arrhythmias, cardiac arrest** (with rapid I.V. injection)
GI: nausea, vomiting, diarrhea, constipation, epigastric pain or discomfort
GU: urinary frequency, renal calculi
Metabolic: hypercalcemia
Musculoskeletal: joint pain, back pain
Respiratory: dyspnea
Skin: rash
Other: altered or chalky taste, excessive thirst, allergic reactions (including facial flushing, swelling, tingling, tenderness in hands, and **anaphylaxis**)

Interactions
Drug-drug. *Atenolol, fluoroquinolones, tetracycline:* decreased bioavailability of these drugs
Calcium channel blockers: decreased calcium effects
Cardiac glycosides: increased risk of cardiac glycoside toxicity
Iron salts: decreased iron absorption
Sodium polystyrene sulfonate: metabolic alkalosis
Verapamil: reversal of verapamil effects
Drug-diagnostic tests. *Calcium:* increased level
Drug-food. *Foods containing oxalic acid (such as spinach), phytic acid (such as whole grain cereal), or phosphorus (such as dairy products):* interference with calcium absorption

Patient monitoring
- Monitor calcium levels frequently, especially in elderly patients.

Patient teaching
- Instruct patient to consume plenty of milk and dairy products during therapy.
- Refer patient to dietitian for help in meal planning and preparation.
- As appropriate, review all other significant and life-threatening adverse reactions and interactions, especially those related to the drugs, tests, and foods mentioned above.

calcium polycarbophil

Equalactin, FiberCon, Fiber-Lax, FiberNorm, Konsyl, Mitrolan

Pharmacologic class: Bulk-forming agent
Therapeutic class: Laxative
Pregnancy risk category NR

Action

Absorbs water, thereby expanding and increasing bulk and moisture content of stool; increased bulk promotes peristalsis and bowel movement.

Availability

Tablets: 500 mg
Tablets (chewable): 500 mg, 1,250 mg

Indications and dosages

➢ Constipation

Adults and children ages 12 and older: 1 g P.O. q.i.d. as needed. Maximum dosage is 6 g daily.
Children ages 7 to 12: 500 mg P.O. one to three times daily as needed. Maximum dosage is 3 g daily.
Children ages 3 to 6: 500 mg P.O. b.i.d. as needed. Maximum dosage is 1.5 g daily.

➢ Diarrhea; irritable bowel syndrome

Adults and children ages 12 and older: 1 g P.O. q.i.d. as needed. Maximum dosage is 6 g daily.
Children ages 7 to 12: 500 mg P.O. one to three times daily as needed. Maximum dosage is 3 g in a 24-hour period.
Children ages 3 to 6: 500 mg P.O. b.i.d. as needed. Maximum dosage is 1.5 g daily.

Contraindications

- GI obstruction
- Difficulty swallowing

Precautions

Use cautiously in:
- pregnant or breastfeeding patients
- children.

Administration

- Give with at least 8 oz of water or other fluid.
- Administer at least 2 hours before or after other drugs.
- Make sure patient maintains adequate fluid intake.

Route	Onset	Peak	Duration
P.O.	12-24 hr	3 days	Variable

Adverse reactions

CV: chest pain
GI: nausea, vomiting, abdominal pain, flatulence, rectal bleeding, **intestinal obstruction**
Respiratory: difficulty breathing
Other: laxative dependence

Interactions

Drug-drug. *Tetracyclines:* impaired tetracycline absorption
Drug-herbs. *Lily of the valley, pheasant's eye, squill:* increased risk of adverse drug reactions

Patient monitoring

- (Clinical alert) Monitor patient for difficulty breathing and signs and symptoms of intestinal obstruction.
- Assess for rectal bleeding and for failure to respond to drug.
- Monitor fluid intake and output, and assess hydration status regularly.

Patient teaching

- Instruct patient to take each dose with at least 8 oz of water or other fluid.
- Advise patient to space doses at least 2 hours apart from other drugs.
- (Clinical alert) Urge patient to seek immediate medical attention if he experiences chest pain, vomiting, difficulty breathing, or rectal bleeding.

• Advise patient to tell prescriber if he's taking other drugs or if he has abdominal pain, nausea, vomiting, or a sudden change in bowel habits lasting 2 weeks or longer.
• As appropriate, review all other significant and life-threatening adverse reactions and interactions, especially those related to the drugs and herbs mentioned above.

calfactant

Infasurf

Pharmacologic class: Natural lung surfactant
Therapeutic class: Lung surfactant
Pregnancy risk category NR

Action

Adsorbs rapidly to air: liquid interface of lung alveoli, stabilizing and modifying surface tension. Restores adequate pressure volumes, gas exchange, and overall lung compliance.

Availability

Suspension for intratracheal injection: 6 ml in single-dose vials

Indications and dosages

➢ To prevent respiratory distress syndrome (RDS) in at-risk premature infants; treatment of infants who develop RDS
Premature infants: 3 ml/kg at birth intratracheally q 12 hours, up to three doses. Initial dose must be administered as two 1.5-ml doses.

Contraindications

None

Precautions

Use cautiously in:
• altered ventilation requirements
• risk of cyanosis, bradycardia, or airway obstruction.

Administration

Clinical alert: Know that drug is intended for intratracheal administration and should be given only by neonatologists or other clinicians experienced in neonatal intubation and ventilatory management in facilities with adequate personnel, equipment, and drugs.
Clinical alert: Don't dilute drug or shake vial.
• Be aware that drug must be drawn into syringe through 20G or larger needle, taking care to avoid excessive foaming. Needle must be removed before drug is delivered through endotracheal tube.
Clinical alert: Know that infant must receive continuous monitoring before, during, and after drug administration.

Route	Onset	Peak	Duration
Intratrach.	Rapid	Unknown	Unknown

Adverse reactions

CV: bradycardia
Respiratory: requirement for manual ventilation or reintubation, **airway obstruction, reflux of drug into endotracheal tube, cyanosis**

Interactions

None significant

Patient monitoring

Clinical alert: Monitor infant's respiratory status continuously during and after drug administration.

Patient teaching

• Teach parents about treatment and assure them that infant will be monitored carefully.

C

candesartan cilexetil
Atacand

Pharmacologic class: Angiotensin II receptor antagonist
Therapeutic class: Antihypertensive
Pregnancy risk category C (first trimester), ***D*** (second and third trimesters)

Action
Blocks aldosterone-producing and vasoconstrictive effects of angiotensin II at various receptor sites, including vascular smooth muscle and adrenal glands

Availability
Tablets: 4 mg, 8 mg, 16 mg, 32 mg

Indications and dosages
➢ Hypertension
Adults: 16 mg P.O. daily. Start at lower dosage if patient is receiving diuretics or is volume depleted. Range is 2 to 32 mg/day as a single dose or divided in two doses.

Dosage adjustment
• Renal impairment
• Hepatic insufficiency

Contraindications
• Hypersensitivity to drug
• Pregnancy or breastfeeding
• Children (safety and efficacy not established)

Precautions
Use cautiously in:
• heart failure, renal or hepatic impairment, obstructive biliary disorders
• volume- or salt-depleted patients receiving high doses of diuretics
• black patients
• females of childbearing age.

Administration
• Give with or without food.
Supervise patient closely if he is receiving concurrent diuretics or is otherwise at risk for intravascular volume depletion.
• Know that diuretic may be added to regimen if candesartan alone doesn't control blood pressure.

Route	Onset	Peak	Duration
P.O.	2-4 hr	6-8 hr	24 hr

Adverse reactions
CNS: dizziness, syncope, fatigue, headache
CV: hypotension, chest pain, peripheral edema, **mitral or aortic valve stenosis**
EENT: ear congestion or pain, sinus disorders, sore throat
GI: nausea, diarrhea, constipation, abdominal pain, dry mouth
GU: albuminuria, **renal failure**
Hepatic: hepatitis
Metabolic: gout, **hyperkalemia**
Musculoskeletal: arthralgia, back pain, muscle weakness
Respiratory: upper respiratory tract infection, cough, bronchitis
Other: dental pain, fever

Interactions
Drug-drug. *Diuretics, other antihypertensives:* increased risk of hypotension
Lithium: increased lithium blood level
Nonsteroidal anti-inflammatory drugs: decreased antihypertensive effect
Potassium-sparing diuretics, potassium supplements: increased risk of hyperkalemia
Drug-food. *Salt substitutes containing potassium:* increased risk of hyperkalemia
Drug-herbs. *Ephedra (ma huang), licorice, yohimbine:* decreased antihypertensive effect

Patient monitoring

- Monitor electrolyte levels and kidney and liver function test results.
- Assess blood pressure regularly to gauge drug efficacy.
- Closely monitor patient with renal dysfunction who is receiving concurrent diuretics.

Patient teaching

- Teach patient about lifestyle changes that help control blood pressure, such as proper diet, exercise, stress reduction, smoking cessation, and moderation of alcohol intake.
- Instruct patient to use reliable birth control method and to contact prescriber if she suspects she's pregnant.
- Caution patient not to take herbs without consulting prescriber.
- As appropriate, review all other significant and life-threatening adverse reactions and interactions, especially those related to the drugs, foods, and herbs mentioned above.

capecitabine

Xeloda

Pharmacologic class: Fluoropyrimidine, antimetabolite (pyrimidine analog)

Therapeutic class: Antineoplastic

Pregnancy risk category D

Action

Enzymatically converts to 5-fluorouracil, which injures cells by interfering with DNA synthesis, cell division, RNA processing, and protein synthesis

Availability

Tablets: 150 mg, 500 mg

Indications and dosages

➢ Metastatic breast cancer resistant to both paclitaxel and a chemotherapy regimen that includes anthracycline; metastatic colorectal cancer when treatment with fluoropyrimidine therapy alone is preferred

Adults: Initially, 2,500 mg/m^2/day P.O. in two divided doses for 2 weeks, followed by a 1-week rest period; administered in 3-week cycles

Dosage adjustment

- Renal impairment
- Hepatic impairment
- Elderly patients

Contraindications

- Hypersensitivity to drug
- Severe renal impairment
- Pregnancy or breastfeeding

Precautions

Use cautiously in:

- mild to moderate renal impairment, hepatic impairment, severe diarrhea, coronary artery disease, intestinal disease, infection, coagulopathy
- children younger than age 18.

Administration

- Give with water within 30 minutes after a meal.
- If dosage must be lowered because of toxicity, don't increase dosage later.

Route	Onset	Peak	Duration
P.O.	Unknown	1.5-2 hr	Unknown

Adverse reactions

CNS: dizziness, fatigue, headache, insomnia, paresthesia

CV: edema

EENT: eye irritation

GI: nausea, vomiting, diarrhea, constipation, abdominal pain, dyspepsia, anorexia, stomatitis, **intestinal obstruction**

Hematologic: anemia, lymphopenia, **neutropenia, thrombocytopenia**

Metabolic: dehydration
Musculoskeletal: myalgia, limb pain
Skin: dermatitis, alopecia, nail disorder, hand and foot syndrome (palmar-plantar erythrodysesthesia)
Other: fever

Interactions

Drug-drug. *Antacids:* increased capecitabine blood level
Leucovorin: increased cytotoxicity
Live-virus vaccines: impaired ability to mount an immune response to vaccine
Phenytoin: increased phenytoin blood level
Warfarin: increased risk of bleeding
Drug-diagnostic tests. *Bilirubin:* increased level
Hemoglobin, neutrophils, platelets, white blood cells: decreased levels

Patient monitoring

- Monitor patient for signs and symptoms of toxicity. Be prepared to reduce dosage or withhold drug when indicated.
- Stay alert for signs and symptoms of infection.
- Carefully assess fluid and electrolyte status if patient has severe diarrhea.
- Monitor weight, CBC, International Normalized Ratio, prothrombin time, and kidney and liver function test results.
- Evaluate closely for adverse reactions in patients older than age 80.

Patient teaching

- Advise patient to take drug with water within 30 minutes after a meal.

Clinical alert: Instruct patient to immediately report nausea, vomiting, diarrhea, mouth ulcers, swollen joints, temperature above 100.5° F (38° C), and other signs or symptoms of infection.

- Tell patient to expect dosage adjustments during therapy.
- Urge patient to use reliable birth control method because drug may harm fetus if she becomes pregnant.
- Caution patient not to breastfeed during therapy.
- As appropriate, review all other significant and life-threatening adverse reactions and interactions, especially those related to the drugs and tests mentioned above.

captopril

Apo-Capto✱, Capoten, Gen-Captopril✱, Novo-Captopril✱, Nu-Capto✱

Pharmacologic class: Angiotensin-converting enzyme (ACE) inhibitor
Therapeutic class: Antihypertensive
Pregnancy risk category C (first trimester), ***D*** (second and third trimesters)

Action

Prevents conversion of angiotensin I to angiotensin II, which leads to decreased vasoconstriction and, ultimately, to lower blood pressure. Also decreases blood pressure by increasing plasma renin secretion from kidney and reducing aldosterone secretion from adrenal cortex. Decreased aldosterone secretion prevents sodium and water retention.

Availability

Tablets: 12.5 mg, 25 mg, 50 mg, 100 mg

Indications and dosages

➢ Hypertension

Adults: 12.5 to 25 mg P.O. two to three times daily; may be increased up to 150/mg/day at 1- to 2-week intervals. Usual dosage is 50 mg t.i.d. If patient is receiving diuretics, start with 6.25 to 12.5 mg P.O. two to three times daily. If blood pressure isn't adequately controlled after 1 to 2 weeks, add diuretic, as prescribed. If further blood pressure decrease is needed, dosage may be raised to 150 mg P.O. t.i.d. while patient continues on diuretic. Maximum dosage is 450 mg/day.

➢ Heart failure

Adults: Usual initial dosage is 25 mg P.O. t.i.d. After increasing to 50 mg P.O. t.i.d. (if indicated), do not increase dosage further for 2 weeks, to determine satisfactory response. Don't exceed 450 mg/day.

➢ Left ventricular dysfunction after myocardial infarction

Adults: 6.25 mg P.O. as a test dose, followed by 12.5 mg t.i.d. May increase up to 50 mg t.i.d.

➢ Diabetic nephropathy

Adults: 25 mg P.O. t.i.d.

Dosage adjustment

- Renal impairment

Off-label uses

- Bartter's syndrome
- Hypertension associated with scleroderma
- Management of hypertensive crisis
- Raynaud's syndrome
- Rheumatoid arthritis
- Severe childhood hypertension

Contraindications

- Hypersensitivity to drug or other ACE inhibitors
- Angioedema (hereditary or idiopathic)
- Pregnancy

Precautions

Use cautiously in:

- renal or hepatic impairment, hypovolemia, hyponatremia, aortic stenosis and hypertrophic cardiomyopathy, cardiac or cerebrovascular insufficiency, systemic lupus erythematous
- family history of angioedema
- black patients with hypertension
- elderly patients
- breastfeeding patients
- children.

Administration

- Discontinue other antihypertensives 1 week before starting captopril, if possible.
- Give 1 hour before meals on empty stomach.

Route	Onset	Peak	Duration
P.O.	0.25-1 hr	1-1.5 hr	6-12 hr

Adverse reactions

CNS: headache, dizziness, drowsiness, fatigue, weakness, insomnia
CV: angina pectoris, tachycardia, **hypotension**
EENT: sinusitis
GI: nausea, diarrhea, anorexia
GU: proteinuria, erectile dysfunction, decreased libido, gynecomastia, **renal failure**
Hematologic: anemia, **agranulocytosis, leukopenia, pancytopenia, thrombocytopenia**
Metabolic: hyperkalemia
Respiratory: cough, asthma, bronchitis, dyspnea, **eosinophilic pneumonitis**
Skin: rash, **angioedema**
Other: altered taste, fever

Interactions

Drug-drug. *Allopurinol:* increased risk of hypersensitivity reaction
Antacids: decreased captopril absorption
Antihypertensives, general anesthetics that lower blood pressure, nitrates, phenothiazines: additive hypotension
Cyclosporine: hyperkalemia
Digoxin, lithium: increased blood levels of these drugs, increased risk of toxicity
Epoetin alfa: additive hyperkalemia
Indomethacin: reduced antihypertensive effect of captopril
Nonsteroidal anti-inflammatory drugs: decreased antihypertensive response
Potassium-sparing diuretics, potassium supplements: hyperkalemia
Probenecid: decreased elimination and increased blood level of captopril

Drug-diagnostic tests. *Alanine aminotransferase, alkaline phosphatase, aspartate aminotransferase, bilirubin, blood urea nitrogen, creatinine, potassium:* increased levels
Granulocytes, hemoglobin, platelets, red blood cells, sodium, white blood cells: decreased levels
Urine acetone: false-positive result
Drug-food. *Any food:* decreased captopril absorption
Salt substitutes containing potassium: hyperkalemia
Drug-herbs. *Capsaicin, yohimbine:* cough
Drug-behaviors. *Acute alcohol ingestion:* additive hypotension

Patient monitoring

🔊 Monitor for sudden blood pressure drop within 3 hours of initial dose if patient is receiving concurrent diuretics and on a low-sodium diet.
- Monitor hematologic, kidney, and liver function test results.
- Check for proteinuria monthly and after first 9 months of therapy.

Patient teaching

- Tell patient to take drug 1 hour before meals on empty stomach.
- Advise patient to report fever, rash, sore throat, mouth sores, fast or irregular heartbeat, chest pain, or cough.
- Inform patient that dizziness, fainting, and light-headedness usually disappear once his body adjusts to drug.
- Tell patient his ability to taste may decrease during first 2 to 3 months of therapy.
- Caution patient to avoid over-the-counter medications unless approved by prescriber.
- As appropriate, review all other significant and life-threatening adverse reactions and interactions, especially those related to the drugs, tests, foods, herbs, and behaviors mentioned above.

carbamazepine

Apo-Carbamazepine✱, Atretol, Carbamaz✱, Carbatrol, Epitol, Novo-Tegretol✱, Tegretol, Tegretol-XR

Pharmacologic class: Iminostilbene derivative
Therapeutic class: Anticonvulsant
Pregnancy risk category D

Action

Unclear. Chemically related to tricyclic antidepressants (TCAs). Anticonvulsant action may result from reduction in polysynaptic responses and blocking of post-tetanic potentiation.

Availability

Capsules (extended-release): 200 mg, 300 mg
Oral suspension: 100 mg/5 ml
Tablets: 200 mg
Tablets (chewable): 100 mg, 200 mg
Tablets (extended-release): 100 mg, 200 mg, 400 mg

Indications and dosages

➤ Prophylaxis of generalized tonic-clonic, mixed, and complex-partial seizures
Adults and children ages 12 and older: Initially, 200 mg P.O. b.i.d. (tablets) or 100 mg q.i.d. (oral suspension). Increase by up to 200 mg/day q 7 days until therapeutic blood levels are reached. Usual maintenance dosage is 600 to 1,200 mg/day in divided doses q 6 to 8 hour. In children ages 12 to 15, don't exceed 1 g/day. Give extended-release forms b.i.d.
Children ages 6 to 12: Initially, 100 mg P.O. b.i.d. (tablets) or 50 mg q.i.d. (oral suspension). Increase by up to 100 mg weekly until therapeutic levels are reached. Usual maintenance dosage is

400 to 800 mg/day. Don't exceed 1 g/day. Give extended-release forms b.i.d.
Children younger than age 6: Initially, 10 to 20 mg/kg/day P.O. in two or three divided doses. May increase by up to 100 mg/day at weekly intervals. Usual maintenance dosage is 250 to 350 mg/day. Don't exceed 400 mg/day.
➢ Trigeminal neuralgia
Adults: Initially, 100 mg b.i.d. (tablets) or 50 mg q.i.d. (oral suspension). Increase by up to 200 mg/day until pain relief occurs; then give maintenance dosage of 200 to 1,200 mg/day in divided doses. Usual maintenance range is 400 to 800 mg/day.

Off-label uses

- Alcohol, cocaine, or benzodiazepine withdrawal
- Atypical psychoses
- Central diabetes insipidus
- Mood disorders
- Neurogenic pain

Contraindications

- Hypersensitivity to drug or TCAs
- MAO inhibitor use within past 14 days
- Bone marrow depression
- Pregnancy or breastfeeding

Precautions

Use cautiously in:

- cardiac disease, hepatic disease, increased intraocular pressure, mixed seizure disorders, glaucoma
- elderly males with prostatic hypertrophy
- psychiatric patients.

Administration

- Don't give within 14 days of MAO inhibitor.
- Give tablets with meals; may give extended-release capsules without regard to meals.
- Don't give with grapefruit juice.
- If desired, contents of extended-release capsules may be sprinkled over food; however, capsule and contents shouldn't be crushed or chewed.

Route	Onset	Peak	Duration
P.O.	Up to 1 mo	4-5 hr	6-12 hr
P.O. (extended)	Up to 1 mo	2-12 hr	12 hr

Adverse reactions

CNS: ataxia, drowsiness, fatigue, psychosis, syncope, vertigo, headache, **worsening of seizures**
CV: hypertension, hypotension, **arrhythmias, atrioventricular block, aggravation of coronary artery disease, heart failure**
EENT: blurred vision, diplopia, nystagmus, corneal opacities, conjunctivitis, pharyngeal dryness
GI: nausea, vomiting, diarrhea, abdominal pain, stomatitis, glossitis, dry mouth, anorexia
GU: urinary hesitancy, retention, or frequency; albuminuria; glycosuria; erectile dysfunction
Hematologic: eosinophilia, lymphadenopathy, **agranulocytosis, aplastic anemia, thrombocytopenia, leukopenia**
Hepatic: hepatitis
Metabolic: syndrome of inappropriate antidiuretic hormone secretion
Respiratory: pneumonitis
Skin: photosensitivity, rash, urticaria, diaphoresis, **erythema multiforme, Stevens-Johnson syndrome**
Other: weight gain, chills, fever

Interactions

Drug-drug. *Acetaminophen:* increased risk of acetaminophen-induced hepatotoxicity, decreased acetaminophen efficacy
Anticoagulants, bupropion: increased metabolism of these drugs, causing decreased efficacy

Barbiturates: decreased barbiturate blood level, increased carbamazepine blood level
Charcoal: decreased carbamazepine absorption
Cimetidine, danazol, diltiazem: increased carbamazepine blood level
Cyclosporine, felbamate, felodipine, haloperidol: decreased blood levels of these drugs
Doxycycline: shortened doxycycline half-life and reduced antimicrobial effect
Hormonal contraceptives: decreased contraceptive efficacy, possibly leading to pregnancy
Hydantoins: increased or decreased hydantoin blood level, decreased carbamazepine blood level
Isoniazid: increased risk of carbamazepine toxicity and isoniazid hepatotoxicity
Lithium: increased risk of CNS toxicity
Macrolide antibiotics (such as clarithromycin and erythromycin), propoxyphene, selective serotonin reuptake inhibitors (such as fluoxetine and fluvoxamine), verapamil: increased carbamazepine blood level, greater risk of toxicity
MAO inhibitors: high fever, hypertension, seizures, and possibly death
Nondepolarizing neuromuscular blockers: shortened carbamazepine duration of action
TCAs: increased carbamazepine blood level and greater risk of toxicity, decreased TCA blood level
Valproic acid: decreased valproic acid blood level with possible loss of seizure control, variable changes in carbamazepine blood level
Drug-diagnostic tests. *Blood urea nitrogen, eosinophils, liver function tests:* increased values
Granulocytes, hemoglobin, platelets, thyroid function tests, white blood cells: decreased values
Drug-food. *Grapefruit juice:* increased drug blood level and effects
Drug-herbs. *Plantain (psyllium seed):* inhibited GI absorption of drug

Patient monitoring

Monitor patient closely. Institute seizure precautions if drug must be withdrawn suddenly.
- Assess for history of psychosis; drug may activate symptoms.
- Monitor baseline hematologic, kidney, and liver function test results.
- During dosage adjustments, monitor vital signs and fluid intake and output. Stay alert for fluid retention, renal failure, and cardiovascular complications.
- With high doses, monitor CBC weekly for first 3 months and then monthly to detect bone marrow depression.

Patient teaching

- Tell patient that he may sprinkle contents of extended-release capsules over food, but that he shouldn't crush or chew capsule or contents.
- Advise patient that coating on extended-release capsules may be visible in stools because it isn't absorbed.
- Tell patient to take drug with meals to minimize GI upset.
- Caution patient to avoid driving and other hazardous activities until he knows how drug affects concentration, alertness, and vision.
- Advise patient to avoid excessive sun exposure and to wear protective clothing and sunscreen.
- Inform female patient that drug may interfere with hormonal contraception. Advise her to use alternative birth-control method.
- As appropriate, review all other significant and life-threatening adverse reactions and interactions, especially those related to the drugs, tests, foods, and herbs mentioned above.

carbidopa-levodopa

Sinemet, Sinemet CR

Pharmacologic class: Dopamine agonist
Therapeutic class: Antiparkinsonian
Pregnancy risk category C

Action

After conversion to dopamine in CNS, levodopa acts as a neurotransmitter, relieving symptoms of Parkinson's disease. Carbidopa prevents destruction of levodopa, making more levodopa available to be decarboxylated to dopamine in brain.

Availability

Tablets: 10 mg carbidopa/100 mg levodopa, 25 mg carbidopa/100 mg levodopa, 25 mg carbidopa/250 mg levodopa
Tablets (extended-release): 25 mg carbidopa/100 mg levodopa, 50 mg carbidopa/200 mg levodopa

Indications and dosages

➤ Idiopathic Parkinson's disease; parkinsonism; symptomatic parkinsonism

Conventional tablets—

Adults not currently receiving levodopa: Initially, 10 mg carbidopa/100 mg levodopa P.O. three to four times daily or 25 mg carbidopa/100 mg levodopa t.i.d.; may be increased q 1 to 2 days until desired effect occurs

Adults converting from levodopa alone (less than 1.5 g/day): Initially, 25 mg carbidopa/100 mg levodopa three to four times daily; may be increased q 1 to 2 days until desired effect occurs

Adults converting from levodopa alone (more than 1.5 g/day): Initially, 25 mg carbidopa/250 mg levodopa three to four times daily; may be increased q 1 to 2 days until desired effect occurs

Extended-release tablets—

Adults not currently receiving levodopa: Initially, 50 mg carbidopa/200 mg levodopa P.O. b.i.d., with doses spaced at least 6 hours apart

Adults converting from standard carbidopa-levodopa: Initiate therapy with at least 10% more levodopa content/day (may need up to 30% more) given at 4- to 8-hour intervals while awake; wait 3 days between dosage changes. Some patients may need higher dosages and shorter dosing intervals.

Contraindications

- Hypersensitivity to drug or tartrazine
- Angle-closure glaucoma
- MAO inhibitor use within past 14 days
- Malignant melanoma
- Breastfeeding

Precautions

Use cautiously in:

- cerebrovascular, renal, hepatic, or endocrine disease
- history of cardiac, psychiatric, or ulcer disease
- abrupt drug discontinuation or dosage
- pregnant patients
- children ages 18 and under (safety not established).

Administration

- Give dose as close as possible to time ordered to ensure stable drug blood level.
- Know that giving extended-release form with food increases drug bioavailability.
- If patient needs general anesthesia, continue drug therapy as appropriate (if he's allowed to have oral fluids and drugs).

Be aware that drug shouldn't be withdrawn abruptly.

Route	Onset	Peak	Duration
P.O.	Unknown	40-120 min	Unknown

Adverse reactions

CNS: anxiety, dizziness, hallucinations, memory loss, headache, numbness, confusion, insomnia, nightmares, delusions, psychotic changes, depression, dementia, poor coordination, worsening hand tremor
CV: cardiac irregularities, palpitations, orthostatic hypotension
EENT: blurred vision, diplopia, mydriasis, eyelid twitching, difficulty swallowing
GI: nausea, vomiting, diarrhea, constipation, abdominal pain or discomfort, flatulence, excessive salivation, dry mouth, anorexia, **upper GI hemorrhage** (with history of peptic ulcer)
GU: urinary retention, urinary incontinence, dark urine
Hematologic: **hemolytic anemia, leukopenia**
Hepatic: hepatotoxicity
Musculoskeletal: muscle twitching, involuntary or spasmodic movements
Respiratory: hyperventilation
Skin: melanoma, flushing, rash, abnormally dark sweat
Other: altered or bitter taste, burning sensation of tongue, tooth grinding (especially at night), weight changes, hot flashes, hiccups

Interactions

Drug-drug. *Anticholinergics:* decreased carbidopa-levodopa absorption
Antihypertensives: additive hypotension
Haloperidol, papaverine, phenothiazines, phenytoin, reserpine: reversal of carbidopa-levodopa effects
Inhalation hydrocarbon anesthetics: increased risk of arrhythmias
MAO inhibitors: hypertensive reactions
Methyldopa: altered efficacy of carbidopa-levodopa, increased risk of adverse CNS reactions
Pyridoxine: antagonism of carbidopa-levodopa effects
Selegiline: increased risk of adverse reactions
Drug-diagnostic tests. *Alanine aminotransferase, alkaline phosphatase, aspartate aminotransferase, bilirubin, blood urea nitrogen, lactate dehydrogenase, low-density lipoproteins, protein-bound iodine, uric acid:* increased levels
Coombs' test: false-positive result
Granulocytes, hemoglobin, platelets, white blood cells: decreased values
Urine glucose, urine ketones: test interference
Drug-food. *Foods rich in pyridoxine (liver, yeast, cereals)*: reversal of carbidopa-levodopa effects
Drug-herbs. *Kava:* decreased carbidopa-levodopa efficacy
Octacosanol: worsening of dyskinesia
Drug-behaviors. *Cocaine use:* increased risk of adverse reactions to carbidopa-levodopa

Patient monitoring

- Monitor patient for orthostatic hypotension.
- Assess patient's need for drug "holiday" if his response to drug decreases.

Patient teaching

Inform patient that muscle and eyelid twitching may indicate toxicity. Tell him to report these symptoms immediately.

Caution patient not to stop taking drug abruptly.

- Instruct patient to swallow extended-release tablets whole without crushing or chewing them.
- Advise patient to move slowly when sitting up or standing, to avoid dizziness or light-headedness caused by sudden blood pressure drop.
- Tell patient that drug may darken or discolor his urine and sweat.

• As appropriate, review all other significant and life-threatening adverse reactions and interactions, especially those related to the drugs, tests, foods, herbs, and behaviors mentioned above.

carbidopa-levodopa-entacapone
Stalevo

Pharmacologic class: Dopamine agonist
Therapeutic class: Antiparkinsonian
Pregnancy risk category C

Action
After conversion to dopamine in CNS, levodopa acts as a neurotransmitter, relieving symptoms of Parkinson's disease. Carbidopa prevents destruction of levodopa, making more levodopa available to be decarboxylated to dopamine in brain. Entacapone increases levodopa blood level by more than 30% and prolongs levodopa's effects.

Availability
Tablets: 12.5 mg carbidopa/50 mg levodopa/200 mg entacapone; 25 mg carbidopa/100 mg levodopa/200 mg entacapone; 37.5 mg carbidopa/150 mg levodopa/200 mg entacapone

Indications and dosages
➣ Idiopathic Parkinson's disease; postencephalitic parkinsonism; symptomatic parkinsonism resulting from carbon monoxide or manganese intoxication
Adults: Optimal daily dosage determined by careful individual titration. Target carbidopa dosage is 70 mg to 100 mg P.O. daily, not to exceed 200 mg; maximum entacapone dosage is 1,600 mg P.O. daily. Patients should receive no more than eight tablets daily.

Contraindications
• Hypersensitivity to drug
• Malignant melanoma (or history of this disease)
• MAO inhibitor use within 14 days
• Angle-closure glaucoma
• Undiagnosed skin lesions
• Breastfeeding

Precautions
Use cautiously in:
• biliary obstruction, renal disease, cerebrovascular disease, endocrine disorders, hepatic impairment, psychiatric disorders
• history of cardiac disease or GI ulcers
• pregnant patients
• children younger than age 18 (safety not established).

Administration
• Give with meals if GI upset occurs.
• Don't crush or break tablets.

Route	Onset	Peak	Duration
P.O.	Unknown	2-3 hr	12 hr

Adverse reactions
CNS: involuntary movements, bradykinesia, anxiety, dizziness, hallucinations, memory loss, psychiatric problems, trismus, increased hand tremor, headache, numbness, weakness, confusion, insomnia, nightmares, delusions, psychotic changes, depression, dementia
CV: cardiac irregularities, palpitations, orthostatic hypotension, **arrhythmias**
EENT: blurred vision, blepharospasm, mydriasis, diplopia
GI: nausea, vomiting, diarrhea, constipation, abdominal pain, dysphagia, burning sensation, flatulence, anorexia, **upper GI hemorrhage**
GU: urinary retention, urinary incontinence, dark urine

Hematologic: hemolytic anemia, leukopenia
Hepatic: hepatotoxicity
Musculoskeletal: muscle twitching
Respiratory: hiccups, hyperventilation, **pulmonary infiltrates**
Skin: melanoma, rash, flushing, abnormally dark sweat
Other: sialorrhea, weight changes, hot flashes

Interactions

Drug-drug. *Ampicillin, chloramphenicol, cholestyramine, erythromycin, probenecid, rifampin:* interference with biliary excretion, additive increase in entacapone blood level
Anticholinergics: decreased levodopa absorption
Antihypertensives: additive hypotension
Haloperidol, papaverine, phenothiazines, phenytoin, reserpine: reversal of levodopa effects
Inhalation hydrocarbon anesthetics: increased risk of arrhythmias
MAO inhibitors: severe hypertension
Methyldopa: altered levodopa efficacy, increased risk of adverse CNS effects
Pyridoxine: antagonism of levodopa's beneficial effects
Drug-diagnostic tests. *Alanine aminotransferase, alkaline phosphatase, aspartame aminotransferase, bilirubin, blood urea nitrogen, lactate dehydrogenase, protein-bound iodine, uric acid:* increased levels
Coombs' test: false-positive result
Granulocytes, hemoglobin, platelets, white blood cells: decreased values
Urine glucose and ketone tests: test interference
Drug-food. *Foods high in pyridoxine:* reversal of levodopa effects
Drug-herbs. *Kava:* decreased levodopa efficacy
Octacosanol: worsening of dyskinesia

Patient monitoring

- Monitor patient closely for mental changes, especially psychosis and depression. Report suicidal ideation immediately.
- Assess neurologic status closely to evaluate drug efficacy and identify adverse effects.
- Monitor CBC with white cell differential; also monitor liver function test results.
- Evaluate vital signs. Watch for arrhythmias, orthostatic hypotension, and respiratory problems.
- Assess fluid intake and output. Check for urinary problems.

Patient teaching

- Inform patient or caregiver that drug may cause significant neurologic effects. Instruct him to report anxiety, dizziness, hallucinations, memory loss, increased hand tremor, headache, confusion, nightmares, and depression.
- Tell patient or caregiver to report breathing problems.
- Teach patient or caregiver about recommended home modifications and other safety measures to reduce risk of injury.
- Advise patient to rise slowly and carefully. Drug may cause blood pressure to drop if he sits up or stands suddenly.
- Caution patient to avoid hazardous activities until disease is well controlled and he knows how drug affects concentration, alertness, vision, and motor function.
- Advise patient to minimize GI upset by eating small, frequent servings of healthy food and ensuring adequate fluid intake.
- Tell patient he'll undergo regular blood testing while taking this drug.
- As appropriate, review all other significant and life-threatening adverse reactions and interactions, especially those related to the drugs, tests, foods, and herbs mentioned above.

carboplatin

Paraplatin, Paraplatin-AQ✤

Pharmacologic class: Alkylating agent
Therapeutic class: Antineoplastic
Pregnancy risk category D

Action

Inhibits DNA synthesis by causing cross-linking of parent DNA strands; interferes with RNA transcription, causing growth imbalance that leads to cell death. Cell-cycle-phase nonspecific.

Availability

Injection: 50-mg, 150-mg, and 450-mg vials

Indications and dosages

➢ Initial treatment of advanced ovarian cancer or palliative treatment of ovarian cancer unresponsive to other chemotherapeutic modalities

Adults: Initially, 300 mg/m^2 I.V. (given with cyclophosphamide) at 4-week intervals. For refractory tumors, 360 mg/m^2 I.V. as a single dose; may be repeated at 4-week intervals, depending on response. However, single dose shouldn't be repeated until neutrophil count is at least 2,000/mm^3 and platelet count at least 100,000/mm^3. Subsequent dosages are based on blood counts.

Dosage adjustment

- Renal impairment
- Reduced bone marrow reserve

Off-label uses

- Advanced endometrial cancer
- Advanced or recurrent squamous cell carcinoma of head and neck
- Relapsed and refractory acute leukemia
- Small-cell lung cancer
- Testicular cancer

Contraindications

- Hypersensitivity to drug, cisplatin, or mannitol
- Pregnancy or breastfeeding

Precautions

Use cautiously in:

- hearing loss, electrolyte imbalances, renal impairment, active infections, diminished bone marrow reserve
- females of childbearing age.

Administration

- Premedicate with antiemetics, as prescribed.
- When preparing and administering drug, follow facility protocol for handling cytotoxic drugs.
- Reconstitute powder for injection by adding sterile water for injection, 0.9% sodium chloride injection, or 5% dextrose injection, as appropriate, to provide 10-mg/ml solution. Drug may be further diluted to concentrations as low as 0.5 mg/ml.
- Don't use with needles or I.V. sets containing aluminum.
- Administer I.V. infusion over at least 15 minutes.
- Make sure patient maintains adequate fluid intake.
- Know that drug is given in combination with other agents.

Route	Onset	Peak	Duration
I.V.	Rapid	21 days	28 days

Adverse reactions

CNS: weakness, dizziness, confusion, peripheral neuropathy, **cerebrovascular accident**
CV: heart failure, embolism
EENT: visual disturbances, ototoxicity
GI: nausea, vomiting, constipation, diarrhea, abdominal pain, stomatitis
GU: gonadal suppression, **nephrotoxicity**

Hematologic: anemia, **leukopenia, thrombocytopenia, neutropenia**
Hepatic: hepatitis
Metabolic: hypocalcemia, hypokalemia, hypomagnesemia, hyponatremia
Respiratory: bronchospasm
Skin: alopecia, rash, urticaria, erythema, pruritus
Other: altered taste, hypersensitivity reactions, **anaphylaxis**

Interactions

Drug-drug. *Live-virus vaccines:* decreased antibody response to vaccine, increased risk of adverse reactions
Myelosuppressants: additive bone marrow depression
Nephrotoxic or ototoxic drugs (such as aminoglycosides, loop diuretics): additive nephrotoxicity or ototoxicity
Phenytoin: decreased phenytoin blood level
Drug-diagnostic tests. *Alkaline phosphatase (ALP), aspartate aminotransferase (AST), blood urea nitrogen, creatinine:* increased values
Electrolytes, hematocrit, hemoglobin. neutrophils, platelets, red blood cells, white blood cells: decreased values

Patient monitoring

- Assess for signs and symptoms of hypersensitivity reactions.
- Monitor CBC to help detect drug-induced anemia and other hematologic reactions.
- Monitor ALP, AST, and total bilirubin levels.
- Evaluate fluid and electrolyte balance.

Patient teaching

- Instruct patient to report signs and symptoms of allergic response and other adverse reactions, such as breathing problems, mouth sores, rash, itching, and reddened skin.
- Advise patient to report unusual bleeding or bruising.
- Caution patient to avoid driving and other hazardous activities until he knows how drug affects concentration and alertness.
- Urge patient to avoid activities that can cause injury. Advise him to use soft toothbrush and electric razor to avoid gum and skin injury.
- Instruct patient to drink plenty of fluids to ensure adequate urinary output.
- Provide dietary counseling and refer patient to dietitian as needed if GI adverse effects significantly limit food intake.
- As appropriate, review all other significant and life-threatening adverse reactions and interactions, especially those related to the drugs and tests mentioned above.

C

carisoprodol

Soma, Vanadom

Pharmacologic class: Carbamate derivative

Therapeutic class: Centrally acting skeletal muscle relaxant

Controlled substance schedule IV (in some states)

Pregnancy risk category C

Action

Unknown. May modify central perception of pain without modifying pain reflexes. Skeletal muscle relaxation may result from sedative properties or from inhibition of activity in descending reticular formation and spinal cord.

Availability

Tablets: 350 mg

Indications and dosages

➢ Adjunctive treatment of muscle spasms associated with acute painful musculoskeletal conditions
Adults: 350 mg P.O. q.i.d.

Contraindications
- Hypersensitivity to drug or meprobamate
- Porphyria or suspected porphyria

Precautions
Use cautiously in:
- severe hepatic or renal disease
- history of substance abuse
- pregnant or breastfeeding patients
- children ages 12 and younger.

Administration
- Give last daily dose at bedtime.
- Administer with food if GI upset occurs.
- If patient can't swallow tablets, mix with syrup, chocolate, or jelly.

Route	Onset	Peak	Duration
P.O.	30 min	1-2 hr	4-6 hr

Adverse reactions
CNS: dizziness, drowsiness, agitation, ataxia, depression, headache, insomnia, vertigo, tremor, depression
CV: hypotension, tachycardia
GI: nausea, vomiting, epigastric distress
Hematologic: eosinophilia, **leukopenia**
Respiratory: asthma attacks
Skin: flushing (especially of face), rash, pruritus, **erythema multiforme**
Other: hiccups, fever, psychological drug dependence, **anaphylactic shock**

Interactions
Drug-drug. *Antihistamines, opioids, sedative-hypnotics:* additive CNS depression
Drug-diagnostic tests. *Eosinophils:* increased count
Drug-herbs. *Chamomile, hops, kava, skullcap, valerian:* increased CNS depression
Drug-behaviors. *Alcohol use:* increased CNS depression

Patient monitoring
- When giving to breastfeeding patient, watch for signs of sedation and GI upset in infant.
- Monitor range of motion, stiffness, and discomfort level.
- Know that drug is metabolized to meprobamate. Monitor for drug dependence, especially in patients with history of substance abuse.

Patient teaching
- Tell patient that psychological drug dependence may occur.
- Instruct patient to avoid over-the-counter drugs and alcohol, because they may increase CNS depression.
- Caution patient to avoid driving and other hazardous activities until he knows how drug affects concentration and alertness.
- As appropriate, review all other significant and life-threatening adverse reactions and interactions, especially those related to the drugs, tests, herbs, and behaviors mentioned above.

carmustine
BCNU, BiCNU, Gliadel Wafer

Pharmacologic class: Alkylating agent
Therapeutic class: Antineoplastic
Pregnancy risk category D

Action
Unclear. Thought to interfere with bacterial cell-wall synthesis by cross-linking strands of DNA and disrupting RNA transcription, causing cell to rupture and die. Exhibits minimal immunosuppressant activity.

Availability
Intracavitary wafer implant: 7.7 mg (available in packages of eight wafers)
Powder for injection: 100-mg vials

Indications and dosages

➢ Brain tumor; multiple myeloma; Hodgkin's disease; other lymphomas

Adults and children: 150 to 200 mg/m^2 I.V. as a single dose q 6 to 8 weeks, or 75 to 100 mg/m^2/day for 2 days q 6 weeks, or 40 mg/m^2/day for 5 days q 6 weeks. Repeat dose q 6 weeks if platelet count exceeds 100,000/mm^3 and white blood cell (WBC) count exceeds 4,000/mm^3.

➢ Adjunct to brain surgery

Adults: Up to 61.6 mg (eight wafers) implanted in surgical cavity created during brain tumor resection

Dosage adjustment

- Based on WBC and platelet counts

Off-label uses

- Mycosis fungoides

Contraindications

- Hypersensitivity to drug
- Radiation therapy
- Chemotherapy
- Pregnancy or breastfeeding

Precautions

Use cautiously in:

- infection; depressed bone marrow reserve; respiratory, hepatic, or renal impairment
- females of childbearing age.

Administration

- Know that drug may be used alone or in conjunction with other treatments, such as surgery or radiation.
- Follow facility policy when preparing, administering, and handling drug.
- Reconstitute drug by dissolving vial of 100 mg with 3 ml of sterile dehydrated alcohol (provided with drug), followed by 27 ml of sterile water for injection; yields solution with concentration of 3.3 mg carmustine/ml. Solution may be further diluted with 5% dextrose injection and delivered by I.V. infusion over 1 to 2 hours.
- Know that infusion lasting less than 1 hour causes intense pain and burning at I.V. site.
- Infuse solution in glass containers only; drug is unstable in plastic I.V. bags.
- Know that skin contact with reconstituted drug may cause transient hyperpigmentation. If contact occurs, wash skin thoroughly with soap and water.
- Be aware that oxidized regenerated cellulose may be placed over wafers to secure them against surgical cavity surface.
- Know that resection cavity should be irrigated after wafer placement and that dura should be closed in watertight fashion.

Route	Onset	Peak	Duration
I.V.	Immediate	15 min	6 wk
Intracavitary	Unknown	Unknown	Unknown

Adverse reactions

CNS: ataxia, drowsiness

GI: nausea, vomiting, diarrhea, esophagitis, stomatitis, anorexia

GU: azotemia, **renal failure, nephrotoxicity**

Hematologic: anemia, **leukopenia, thrombocytopenia, cumulative bone marrow depression, bone marrow dysplasia**

Hepatic: hepatotoxicity

Respiratory: pulmonary fibrosis, pulmonary infiltrates

Skin: alopecia, hyperpigmentation, facial flushing, abnormal bruising

Other: I.V. site pain, **secondary malignancies**

Interactions

Drug-drug. *Anticoagulants, aspirin, nonsteroidal anti-inflammatory drugs:* increased risk of bleeding

Antineoplastics: additive bone marrow depression
Cimetidine: potentiation of bone marrow depression
Digoxin, phenytoin: decreased blood levels of these drugs
Live-virus vaccines: decreased antibody response to vaccines, increased risk of adverse reactions
Drug-diagnostic tests. *Alkaline phosphatase, aspartate aminotransferase, bilirubin, nitrogenous compounds (urea):* increased levels
Hemoglobin, WBCs: decreased values
Drug-behaviors. *Smoking:* increased risk of respiratory toxicity

Patient monitoring

- Assess baseline kidney and liver function tests.
- Monitor CBC for up to 6 weeks after giving dose to detect delayed bone marrow toxicity.
- Know that pulmonary function tests should be performed before therapy begins and regularly throughout therapy to assess for toxicity.

Patient teaching

- Instruct patient to report signs and symptoms of allergic response and other adverse reactions.
- Inform patient that severe flushing may follow I.V. dose but should subside in 2 to 4 hours.
- Tell patient to avoid activities that can cause injury. Advise him to use soft toothbrush and electric razor to avoid gum and skin injury.
- Advise patient to minimize GI upset by eating small, frequent servings of food and drinking plenty of fluids.
- Instruct patient to monitor urinary output and report significant changes.
- Inform patient that drug may cause hair loss.
- Advise patient that he'll undergo regular blood testing during therapy.
- As appropriate, review all other significant and life-threatening adverse reactions and interactions, especially those related to the drugs, tests, and behaviors mentioned above.

carteolol hydrochloride

Cartrol, Ocupress

Pharmacologic class: Beta-adrenergic blocker (nonselective)

Therapeutic class: Antianginal, antihypertensive

Pregnancy risk category C

Action

Blocks stimulation of cardiac $beta_1$-adrenergic receptor sites and pulmonary $beta_2$-adrenergic receptor sites. Shows intrinsic sympathomimetic activity, causing slowing of heart rate, decreased myocardial excitability, reduced cardiac output, and decreased renin release from kidney. Also reduces intraocular pressure.

Availability

Tablets: 2.5 mg, 5 mg
Ophthalmic solution: 1%

Indications and dosages

➤ Hypertension
Adults: 2.5 mg P.O. daily, given alone or with diuretic; may be increased up to 10 mg daily. (Dosages above 10 mg may produce no further response or may decrease response.) Maintenance dosage is 2.5 to 5 mg P.O. daily.
➤ Open-angle glaucoma; ocular hypertension
Adults: One drop (1% solution) in affected eye(s) b.i.d.

Dosage adjustment

- Renal impairment
- Elderly patients

Off-label uses

- Angina pectoris

Contraindications

- Hypersensitivity to drug, its components, or beta-adrenergic blockers
- Uncompensated heart failure
- Pulmonary edema
- Cardiogenic shock, bradycardia, second- or third-degree atrioventricular block
- Bronchial asthma, severe obstructive pulmonary disease
- Overt heart failure (ophthalmic form only)

Precautions

Use cautiously in:
- renal or hepatic impairment, pulmonary disease, diabetes mellitus, hypoglycemia, thyrotoxicosis, hypotension, respiratory depression
- elderly patients
- pregnant or breastfeeding patients
- children.

Administration

- Give with or without food.
- Check apical pulse before giving. If it's slower than 60 beats/minute, withhold dose and call prescriber.

Don't withdraw oral drug abruptly. Doing so may lead to withdrawal phenomenon (angina exacerbation, myocardial infarction, ventricular arrhythmias, and even death).

Route	Onset	Peak	Duration
P.O.	Variable	1-3 hr	24-48 hr
Ophthalmic	Unknown	Unknown	Unknown

Adverse reactions

CNS: fatigue, weakness, anxiety, depression, dizziness, insomnia, memory loss, nightmares, paresthesia, hallucinations, disorientation, slurred speech
CV: orthostatic hypotension, peripheral vasoconstriction, conduction disturbances, **bradycardia, heart failure**
EENT: decreased night vision and stinging (ophthalmic form), blurred vision, dry eyes, tinnitus, stuffy nose, nasal congestion, pharyngitis, **laryngospasm**
GI: nausea, vomiting, diarrhea, constipation, abdominal pain, dry mouth, anorexia
GU: dysuria, polyuria, nocturia, dark urine, erectile dysfunction, decreased libido, Peyronie's disease
Metabolic: hyperglycemia, **hypoglycemia**
Musculoskeletal: arthralgia, back or leg pain, muscle cramps
Respiratory: wheezing, **bronchospasm, respiratory distress, pulmonary edema**
Skin: pruritus, rash, sweating
Other: drug-induced lupuslike syndrome, **anaphylaxis**

Interactions

Drug-drug. *Adrenergics:* antagonism of carteolol effects
Allergen immunotherapy: increased risk of anaphylaxis
Amphetamines, ephedrine, epinephrine, norepinephrine, phenylephrine, pseudoephedrine: unopposed alpha-adrenergic stimulation, causing excessive hypertension and bradycardia
Antihypertensives, nitrates: additive hypotension
Clonidine: increased hypotension and bradycardia, exaggerated withdrawal phenomenon
Digoxin: additive bradycardia
Dobutamine, dopamine: decrease in beneficial cardiovascular effects
General anesthetics, I.V. phenytoin, verapamil: additive myocardial depression
Insulin, oral hypoglycemics: altered efficacy of these drugs
MAO inhibitors: hypertension
Nonsteroidal anti-inflammatory drugs: decreased antihypertensive effect
Thyroid preparations: decreased carteolol efficacy
Drug-diagnostic tests. *Blood urea nitrogen, lipoproteins, potassium, triglycerides, uric acid:* increased levels

Glucose or insulin tolerance test: test interference

Drug-behaviors. *Acute alcohol ingestion:* additive hypotension

Cocaine use: unopposed alpha-adrenergic stimulation, causing excessive hypertension and bradycardia

Sun exposure: photophobia

Patient monitoring

- Monitor vital signs (especially blood pressure) and ECG. Drug may alter cardiac output and cause ineffective airway clearance.
- Weigh patient daily and measure fluid intake and output to detect fluid retention.
- Evaluate renal function.
- Assess blood glucose level regularly if patient has diabetes mellitus.

Patient teaching

Caution patient not to stop using oral drug abruptly, because doing so may cause serious reactions.

Instruct patient to report breathing problems immediately.

- Tell patient to report dizziness, confusion, depression, respiratory problems, or rash.
- Advise patient to move slowly when sitting up or standing to avoid dizziness or light-headedness from sudden blood pressure drop.
- Caution patient to avoid driving and other hazardous activities until he knows how drug affects concentration and alertness.
- Inform male patient that drug may cause erectile dysfunction. Advise him to discuss this issue with prescriber.
- Teach patient proper use of eyedrops. Tell him to wash hands first, not to touch dropper tip to any surface, and not to use drops when contact lenses are in eyes.
- Inform patient that although eyedrops commonly cause stinging and blurred vision, he should notify prescriber if these symptoms are severe.
- As appropriate, review all other significant and life-threatening adverse reactions and interactions, especially those related to the drugs, tests, and behaviors mentioned above.

carvedilol

Coreg

Pharmacologic class: Beta-adrenergic blocker (nonselective)

Therapeutic class: Antihypertensive

Pregnancy risk category C

Action

Blocks stimulation of cardiac $beta_1$-adrenergic receptor sites and pulmonary $beta_2$-adrenergic receptor sites. Shows intrinsic sympathomimetic activity, causing slowing of heart rate, decreased myocardial excitability, reduced cardiac output, and decreased renin release from kidney.

Availability

Tablets: 3.125 mg, 6.25 mg, 12.5 mg, 25 mg

Indications and dosages

➢ Hypertension

Adults: Initially, 6.25 mg P.O. b.i.d. May be increased q 7 to 14 days to a maximum dosage of 25 mg b.i.d.

➢ Heart failure caused by ischemia or cardiomyopathy

Adults: Initially, 3.125 mg P.O. b.i.d. for 2 weeks. May increase to 6.25 mg b.i.d. Dosage may be doubled q 2 weeks as tolerated, not to exceed 25 mg b.i.d. in patients weighing less than 85 kg (187 lb) or 50 mg b.i.d. in patients weighing more than 85 kg.

Off-label uses

- Angina pectoris
- Idiopathic cardiomyopathy

Contraindications
- Hypersensitivity to drug
- Uncompensated heart failure
- Pulmonary edema
- Cardiogenic shock
- Bradycardia or heart block
- Severe hepatic impairment
- Bronchial asthma, bronchospasm

Precautions
Use cautiously in:
- renal or hepatic impairment, pulmonary disease, diabetes mellitus, hypoglycemia, thyrotoxicosis, peripheral vascular disease, hypotension, respiratory depression
- elderly patients
- pregnant or breastfeeding patients
- children.

Administration
- Give with food to slow absorption and minimize orthostatic hypotension.
- Check apical pulse before administering. If it's below 60 beats/minute, withhold dosage and contact prescriber.
- Be aware that addition of diuretic may cause additive effects and may worsen orthostatic hypotension.
- Know that full antihypertensive effect takes 7 to 14 days.

🔊 Don't withdraw drug abruptly, because this may lead to withdrawal phenomenon (angina exacerbation, myocardial infarction, ventricular arrhythmias, and even death).
- Know that drug may be given with digoxin, diuretic, or angiotensin-converting enzyme inhibitor.

Route	Onset	Peak	Duration
P.O.	Within 1 hr	1-2 hr	12 hr

Adverse reactions
CNS: dizziness, fatigue, anxiety, depression, insomnia, memory loss, nightmares, headache, pain
CV: orthostatic hypotension, peripheral vasoconstriction, angina pectoris, chest pain, hypertension, **bradycardia, heart failure, atrioventricular block**
EENT: blurred or abnormal vision, dry eyes, stuffy nose, rhinitis, sinusitis, pharyngitis
GI: nausea, diarrhea, constipation
GU: urinary tract infection, hematuria, albuminuria, decreased libido, erectile dysfunction, **renal dysfunction**
Hematologic: bleeding, **purpura, thrombocytopenia**
Metabolic: hypovolemia, hypervolemia, hyperglycemia, hyponatremia, hyperuricemia, glycosuria, gout, **hypoglycemia**
Musculoskeletal: arthralgia, back pain, muscle cramps
Respiratory: wheezing, upper respiratory tract infection, dyspnea, bronchitis, **bronchospasm, pulmonary edema**
Skin: pruritus, rash
Other: weight gain, lupuslike syndrome, viral infection, **anaphylaxis**

Interactions
Drug-drug. *Antihypertensives:* additive hypotension
Calcium channel blockers, general anesthetics, I.V. phenytoin: additive myocardial depression
Cimetidine: increased carvedilol toxicity
Clonidine: increased hypotension and bradycardia, exaggerated withdrawal phenomenon
Digoxin: additive bradycardia
Dobutamine, dopamine: decrease in beneficial cardiovascular effects
Insulin, oral hypoglycemics: altered efficacy of these drugs
MAO inhibitors: hypertension
Nonsteroidal anti-inflammatory drugs: decreased antihypertensive action
Rifampin, thyroid preparations: decreased carvedilol efficacy
Theophyllines: reduced theophylline elimination, antagonistic effect that decreases theophylline or carteolol efficacy

Drug-diagnostic tests. *Antinuclear antibodies:* increased titers
Blood urea nitrogen, glucose, lipoproteins, potassium, triglycerides, uric acid: increased levels
Drug-food. *Any food:* delayed drug absorption
Drug-behaviors. *Acute alcohol ingestion:* additive hypotension

Patient monitoring

- Watch for signs and symptoms of hypersensitivity reaction.
- Assess baseline CBC and kidney and liver function test results.
- Monitor vital signs (especially blood pressure), ECG, and exercise tolerance. Drug may alter cardiac output and cause ineffective airway clearance.
- Weigh patient daily and measure fluid intake and output to detect fluid retention.
- Measure blood glucose regularly if patient has diabetes mellitus. Drug may mask signs and symptoms of hypoglycemia.

Patient teaching

- Instruct patient to take drug with food exactly as prescribed.

Caution patient not to stop taking drug abruptly, because serious reactions may result.

- Advise patient to move slowly when sitting up or standing, to avoid dizziness or light-headedness from sudden blood pressure drop.
- Caution patient to avoid driving and other hazardous activities until he knows how drug affects concentration and alertness.
- Inform male patient that drug may cause erectile dysfunction. Advise him to discuss this issue with prescriber.
- Advise patient to use soft-bristled toothbrush and electric razor to avoid gum and skin injury.
- As appropriate, review all other significant and life-threatening adverse reactions and interactions, especially those related to the drugs, tests, foods, and behaviors mentioned above.

caspofungin acetate

Cancidas

Pharmacologic class: Glucan synthesis inhibitor
Therapeutic class: Antifungal
Pregnancy risk category C

Action

Inhibits synthesis of beta (1, 3)-D-glucan, an important component of cell wall in *Aspergillus* and other fungal cells. This inhibition leads to cell rupture and death.

Availability

Lyophilized powder for injection: 50 mg and 75 mg in single-use vials

Indications and dosages

➢ Invasive aspergillosis
Adults: 70 mg I.V. as a single loading dose on first day, followed by 50 mg/day thereafter
➢ Esophageal candidiasis
Adults: 50 mg daily by slow I.V. infusion

Contraindications

- Hypersensitivity to drug

Precautions

Use cautiously in:

- hepatic impairment
- bone marrow depression
- renal insufficiency
- pregnant or breastfeeding patients.

Administration

Don't mix with other drugs or with diluents containing dextrose.

- Reconstitute powder using 0.9% sodium chloride for injection or bacteriostatic water for injection. Mix gently

until solution is clear; further dilute with sodium chloride or lactated Ringer's solution.
• Administer by slow I.V. infusion over 1 hour.
• Know that in patients with human immunodeficiency virus, oral therapy may be given to help prevent relapse of oropharyngeal candidiasis.

Route	Onset	Peak	Duration
I.V.	Immediate	9-11 hr	40-50 hr

Adverse reactions

CNS: headache, paresthesia
CV: tachycardia, phlebitis
GI: nausea, vomiting, diarrhea, abdominal pain, anorexia
Hematologic: eosinophilia, anemia
Metabolic: hypokalemia
Musculoskeletal: pain, myalgia
Respiratory: tachypnea
Skin: histamine-mediated symptoms (including rash, facial swelling, pruritus, and warm sensation)

Interactions

Drug-drug. *Cyclosporine:* markedly increased caspofungin blood level
Inducers of drug clearance, mixed inducers-inhibitors (carbamazepine, dexamethasone, efavirenz, nelfinavir, nevirapine, phenytoin, rifampin): reduced caspofungin blood level
Tacrolimus: possible alteration in tacrolimus blood level
Drug-diagnostic tests. *Alkaline phosphatase, eosinophils:* increased levels
Hemoglobin, potassium: decreased levels

Patient monitoring

• Monitor I.V. site carefully for phlebitis and other complications.
• Monitor CBC and serum electrolyte levels. Watch for signs and symptoms of hypokalemia.
• Stay alert for histamine-mediated signs and symptoms (rash, facial swelling, pruritus, and sensation of warmth).
• Monitor vital signs, especially for tachycardia and tachypnea.
• Monitor nutritional and hydration status.

Patient teaching

• Teach patient about histamine-mediated signs and symptoms. Tell him when to notify prescriber.
• Advise patient to minimize GI adverse effects by eating small, frequent servings of healthy food and ensuring adequate fluid intake.
🔊 Tell patient that drug may irritate vein used for infusion. Encourage him to immediately report pain, swelling, or other symptoms.
• As appropriate, review all other significant adverse reactions and interactions, especially those related to the drugs and tests mentioned above.

cefaclor

Apo-Cefaclor✤ Ceclor, Ceclor CD, Ceclor Pulvules, PMS-Cefaclor✤

Pharmacologic class: Second-generation cephalosporin
Therapeutic class: Anti-infective
Pregnancy risk category B

Action

Interferes with bacterial cell-wall synthesis, causing cell to rupture and die

Availability

Capsules: 250 mg, 500 mg
Oral suspension: 125 mg/5 ml, 187 mg/5 ml, 250 mg/5 ml, 375 mg/5 ml
Tablets (extended-release): 375 mg, 500 mg

Indications and dosages

➢ Uncomplicated skin infections caused by *Staphylococcus aureus*
Adults and children ages 16 and older: 375 mg P.O. (extended-release tablet) q 12 hours for 7 to 10 days

➢ Pharyngitis and tonsillitis not caused by *Haemophilus influenzae*
Adults and children ages 16 and older: 375 mg P.O. (extended-release tablet) q 12 hours for 10 days

➢ Chronic bronchitis and acute bronchitis not caused by *H. influenzae*
Adults and children ages 16 and older: 500 mg P.O. (extended-release tablet) q 12 hours for 7 days

➢ Otitis media caused by staphylococci; lower respiratory tract infections caused by *H. influenzae, S. pyogenes,* and *S. pneumoniae;* pharyngitis and tonsillitis caused by *S. pyogenes;* urinary tract infections caused by *Klebsiella* species, *Escherichia coli, Proteus mirabilis,* and coagulase-negative staphylococci
Adults and children ages 13 to 17: 250 mg P.O. q 8 hours. For severe infections, 500 mg P.O. q 8 hours.
Children: 20 mg/kg/day P.O. in divided doses q 8 hours. For serious infections, 40 mg/kg/day P.O. in divided doses q 8 hours. Maximum dosage is 1 g/day.

Dosage adjustment

- Renal insufficiency
- Elderly patients

Contraindications

- Hypersensitivity to cephalosporins or penicillins

Precautions

Use cautiously in:

- renal impairment, phenylketonuria
- history of GI disease (especially colitis)
- emaciated patients
- elderly patients
- pregnant or breastfeeding patients
- children.

Administration

- Obtain specimens for culture and sensitivity testing as necessary before starting therapy.
- Be aware that cross-sensitivity to penicillins may occur.
- Give extended-release tablets with food to enhance absorption.
- Don't give antacids within 2 hours of extended-release form.

Route	Onset	Peak	Duration
P.O.	Rapid	30-60 min	6-12 hr
P.O. (extended)	Unknown	1.5-2.5 hr	12 hr

Adverse reactions

CNS: headache, lethargy, paresthesia, syncope, **seizures**
CV: hypotension, palpitations, chest pain, vasodilation
EENT: hearing loss
GI: nausea, vomiting, diarrhea, abdominal cramps, oral candidiasis, **pseudomembranous colitis**
GU: vaginal candidiasis, **nephrotoxicity**
Hematologic: lymphocytosis, eosinophilia, **bleeding tendency, hemolytic anemia, hypoprothrombinemia, neutropenia, thrombocytopenia, agranulocytosis, bone marrow depression**
Hepatic: hepatic failure, hepatomegaly
Musculoskeletal: arthralgia
Respiratory: dyspnea
Skin: urticaria, maculopapular or erythematous rash
Other: chills, fever, superinfection, **anaphylaxis, serum sickness**

Interactions

Drug-drug. *Aminoglycosides, loop diuretics:* increased risk of nephrotoxicity
Antacids: decreased absorption of extended-release cefaclor tablets

Chloramphenicol: antagonistic effect
Probenecid: decreased excretion and increased blood level of cefaclor
Drug-diagnostic tests. *Alanine aminotransferase, alkaline phosphatase, aspartate aminotransferase, bilirubin, blood urea nitrogen, creatinine, eosinophils, gamma-glutamyltransferase, lactate dehydrogenase:* increased levels
Coombs' test, urinary 17-ketosteroids, nonenzyme-based urine glucose tests (such as Clinitest): false-positive results
Hemoglobin, platelets, white blood cells: decreased values

Patient monitoring

- Assess CBC and kidney and liver function test results.
- With long-term therapy, obtain monthly Coombs' test.
- Monitor for signs and symptoms of superinfection and other serious adverse reactions.

Patient teaching

- Instruct patient to take drug with food or milk to reduce GI upset.
- Advise patient to complete entire course of therapy even if he feels better.
- Tell patient to report signs and symptoms of allergic response and other adverse reactions, such as rash, easy bruising, bleeding, severe GI problems, or difficulty breathing.
- Instruct patient to avoid taking antacids within 2 hours of extended-release cefaclor.
- As appropriate, review all other significant and life-threatening adverse reactions and interactions, especially those related to the drugs and tests mentioned above.

cefadroxil

Duricef, Novo-Cefadroxil✦

Pharmacologic class: First-generation cephalosporin
Therapeutic class: Anti-infective
Pregnancy risk category B

Action

Interferes with bacterial cell-wall synthesis, causing cell to rupture and die

Availability

Capsules: 500 mg
Oral suspension: 125 mg/5 ml, 250 mg/5 ml, 500 mg/5 ml
Tablets: 1 g

Indications and dosages

➤ Pharyngitis and tonsillitis caused by beta-hemolytic streptococci
Adults: 1 g/day P.O. or 500 mg P.O. b.i.d. for 10 days
Children: 30 mg/kg/day P.O. in divided doses q 12 hours for 10 days
➤ Skin infections caused by staphylococci and streptococci
Adults: 1 g/day P.O. or 500 mg P.O. q 12 hours
Children: 30 mg/kg/day P.O. in divided doses q 12 hours
➤ Urinary tract infections caused by *Proteus mirabilis, Escherichia coli,* and *Klebsiella* species
Adults: 1 to 2 g/day P.O. in divided doses q 12 hours
Children: 30 mg/kg/day P.O. in divided doses q 12 hours

Dosage adjustment

- Renal insufficiency
- Elderly patients

Off-label uses

- Bone and joint infections
- Unspecified respiratory infections

Contraindications
• Hypersensitivity to cephalosporins or penicillins

Precautions
Use cautiously in:
• renal impairment, phenylketonuria
• history of GI disease (especially colitis)
• elderly patients
• pregnant or breastfeeding patients
• children.

Administration
• Obtain specimens for culture and sensitivity testing as necessary before starting therapy.
• Give with or without food.

Route	Onset	Peak	Duration
P.O.	Rapid	1.5-2 hr	12-24 hr

Adverse reactions
CNS: headache, lethargy, paresthesia, syncope, **seizures**
CV: hypotension, palpitations, chest pain, vasodilation
EENT: hearing loss
GI: nausea, vomiting, diarrhea, cramps, oral candidiasis, **pseudomembranous colitis**
GU: vaginal candidiasis, **nephrotoxicity**
Hematologic: lymphocytosis, eosinophilia, **bleeding tendency, hemolytic anemia, hypoprothrombinemia, neutropenia, thrombocytopenia, agranulocytosis, bone marrow depression**
Hepatic: hepatic failure, hepatomegaly
Musculoskeletal: arthralgia
Respiratory: dyspnea
Skin: urticaria, maculopapular or erythematous rash
Other: chills, fever, superinfection, **anaphylaxis**

Interactions
Drug-drug. *Aminoglycosides, loop diuretics:* increased risk of nephrotoxicity
Probenecid: decreased excretion and increased blood level of cefadroxil
Drug-diagnostic tests. *Alanine aminotransferase, alkaline phosphatase, aspartate aminotransferase, bilirubin, blood urea nitrogen, creatinine, eosinophils, gamma-glutamyltransferase, lactate dehydrogenase:* increased levels
Coombs' test, urinary 17-ketosteroids, nonenzyme-based urine glucose tests (such as Clinitest): false-positive results
Hemoglobin, platelets, white blood cells: decreased values

Patient monitoring
• Assess baseline CBC and kidney and liver function test results.
• Monitor for signs and symptoms of superinfection and other serious adverse reactions.
• Be aware that cross-sensitivity to penicillins may occur.
• With long-term therapy, obtain monthly Coombs' test.

Patient teaching
• Advise patient to take drug with food or milk if GI upset occurs.
• Instruct patient to complete entire course of therapy even if he feels better.
• Tell patient to report signs and symptoms of allergic response and other adverse reactions, such as rash, easy bruising, bleeding, severe GI problems, or difficulty breathing.
• As appropriate, review all other significant and life-threatening adverse reactions and interactions, especially those related to the drugs and tests mentioned above.

cefazolin sodium

Ancef, Kefzol

Pharmacologic class: First-generation cephalosporin
Therapeutic class: Anti-infective
Pregnancy risk category B

Action

Interferes with bacterial cell-wall synthesis, causing cell to rupture and die

Availability

Powder for injection: 250 mg, 500 mg, 1 g, 5 g, 10 g, 20 g
Premixed containers: 500 mg/50 ml in dextrose 5% in water (D_5W), 1 g/50 ml in D_5W

Indications and dosages

➢ Respiratory tract infections caused by group A beta-hemolytic streptococci, *Klebsiella* species, *Haemophilus influenzae,* and *Staphylococcus aureus;* skin infections caused by *S. aureus* and beta-hemolytic streptococci; biliary tract infections caused by *Escherichia coli, Klebsiella* species, *Proteus mirabilis,* and *S. aureus;* bone and joint infections caused by *S. aureus;* genital infections caused by *E. coli, Klebsiella* species, *P. mirabilis,* and strains of enterococci; septicemia caused by *E. coli, Klebsiella* species, *P. mirabilis, S. aureus,* and *S. pneumoniae;* endocarditis caused by *S. aureus* or beta-hemolytic streptococci
Adults: For mild infections, 250 to 500 mg q 8 hours I.V. or I.M. For moderate to severe infections, 500 to 1,000 mg I.V. or I.M. q 6 to 8 hours. For life-threatening infections, 1,000 to 1,500 mg I.M. or I.V. q 6 hours, to a maximum dosage of 6 g/day.
Children: For mild to moderate infections, 25 to 50 mg/kg/day I.V. or I.M. in divided doses t.i.d. or q.i.d. For severe infections, 100 mg/kg/day I.V. or I.M. in divided doses t.i.d. or q.i.d.
➢ Acute uncomplicated urinary tract infections (UTIs) caused by *E. coli, Klebsiella* species, *P. mirabilis,* and strains of *Enterococcus* and *Enterobacter* species
Adults: 1 g I.V. or I.M. q 12 hours
➢ Surgical prophylaxis
Adults: 1g I.V. or I.M. 30 to 60 minutes before surgery, then 0.5 to 1 g I.V. or I.M. q 6 to 8 hours for 24 hours. If surgery exceeds 2 hours, another 0.5- to 1-g dose I.M. or I.V. may be given intraoperatively.
➢ Pneumococcal pneumonia
Adults: 500 mg I.M. or I.V. infusion q 12 hours

Dosage adjustment

- Renal impairment
- Elderly patients

Contraindications

- Hypersensitivity to cephalosporins or penicillins

Precautions

Use cautiously in:

- renal impairment, phenylketonuria
- history of GI disease (especially colitis)
- emaciated patients
- elderly patients
- pregnant or breastfeeding patients
- children.

Administration

- Obtain specimens for culture and sensitivity testing as needed before starting therapy.
- For intermittent I.V. infusion, administer in volume-control set or in separate, secondary I.V. container over 30 to 60 minutes.
- For direct I.V. injection, dilute reconstituted dose in 5 ml of sterile water for injection and administer slowly over 3 to 5 minutes.

• For I.M. use, reconstitute with sterile water for injection, bacteriostatic water, or normal saline solution for injection. Shake well until dissolved.
• Inject I.M. into large muscle mass.

Route	Onset	Peak	Duration
I.V.	Rapid	End of infusion	6-12 hr
I.M.	Rapid	1-2 hr	6-12 hr

Adverse reactions

CNS: headache, lethargy, confusion, hemiparesis, paresthesia, syncope, **seizures**
CV: hypotension, palpitations, chest pain, vasodilation
EENT: hearing loss
GI: nausea, vomiting, diarrhea, abdominal cramps, oral candidiasis, **pseudomembranous colitis**
GU: vaginal candidiasis, **nephrotoxicity**
Hematologic: lymphocytosis, eosinophilia, **bleeding tendency, hemolytic anemia, hypoprothrombinemia, neutropenia, thrombocytopenia, agranulocytosis, bone marrow depression**
Hepatic: hepatic failure, hepatomegaly
Musculoskeletal: arthralgia
Respiratory: dyspnea
Skin: urticaria, maculopapular or erythematous rash
Other: chills, fever, superinfection, **anaphylaxis, serum sickness**

Interactions

Drug-drug. *Aminoglycosides, loop diuretics:* increased risk of nephrotoxicity
Anticoagulants: increased anticoagulant effect
Chloramphenicol: antagonistic effect
Probenecid: decreased excretion and increased blood level of cefazolin
Drug-diagnostic tests. *Alanine aminotransferase, alkaline phosphatase, aspartate aminotransferase, bilirubin, blood urea nitrogen, creatinine, eosinophils, gamma-glutamyltransferase, lactate dehydrogenase:* increased levels
Coombs' test, urinary 17-ketosteroids, nonenzyme-based urine glucose tests (such as Clinitest): false-positive results
Hemoglobin, platelets, white blood cells: decreased values
Drug-behaviors. *Alcohol use:* acute alcohol intolerance (disulfiram-like reaction) if alcohol is consumed within 72 hours of drug administration

Patient monitoring

🔊 If patient is receiving high doses, monitor for extreme confusion, tonic-clonic seizures, and mild hemiparesis.
• Monitor CBC, prothrombin time, and kidney and liver function test results.
• Watch for signs and symptoms of superinfection and other serious adverse reactions.
• Be aware that cross-sensitivity to penicillins may occur.

Patient teaching

• Tell patient to report reduced urinary output, persistent diarrhea, bruising, or bleeding.
• Instruct patient to take drug exactly as prescribed and to complete full course of therapy even when he feels better.
• As appropriate, review all other significant and life-threatening adverse reactions and interactions, especially those related to the drugs, tests, and behaviors mentioned above.

cefdinir

Omnicef

Pharmacologic class: Third-generation cephalosporin
Therapeutic class: Anti-infective
Pregnancy risk category B

C

Action
Interferes with bacterial cell-wall synthesis and division by binding to cell wall, causing cell to die. Active against gram-negative and gram-positive bacteria, with expanded activity against gram-negative bacteria. Exhibits minimal immunosuppressant activity.

Availability
Capsules: 300 mg
Oral suspension: 125 mg/5 ml in 60- and 100-ml bottles

Indications and dosages
➢ Acute bacterial otitis media caused by *Haemophilus influenzae, Streptococcus pneumoniae,* and *Moraxella catarrhalis*
Adults and children ages 13 and older: 300 mg P.O. q 12 hours or 600 mg P.O. q 24 hours for 10 days
Children ages 6 months to 12 years: 7 mg/kg P.O. q 12 hours for 5 to 10 days or 14 mg/kg P.O. q 24 hours for 10 days
➢ Uncomplicated skin and soft-tissue infections caused by *Staphylococcus aureus* and *Streptococcus pyogenes*
Adults and children ages 13 and older: 300 mg P.O. q 12 hours for 10 days. Maximum dosage is 600 mg/day.
➢ Acute maxillary sinusitis caused by *H. influenzae, S. pneumoniae,* and *M. catarrhalis*
Adults and children ages 13 and older: 300 mg P.O. q 12 hours or 600 mg P.O. q 24 hours for 10 days. Maximum dosage is 600 mg/day.
Children ages 6 months to 12 years: 7 mg/kg P.O. q 12 hours or 14 mg/kg P.O. q 24 hours for 10 days
➢ Pharyngitis or tonsillitis caused by *S. pyogenes*, chronic bronchitis caused by *H. influenzae, S. pneumoniae,* and *M. catarrhalis*
Adults and children ages 13 and older: 300 mg P.O. q 12 hours for 5 to 10 days or 600 mg P.O. q 24 hours for 10 days. Maximum dosage is 600 mg/day.
➢ Community-acquired pneumonia caused by *H. influenzae, Haemophilus parainfluenzae, S. pneumoniae,* and *M. catarrhalis*
Adults and children ages 13 and older: 300 mg P.O. q 12 hours for 10 days. Maximum dosage is 600 mg/day.

Dosage adjustment
- Renal impairment

Contraindications
- Hypersensitivity to cephalosporins or penicillins

Precautions
Use cautiously in:
- renal impairment, phenylketonuria
- history of GI disease (especially colitis)
- elderly patients
- pregnant or breastfeeding patients
- children.

Administration
- Obtain specimens for culture and sensitivity tests as necessary before starting therapy.
- Give with or without food.
- Administer 2 hours before or after iron supplements or antacids containing aluminum or magnesium.
- Give capsules, if possible, to diabetic patients (oral suspension contains 2.86 g of sucrose per teaspoon).

Route	Onset	Peak	Duration
P.O.	Rapid	2-4 hr	12-24 hr

Adverse reactions
CNS: headache, lethargy, paresthesia, syncope, **seizures**
CV: hypotension, palpitations, chest pain, vasodilation
EENT: hearing loss
GI: nausea, vomiting, diarrhea, abdominal cramps, oral candidiasis, **pseudomembranous colitis**
GU: vaginal candidiasis, **nephrotoxicity**

Hematologic: lymphocytosis, eosinophilia, **bleeding tendency, hemolytic anemia, hypoprothrombinemia, neutropenia, thrombocytopenia, agranulocytosis, bone marrow depression**
Hepatic: hepatomegaly, hepatic failure
Musculoskeletal: arthralgia
Respiratory: dyspnea
Skin: chills, fever, urticaria, maculopapular or erythematous rash
Other: superinfection, **anaphylaxis, serum sickness**

Interactions

Drug-drug. *Aminoglycosides, loop diuretics:* increased risk of nephrotoxicity
Antacids, iron-containing preparations: decreased cefdinir absorption
Probenecid: decreased excretion and increased blood level of cefdinir
Drug-diagnostic tests. *Alanine aminotransferase, alkaline phosphatase, aspartate aminotransferase, bilirubin, blood urea nitrogen, creatinine, eosinophils, gamma-glutamyltransferase, lactate dehydrogenase:* increased levels
Coombs' test, urinary 17-ketosteroids, nonenzyme-based urine glucose tests (such as Clinitest): false-positive results
Hemoglobin, platelets, white blood cells: decreased values
Drug-herbs. *Angelica, anise, arnica, asafetida, bogbean, boldo, celery, chamomile, clove, danshen, fenugreek, feverfew, garlic, ginger, ginkgo, horse chestnut, horseradish, licorice, meadowsweet, onion, ginseng, papain, passionflower, poplar, prickly ash, quassia, red clover, turmeric, wild carrot, wild lettuce, willow:* increased risk of bleeding

Patient monitoring

- Monitor CBC and kidney and liver function test results.
- Monitor for signs and symptoms of superinfection and other serious adverse reactions.

Patient teaching

- Tell patient he may take drug with or without food.
- Instruct patient to report persistent diarrhea (more than four episodes daily) and other adverse effects.
- If patient uses antacids or iron-containing preparations (such as iron supplements), tell him to take these 2 hours before or after cefdinir.
- Inform patient that drug may temporarily discolor stools.
- As appropriate, review all other significant and life-threatening adverse reactions and interactions, especially those related to the drugs, tests, and herbs mentioned above.

cefditoren pivoxil

Spectracef

Pharmacologic class: Third-generation cephalosporin
Therapeutic class: Anti-infective
Pregnancy risk category B

Action

Interferes with bacterial cell-wall synthesis and division by binding to cell wall, causing cell to die. Active against gram-negative and gram-positive bacteria, with expanded activity against gram-negative bacteria. Exhibits minimal immunosuppressant activity.

Availability

Tablets: 200 mg

Indications and dosages

➢ Mild to moderate pharyngitis and tonsillitis caused by *Streptococcus pyogenes*
Adults and children ages 12 and older: 200 mg P.O. b.i.d. for 10 days

➢ Mild to moderate uncomplicated skin and soft-tissue infections caused by *S. pyogenes* and *Staphylococcus aureus*
Adults and children ages 12 and older: 200 mg P.O. b.i.d. for 10 days
➢ Mild to moderate chronic bronchitis caused by *Haemophilus influenzae, Haemophilus parainfluenzae, Streptococcus pneumoniae,* and *Moraxella catarrhalis*
Adults and children ages 12 and older: 400 mg P.O. b.i.d. for 10 days

Dosage adjustment

• Renal impairment

Contraindications

• Hypersensitivity to cephalosporins, drug components, penicillins, or milk protein
• Carnitine deficiency

Precautions

Use cautiously in:
• renal impairment, phenylketonuria
• history of GI disease (especially colitis)
• emaciated patients
• elderly patients
• pregnant or breastfeeding patients
• children.

Administration

• Obtain specimens for culture and sensitivity testing as needed before starting therapy.
• Administer with meals to increase drug's bioavailability.
• Give 2 hours before antacids or other drugs that reduce stomach acid.

Route	Onset	Peak	Duration
P.O.	Unknown	1.5-3 hr	8-10 hr

Adverse reactions

CNS: headache, lethargy, paresthesia, syncope, **seizures**
CV: hypotension, palpitations, chest pain, vasodilation
EENT: hearing loss
GI: nausea, vomiting, diarrhea, abdominal cramps, oral candidiasis, **pseudomembranous colitis**
GU: vaginal candidiasis, **nephrotoxicity**
Hematologic: lymphocytosis, eosinophilia, **bleeding tendency, hemolytic anemia, hypoprothrombinemia, neutropenia, thrombocytopenia, agranulocytosis, bone marrow depression**
Hepatic: hepatic failure, hepatomegaly
Metabolic: carnitine deficiency
Musculoskeletal: arthralgia
Respiratory: dyspnea
Skin: urticaria, maculopapular or erythematous rash
Other: chills, fever, drug fever, superinfection, **anaphylaxis, serum sickness**

Interactions

Drug-drug. *Aminoglycosides, loop diuretics:* increased risk of nephrotoxicity
Antacids, histamine$_2$-receptor antagonists: decreased cefditoren absorption
Probenecid: decreased excretion and increased blood level of cefditoren
Drug-diagnostic tests. *Alanine aminotransferase, alkaline phosphatase, aspartate aminotransferase, bilirubin, blood urea nitrogen, creatinine, eosinophils, gamma-glutamyltransferase, lactate dehydrogenase:* increased levels
Coombs' test, urinary 17-ketosteroids, nonenzyme-based urine glucose tests (such as Clinitest): false-positive results
Hemoglobin, platelets, white blood cells: decreased values
Drug-food. *Moderate- or high-fat meal:* increased drug bioavailability

Patient monitoring

• Monitor CBC and kidney and liver function test results.

• Monitor for signs and symptoms of superinfection and other serious adverse reactions.
• Be aware that cross-sensitivity to penicillins may occur.

Patient teaching
• Advise patient to take drug with food to promote drug absorption.
• Instruct patient to continue to take full amount prescribed even when he feels better.
• Tell patient to avoid taking antacids within 2 hours of drug.
• Instruct patient to report signs and symptoms of allergic response and other adverse reactions, such as rash, easy bruising, bleeding, severe GI problems, or difficulty breathing.
• Caution patient not to take drug with other medications unless prescriber approves.
• As appropriate, review all other significant and life-threatening adverse reactions and interactions, especially those related to the drugs, tests, and foods mentioned above.

cefepime hydrochloride
Maxipime

Pharmacologic class: Fourth-generation cephalosporin
Therapeutic class: Anti-infective
Pregnancy risk category B

Action
Interferes with bacterial cell-wall synthesis and division by binding to cell wall, causing cell to die. Active against gram-negative and gram-positive bacteria, with expanded activity against gram-negative bacteria. Exhibits minimal immunosuppressant activity.

Availability
Powder for injection: 500-mg vial, 1-g vial, 2-g vial; 1-g and 2-g piggyback bottles; 1 g/15 ml vial

Indications and dosages
➢ Urinary tract infections (UTIs) caused by *Escherichia coli, Klebsiella pneumoniae,* and *Proteus mirabilis*
Adults: 500 mg to 1g by I.V. infusion or I.M. q 12 hours for 7 to 10 days
➢ Severe UTIs caused by *E. coli* or *K. pneumoniae;* moderate to severe skin infections caused by *Staphylococcus aureus* or *Streptococcus pyogenes*
Adults: 2 g by I.V. infusion q 12 hours for 10 days
➢ Febrile neutropenia
Adults and children ages 2 months to 16 years: 2 g by I.V. infusion q 8 hours for 7 days
➢ Complicated intra-abdominal infections caused by alpha-hemolytic streptococci, *E. coli, K. pneumoniae, Pseudomonas aeruginosa, Enterobacter* species, *or Bacteroides fragilis*
Adults: 2 g by I.V. infusion q 12 hours for 7 to 10 days (given with metronidazole)
➢ Moderate to severe pneumonia caused by *K. pneumoniae, P. aeruginosa, Enterobacter* species, or *Streptococcus pneumoniae*
Adults: 1 to 2 g by I.V. infusion q 12 hours for 10 days

Dosage adjustment
• Renal impairment

Contraindications
• Hypersensitivity to cephalosporins or penicillins

Precautions
Use cautiously in:
• renal impairment, phenylketonuria
• history of GI disease
• elderly patients
• pregnant or breastfeeding patients
• children.

Administration

- Obtain specimens for culture and sensitivity testing as needed before starting therapy.
- Don't mix with ampicillin (at concentrations above 40 mg/ml), metronidazole, aminoglycosides, or aminophylline if ordered concurrently. Give each drug separately.
- For I.V. infusion, use small I.V. needle and infuse into large vein over 30 to 60 minutes.
- For I.M. administration, inject deep into large muscle.

Route	Onset	Peak	Duration
I.V.	Rapid	End of infusion	12 hr
I.M.	Rapid	1-2 hr	12 hr

Adverse reactions

CNS: headache, lethargy, paresthesia, syncope, **seizures**
CV: phlebitis, hypotension, palpitations, chest pain, vasodilation, **thrombophlebitis**
EENT: hearing loss
GI: nausea, vomiting, diarrhea, abdominal cramps, oral candidiasis, **pseudomembranous colitis**
GU: vaginal candidiasis, **nephrotoxicity**
Hematologic: lymphocytosis, eosinophilia, **bleeding tendency, hemolytic anemia, hypoprothrombinemia, neutropenia, thrombocytopenia, agranulocytosis, bone marrow depression**
Hepatic: hepatic failure, hepatomegaly
Musculoskeletal: arthralgia
Respiratory: dyspnea
Skin: urticaria, maculopapular or erythematous rash, redness, swelling, induration
Other: chills, fever, superinfection, pain at I.M. site, phlebitis at I.V. site, **anaphylaxis, serum sickness**

Interactions

Drug-drug. *Aminoglycosides, loop diuretics:* increased risk of nephrotoxicity
Probenecid: decreased excretion and increased blood level of cefepime
Drug-diagnostic tests. *Alanine aminotransferase, alkaline phosphatase, aspartate aminotransferase, bilirubin, blood urea nitrogen, creatinine, eosinophils, gamma-glutamyltransferase, lactate dehydrogenase:* increased levels
Coombs' test, urinary 17-ketosteroids, nonenzyme-based urine glucose tests (such as Clinitest): false-positive results
Hemoglobin, platelets, white blood cells: decreased values
Drug-herbs. *Angelica, anise, arnica, asafetida, bogbean, boldo, celery, chamomile, clove, danshen, fenugreek, feverfew, garlic, ginger, ginkgo, ginseng, horse chestnut, horseradish, licorice, meadowsweet, onion, papain, passionflower, poplar, prickly ash, quassia, red clover, turmeric, wild carrot, wild lettuce, willow:* increased risk of bleeding

Patient monitoring

- Assess baseline CBC and kidney and liver function test results.
- Monitor for signs and symptoms of superinfection and other serious adverse reactions.
- Monitor for inflammation at infusion site.
- Be aware that cross-sensitivity to penicillins may occur.

Patient teaching

- Instruct patient to report reduced urinary output, persistent diarrhea, bruising, or bleeding.
- Caution patient not to take herbs without consulting prescriber.
- As appropriate, review all other significant and life-threatening adverse reactions and interactions, especially those related to the drugs, tests, and herbs mentioned above.

cefixime

Suprax

Pharmacologic class: Third-generation cephalosporin
Therapeutic class: Anti-infective
Pregnancy risk category B

Action

Interferes with bacterial cell-wall synthesis and division by binding to cell wall, causing cell to die. Active against gram-negative and gram-positive bacteria, with expanded activity against gram-negative bacteria. Exhibits minimal immunosuppressant activity.

Availability

Oral suspension: 100 mg/5 ml
Tablets: 200 mg, 400 mg

Indications and dosages

➢ Uncomplicated gonorrhea caused by *Neisseria gonorrhoeae*
Adults and children weighing more than 50 kg (110 lb): 400 mg P.O. daily
➢ Uncomplicated urinary tract infections caused by *Escherichia coli* and *Proteus mirabilis;* otitis media caused by *Haemophilus influenzae, Moraxella catarrhalis,* and *Streptococcus pyogenes;* pharyngitis and tonsillitis caused by *S. pyogenes;* acute bronchitis and acute exacerbation of chronic bronchitis caused by *H. influenzae* and *Streptococcus pneumoniae*
Adults and children older than age 12 or weighing more than 50 kg (110 lb): 400 mg P.O. daily or 200 mg P.O. q 12 hours
Children ages 12 and younger or weighing 50 kg (110 lb) or less: 8 mg/kg P.O. daily or 4 mg/kg P.O. q 12 hours

Dosage adjustment

- Renal impairment

Contraindications

- Hypersensitivity to cephalosporins or penicillins

Precautions

Use cautiously in:

- renal impairment, phenylketonuria
- history of GI disease
- elderly patients
- pregnant or breastfeeding patients
- children.

Administration

- Obtain specimens for culture and sensitivity testing as necessary before starting therapy.
- Know that drug may be taken with food.
- Be aware that suspension should be given for otitis media because it provides higher serum concentration.

Route	Onset	Peak	Duration
P.O.	Rapid	2-6 hr	24 hr

Adverse reactions

CNS: headache, lethargy, paresthesia, syncope, **seizures**
CV: hypotension, palpitations, chest pain, vasodilation
EENT: hearing loss
GI: nausea, vomiting, diarrhea, abdominal cramps, oral candidiasis, **pseudomembranous colitis**
GU: vaginal candidiasis, **nephrotoxicity**
Hematologic: lymphocytosis, eosinophilia, **bleeding tendency, hemolytic anemia, hypoprothrombinemia, neutropenia, thrombocytopenia, agranulocytosis, bone marrow depression**
Hepatic: hepatic failure, hepatomegaly
Musculoskeletal: arthralgia
Respiratory: dyspnea
Skin: urticaria, maculopapular or erythematous rash

Other: chills, fever, superinfection, **anaphylaxis, serum sickness**

Interactions

Drug-drug. *Aminoglycosides, loop diuretics:* increased risk of nephrotoxicity
Probenecid: decreased excretion and increased blood level of cefixime
Drug-diagnostic tests. *Alanine aminotransferase, alkaline phosphatase, aspartate aminotransferase, bilirubin, blood urea nitrogen, creatinine, eosinophils, gamma-glutamyltransferase, lactate dehydrogenase:* increased levels
Coombs' test, urinary 17-ketosteroids, nonenzyme-based urine glucose tests (such as Clinitest): false-positive results
Hemoglobin, platelets, white blood cells: decreased values
Drug-herbs. *Angelica, anise, arnica, asafetida, bogbean, boldo, celery, chamomile, clove, danshen, fenugreek, feverfew, garlic, ginger, ginkgo, ginseng, horse chestnut, horseradish, licorice, meadowsweet, onion, papain, passionflower, poplar, prickly ash, quassia, red clover, turmeric, wild carrot, wild lettuce, willow:* increased risk of bleeding

Patient monitoring

- Monitor baseline CBC and kidney and liver function test results.
- Monitor for signs and symptoms of superinfection and other serious adverse reactions.
- Be aware that cross-sensitivity to penicillins may occur.

Patient teaching

- Tell patient to take once-daily doses at same time each day.
- Advise patient to take drug exactly as prescribed and to continue to take full amount prescribed even when he feels better.
- Instruct patient to report signs and symptoms of allergic response and other adverse reactions, such as rash, easy bruising, bleeding, severe GI problems, or difficulty breathing.
- Caution patient not to take herbs without consulting prescriber.
- As appropriate, review all other significant and life-threatening adverse reactions and interactions, especially those related to the drugs, tests, and herbs mentioned above.

cefmetazole sodium

Zefazone

Pharmacologic class: Second-generation cephalosporin
Therapeutic class: Anti-infective
Pregnancy risk category B

Action

Interferes with bacterial cell-wall synthesis, causing cell to rupture and die

Availability

Powder for injection: 1 g/50 ml, 2 g/ 50 ml

Indications and dosages

➤ Respiratory tract infections; skin infections; urinary tract infections; gynecologic infections; gonorrhea; preoperative prophylaxis
Adults: 2 g I.V. q 6 to 12 hours. For gonorrhea, give 1 g I.M. with or 30 minutes after 1 g probenecid P.O.

Dosage adjustment

- Renal impairment

Contraindications

- Hypersensitivity to cephalosporins or penicillins

Precautions

Use cautiously in:

- renal impairment, phenylketonuria

- history of GI disease
- elderly patients
- pregnant or breastfeeding patients
- children.

Administration

- Obtain specimens for culture and sensitivity testing as necessary before starting therapy.
- Don't give with products containing alcohol.
- Reconstitute powder for injection with sterile water for injection, bacteriostatic water, or normal saline solution for injection. As directed, drug may be diluted further and given as I.V. infusion over 10 to 60 minutes.
- Administer in volume-control set or separate secondary I.V. container.
- For I.M. administration, inject deep into large muscle.
- Be aware that cross-sensitivity to penicillins may occur.

Route	Onset	Peak	Duration
I.V.	Unknown	Immediate	Unknown
I.M.	Unknown	90 min	Unknown

Adverse reactions

CNS: headache, confusion, hemiparesis, lethargy, paresthesia, syncope, **seizures**
CV: hypotension, palpitations, chest pain, vasodilation
EENT: hearing loss
GI: nausea, vomiting, diarrhea, abdominal cramps, oral candidiasis, **pseudomembranous colitis**
GU: vaginal candidiasis, **nephrotoxicity**
Hematologic: lymphocytosis, eosinophilia, **bleeding tendency, hemolytic anemia, hypoprothrombinemia, neutropenia, thrombocytopenia, agranulocytosis, bone marrow depression**
Hepatic: hepatic failure, hepatomegaly
Musculoskeletal: arthralgia
Respiratory: dyspnea
Skin: urticaria, maculopapular or erythematous rash
Other: chills, fever, superinfection, **anaphylaxis, serum sickness**

Interactions

Drug-drug. *Anticoagulants:* increased risk of bleeding
Probenecid: increased cefmetazole blood level
Drug-diagnostic tests. *Blood urea nitrogen:* increased
Coombs' test, urine glucose tests using Benedict's reagent: false-positive results
Glucose, hematocrit: decreased levels
Drug-behaviors. *Alcohol use:* disulfiram-like reaction when alcohol is used within 48 to 72 hours of drug administration

Patient monitoring

- 🔊 Monitor for extreme confusion, tonic-clonic seizures, and mild hemiparesis when giving high doses.
- Evaluate baseline CBC and kidney and liver function test results.
- Monitor for signs and symptoms of superinfection and other serious adverse reactions.
- Be aware that cross-sensitivity to penicillins may occur.

Patient teaching

- Instruct patient to report reduced urinary output, persistent diarrhea, bruising, and bleeding.
- As appropriate, review all other significant and life-threatening adverse reactions and interactions, especially those related to the drugs, tests, and behaviors mentioned above.

cefoperazone sodium

Cefobid

Pharmacologic class: Third-generation cephalosporin
Therapeutic class: Anti-infective
Pregnancy risk category B

Action

Interferes with bacterial cell-wall synthesis and division by binding to cell wall, causing cell to die. Active against gram-negative and gram-positive bacteria, with expanded activity against gram-negative bacteria. Exhibits minimal immunosuppressant activity.

Availability

Powder for injection: 1 g, 2 g, 10 g
Premixed containers: 1 g/50 ml, 2 g/50 ml

Indications and dosages

➤ Respiratory tract infections caused by *Escherichia coli, Haemophilus influenzae, Enterobacter* species, *Klebsiella* species, *Proteus mirabilis,* staphylococci, streptococci, and *Pseudomonas aeruginosa;* urinary tract infections caused by *E. coli* and *P. aeruginosa*; uncomplicated gonorrhea caused by *Neisseria gonorrhoeae;* gynecologic infections caused by gram-positive cocci; bacterial septicemia caused by *E. coli, Klebsiella* species, *Serratia marcescens, Staphylococcus aureus,* and streptococci; skin and soft-tissue infections caused by *P. aeruginosa, S. aureus,* and *Streptococcus pyogenes*; intra-abdominal infections caused by gram-negative bacilli

Adults: 1 to 2 g I.V. or I.M. q 12 hours; maximum dosage is 12 g/day. For severe infections, 6 to 12 g/day I.V. in divided doses two, three, or four times daily.

Dosage adjustment

- Renal impairment
- Hepatic impairment

Contraindications

- Hypersensitivity to cephalosporins or penicillins

Precautions

Use cautiously in:

- renal impairment, phenylketonuria
- history of GI disease
- elderly patients
- pregnant or breastfeeding patients
- children.

Administration

- Obtain specimens for culture and sensitivity testing as necessary before starting therapy.
- Reconstitute powder for injection with at least 2.8 ml diluent per gram of cefoperazone, using a compatible solution, such as dextrose 5% in water (D_5W), D_5W and lactated Ringer's injection, normal saline solution, or D_5W and normal saline solution.
- For intermittent I.V. infusion, further dilute reconstituted drug with 20 to 40 ml of diluent per gram of cefoperazone; give over 15 to 30 minutes. Use large veins, and rotate infusion sites.
- For continuous I.V. infusion, dilute to final concentration of 2 to 25 mg/ml and give over 6 to 24 hours.
- For I.M. injection, dilute with bacteriostatic water or sterile water. For concentrations of 250 mg/ml or more, prepare solution using 0.5% lidocaine hydrochloride.
- Administer I.M. injection into large muscle mass.
- Don't mix with aminoglycosides. If both drugs are prescribed, give cefoperazone before aminoglycoside.

Route	Onset	Peak	Duration
I.V.	Rapid	End of infusion	12 hr
I.M.	Rapid	1-2 hr	12 hr

Adverse reactions

CNS: headache, lethargy, paresthesia, syncope, **seizures**
CV: hypotension, palpitations, chest pain, vasodilation
EENT: hearing loss
GI: nausea, vomiting, diarrhea, abdominal cramps, oral candidiasis, **pseudomembranous colitis**
GU: vaginal candidiasis, **nephrotoxicity**
Hematologic: lymphocytosis, eosinophilia, **bleeding tendency, hemolytic anemia, hypoprothrombinemia, neutropenia, thrombocytopenia, agranulocytosis, bone marrow depression**
Hepatic: hepatic failure, hepatomegaly
Musculoskeletal: arthralgia
Respiratory: dyspnea
Skin: urticaria, maculopapular or erythematous rash
Other: chills, fever, superinfection, I.M. injection site pain, vitamin K deficiency, **anaphylaxis, serum sickness**

Interactions

Drug-drug. *Aminoglycosides, loop diuretics:* increased risk of nephrotoxicity
Anticoagulants: increased anticoagulant effect
Probenecid: decreased excretion and increased blood level of cefoperazone
Drug-diagnostic tests. *Alanine aminotransferase, alkaline phosphatase, aspartate aminotransferase, bilirubin, blood urea nitrogen, creatinine, eosinophils, gamma-glutamyltransferase, lactate dehydrogenase:* increased levels
Coombs' test, urinary 17-ketosteroids, nonenzyme-based urine glucose tests (such as Clinitest): false-positive results
Hemoglobin, platelets, white blood cells: decreased values
Drug-herbs. *Angelica, anise, arnica, asafetida, bogbean, boldo, celery, chamomile, clove, danshen, fenugreek, feverfew, garlic, ginger, ginkgo, ginseng, horse chestnut, horseradish, licorice, meadowsweet, onion, papain, passionflower, poplar, prickly ash, Quassia, red clover, turmeric, wild carrot, wild lettuce, willow:* increased risk of bleeding
Drug-behaviors. *Alcohol use:* disulfiram-like reactions when alcohol is consumed within 72 hours of drug administration

Patient monitoring

- Monitor kidney and liver function test results.
- Monitor CBC with white cell differential, prothrombin time, and bleeding times. Watch for signs and symptoms of blood dyscrasias, especially hypoprothrombinemia.
- Monitor for signs and symptoms of superinfection and other serious adverse reactions.
- Be aware that cross-sensitivity to penicillin may occur.

Patient teaching

- Advise patient to report reduced urinary output, persistent diarrhea, bruising, or bleeding.

◀⁝ Caution patient not to consume alcohol while taking drug and for 72 hours after discontinuation, because alcohol withdrawal-like symptoms may occur.

- Tell patient not to use herbs without consulting prescriber.
- As appropriate, review all other significant and life-threatening adverse reactions and interactions, especially those related to the drugs, tests, herbs, and behaviors mentioned above.

cefotaxime sodium

Claforan

Pharmacologic class: Third-generation cephalosporin
Therapeutic class: Anti-infective
Pregnancy risk category B

Action

Interferes with bacterial cell-wall synthesis and division by binding to cell wall, causing cell to die. Active against gram-negative and gram-positive bacteria, with expanded activity against gram-negative bacteria. Exhibits minimal immunosuppressant activity.

Availability

Powder for injection: 1 g, 2 g, 10 g
Premixed containers: 1 g/50 ml, 2 g/50 ml

Indications and dosages

➢ Perioperative prophylaxis
Adults and children weighing more than 50 kg (110 lb): 1 g I.V. or I.M. 30 to 90 minutes before surgery
➢ Prophylaxis in patients undergoing cesarean delivery
Adults: 1 g I.V. or I.M. as soon as umbilical cord is clamped
➢ Gonococcal urethritis and cervicitis
Adults weighing more than 50 kg (110 lb): 500 mg I.M. as a single dose
➢ Rectal gonorrhea (females)
Adults weighing more than 50 kg (110 lb): 500 mg I.M. as a single dose
➢ Rectal gonorrhea (males)
Adults weighing more than 50 kg (110 lb): 1 g I.M. as a single dose
➢ Disseminated gonorrhea
Adults and children weighing 50 kg (110 lb) or more: 1 g by I.V. infusion q 8 hours
➢ Uncomplicated infections caused by susceptible organisms
Adults and children weighing 50 kg (110 lb) or more: 1 g I.V. or I.M. q 12 hours
Children ages 1 month to 12 years weighing less than 50 kg (110 lb): 50 to 180 mg/kg/day I.V. or I.M. in four to six divided doses
➢ Moderate to severe infections caused by susceptible organisms
Adults and children weighing 50 kg (110 lb) or more: 1 to 2 g I.V. or I.M. q 8 hours
➢ Life-threatening infections caused by susceptible organisms
Adults and children weighing 50 kg (110 lb) or more: 2 g by I.V. infusion q 4 hours. Maximum dosage is 12 g/day.
➢ Septicemia and other infections that commonly require antibiotics in higher doses
Adults and children weighing 50 kg (110 lb) or more: 2 g by I.V. infusion q 6 to 8 hours

Dosage adjustment

- Renal impairment

Contraindications

- Hypersensitivity to cephalosporins or penicillins

Precautions

Use cautiously in:
- renal impairment, phenylketonuria
- history of GI disease
- elderly patients
- pregnant or breastfeeding patients
- children.

Administration

- Obtain specimens for culture and sensitivity testing as necessary before starting therapy.
- Reconstitute powder for I.V. injection with at least 10 ml of sterile water, and give over 3 to 5 minutes. For intermittent infusion, drug may be diluted

further with 50 or 100 ml of normal saline solution or dextrose 5% in water (D_5W) and given over 30 minutes.

• Reconstituted drug may be diluted further for a continuous I.V. infusion of up to 1,000 ml with a compatible solution, such as normal saline solution, dextrose 5% or 10% in water, or D_5W and normal saline solution. Give over 6 to 24 hours, depending on concentration.

• Don't use diluents with pH above 7.5 (such as sodium bicarbonate).

• Rotate infusion sites.

• Inject I.M. deep into large muscle mass. Divide 2-g dose in half and inject into separate large muscle masses.

Route	Onset	Peak	Duration
I.V.	Rapid	End of infusion	4-12 hr
I.M.	Rapid	0.5 hr	4-12 hr

Adverse reactions

CNS: headache, lethargy, paresthesia, syncope, **seizures**
CV: hypotension, palpitations, chest pain, vasodilation
EENT: hearing loss
GI: nausea, vomiting, diarrhea, abdominal cramps, oral candidiasis, **pseudomembranous colitis**
GU: vaginal candidiasis, **nephrotoxicity**
Hematologic: lymphocytosis, eosinophilia, **bleeding tendency, hemolytic anemia, hypoprothrombinemia, neutropenia, thrombocytopenia, agranulocytosis, bone marrow depression**
Hepatic: hepatic failure, hepatomegaly
Musculoskeletal: arthralgia
Respiratory: dyspnea
Skin: urticaria, maculopapular or erythematous rash
Other: chills, fever, superinfection, pain at I.M. injection site, **anaphylaxis, serum sickness**

Interactions

Drug-drug. *Aminoglycosides, loop diuretics:* increased risk of nephrotoxicity
Probenecid: decreased excretion and increased blood level of cefotaxime
Drug-diagnostic tests. *Alanine aminotransferase, alkaline phosphatase, aspartate aminotransferase, bilirubin, blood urea nitrogen, creatinine, eosinophils, gamma-glutamyltransferase, lactate dehydrogenase:* increased levels
Coombs' test, urinary 17-ketosteroids, nonenzyme-based urine glucose tests (such as Clinitest): false-positive results
Hemoglobin, platelets, white blood cells: decreased values
Drug-herbs. *Angelica, anise, arnica, asafetida, bogbean, boldo, celery, chamomile, clove, danshen, fenugreek, feverfew, garlic, ginger, ginkgo, ginseng, horse chestnut, horseradish, licorice, meadowsweet, onion, papain, passionflower, poplar, prickly ash, quassia, red clover, turmeric, wild carrot, wild lettuce, willow:* increased risk of bleeding

Patient monitoring

• Monitor CBC and kidney and liver function test results.

• Monitor for signs and symptoms of superinfection and other serious adverse reactions.

• Be aware that cross-sensitivity to penicillins may occur.

Patient teaching

• Advise patient to report reduced urinary output, persistent diarrhea, bruising, and bleeding.

• As appropriate, review all other significant and life-threatening adverse reactions and interactions, especially those related to the drugs, tests, and herbs mentioned above.

C

cefotetan disodium

Cefotan

Pharmacologic class: Second-generation cephalosporin
Therapeutic class: Anti-infective
Pregnancy risk category B

Action

Interferes with bacterial cell-wall synthesis and division by binding to cell wall, causing cell to die. Active against gram-negative and gram-positive bacteria, with expanded activity against gram-negative bacteria. Exhibits minimal immunosuppressant activity.

Availability

Powder for injection: 1 g, 2 g

Indications and dosages

➤ Post-cesarean prophylaxis
Adults: 1 to 2 g I.V. as soon as umbilical cord is clamped
➤ Urinary tract infections caused by *Escherichia coli, Proteus* species, and *Klebsiella* species
Adults: 0.5 to 2 g I.V. or I.M. q 12 hours, or 1 to 2 g I.V. or I.M. q 24 hours
➤ Skin and soft-tissue infections caused by *E. coli, Klebsiella pneumoniae, Peptostreptococcus* species, *Staphylococcus aureus,* and *Staphylococcus epidermidis*
Adults: For mild to moderate infections, 1 to 2 g I.V. or I.M. q 12 hours. For severe infections, 2 g I.V. q 12 hours.
➤ Lower respiratory tract infections caused by *E. coli, Haemophilus influenzae, Klebsiella* species, *Proteus mirabilis,* and *Serratia marcescens*
Adults: For mild to moderate infections, 1 to 2 g I.V. or I.M. q 12 hours. For severe infections, 2 g I.V. q 12 hours. For life-threatening infections, 3 g I.V. q 12 hours.

Dosage adjustment

• Renal impairment

Contraindications

• Hypersensitivity to cephalosporins or penicillins

Precautions

Use cautiously in:
• renal impairment, phenylketonuria
• history of GI disease
• elderly patients
• pregnant or breastfeeding patients
• children.

Administration

• Obtain specimens for culture and sensitivity testing as necessary before starting therapy.
• For I.V. administration, reconstitute with sterile water.
• For intermittent I.V. infusion, give 1 or 2 g in 10 ml of sterile water over 3 to 5 minutes. If patient has I.V. line in place, give over 30-minute period through I.V. tubing.
• For I.M. injection, reconstitute with sterile water, bacteriostatic water, 0.5% or 1% lidocaine hydrochloride, or normal saline solution.
• Inject I.M. deep into large muscle mass; divide 2-g dose in half and inject into separate large muscle masses.

Route	Onset	Peak	Duration
I.V.	Rapid	End of infusion	12 hr
I.M.	Rapid	1-3 hr	12 hr

Adverse reactions

CNS: headache, confusion, hemiparesis, lethargy, paresthesia, syncope, **seizures**
CV: hypotension, palpitations, chest pain, vasodilation

EENT: hearing loss
GI: nausea, vomiting, diarrhea, abdominal cramps, oral candidiasis, **pseudomembranous colitis**
GU: vaginal candidiasis, **nephrotoxicity**
Hematologic: lymphocytosis, eosinophilia, **bleeding tendency, hemolytic anemia, hypoprothrombinemia, neutropenia, thrombocytopenia, agranulocytosis, bone marrow depression**
Hepatic: hepatic failure, hepatomegaly
Musculoskeletal: arthralgia
Respiratory: dyspnea
Skin: urticaria, maculopapular or erythematous rash
Other: chills, fever, allergic reactions (including superinfection), pain at I.M. injection site, phlebitis at I.V. site, **anaphylaxis, serum sickness**

Interactions

Drug-drug. *Aminoglycosides, loop diuretics:* increased risk of nephrotoxicity
Antacids: decreased absorption
Anticoagulants: increased anticoagulant effect
Probenecid: decreased excretion and increased blood level of cefotetan
Drug-diagnostic tests. *Alanine aminotransferase, alkaline phosphatase, aspartate aminotransferase, bilirubin, blood urea nitrogen, creatinine, eosinophils, gamma-glutamyltransferase, lactate dehydrogenase:* increased levels
Coombs' test, urinary 17-ketosteroids, nonenzyme-based urine glucose tests (such as Clinitest): false-positive results
Hemoglobin, platelets, white blood cells: decreased values
Drug-food. *Moderate- or high-fat meal:* increased drug bioavailability
Drug-behaviors. *Alcohol use:* disulfiram-like reaction when alcohol is consumed within 48 to 72 hours of drug administration

Patient monitoring

Monitor for extreme confusion, tonic-clonic seizures, and mild hemiparesis when giving high doses.
- Monitor CBC with white cell differential, prothrombin time, and bleeding times. Watch for signs and symptoms of blood dyscrasias, especially hypoprothrombinemia.
- Assess kidney and liver function test results.
- Monitor for signs and symptoms of superinfection and other serious adverse reactions.
- Be aware that cross-sensitivity to penicillins may occur.

Patient teaching

- Instruct patient to report reduced urinary output, persistent diarrhea, bruising, or bleeding.
- Caution patient to avoid alcohol in any form.
- As appropriate, review all other significant and life-threatening adverse reactions and interactions, especially those related to the drugs, tests, foods, and behaviors mentioned above.

cefoxitin sodium

Mefoxin

Pharmacologic class: Second-generation cephalosporin
Therapeutic class: Anti-infective
Pregnancy risk category B

Action

Interferes with bacterial cell-wall synthesis and division by binding to cell wall, causing cell to die. Active against gram-negative and gram-positive bacteria, with expanded activity against gram-negative bacteria. Exhibits minimal immunosuppressant activity.

Availability

Powder for injection: 1 g, 2 g
Premixed containers: 1 g/50 ml in dextrose 5% in water (D_5W), 2 g/50 ml in D_5W

Indications and dosages

➢ Respiratory tract infections, skin infections, bone and joint infections, urinary tract infections, gynecologic infections, septicemia
Adults: For most infections, 1 g I.M. or I.V. q 6 to 8 hours. For severe infections, 1 g I.M. or I.V. q 4 hours or 2 g I.M. or I.V. q 6 to 8 hours. For life-threatening infections, 2 g I.V. q 4 hours or 3 g I.V. q 6 hours.
Children ages 3 months and older: For most infections, 13.3 to 26.7 mg/kg I.M. or I.V. q 4 hours or 20 to 40 mg/kg q 6 hours.
➢ Preoperative prophylaxis
Adults: 1 to 2 g I.V. within 60 minutes of incision, then q 6 hours for up to 24 hours

Dosage adjustment

- Renal failure

Contraindications

- Hypersensitivity to cephalosporins or penicillins

Precautions

Use cautiously in:
- renal impairment, hepatic disease, or biliary obstruction
- history of GI disease
- elderly patients
- children.

Administration

- Obtain specimens for culture and sensitivity testing as necessary before starting therapy.
- Reconstitute 1-g dose with 10 ml of sterile water; reconstitute 2-g dose with 10 to 20 ml.
- For direct I.V. injection, give 10 ml of sterile water with each gram of cefoxitin over 3 to 5 minutes. Inject into large vein and rotate sites, or give through existing I.V. tubing.
- For intermittent or continuous I.V. infusion, add reconstituted drug to compatible solution, such as D_5W, normal saline solution, or D_5W and normal saline solution.
- For I.M. injection, reconstitute each gram with 2 ml of sterile water or 2 ml of 0.5% lidocaine hydrochloride (without epinephrine).
- Inject I.M. deep into large muscle mass; divide 2-g dose in half and inject into separate large muscle masses.
- Know that dry powder and solution may darken, but this does not alter drug efficacy.

Route	Onset	Peak	Duration
I.V.	Rapid	End of infusion	4-8 hr
I.M.	Rapid	30 min	4-8 hr

Adverse reactions

CNS: headache, lethargy, paresthesia, syncope, **seizures**
CV: hypotension, palpitations, chest pain, vasodilation, **thrombophlebitis**
EENT: hearing loss
GI: nausea, vomiting, diarrhea, abdominal cramps, oral candidiasis, **pseudomembranous colitis**
GU: vaginal candidiasis, **nephrotoxicity**
Hematologic: lymphocytosis, eosinophilia, **bleeding tendency, hemolytic anemia, hypoprothrombinemia, neutropenia, thrombocytopenia, agranulocytosis, bone marrow depression**
Hepatic: hepatic failure, hepatomegaly
Musculoskeletal: arthralgia
Respiratory: dyspnea
Skin: urticaria, maculopapular or erythematous rash
Other: chills, fever, superinfection, pain at I.M. site, **anaphylaxis, serum sickness**

Interactions

Drug-drug. *Aminoglycosides, loop diuretics:* increased risk of nephrotoxicity
Probenecid: decreased excretion and increased blood level of cefoxitin
Drug-diagnostic tests. *Alanine aminotransferase, alkaline phosphatase, aspartate aminotransferase, bilirubin, blood urea nitrogen, creatinine, eosinophils, gamma-glutamyltransferase, lactate dehydrogenase:* increased levels
Coombs' test, urinary 17-ketosteroids, nonenzyme-based urine glucose tests (such as Clinitest): false-positive results
Hemoglobin, platelets, white blood cells: decreased values

Patient monitoring

- Assess CBC and kidney and liver function test results.
- Monitor fluid intake and output. Report significant decrease in output.
- Monitor for signs and symptoms of superinfection and other serious adverse reactions.
- Be aware that cross-sensitivity to penicillins may occur.

Patient teaching

- Instruct patient to report reduced urinary output, persistent diarrhea, bruising, and bleeding.
- As appropriate, review all other significant and life-threatening adverse reactions and interactions, especially those related to the drugs and tests mentioned above.

cefpodoxime proxetil

Vantin

Pharmacologic class: Third-generation cephalosporin
Therapeutic class: Anti-infective
Pregnancy risk category B

Action

Interferes with bacterial cell-wall synthesis and division by binding to cell wall, causing cell to die. Active against gram-negative and gram-positive bacteria, with expanded activity against gram-negative bacteria. Exhibits minimal immunosuppressant activity.

Availability

Oral suspension: 50 mg/5 ml, 100 mg/5 ml
Tablets: 100 mg, 200 mg

Indications and dosages

➤ Acute community-acquired pneumonia caused by *Haemophilus influenzae* or *Streptococcus pneumoniae*
Adults and children ages 13 and older: 200 mg P.O. q 12 hours for 14 days
➤ Acute bacterial or chronic bronchitis
Adults and children ages 13 and older: 200 mg P.O. q 12 hours for 10 days
➤ Uncomplicated gonorrhea; rectal gonococcal infection caused by *Neisseria gonorrhoeae*
Adults: 200 mg P.O. as a single dose
➤ Uncomplicated urinary tract infections caused by *Escherichia coli, Klebsiella pneumoniae, Proteus mirabilis,* and *Staphylococcus saprophyticus*
Adults: 100 mg P.O. q 12 hours for 7 days
➤ Skin and soft-tissue infections caused by *Staphylococcus aureus* and *Streptococcus pyogenes*
Adults and children ages 13 and older: 400 mg P.O. q 12 hours for 7 to 14 days
➤ Acute otitis media caused by *H. influenzae, S. pneumoniae,* and *Moraxella catarrhalis*
Children ages 5 months to 12 years: 5 mg/kg P.O. q 12 hours (maximum of 200 mg/dose) or 10 mg/kg q 24 hours (maximum of 400 mg/dose) for 10 days
➤ Tonsillitis and pharyngitis caused by *S. pyogenes*
Adults and children ages 13 and older: 100 mg P.O. q 12 hours for 5 to 10 days

Children ages 2 months to 12 years: 5 mg/kg P.O. q 12 hours for 5 to 10 days

Dosage adjustment

- Renal impairment

Contraindications

- Hypersensitivity to cephalosporins or penicillins

Precautions

Use cautiously in:

- renal impairment, phenylketonuria
- history of GI disease
- elderly patients
- pregnant or breastfeeding patients
- children.

Administration

- Obtain specimens for culture and sensitivity testing as necessary before starting therapy.
- Give tablets with food to enhance absorption. Oral suspension may be given with or without food.
- Don't give antacids within 2 hours of cefpodoxime.

Route	Onset	Peak	Duration
P.O.	Unknown	2-3 hr	12 hr

Adverse reactions

CNS: headache, lethargy, paresthesia, syncope, **seizures**
CV: hypotension, palpitations, chest pain, vasodilation
EENT: hearing loss
GI: nausea, vomiting, diarrhea, abdominal cramps, oral candidiasis, **pseudomembranous colitis**
GU: vaginal candidiasis, **nephrotoxicity**
Hematologic: lymphocytosis, eosinophilia, **bleeding tendency, hemolytic anemia, hypoprothrombinemia, neutropenia, thrombocytopenia, agranulocytosis, bone marrow depression**
Hepatic: hepatic failure, hepatomegaly
Musculoskeletal: arthralgia
Respiratory: dyspnea
Skin: urticaria, maculopapular or erythematous rash
Other: chills, fever, superinfection, **anaphylaxis, serum sickness**

Interactions

Drug-drug. *Aminoglycosides, loop diuretics:* increased risk of nephrotoxicity
Antacids: decreased cefpodoxime absorption
Probenecid: decreased excretion and increased blood level of cefpodoxime
Drug-diagnostic tests. *Alanine aminotransferase, alkaline phosphatase, aspartate aminotransferase, bilirubin, blood urea nitrogen, creatinine, eosinophils, gamma-glutamyltransferase, lactate dehydrogenase:* increased levels
Coombs' test, urinary 17-ketosteroids, nonenzyme-based urine glucose tests (such as Clinitest): false-positive results
Hemoglobin, platelets, white blood cells: decreased values
Drug-herbs. *Angelica, anise, arnica, asafetida, bogbean, boldo, celery, chamomile, clove, danshen, fenugreek, feverfew, garlic, ginger, ginkgo, ginseng, horse chestnut, horseradish, licorice, meadowsweet, onion, papain, passionflower, poplar, prickly ash, quassia, red clover, turmeric, wild carrot, wild lettuce, willow:* increased risk of bleeding

Patient monitoring

- Assess CBC and kidney and liver function test results.
- Monitor for signs and symptoms of superinfection and other serious adverse reactions.
- Be aware that cross-sensitivity to penicillins may occur.

Patient teaching

- Instruct patient to take drug with food or milk to reduce GI distress and enhance absorption.

• Advise patient not to take antacids within 2 hours of drug.
• Tell patient to continue to take full amount prescribed even when he feels better.
• Instruct patient to report signs and symptoms of allergic response and other adverse reactions, such as rash, easy bruising, bleeding, severe GI problems, or difficulty breathing.
• If patient is being treated for gonorrhea, instruct him to have partner tested and treated (as needed) and to use barrier contraception to prevent reinfection.
• As appropriate, review all other significant and life-threatening adverse reactions and interactions, especially those related to the drugs, tests, and herbs mentioned above.

cefprozil
Cefzil

Pharmacologic class: Second-generation cephalosporin
Therapeutic class: Anti-infective
Pregnancy risk category B

Action
Interferes with bacterial cell-wall synthesis and division by binding to cell wall, causing cell to die. Active against gram-negative and gram-positive bacteria, with expanded activity against gram-negative bacteria. Exhibits minimal immunosuppressant activity.

Availability
Powder for suspension: 125 mg/5 ml, 250 mg/5 ml
Tablets: 250 mg, 500 mg

Indications and dosages
➢ Uncomplicated skin infections caused by *Staphylococcus aureus* and *Streptococcus pyogenes*
Adults and children ages 13 and older: 250 to 500 mg P.O. q 12 hours or 500 mg P.O. daily for 10 days
➢ Pharyngitis or tonsillitis caused by *S. pyogenes*
Adults and children ages 13 and older: 500 mg P.O. daily for at least 10 days
➢ Acute bronchitis; acute bacterial chronic bronchitis caused by *Streptococcus pneumoniae, Haemophilus influenzae,* and *Moraxella catarrhalis*
Adults and children ages 13 and older: 500 mg P.O. q 12 hours for 10 days
➢ Acute sinusitis caused by *S. pneumoniae, H. influenzae,* and *M. catarrhalis*
Adults and children ages 13 and older: 250 mg P.O. q 12 hours for 10 days; for moderate to severe infections, 500 mg P.O. q 12 hours for 10 days
Children ages 6 months to 12 years: 7.5 mg/kg P.O. q 12 hours for 10 days; for moderate to severe infections, 15 mg/kg P.O. q 12 hours for 10 days
➢ Otitis media caused by *S. pneumoniae, H. influenzae,* and *M. catarrhalis*
Children ages 6 months to 12 years: 15 mg/kg P.O. q 12 hours for 10 days

Dosage adjustment
• Renal impairment

Contraindications
• Hypersensitivity to cephalosporins or penicillins
• Renal failure

Precautions
Use cautiously in:
• renal or hepatic impairment
• pregnant or breastfeeding patients
• children.

Administration
• Obtain specimens for culture and sensitivity testing as necessary before starting therapy.
• Give drug with food.

Route	Onset	Peak	Duration
P.O.	Unknown	6-10 hr	24-28 hr

Adverse reactions

CNS: headache, dizziness, drowsiness, hyperactivity, hypotonia, insomnia, confusion, **seizures**
GI: nausea, vomiting, diarrhea, abdominal pain, dyspepsia, **pseudomembranous colitis**
GU: hematuria, vaginal candidiasis, genital pruritus, **renal dysfunction, toxic nephropathy**
Hematologic: eosinophilia, **aplastic anemia, hemolytic anemia, hemorrhage, bone marrow depression, hypoprothrombinemia**
Hepatic: hepatic dysfunction
Skin: toxic epidermal necrolysis, diaper rash, **erythema multiforme, Stevens-Johnson syndrome**
Other: allergic reactions, carnitine deficiency, drug fever, superinfection, **serum sickness–like reaction, anaphylaxis**

Interactions

Drug-drug. *Aminoglycosides:* increased risk of nephrotoxicity
Antacids containing aluminum or magnesium, histamine$_2$-receptor antagonists: increased cefprozil absorption
Probenecid: decreased excretion and increased blood level of cefprozil
Drug-diagnostic tests. *Alanine aminotransferase, alkaline phosphatase, aspartate aminotransferase, bilirubin, blood urea nitrogen, creatinine, eosinophils, gamma-glutamyltransferase, lactate dehydrogenase, white blood cells in urine:* increased levels
Blood glucose, Coombs' test, urine glucose tests using Benedict's solution: false-positive results
Platelets, white blood cells: decreased counts
Drug-food. *Moderate- or high-fat meal:* increased drug bioavailability

Patient monitoring

- Stay alert for life-threatening reactions, including anaphylaxis, serum sickness–like reaction, Stevens-Johnson syndrome, and pseudomembranous colitis.
- Monitor neurologic status, particularly for signs and symptoms of impending seizures.
- Monitor kidney and liver function test results and assess fluid intake and output.
- Monitor CBC with white cell differential, prothrombin time, and bleeding time. Watch for signs and symptoms of blood dyscrasias, especially hypoprothrombinemia.
- Monitor temperature. Stay alert for signs and symptoms of superinfection.

Patient teaching

- Advise patient to immediately report rash, bleeding tendency, or CNS changes.
- Teach patient to recognize signs and symptoms of superinfection, and instruct him to report these right away.
- Tell patient to take drug with food.
- As appropriate, review all other significant and life-threatening adverse reactions and interactions, especially those related to the drugs, tests, and foods mentioned above.

ceftazidime

Ceptaz, Fortaz, Tazicef, Tazidime

Pharmacologic class: Third-generation cephalosporin
Therapeutic class: Anti-infective
Pregnancy risk category B

Action

Interferes with bacterial cell-wall synthesis and division by binding to cell wall, causing cell to die. Active against gram-negative and gram-positive bacteria, with expanded activity against gram-negative bacteria. Exhibits minimal immunosuppressant activity.

Availability

Powder for injection: 500 mg, 1 g, 2 g, 6 g, 10 g
Premixed containers: 1 g/50 ml, 2 g/50 ml

Indications and dosages

➢ Skin infections; bone and joint infections; urinary tract and gynecologic infections, including gonorrhea; respiratory tract infections; intra-abdominal infections; septicemia
Adults and children ages 12 and older: For most infections, 500 mg to 2 g I.V. or I.M. q 8 to 12 hours. For pneumonia and skin infections, 0.5 to 1 g I.V. or I.M. q 8 to 12 hours. For bone and joint infections, 2 g I.V. or I.M. q 12 hours. For severe and life-threatening infections, 2 g I.V. q 8 hours. For complicated urinary tract infections (UTIs), 500 mg q 8 to 12 hours. For uncomplicated UTIs, 250 mg I.M. or I.V. q 12 hours.
Children ages 1 month to 12 years: 30 to 50 mg/kg I.V. q 8 hours
Neonates younger than 4 weeks: 30 mg/kg I.V. q 12 hours

Dosage adjustment

• Renal impairment

Off-label uses

• Febrile neutropenia
• Prophylaxis of perinatal infections

Contraindications

• Hypersensitivity to cephalosporins or penicillins

Precautions

Use cautiously in:
• renal impairment, hepatic disease, biliary obstruction, phenylketonuria
• history of GI disease
• elderly patients
• pregnant or breastfeeding patients
• children.

Administration

• Obtain specimens for culture and sensitivity testing as necessary before starting therapy.
• Reconstitute powder for injection with sterile water, following manufacturer's directions for amount of diluent to use.
• For I.V. injection, dilute in sterile water as directed, and give single dose over 3 to 5 minutes. Inject into large vein; rotate injection sites.
• For intermittent I.V. infusion, dilute further with 100 ml of sterile water or another compatible fluid, such as normal saline solution or dextrose 5% in water. Infuse over 30 minutes.
• Don't dilute with sodium bicarbonate.
• For I.M. injection, reconstitute with sterile water, bacteriostatic water, or 0.5% or 1% lidocaine hydrochloride.
• When giving I.M., inject deep into large muscle mass.

Route	Onset	Peak	Duration
I.V.	Rapid	End of infusion	6-12 hr
I.M.	Rapid	1 hr	6-12 hr

Adverse reactions

CNS: headache, confusion, hemiparesis, lethargy, paresthesia, syncope, asterixis, neuromuscular excitability (with increased drug blood levels in renally impaired patients), **seizures, encephalopathy**
CV: hypotension, palpitations, chest pain, vasodilation
EENT: hearing loss
GI: nausea, vomiting, diarrhea, abdominal cramps, oral candidiasis, **pseudomembranous colitis**
GU: vaginal candidiasis, **nephrotoxicity**

Hematologic: lymphocytosis, eosinophilia, **bleeding tendency, hemolytic anemia, hypoprothrombinemia, neutropenia, thrombocytopenia, agranulocytosis, bone marrow depression**
Hepatic: hepatic failure, hepatomegaly
Musculoskeletal: arthralgia
Respiratory: dyspnea
Skin: urticaria, maculopapular or erythematous rash
Other: chills, fever, superinfection, I.M. site pain, **anaphylaxis, serum sickness**

Interactions

Drug-drug. *Aminoglycosides, loop diuretics:* increased risk of nephrotoxicity
Chloramphenicol: antagonism of ceftazidime's effects
Probenecid: decreased excretion and increased blood level of ceftazidime
Drug-diagnostic tests. *Alanine aminotransferase, alkaline phosphatase, aspartate aminotransferase, bilirubin, blood urea nitrogen, creatinine, eosinophils, gamma-glutamyltransferase, lactate dehydrogenase:* increased levels
Hemoglobin, platelets, white blood cells: decreased values
Coombs' test, urinary 17-ketosteroids, nonenzyme-based urine glucose tests (such as Clinitest): false-positive results
Drug-herbs. *Angelica, anise, arnica, asafetida, bogbean, boldo, celery, chamomile, clove, danshen, fenugreek, feverfew, garlic, ginger, ginkgo, ginseng, horse chestnut, horseradish, licorice, meadowsweet, onion, papain, passionflower, poplar, prickly ash, quassia, red clover, turmeric, wild carrot, wild lettuce, willow:* increased risk of bleeding

Patient monitoring

🔊 Monitor for extreme confusion, tonic-clonic seizures, and mild hemiparesis when giving high doses.
- Assess CBC and kidney and liver function test results.
- Monitor for signs and symptoms of superinfection and other serious adverse reactions.
- Be aware that cross-sensitivity to penicillins may occur.

Patient teaching

- Instruct patient to report reduced urine output, persistent diarrhea, bruising, and bleeding.
- As appropriate, review all other significant and life-threatening adverse reactions and interactions, especially those related to the drugs, tests, and herbs mentioned above.

ceftibuten

Cedax

Pharmacologic class: Third-generation cephalosporin
Therapeutic class: Anti-infective
Pregnancy risk category B

Action

Interferes with bacterial cell-wall synthesis and division by binding to cell wall, causing cell to die. Active against gram-negative and gram-positive bacteria, with expanded activity against gram-negative bacteria. Exhibits minimal immunosuppressant activity.

Availability

Capsules: 400 mg
Oral suspension: 90 mg/5 ml, 180 mg/5 ml

Indications and dosages

➤ Acute bacterial exacerbations of chronic bronchitis caused by *Haemophilus influenzae, Moraxella catarrhalis,* and *Streptococcus pneumoniae;* pharyngitis and tonsillitis caused by *Streptococcus pyogenes;* acute bacterial otitis media caused by *H. influenzae, M. catarrhalis,* and *S. pyogenes*

Adults and children ages 12 and older: 400 mg P.O. q 24 hours for 10 days
Children ages 12 and younger: 9 mg/kg P.O. daily for 10 days. Maximum dosage shouldn't exceed 400 mg daily.

Dosage adjustment
• Renal impairment

Off-label uses
• Urinary tract infections

Contraindications
• Hypersensitivity to cephalosporins and penicillins

Precautions
Use cautiously in:
• renal impairment, hepatic disease, biliary obstruction, phenylketonuria
• history of GI disease
• elderly patients
• pregnant or breastfeeding patients
• children.

Administration
• Obtain specimens for culture and sensitivity testing as necessary before starting therapy.
• Give oral suspension at least 1 hour before or 2 hours after a meal.

Route	Onset	Peak	Duration
P.O.	Rapid	3 hr	24 hr

Adverse reactions
CNS: headache, lethargy, paresthesia, syncope, **seizures**
CV: hypotension, palpitations, chest pain, vasodilation
EENT: hearing loss
GI: nausea, vomiting, diarrhea, abdominal cramps, oral candidiasis, **pseudomembranous colitis**
GU: vaginal candidiasis, **nephrotoxicity**
Hematologic: lymphocytosis, eosinophilia, **bleeding tendency, hemolytic anemia, hypoprothrombinemia, neutropenia, thrombocytopenia, agranulocytosis, bone marrow depression**
Hepatic: hepatic failure, hepatomegaly
Musculoskeletal: arthralgia
Respiratory: dyspnea
Skin: urticaria, easy bruising, maculopapular or erythematous rash
Other: chills, fever, superinfection, **anaphylaxis, serum sickness**

Interactions
Drug-drug. *Aminoglycosides, loop diuretics:* increased risk of nephrotoxicity
Probenecid: decreased excretion and increased blood level of ceftibuten
Drug-diagnostic tests. *Alanine aminotransferase, alkaline phosphatase, aspartate aminotransferase, bilirubin, blood urea nitrogen, creatinine, eosinophils, gamma-glutamyltransferase, lactate dehydrogenase:* increased levels
Coombs' test, urinary 17-ketosteroids, nonenzyme-based urine glucose tests (such as Clinitest): false-positive results
Hemoglobin, platelets, white blood cells: decreased values
Drug-herbs. *Angelica, anise, arnica, asafetida, bogbean, boldo, celery, chamomile, clove, danshen, fenugreek, feverfew, garlic, ginger, ginkgo, ginseng, horse chestnut, horseradish, licorice, meadowsweet, onion, papain, passionflower, poplar, prickly ash, quassia, red clover, turmeric, wild carrot, wild lettuce, willow:* increased risk of bleeding

Patient monitoring
• Assess CBC and kidney and liver function test results.
• Monitor for signs and symptoms of superinfection and other serious adverse reactions.
• Be aware that cross-sensitivity to penicillins may occur.

Patient teaching

- Instruct patient to take oral suspension at least 1 hour before or 2 hours after a meal.
- Advise patient to continue to take full amount prescribed even when he feels better.
- Tell patient to report signs and symptoms of allergic response and other adverse reactions, such as rash, easy bruising, bleeding, severe GI problems, or difficulty breathing.
- As appropriate, review all other significant and life-threatening adverse reactions and interactions, especially those related to the drugs, tests, and herbs mentioned above.

ceftizoxime sodium

Cefizox

Pharmacologic class: Third-generation cephalosporin

Therapeutic class: Anti-infective

Pregnancy risk category B

Action

Interferes with bacterial cell-wall synthesis and division by binding to cell wall, causing cell to die. Active against gram-negative and gram-positive bacteria, with expanded activity against gram-negative bacteria. Exhibits minimal immunosuppressant activity.

Availability

Powder for injection: 500 mg, 1 g, 2 g, 10 g

Premixed containers: 1 g/50 ml, 2 g/50 ml

Indications and dosages

➢ Skin infections; bone and joint infections; urinary tract and gynecologic infections; respiratory tract infections; intra-abdominal infections; septicemia

Adults: For mild or moderate infections, 1g I.V. or I.M. q 8 to 12 hours. For uncomplicated urinary tract infections, 500 mg I.V. or I.M. q 12 hours. For severe infections, 2 g I.V. q 8 to 12 hours. For life-threatening infections, 4 g I.V. q 8 hours.

Children age 6 months and older: 50 mg/kg I.M. or I.V. q 6 to 8 hours

Dosage adjustment

- Renal impairment

Contraindications

- Hypersensitivity to cephalosporins or penicillins

Precautions

Use cautiously in:

- renal impairment, hepatic disease, biliary obstruction, phenylketonuria
- history of GI disease
- elderly patients
- pregnant or breastfeeding patients
- children.

Administration

- Obtain specimens for culture and sensitivity testing as necessary before starting therapy.
- Reconstitute powder with sterile water, following manufacturer's guidelines for amount of diluent to use.
- For single I.V. injection, give in at least 10 ml of solution per gram; inject over 3 to 5 minutes. Use large vein, and rotate injection sites.
- For intermittent, piggyback, or continuous I.V. administration, dilute reconstituted drug in compatible solution, such as normal saline solution, dextrose 5% in water (D_5W), dextrose 10% in water, D_5W and normal saline solution, half-normal saline solution, or lactated Ringer's injection. Infuse over at least 30 minutes.
- Divide large I.M. doses equally and administer in two separate sites. Inject deep into large muscle mass.

Route	Onset	Peak	Duration
I.V.	Rapid	End of infusion	6-12 hr
I.M.	Rapid	0.5-1.5 hr	6-12 hr

Adverse reactions

CNS: headache, confusion, hemiparesis, lethargy, paresthesia, syncope, **seizures**
CV: hypotension, palpitations, chest pain, vasodilation
EENT: hearing loss
GI: nausea, vomiting, diarrhea, abdominal cramps, oral candidiasis, **pseudomembranous colitis**
GU: vaginal candidiasis, **nephrotoxicity**
Hematologic: lymphocytosis, eosinophilia, **bleeding tendency, hemolytic anemia, hypoprothrombinemia, neutropenia, thrombocytopenia, agranulocytosis, bone marrow depression**
Hepatic: hepatic failure, hepatomegaly
Musculoskeletal: arthralgia
Respiratory: dyspnea
Skin: urticaria, maculopapular or erythematous rash
Other: chills, fever, superinfection, pain at I.M. injection site, **anaphylaxis, serum sickness**

Interactions

Drug-drug. *Aminoglycosides, loop diuretics:* increased risk of nephrotoxicity
Probenecid: decreased excretion and increased blood level of ceftizoxime
Drug-diagnostic tests. *Alanine aminotransferase, alkaline phosphatase, aspartate aminotransferase, bilirubin, blood urea nitrogen, creatinine, eosinophils, gamma-glutamyltransferase, lactate dehydrogenase:* increased levels
Coombs' test, urinary 17-ketosteroids, nonenzyme-based urine glucose tests (such as Clinitest): false-positive results
Hemoglobin, platelets, white blood cells: decreased values
Drug-herbs. *Angelica, anise, arnica, asafetida, bogbean, boldo, celery, chamomile, clove, danshen, fenugreek, feverfew, garlic, ginger, ginkgo, ginseng, horse chestnut, horseradish, licorice, meadowsweet, onion, papain, passionflower, poplar, prickly ash, quassia, red clover, turmeric, wild carrot, wild lettuce, willow:* increased risk of bleeding.

Patient monitoring

- Monitor for extreme confusion, tonic-clonic seizures, and mild hemiparesis when giving high doses.
- Assess CBC and kidney and liver function test results.
- Monitor for signs and symptoms of superinfection and other serious adverse reactions.
- Be aware that cross-sensitivity to penicillins may occur.

Patient teaching

- Advise patient to report reduced urine output, persistent diarrhea, bruising, and bleeding.
- As appropriate, review all other significant and life-threatening adverse reactions and interactions, especially those related to the drugs, tests, and herbs mentioned above.

ceftriaxone sodium

Rocephin

Pharmacologic class: Third-generation cephalosporin

Therapeutic class: Anti-infective

Pregnancy risk category B

Action

Interferes with bacterial cell-wall synthesis and division by binding to cell wall, causing cell to die. Active against gram-negative and gram-positive bacteria, with expanded activity against gram-negative bacteria. Exhibits minimal immunosuppressant activity.

Availability
Powder for injection: 250 mg, 500 mg, 1 g, 2 g
Premixed containers: 1 g/50 ml, 2 g/50 ml

Indications and dosages
➤ Infections of respiratory system, bones, joints, and skin; septicemia
Adults: 1 to 2 g/day I.M. or I.V. or in equally divided doses q 12 hours. Maximum daily dosage is 4 g.
➤ Uncomplicated gonorrhea
Adults: 250 mg I.M. as a single dose
➤ Surgical prophylaxis
Adults: 1 g I.V. as a single dose 30 minutes to 2 hours before start of surgical procedure
➤ Meningitis
Adults: 1 g to 2 g I.V. q 12 hours for 10 to 14 days
Children: Initially, 100 mg/kg/day I.M. or I.V. (not to exceed 4 g). Then 100 mg/kg/day I.M. or I.V. once daily or in equally divided doses q 12 hours (not to exceed 4 g) for 7 to 14 days.
➤ Otitis media
Children: 50 mg/kg I.M. as a single dose; maximum of 1 g/dose.
➤ Skin and skin-structure infections
Children: 50 to 75 mg/kg/day I.V. or I.M. once or twice daily. Maximum dosage is 2 g daily.
➤ Other serious infections
Children: 50 to 75 mg/kg/day I.V. or I.M. once or twice daily

Off-label uses
- Disseminated gonorrhea
- Endocarditis
- Epididymitis
- Gonorrhea-associated meningitis
- Lyme disease
- *Neisseria meningitides* carriers
- Pelvic inflammatory disease

Contraindications
- Hypersensitivity to cephalosporins or penicillins

Precautions
Use cautiously in:
- renal impairment, hepatic disease, biliary obstruction, phenylketonuria
- history of GI disease
- elderly patients
- pregnant or breastfeeding patients.

Administration
- Obtain specimens for culture and sensitivity testing as necessary before starting therapy.
- Know that drug for I.V. injection is compatible with sterile water, normal saline solution, dextrose 5% in water (D_5W), half-normal saline solution, and D_5W and normal saline solution.
- After reconstituting, dilute further to desired concentration for intermittent I.V. infusion. Infuse over 30 minutes.
- For I.M. use, reconstitute powder for injection with compatible solution by adding 0.9 ml of diluent to 250-mg vial, 1.8 ml to 500-mg vial, 3.6 ml to 1-g vial, or 7.2 ml to 2-g vial, to yield a concentration averaging 250 mg/ml.
- Divide high I.M. doses equally and administer in two separate sites. Inject deep into large muscle mass.

Route	Onset	Peak	Duration
I.V.	Rapid	End of infusion	12-24 hr
I.M.	Rapid	1-2 hr	12-24 hr

Adverse reactions
CNS: headache, confusion, hemiparesis, lethargy, paresthesia, syncope, **seizures**
CV: hypotension, palpitations, chest pain, vasodilation
EENT: hearing loss
GI: nausea, vomiting, diarrhea, abdominal cramps, oral candidiasis, **pseudomembranous colitis**

GU: vaginal candidiasis, **nephrotoxicity**
Hematologic: lymphocytosis, eosinophilia, **bleeding tendency, hemolytic anemia, hypoprothrombinemia, neutropenia, thrombocytopenia, agranulocytosis, bone marrow depression**
Hepatic: hepatic failure, hepatomegaly
Musculoskeletal: arthralgia
Respiratory: dyspnea
Skin: urticaria, maculopapular or erythematous rash
Other: chills, fever, superinfection, pain at I.M. injection site, **anaphylaxis, serum sickness**

Interactions

Drug-drug. *Aminoglycosides, loop diuretics:* increased risk of nephrotoxicity
Probenecid: decreased excretion and increased blood level of ceftriaxone
Drug-diagnostic tests. *Alanine aminotransferase, alkaline phosphatase, aspartate aminotransferase, bilirubin, blood urea nitrogen, creatinine, eosinophils, gamma-glutamyltransferase, lactate dehydrogenase:* increased levels
Coombs' test, urinary 17-ketosteroids, nonenzyme-based urine glucose tests (such as Clinitest): false-positive results
Hemoglobin, platelets, white blood cells: decreased values
Drug-herbs. *Angelica, anise, arnica, asafetida, bogbean, boldo, celery, chamomile, clove, danshen, fenugreek, feverfew, garlic, ginger, ginkgo, ginseng, horse chestnut, horseradish, licorice, meadowsweet, onion, papain, passionflower, poplar, prickly ash, quassia, red clover, turmeric, wild carrot, wild lettuce, willow:* increased risk of bleeding.

Patient monitoring

- Monitor for extreme confusion, tonic-clonic seizures, and mild hemiparesis when giving high doses.
- Monitor coagulation studies.
- Assess CBC and kidney and liver function test results.
- Monitor for signs and symptoms of superinfection and other serious adverse reactions.
- Be aware that cross-sensitivity to penicillins may occur.

Patient teaching

- Instruct patient to report reduced urine output, persistent diarrhea, bruising, or bleeding.
- Caution patient not to use herbs unless prescriber approves.
- As appropriate, review all other significant and life-threatening adverse reactions and interactions, especially those related to the drugs, tests, and herbs mentioned above.

cefuroxime axetil
Ceftin

cefuroxime sodium
Zinacef

Pharmacologic class: Second-generation cephalosporin
Therapeutic class: Anti-infective
Pregnancy risk category B

Action

Interferes with bacterial cell-wall synthesis and division by binding to cell wall, causing cell to die. Active against gram-negative and gram-positive bacteria, with expanded activity against gram-negative bacteria. Exhibits minimal immunosuppressant activity.

Availability

Oral suspension: 125 mg/5 ml
Powder for injection: 750 mg, 1.5 g, 7.5 g

Premixed containers: 750 mg/50 ml, 1.5 g/50 ml
Tablets: 125 mg, 250 mg, 500 mg

Indications and dosages

➢ Moderate to severe infections, including those of skin, bone, joints, urinary or respiratory tract, gynecologic infections, and septicemia
Adults and children ages 12 and older: 750 mg to 1.5 g I.M. or I.V. q 8 hours for 5 to 10 days or 250 to 500 mg P.O. q 12 hours
Children ages 3 months to 12 years: 50 to 100 mg/kg/day I.V. or I.M. in divided doses q 6 to 8 hours
➢ Gonorrhea
Adults: 750 mg to 1.5 g I.M. or I.V. as a single dose, or 1.5 g I.M. (750 mg in two separate sites), given with 1 g probenecid P.O.
➢ Bacterial meningitis
Adults and children ages 12 and older: Up to 3 g I.V. or I.M. q 8 hours
Children ages 3 months to 12 years: 200 to 240 mg/kg I.V. daily in divided doses q 6 to 8 hours
➢ Otitis media
Children ages 3 months to 12 years: 15 mg/kg P.O. q 12 hours (oral suspension) for 10 days, or 250 mg (tablets) P.O. q 12 hours for 10 days
➢ Pharyngitis; tonsillitis
Adults and children ages 13 and older: 250 mg P.O. b.i.d. for 10 days
Children ages 3 months to 12 years: 125 mg P.O. q 12 hours for 10 days, or 20 mg/kg/day P.O. in two divided doses for 10 days as oral suspension (maximum 500 mg/day)

Dosage adjustment

- Renal impairment

Contraindications

- Hypersensitivity to cephalosporins or penicillins
- Carnitine deficiency

Precautions

Use cautiously in:
- renal or hepatic impairment
- pregnant or breastfeeding patients
- children.

Administration

- Reconstitute drug in vial with sterile water for injection.
- Give by direct I.V. injection over 3 to 5 minutes into large vein or flowing I.V. line.
- For intermittent I.V. infusion, reconstitute drug with 100 ml of dextrose 5% in water or normal saline solution; administer over 15 minutes to 1 hour. For continuous infusion, give in 500 to 1,000 ml of compatible solution; infuse over 6 to 24 hours.
- Inject I.M. doses deep into large muscle mass.
- Give oral form with food.
- Be aware that tablets and oral suspension are exchangeable on a milligram-for-milligram basis.

Route	Onset	Peak	Duration
P.O.	Unknown	2 hr	8-12 hr
I.V., I.M.	Rapid	End of infusion	6-12 hr

Adverse reactions

CNS: headache, hyperactivity, hypertonia, **seizures**
GI: nausea, vomiting, diarrhea, abdominal pain, dyspepsia, **pseudomembranous colitis**
GU: hematuria, vaginal candidiasis, **renal dysfunction, toxic nephropathy**
Hematologic: hemolytic anemia, aplastic anemia, hemorrhage
Hepatic: hepatic dysfunction
Metabolic: hyperglycemia
Skin: toxic epidermal necrolysis, **erythema multiforme, Stevens-Johnson syndrome**
Other: allergic reaction, drug fever, superinfection, **anaphylaxis**

Interactions

Drug-drug. *Antacids containing aluminum or magnesium, histamine$_2$-receptor antagonists:* increased cefuroxime absorption
Probenecid: decreased excretion and increased blood level of cefuroxime
Drug-diagnostic tests. *Blood glucose, Coombs' test, urine glucose tests using Benedict's solution:* false-positive results
Glucose, hematocrit: decreased levels
White blood cells in urine: increased level
Drug-food. *Moderate- or high-fat meal:* increased drug bioavailability

Patient monitoring

- Monitor patient for life-threatening adverse effects, including anaphylaxis, Stevens-Johnson syndrome, and pseudomembranous colitis.
- Monitor neurologic status, particularly for signs of impending seizures.
- Monitor kidney and liver function test results and intake and output.
- Monitor CBC with differential and prothrombin time; watch for signs and symptoms of blood dyscrasias.
- Monitor temperature; watch for signs and symptoms of superinfection.

Patient teaching

- Advise patient to immediately report rash or bleeding tendency.
- Instruct patient to take drug with food every 12 hours as prescribed.
- Teach patient how to recognize signs and symptoms of superinfection. Instruct him to report these right away.
- Advise patient to report CNS changes.
- As appropriate, review all other significant and life-threatening adverse reactions and interactions, especially those related to the drugs, tests, and foods mentioned above.

celecoxib

Celebrex

Pharmacologic class: Nonsteroidal cyclooxygenase-2 (COX-2) inhibitor, nonsteroidal anti-inflammatory drug (NSAID)
Therapeutic class: Antirheumatic
Pregnancy risk category C

Action

Exhibits anti-inflammatory, analgesic, and antipyretic action due to inhibition of COX-2 enzyme

Availability

Capsules: 100 mg, 200 mg

Indications and dosages

➢ Osteoarthritis
Adults: 200 mg/day P.O. as a single dose or 100 mg P.O. b.i.d.
➢ Rheumatoid arthritis
Adults: 100 to 200 mg P.O. b.i.d.
➢ Adjunctive treatment in familial adenomatous polyposis to decrease the number of adenomatous colorectal polyps
Adults: 400 mg P.O. b.i.d.
➢ Acute pain or primary dysmenorrhea
Adults: 400 mg P.O. once, plus one additional 200 mg-dose as needed on first day; then 200 mg b.i.d. as needed

Dosage adjustment

- Hepatic impairment
- Patients weighing less than 50 kg (110 lb)

Contraindications

- Hypersensitivity to drug, sulfonamides, or other NSAIDs
- Advanced renal disease
- Severe hepatic impairment
- Sensitivity precipitated by aspirin

• Third trimester of pregnancy
• Breastfeeding

Precautions

Use cautiously in:
• renal insufficiency, hypertension
• history of asthma, urticaria, renal disease, hepatic dysfunction, heart failure
• patients on long-term NSAID therapy
• elderly patients
• pregnant patients in first or second trimester
• children younger than age 18 (safety not established).

Administration

• When administering doses higher than 200/mg daily, give with food or milk to improve drug absorption.

Route	Onset	Peak	Duration
P.O.	Unknown	3 hr	Unknown

Adverse reactions

CNS: dizziness, drowsiness, headache, insomnia, fatigue
CV: angina, tachycardia, peripheral edema, **myocardial infarction**
EENT: ophthalmic effects, tinnitus, epistaxis, pharyngitis, rhinitis, sinusitis
GI: nausea, diarrhea, constipation, abdominal pain, dyspepsia, flatulence, dry mouth, **GI bleeding**
GU: menorrhagia
Hematologic: eosinophilia, ecchymosis, **neutropenia, leukopenia, pancytopenia, thrombocytopenia, agranulocytosis, granulocytopenia, aplastic anemia, bone marrow depression**
Hepatic: hepatotoxicity
Metabolic: hyperchloremia, hypophosphatemia
Musculoskeletal: back pain, leg cramps
Respiratory: upper respiratory tract infection
Skin: rash
Other: anaphylaxis

Interactions

Drug-drug. *Angiotensin-converting enzyme inhibitors, furosemide, thiazides:* reduced celecoxib efficacy
Antacids containing aluminum and magnesium: decreased celecoxib blood level
Aspirin (regular doses): increased risk of GI bleeding and GI ulcers
Fluconazole, lithium: increased blood levels of these drugs
Warfarin: increased risk of bleeding
Drug-diagnostic tests. *Alanine aminotransferase, aspartate aminotransferase, blood urea nitrogen:* increased levels
Hematocrit, hemoglobin: decreased values
Drug-herbs. *Dong quai, feverfew, garlic, ginger, horse chestnut, red clover:* increased risk of bleeding
White willow: increased risk of GI ulcers
Drug-behaviors. *Long-term alcohol use, smoking:* GI irritation and bleeding

Patient monitoring

• Monitor CBC, electrolyte levels, creatinine clearance, occult fecal blood test, and liver function test results every 6 to 12 months.

Patient teaching

🔊 Advise patient to immediately report bloody stools, vomiting of blood, or signs or symptoms of liver damage (nausea, fatigue, lethargy, pruritus, yellowing of eyes or skin, tenderness in upper right abdomen, or flulike symptoms).
• Instruct patient to take drug with food or milk.
• Tell patient to avoid aspirin and other NSAIDs (such as ibuprofen and naproxen) during therapy.
• As appropriate, review all other significant and life-threatening adverse reactions and interactions, especially those related to the drugs, tests, herbs, and behaviors mentioned above.

cephalexin hydrochloride
Keftab

cephalexin monohydrate
Apo-Cephalex✤, Biocef, Keflex, Novo-Lexin✤, Nu-Cephalex✤, Panixine DisperDose, PMS-Cephalexin✤

Pharmacologic class: First-generation cephalosporin
Therapeutic class: Anti-infective
Pregnancy risk category B

Action
Interferes with bacterial cell-wall synthesis, causing cell to rupture and die. Active against many gram-positive bacteria; shows limited activity against gram-negative bacteria.

Availability
Capsules: 250 mg, 500 mg
Oral suspension: 100 mg/ml, 125 mg/5 ml, 250 mg/5 ml
Tablets: 250 mg, 500 mg
Tablets for oral suspension (DisperDose): 125 mg, 250 mg

Indications and dosages
➢ Respiratory tract infections caused by streptococci; skin and skin-structure infections caused by staphylococci and streptococci; bone infections caused by staphylococci or *Proteus mirabilis;* genitourinary infections caused by *Escherichia coli, P. mirabilis,* and *Klebsiella* species; *Haemophilus influenzae,* staphylococcal, streptococcal, and *Moraxella catarrhalis* infections
Adults: 1 to 4 g P.O. daily in divided doses (usually 250 mg P.O. q 6 hours). For uncomplicated cystitis, skin and soft-tissue infections, and streptococcal pharyngitis, 500 mg P.O. q 12 hours.
Children: 25 to 50 mg/kg/day P.O. in divided doses
➢ Otitis media caused by *S. pneumoniae*
Children: 75 to 100 mg/kg/day P.O. in four divided doses

Dosage adjustment
- Renal impairment

Contraindications
- Hypersensitivity to cephalosporins or penicillin

Precautions
Use cautiously in:
- renal impairment, phenylketonuria
- history of GI disease
- debilitated or emaciated patients
- elderly patients
- pregnant or breastfeeding patients.

Administration
- Give with or without food.
- Be aware that DisperDose tablet is intended for suspension. Mix with water before administering.
- Refrigerate oral suspension.

Route	Onset	Peak	Duration
P.O.	Rapid	1 hr	6-12 hr

Adverse reactions
CNS: fever, headache, lethargy, paresthesia, syncope, **seizures**
CV: edema, hypotension, vasodilation, palpitations, chest pain
EENT: hearing loss
GI: nausea, vomiting, diarrhea, abdominal cramps, oral candidiasis, **pseudomembranous colitis**
GU: vaginal candidiasis, **nephrotoxicity**
Hematologic: lymphocytosis, eosinophilia, **bleeding tendency, hemolytic anemia, neutropenia, thrombocytopenia, agranulocytosis, bone marrow depression**
Musculoskeletal: joint pain
Respiratory: dyspnea

Skin: rash, maculopapular and erythematous urticaria
Other: superinfection, chills, pain, allergic reaction, hypersensitivity reactions including **anaphylaxis, serum sickness**

Interactions

Drug-drug. *Aminoglycosides, loop diuretics:* increased risk of nephrotoxicity
Chloramphenicol: antagonistic effect
Probenecid: increased cephalexin blood level
Drug-diagnostic tests. *Alanine aminotransferase, alkaline phosphatase, aspartate aminotransferase, bilirubin, blood urea nitrogen, creatinine, eosinophils, lactate dehydrogenase, lymphocytes:* increased values
Coombs' test: false-positive result (especially in neonates whose mothers received drug before delivery)
Granulocytes, neutrophils, white blood cells: decreased counts

Patient monitoring

- Assess for signs and symptoms of serious adverse reactions, including hypersensitivity, severe diarrhea, and bleeding.
- During long-term therapy, monitor CBC and liver and kidney function test results.

Patient teaching

Instruct patient to stop taking drug and contact prescriber immediately if he develops rash or difficulty breathing.
- Tell patient to take drug with full glass of water.
- Instruct patient to mix DisperDose tablet with water before taking.
- Advise patient to report severe diarrhea.
- As appropriate, review all other significant and life-threatening adverse reactions and interactions, especially those related to the drugs and tests mentioned above.

cephradine

Velosef

Pharmacologic class: First-generation cephalosporin
Therapeutic class: Anti-infective
Pregnancy risk category B

Action

Interferes with bacterial cell-wall synthesis, causing cell to rupture and die. Active against many gram-positive bacteria; shows limited activity against gram-negative bacteria.

Availability

Capsules: 250 mg, 500 mg
Oral suspension: 125 mg/5 ml, 250 mg/5 ml

Indications and dosages

➤ Respiratory, skin, and other infections
Adults: 250 to 1,000 mg P.O. q 6 to 12 hours. For severe or chronic infection, dosage may be increased up to 1 g q 6 hours.
Children older than age 9 months: 25 to 50 mg/kg/day P.O. q 6 hours in divided doses. For otitis media, usual dosage is 75 to 100 mg/kg/day P.O. q 6 to 12 hours in divided doses.

Dosage adjustment

- Renal impairment

Contraindications

- Hypersensitivity to cephalosporins or penicillin

Precautions

Use cautiously in:
- renal impairment, phenylketonuria
- history of GI disease
- debilitated or emaciated patients
- elderly patients
- pregnant or breastfeeding patients.

Administration
• Give drug with food if it causes GI upset.

Route	Onset	Peak	Duration
P.O.	Rapid	1-2 hr	6-12 hr

Adverse reactions
CNS: headache, lethargy, paresthesia, syncope, **seizures**
CV: hypotension, vasodilation, palpitations, chest pain, phlebitis, **thrombophlebitis**
EENT: hearing loss, scleral yellowing
GI: nausea, vomiting, constipation, abdominal cramps, oral candidiasis, **pseudomembranous colitis**
GU: vaginal candidiasis, **nephrotoxicity**
Hematologic: anemia, lymphocytosis, eosinophilia, **bleeding tendency, leukopenia, bone marrow depression, hypoprothrombinemia, neutropenia, thrombocytopenia, agranulocytosis**
Hepatic: hepatomegaly
Musculoskeletal: joint pain
Respiratory: dyspnea
Skin: rash, maculopapular and erythematous urticaria, yellow skin discoloration
Other: chills, fever, edema, allergic reactions including **anaphylaxis, serum sickness**

Interactions
Drug-drug. *Aminoglycosides, loop diuretics:* increased risk of nephrotoxicity
Probenecid: increased cephradine blood level
Drug-diagnostic tests. *Alanine aminotransferase, alkaline phosphatase, aspartate aminotransferase, bilirubin, blood urea nitrogen, creatinine, eosinophils, lactate dehydrogenase, lymphocytes:* increased levels
Coombs' test: false-positive result (especially in neonates whose mothers received drug before delivery)
Granulocytes, neutrophils, white blood cells: decreased counts

Patient monitoring
• Assess for signs and symptoms of serious adverse reactions, including hypersensitivity, jaundice, and bleeding.
• Monitor liver and kidney function test results.

Patient teaching
• Tell patient to take drug with full glass of water.
🔊 Instruct patient to immediately report severe diarrhea, abdominal pain, or vomiting.
🔊 Advise patient to stop taking drug and contact prescriber immediately if rash occurs.
• As appropriate, review all other significant and life-threatening adverse reactions and interactions, especially those related to the drugs and tests mentioned above.

cetirizine hydrochloride
Reactine✱, Zyrtec

Pharmacologic class: Histamine$_1$-receptor antagonist (peripherally selective)
Therapeutic class: Allergy, cold, and cough agent; antihistamine
Pregnancy risk category B

Action
Antagonizes histamine's effects at histamine$_1$-receptor sites, preventing allergic response. Also has mild bronchodilatory effects and blocks histamine-induced bronchoconstriction in asthma.

Availability
Syrup: 5 mg/5 ml
Tablets: 5 mg, 10 mg

Indications and dosages

➢ Allergic symptoms caused by histamine release

Adults and children older than age 6: 5 to 10 mg P.O. daily

Children ages 2 to 5: 2.5 mg to 5 mg P.O. daily

Dosage adjustment

- Renal impairment
- Hepatic impairment

Off-label uses

- Bronchial asthma

Contraindications

- Hypersensitivity to drug or hydroxyzine
- Acute asthma attacks
- Angle-closure glaucoma
- Pyloroduodenal obstruction
- Breastfeeding

Precautions

Use cautiously in:

- renal impairment, significant hepatic dysfunction
- elderly patients
- pregnant patients
- children younger than age 2 (safety not established).

Administration

- Give with or without food.
- Administer at same time each day.

Route	Onset	Peak	Duration
P.O.	30 min	1-4 hr	24 hr

Adverse reactions

CNS: dizziness, drowsiness, fatigue
CV: palpitations, edema
EENT: pharyngitis
GI: nausea, vomiting, abdominal distress, dry mouth
Musculoskeletal: myalgia, joint pain
Respiratory: bronchospasm
Skin: photosensitivity, rash, **angioedema**
Other: fever

Interactions

Drug-drug. *CNS depressants:* additive CNS effects

Theophylline: decreased cetirizine clearance

Drug-diagnostic tests. *Allergy skin tests:* false-negative results

Drug-behaviors. *Alcohol use:* additive CNS effects

Sun exposure: photosensitivity

Patient monitoring

- Monitor creatinine levels in patients with renal dysfunction.
- Assess hepatic enzyme levels in patients with hepatic disease.

Patient teaching

- Tell patient to take with full glass of water.
- Inform patient that drug may impair alertness and that alcohol may exaggerate this effect.
- Caution patient to avoid driving and other hazardous activities until he knows how drug affects concentration and alertness.
- As appropriate, review all other significant and life-threatening adverse reactions and interactions, especially those related to the drugs, tests, and behaviors mentioned above.

chloral hydrate

Aquachloral, Novo-Chloralhydrate✦, PMS-Chloral Hydrate✦

Pharmacologic class: CNS agent
Therapeutic class: Sedative-hypnotic
Controlled substance schedule IV
Pregnancy risk category C

Action

Unclear. Thought to produce CNS depression by converting into its metabolite, trichloroethanol.

Availability

Capsules: 250 mg, 500 mg
Suppositories: 324 mg, 500 mg, 648 mg
Syrup: 250 mg/ml, 500 mg/ml

Indications and dosages

➢ Nighttime sedation

Adults: 500 mg to 1 g P.O. or P.R. 15 to 30 minutes before bedtime, not to exceed 2 g

Children: 50 mg/kg/day P.O., to a maximum dosage of 1 g given as a single dose or in divided doses

➢ Sedation

Adults: 250 mg P.O. or P.R. t.i.d. after meals

Children: 25 mg/kg/day P.O. or P.R., to a maximum daily dosage of 500 mg, given as a single dose or in divided doses

Contraindications

- Hypersensitivity to drug or tartrazine
- Coma, CNS depression, esophagitis, ulcer disease
- Pregnancy or breastfeeding

Precautions

Use cautiously in:
- hepatic dysfunction, severe renal impairment
- elderly patients.

Administration

- Know that drug may take 45 to 60 minutes to achieve adequate preprocedural sedation in children.

When giving to children for preprocedural sedation, be aware that drug may cause unpredictable or paradoxical effects.

Route	Onset	Peak	Duration
P.O.	30 min	1 hr	4-8 hr
P.R.	0.5-1 hr	Unknown	4-8 hr

Adverse reactions

CNS: dizziness, drowsiness, nightmares, ataxia, paradoxical stimulation, hangover, delirium, light-headedness, hallucinations, confusion

GI: nausea, vomiting, diarrhea, flatulence

Hematologic: eosinophilia, **leukopenia**

Skin: hypersensitivity reactions

Other: physical and psychological drug dependence

Interactions

Drug-drug. *CNS depressants (including antidepressants, antihistamines, narcotics, sedating antipsychotic drugs, and other sedative-hypnotics):* excessive CNS depression

Furosemide: diaphoresis, flushing, nausea, uneasiness, variable blood pressure

Oral anticoagulants: increased risk of bleeding

Phenytoin: decreased phenytoin blood level

Drug-diagnostic tests. *Eosinophils:* increased count

Urinary 17-hydroxycorticosteroids: interference with test interpretation

White blood cells: decreased count

Drug-behaviors. *Alcohol use:* excessive CNS and respiratory depression

Patient monitoring

- Monitor respiratory status, including oxygen saturation (using pulse oximetry), especially in children.
- Assess creatinine levels in patients with chronic renal disease.
- Monitor hepatic enzyme levels in patients with chronic hepatic disease.
- After giving drug to child, turn down room lights and minimize other stimulation.

Patient teaching

- Instruct patient to avoid driving and other hazardous activities until he knows how drug affects concentration and alertness.
- Caution patient not to drink alcohol during therapy.

• When administering to a child, instruct parents to minimize stimulation to decrease risk of paradoxical reaction.
• As appropriate, review all other significant and life-threatening adverse reactions and interactions, especially those related to the drugs, tests, and behaviors mentioned above.

chlorambucil

Leukeran

Pharmacologic class: Alkylating agent, nitrogen mustard
Therapeutic class: Antineoplastic, immunosuppressant
Pregnancy risk category D

Action
Interacts with cellular DNA to produce cytotoxic cross-linkage, which disrupts cell function. Cell-cycle-phase nonspecific.

Availability
Tablets: 2 mg

Indications and dosages
➢ Chronic lymphocytic leukemia, malignant lymphoma
Adults: Initially, 0.1 to 0.2 mg/kg/day P.O. for 3 to 6 weeks as a single dose or in divided doses. Maintenance dosage is based on CBC but shouldn't exceed 0.1 mg/kg/day.

Off-label uses
• Idiopathic membranous nephropathy
• Meningoencephalitis associated with Behçet's disease
• Rheumatoid arthritis

Contraindications
• Hypersensitivity to drug or other alkylating agents
• Pregnancy or breastfeeding

Precautions
Use cautiously in:
• hematopoietic depression, infection, other chronic debilitating diseases
• history of seizures or head trauma
• patients who have undergone radiation or other chemotherapy
• elderly patients
• females of childbearing age
• children (safety and efficacy not established).

Administration
• Before starting therapy, assess for history of seizures or head trauma.
• After full-course radiation or chemotherapy, wait 4 weeks before giving full doses (because of bone marrow vulnerability).
• To minimize GI effects, drug may be given at bedtime with antiemetic, especially if high dosage is prescribed.

Route	Onset	Peak	Duration
P.O.	Unknown	1 hr	Unknown

Adverse reactions
CNS: peripheral neuropathy, tremor, confusion, agitation, ataxia, flaccid paresis, **seizures**
EENT: keratitis
GI: nausea, vomiting, diarrhea
GU: sterile cystitis, amenorrhea, sterility, decreased sperm count
Hematologic: anemia, **leukopenia, thrombocytopenia, neutropenia, bone marrow depression**
Hepatic: jaundice, **hepatotoxicity**
Metabolic: hyperuricemia
Musculoskeletal: muscle twitching
Respiratory: interstitial pneumonitis, pulmonary fibrosis
Skin: rash, **erythema multiforme, epidermal necrolysis, Stevens-Johnson syndrome**
Other: drug fever, allergic reaction, **secondary malignancies**

Interactions

Drug-drug. *Anticoagulants, aspirin:* increased risk of bleeding
Immunosuppressants, myelosuppressants: additive bone marrow depression
Live-virus vaccines: decreased antibody response to vaccine, increased risk of adverse reactions
Drug-diagnostic tests. *Alanine aminotransferase, alkaline phosphatase, aspartate aminotransferase, uric acid:* increased levels (may reflect hepatotoxicity)
Granulocytes, hemoglobin, neutrophils, platelets, red blood cells, white blood cells (WBCs): decreased counts
Drug-herbs. *Astragalus, echinacea, melatonin:* interference with immunosuppressant action

Patient monitoring

🔊 Monitor CBC with white cell differential and platelet count weekly.
- Monitor WBC count every 3 to 4 days.
- Assess liver function test results.

Patient teaching

- Instruct patient to immediately report unusual bleeding or bruising, fever, nausea, vomiting, rash, chills, sore throat, cough, shortness of breath, seizures, amenorrhea, unusual lumps or masses, flank or stomach pain, joint pain, lip or mouth sores, or yellowing of skin or sclera.
- Tell patient to take drug with full glass of water.
- Inform patient that drug may increase his risk for infection. Advise him to wash hands frequently, wear a mask in public places, and avoid people with infections.
- Instruct patient to contact prescriber before receiving vaccines.
- Advise female patient to use reliable contraception.
- As appropriate, review all other significant and life-threatening adverse reactions and interactions, especially those related to the drugs, tests, and herbs mentioned above.

chloramphenicol

AK-Chlor, Chloromycetin Ophthalmic, Chloroptic, Chloroptic S.O.P., Novochlorocap🍁, Pentamycetin🍁

Pharmacologic class: Dichloroacetic acid derivative
Therapeutic class: Anti-infective
Pregnancy risk category NR

Action

Exerts bacteriostatic activity by binding with 50S subunit of ribosome and inhibiting protein synthesis

Availability

Injection: 1-g vial
Ointment (ophthalmic): 10 mg/g
Powder for solution (ophthalmic): 25 mg/vial
Solution (ophthalmic): 5 mg/ml

Indications and dosages

➢ Serious infections when less potentially dangerous drugs are ineffective or contraindicated
Adults: 50 to 100 mg/kg/day I.V. in divided doses q 6 hours, to a maximum dosage of 4 g/day
Children: 50 to 75 mg/kg/day I.V. in divided doses q 6 hours
➢ Bacteremia or meningitis
Children: 50 to 100 mg/kg/day I.V. in divided doses q 6 hours
➢ Ocular infections
Adults and children: Instill two drops of ophthalmic solution in each eye q.i.d. As supplement to solution, apply small amount of ophthalmic ointment to conjunctival sac at bedtime. (Solution and ointment may be used together or alone.)

Dosage adjustment
- Hepatic or renal impairment

Off-label uses
- Unspecified acne

Contraindications
- Hypersensitivity to drug
- Severe renal or hepatic impairment
- Prophylaxis for bacterial infections
- Acute porphyria

Precautions
Use cautiously in:
- hepatic disease, renal disease, bone marrow depression
- pregnant or breastfeeding patients
- infants and children.

Administration
- Dilute parenteral dose with aqueous solution (for example, water for injection or dextrose 5% in water injection) to at least 100 mg/ml.
- Give parenteral form by I.V. injection over at least 2 minutes. For intermittent infusion, drug may be diluted further in 50 to 100 ml of dextrose 5% in wate and given over 10 to 30 minutes.
- Don't give drug I.M.

🔊 Know that drug may cause serious reactions (because of its narrow therapeutic window) and should be used only when safer anti-infectives are ineffective or contraindicated.

Route	Onset	Peak	Duration
I.V.	Immediate	1-2 hr	8 hr
Ophthalmic	Unknown	Unknown	Unknown

Adverse reactions
CNS: confusion, delirium, depression, headache, peripheral neuropathy
EENT: optic neuritis, vision loss
GI: nausea, vomiting, diarrhea, abdominal pain, glossitis, colitis, pruritus ani, dry mouth
Hematologic: reticulocytopenia, aplastic anemia, bone marrow depression, granulocytopenia, hypoplastic anemia, leukopenia, thrombocytopenia
Skin: rash, itching, urticaria, contact dermatitis, **angioedema**
Other: fever, **anaphylaxis, gray syndrome in neonates**

Interactions
Drug-drug. *Aminoglycosides, penicillins:* decreased activity of these drugs
Barbiturates: increased barbiturate level, decreased chloramphenicol blood level
Hepatic enzyme inducers: decreased chloramphenicol blood level
Hydantoins: increased hydantoin blood level
Iron salts: increased iron level
Myelosuppressants, drugs that cause blood dyscrasias: increased bone marrow depression
Vitamin B_{12}: antagonism of hematopoietic response
Warfarin: enhanced warfarin action
Drug-diagnostic tests. *Alanine aminotransferase, aspartate aminotransferase, hemoglobin, platelets, red blood cells, white blood cells:* altered values

Patient monitoring
🔊 Monitor patient for signs and symptoms of aplastic anemia, which may occur weeks or months after therapy ends.
- Monitor CBC count closely.
- Assess hepatic enzyme levels in patients with hepatic disease.
- Monitor creatinine levels in patients with renal insufficiency or failure.

Patient teaching
🔊 Instruct patient to report bleeding or bruising, even if therapy ended several weeks or months earlier.
- Tell patient to report rash or itching.
- Caution patient to avoid pregnancy during therapy. If she's using hormonal contraceptives, advise her to use additional birth control method (drug

may make hormonal contraceptives ineffective).
• As appropriate, review all other significant and life-threatening adverse reactions and interactions, especially those related to the drugs and tests mentioned above.

chlordiazepoxide hydrochloride

Apo-Chlordiazepoxide✱, Librium, Mitran, Novo-Poxide✱, Reposans-10

Pharmacologic class: Benzodiazepine
Therapeutic class: Anxiolytic, sedative-hypnotic
Controlled substance schedule IV
Pregnancy risk category D

Action

Unknown. May potentiate effects of gamma-aminobutyric acid (an inhibitory neurotransmitter) by increasing neuronal membrane permeability; may depress CNS at limbic and subcortical levels of brain. Anxiolytic effect occurs at doses well below those that cause sedation or ataxia.

Availability

Capsules: 5 mg, 10 mg, 25 mg
Injection: 100-mg ampules

Indications and dosages

➢ Mild to moderate anxiety
Adults: 5 to 10 mg P.O. three to four times daily
➢ Severe anxiety
Adults: Initially, 50 to 100 mg I.M. or I.V.; then 25 to 50 mg P.O. three to four times daily as needed
➢ Preoperative apprehension or anxiety
Adults: 5 to 10 mg P.O. three to four times daily for several days before surgery or 50 to 100 mg I.M. 1 hour before surgery
➢ Acute alcohol withdrawal
Adults: Initially, 50 to 100 mg I.V. or I.M. Repeat dose as needed up to 300 mg/day.

Dosage adjustment

• Renal impairment
• Age 65 or older

Contraindications

• Hypersensitivity to drug, other benzodiazepines, or tartrazine
• CNS depression
• Uncontrolled severe pain
• Porphyria
• Pregnancy or breastfeeding
• Children younger than age 6

Precautions

Use cautiously in:
• hepatic dysfunction, severe renal impairment
• debilitated or elderly patients.

Administration

• Dilute I.V. preparation with 5 ml of normal saline solution. Administer slowly over at least 1 minute.
• When giving I.M., use 2 ml of special I.M. diluent. Inject slowly and deeply into gluteus muscle.
• Don't use I.M. diluent for I.V. preparation.
• After I.V. or I.M. administration, observe patient closely and enforce bedrest for at least 3 hours.

Route	Onset	Peak	Duration
P.O.	Rapid	0.5-4 hr	Up to 24 hr
I.V.	1-5 min	Unknown	0.25-1 hr
I.M.	15-30 min	Unknown	Unknown

Adverse reactions

CNS: dizziness, drowsiness, hangover, headache, depression, paradoxical stimulation
EENT: blurred vision

GI: nausea, vomiting, constipation, diarrhea
Hematologic: agranulocytosis
Hepatic: jaundice
Skin: rash
Other: physical or psychological drug dependence, drug tolerance, pain at I.M. site

Interactions

Drug-drug. *Antidepressants, antihistamines, opioids:* additive CNS depression
Barbiturates, rifampin: decreased chlordiazepoxide efficacy
Cimetidine, disulfiram, fluoxetine, hormonal contraceptives, isoniazid, ketoconazole, metoprolol, propoxyphene, propranolol, valproic acid: enhanced chlordiazepoxide effect
Levodopa: decreased levodopa efficacy
Drug-diagnostic tests. *Alanine aminotransferase, aspartate aminotransferase, bilirubin:* increased levels
Granulocytes: decreased count
Metyrapone test: decreased response
Radioactive iodine uptake test (^{123}I or ^{131}I): decreased uptake
Urine 17-ketogenic steroids, urine 17-ketosteroids: altered test results
Drug-herbs. *Chamomile, hops, kava, skullcap, valerian:* increased CNS depression
Drug-behaviors. *Alcohol use:* increased CNS depression

Patient monitoring

- Monitor CBC and hepatic enzyme levels in prolonged therapy.
- Monitor renal and hepatic studies.
- Assess patient for apnea, bradycardia, and hypotension.

Patient teaching

- Caution patient to avoid driving and other hazardous activities until he knows how drug affects concentration and alertness.
- Advise patient to avoid alcohol during therapy.
- Tell patient not to stop taking drug abruptly. Instruct him to discuss dosage-tapering schedule with prescriber.
- Caution female patient not to take drug if she's pregnant or might become pregnant during therapy. Advise her to use reliable contraception.
- As appropriate, review all other significant and life-threatening adverse reactions and interactions, especially those related to the drugs, tests, herbs, and behaviors mentioned above.

chloroquine phosphate

Aralen

Pharmacologic class: 4-aminoquinolone derivative
Therapeutic class: Antimalarial, amebicide
Pregnancy risk category C

Action

Unknown. Antimalarial action may occur through inhibition of protein synthesis and alteration of DNA in susceptible parasites.

Availability

Tablets: 250 mg (150-mg base), 500 mg (300-mg base)

Indications and dosages

➤ Uncomplicated acute malarial attacks

Adults: Initially, 1 g (600-mg base) P.O., then an additional 500 mg (300-mg base) P.O. 6 hours later and a single dose of 500 mg (300-mg base) P.O. on second and third days. Or initially, 160- to 200-mg base I.M., repeated in 6 hours (800-mg base maximum dosage during first 24 hours); continue for 3 days until total dosage of 1.5-g base has been given. Switch to oral therapy as soon as possible.

Children: Initially, 10 mg (base)/kg P.O., then 5 mg (base)/kg 6 hours, 24 hours, and 36 hours later; don't exceed recommended adult dosage. Or initially, 5 mg (base)/kg I.M. repeated 6 hours later, 18 hours after second dose, and then 24 hours after third dose; don't exceed recommended adult dosage.

➢ Malaria prophylaxis

Adults: 500 mg (300-mg base) P.O. weekly 1 to 2 weeks before visiting endemic area and continued for 4 weeks after leaving area. If therapy starts after malaria exposure, initial dosage is 600-mg base P.O. in two divided doses given 6 hours apart.

Children: 5 mg (base)/kg P.O. weekly for 1 to 2 weeks before visiting endemic area and continued for 4 weeks after leaving area, to a maximum dosage of 300 mg weekly. If treatment starts after exposure, 10 mg (base)/kg P.O. in two divided doses 6 hours apart and continued for 8 weeks after leaving area.

➢ Extraintestinal amebiasis

Adults: Initially, 1 g (600-mg base) P.O. daily for 2 days, then 500 mg (300-mg base) daily for 2 to 3 weeks. When oral therapy isn't tolerated, give 160- to 200-mg base I.M. daily for 10 to 12 days; switch to oral therapy as soon as possible.

Children: 10 mg (base)/kg P.O. once daily for 2 to 3 weeks, to a maximum dosage of 300 mg (base) daily

Off-label uses

- Lupus erythematosus
- Rheumatoid arthritis

Contraindications

- Hypersensitivity to drug
- Retinal and visual field changes
- Porphyria

Precautions

Use cautiously in:

- severe GI, neurologic, or blood disorders; hepatic impairment; G6PD deficiency; neurologic disease; eczema; alcoholism
- pregnant patients
- children.

Administration

- For obese patient, determine weight-based dosages from lean body weight. (Drug is stored in body tissues and eliminated slowly.)

Route	Onset	Peak	Duration
P.O.	Unknown	1-3 hr	Unknown

Adverse reactions

CNS: mild and transient headache, personality changes, dizziness, vertigo neuropathy, **seizures**

CV: hypotension, ECG changes

EENT: blurred vision, difficulty focusing, reversible corneal changes, irreversible retinal damage leading to vision loss, scotomas, ototoxicity, tinnitus, nerve deafness

GI: nausea, vomiting, diarrhea, abdominal pain, stomatitis, anorexia

Hematologic: agranulocytosis, aplastic anemia, hemolytic anemia, thrombocytopenia

Skin: lichen planus eruptions, skin and mucosal pigmentation changes, pruritus, pleomorphic skin eruptions

Interactions

Drug-drug. *Aluminum and magnesium salts, kaolin:* decreased GI absorption of chloroquine

Ampicillin: reduced ampicillin bioavailability

Cimetidine: decreased hepatic metabolism of chloroquine

Cyclosporine: sudden increase in cyclosporine blood level

Drug-diagnostic tests. *Granulocytes, hemoglobin, platelets:* decreased values

Drug-behaviors. *Sun exposure:* exacerbation of drug-induced dermatoses

Patient monitoring

- Monitor hepatic enzyme levels in patients with hepatic disease.
- Assess creatinine levels in patients with renal insufficiency or failure.
- In long-term therapy (as for lupus or rheumatoid arthritis), be aware that desired effects may be delayed for up to 6 months.
- Be aware that drug is secreted in breast milk but not in sufficient amounts to prevent malaria in infant.

Patient teaching

- Tell patient to take drug with food at evenly spaced intervals.
- Instruct patient to immediately report blurred vision or hearing changes.
- In areas where malaria is endemic, advise pregnant patient to consult prescriber about taking drug.
- Inform patient on long-term therapy that beneficial effects may take up to 6 months.
- As appropriate, review all other significant and life-threatening adverse reactions and interactions, especially those related to the drugs, tests, and behaviors mentioned above.

chlorothiazide

Diuril

Pharmacologic class: Thiazide
Therapeutic class: Diuretic, antihypertensive
Pregnancy risk category B

Action

Increases sodium and water excretion and inhibits sodium reabsorption in distal tubule, thereby promoting excretion of chloride, potassium, magnesium, and bicarbonate

Availability

Oral suspension: 250 mg/5 ml
Powder for injection: 500 mg
Tablets: 250 mg, 500 mg

C

Indications and dosages

➤ Edema associated with heart failure, renal dysfunction, cirrhosis, corticosteroid therapy, or estrogen therapy
Adults: 0.5 to 1 g P.O. daily as a single dose or in two divided doses
Children ages 3 to 6 months: 10 to 20 mg/kg P.O. daily as a single dose or in two divided doses

➤ Mild to moderate hypertension
Adults: 0.5 to 1 g P.O. daily as a single dose or in divided doses. Adjust dosage to blood pressure response.
Children: 10 to 20 mg/kg P.O. daily as a single dose or in two divided doses, not to exceed 375 mg/day (2.5 to 7.5 ml or ½ to 1½ tsp of oral suspension) in infants up to age 2, or 1 g/day in children ages 2 to 12. Infants younger than 6 months may require up to 30 mg/kg daily in two divided doses.

Contraindications

- Hypersensitivity to drug, other thiazides, benzodiazepines, sulfonamides, or tartrazine
- Anuria
- Gout
- Systemic lupus erythematosus
- Glucose tolerance abnormalities
- Hyperparathyroidism
- Bipolar disorder
- Breastfeeding

Precautions

Use cautiously in:
- renal or severe hepatic impairment
- pregnant patients.

Administration

- Be aware that drug is given I.V. in emergency use and for patients unable to receive oral form. I.V. dosage is individualized; use smallest dosage needed to achieve response.

• Know that drug is not safe for I.M. or subcutaneous use, and that I.V. use in children is not recommended.
• Be aware that drug may be ineffective in patients with renal insufficiency.
• Rarely, patients may require up to 2 g/day in divided doses.

Route	Onset	Peak	Duration
P.O.	2 hr	4 hr	6-12 hr
I.V.	15 min	30 min	Unknown

Adverse reactions

CNS: dizziness, drowsiness, lethargy, headache, insomnia, nervousness, vertigo, paresthesia, confusion, fatigue, asterixis, **encephalopathy**
CV: hypotension, ECG changes, chest pain, **thrombophlebitis, arrhythmias**
EENT: nystagmus
GI: nausea, vomiting, abdominal cramps, pancreatitis, anorexia
GU: polyuria, nocturia, erectile dysfunction, loss of libido
Hematologic: blood dyscrasias
Hepatic: jaundice, **hepatitis**
Metabolic: dehydration, hypovolemia, hyperglycemia, hypokalemia, hypocalcemia, hypomagnesemia, hyponatremia, hypophosphatemia, hyperuricemia, gout attack, **hypochloremic alkalosis**
Musculoskeletal: muscle cramps or spasms
Skin: photosensitivity, rash, urticaria, flushing
Other: fever, weight loss, hypersensitivity reactions

Interactions

Drug-drug. *Allopurinol:* increased risk of hypersensitivity reaction
Amphotericin B, corticosteroids, mezlocillin, piperacillin, ticarcillin: additive hypokalemia
Antihypertensives, barbiturates, nitrates, opiates: increased hypotension
Cholestyramine, colestipol: increased chlorothiazide absorption
Digoxin: increased risk of hypokalemia
Lithium: decreased lithium excretion, lithium toxicity
Nonsteroidal anti-inflammatory drugs: decreased chlorothiazide efficacy
Drug-diagnostic tests. *Bilirubin, serum and urine glucose (in diabetic patients), calcium, creatinine, uric acid:* increased levels
Cholesterol, low-density lipoproteins (LDLs), triglycerides: decreased levels
Magnesium, potassium, protein-bound iodine, sodium: decreased levels
Urine calcium: decreased level
Drug-herbs. *Ginkgo:* decreased antihypertensive effect
Licorice, stimulant laxative herbs (aloe, cascara sagrada, senna): increased risk of hypokalemia
Drug-behaviors. *Acute alcohol ingestion:* additive hypotension
Sun exposure: increased risk of photosensitivity

Patient monitoring

• Monitor blood pressure.
• Assess electrolyte, bilirubin, creatinine, uric acid, magnesium, cholesterol, LDL, and triglyceride levels.
• Monitor urine calcium level.
• Evaluate blood and urine glucose levels in patients with diabetes.

Patient teaching

• Advise patient to take drug in morning to avoid sleep interruptions caused by nighttime voiding.
🔊 Instruct patient to immediately report yellowing of eyes or skin, nausea, vomiting, diarrhea, fatigue, or lethargy.
• Advise patient not to stop taking drug abruptly. Advise him to discuss dosage-tapering schedule with prescriber.
• Caution patient to use alcohol cautiously, if at all.
• Inform patient that drug makes him prone to dehydration. Tell him to stay indoors in hot weather and to increase fluid intake if he sweats more than usual.

• As appropriate, review all other significant and life-threatening adverse reactions and interactions, especially those related to the drugs, tests, herbs, and behaviors mentioned above.

chlorpheniramine maleate

Aller-Chlor, Allergy Chlo-Amine, Chlorate, Chlor-Trimeton, Chlor-Trimeton Allergy 4 Hour, Chlor-Trimeton Allergy 8 Hour, Chlor-Trimeton Allergy 12 Hour, Chlor-Tripolon✤, Novo-Pheniram✤, PediaCare Allergy Formula, Phenetron, Teldrin, Telachlor

Pharmacologic class: Propylamine (nonselective)
Therapeutic class: Antihistamine; allergy, cold, and cough remedy
Pregnancy risk category B

Action
Antagonizes effects of histamine at histamine$_2$-receptor sites, preventing histamine-mediated responses

Availability
Capsules (sustained-release): 8 mg, 12 mg
Syrup: 1 mg/5 ml, 2 mg/5 ml, 2.5 mg/5 ml
Tablets: 4 mg, 8 mg, 12 mg
Tablets (chewable): 2 mg
Tablets (timed-release): 8 mg, 12 mg

Indications and dosages
➢ Allergy symptoms; management of anaphylaxis and transfusion reactions
Adults: 4 mg q 4 to 6 hours P.O. or 8 to 12 mg P.O. of sustained-release form q 8 to 12 hours. Maximum dosage is 24 mg/day.
Children ages 6 to 12: 2 mg P.O. q 4 to 6 hours daily. Maximum dosage is 12 mg/day.

Dosage adjustment
• Glaucoma
• Gastric ulcer
• Hyperthyroidism
• Heart disease

Contraindications
• Hypersensitivity to drug
• Acute asthma attacks
• Stenosing peptic ulcer
• Breastfeeding

Precautions
Use cautiously in:
• hepatic or renal disease, asthma, angle-closure glaucoma, prostatic hypertrophy
• elderly patients
• pregnant patients (safety not established).

Administration
• Don't crush or break timed-release tablets or sustained-release capsules.
• Discontinue drug 4 days before allergy skin tests. (Drug may cause false-negative reactions.)

Route	Onset	Peak	Duration
P.O.	15-30 min	1-2 hr	4-12 hr
P.O. (sustained)	Unknown	Unknown	Unknown

Adverse reactions
CNS: dizziness, drowsiness, excitation (in children), sedation, poor coordination, fatigue, confusion, restlessness, nervousness, tremor, headache, hysteria, tingling sensation, sensation of heaviness and weakness in hands
CV: palpitations, hypotension, bradycardia, tachycardia, extrasystoles, **arrhythmias**
EENT: blurred vision, diplopia, vertigo, tinnitus, acute labyrinthitis, nasal congestion, dry nose, dry throat, sore throat
GI: nausea, vomiting, diarrhea, constipation, epigastric distress, anorexia, dry mouth, **GI obstruction**

GU: urinary retention, urinary hesitancy, dysuria, early menses, decreased libido, erectile dysfunction
Hematologic: hemolytic anemia, hypoplastic anemia, thrombocytopenia, leukopenia, pancytopenia, agranulocytosis
Respiratory: thickened bronchial secretions, chest tightness, wheezing
Skin: urticaria, rash, photosensitivity, diaphoresis
Other: chills, increased appetite, weight gain, **anaphylactic shock**

Interactions

Drug-drug. *Anticholinergics, anticholinergic-like drugs (such as some antidepressants, atropine, haloperidol, phenothiazines, quinidine, disopyramide):* additive anticholinergic effects
CNS depressants (such as opioids, sedative-hypnotics): additive CNS depression
MAO inhibitors: intensified, prolonged anticholinergic effects
Drug-diagnostic tests. *Allergy skin tests:* false-negative reactions
Drug-behaviors. *Alcohol use:* additive CNS depression
Sun exposure: photosensitivity

Patient monitoring

- Assess for urinary retention and frequency.
- Monitor respiratory status throughout therapy.

Patient teaching

- Advise patient to take with full glass of water.
- Tell patient not to crush timed-release tablets or sustained-release capsules. Instruct him to swallow them whole.
- Caution patient to avoid driving and other hazardous activities until he knows how drug affects concentration and alertness.
- Advise parents to give dose to children in evening, because morning doses may cause inattention in school.
- As appropriate, review all other significant and life-threatening adverse reactions and interactions, especially those related to the drugs, tests, and behaviors mentioned above.

chlorpromazine hydrochloride

Chlorpromanyl✦, Largactil✦, Novo-Chlorpromazine✦, Thorazine, Thorazine Spansule

Pharmacologic class: Phenothiazine
Therapeutic class: Antipsychotic, anxiolytic, antiemetic
Pregnancy risk category C

Action

Unknown. May block postsynaptic dopamine receptors in brain and depress areas involved in wakefulness and emesis. Also possesses anticholinergic, antihistaminic, and adrenergic-blocking properties.

Availability

Capsules (sustained-release): 30 mg, 75 mg, 150 mg, 200 mg, 300 mg
Injection: 25 mg/ml
Oral concentrate: 30 mg/ml, 40 mg/ml, 100 mg/ml
Suppositories: 25 mg, 100 mg
Syrup: 10 mg/5 ml, 25 mg/5 ml, 100 mg/5 ml
Tablets: 10 mg, 25 mg, 50 mg, 100 mg, 200 mg

Indications and dosages

➢ Acute schizophrenia or mania
Adults: *Hospitalized patients*—Initially, 25 mg I.M; if necessary, give an additional 25 to 50 mg in 1 hour. Increase dosage gradually, as needed, for several

days (up to 400 mg q 4 to 6 hours in exceptionally severe cases) until symptoms are controlled; then give 500 mg P.O. daily. In less acutely disturbed patients, 25 mg P.O. t.i.d., increased gradually until effective dosage is reached (usually 400 mg P.O. daily). *Acutely disturbed outpatients*—Initially, 10 mg P.O. three or four times daily or 25 mg P.O. two or three times daily. In more severe cases, 25 mg P.O. t.i.d.; after 1 or 2 days, increase daily dosage by 20 to 50 mg at semiweekly intervals until effective dosage is reached.
Children ages 6 months to 12 years: 0.55 mg/kg P.O. (15 mg/m^2) q 4 to 6 hours as needed, or 0.55 mg/kg I.M. (15 mg/m^2) q 6 to 8 hours (not to exceed 40 mg/day in children ages 6 months to 5 years, or 75 mg/day in children ages 6 to 12), or 1 mg/kg P.R. q 6 to 8 hours p.r.n.

➢ Nausea and vomiting
Adults: 10 to 25 mg P.O. q 4 to 6 hours, increased if necessary; or 25 mg I.M. If no hypertension occurs, give 25 to 50 mg I.M. q 3 to 4 hours as needed until vomiting stops; then switch to oral dosing or one 100-mg suppository q 6 to 8 hours p.r.n.

➢ Nausea and vomiting during surgery
Adults: 12.5 mg I.M., repeated in 30 minutes p.r.n. if no hypotension occurs; or 2 mg I.V. at 2-minute intervals (not to exceed 25 mg)
Children ages 6 months to 12 years: 0.275 mg/kg I.M.; may repeat in 30 minutes as needed

➢ Preoperative sedation
Adults: 25 to 50 mg P.O. 2 to 3 hours before surgery, or 12.5 to 25 mg I.M. 1 to 2 hours before surgery
Children ages 6 months to 12 years: 0.55 mg/kg P.O. (15 mg/m^2) 2 to 3 hours before surgery, or 0.55 mg/kg I.M. 1 to 2 hours before surgery

➢ Intractable hiccups
Adults: 25 to 50 mg P.O. three to four times daily. If symptoms continue for 2 to 3 days, give 25 to 50 mg I.M.; if symptoms still persist, give 25 to 50 mg by slow I.V. infusion with patient positioned flat in bed.

➢ Acute intermittent porphyria
Adults: 25 to 50 mg P.O. three to four times daily. Drug usually is discontinued after several weeks, but some patients require maintenance doses. Or 25 mg I.M. t.i.d. until patient can tolerate oral doses.

➢ Tetanus
Adults: 25 to 50 mg P.O. three to four times daily (given with barbiturates, as prescribed). Total dosage and frequency determined by patient response.
Children ages 6 months to 12 years: 0.55 mg/kg I.M. or 0.55 mg/kg I.V. q 6 to 8 hours

Dosage adjustment
- Age over 60

Off-label uses
- Anxiety disorders
- Migraine
- Phencyclidine (PCP) psychosis

Contraindications
- Hypersensitivity to drug, other phenothiazines, sulfites (injection), benzyl alcohol (sustained-release capsules)
- Angle-closure glaucoma
- Bone marrow depression
- Severe hepatic or cardiovascular disease

Precautions
Use cautiously in:
- diabetes mellitus, respiratory disease, prostatic hypertrophy, CNS tumors, epilepsy, intestinal obstruction
- elderly patients
- pregnant or breastfeeding patients
- children.

Administration
Know that I.V. infusion is recommended only for severe hiccups.

• When giving by I.V. infusion for intractable hiccups, dilute in 500 to 1,000 ml of normal saline solution and infuse slowly.
• For direct I.V. injection, dilute to 1 mg/ml using normal saline solution. Administer at a rate of at least 1 mg/minute for adults or 2 mg/minute for children.
• When giving I.M., use Z-track injection method to minimize tissue irritation.
• Don't inject subcutaneously.
• Know that in preoperative use, drug increases risk of neuromuscular excitation and hypotension when followed by barbiturate anesthetics.

Route	Onset	Peak	Duration
P.O.	30-60 min	Unknown	4-6 hr
P.O. (sustained)	30-60 min	Unknown	10-12 hr
I.V.	Rapid	Unknown	Unknown
I.M.	Unknown	Unknown	4-8 hr
P.R.	1-2 hr	Unknown	3-4 hr

Adverse reactions

CNS: sedation, drowsiness, extrapyramidal reactions, tardive dyskinesia, pseudoparkinsonism, **neuroleptic malignant syndrome, seizures**
CV: tachycardia, hypotension (especially with I.M. or I.V. use)
EENT: blurred vision, dry eyes, lens opacities, nasal congestion
GI: constipation, ileus, anorexia, dry mouth
GU: urinary retention, menstrual irregularities, galactorrhea, gynecomastia, inhibited ejaculation, priapism
Hematologic: eosinophilia, **agranulocytosis, leukopenia, hemolytic anemia, aplastic anemia, thrombocytopenia**
Hepatic: jaundice, **hepatitis**
Skin: rash, photosensitivity, pigmentation changes, sterile abscess
Other: allergic reactions, hyperthermia, pain at injection site

Interactions

Drug-drug. *Activated charcoal, adsorbent antidiarrheals, antacids:* decreased chlorpromazine absorption
Antidepressants, antihistamines, general anesthetics, MAO inhibitors, opioids, sedative-hypnotics: additive CNS depression
Antihistamines, disopyramide, quinidine, tricyclic antidepressants (TCAs): increased anticholinergic effects
Antihypertensives: additive hypotension
Barbiturates: increased metabolism and decreased efficacy of chlorpromazine
Bromocriptine: decreased bromocriptine efficacy
Epinephrine: antagonism of peripheral vasoconstriction, epinephrine reversal
Guanethidine: inhibition of antihypertensive effects
Lithium: disorientation, loss of consciousness, extrapyramidal symptoms
Meperidine: excessive sedation and hypotension
Norepinephrine: reduced pressor effect, elimination of bradycardia
Phenytoin: altered phenytoin blood level, lowered seizure threshold
Pimozide: increased risk of potentially serious CV reactions
Propranolol: increased blood levels of both drugs
TCAs: increased TCA blood levels and effects
Valproic acid: decreased elimination and increased effects of valproic acid
Drug-diagnostic tests. *Alanine aminotransferase, alkaline phosphatase, aspartate aminotransferase, bilirubin:* increased levels
Granulocytes, hematocrit, hemoglobin, platelets, white blood cells: decreased values
Pregnancy tests: false-positive or false-negative result
Urine bilirubin: false-positive result

Drug-herbs. *Angel's trumpet, jimsonweed, scopolia:* increased anticholinergic effects
Chamomile, hops, kava, skullcap, valerian: increased CNS depression
St. John's wort: photosensitivity
Yohimbe: increased risk of toxicity
Drug-behaviors. *Alcohol use:* increased CNS depression
Sun exposure: increased risk of photosensitivity

Patient monitoring

- Monitor blood pressure closely during I.V. infusion.

🔊 Stay alert for signs and symptoms of neuroleptic malignant syndrome (hyperpyrexia, muscle rigidity, altered mental status, irregular pulse or blood pressure, tachycardia, diaphoresis, and arrhythmias). Stop drug immediately if these occur.

- Assess for extrapyramidal symptoms.

Patient teaching

- Tell patient to take capsules or tablets with a full glass of water, with or without food.
- Instruct patient not to crush sustained-release capsules.
- Tell patient to mix oral concentrate in juice, soda, applesauce, or pudding.
- Caution patient to avoid driving and other hazardous activities until he knows how drug affects concentration and alertness.
- As appropriate, review all other significant and life-threatening adverse reactions and interactions, especially those related to the drugs, tests, herbs, and behaviors mentioned above.

chlorpropamide

Apo-Chlorpropamide♣, Chloronase♣, Diabinese, Novo-Propamide♣

Pharmacologic class: Sulfonylurea
Therapeutic class: Hypoglycemic
Pregnancy risk category C

Action

Unclear. Thought to reduce blood glucose level primarily by stimulating secretion of endogenous insulin from pancreatic beta cells.

Availability

Tablets: 100 mg, 250 mg

Indications and dosages

➤ To lower glucose level in patients with non-insulin-dependent (type 2) diabetes mellitus
Adults: 250 mg P.O. daily with breakfast, increased as necessary to a maximum dosage of 750 mg daily
➤ To convert from insulin therapy to oral hypoglycemic therapy
Adults: For patient on 40 units of insulin or less, stop insulin and start chlorpropamide at 250 mg P.O. daily. If patient is receiving more than 40 units of insulin, start chlorpropamide at 250 mg P.O. daily, with insulin dosage reduced 50%; further insulin decreases depend on patient response.

Dosage adjustment

- Renal impairment
- Debilitated patients
- Elderly patients

Off-label uses

- Diabetes insipidus

Contraindications

- Hypersensitivity to drug

- Diabetic ketoacidosis
- Insulin-dependent (type 1) diabetes mellitus

Precautions

Use cautiously in:

- insulin hypersensitivity, hepatic or renal impairment, severe infection, trauma, major surgery
- elderly patients
- pregnant or breastfeeding patients.

Administration

- Give before meals for best results.
- If drug causes GI upset, give with food.
- To prevent hypoglycemia, adjust dosage during times of stress, illness, or decreased caloric intake.

Route	Onset	Peak	Duration
P.O.	1 hr	2-4 hr	24 hr

Adverse reactions

CNS: paresthesia, fatigue, dizziness, vertigo, malaise, headache
CV: increased risk of CV mortality
EENT: tinnitus
GI: nausea, heartburn, epigastric distress
GU: tea-colored urine
Hematologic: leukopenia, thrombocytopenia, aplastic anemia, agranulocytosis, hemolytic anemia
Hepatic: cholestatic jaundice
Metabolic: dilutional hyponatremia, **prolonged hypoglycemia**
Skin: rash, pruritus, erythema, urticaria
Other: hypersensitivity reaction, **disulfiram-like reaction**

Interactions

Drug-drug. *Anabolic steroids, chloramphenicol, clofibrate, guanethidine, MAO inhibitors, salicylates, sulfonamides:* increased hypoglycemia
Beta-adrenergic blockers: prolonged hypoglycemia
Corticosteroids, glucagons, rifampin, thiazide diuretics: decreased hypoglycemic response
Hydantoins: increased hydantoin blood level
Oral anticoagulants: increased hypoglycemic activity
Drug-diagnostic tests. *Alanine aminotransferase, alkaline phosphatase, aspartate aminotransferase, bilirubin, blood urea nitrogen, cholesterol, creatinine, lactate dehydrogenase:* increased levels
Glucose, granulocytes, hemoglobin, platelets, sodium, white blood cells: decreased values
Drug-herbs. *Bitter melon, burdock, dandelion, eucalyptus, ginkgo, marshmallow:* increased hypoglycemic activity
Drug-behaviors. *Alcohol use:* altered glycemic control (most commonly leading to hypoglycemia), disulfiram-like reaction

Patient monitoring

- Assess serum electrolyte levels before starting therapy.
- Watch for signs and symptoms of jaundice.
- Monitor patient for fluid and electrolyte imbalances.
- Check blood pressure frequently.
- Monitor urine for ketones and glucose.

Patient teaching

- If patient takes drug once daily, instruct him to take dose before breakfast. If he takes it more than once daily, advise him to take doses before meals.
- Teach patient how to recognize signs and symptoms of hypoglycemia (such as shaking, irritability, flushed skin, and inability to think clearly). Tell him to keep orange juice or other high-energy food available at all times to raise blood glucose level quickly. Instruct him to report hypoglycemia promptly.
- Advise patient to immediately report yellowing of eyes or skin.

• Teach patient how to test urine or blood for glucose. Stress the need for regular testing.

Clinical alert: If patient is switching from insulin, instruct him to test his urine three times a day for glucose and ketones and to immediately report positive results.

• Emphasize importance of following recommendations regarding diet, exercise, and weight loss (if needed) to help control diabetes.

• Urge patient to consult prescriber before breastfeeding. Drug may cause hypoglycemia in infant.

• Caution patient not to take over-the-counter weight-loss, cough, cold, or allergy preparations without consulting prescriber.

• As appropriate, review all other significant and life-threatening adverse reactions and interactions, especially those related to the drugs, tests, herbs, and behaviors mentioned above.

chlorthalidone

Apo-Chlorthalidone✱, Hygroton, Novo-Thalidone✱, Thalitone, Uridon✱

Pharmacologic class: Thiazide-like diuretic

Therapeutic class: Diuretic, antihypertensive

Pregnancy risk category B

Action

Unclear. Enhances excretion of sodium, chloride, and water by interfering with transport of sodium ions across renal tubular epithelium. Also may dilate arterioles.

Availability

Tablets: 15 mg, 25 mg, 50 mg, 100 mg

Indications and dosages

➢ Edema associated with heart failure, renal dysfunction, cirrhosis, corticosteroid therapy, and estrogen therapy

Adults: 50 to 100 mg/day (30 to 60 mg Thalitone) P.O. or 100 mg every other day (60 mg Thalitone) P.O., up to 200 mg/day (120 mg Thalitone) P.O.

➢ Management of mild to moderate hypertension

Adults: 25 mg/day (15 mg Thalitone) P.O. Based on patient response, may increase to 50 mg/day (30 to 50 mg Thalitone) P.O., then up to 100 mg/day (except Thalitone) P.O.

Contraindications

• Hypersensitivity to drug, other thiazides, sulfonamides, or tartrazine

• Renal decompensation

Precautions

Use cautiously in:

• renal or severe hepatic disease, abnormal glucose tolerance, gout, systemic lupus erythematosus, hyperparathyroidism, bipolar disorder

• elderly patients

• pregnant or breastfeeding patients.

Administration

• Know that dosages above 25 mg/day are likely to increase potassium excretion without further increasing sodium excretion or reducing blood pressure.

Route	Onset	Peak	Duration
P.O.	2 hr	4 hr	48-72 hr

Adverse reactions

CNS: dizziness, vertigo, drowsiness, lethargy, confusion, headache, insomnia, nervousness, paresthesia, asterixis, nystagmus, **encephalopathy**

CV: hypotension, ECG changes, chest pain, **arrhythmias, thrombophlebitis**

GI: nausea, vomiting, cramping, anorexia, pancreatitis

GU: polyuria, nocturia, erectile dysfunction, loss of libido

Hematologic: blood dyscrasias
Metabolic: gout attack, dehydration, hyperglycemia, hypokalemia, hypocalcemia, hypomagnesemia, hyponatremia, hypophosphatemia, hyperuricemia, hyperlipidemia, **hypochloremic alkalosis**
Musculoskeletal: muscle cramps, muscle spasms
Skin: flushing, photosensitivity, hives, rash, exfoliative dermatitis, **toxic epidermal necrolysis**
Other: fever, weight loss, hypersensitivity reactions

Interactions

Drug-drug. *Allopurinol:* increased risk of hypersensitivity reaction
Amphotericin B, corticosteroids, mezlocillin, piperacillin, ticarcillin: additive hypokalemia
Antihypertensives, barbiturates, nitrates, opiates: increased hypotension
Cholestyramine, colestipol: decreased chlorthalidone blood level
Digoxin: increased risk of hypokalemia
Lithium: increased risk of lithium toxicity
Nonsteroidal anti-inflammatory drugs: decreased diuretic effect
Drug-diagnostic tests. *Bilirubin, calcium, creatinine, uric acid:* increased levels
Glucose (in diabetic patients): increased blood and urine levels
Magnesium, potassium, protein-bound iodine, sodium, urine calcium: decreased levels
Drug-herbs. *Ginkgo:* decreased antihypertensive effects
Licorice, stimulant laxative herbs (aloe, cascara sagrada, senna): increased risk of potassium depletion
Drug-behaviors. *Acute alcohol ingestion:* additive hypotension
Sun exposure: increased risk of photosensitivity

Patient monitoring

- Closely monitor patient with renal insufficiency.
- Assess for signs and symptoms of hematologic disorders.
- Monitor CBC with white cell differential and serum uric acid and electrolyte levels.
- Assess for signs and symptoms of hypersensitivity reactions, especially dermatitis.
- Watch for fluid and electrolyte imbalances.

Patient teaching

- Instruct patient to consume a low-sodium diet containing plenty of potassium-rich foods and beverages (such as bananas, green leafy vegetables, and citrus juice).
- Caution patient to avoid driving and other hazardous activities until he knows whether drug makes him dizzy or affects concentration and alertness.
- Tell patient with diabetes to check urine or blood glucose level frequently.
- As appropriate, review all other significant and life-threatening adverse reactions and interactions, especially those related to the drugs, tests, herbs, and behaviors mentioned above.

chlorzoxazone

EZE-DS, Parafon Forte DSC, Relaxazone, Remular, Remular-S, Strifon Forte DSC

Pharmacologic class: Autonomic nervous system agent
Therapeutic class: Skeletal muscle relaxant (centrally acting)
Pregnancy risk category C

Action

Unclear. Thought to act on spinal cord and subcortical levels of brain, inhibiting multisynaptic reflex arcs responsible for skeletal muscle activity.

Availability

Caplets: 250 mg, 500 mg
Tablets: 250 mg, 500 mg

Indications and dosages

➤ Adjunct to rest and physical therapy in treatment of muscle spasms associated with acute, painful musculoskeletal conditions
Adults: 250 to 750 mg P.O. three to four times daily

Contraindications

- Hypersensitivity to drug
- Hepatic impairment

Precautions

Use cautiously in:
- underlying cardiovascular disease, renal impairment
- children (safety not established).

Administration

- If desired, crush tablets and mix contents with food or water.
- Don't withdraw drug abruptly.

Route	Onset	Peak	Duration
P.O.	30-60 min	1-2 hr	3-4 hr

Adverse reactions

CNS: dizziness, drowsiness, lightheadedness, malaise, headache, overstimulation, tremor
GI: nausea, vomiting, constipation, diarrhea, heartburn, abdominal distress, anorexia
GU: orange or purplish-red urine
Hepatic: hepatic dysfunction
Skin: allergic dermatitis, urticaria, erythema, pruritus, petechiae, ecchymosis, **angioedema**
Other: allergic reactions

Interactions

Drug-drug. *CNS depressants (including antihistamines, antidepressants, opioids, sedative-hypnotics):* increased risk of CNS depression
Drug-diagnostic tests. *Alanine aminotransferase, alkaline phosphatase, bilirubin:* increased levels
Drug-herbs. *Chamomile, hops, kava, skullcap, valerian:* increased CNS depression
Drug-behaviors. *Alcohol use:* increased sedation

Patient monitoring

🔊 Stay alert for signs and symptoms of hepatic dysfunction. Withhold drug and notify prescriber if these occur.
- Monitor hepatic enzyme and serum electrolyte levels.

Patient teaching

🔊 Instruct patient to promptly report yellowing of eyes or skin.
- Caution patient not to consume alcohol during therapy.
- Instruct patient to avoid driving and other hazardous activities until he knows how drug affects concentration and alertness.
- Tell patient that drug may turn his urine orange or purplish-red.
- As appropriate, review all other significant and life-threatening adverse reactions and interactions, especially those related to the drugs, tests, herbs, and behaviors mentioned above.

cholestyramine

LoCHOLEST, LoCHOLEST Light, Novo-Cholamine✱, Novo-Cholamine Light✱, Prevalite, Questran, Questran Light

Pharmacologic class: Bile acid sequestrant
Therapeutic class: Lipid-lowering agent
Pregnancy risk category C

Action

Combines with bile acid in GI tract to form insoluble complex excreted in feces. Complex regulates and increases cholesterol synthesis, thereby decreasing serum cholesterol and low-density lipoprotein levels.

Availability

Powder for suspension; powder for suspension with aspartame: 4 g cholestyramine/packet or scoop

Indications and dosages

➤ Primary hypercholesterolemia and pruritus caused by biliary obstruction; primary hyperlipidemia

Adults: Initially, 4 g P.O. once or twice daily. May increase as needed and tolerated, up to 24 g/day in six divided doses.

Off-label uses

- Antibiotic–induced pseudomembranous colitis
- Adjunct in infantile diarrhea
- Digoxin toxicity

Contraindications

- Hypersensitivity to drug, its components, or other bile-acid sequestering resins
- Complete biliary obstruction
- Phenylketonuria (suspension containing aspartame)

Precautions

Use cautiously in:

- history of constipation or abnormal intestinal function
- pregnant patients
- children.

Administration

- Mix powder with soup, cereal, pulpy fruit, juice, milk, or water.
- Administer 1 hour before or 4 to 6 hours after other drugs.
- Be aware that fat-soluble vitamin supplements may be necessary with long-term drug use.

Route	Onset	Peak	Duration
P.O.	24-48 hr	1-3 wk	2-4 wk

Adverse reactions

CNS: headache, anxiety, vertigo, dizziness, insomnia, fatigue, syncope
EENT: tinnitus
GI: nausea, vomiting, constipation, abdominal discomfort, fecal impaction, flatulence, hemorrhoids, perianal irritation, steatorrhea
GU: hematuria, dysuria, diuresis, burnt odor to urine
Hematologic: anemia, ecchymosis
Hepatic: hepatic dysfunction
Metabolic: vitamin A, D, E, and K deficiencies; **hyperchloremic acidosis**
Musculoskeletal: joint pain, arthritis, back pain, muscle pain
Respiratory: wheezing, asthma
Skin: hypersensitivity reaction (irritation, rash, urticaria)
Other: tongue irritation

Interactions

Drug-drug. *Acetaminophen, amiodarone, clindamycin, clofibrate, corticosteroids, digoxin, diuretics, fat-soluble vitamins (A, D, E, and K), gemfibrozil, glipizide, imipramine, methotrexate, methyldopa, mycophenolate, niacin, nonsteroidal anti-inflammatory drugs, penicillin, phenytoin, phosphates, propranolol, tetracyclines, tolbutamide, thyroid preparations, ursodiol, warfarin:* decreased absorption and effects of these drugs

Drug-diagnostic tests. *Alkaline phosphatase:* increased level
Hemoglobin: decreased value
Prothrombin time: increased

Patient monitoring

- Monitor CBC with white cell differential and liver function test results.

• If bleeding or bruising occurs, monitor prothrombin time. Drug may reduce vitamin K absorption.
• Watch for constipation, especially in patients with coronary artery disease. Take appropriate steps to prevent this problem.

Patient teaching

• Instruct patient to immediately report yellowing of skin or eyes or easy bruising or bleeding.
• Tell patient to take drug 1 hour before or 4 to 6 hours after other drugs.
• Teach patient about role of diet in controlling cholesterol level and preventing constipation.
• Instruct patient to avoid inhaling or ingesting raw powder. Tell him to mix powder with food, juice, or milk before consuming.
• As appropriate, review all other significant and life-threatening adverse reactions and interactions, especially those related to the drugs and tests mentioned above.

cidofovir

Vistide

Pharmacologic class: Purine nucleotide cytosine analog
Therapeutic class: Antiviral
Pregnancy risk category C

Action

Exerts antiviral effect by interfering with DNA synthesis of cytomegalovirus (CMV), thereby inhibiting viral replication

Availability

Solution for injection: 75 mg/ml in 5-ml, single-use vials

Indications and dosages

➢ CMV retinitis in AIDS patients
Adults: 5 mg/kg I.V. infused over 1 hour q week for 2 continuous weeks; then 5 mg/kg I.V. once q 2 weeks as a maintenance dose

Dosage adjustment

• Renal impairment

Contraindications

• Hypersensitivity to drug, probenecid, or other sulfa-containing agents
• Creatinine level above 1.5 mg/dl, calculated creatinine clearance of 55 ml/minute or less, or urine protein level of 100 mg/dl or higher
• Concurrent use of nephrotoxic drugs

Precautions

Use cautiously in:
• mild renal impairment
• elderly patients
• pregnant or breastfeeding patients
• children younger than age 12 (safety and efficacy not established).

Administration

• Be aware that drug carries a high risk of nephrotoxicity. Follow administration instructions carefully, including preinfusion and postinfusion hydration with I.V. normal saline solution.
• Premedicate with probenecid 2 g P.O., as prescribed, 3 hours before starting cidofovir infusion.
• Before starting infusion, give 1 L of normal saline solution over 1 to 2 hours.
• Mix I.V. dose in 100 ml of normal saline solution and infuse over 1 hour using infusion pump.
• Give 1 L of normal saline solution during or immediately after cidofovir infusion (unless contraindicated).
• Administer probenecid 1 g 2 hours and 8 hours after infusion ends, as prescribed.

If drug touches skin, flush thoroughly with water.

Route	Onset	Peak	Duration
I.V.	Rapid	End of infusion	Unknown

Adverse reactions

CNS: headache, **seizures, coma**
EENT: decreased intraocular pressure
GI: nausea, vomiting, diarrhea, anorexia, oral candidiasis
GU: proteinuria, **nephrotoxicity**
Hematologic: neutropenia
Hepatic: hepatomegaly
Metabolic: metabolic acidosis
Musculoskeletal: muscle contractions
Respiratory: dyspnea, increased cough
Skin: rash, alopecia
Other: pain, fever, chills, infection, pain at I.V. site

Interactions

Drug-drug. *Nephrotoxic drugs:* increased risk of nephrotoxicity
Drug-diagnostic tests. *Alanine aminotransferase, alkaline phosphatase, aspartate aminotransferase, blood urea nitrogen, creatinine, lactate dehydrogenase:* increased values
Bicarbonate, creatinine clearance, hemoglobin, neutrophils, platelets: decreased values

Patient monitoring

- Assess white blood cell count and creatinine and urine protein levels within 48 hours of each dose.
- Closely monitor intraocular pressure and visual acuity.
- Monitor hepatic enzyme levels in patients with hepatic disease.

Patient teaching

Tell patient to immediately report fever, vision changes, nausea, vomiting, rash, or urinary output changes.
- Instruct patient to take probenecid, as prescribed, before each dose and to have regular eye examinations.
- Urge female patient of childbearing age to use effective contraception during and for 1 month after therapy.
- Instruct male patients to use barrier contraception during and for 3 months after therapy.
- As appropriate, review all other significant and life-threatening adverse reactions and interactions, especially those related to the drugs and tests mentioned above.

cilostazol
Pletal

Pharmacologic class: Quinolone derivative
Therapeutic class: Antiplatelet agent
Pregnancy risk category C

Action

Unclear. Thought to inhibit phosphodiesterase III by increasing cyclic adenosine monophosphate in platelets and blood vessels, causing vasodilation and enhancing cardiac contractility and coronary blood flow

Availability

Tablets: 50 mg, 100 mg

Indications and dosages

➢ Intermittent claudication
Adults: 100 mg P.O. b.i.d. at least 30 minutes before or 2 hours after breakfast and dinner

Dosage adjustment

- Concurrent use of diltiazem, erythromycin, itraconazole, ketoconazole, or omeprazole

Contraindications

- Hypersensitivity to drug
- Heart failure

Precautions

Use cautiously in:
- cardiovascular disorders
- patients receiving other antiplatelet agents concurrently
- pregnant or breastfeeding patients
- children (safety and efficacy not established).

Administration

- Give with water 30 minutes before or 2 hours after patient consumes food or milk.
- Don't give with grapefruit juice.
- Be aware that although response may occur within 2 to 3 weeks, patient should continue therapy for up to 12 weeks or as prescribed.

Route	Onset	Peak	Duration
P.O.	Gradual	4-6 hr	Unknown

Adverse reactions

CNS: dizziness, headache, vertigo
CV: tachycardia
GI: abdominal pain, abnormal stools, dyspepsia, flatulence
EENT: rhinitis, pharyngitis
Musculoskeletal: back pain, myalgia
Respiratory: increased cough
Other: infection

Interactions

Drug-drug. *CYP3A4 and CYP2C19 inhibitors, diltiazem, erythromycin, macrolides, omeprazole:* increased cilostazol blood level
Drug-food. *Grapefruit juice, high-fat meals:* increased cilostazol blood level
Drug-behaviors. *Smoking:* decreased exposure to cilostazol

Patient monitoring

- Monitor cardiovascular status.
- Closely monitor patient if he's receiving other antiplatelet drugs.

Patient teaching

- Instruct patient to take drug with full glass of water, 30 minutes before or 2 hours after food or milk.
- Tell patient not to drink grapefruit juice during therapy.
- Advise patient to report nausea, vomiting, or abdominal pain.
- Instruct patient not to smoke, because smoking impedes drug effects.
- As appropriate, review all other significant adverse reactions and interactions, especially those related to the drugs, foods, and behaviors mentioned above.

cimetidine

Apo-Cimetidine✦, Gen-Cimetidine✦, Novo-Cimetine✦, Nu-Cimet✦, Tagamet, Tagamet HB, Tagamet HB 200 Suspension

Pharmacologic class: Histamine$_2$-receptor antagonist
Therapeutic class: Antiulcer drug
Pregnancy risk category B

Action

Competitively inhibits histamine action at histamine$_2$-receptor sites of gastric parietal cells, thereby inhibiting gastric acid secretion

Availability

Oral liquid: 200 mg/5 ml, 300 mg/5 ml
Solution for injection: 300 mg/2-ml vials, 300 mg/50 ml premixed in normal saline solution
Tablets: 100 mg, 200 mg, 300 mg, 400 mg, 600 mg, 800 mg

Indications and dosages

➢ Active duodenal ulcer (short-term therapy)
Adults and children older than age 16: 800 mg P.O. at bedtime, or 300 mg P.O.

q.i.d. with meals and at bedtime, or 400 mg P.O. b.i.d. Maintenance dosage is 400 mg P.O. at bedtime.

➤ Active benign gastric ulcer (short-term therapy)

Adults and children older than age 16: 800 mg P.O. at bedtime or 300 mg P.O. q.i.d. with meals and at bedtime

➤ Gastric hypersecretory conditions (such as Zollinger-Ellison syndrome); intractable ulcers

Adults and children older than age 16: 300 mg P.O. q.i.d. with meals and at bedtime; in hospitalized patients, 300 mg I.M. or I.V. q 6 hours

➤ Erosive gastroesophageal reflux disease

Adults and children older than age 16: 1,600 mg P.O. daily in divided doses (800 mg b.i.d. or 400 mg q.i.d.) for 12 weeks

➤ Prevention of stress-induced upper GI bleeding in critically ill patients

Adults and children older than age 16: 50 mg/hour as a continuous I.V. infusion

➤ Heartburn; acid indigestion

Adults and children older than age 16: 200 mg (two tablets of over-the-counter product only) P.O. up to b.i.d. Give maximum dosage no longer than 2 weeks continuously, unless directed by prescriber.

Dosage adjustment

- Renal impairment

Off-label uses

- Acetaminophen overdose
- Adjunctive therapy in burns
- Barrett's esophagus
- Renal cancer
- Anaphylaxis

Contraindications

- Hypersensitivity to drug
- Alcohol intolerance (oral drug forms)

Precautions

Use cautiously in:

- renal impairment
- elderly patients
- pregnant or breastfeeding patients.

Administration

- Give P.O. doses with meals.
- Give I.M. doses undiluted.
- Dilute I.V. doses in normal saline solution or other compatible solution.
- Administer I.V. injection over at least 5 minutes; may give intermittent infusion over 15 to 20 minutes.
- Give continuous I.V. infusion at a rate of 37.5 mg/hour over 24 hours, using an infusion pump.
- When giving drug to prevent stress ulcers, administer by continuous I.V. infusion at a rate of 50 mg/hour.

Route	Onset	Peak	Duration
P.O.	30 min	45-90 min	4-5 hr
I.V., I.M.	10 min	30 min	4-5 hr

Adverse reactions

CNS: confusion, dizziness, drowsiness, hallucinations, agitation, psychosis, depression, anxiety, headache

GI: diarrhea

GU: reversible erectile dysfunction, gynecomastia

Other: pain at I.M. injection site

Interactions

Drug-drug. *Calcium channel blockers, carbamazepine, chloroquine, lidocaine, metformin, metronidazole, moricizine, pentoxifylline, phenytoin, propafenone, quinidine, quinine, some benzodiazepines, some beta-adrenergic blockers (chlordiazepoxide, diazepam, midazolam), sulfonylureas, tacrine, theophylline, triamterene, tricyclic antidepressants, valproic acid, warfarin:* decreased metabolism of these drugs, possible toxicity

Drug-diagnostic tests. *Creatinine, transaminases:* increased levels
Parathyroid hormone: decreased level
Prolactin (after I.V. bolus of cimetidine): increased level
Skin tests using allergenic extracts: false-negative results (drug should be discontinued 24 hours before testing)
Drug-food. *Caffeine-containing foods and beverages (such as coffee, chocolate):* increased cimetidine blood level, increased risk of toxicity
Drug-herbs. *Pennyroyal:* change in formation rate of herb's toxic metabolite
Yerba maté: decreased yerba maté clearance, possible toxicity
Drug-behaviors. *Alcohol use:* increased blood alcohol level

Patient monitoring

- Monitor creatinine levels in patients with renal insufficiency or failure.
- Assess elderly or chronically ill patients for confusion (which usually resolves once drug therapy ends).

Patient teaching

- Inform patient with gastric ulcer that ulcer may take up to 2 months to heal. Advise him not to discontinue therapy, even if he feels better, without first consulting prescriber. Ulcer may recur if therapy ends too soon.
- Advise patient not to take over-the-counter cimetidine for more than 2 weeks continuously, except with prescriber's advice and supervision.
- As appropriate, review all other significant adverse reactions and interactions, especially those related to the drugs, tests, foods, herbs, and behaviors mentioned above.

ciprofloxacin hydrochloride

Ciloxam, Cipro, Cipro HC Otic, Cipro I.V., Cipro XR

Pharmacologic class: Fluoroquinolone
Therapeutic class: Anti-infective
Pregnancy risk category C

Action

Inhibits bacterial DNA synthesis by inhibiting DNA gyrase in susceptible gram-negative and gram-positive organisms

Availability

Injection: 200 mg/20 ml, 400 mg/40 ml, 200 mg/100 ml premixed in dextrose 5% in water (D_5W), 400 mg/200 ml premixed in D_5W, 1,200 mg/120-ml bulk package
Ophthalmic ointment: 3.5-g tube
Ophthalmic solution: 2.5-ml and 5-ml plastic dispensers
Oral suspension: 5 g/100 ml (5%), 10 g/100 ml (10%)
Tablets: 250 mg, 500 mg, 750 mg
Tablets (extended-release): 500 mg, 1,000 mg

Indications and dosages

➢ Acute sinusitis
Adults: 500 mg P.O. q 12 hours or 400 mg I.V. for 10 days
➢ Prostatitis
Adults: 500 mg P.O. q 12 hours or 400 mg I.V. for 28 days
➢ Intra-abdominal infections
Adults: 500 mg P.O. q 12 hours or 400 mg I.V. for 7 to 14 days
➢ Febrile neutropenic patients
Adults: 400 mg I.V. q 8 hours for 7 to 14 days
➢ Gonorrhea
Adults: 500 mg P.O. as a single dose

➢ Infectious diarrhea
Adults: 500 mg P.O. q 12 hours for 5 to 7 days
➢ Inhalation anthrax (postexposure)
Adults: 500 mg P.O. q 12 hours for 60 days or 400 mg I.V. q 12 hours for 60 days
Children: 15 mg/kg P.O. q 12 hours for 60 days (not to exceed 500 mg/dose), or 10 mg/kg I.V. q 12 hours for 60 days, not to exceed 400 mg/dose
➢ Infections of lower respiratory tract, skin and skin structures, bones, and joints
Adults: 500 to 750 mg P.O. q 12 hours or 400 mg I.V. q 8 hours for 7 to 14 days. Severe bone and joint infections may necessitate up to 6 weeks of therapy.
➢ Nosocomial pneumonia
Adults: 400 mg I.V. q 8 hours for 10 to 14 days
➢ Typhoid fever
Adults: 500 mg P.O. q 12 hours for 10 days
➢ Urinary tract infections
Adults: 250 to 500 mg P.O. q 12 hours, or 500 to 1,000 mg Cipro XR P.O. daily, or 200 to 400 mg I.V. q 12 hours for 3 days in acute uncomplicated infection or for 7 to 14 days in mild to severe complicated infection
➢ Pyelonephritis
Adults: 1,000 mg Cipro XR P.O. daily for 7 to 14 days
➢ Bacterial conjunctivitis caused by susceptible organisms
Adults: 0.5" ribbon of ophthalmic ointment applied to conjunctival sac t.i.d. on first 2 days, then 0.5" ribbon b.i.d. for 5 days. Or one to two drops of ophthalmic solution applied to conjunctival sac q 2 hours while awake for 2 days, then one or two drops q 4 hours while awake for 5 days.
➢ Corneal ulcers caused by susceptible organisms
Adults: Two drops of ophthalmic solution instilled into affected eye q 15 minutes for first 6 hours, then two drops into affected eye q 30 minutes for remainder of first day. On second day, two drops of ophthalmic solution hourly; on days 3 through 14, two drops q 4 hours.

Dosage adjustment

• Renal impairment or insufficiency

Off-label uses

• Chancroid
• Cystic fibrosis
• Pseudomembranous colitis caused by anti-infectives

Contraindications

• Hypersensitivity to drug or other fluoroquinolones

Precautions

Use cautiously in:
• cirrhosis, renal impairment, underlying CNS disease
• elderly patients
• pregnant or breastfeeding patients
• children younger than age 18.

Administration

• Infuse I.V. dose over at least 1 hour, using pump to ensure 1-hour duration.
(Clinical alert) Know that too-rapid I.V. infusion increases risk of anaphylaxis and other adverse reactions.
• Be aware that oral suspension isn't suitable for use in nasogastric tube.
• Know that treatment with ophthalmic solution may be continued after 14 days if corneal re-epithelialization hasn't occurred.

Route	Onset	Peak	Duration
P.O.	Rapid	1-2 hr	12 hr
I.V.	Rapid	End of infusion	12 hr
Ophthal.	Unknown	Unknown	Unknown

Adverse reactions

CNS: agitation, headache, restlessness, confusion, delirium, **toxic psychosis**
CV: orthostatic hypotension, vasculitis
EENT: nystagmus; with ophthalmic use—blurred vision; burning, stinging, irritation, itching, tearing, and redness of eyes; eyelid itching, swelling, or crusting; sensitivity to light
GI: nausea, vomiting, diarrhea, constipation, abdominal pain or discomfort, dyspepsia, dysphagia, flatulence, pancreatitis, **pseudomembranous colitis**
GU: albuminuria, candiduria, renal calculi
Hematologic: methemoglobinemia, agranulocytosis, hemolytic anemia
Hepatic: jaundice, **hepatic necrosis**
Metabolic: hyperglycemia, **hyperkalemia**
Musculoskeletal: myalgia, myoclonus, tendinitis, tendon rupture
Skin: rash, exfoliative dermatitis, toxic epidermal necrolysis, **erythema multiforme**
Other: altered taste, anosmia, exacerbation of myasthenia gravis, overgrowth of nonsusceptible organisms, hypersensitivity reactions including **anaphylaxis** and **Stevens-Johnson syndrome**

Interactions

Drug-drug. *Antacids, bismuth subsalicylate, iron salts, sucralfate, zinc salts:* decreased ciprofloxacin absorption
Cyclosporine: transient creatinine increase
Hormonal contraceptives: reduced contraceptive efficacy
Oral anticoagulants: increased anticoagulant effects
Phenytoin: increased or decreased phenytoin blood level
Probenecid: decreased renal elimination of ciprofloxacin, causing increased blood level
Theophylline: increased theophylline blood level, greater risk of toxicity
Drug-diagnostic tests. *Alanine aminotransferase, alkaline phosphatase, aspartate aminotransferase, bilirubin, cholesterol, glucose, lactate dehydrogenase, potassium, triglycerides:* increased levels
Prothrombin time: prolonged
Drug-food. *Caffeine:* interference with caffeine clearance
Concurrent tube feedings, milk or yogurt (when consumed alone with ciprofloxacin): impaired drug absorption
Drug-herbs. *Fennel:* decreased drug absorption

Patient monitoring

- In patients with renal insufficiency, assess creatinine level before giving first dose and at least once a week during prolonged therapy. Monitor drug blood level closely.
- Watch for signs and symptoms of serious adverse reactions, including GI problems, jaundice, and hypersensitivity reactions.

Patient teaching

- Tell patient to take drug 2 hours after a meal.
- Advise patient not to take drug with dairy products alone or with caffeinated beverages.
- Instruct patient to swallow microcapsules in oral suspension whole without chewing.
- Advise patient to drink 8 oz of water every hour while awake to ensure adequate hydration.

Instruct patient to stop taking drug and notify prescriber at first sign of rash.

- Advise patient taking hormonal contraceptives to use supplemental birth control method, such as condoms, because drug reduces contraceptive efficacy.
- Inform breastfeeding patient that drug is excreted in breast milk and can affect infant's bone growth. Advise her to consult prescriber before using drug.

• Teach patient how to use eye ointment or solution.
• Tell patient not to touch eye dropper tip to any surface, to avoid contamination.
• Caution patient with bacterial conjunctivitis not to wear contact lenses.
• As appropriate, review all other significant and life-threatening adverse reactions and interactions, especially those related to the drugs, tests, foods, and herbs mentioned above.

cisatracurium besylate

Nimbex

Pharmacologic class: Neuromuscular blocker
Therapeutic class: Skeletal muscle relaxant
Pregnancy risk category B

Action

Competitively binds to cholinergic receptors on motor endplate, antagonizing the action of acetylcholine and blocking neuromuscular transmission

Availability

Injection: 2 mg/ml, 10 mg/ml

Indications and dosages

➢ Adjunct to general anesthesia; skeletal muscle relaxation during mechanical ventilation
Adults: Initially, 0.15 mg/kg I.V., then maintain on dosage of 0.03 mg/kg I.V. q 40 to 50 minutes; or initially, 0.2 mg/kg I.V., then maintain on dosage of 0.03 mg/kg I.V. q 50 to 60 minutes. Or initially, maintenance I.V. infusion of 3 mcg/kg/minute, titrated to 1 to 2 mcg/kg/minute p.r.n.
Children ages 2 to 12: 0.1 mg/kg I.V. over 5 to 10 seconds; then give maintenance infusion at 3 mcg/kg/minute, titrating to 1 to 2 mcg/kg/minute p.r.n.

Contraindications

• Hypersensitivity to drug

Precautions

Use cautiously in:
• neuromuscular disease, peripheral neuropathy
• concurrent anticonvulsant therapy
• pregnant or breastfeeding patients.

Administration

Clinical alert: Don't give drug unless mechanical ventilation support and emergency equipment are readily available.
• Know that initial dose may be given as I.V. bolus over 5 to 10 seconds, followed by continuous infusion at prescribed rate.
• Always use volume infusion pump or microdrip (60 gtt/ml).

Route	Onset	Peak	Duration
I.V.	1-2 min	2-5 min	25-44 min

Adverse reactions

CV: hypotension, flushing, **bradycardia**
Respiratory: bronchospasm, prolonged apnea
Skin: rash

Interactions

Drug-drug. *Aminoglycosides, bacitracin, clindamycin, colistimethate sodium, colistin, lincomycin, lithium, local anesthetics, magnesium salts, polymyxins, procainamide, quinidine, tetracyclines:* enhanced neuromuscular blockade
Carbamazepine, phenytoin: shortened duration of neuromuscular blockade
Enflurane or isoflurane given with nitrous oxide or oxygen: prolonged duration of cisatracurium action
Succinylcholine: faster onset of maximal neuromuscular blockade
Drug-herbs. *St. John's wort:* increased risk of cardiovascular collapse, delayed emergence from anesthesia

Patient monitoring

- Monitor vital signs and ECG. Stay alert for respiratory depression, bradycardia, and hypotension.
- Use peripheral nerve stimulator to monitor degree of neuromuscular blockade during administration. Continue to use nerve stimulator to monitor recovery from neuromuscular blockade after drug therapy ends.

Patient teaching

- Be aware that patient's hearing is intact during neuromuscular blockade. Continue to provide explanations and reassurance during this time.

cisplatin

Platinol, Platinol-AQ

Pharmacologic class: Alkylating agent, platinum coordination complex

Therapeutic class: Antineoplastic

Pregnancy risk category D

Action

Inhibits DNA synthesis by causing intrastrand and interstrand cross-linking of DNA

Availability

Injection: 1 mg/ml in 50-mg and 100-mg vials

Indications and dosages

➢ Metastatic testicular tumors

Adults: 20 mg/m² I.V. daily for 5 days/cycle, repeated q 3 to 4 weeks

➢ Metastatic ovarian cancer

Adults: 75 to 100 mg/m² I.V., repeated q 4 weeks in combination with cyclophosphamide; or 100 mg/m² q 4 weeks as a single agent

➢ Advanced bladder cancer

Adults: 50 to 70 mg/m² I.V. q 3 to 4 weeks as a single agent; dosage depends on whether patient has undergone radiation or chemotherapy.

Off-label uses

- Cervical cancer

Contraindications

- Hypersensitivity to drug or other platinum-containing compounds
- Severe impairment of renal function
- Severe myelosuppression
- Hearing impairment
- Pregnancy or breastfeeding

Precautions

Use cautiously in:

- mild to moderate renal impairment, active infection, myelosuppression, chronic debilitating illness, heart failure, electrolyte abnormalities
- females of childbearing age.

Administration

- Prepare drug with equipment that doesn't contain aluminum.
- Give 2 L of I.V. fluids, as prescribed, 8 to 12 hours before drug infusion to help prevent toxicity.
- Dilute each dose in 2 L of dextrose 5% in 1/4 or 1/2 saline solution or 0.9% normal saline solution. Do not use dextrose 5% in water.
- Infuse each liter over 3 to 4 hours to minimize toxicity. In well-hydrated patients with good renal function, infusions of 100 to 500 ml may be given over 30 minutes.
- Follow facility policy for handling and disposal of antineoplastics.

If solution contacts skin, wash immediately and thoroughly with soap and water. If solution contacts mucosa, flush with water immediately.

- Protect drug from light.

Route	Onset	Peak	Duration
I.V.	Unknown	18-23 days	39 days

Adverse reactions

CNS: malaise, weakness, **seizures**

EENT: ototoxicity, tinnitus
GI: severe nausea, vomiting, diarrhea
GU: sterility, **nephrotoxicity**
Hematologic: anemia, **leukopenia, thrombocytopenia**
Hepatic: hepatotoxicity
Metabolic: hypocalcemia, hypokalemia, hypomagnesemia, hyperuricemia
Skin: alopecia
Other: phlebitis at I.V. site, **anaphylaxis**

Interactions

Drug-drug. *Amphotericin B, loop diuretics:* increased risk of hypokalemia and hypomagnesemia
Antineoplastics: additive bone marrow depression
Live-virus vaccines: decreased antibody response to vaccine, increased risk of adverse reactions
Nephrotoxic drugs (such as aminoglycosides): additive nephrotoxicity
Ototoxic drugs (such as loop diuretics): additive ototoxicity
Phenytoin: reduced phenytoin blood level
Drug-diagnostic tests. *Aspartate aminotransferase, bilirubin, blood urea nitrogen, creatinine, uric acid:* increased levels
Calcium, magnesium, phosphate, potassium, sodium: decreased levels
Coombs' test: positive result

Patient monitoring

- Before starting therapy and before each subsequent dose, assess renal function test results and CBC with white cell differential.
- Monitor neurologic status, hepatic enzyme and uric acid levels, and audiogram results.
- Monitor urine output closely.

Patient teaching

- Instruct patient to drink 8 oz of water every hour while awake.

◀ Advise patient to promptly report bleeding, bruising, hearing loss, yellowing of skin or eyes, decreased urine output, or suspected infection.

- Tell patient that drug may cause hair loss.
- Instruct female patient to use reliable contraception; drug can harm fetus.
- As appropriate, review all other significant and life-threatening adverse reactions and interactions, especially those related to the drugs and tests mentioned above.

citalopram hydrobromide

Celexa

Pharmacologic class: Selective serotonin reuptake inhibitor
Therapeutic class: Antidepressant
Pregnancy risk category C

Action

Unclear. Thought to potentiate serotonergic activity in CNS by inhibiting neuronal uptake of serotonin.

Availability

Oral solution: 10 mg/5 ml
Tablets: 10 mg, 20 mg, 40 mg

Indications and dosages

➢ Depression
Adults: Initially, 20 mg P.O. daily; may increase by 20 mg/day at weekly intervals, up to 60 mg/day. Usual dosage is 40 mg/day.

Dosage adjustment

- Hepatic impairment
- Elderly patients

Off-label uses

- Alcoholism
- Panic disorder
- Premenstrual dysphoria
- Social phobia

Contraindications
- Hypersensitivity to drug
- MAO inhibitor use within 14 days

Precautions
Use cautiously in:
- severe renal impairment, hepatic impairment, conditions likely to cause altered metabolism or hemodynamic responses
- history of mania or seizure disorder
- elderly patients
- pregnant patients
- children (safety not established).

Administration
Don't give within 14 days of MAO inhibitor; life-threatening interactions may occur.

Route	Onset	Peak	Duration
P.O.	1-4 wk	Unknown	Unknown

Adverse reactions
CNS: apathy, confusion, drowsiness, insomnia, migraine, weakness, agitation, amnesia, anxiety, dizziness, fatigue, poor concentration, tremor, paresthesia, deepening of depression, **suicide attempt**
CV: orthostatic hypotension, tachycardia
EENT: abnormal visual accommodation
GI: nausea, vomiting, diarrhea, abdominal pain, dyspepsia, flatulence, ncreased saliva, dry mouth, increased appetite, anorexia
GU: polyuria, amenorrhea, dysmenorrhea, ejaculatory delay, erectile dysfunction, decreased libido
Musculoskeletal: joint pain, myalgia
Respiratory: cough
Skin: rash, pruritus, diaphoresis, photosensitivity
Other: altered taste, fever, yawning, weight changes

Interactions
Drug-drug. *Carbamazepine:* decreased citalopram blood level
Centrally acting drugs (such as antihistamines, opioids, sedative-hypnotics): additive CNS effects
Erythromycin, itraconazole, ketoconazole, omeprazole: increased citalopram blood level
5-hydroxytryptamine$_1$ receptor agonists (such as sumatriptan, zolmitriptan): increased risk of adverse reactions
Lithium: potentiation of serotonergic effects
MAO inhibitors: life-threatening reactions
Tricyclic antidepressants (TCAs): altered TCA pharmacokinetics
Drug-herbs. *St. John's wort, S-adenosylmethionine (SAM-e):* increased risk of serotonergic reactions, including serotonin syndrome
Drug-behaviors. *Alcohol use:* additive CNS depression
Sun exposure: photosensitivity

Patient monitoring
- If patient is receiving lithium concurrently, watch closely for potentiation of serotonergic effects.
- Assess for evidence of drug efficacy.

Patient teaching
- Instruct patient to take drug with full glass of water at same time every day.

Advise patient (especially child or adolescent) to immediately report suicidal thoughts or extreme depression.
- Instruct patient to move slowly when sitting up or standing, to avoid dizziness or light-headedness caused by sudden blood pressure decrease.
- Tell patient several weeks may pass before he starts to feel better.
- Advise patient to avoid alcohol during therapy.
- Tell male patient he may experience inadequate filling of penile erectile tissue. Advise him to consult prescriber if he experiences adverse sexual effects.

• As appropriate, review all other significant and life-threatening adverse reactions and interactions, especially those related to the drugs, herbs, and behaviors mentioned above.

clarithromycin

Biaxin Filmtab, Biaxin Granules, Biaxin XL Filmtab

Pharmacologic class: Macrolide
Therapeutic class: Anti-infective, antiulcer drug
Pregnancy risk category B

Action

Reversibly binds to 50S ribosomal subunit of susceptible bacterial organisms, blocking protein synthesis

Availability

Granules for oral suspension: 125 mg/5 ml, 250 mg/5 ml
Tablets: 250 mg, 500 mg
Tablets (extended-release): 500 mg

Indications and dosages

➢ Pharyngitis or tonsillitis caused by *Streptococcus pyogenes*
Adults: 250 mg P.O. q 12 hours for 10 days

➢ Acute maxillary sinusitis caused by *Haemophilus influenzae, Moraxella catarrhalis, or Streptococcus pneumoniae*
Adults: 500 mg P.O. q 12 hours for 14 days or two 500-mg extended-release tablets P.O. q 24 hours for 14 days

➢ Acute exacerbation of chronic bronchitis caused by *H. influenzae, Haemophilus parainfluenzae, M. catarrhalis, or S. pneumoniae*
Adults: 500 mg P.O. q 12 hours for 7 to 14 days or two 500-mg extended-release tablets P.O. q 24 hours for 7 days

➢ Community-acquired pneumonia caused by *S. pneumoniae, Mycoplasma pneumoniae,* or *Chlamydia pneumoniae;* acute exacerbation of chronic bronchitis caused by *S. pneumoniae or M. catarrhalis*
Adults: 250 mg P.O. q 12 hours for 7 to 14 days or two 500-mg extended-release tablets P.O. q 24 hours for 7 days

➢ Community-acquired pneumonia caused by *H. influenzae*
Adults: 250 mg P.O. q 12 hours for 7 days or two 500-mg extended-release tablets P.O. q 24 hours for 7 days

➢ Community-acquired pneumonia caused by *H. parainfluenzae* or *M. catarrhalis*
Adults: Two 500-mg extended-release tablets P.O. q 24 hours for 7 days

➢ Uncomplicated skin and skin-structure infections
Adults: 250 mg P.O. q 12 hours for 7 to 14 days

➢ Eradication of *Helicobacter pylori* as part of triple therapy with amoxicillin and omeprazole or lansoprazole
Adults: 500 mg P.O. q 12 hours for 10 to 14 days

➢ Eradication of *H. pylori* as part of dual therapy with omeprazole or ranitidine
Adults: 500 mg P.O. t.i.d. for 14 days

➢ Mycobacterial infections
Adults: 500 mg P.O. b.i.d.
Children: 7.5 mg/kg P.O. b.i.d., up to 500 mg b.i.d.

Dosage adjustment

• Renal or hepatic impairment

Off-label uses

• *Borrelia burgdorferi* infection

Contraindications

• Hypersensitivity to drug, erythromycin, or other macrolide anti-infectives
• Concurrent use of astemizole, cisapride, or pimozide
• Cardiac disease

Precautions

Use cautiously in:
- severe renal or hepatic impairment
- pregnant or breastfeeding patients.

Administration

- Obtain specimens for culture and sensitivity testing as appropriate before starting therapy.
- Give with or without food.

(Clinical alert) Don't give concurrently with astemizole (no longer available in U.S.), cisapride, or pimozide.
- Don't refrigerate oral suspension.

Route	Onset	Peak	Duration
P.O.	Unknown	2 hr	12 hr
P.O. (extended)	Unknown	4 hr	24 hr

Adverse reactions

CNS: headache
CV: ventricular arrhythmias
GI: nausea, diarrhea, abdominal pain or discomfort, dyspepsia
Other: abnormal taste

Interactions

Drug-drug. *Astemizole, cisapride, pimozide:* increased risk of arrhythmias and sudden death
Carbamazepine, digoxin, theophylline: increased blood levels of these drugs, greater risk of toxicity
Digoxin: increased digoxin blood level, causing digoxin toxicity
HMG-CoA reductase inhibitors (such as lovastatin, simvastatin): rhabdomyolysis
Zidovudine: increased or decreased peak zidovudine blood level
Drug-diagnostic tests. *Alkaline phosphatase, blood urea nitrogen:* increased values
Prothrombin time: increased
White blood cells: decreased count

Patient monitoring

- Monitor hepatic enzyme and creatinine levels during long-term therapy.
- Assess cardiovascular status.

Patient teaching

- Advise patient to take drug with full glass of water, either with food or on an empty stomach.
- Tell patient using oral suspension not to refrigerate it, and to discard it 14 days after mixing.
- Tell patient to swallow extended-release tablets whole.
- As appropriate, review all other significant and life-threatening adverse reactions and interactions, especially those related to the drugs and tests mentioned above.

clindamycin hydrochloride

Alti-Clindamycin✤, Cleocin, Dalacin C

clindamycin palmitate hydrochloride

Cleocin Pediatric, Dalacin C Flavored Granules✤

clindamycin phosphate

Cleocin Phosphate, Cleocin T, Clinda-Derm, Clindagel, ClindaMax, Clindets, C/T/S, Dalacin C Phosphate✤, Dalacin T✤

Pharmacologic class: Lincosamide
Therapeutic class: Anti-infective
Pregnancy risk category B

Action

Inhibits protein synthesis in susceptible bacteria at level of 50S ribosome, thereby inhibiting peptide bond formation and causing cell death

Availability

Capsules: 75 mg, 150 mg, 300 mg
Granules for oral suspension: 75 mg/5 ml
Injection: 150 mg base/ml
Topical: 1% gel, lotion, single-use applicators, solution, and suspension
Vaginal cream: 2%
Vaginal suppositories (ovules): 100 mg

Indications and dosages

➢ Severe infections caused by sensitive organisms (such as *Bacteroides fragilis, Clostridium perfringens, Fusobacterium,* pneumococci, staphylococci, and streptococci)
Adults: 300 to 450 mg P.O. q 6 hours, or (for other than *C. perfringens)* 1.2 to 2.7 g/day I.M. or I.V. in two to four equally divided doses
Children: 16 to 20 mg/kg/day P.O. (hydrochloride) in three to four equally divided doses, or 13 to 25 mg/kg/day P.O. (palmitate hydrochloride) in three to four equally divided doses
Neonates younger than 1 month: 15 to 20 mg/kg/day I.M. or I.V. in three to four equally divided doses
➢ Acute pelvic inflammatory disease
Adults: 900 mg I.V. q 8 hours (given with gentamicin)
➢ Acne vulgaris
Adults and children older than age 12: Apply a thin film of topical gel, lotion, or solution locally to affected area b.i.d.

Off-label uses

- Bacterial vaginosis (phosphate)
- *Chlamydia trachomatis* infection in females
- CNS toxoplasmosis in AIDS patients (given with pyrimethamine)
- *Pneumocystis jiroveci* pneumonia (given with primaquine)
- Rosacea (lotion)

Contraindications

- Hypersensitivity to drug or lincomycin

Precautions

Use cautiously in:
- renal or hepatic impairment
- known alcohol intolerance
- pregnant patients
- neonates.

Administration

- Give oral doses with full glass of water, with or without food.

Don't give as I.V. bolus injection.
- Dilute I.V. solution to a concentration of 18 mg/ml using normal saline solution, dextrose 5% in water, or lactated Ringer's solution. Infuse no faster than 30 mg/minute.
- Don't administer I.M. dosages above 600 mg.
- Inject I.M. doses deep into large muscle mass to prevent induration and sterile abscess.

Route	Onset	Peak	Duration
P.O.	Rapid	45 min	6-8 hr
I.V.	Rapid	End of infusion	6-8 hr
I.M.	Rapid	1-3 hr	6-8 hr
Topical, vaginal	Unknown	Unknown	Unknown

Adverse reactions

GI: nausea, vomiting, diarrhea, abdominal pain, esophagitis, **pseudomembranous colitis**
Hematologic: neutropenia, leukopenia, agranulocytosis, thrombocytopenia purpura
Hepatic: jaundice, **hepatic dysfunction**
Skin: maculopapular rash, generalized morbilliform-like rash
Other: bitter taste (with I.V. use), phlebitis at I.V. site, induration and sterile abscess (with I.M. use), **anaphylaxis**

Interactions

Drug-drug. *Erythromycin:* antagonistic effect

Kaolin/pectin: decreased GI absorption of clindamycin
Hormonal contraceptives: decreased contraceptive efficacy
Neuromuscular blockers: enhanced neuromuscular blockade
Drug-diagnostic tests. *Alanine aminotransferase, alkaline phosphatase, aspartate aminotransferase, bilirubin, creatine kinase:* increased levels
Platelets, white blood cells: transient decrease in counts

Patient monitoring
- Monitor creatinine level closely in patients with renal insufficiency.
- Monitor hepatic enzyme levels in patients with hepatic disease.
- Assess for signs and symptoms of hypersensitivity reactions, including anaphylaxis.
- Assess for diarrhea and signs and symptoms of colitis.

Patient teaching
- Tell patient to take drug with food if it causes stomach upset.
- Urge patient to contact prescriber immediately if he develops rash, unusual fatigue, or yellowing of skin or eyes or if diarrhea occurs during or after treatment.
- Tell patient that I.V. use may cause bitter taste. Reassure him that this effect will resolve on its own.
- Caution patient not to rely on condoms or diaphragm for contraception for 72 hours after using vaginal preparation; drug may weaken latex products and cause breakage.
- Instruct patient taking hormonal contraceptives to use supplemental birth control method, such as condoms (unless she's using a vaginal preparation); drug may reduce hormonal contraceptive efficacy.
- As appropriate, review all other significant and life-threatening adverse reactions and interactions, especially those related to the drugs and tests mentioned above.

C

clomiphene citrate
Clomid, Milophene, Serophene

Pharmacologic class: Chlorotrianisene derivative
Therapeutic class: Fertility drug, ovulation stimulant
Pregnancy risk category X

Action
Binds with estrogen receptors in cytoplasm, increasing secretion of follicle-stimulating hormone, luteinizing hormone, and gonadotropin in hypothalamus and pituitary gland. These actions induce ovulation.

Availability
Tablets: 50 mg

Indications and dosages
➢ Ovarian failure
Adults: 50 mg/day P.O. for 5 days starting any time in patients with no recent uterine bleeding; or 50 mg/day P.O. starting on fifth day of menstrual cycle. If ovulation doesn't occur, increase to 100 mg/day P.O. for 5 days. Start next course of therapy as early as 30 days after previous course. If patient doesn't respond after three courses, no further doses are recommended.

Off-label uses
- Male sterility (controversial)

Contraindications
- Hepatic disease
- Organic intracranial lesions
- Uncontrolled thyroid or adrenal dysfunction
- Ovarian cyst

• Abnormal uterine bleeding or bleeding of undetermined origin
• Pregnancy

Precautions
None

Administration
• Obtain pregnancy test before therapy begins.
• Be aware that patient should undergo pelvic and eye examinations before starting therapy.

Route	Onset	Peak	Duration
P.O.	5-8 days	Unknown	6 wk

Adverse reactions
CNS: nervousness, insomnia, dizziness, light-headedness
CV: vasomotor flushing
EENT: visual disturbances
GI: nausea; vomiting; abdominal discomfort, distention, and bloating
GU: breast tenderness, ovarian enlargement, multiple pregnancies, birth defects in resulting pregnancies, **ovarian hyperstimulation syndrome, uterine bleeding**

Interactions
None significant

Patient monitoring
• Monitor patient for bleeding and other adverse reactions.

Patient teaching
Instruct patient to immediately report signs and symptoms of ovarian hyperstimulation syndrome, including nausea, vomiting, diarrhea, abdominal or pelvic pain, and swelling in hands or legs.
• Tell patient to report bleeding.
• Advise patient not to take drug if she is or may become pregnant.
• Inform patient that drug increases risk of multiple births, which heightens maternal risk.
• As appropriate, review all other significant and life-threatening adverse reactions.

clomipramine hydrochloride
Anafranil, Apo-Clomipramine*, Gen-Clomipramine*, Novo-Clopamine*

Pharmacologic class: Tricyclic antidepressant (TCA)
Therapeutic class: Antiobsessional agent, antidepressant
Pregnancy risk category C

Action
Unknown. Selectively inhibits norepinephrine and serotonin reuptake at presynaptic neurons in brain; also possesses moderate anticholinergic properties.

Availability
Capsules: 25 mg, 50 mg, 75 mg

Indications and dosages
➢ Obsessive-compulsive disorder
Adults: Initially, 25 mg/day P.O., increased over 2 weeks to 100 mg/day given in divided doses. May be increased further over several weeks, up to 250 mg/day given in divided doses.
Children ages 10 to 17: Initially, 25 mg/day P.O., increased over 2 weeks to 3 mg/kg/day or 100 mg/day (whichever is smaller) given in divided doses. May be increased further to 3 mg/kg/day or 200 mg/day (whichever is smaller) given in divided doses.

Dosage adjustment
• Elderly patients

Off-label uses
• Panic disorder

Contraindications

- Hypersensitivity to drug or other TCAs
- Recent myocardial infarction (MI)
- Concurrent MAO inhibitor or clonidine use

Precautions

Use cautiously in:

- glaucoma, hyperthyroidism, prostatic hypertrophy, preexisting cardiovascular disease
- elderly patients
- pregnant or breastfeeding patients
- children younger than age 10 (safety not established).

Administration

- Don't give with grapefruit juice.
- Once stabilizing dosage is reached, entire daily dose may be given at bedtime.

Route	Onset	Peak	Duration
P.O.	Unknown	2-6 hr	Unknown

Adverse reactions

CNS: lethargy, sedation, weakness, aggressive behavior, extrapyramidal reactions, poor concentration, feeling of unreality, delusions, anxiety, restlessness, panic, asthenia, syncope, insomnia, **seizures, suicidal ideation or behavior (especially in child or adolescent)**
CV: orthostatic hypotension, hypertension, ECG changes, tachycardia, palpitations, vasculitis, **arrhythmias, MI, precipitation of heart block**
EENT: blurred vision, dry eyes, vestibular disorder, nasal congestion, laryngitis
GI: nausea, vomiting, constipation, abdominal cramps, belching, epigastric distress, flatulence, dysphagia, increased salivation, stomatitis, parotid gland swelling, black tongue, dry mouth, **paralytic ileus**
GU: urinary retention, urinary hesitancy, urinary tract dilation, male sexual dysfunction, testicular swelling, gynecomastia, breast enlargement, menstrual irregularities, galactorrhea, libido changes
Hematologic: eosinophilia, purpura, anemia, **bone marrow depression, agranulocytosis, thrombocytopenia, leukopenia**
Metabolic: hyperthermia, hypothermia, **syndrome of inappropriate antidiuretic hormone secretion**
Musculoskeletal: muscle weakness
Skin: sweating, dry skin, photosensitivity, rash, pruritus, petechiae, flushing
Other: abnormal taste, chills, edema, increased appetite, weight gain

Interactions

Drug-drug. *Adrenergics, anticholinergics:* additive adrenergic or anticholinergic effects
Cimetidine, hormonal contraceptives, phenothiazines, selective serotonin reuptake inhibitors: increased clomipramine effects, greater risk of toxicity
Clonidine: hypertensive crisis
CNS depressants (including antihistamines, opioid analgesics, sedative-hypnotics): additive CNS depression
Disulfiram: transient delirium
Guanethidine: interference with antihypertensive response
MAO inhibitors: severe or life-threatening adverse reactions
Sparfloxacin: increased risk of adverse cardiovascular reactions
Drug-diagnostic tests. *Blood glucose, prolactin:* elevated levels
Drug-food. *Grapefruit juice:* increased clomipramine blood level and effects
Drug-herbs. *Chamomile, hops, kava, skullcap, valerian:* increased CNS depression
S-adenosylmethionine (SAM-e), St. John's wort: increased serotonergic effects, possibly causing serotonin syndrome
Drug-behaviors. *Alcohol use:* additive CNS depression

Nicotine use: increased metabolism and decreased efficacy of clomipramine
Sun exposure: photosensitivity

Patient monitoring

- Monitor patient for cardiovascular, CNS, and hematologic adverse reactions.

🔊 Assess for suicidal ideation. If necessary, institute suicide precautions.

Patient teaching

🔊 Advise patient (especially children or their parents) to immediately report suicidal thoughts or severe depression.

- Instruct patient not to drink grapefruit juice during therapy.
- Caution patient to avoid driving and other hazardous activities until he knows how drug affects concentration and alertness.
- Instruct patient to avoid alcohol, because it increases drowsiness.
- Tell patient to move slowly when sitting up or standing, to avoid dizziness or light-headedness caused by sudden blood pressure drop.
- Caution patient not to stop taking drug abruptly, because this may cause nausea, headache, or malaise.
- As appropriate, review all other significant and life-threatening adverse reactions and interactions, especially those related to the drugs, tests, foods, herbs, and behaviors mentioned above.

clonazepam

Alti-Clonazepam✤, Apo-Clonazepam✤, Clonapam✤, Gen-Clonazepam✤, Klonopin, Klonopin Wafer, Rivotril✤

Pharmacologic class: Benzodiazepine
Therapeutic class: Anticonvulsant
Controlled substance schedule IV
Pregnancy risk category D

Action

Unknown. May enhance activity of gamma-aminobutyric acid, an inhibitory neurotransmitter in CNS.

Availability

Rapidly disintegrating tablets (wafers): 0.125 mg, 0.25 mg, 0.5 mg, 1 mg, 2 mg
Tablets: 0.5 mg, 1 mg, 2 mg

Indications and dosages

➢ Absence seizures (Lennox-Gastaut syndrome); akinetic and myoclonic seizures

Adults: Initially, 1.5 mg/day P.O. in three divided doses; may increase by 0.5 to 1 mg q 3 days until seizures are adequately controlled or drug intolerance occurs. Maximum dosage is 20 mg/day.

Infants and children ages 10 and younger or weighing 30 kg (66 lb) or less: Initially, 0.01 to 0.03 mg/kg/day P.O. Give total dosage (not to exceed 0.05 mg/kg/day) in two to three equally divided doses. Increase by no more than 0.25 to 0.5 mg q 3 days until dosage of 0.1 to 0.2 mg/kg/day is reached, seizures are adequately controlled, or drug intolerance occurs.

Off-label uses

- Acute manic episodes of bipolar disorder
- Multifocal tic disorders
- Neuralgias
- Parkinsonian dysarthria
- Periodic leg movements occurring during sleep
- Adjunctive treatment of schizophrenia

Contraindications

- Hypersensitivity to drug or other benzodiazepines
- Severe hepatic disease
- Acute angle-closure glaucoma

Precautions

Use cautiously in:
- renal impairment, chronic respiratory disease, open-angle glaucoma
- history of porphyria
- pregnant or breastfeeding patients
- children.

Administration

Be aware that overdose may cause fatal respiratory depression or cardiovascular collapse.
- Give tablets with water, and make sure patient swallows them whole.
- Administer orally disintegrating tablet (wafer) as follows: After opening pouch, peel back foil on blister, but don't push tablet through foil. Immediately after opening blister, use dry hands to remove tablet, and place it in patient's mouth. Wafer can be easily swallowed with or without water because it disintegrates rapidly in saliva.

Route	Onset	Peak	Duration
P.O.	20-60 min	1-2 hr	6-12 hr
P.O. (wafer)	Rapid	Unknown	Unknown

Adverse reactions

CNS: ataxia, fatigue, drowsiness, behavioral changes, depression, dizziness, nervousness, reduced intellectual ability
CV: palpitations
EENT: abnormal eye movements, blurred vision, diplopia, nystagmus, sinusitis, rhinitis, pharyngitis
GI: constipation, diarrhea, hypersalivation
GU: dysuria, nocturia, urinary retention, dysmenorrhea, delayed ejaculation, erectile dysfunction
Hematologic: anemia, eosinophilia, **leukopenia, thrombocytopenia**
Hepatic: hepatitis
Musculoskeletal: myalgia
Respiratory: increased respiratory secretions, upper respiratory tract infection, cough, bronchitis, **respiratory depression**
Other: appetite changes, fever, physical or psychological drug dependence, drug tolerance, allergic reaction

Interactions

Drug-drug. *Antidepressants, antihistamines, opioids, other benzodiazepines:* additive CNS depression
Barbiturates, rifampin: increased metabolism and decreased efficacy of clonazepam
Cimetidine, disulfiram, fluoxetine, hormonal contraceptives, isoniazid, ketoconazole, metoprolol, propoxyphene, propranolol, valproic acid: decreased clonazepam metabolism
Phenytoin: decreased clonazepam blood level
Drug-diagnostic tests. *Eosinophils, liver function tests:* increased values
Platelets, white blood cells: decreased counts
Drug-herbs. *Chamomile, hops, kava, skullcap, valerian:* increased CNS depression
Drug-behaviors. *Alcohol use:* increased CNS depression

Patient monitoring

- Monitor patient for respiratory depression. Assess respiratory rate and quality, oxygen saturation (using pulse oximetry), and mental status.
- Monitor hematologic and liver function test results.

Patient teaching

Instruct patient to immediately report easy bleeding or bruising or yellowing of skin or eyes.
- Teach patient how to take rapidly disintegrating wafer.
- Advise patient to avoid driving and other hazardous activities until he knows how drug affects concentration and alertness.

Caution patient not to stop taking drug abruptly. Advise him to consult

prescriber for dosage-tapering schedule if he wishes to discontinue drug.
• Advise patient not to drink alcohol, which may increase drowsiness, dizziness, and risk of seizures.
• As appropriate, review all other significant and life-threatening adverse reactions and interactions, especially those related to the drugs, tests, herbs, and behaviors mentioned above.

clonidine
Catapres-TTS

clonidine hydrochloride
Apo-Clonidine✤, Catapres, Dixarit✤, Duraclon, Novo-Clonidine✤, Nu-Clonidine✤

Pharmacologic class: Centrally acting sympatholytic
Therapeutic class: Antihypertensive
Pregnancy risk category C

Action
Stimulates alpha-adrenergic receptors in CNS, decreasing sympathetic outflow, inhibiting vasoconstriction, and ultimately reducing blood pressure. Also prevents transmission of pain impulses by inhibiting pain pathway signals in brain.

Availability
Solution for epidural injection: 100 mcg/ml in 10-ml vials, 500 mcg/ml in 10-ml vials
Tablets: 25 mcg (0.025 mg), 100 mcg (0.1 mg), 200 mcg (0.2 mg), 300 mcg (0.3 mg)
Transdermal systems: 2.5 mg total released as 0.1 mg/24 hours (TTS 1), 5 mg total released as 0.2 mg/24 hours (TTS 2), 7.5 mg total released as 0.3 mg/24 hours (TTS 3)

Indications and dosages
➢ Mild to moderate hypertension
Adults: 0.1 mg P.O. b.i.d. (morning and bedtime) alone or with other antihypertensives; increase in increments of 0.1 mg/day q week until desired response occurs. Or, one transdermal system applied once q 7 days to hairless area of intact skin on upper outer arm or chest.
➢ Severe pain in cancer patients unresponsive to opioids alone
Adults: Initially, 30 mcg/hour by continuous epidural infusion, titrated upward or downward depending on patient response

Dosage adjustment
• Renal impairment

Off-label uses
• Acute alcohol withdrawal
• Akathisia
• Diarrhea
• Prolonged surgical anesthesia

Contraindications
• Hypersensitivity to drug
• Hypersensitivity to components of adhesive layer (transdermal form)
• Infection at epidural injection site, bleeding problems (epidural use)
• Concurrent anticoagulant therapy

Precautions
Use cautiously in:
• renal insufficiency, serious cardiac or cerebrovascular disease
• elderly patients
• pregnant or breastfeeding patients.

Administration
• For epidural use, dilute drug solution in normal saline solution, as ordered.
• To minimize sedative effects, give largest portion of maintenance P.O. dose at bedtime.

Route	Onset	Peak	Duration
P.O.	30-60 min	2-4 hr	8-12 hr
Epidural	Rapid	19 min	Variable
Transdermal	Slow	2-3 days	7 days

Adverse reactions

CNS: drowsiness, depression, dizziness, nervousness, nightmares
CV: hypotension (especially with epidural use), palpitations, bradycardia
GI: nausea, vomiting, constipation, dry mouth
GU: urinary retention, nocturia, erectile dysfunction
Metabolic: sodium retention
Skin: rash, sweating, pruritus, dermatitis
Other: weight gain, withdrawal phenomenon

Interactions

Drug-drug. *Amphetamines, beta-adrenergic blockers, MAO inhibitors, prazosin, tricyclic antidepressants:* decreased antihypertensive effect
Beta-adrenergic blockers: increased withdrawal phenomenon
CNS depressants (including antihistamines, opioids, sedative-hypnotics): additive sedation
Epidurally administered local anesthetics: prolonged clonidine effects
Levodopa: decreased levodopa efficacy
Myocardial depressants (including beta-adrenergic blockers): additive bradycardia
Other antihypertensives, nitrates: additive hypotension
Verapamil: increased risk of adverse cardiovascular reactions
Drug-herbs. *Capsicum:* reduced antihypertensive effect
Drug-behaviors. *Alcohol use:* increased sedation

Patient monitoring

- Monitor patient for signs and symptoms of adverse cardiovascular reactions.
- Frequently assess vital signs, especially blood pressure and pulse.
- Monitor patient for drug tolerance and efficacy.

Patient teaching

- Instruct patient to move slowly when sitting up or standing, to avoid dizziness or light-headedness caused by sudden blood pressure decrease.

Caution patient not to stop taking drug abruptly.

- As appropriate, review all other significant adverse reactions and interactions, especially those related to the drugs, herbs, and behaviors mentioned above.

clopidogrel bisulfate

Plavix

Pharmacologic class: Platelet aggregation inhibitor
Therapeutic class: Antiplatelet drug
Pregnancy risk category B

Action

Inhibits platelet aggregation by blocking binding of adenosine diphosphate to platelets, thereby preventing thrombus formation

Availability

Tablets: 75 mg

Indications and dosages

➤ To reduce atherosclerotic events in patients with recent myocardial infarction (MI) or cerebrovascular accident and in those with established peripheral arterial disease or acute coronary syndrome
Adults: 75 mg/day P.O.
➤ Acute coronary syndrome (unstable angina or non-Q-wave MI)
Adults: 300 mg P.O. as a loading dose, then 75 mg/day P.O.

Contraindications

- Hypersensitivity to drug
- Active pathologic bleeding

Precautions

Use cautiously in:

- severe hepatic impairment, GI bleeding, ulcer disease
- increased risk of bleeding
- pregnant or breastfeeding patients
- children.

Administration

- Give with or without food.
- Know that drug may need to be discontinued 5 days before surgery.

Route	Onset	Peak	Duration
P.O.	Variable	60 min	3-4 hr

Adverse reactions

CNS: depression, dizziness, fatigue, headache
CV: chest pain, hypertension
EENT: epistaxis, rhinitis
GI: diarrhea, abdominal pain, dyspepsia, gastritis, **GI bleeding**
Hematologic: bleeding, neutropenia, thrombotic thrombocytopenic purpura
Metabolic: hypercholesterolemia, gout
Musculoskeletal: joint pain, back pain
Respiratory: cough, dyspnea, bronchitis, upper respiratory tract infection, **bronchospasm**
Skin: pruritus, rash, angioedema
Other: hypersensitivity reactions, **anaphylactic reactions**

Interactions

Drug-drug. *Abciximab, aspirin, eptifibatide, heparin, heparinoids, nonsteroidal anti-inflammatory drugs (NSAIDs), thrombolytics, ticlopidine, tirofiban, warfarin:* increased risk of bleeding
Fluvastatin, many NSAIDs, phenytoin, tamoxifen, tolbutamide, torsemide: interference with metabolism of these drugs
Drug-diagnostic tests. *Bilirubin, hepatic enzymes, nonprotein nitrogen, total cholesterol, uric acid:* increased levels
Platelets: decreased count
Drug-herbs. *Anise, arnica, chamomile, clove, fenugreek, feverfew, garlic, ginger, ginkgo, ginseng:* increased risk of bleeding

Patient monitoring

- Monitor hemoglobin and hematocrit periodically.
- Monitor patient for unusual bleeding or bruising; drug significantly increases risk of bleeding.
- Assess for occult GI blood loss if patient is receiving naproxen concurrently with clopidogrel.

Patient teaching

[Clinical alert] Advise patient to immediately report unusual or acute chest pain, respiratory difficulty, rash, unresolved bleeding, diarrhea, GI distress, nosebleed, or acute headache.

- Instruct patient to tell all health care providers that he's taking clopidogrel, especially if surgery is scheduled or new drugs are prescribed.
- Tell patient drug may cause headache and dizziness. Caution him to avoid driving and other hazardous activities until he knows how drug affects concentration and alertness.
- Advise patient to minimize adverse GI effects by eating small, frequent meals or chewing gum.
- As appropriate, review all other significant and life-threatening adverse reactions and interactions, especially those related to the drugs, tests, and herbs mentioned above.

clorazepate dipotassium

Apo-Clorazepate*, Novo-Clopate*, Tranxene, Tranxene-SD, Tranxene-SD Half Strength, Tranxene-T

Pharmacologic class: Benzodiazepine
Therapeutic class: Anticonvulsant, anxiolytic
Controlled substance schedule IV
Pregnancy risk category D

Action

Unclear. Thought to potentiate effects of gamma-aminobutyric acid and other neurotransmitters, promoting inhibitory neurotransmission at excitatory synapses.

Availability

Capsules: 3.75 mg, 7.5 mg, 15 mg
Tablets: 3.75 mg, 7.5 mg, 11.25 mg, 15 mg, 22.5 mg

Indications and dosages

➢ Anxiety
Adults: 7.5 to 15 mg P.O. two to four times daily
➢ Adjunctive therapy in partial seizure disorder
Adults and children older than age 12: Initially, 7.5 mg P.O. t.i.d.; increase by no more than 7.5 mg/week. Don't exceed 90 mg/day.
Children ages 9 to 12: Initially, 7.5 mg P.O. b.i.d; increase by no more than 7.5 mg/week. Don't exceed 60 mg/day.
➢ Management of alcohol withdrawal
Adults: Initially, 30 mg P.O., followed by 15 mg P.O. two to four times daily on first day. On second day, give 45 to 90 mg P.O. in divided doses, then decrease gradually over subsequent days to 7.5 mg to 15 mg P.O. daily.

Dosage adjustment

- Elderly or debilitated patients

Contraindications

- Benzodiazepine hypersensitivity
- Acute angle-closure glaucoma
- Psychosis
- Concurrent ketoconazole or itraconazole therapy
- Children younger than age 9

Precautions

Use cautiously in:
- depression or suicidal ideation
- psychotic reaction
- elderly patients
- females of childbearing age
- pregnant or breastfeeding patients.

Administration

- If GI upset occurs, give with food.
- When discontinuing therapy after long-term use, taper dosage gradually over 4 to 8 weeks to avoid withdrawal symptoms.
- Take suicide precautions if patient is depressed or anxious.

Route	Onset	Peak	Duration
P.O.	Rapid	1-2 hr	Days

Adverse reactions

CNS: dizziness, drowsiness, lethargy, sedation, depression, fatigue, nervousness, confusion, irritability, headache, slurred speech, difficulty articulating words, stupor, rigidity, tremor, poor coordination
CV: hypertension, hypotension, palpitations
EENT: blurred or double vision
GI: dry mouth
Hematologic: neutropenia
Hepatic: jaundice
Skin: rash, diaphoresis
Other: weight gain or loss, drug dependence or tolerance

Interactions

Drug-drug. *Antacids:* altered clorazepate absorption rate
Antidepressants, antihistamines, opioids: additive CNS depression

Barbiturates, MAO inhibitors, other antidepressants, phenothiazines: potentiation of clorazepate effects
Cimetidine, disulfiram, fluoxetine, hormonal contraceptives, isoniazid, itraconazole, ketoconazole, metoprolol, propoxyphene, propranolol, valproic acid: decreased clorazepate metabolism, causing enhanced drug action or markedly increased CNS effects
Levodopa: decreased antiparkinsonian effect
Probenecid: rapid onset or prolonged action of clorazepate
Rifampin: increased metabolism and decreased efficacy of clorazepate
Theophylline: decreased sedative effect of clorazepate
Drug-diagnostic tests. *Alanine aminotransferase, alkaline phosphatase, aspartate aminotransferase:* increased levels
Drug-herbs. *Chamomile, hops, kava, skullcap, valerian:* increased CNS depression
Drug-behaviors. *Alcohol use:* increased CNS depression
Smoking: decreased drug absorption

Patient monitoring

- Assess for pregnancy before initiating therapy.
- Evaluate patient for depression, drug dependence, and drug tolerance.
- Monitor blood counts and liver function test results during long-term therapy; drug may cause neutropenia and jaundice.

Patient teaching

- Instruct patient to avoid driving and other hazardous activities until he knows how drug affects concentration and alertness.
- Tell patient to avoid smoking and use of alcohol or other CNS depressants.
- Caution patient not to stop therapy abruptly, because withdrawal symptoms may occur.
- As appropriate, review all other significant and life-threatening adverse reactions and interactions, especially those related to the drugs, tests, herbs, and behaviors mentioned above.

clozapine

Clozaril, Fazalco

Pharmacologic class: Dibenzodiazepine derivative
Therapeutic class: Antipsychotic agent
Pregnancy risk category B

Action

Unclear. Thought to interfere with dopamine binding in limbic system of CNS, with high affinity for $dopamine_4$ receptors. May antagonize adrenergic, cholinergic, histaminergic, and serotonergic receptors.

Availability

Tablets: 25 mg, 100 mg
Tablets (orally disintegrating): 25 mg, 100 mg

Indications and dosages

➢ Schizophrenia in patients unresponsive to other therapies
Adults: 12.5 mg P.O. daily or b.i.d.; increase daily in 25- to 50-mg increments, as tolerated, to target dosage of 300 to 450 mg/day by end of second week. Make subsequent dosage increases once or twice weekly in increments of 100 mg or less, to a maximum dosage of 900 mg/day P.O. in divided doses.

Dosage adjustment

- Renal impairment
- Elderly patients

Contraindications

- Hypersensitivity to drug
- Uncontrolled seizures
- Severe CNS depression or coma

• Concurrent use of drugs that cause agranulocytosis or bone marrow depression

Precautions

Use cautiously in:
• hypersensitivity to phenothiazines
• cardiac, hepatic, or renal impairment; CNS tumors; diabetes mellitus; history of seizures; prostatic hypertrophy; intestinal obstruction; paralytic ileus; angle-closure glaucoma
• elderly patients
• pregnant or breastfeeding patients
• children.

Administration

Obtain white blood cell (WBC) count before starting therapy. Don't give drug if WBC count is below 3,500/mm^3.
• When discontinuing drug, taper dosage gradually over 1 to 2 weeks.
• Be aware that orally disintegrating tablets are meant to dissolve in mouth.

Route	Onset	Peak	Duration
P.O.	Unknown	2.5 hr	4-12 hr
P.O. (orally disint.)	Unknown	Unknown	Unknown

Adverse reactions

CNS: sedation, drowsiness, dizziness, vertigo, headache, tremor, insomnia, disturbed sleep, nightmares, agitation, lethargy, fatigue, weakness, confusion, anxiety, parkinsonism, slurred speech, depression, restlessness, extrapyramidal reactions, tardive dyskinesia, akathisia, syncope, **neuroleptic malignant syndrome, autonomic disturbances, seizures**
CV: hypotension, tachycardia, ECG changes, chest pain, **myocarditis**
EENT: blurred vision, dry eyes, nasal congestion, sinusitis
GI: nausea, vomiting, constipation, dyspepsia, salivation, dry mouth, anorexia
GU: urinary retention, urinary incontinence, urinary frequency and urgency, inhibited ejaculation
Musculoskeletal: muscle spasms, rigidity, back and muscle pain
Hematologic: agranulocytosis, leukopenia, hemolytic anemia, aplastic anemia, thrombocytopenia, neutropenia, eosinophilia
Respiratory: dyspnea
Skin: rash, sweating
Other: weight gain, fever

Interactions

Drug-drug. *Anticholinergics, antihypertensives, digoxin, warfarin:* increased effects of these drugs
Cimetidine, erythromycin: increased therapeutic and toxic effects of clozapine
Epinephrine: increased hypotension
Fluoxetine, fluvoxamine, paroxetine, sertraline: increased clozapine blood level
Phenytoin, rifampin: decreased clozapine blood level
Psychoactive drugs: additive psychoactive effect
Drug-diagnostic tests. *Granulocytes, hematocrit, hemoglobin, platelets, white blood cells:* decreased values
Liver function tests: abnormal values
Pregnancy test: false-positive result
Drug-food. *Caffeine:* increased clozapine blood level
Drug-herbs. *Angel's trumpet, jimsonweed, scopolia:* increased anticholinergic effects
Nutmeg: decreased clozapine efficacy
St. John's wort: decreased clozapine blood level
Drug-behaviors. *Alcohol use:* increased CNS depression
Smoking: decreased clozapine blood level

Patient monitoring

Monitor WBC count weekly for first 6 months of therapy; if it's normal, WBC testing can be reduced to

every other week. Notify prescriber immediately if WBC count decreases or agranulocytosis occurs.
• Monitor ECG and liver function test results.
• If drug must be withdrawn abruptly, monitor patient for psychosis and cholinergic rebound (headache, nausea, vomiting, diarrhea).
• Continue to monitor WBC count weekly for 4 weeks after therapy ends.

Patient teaching

• Tell patient to allow orally disintegrating tablet to dissolve in mouth.
• Teach patient about significant risk of agranulocytosis; tell him he'll need to undergo weekly blood testing to check for this blood disorder. Mention that clozapine tablets are available only through a special program that ensures required blood monitoring.
Advise patient to immediately report new onset of lethargy, weakness, fever, sore throat, malaise, mucous membrane ulcers, flulike symptoms, or other signs and symptoms of infection.
• As appropriate, review all other significant and life-threatening adverse reactions and interactions, especially those related to the drugs, tests, foods, herbs, and behaviors mentioned above.

coagulation factor VIIa (recombinant)

NovoSeven

Pharmacologic class: Coagulation factor VIIa
Therapeutic class: Antihemophilic agent
Pregnancy risk category C

Action

Promotes hemostasis by activating intrinsic pathway of coagulation cascade to form fibrin

Availability

Lyophilized powder for injection: 1.2 mg/vial, 2.4 mg/vial, 4.8 mg/vial

Indications and dosages

➤ Bleeding episodes in patients with hemophilia A or B who have inhibitors to factor VIII or IX
Adults: 90 mcg/kg I.V. bolus q 2 hours until hemostasis occurs or therapy is deemed ineffective

Contraindications

• Hypersensitivity to drug or to mouse, hamster, or bovine products

Precautions

Use cautiously in:
• pregnant or breastfeeding patients
• children.

Administration

Give by I.V. bolus only over 2 to 5 minutes, depending on dosage.
• Reconstitute only with specified volume of sterile water for injection.
Don't mix with infusion solutions.
• Administer within 3 hours of reconstituting.

Route	Onset	Peak	Duration
I.V.	Unknown	Unknown	Unknown

Adverse reactions

CNS: headache
CV: hypertension, hypotension, bradycardia
GU: renal dysfunction
Hematologic: purpura, **hemorrhage, hemarthrosis, disseminated intravascular coagulation, coagulation disorders, decreased fibrinogen plasma, thrombosis**
Musculoskeletal: arthrosis
Skin: pruritus, rash

Other: fever, edema, pain, redness or reaction at injection site, hypersensitivity reaction

Interactions

Drug-drug. *Activated prothrombin complex concentrates, prothrombin complex concentrates:* risk of potential interaction (though not evaluated)

Patient monitoring

- Monitor for signs and symptoms of coagulation activation or thrombosis.
- Be aware that laboratory coagulation parameters may be used as adjunct to clinical evaluation of hemostasis to monitor drug efficacy and treatment schedule. However, these parameters lack direct correlation with achievement of hemostasis.

Patient teaching

- Instruct patient to report swelling, pain, burning, or itching at infusion site.
- Tell patient to inform prescriber if she's pregnant or intends to become pregnant.
- As appropriate, review all other significant and life-threatening adverse reactions and interactions, especially those related to the drugs mentioned above.

codeine phosphate

codeine sulfate

Pharmacologic class: Opioid agonist
Therapeutic class: Opioid analgesic, antitussive
Controlled substance schedule II
Pregnancy risk category C

Action

Binds to opioid receptors in CNS, altering perception of painful stimuli. Causes generalized CNS depression, decreases cough reflex, and reduces GI motility.

Availability

Injection (phosphate): 30 mg/ml, 60 mg/ml
Oral solution (phosphate): 10 mg/5 ml, 15 mg/5 ml
Tablets (sulfate): 15 mg, 30 mg, 60 mg; 30 mg, 60 mg (soluble)

Indications and dosages

➢ Pain
Adults: 15 to 60 mg P.O. or 15 to 60 mg (phosphate) I.M., I.V., or subcutaneously q 4 to 6 hours. Usual daily dosage is 30 mg; maximum daily dosage is 360 mg.
Children ages 1 and older: 0.5 mg/kg or 15 mg/m^2 P.O., I.M., or subcutaneously q 4 to 6 hours
➢ Cough
Adults: 10 to 20 mg P.O. q 4 to 6 hours as needed. Don't exceed 120 mg/day.
Children ages 6 to 12: 5 to 10 mg P.O. q 4 to 6 hours as needed. Don't exceed 60 mg/day.
Children ages 2 to 6: 2.5 to 5 mg P.O. q 4 to 6 hours as needed. Don't exceed 30 mg/day.

Dosage adjustment

- Elderly or debilitated patients

Contraindications

- Hypersensitivity to narcotics
- Labor and delivery of premature neonate
- Premature neonates

Precautions

Use cautiously in:
- severe renal, hepatic, or pulmonary disease
- adrenal insufficiency, head trauma, hypothyroidism, increased intracranial pressure, prostatic hypertrophy, undiagnosed abdominal pain, alcoholism

- elderly patients
- pregnant or breastfeeding patients.

Administration

- If GI upset occurs, give with food.
- Titrate dosage for appropriate analgesic effect.
- When changing administration route, be aware that oral dose is two-thirds as effective as parenteral dose.

🔊 Don't give I.V. to children.

🔊 If overdose occurs, give naloxone I.V. as prescribed. Repeat administration as needed (up to manufacturer's recommended maximum dosage) to reverse toxic effects.

🔊 Don't mix with other solutions; drug is incompatible with other drugs.

Route	Onset	Peak	Duration
P.O.	30-45 min	1-2 hr	4 hr
I.M.	10-30 min	30-60 min	4 hr
Subcut.	10-30 min	Unknown	4 hr

Adverse reactions

CNS: confusion, sedation, malaise, agitation, euphoria, floating feeling, headache, hallucinations, unusual dreams, apathy, mood changes
CV: hypotension, bradycardia, peripheral vasodilation, reduced peripheral resistance
EENT: blurred or double vision, miosis, reddened sclera
GI: nausea, vomiting, constipation, decreased gastric motility
GU: urinary retention, urinary tract spasms, urinary urgency
Respiratory: suppressed cough reflex, **respiratory depression**
Skin: flushing, sweating
Other: physical or psychological drug dependence, drug tolerance

Interactions

Drug-drug. *Antidepressants, antihistamines, sedative-hypnotics:* additive CNS depression
Nalbuphine, pentazocine: decreased analgesic effect
Opioid partial agonists (buprenorphine, butorphanol, nalbuphine, pentazocine): precipitation of opioid withdrawal in physically dependent patients
Drug-herbs. *Chamomile, hops, kava, skullcap, valerian:* increased CNS depression
Drug-behaviors. *Alcohol use:* increased CNS depression

Patient monitoring

- Monitor vital signs and CNS status.
- Assess pain level and efficacy of pain relief.
- Evaluate patient for adverse reactions.

🔊 Stay alert for overdose signs and symptoms, such as CNS and respiratory depression, GI cramping, and constipation.

- Assess other drugs in patient's drug regimen for those that could cause additive or adverse interactions.
- Monitor patient for signs and symptoms of drug dependence or tolerance.

Patient teaching

- With oral use, advise patient to minimize adverse GI effects by taking doses with food or milk.

🔊 Tell patient to notify prescriber promptly if he experiences shortness of breath or difficulty breathing or if nausea, vomiting, or constipation become pronounced.

- Caution patient to avoid driving and other hazardous activities until he knows how drug affects concentration, alertness, vision, coordination, and physical dexterity.
- Instruct patient to move slowly when sitting up or standing, to avoid dizziness or light-headedness from sudden blood pressure decrease.
- As appropriate, review all other significant and life-threatening adverse reactions and interactions, especially those related to the drugs, herbs, and behaviors mentioned above.

C

colchicine

Pharmacologic class: Colchicum alkaloid

Therapeutic class: Antigout drug

Pregnancy risk category C

Action

Unclear. Antigout action may occur through white blood cell (WBC) migration and reduced lactic acid production by WBCs. This action in turn decreases uric acid deposition, kinetin formation, and phagocytosis, leading to reduction in inflammatory response.

Availability

Injection: 0.5 mg/ml
Tablets: 0.5 mg, 0.6 mg

Indications and dosages

➢ Acute gouty arthritis

Adults: Initially, 0.6 to 1.2 mg P.O.; then 0.6 to 1.2 mg P.O. q 1 to 2 hours or until relief occurs, adverse GI reactions occur, or patient has received a total cumulative dosage of 8 mg. Or 2 mg I.V., followed by 0.5 mg I.V. q 6 hours p.r.n., not to exceed 4 mg daily.

➢ Prophylaxis for recurrent gouty arthritis

Adults: In patients who have one yearly attack or less, 0.6 mg P.O. daily 3 days per week. In patients who have more than one yearly attack, 0.6 mg P.O. daily; in severe cases, 1 to 1.8 mg P.O. daily.

Dosage adjustment

- Mild hepatic or renal impairment

Off-label uses

- Hepatic cirrhosis
- Chronic progressive multiple sclerosis
- Pyoderma gangrenosum associated with Crohn's disease
- Psoriasis
- Dermatitis herpetiformis

Contraindications

- Hypersensitivity to drug
- Blood dyscrasias
- Serious GI, renal, hepatic, or cardiac disorders

Precautions

Use cautiously in:

- renal impairment
- elderly or debilitated patients
- pregnant or breastfeeding patients
- children (safety not established).

Administration

◀ Know that I.V. colchicine is a high-alert drug.

- Initiate therapy at first sign of acute gout attack.

◀ Don't administer I.M. or subcutaneously, because severe local irritation may occur.

◀ Don't dilute with 5% dextrose in water. If dilution is required, use normal saline solution injection.

- For I.V. injection, give by slow I.V. push over 2 to 5 minutes.
- Know that GI reactions may be troublesome in patients with peptic ulcer or irritable bowel.

Route	Onset	Peak	Duration
P.O.	12 hr	24-72 hr	Unknown
I.V.	Rapid	Rapid	Rapid

Adverse reactions

CNS: peripheral neuritis, neuropathy
GI: nausea, vomiting, diarrhea, abdominal pain
GU: anuria, hematuria, reversible azoospermia, renal impairment
Hematologic: purpura, **agranulocytosis, aplastic anemia, thrombocytopenia**
Metabolic: vitamin B_{12} malabsorption
Musculoskeletal: myopathy

Skin: dermatosis, alopecia
Other: hypersensitivity reactions

Interactions

Drug-drug. *Cyclosporine:* colchicine-induced myopathy
Vitamin B_{12}: reversible vitamin malabsorption
Drug-diagnostic tests. *Alkaline phosphatase, aspartate aminotransferase:* increased levels
Hematocrit, hemoglobin, platelets: decreased values
Urine hemoglobin, urinary red blood cells: false-positive results
Drug-food. *Caffeine-containing foods and beverages:* decreased colchicine effect
Drug-herbs. *Herbal teas, St. John's wort:* decreased drug effect
Drug-behaviors. *Alcohol use:* increased uric acid level

Patient monitoring

Monitor patient for signs and symptoms of toxicity (nausea, vomiting, abdominal pain, bloody diarrhea, burning sensation, muscle weakness, oliguria, hematuria, ascending paralysis, delirium, and seizures). Discontinue drug if these occur.
• Monitor CBC and renal function test results regularly.
• Be aware that patient may need opioids to control drug-induced diarrhea (especially if he's receiving maximum colchicine dosage).

Patient teaching

• Instruct patient to report rash, sore throat, fever, tiredness, weakness, numbness, or tingling.
Tell patient to immediately report muscle tremors, weakness, fatigue, bruising, bleeding, yellowing of eyes or skin, pale stools, dark urine, severe vomiting, watery or bloody diarrhea, or abdominal pain.
• Advise patient to increase fluid intake to prevent renal calculi (unless prescriber wants him to restrict fluids).
• Instruct patient to avoid alcohol, herbal teas, and caffeine during therapy.
• As appropriate, review all other significant and life-threatening adverse reactions and interactions, especially those related to the drugs, tests, foods, herbs, and behaviors mentioned above.

colesevelam hydrochloride

Welchol

Pharmacologic class: Bile acid sequestrant
Therapeutic class: Antihyperlipidemic
Pregnancy risk category B

Action

Binds bile acids in GI tract and forms insoluble complex, impeding bile acid reabsorption and promoting its excretion. As a result, cholesterol and low-density lipoprotein (LDL) levels decrease.

Availability

Tablets: 625 mg

Indications and dosages

➤ Adjunct to diet and exercise to reduce LDL cholesterol in patients with primary hypercholesterolemia
Adults: Three tablets P.O. b.i.d., or six tablets P.O. once daily. Maximum daily dosage is 4,375 mg.

Contraindications

• Hypersensitivity to drug
• Bowel obstruction
• Vitamin K deficiency

Precautions

Use cautiously in:
• serum triglyceride level above 300 mg/dl
• children (safety and efficacy not established).

Administration
- Give with meals and fluids.
- Ensure that patient swallows tablets whole without crushing or chewing.
- Know that drug may be used alone or with HMG-CoA reductase inhibitor.
- Store tablets at room temperature.

Route	Onset	Peak	Duration
P.O.	Unknown	2 wk	Unknown

Adverse reactions
CNS: headache, anxiety, vertigo, dizziness, insomnia, fatigue, syncope
EENT: tinnitus
GI: nausea, vomiting, diarrhea, constipation, abdominal discomfort, flatulence, fecal impaction, loose stools, fatty stools, rectal or hemorrhoidal bleeding, **other GI bleeding**
GU: increased libido
Hematologic: anemia, **bleeding tendency**
Metabolic: malabsorption of vitamins A, D, E, and K
Musculoskeletal: back, muscle, or joint pain
Skin: bruising

Interactions
Drug-drug. *Fat-soluble vitamins (A, D, E, and K):* decreased vitamin absorption

Patient monitoring
- Monitor lipid levels before starting therapy and periodically thereafter.

Patient teaching
- Instruct patient to take drug with meals as directed.
- Tell patient to report persistent GI upset, back or muscle pain or weakness, and respiratory problems.
- If drug causes constipation, instruct patient to increase exercise, drink plenty of fluids, consume more fruits and fiber, or take a stool softener.
- As appropriate, review all other significant and life-threatening adverse reactions and interactions, especially those related to the drugs mentioned above.

C

colestipol hydrochloride
Colestid

Pharmacologic class: Bile acid sequestrant
Therapeutic class: Antihyperlipidemic
Pregnancy risk category NR

Action
Binds bile acids in GI tract and forms insoluble complex, impeding bile acid reabsorption and promoting its excretion. As a result, cholesterol and low-density lipoprotein levels decrease.

Availability
Granules for suspension: 5 g/packet or scoop
Tablets: 1 g

Indications and dosages
➤ Primary hypercholesterolemia
Adults: *Granules*—5 g P.O. once or twice daily; may increase q 1 to 2 months up to 30 g/day P.O. given in one or two divided doses. *Tablets*—2 g P.O. once or twice daily; may increase q 1 to 2 months up to 16 g/day P.O. given in one or two divided doses.

Off-label uses
- Digoxin toxicity

Contraindications
- Hypersensitivity to drug

Precautions
Use cautiously in:
- history of constipation
- breastfeeding patients

• children (safety and efficacy not established).

Administration

• Mix granules with at least 90 ml of liquid, and stir until completely mixed.
• Give tablets with large amount of water.
• Administer other drugs 1 hour before or 4 hours after colestipol.

Route	Onset	Peak	Duration
P.O.	24-48 hr	1 mo	1 mo

Adverse reactions

CNS: dizziness, headache, vertigo, anxiety, syncope, fatigue
CV: chest pain
GI: nausea, vomiting, constipation, abdominal discomfort, fecal impaction, flatulence, fatty stools, hemorrhoids, perianal irritation, tongue irritation
Metabolic: deficiency of vitamins A, D, E, and K and folic acid, **hyperchloremic acidosis**
Musculoskeletal: osteoporosis, backache, muscle and joint pain, arthritis
Skin: irritation, rashes

Interactions

Drug-drug. *Amiodarone, corticosteroids, digoxin, diuretics, fat-soluble vitamins (A, D, E, K), folic acid, gemfibrozil, imipramine, methotrexate, mycophenolate, nonsteroidal anti-inflammatory drugs, penicillin G, phosphates, propranolol, tetracyclines, thyroid preparations, ursodiol:* decreased absorption of these drugs (when given orally)
Drug-diagnostic tests. *Alanine aminotransferase, alkaline phosphatase, aspartate aminotransferase, phosphorus:* increased levels
Prothrombin time: prolonged

Patient monitoring

• Monitor lipid levels frequently during first few months of therapy and periodically thereafter.
• Evaluate patient for signs and symptoms of abnormal bleeding.
• Be aware that prolonged use may increase bleeding tendency (from hypoprothrombinemia resulting from vitamin K deficiency). As prescribed and needed, give oral or parenteral vitamin K to reverse this effect.

Patient teaching

• Instruct patient to take granules with 3 to 4 oz of water, fruit juice, soup with high fluid content, cereal, or pulpy fruits (crushed).
• Tell patient to swallow tablets whole, one at a time, and not to crush, cut, or chew them.
• Inform patient that drug may interfere with absorption of many other drugs. Advise him to take other drugs 1 hour before or 4 hours after colestipol.
• As appropriate, review all other significant and life-threatening adverse reactions and interactions, especially those related to the drugs and tests mentioned above.

cortisone acetate

Pharmacologic class: Glucocorticoid
Therapeutic class: Adrenocorticoid
Pregnancy risk category C

Action

Unclear. Reduces inflammation, possibly by suppressing cell-mediated immune reactions; decreasing white blood cell, monocyte, and eosinophil counts; reducing binding of immunoglobulins to cell surface receptors; and inhibiting interleukin synthesis. Also stabilizes lysosomal membranes, curbs polymorphonuclear leukocyte migration, interrupts phagocytosis, and diminishes antibody formation in infected and injured tissues.

Availability

Injection: 50 mg/ml
Tablets: 5 mg, 10 mg, 25 mg

Indications and dosages

➤ Asthma; adrenal insufficiency; chronic inflammatory, allergic, hematologic, neoplastic, and autoimmune disorders; prevention of organ rejection in organ transplant recipients (given with other immunosuppressants)
Adults: 25 to 300 mg P.O. daily, or 20 to 300 mg I.M. daily or on alternate days. Individualize dosage based on disease and patient response.

Dosage adjustment

- Renal impairment
- Elderly patients

Contraindications

- Hypersensitivity to drug
- Systemic fungal infections

Precautions

Use cautiously in:
- renal insufficiency, cirrhosis, diabetes mellitus, diverticulitis, nonspecific ulcerative colitis, recent intestinal anastomoses, peptic ulcer (active or latent), heart failure, hypertension, thromboembolic disorders, hypoprothrombinemia, hypothyroidism, myasthenia gravis, glaucoma, ocular herpes simplex, osteoporosis, seizures, underlying immunosuppression, systemic infections, active untreated infections
- emotional instability or psychotic tendency
- pregnant or breastfeeding patients
- children.

Administration

- To help prevent peptic ulcer, give large doses between meals with antacids.
- If possible, administer before 9 A.M. (Exogenous corticosteroids are less likely to suppress adrenocortical activity when given at time of maximal activity.)

Route	Onset	Peak	Duration
P.O.	Rapid	2 hr	1.25-1.5 days
I.M.	24-48 hr	Variable	Variable

Adverse reactions

CNS: depression, euphoria, psychosis, vertigo, headache, **increased intracranial pressure, seizures**
CV: hypertension, **thrombophlebitis, thromboembolism**
EENT: cataracts, glaucoma, exophthalmos, increased intraocular pressure
GI: nausea, abdominal distention, **pancreatitis, peptic ulcers, ulcerative esophagitis**
GU: menstrual irregularities
Metabolic: sodium retention, fluid retention, potassium loss, carbohydrate intolerance, negative nitrogen balance, hyperglycemia, cushingoid appearance (moon face, buffalo hump), **hypokalemic acidosis**
Musculoskeletal: muscle wasting, osteoporosis, aseptic joint necrosis, muscle pain or weakness, vertebral compression fractures, steroid myopathy, tendon rupture, decreased growth (in children)
Skin: decreased wound healing, bruising, fragile skin, petechiae, urticaria, facial erythema, diaphoresis, hirsutism
Other: weight gain or loss, facial edema, increased susceptibility to or masking of infection, hypersensitivity reactions

Interactions

Drug-drug. *Anticoagulants:* increased or decreased anticoagulant blood level
Barbiturates, phenytoin, rifampin: decreased cortisone effects
Digoxin: increased risk of digitalis toxicity
Estrogens, hormonal contraceptives: increased cortisone effects

Fluoroquinolones: increased risk of tendon rupture
Itraconazole, ketoconazole: increased cortisone blood level
Live-virus vaccines: decreased antibody response to vaccine, increased risk of adverse reactions
Somatrem, somatropin: inhibition of growth-promoting effect
Thiazide and loop diuretics: additive hypokalemia
Drug-diagnostic tests. *Alanine aminotransferase, alkaline phosphatase, aspartate aminotransferase, cholesterol, glucose:* increased levels
Calcium, potassium: decreased levels
Nitroblue tetrazolium test: false-negative result
Drug-herbs. *Echinacea:* increased immune-stimulating effects
Ginseng: increased immune-modulating response

Patient monitoring

- Monitor patient closely for signs and symptoms of infection. Be aware that drug may mask these.
- Watch for weight gain, edema, and signs and symptoms of hypokalemia.
- Measure blood pressure regularly to detect hypertension.

◀ When discontinuing drug after long-term therapy, taper dosage gradually. Abrupt withdrawal may be fatal.

- With long-term therapy, evaluate patient for negative nitrogen balance; drug may cause protein catabolism. Also check vital signs and evaluate laboratory findings (including 2-hour postprandial blood glucose level, potassium level, and chest X-ray) at regular intervals.
- Monitor upper GI X-rays in patients with suspected peptic ulcer disease or significant dyspepsia or gastric distress.

Patient teaching

- Advise patient to take drug with meal or snack.
- Tell patient taking single daily dose or alternate-day doses to take drug in morning before 9 A.M. Instruct patient taking multiple daily doses to take doses at evenly spaced intervals throughout day.
- Instruct patient to carry identification stating that he's on long-term steroid therapy.
- Tell patient to report unusual weight gain, leg or foot swelling, muscle weakness, puffy face, cold, or infection.

◀ Caution patient never to stop therapy abruptly, because doing so may cause life-threatening adrenal insufficiency.

◀ Tell patient to contact prescriber immediately if signs or symptoms of adrenal insufficiency follow dosage reduction or drug discontinuation.

- Inform patient that he'll require continued supervision after discontinuing drug, because his disease or disorder may suddenly recur.
- As appropriate, review all other significant and life-threatening adverse reactions and interactions, especially those related to the drugs, tests, and herbs mentioned above.

cromolyn sodium

Crolom, Gastrocrom, Intal, Nalcrom♣, Nasalcrom

Pharmacologic class: Chromone derivative

Therapeutic class: Mast cell stabilizer, antiasthmatic, ophthalmic decongestant

Pregnancy risk category B

Action

Inhibits release of histamine and reacting substances of anaphylaxis from mast cells, stabilizing the cell membrane and reducing the allergic response and inflammatory reaction

Availability
Aerosol spray for inhalation: 800 mcg/ spray in 8.1-g container (112 sprays) or 14.2-g container (200 sprays)
Nasal solution: 40 mg/ml (5.2 mg/ spray) in 13-ml container (100 sprays) or 26-ml container (200 sprays)
Ophthalmic solution: 4%
Oral solution: 100 mg/5 ml
Solution for nebulization: 10 mg/ml

Indications and dosages
➢ Prevention of exercise-induced bronchospasm; adjunct in prevention of allergic disorders, including rhinitis and asthma
Adults and children ages 5 and older: One aerosol spray in each nostril (5.2 mg/spray) q.i.d., or two metered-dose sprays using inhaler at regular intervals or shortly before exposure to triggering event
Children ages 2 to 5: 20 mg q.i.d. via nebulization at regular intervals or no more than 1 hour before exposure to triggering event
➢ Mastocytosis
Adults and children ages 13 and older: 200 mg P.O. q.i.d.
Children ages 2 to 12: 100 mg P.O. q.i.d.
➢ Vernal keratoconjunctivitis, vernal conjunctivitis, and vernal keratitis
Adults and children ages 4 and older: One to two drops of ophthalmic solution in each eye four to six times daily at regular intervals

Off-label uses
- Proctitis
- Ulcerative colitis
- Urticaria

Contraindications
- Hypersensitivity to drug
- Status asthmaticus

Precautions
Use cautiously in:
- renal or hepatic impairment, acute bronchospasm attacks
- pregnant or breastfeeding patients
- children younger than age 5.

Administration
- Administer oral form 30 minutes before meals and at bedtime.
- Before giving by inhalation, shake canister gently.
- Don't immerse canister in water.
- Before using nasal spray, have patient clear nasal passages by blowing nose.
- Don't expose solutions to direct sunlight.

Route	Onset	Peak	Duration
P.O., inhalation, nasal, ophthalmic	<1 wk	2-4 wk	Unknown

Adverse reactions
CNS: headache, drowsiness, dizziness
EENT: nasal irritation, sneezing, epistaxis, postnasal drip (with nasal solution); stinging of eyes, lacrimation (with ophthalmic solution)
GI: nausea, diarrhea, stomachache, swollen parotid glands
GU: difficult or painful urination, urinary frequency
Musculoskeletal: myopathy
Respiratory: wheezing, cough, **bronchospasm**
Skin: erythema, rash, urticaria, angioedema
Other: altered taste, substernal burning, allergic reactions including **anaphylaxis, serum sickness**

Interactions
None significant

Patient monitoring
- Monitor pulmonary function periodically.

• Evaluate patient for signs and symptoms of overdose, including bronchospasm and difficult or painful urination.

Patient teaching

With nebulizer—

• Instruct patient to prepare nebulizer according to package instructions, to clear as much mucus as possible before use, and to rinse mouth after each use (to help prevent opportunistic infections and reduce unpleasant aftertaste).

With nasal form—

• Teach patient how to instill nasal spray as directed.

• Tell patient that drug may cause unpleasant taste, but that rinsing mouth and performing frequent oral care may help. Also inform him that drug may cause headache.

• Advise patient to report increased sneezing; nasal burning, stinging, or irritation; sore throat; hoarseness; or nosebleed.

With oral form—

• Tell patient to take oral form 30 minutes before meals.

With ophthalmic form—

• Instruct patient to wash hands before using.

• Teach patient how to instill drops: Instruct him to tilt his head back and look up, place drops inside lower eyelid, close his eye, and roll eyeball in all directions. Tell him not to blink for about 30 seconds, and then to apply gentle pressure to inner corner of eye for 30 seconds.

• Caution patient not to let applicator tip touch eye or any other surface.

• Tell patient drug may cause temporary stinging of eye or blurred vision.

• Advise patient not to wear contact lenses during therapy.

With all forms—

• As appropriate, review all other significant adverse reactions.

cyclobenzaprine hydrochloride

Apo-Cyclobenzaprine✤, Flexeril, Novo-Cycloprine✤

Pharmacologic class: Autonomic nervous system drug

Therapeutic class: Skeletal muscle relaxant (centrally acting)

Pregnancy risk category B

Action

Unclear. Thought to act primarily at brain stem (and to a lesser extent at spinal cord level) to relieve skeletal muscle spasms of local origin without altering muscle function.

Availability

Tablets: 5 mg, 10 mg

Indications and dosages

➤ Adjunct to physical therapy to relieve muscle spasms

Adults: 5 mg P.O. t.i.d. May increase to 10 mg P.O. t.i.d. as needed.

Contraindications

• Hypersensitivity to drug
• Acute recovery phase after myocardial infarction (MI)
• Heart failure
• Arrhythmias
• Hyperthyroidism
• MAO inhibitor use within past 14 days

Precautions

Use cautiously in:

• cardiovascular disease, closed-angle glaucoma, hepatic impairment, increased intraocular pressure, urinary retention
• elderly patients
• pregnant or breastfeeding patients
• children younger than age 15.

Administration

Don't give within 14 days of MAO inhibitor. Drug interaction may cause hypertensive crisis and severe seizures.
- Know that drug shouldn't be used for more than 3 weeks.
- Be aware that drug may not be first-line agent for elderly patients because of its anticholinergic effects.

Route	Onset	Peak	Duration
P.O.	1 hr	4-6 hr	12-24 hr

Adverse reactions

CNS: dizziness, drowsiness, syncope, confusion, fatigue, headache, nervousness, decreased mental acuity, irritability, weakness, insomnia, depression, disorientation, delusions, peripheral neuropathy, abnormal gait, Bell's palsy, EEG changes, extrapyramidal symptoms, **cerebrovascular accident**
CV: vasodilation, tachycardia, chest pain, hypotension, **MI, heart block**
EENT: blurred vision
GI: nausea, constipation, dyspepsia, swollen parotid glands, mouth inflammation, discolored tongue, dry mouth, **paralytic ileus**
GU: galactorrhea, urinary retention, urinary frequency, gynecomastia, testicular swelling, libido changes, erectile dysfunction
Hematologic: purpura, eosinophilia, **bone marrow depression, leukopenia, thrombocytopenia**
Metabolic: hyperglycemia, **hypoglycemia, syndrome of inappropriate diuretic hormone secretion**
Musculoskeletal: muscle ache
Respiratory: dyspnea
Skin: photosensitization, alopecia, angioedema
Other: unpleasant taste, weight gain or loss, edema

Interactions

Drug-drug. *Anticholinergics, anticholinergic-like drugs (including antidepressants, antihistamines, disopyramide, haloperidol, phenothiazines):* additive anticholinergic effects
Antihistamines, CNS depressants, opioids, sedative-hypnotics: additive CNS depression
Guanadrel, guanethidine: reduction in or blockage of these drugs' actions
MAO inhibitors: hyperpyretic crisis, seizures, death
Drug-herbs. *Chamomile, hops, kava, skullcap, valerian:* increased CNS depression
Drug-behaviors. *Alcohol use:* increased CNS depression

Patient monitoring

- Assess for adverse CNS effects, such as drowsiness, dizziness, and decreased mental acuity.
- Monitor patient for evidence of drug interactions, especially when giving drug with CNS depressants.

Patient teaching

- Tell patient that drug may cause dry mouth.
- Caution patient to avoid driving and other hazardous activities until he knows how drug affects concentration, alertness, and vision.
- Advise patient not to use alcohol, sedatives, pain medications, over-the-counter preparations, or herbs without consulting prescriber.
- As appropriate, review all other significant and life-threatening adverse reactions and interactions, especially those related to the drugs, herbs, and behaviors mentioned above.

cyclophosphamide

Cytoxan, Procytox✦

Pharmacologic class: Alkylating agent, nitrogen mustard

Therapeutic class: Antineoplastic

Pregnancy risk category D

Action

Unclear. Thought to prevent cell division by cross-linking DNA strands, thereby interfering with growth of susceptible cancer cells.

Availability

Powder for injection: 100 mg, 200 mg, 500 mg, 1 g, 2 g

Tablets: 25 mg, 50 mg

Indications and dosages

➢ Hodgkin's disease; malignant lymphoma; multiple myeloma; leukemia; advanced mycosis fungoides; neuroblastoma; ovarian cancer; breast cancer; and certain other tumors

Adults: Initially, 40 to 50 mg/kg I.V. in divided doses over 2 to 5 days, or 10 to 15 mg/kg I.V. q 10 days, or 3 to 5 mg/kg I.V. twice weekly.

Children: Initially, 2 to 8 mg/kg or 60 to 250 mg/m^2 P.O. or I.V. daily in divided doses for 6 or more days. Maintenance dosage is 2 to 5 mg/kg or 50 to 150 mg/m^2 P.O. twice weekly.

➢ Biopsy-proven nephrotic syndrome in children

Children: 2.5 to 3 mg/kg/day P.O. for 60 to 90 days

Off-label uses

- Severe rheumatologic conditions
- Selected cases of severe progressive rheumatoid arthritis and systemic lupus erythematosus

Contraindications

- Hypersensitivity to drug
- Severe bone marrow depression
- Breastfeeding

Precautions

Use cautiously in:

- renal or hepatic impairment, adrenalectomy, mild to moderate bone marrow depression, other chronic debilitating illnesses
- females of childbearing age
- pregnant patients.

Administration

- Verify that patient isn't pregnant before administering.
- Follow facility procedures for safe handling, administration, and disposal of chemotherapeutic drugs.
- Administer tablets on empty stomach. If drug causes severe GI upset, give with food.
- Don't cut or crush tablets.
- Know that dosage may need to be decreased if drug is given with other antineoplastics.
- Dilute each 100 mg of powder with 5 ml of sterile water for injection, to yield 20 mg/ml. Further dilute with compatible fluid, such as 5% dextrose injection, 5% dextrose and normal saline solution for injection, 5% dextrose and Ringer's injection, lactated Ringer's injection, or half-normal saline solution for injection.
- For I.V. injection, give each 100 mg over at least 1 minute. When giving dosages above 500 mg diluted in 100 to 250 ml of compatible solution, administer over 20 to 60 minutes.
- Use solution prepared with bacteriostatic water for injection within 24 hours if stored at room temperature or within 6 days if refrigerated.
- To minimize bladder toxicity, increase patient's fluid intake during therapy and for 1 to 2 days afterward. Most adults require fluid intake of at least 2 L/day.

Route	Onset	Peak	Duration
P.O., I.V.	7 days	7-15 days	21 days

Adverse reactions

CV: cardiotoxicity
GI: nausea, vomiting, diarrhea, abdominal pain or discomfort, stomatitis, oral mucosal ulcers, anorexia, **hemorrhagic colitis**
GU: urinary bladder fibrosis, hematuria, amenorrhea, decreased sperm count, sterility, **acute hemorrhagic cystitis, renal tubular necrosis, hemorrhagic ureteral inflammation**
Hematologic: anemia, **leukopenia, thrombocytopenia, bone marrow depression, neutropenia**
Hepatic: jaundice
Metabolic: hyperuricemia
Respiratory: interstitial pulmonary fibrosis
Skin: nail and pigmentation changes, alopecia
Other: poor wound healing, infections, allergic reactions including **anaphylaxis, secondary cancer**

Interactions

Drug-drug. *Allopurinol, thiazide diuretics:* increased risk of leukopenia
Digoxin: decreased digoxin blood level
Cardiotoxic drugs (such as cytarabine, daunorubicin, doxorubicin): additive cardiotoxicity
Chloramphenicol: prolonged cyclophosphamide half-life
Phenobarbital: increased risk of cyclophosphamide toxicity
Quinolones: decreased antimicrobial effect
Succinylcholine: prolonged neuromuscular blockade
Warfarin: increased anticoagulant effect
Drug-diagnostic tests. *Hemoglobin, platelets, pseudocholinesterase, red blood cells (RBCs), white blood cells:* decreased values
Uric acid: increased level

Patient monitoring

- Assess infusion site for signs of extravasation.
- Monitor hematologic profile to determine degree of hematopoietic suppression. Be aware that leukopenia is an expected drug effect and is used to help determine dosage.
- Monitor urine regularly for RBCs, which may precede hemorrhagic cystitis.

Patient teaching

- Tell patient to take tablets on empty stomach. However, if GI upset occurs, instruct him to take them with food.

(Clinical alert) Advise patient to promptly report unusual bleeding or bruising, fever, chills, sore throat, cough, shortness of breath, seizures, lack of menstrual flow, unusual lumps or masses, flank or stomach pain, joint pain, mouth or lip sores, or yellowing of skin or eyes.

- Instruct patient to drink 2 to 3 L of fluids daily (unless prescriber has told him to restrict fluids).
- Tell patient that drug may cause hair loss, but that hair usually grows back after treatment ends.
- Advise female patient to use barrier contraception during therapy and for 1 month afterward.
- As appropriate, review all other significant and life-threatening adverse reactions and interactions, especially those related to the drugs and tests mentioned above.

cyclosporine

Gengraf, Neoral, Sandimmune

Pharmacologic class: Polypeptide antibiotic
Therapeutic class: Immunosuppressant
Pregnancy risk category C

Action
Unclear. Thought to act by specific, reversible inhibition of immunocompetent lymphocytes in G_0-G_1 phase of cell cycle. Preferentially inhibits T lymphocytes; also inhibits lymphokine production.

Availability
Capsules: 25 mg, 100 mg
Injection: 50 mg/ml
Oral solution: 100 mg/ml

Indications and dosages
➢ Psoriasis
Adults: *Neoral only*—1.25 mg/kg P.O. b.i.d. for 4 weeks. Based on patient response, may increase by 0.5 mg/kg/day once q 2 weeks, to a maximum dosage of 4 mg/kg/day.
➢ Severe active rheumatoid arthritis
Adults: *Neoral only*—1.25 mg/kg P.O. b.i.d. May adjust dosage by 0.5 to 0.75 mg/kg/day after 8 weeks and again after 12 weeks, to a maximum dosage of 4 mg/kg/day. If no response occurs after 16 weeks, discontinue therapy. *Gengraf only*—2.5 mg/kg P.O. daily given in two divided doses; after 8 weeks, may increase to a maximum dosage of 4 mg/kg/day.
➢ To prevent organ rejection in kidney, liver, or heart transplantation
Adults and children: *Sandimmune only*—Initially, 15 mg/kg P.O. 4 to 12 hours before transplantation, then daily for 1 to 2 weeks postoperatively. Reduce dosage by 5% weekly to a maintenance level of 5 to 10 mg/kg/day. Or 5 to 6 mg/kg I.V. as a continuous infusion 4 to 12 hours before transplantation.

Off-label uses
- Aplastic anemia
- Atopic dermatitis

Contraindications
- Hypersensitivity to drug
- Rheumatoid arthritis, psoriasis in patients with abnormal renal function, uncontrolled hypertension, cancer (Gengraf, Neoral)

Precautions
Use cautiously in:
- hepatic impairment, renal dysfunction, active infection, hypertension
- pregnant or breastfeeding patients
- children.

Administration
- For I.V. infusion, dilute as ordered with dextrose 5% in water or 0.9% normal saline solution. Administer over 2 to 6 hours.
- Mix Neoral solution with orange juice or apple juice to improve its taste.
- Dilute Sandimmune oral solution with milk, chocolate milk, or orange juice. Be aware that grapefruit and grapefruit juice affect drug metabolism.
- In postoperative patients, switch to P.O. dosage as tolerance allows.
- Be aware that Sandimmune and Neoral aren't bioequivalent. Don't use interchangeably.

Route	Onset	Peak	Duration
P.O.	Unknown	1.5-3.5 hr	Unknown
I.V.	Rapid	1-2 hr	Unknown

Adverse reactions
CNS: tremor, headache, confusion, paresthesia, insomnia, anxiety, depression, lethargy, weakness
CV: hypertension, chest pain, **myocardial infarction**
EENT: visual disturbances, hearing loss, tinnitus, rhinitis
GI: nausea, vomiting, diarrhea, constipation, abdominal discomfort, gastritis, peptic ulcer, mouth sores, difficulty swallowing, anorexia, **upper GI bleeding, pancreatitis**

GU: gynecomastia, hematuria, **nephrotoxicity, renal dysfunction, glomerular capillary thrombosis**
Hematologic: anemia, **leukopenia, thrombocytopenia**
Metabolic: hyperglycemia, hypomagnesemia, hyperuricemia, **hyperkalemia, metabolic acidosis**
Musculoskeletal: muscle and joint pain
Respiratory: cough, dyspnea, ***Pneumocystis jiroveci* pneumonia, bronchospasm**
Skin: acne, hirsutism, brittle fingernails, hair breakage, night sweats
Other: gum hyperplasia, flulike symptoms, edema, fever, weight loss, hiccups, **anaphylaxis**

Interactions

Drug-drug. *Acyclovir, aminoglycosides, amphotericin B, cimetidine, diclofenac, gentamicin, ketoconazole, melphalan, naproxen, ranitidine, sulindac, sulfamethoxazole, tacrolimus, tobramycin, trimethoprim, vancomycin:* increased risk of nephrotoxicity
Allopurinol, amiodarone, bromocriptine, clarithromycin, colchicine, danazol, diltiazem, erythromycin, fluconazole, imipenem and cilastatin, itraconazole, ketoconazole, methylprednisolone, nicardipine, prednisolone, quinupristin/dalfopristin, verapamil: increased cyclosporine blood level
Azathioprine, corticosteroids, cyclophosphamide: increased immunosuppression
Carbamazepine, isoniazid, nafcillin, octreotide, orlistat, phenobarbital, phenytoin, rifabutin, rifampin, ticlopidine: decreased cyclosporine blood level
Digoxin: decreased digoxin clearance
Live-virus vaccines: decreased antibody response to vaccine
Lovastatin: decreased lovastatin clearance, increased risk of myopathy and rhabdomyolysis
Potassium-sparing diuretics: increased risk of hyperkalemia

Drug-diagnostic tests. *Alanine aminotransferase, aspartate aminotransferase, bilirubin, blood urea nitrogen, creatinine, glucose, low-density lipoproteins:* increased levels
Hemoglobin, platelets, white blood cells: decreased values

Drug-food. *Grapefruit, grapefruit juice:* decreased cyclosporine metabolism, increased cyclosporine blood level
High-fat diet: decreased drug absorption (Neoral)

Drug-herbs. *Alfalfa sprouts, astragalus, echinacea, licorice:* interference with immunosuppressant action
St. John's wort: reduced cyclosporine blood level, possibly leading to organ rejection

Patient monitoring

- Observe patient for first 30 to 60 minutes of infusion. Monitor frequently thereafter.
- Monitor cyclosporine blood level, electrolyte levels, and liver and kidney function test results.
- Assess for signs and symptoms of hyperkalemia in patients receiving concurrent potassium-sparing diuretic.

Patient teaching

- Advise patient to dilute Neoral oral solution with orange or apple juice (preferably at room temperature) to improve its flavor.
- Instruct patient to use glass container when taking oral solution. Tell him not to let solution stand before drinking, to stir solution well and then drink all at once, and to rinse glass with same liquid and then drink again to ensure that he takes entire dose.
- Tell patient taking Neoral to avoid high-fat meals, grapefruit, and grapefruit juice.
- Advise patient to dilute Sandimmune oral solution with milk, chocolate milk, or orange juice to improve its flavor.

• Inform patient that he's at increased risk for infection. Caution him to avoid crowds and exposure to illness.
• Tell patient he'll need to undergo repeated laboratory testing during therapy.
• As appropriate, review all other significant and life-threatening adverse reactions and interactions, especially those related to the drugs, tests, foods, and herbs mentioned above.

cyproheptadine hydrochloride

Periactin, PMS-Cyproheptadine✱

Pharmacologic class: Piperidine (nonselective)
Therapeutic class: Antihistamine
Pregnancy risk category B

Action

Antagonizes effects of histamine at histamine$_1$-receptor sites, preventing histamine-mediated responses. Also blocks effects of serotonin, causing increased appetite.

Availability

Syrup: 2 mg/5 ml
Tablets: 4 mg

Indications and dosages

➢ Allergy symptoms caused by histamine release (including seasonal and perennial allergic rhinitis); chronic urticaria; angioedema; dermographism; cold urticaria; adjunctive therapy for anaphylactic reactions
Adults: Initially, 4 mg P.O. q 8 hours. Maintenance dosage is 4 to 20 mg/day in three divided doses, to a maximum dosage of 0.5 mg/kg/day.
Children ages 7 to 14: 2 to 4 mg P.O. q 12 hours. Don't exceed 16 mg/day.
Children ages 2 to 6: 2 mg P.O. q 12 hours. Don't exceed 12 mg/day.

Off-label uses

• Vascular cluster headaches

Contraindications

• Hypersensitivity to drug
• Alcohol intolerance (syrup only)
• Bladder neck obstruction
• Angle-closure glaucoma
• Ulcer disease
• Symptomatic prostatic hypertrophy
• MAO inhibitor use within past 14 days

Precautions

Use cautiously in:
• hepatic impairment
• elderly patients
• pregnant patients (safety not established)
• breastfeeding patients.

Administration

• Give with food or milk to decrease GI upset.

Route	Onset	Peak	Duration
P.O.	15-60 min	1-2 hr	8 hr

Adverse reactions

CNS: drowsiness, dizziness, excitation (especially in children), fatigue, sedation, hallucinations, disorientation, tremor
CV: palpitations, hypotension, **arrhythmias**
EENT: blurred vision, nasal dryness and congestion, dry throat
GI: constipation, dry mouth
GU: urinary retention, urinary frequency, ejaculatory inhibition, early menses
Respiratory: thickened bronchial secretions
Skin: rash, photosensitivity
Other: weight gain

Interactions

Drug-drug. *CNS depressants (including opioid analgesics, sedative-hypnotics):* increased CNS depression
MAO inhibitors: intensified, prolonged anticholinergic effects
Drug-diagnostic tests. *Allergy skin tests:* false-negative reactions
Drug-behaviors. *Alcohol use:* increased CNS depression

Patient monitoring

- Monitor patient for excessive anticholinergic effects.
- Assess for excessive CNS depression.
- Discontinue drug 4 days before diagnostic skin testing.

Patient teaching

- Advise patient to take drug with food to minimize GI upset.
- Caution patient not to use other CNS depressants, sleep aids, or alcohol during therapy.
- Instruct patient to avoid driving and other hazardous activities until he knows how drug affects concentration and alertness.
- As appropriate, review all other significant and life-threatening adverse reactions and interactions, especially those related to the drugs, tests, and behaviors mentioned above.

cytarabine

Cytosar✱, Cytosar-U, DepoCyt

Pharmacologic class: Antimetabolite, pyrimidine analog
Therapeutic class: Antineoplastic
Pregnancy risk category D

Action

Unclear. Cytotoxic effect may stem from inhibition of DNA polymerase by drug's active metabolite.

Availability

Injection (conventional form): 20 mg
Liposomal injection for intrathecal use (sustained-release): 50 mg/5-ml vial
Powder for injection (conventional form): 100 mg, 500 mg, 1g, 2 g

Indications and dosages

➤ To induce remission of acute nonlymphocytic leukemia
Adults: Injection (conventional form)—100 mg/m²/day by continuous I.V. infusion on days 1 through 7, or 100 mg/m² I.V. q 12 hours on days 1 through 7, given with other antineoplastics
➤ Meningeal leukemia
Adults: Injection (conventional form)—5 to 75 mg/m²/day intrathecally for 4 days, or once q 4 days. Most common dosage is 30 mg/m² q 4 days until cerebrospinal fluid is normal.
➤ Lymphomatous meningitis
Adults: Liposomal injection—50 mg intrathecally q 14 days for two doses (at weeks 1 and 3); then q 14 days for three doses (at weeks 5, 7, and 9), with one additional dose at week 13; then q 28 days for four doses

Contraindications

- Hypersensitivity to drug
- Active meningeal infection (liposomal form)

Precautions

Use cautiously in:
- renal or hepatic disease, active infection, decreased bone marrow reserve, other chronic illnesses
- females of childbearing age
- pregnant or breastfeeding patients
- children.

Administration

- Follow facility procedures for safe handling, administration, and disposal of chemotherapeutic drugs.
- For I.V. injection, reconstitute each 100 mg with 5 ml of diluent (if neces-

sary), and give each 100-mg dose over 1 to 3 minutes. For I.V. infusion, dilute further with 50 to 100 ml of dextrose 5% in water or normal saline solution, and infuse over 30 minutes to 24 hours (depending on dosage and concentration).
• Be aware that conventional and liposomal forms can be administered inthrathecally.
Don't use intrathecal route for formulations containing benzyl alcohol.
• When giving conventional form intrathecally, reconstitute with autologous spinal fluid or preservative-free normal saline solution for injection. Use immediately.
• If patient is receiving liposomal cytarabine concurrently with dexamethasone, provide appropriate care to ease symptoms of chemical arachnoiditis.

Route	Onset	Peak	Duration
I.V.	Unknown	Unknown	Unknown
Intrathecal	Rapid	5 hr	14-28 hr

Adverse reactions
CNS: malaise, dizziness, headache, neuritis, **neurotoxicity, chemical arachnoiditis**
CV: chest pain, **thrombophlebitis**
EENT: conjunctivitis
GI: nausea, vomiting, diarrhea, abdominal pain, anal ulcers, esophagitis, esophageal ulcers, oral ulcers (in 5 to 10 days), anorexia, **bowel necrosis**
GU: urinary retention, **renal dysfunction**
Hematologic: anemia, **megaloblastosis, reticulocytopenia, leukopenia, thrombocytopenia**
Hepatic: hepatic dysfunction
Metabolic: hyperuricemia
Musculoskeletal: muscle ache, bone pain
Respiratory: pneumonia, shortness of breath
Skin: rash, pruritus, freckling, skin ulcers, urticaria, alopecia
Other: flulike symptoms, edema, infection, fever, cellulitis at injection site, **anaphylaxis, infection (mild to fatal)**

Interactions
Drug-drug. *Digoxin:* decreased digoxin blood level
Fluorocytosine: decreased fluorocytosine blood level
Gentamicin: decreased gentamicin effects
Drug-diagnostic tests. *Hemoglobin, platelets, red blood cells, reticulocytes, white blood cells:* decreased values
Megaloblasts, uric acid: increased levels

Patient monitoring
• Observe for signs and symptoms of cytarabine syndrome (malaise, fever, muscle ache, bone pain, occasional chest pain, maculopapular rash, and conjunctivitis).
When giving liposomal form, assess for signs and symptoms of chemical arachnoiditis, such as neck rigidity and pain, nausea, vomiting, headache, fever, and back pain.
• Monitor liver function test results, CBC with differential, platelet count, blood urea nitrogen, and serum creatinine and uric acid levels.
Observe closely for signs and symptoms of infection, which could become severe and fatal.

Patient teaching
Tell patient to contact prescriber immediately if he develops signs or symptoms of infection, cytarabine syndrome (malaise, fever, muscle ache, bone pain, chest pain, rash, eye infection), or chemical arachnoiditis (neck rigidity or pain, nausea, vomiting, headache, fever, or back pain).
Tell patient that drug makes him more susceptible to infection. Advise him to avoid crowds and exposure to illness.
• Advise patient to increase fluid intake, to promote uric acid excretion.

• As appropriate, review all other significant and life-threatening adverse reactions and interactions, especially those related to the drugs and tests mentioned above.

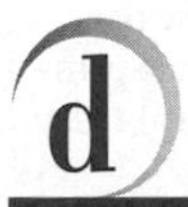

d

dacarbazine

DTIC✤, DTIC-Dome

Pharmacologic class: Alkylating drug, triazene
Therapeutic class: Antineoplastic
Pregnancy risk category C

Action

Unclear. Thought to inhibit DNA synthesis by acting as purine analog. Also causes alkylation and may interact with sulfhydryl groups.

Availability

Injection: 100-mg and 200-mg vials

Indications and dosages

➢ Hodgkin's disease
Adults: 150 mg/m² I.V. daily for 5 days in combination with other drugs, repeated q 4 weeks. Or 375 mg/m² I.V. on first day of combination therapy, repeated q 15 days.
➢ Metastatic malignant melanoma
Adults: 2 to 4.5 mg/kg I.V. daily for 10 days, repeated q 4 weeks. Or 250 mg/m² I.V. daily for 5 days, repeated q 3 weeks.

Off-label uses

• Malignant pheochromocytoma
• Metastatic malignant melanoma

Contraindications

• Hypersensitivity to drug

Precautions

Use cautiously in:
• hepatic dysfunction, impaired bone marrow function
• pregnant or breastfeeding patients.

Administration

• Follow facility procedures for safe handling, administration, and disposal of chemotherapeutic drugs.
• Reconstitute with sterile water for injection according to manufacturer's directions.
• Further dilute reconstituted drug with 5% dextrose in water or normal saline solution.
◀ Administer over 30 to 60 minutes by I.V. infusion only.
◀ Take steps to prevent extravasation, which may cause tissue damage and severe pain.

Route	Onset	Peak	Duration
I.V.	Unknown	Unknown	Unknown

Adverse reactions

CNS: malaise, paresthesia
GI: nausea, vomiting, dyspepsia, anorexia
Hematologic: anemia, **leukopenia, thrombocytopenia, bone marrow depression**
Musculoskeletal: myalgia
Skin: dermatitis, erythematous or urticarial rash, alopecia, flushing, photosensitivity
Others: flulike symptoms, fever, **hypersensitivity reactions** including **anaphylaxis**

Interactions

Drug-diagnostic tests. *Platelets, red blood cells, white blood cells:* decreased counts
Drug-behaviors. *Sun exposure:* photosensitivity reaction

Patient monitoring

Frequently monitor CBC with white cell differential and platelet count. Know that hematopoietic depression is the most common toxicity and can be fatal.

- Assess infusion site closely for extravasation.

Patient teaching

Instruct patient to immediately report pain, burning, or swelling at infusion site; numbness in arms or legs; gait changes; respiratory distress; difficulty breathing; rash; or easy bruising or bleeding.

- Advise patient to minimize GI distress by eating small, frequent servings of healthy food and drinking plenty of fluids.
- Tell patient he'll undergo regular blood testing during therapy.
- As appropriate, review all other significant and life-threatening adverse reactions and interactions, especially those related to the tests and behaviors mentioned above.

daclizumab

Zenapax

Pharmacologic class: Immunomodulator, humanized immunoglobulin G_1 monoclonal antibody

Therapeutic class: Immunosuppressant

Pregnancy risk category C

Action

Binds to alpha subunit of high-affinity interleuken-2 (IL-2) receptor complex, inhibiting IL-2 binding and blocking critical pathway in cellular immune response against allografts. Also impedes immunologic response to antigens.

Availability

Injection: 25 mg/5 ml

Indications and dosages

➢ Prevention of acute organ rejection in kidney transplantation

Adults: 1 mg/kg by I.V. infusion, usually for five doses. Give first dose no more than 24 hours before transplantation; give remaining doses at 14-day intervals.

Contraindications

- Hypersensitivity to drug

Precautions

Use cautiously in:

- elderly patients
- pregnant or breastfeeding patients
- children.

Administration

- Know that drug is given as part of immunosuppressive combination therapy.
- Don't give by direct I.V. injection.
- Mix diluted dose with 50 ml of sterile normal saline solution.
- Deliver through peripheral or central vein over 15 minutes.
- Don't add or infuse other drugs through same I.V. line.
- Administer diluted drug within 4 hours of preparation if stored at room temperature or within 24 hours if refrigerated. Discard prepared solution after 24 hours.
- Protect undiluted solution from direct light.

Route	Onset	Peak	Duration
I.V.	Rapid	After 5th dose	120 days

Adverse reactions

CNS: headache, tremor, dizziness, prickly sensations, insomnia, fatigue, weakness, depression, anxiety

CV: tachycardia, chest pain, hypotension, hypertension, **thrombosis**

EENT: blurred vision, rhinitis, pharyngitis
GI: nausea, vomiting, constipation, diarrhea, abdominal pain, abdominal distention, flatulence, epigastric pain, heartburn, dyspepsia, gastritis, hemorrhoids
GU: kidney enlargement, urinary tract bleeding, dysuria, urinary retention, **renal insufficiency, oliguria, renal tubular necrosis**
Hematologic: bleeding
Metabolic: diabetes mellitus, dehydration, **fluid overload**
Musculoskeletal: myalgia; joint, back, or leg pain
Respiratory: dyspnea, cough, hypoxia, crackles, crepitus, rhonchi, congestion, abnormal or decreased breath sounds, hemoptysis, upper respiratory tract infection, **atelectasis, pleural effusion**
Skin: acne, wound infection, impaired wound healing
Other: lymphocele (cystic mass), pain, edema at injection site, peripheral edema, cellulitis, cytomegalovirus infection, shivering, fever

Interactions
None significant

Patient monitoring
Monitor patient closely. Drug increases risk of infectious complications and secondary cancers.
• Monitor bone marrow function and CBC and platelet count frequently.
• Assess cardiovascular, respiratory, and renal function during infusion and periodically between infusions.
• Monitor blood glucose level, especially in patients receiving high-dose corticosteroids concurrently with daclizumab.

Patient teaching
• Explain that drug's purpose is to prevent transplant rejection.
Instruct patient to immediately report difficulty breathing or swallowing, tightness in jaw or throat, chest pain, or pain at infusion site.
Tell patient to promptly report changes in urinary pattern, unusual bleeding or bruising, rash, fever, and other adverse effects.
• Inform patient that drug increases risk of infection. Caution him to avoid crowds and exposure to illness.
• As appropriate, review all other significant and life-threatening adverse reactions.

dactinomycin (actinomycin D, ACT)
Cosmegen

Pharmacologic class: Anti-infective
Therapeutic class: Antineoplastic
Pregnancy risk category D

Action
Inhibits RNA synthesis, resulting in cell death. Cell-cycle-phase nonspecific.

Availability
Lyophilized powder for injection: 500-mcg vial

Indications and dosages
➢ Wilms' tumor; childhood rhabdomyosarcoma; Ewing's sarcoma
Children: Maximum dosage is 15 mcg/kg/day I.V. for 5 days, or 500 mcg/day or 2.5 mg/m^2 in equally divided doses over 7-day period (given with other chemotherapeutic drugs). Regimen may be repeated in 3 weeks if toxicity signs and symptoms have disappeared.
➢ Metastatic nonseminomatous testicular cancer
Adults: 1,000 mcg/m^2 I.V. on first day as part of combination regimen with cyclophosphamide, bleomycin, vinblastine, and cisplatin

➢ Gestational trophoblastic neoplasia
Adults: 12 mcg/kg/day I.V. for 5 days as monotherapy. Or 500 mcg I.V. on first and second days as part of combination regimen with etoposide, methotrexate, folinic acid, and vincristine.

Dosage adjustment
- Obesity
- Edema

Contraindications
- Hypersensitivity to drug
- Chickenpox
- Herpes zoster
- Infants younger than 12 months old

Precautions
Use cautiously in:
- renal or hepatic disease
- bone marrow depression in patients undergoing radiation therapy
- pregnant or breastfeeding patients.

Administration
🔊 Know that drug is highly toxic, so prepare and administer with care. Don't inhale dust or vapors or let drug contact skin or mucous membranes. If contact occurs, irrigate with copious amounts of water.
- Reconstitute powder by adding 1.1 ml of sterile water for injection (free of preservatives). Add reconstituted solution directly to infusion solution of 5% dextrose injection or sodium chloride injection or add to tubing of running I.V. infusion and infuse over 20 to 30 minutes.
- Be aware that dosages are almost always expressed in micrograms rather than milligrams.

🔊 Keep in mind that drug is an extremely corrosive vesicant. Take care to avoid extravasation because severe tissue damage will result. If extravasation occurs, discontinue drug immediately and apply cold compresses to area.
- Premedicate with antiemetic, as prescribed, because drug usually causes severe nausea and vomiting for up to 24 hours.
- Know that toxic reactions are common and may limit amount of drug that can be given.

Route	Onset	Peak	Duration
I.V.	Unknown	Unknown	Unknown

Adverse reactions
CNS: malaise, fatigue, lethargy
EENT: pharyngitis
GI: nausea, vomiting, diarrhea, dyspepsia, abdominal pain, proctitis, difficulty swallowing, esophagitis, dry mouth, lip inflammation and cracking, stomatitis, anorexia
Hematologic: anemia, **bleeding, thrombocytopenia, leukocytosis, leukopenia, pancytopenia, agranulocytosis, aplastic anemia, reticulocytopenia**
Hepatic: hepatotoxicity
Metabolic: hypocalcemia
Musculoskeletal: joint pain, growth retardation (in children)
Respiratory: pneumonitis
Skin: skin eruptions, petechiae, acne, erythema, increased pigmentation, diaphoresis, alopecia
Other: phlebitis and soft-tissue damage at injection site, fever, infection, edema

Interactions
Drug-drug. *Myelosuppressants:* additive toxicity
Drug-diagnostic tests. *Antibacterial drug assays:* test interference
Calcium, granulocytes, hemoglobin, platelets, red blood cells, white blood cells: decreased values
Liver function tests: abnormal results

Patient monitoring
- Monitor patient for severe nausea and vomiting.
- Watch infusion site closely for irritation and signs of extravasation.

• Monitor daily platelet count and CBC with white cell differential. Be prepared to withhold drug if any of these values drops significantly.
• Check liver and renal function test results frequently.

Patient teaching
• Tell patient he'll be premedicated to help minimize nausea and vomiting.
• Inform patient that drug may cause fatigue, appetite loss, and diarrhea. Advise him to report these symptoms if they persist.
Instruct patient to immediately report pain or swelling at I.V. site.
• Advise patient to minimize GI distress by eating small, frequent servings of healthy food and drinking plenty of fluids.
• Inform patient that drug makes him more susceptible to infections, so he should avoid crowds and exposure to illness.
• Mention that drug may cause hair loss, but that hair usually grows back after therapy.
• Tell patient he'll undergo regular blood testing during therapy.
• As appropriate, review all other significant and life-threatening adverse reactions and interactions, especially those related to the drugs and tests mentioned above.

dalteparin sodium
Fragmin

Pharmacologic class: Low-molecular-weight heparin
Therapeutic class: Anticoagulant
Pregnancy risk category B

Action
Inhibits thrombus and clot formation by blocking factor Xa and thrombin

Availability
Solution for injection (prefilled syringes): 2,500 antifactor Xa international units/0.2 ml; 5,000 antifactor Xa international units/0.2 ml; 7,500 antifactor Xa international units/0.3 ml; 10,000 antifactor Xa international units/1 ml; 25,000 antifactor Xa international units/0.2 ml

d

Indications and dosages
➤ To prevent deep-vein thrombosis and pulmonary embolism in patients undergoing surgery that increases the risk of these complications (abdominal surgery, hip replacement)
Adults: *Abdominal surgery*—2,500 international units subcutaneously 1 to 2 hours before surgery; then once daily for 5 to 10 days. For high-risk patients, 5,000 international units subcutaneously on evening before surgery; then once daily for 5 to 10 days. For cancer patients, 2,500 international units subcutaneously 1 to 2 hours before surgery; repeat dose 12 hours later, then give 5,000 international units subcutaneously every day for 5 to 10 days. *Hip replacement surgery*—5,000 international units subcutaneously 10 to 14 hours before surgery; repeat dose 4 to 8 hours after surgery, then give 5,000 international units daily for 5 to 10 days.
➤ To prevent ischemic complications in patients with unstable angina and non-Q-wave myocardial infarction
Adults: 120 international units/kg (not to exceed 10,000 international units) subcutaneously q 12 hours (concurrently with aspirin P.O.) for 5 to 8 days

Off-label uses
• Systemic anticoagulation

Contraindications
• Hypersensitivity to drug, heparin, pork products, sulfites, or benzyl alcohol

- Active major bleeding
- Thrombocytopenia

Precautions

Use cautiously in:

- bacterial endocarditis, bleeding disorders, hemorrhagic stroke, severe uncontrolled hypertension, GI ulcer, severe renal or hepatic insufficiency, hypertensive or diabetic retinopathy
- history of thrombocytopenia from heparin use
- history of congenital or acquired bleeding disorder
- recent CNS or ophthalmologic surgery
- recent GI disease
- spinal or epidural anesthesia
- pregnant or breastfeeding patients
- children (safety not established).

Administration

🔊 Know that dalteparin sodium is high-alert drug.

🔊 Administer by subcutaneous route only. Don't give by I.M. or I.V. route.

- To minimize bruising at injection site, massage site with ice before giving injection.
- To give subcutaneous injection, have patient either sit up or lie down. Inject in U-shaped area around navel, upper outer side of thigh, or upper outer quadrangle of buttock. Rotate injection sites daily.
- Don't use interchangeably with heparin or other low-molecular-weight heparins.

Route	Onset	Peak	Duration
Subcut.	20-60 min	3-5 hr	12 hr

Adverse reactions

Hematologic: anemia, ecchymosis, **bleeding, thrombocytopenia, hemorrhage**

Skin: rash, urticaria

Other: pain, irritation, and hematoma at injection site; fever; edema

Interactions

Drug-drug. *Antiplatelet drugs (aspirin, clopidogrel, dipyridamole, ticlopidine), thrombolytics, warfarin:* increased risk of bleeding

Drug-diagnostic tests. *Alanine aminotransferase, aspartate aminotransferase:* increased levels

Platelets: decreased count

Drug-herbs. *Anise, arnica, chamomile, clove, feverfew, garlic, ginger, ginkgo, ginseng:* increased risk of bleeding

Patient monitoring

🔊 Monitor patient for increased risk of bleeding if he's receiving concomitant drugs that affect platelet function.

- Monitor CBC and platelet count.
- Monitor stools for occult blood.

Patient teaching

- Tell patient that drug may cause him to bleed easily. To avoid injury, advise him to brush teeth with soft toothbrush, use electric razor, and avoid scissors and sharp knives.

🔊 Advise patient to immediately report bleeding, bruising, dizziness, light-headedness, itching, rash, fever, swelling, or difficulty breathing.

- As appropriate, review all other significant and life-threatening adverse reactions and interactions, especially those related to the drugs, tests, and herbs mentioned above.

danazol

Cyclomen✱, Danocrine

Pharmacologic class: Androgen (synthetic)

Therapeutic class: Sex hormone

Pregnancy risk category X

Action

Suppresses pituitary-ovarian axis, probably through a combination of depressed hypothalamic-pituitary response to reduced estrogen production, altered sex hormone metabolism, and interaction with sex hormone receptors

Availability

Capsules: 50 mg, 100 mg, 200 mg

Indications and dosages

➤ Moderate endometriosis amenable to hormonal management

Adults and adolescents: 400 mg P.O. b.i.d for up to 9 months. In milder cases, 100 to 200 mg P.O. b.i.d. initially, with dosage adjustments based on patient response.

➤ Fibrocystic breast disease

Adults and adolescents: 100 to 200 mg P.O. b.i.d. for 2 to 6 months

➤ Hereditary angioedema

Adults and adolescents: 200 mg P.O. two to three times daily. If possible, decrease dosage by 50% or less q 1 to 3 months. If acute angioedema attack occurs, increase dosage up to 200 mg/ day.

Off-label uses

- Menorrhagia
- Precocious puberty

Contraindications

- Hypersensitivity to drug
- Abnormal GU tract bleeding
- Porphyria
- Severe hepatic, renal, or cardiac disease
- Pregnancy or breastfeeding

Precautions

Use cautiously in:

- coronary artery disease, conditions aggravated by edema
- mild to moderate hepatic disease
- children.

Administration

- Verify that patient isn't pregnant before initiating therapy. Start therapy during menstruation.
- Don't give to female of childbearing age unless she's willing and able to use barrier contraception during therapy.

Route	Onset	Peak	Duration
P.O. (endometriosis)	Unknown	6-8 wk	60-90 days
P.O. (fibrocyst.)	1 mo	2-6 mo	1 yr
P.O. (angioedema)	Unknown	1-3 mo	Unknown

Adverse reactions

CNS: headache, tremor, emotional lability, irritability, nervousness, anxiety, depression, sleep disorders, epilepsy exacerbation, **benign intracranial hypertension**

CV: increased blood pressure, palpitations, tachycardia, **thrombotic events, myocardial infarction**

EENT: cataracts, blurred vision, nasal congestion, **papilledema**

GI: nausea, vomiting, constipation, indigestion, gastroenteritis, anorexia, **pancreatitis**

GU: hematuria; amenorrhea; menstrual cycle disturbances (spotting, altered cycle); anovulation; vaginal dryness; changes in breast size; clitoral enlargement; testicular atrophy; abnormalities in semen volume, viscosity, mobility, and sperm count; decreased libido

Hematologic: reversible erythrocytosis, eosinophilia, polycythemia, thrombocytosis, **leukocytosis, leukopenia, thrombocytopenia**, **splenic peliosis**

Hepatic: cholestatic jaundice, **peliosis hepatitis, hepatic adenoma, malignant hepatic tumor**

Metabolic: increased insulin requirement (in diabetic patients)

Musculoskeletal: muscle cramps, spasms, pain, or fasciculations; joint pain and swelling; joint "lock-up"; pain in back, neck, or limbs; carpal tunnel syndrome

Skin: acne, hirsutism, oily skin, rash, photosensitivity, yellowing of skin and

sclera, pigmentation changes, seborrhea, sweating
Other: weight gain, edema, deepening of voice, **Stevens-Johnson syndrome**

Interactions

Drug-drug. *Carbamazepine:* increased carbamazepine blood level
Cyclosporine, tacrolimus: increased blood levels of these drugs, increased risk of nephrotoxicity
Insulin, oral hypoglycemics: increased blood glucose level and insulin resistance, necessitating adjustment of insulin or oral hypoglycemic dosages
Warfarin: prolonged prothrombin time
Drug-diagnostic tests. *Creatine kinase, glucagon, glucose, hepatic enzymes, low-density lipoproteins, plasma proteins, sex hormone-binding globulins:* increased levels
Glucose tolerance, thyroid function: altered test results
High-density lipoproteins: decreased level

Patient monitoring

Assess for early indications of benign intracranial hypertension, such as headache, nausea, vomiting, and visual disturbances. Screen for papilledema; if present, refer patient to neurologist immediately.
Watch for hepatic problems. Long-term use is linked to peliosis hepatitis and hepatic tumors, which may be silent until complicated by acute, life-threatening intra-abdominal hemorrhage.
- Monitor patient for thromboembolism and thrombophlebitis.
- Check CBC with white cell differential and liver and kidney function test results regularly.

Patient teaching

- Advise female of childbearing age to use barrier contraception, because drug causes fetal abnormalities.
- Inform female patient that drug frequently causes amenorrhea after 6 to 8 weeks of therapy.

Instruct female patient to report masculinizing effects, such as facial hair or deepening of voice.
- Tell male patient that drug may cause sperm reduction during therapy.

Instruct patient to promptly report signs and symptoms of fluid retention (swelling of ankles, feet, or hands; difficulty breathing; sudden weight gain), change in urine or stool color, yellowing of eyes and skin, and easy bruising or bleeding.
- As appropriate, review all other significant and life-threatening adverse reactions and interactions, especially those related to the drugs and tests mentioned above.

dantrolene sodium

Dantrium, Dantrium Intravenous

Pharmacologic class: Hydantoin derivative

Therapeutic class: Skeletal muscle relaxant (direct-acting), malignant hyperthermia agent

Pregnancy risk category C

Action

Relaxes skeletal muscle by affecting excitation-contraction coupling response at site beyond myoneural junction, probably by interfering with calcium release from sarcoplasmic reticulum

Availability

Capsules: 25 mg, 50 mg, 100 mg
Powder for injection: 20 mg/vial

Indications and dosages

➢ Chronic spasticity resulting from upper motor neuron disorders, such as multiple sclerosis, cerebral palsy, or spinal cord injury

Adults: Initially, 25 mg P.O. daily, increased gradually in 25-mg increments, if needed, up to 100 mg two or three times daily, to a maximum dosage of 400 mg P.O. daily. Maintain dosage level for 4 to 7 days to gauge patient response.
Children: Initially, 0.5 mg/kg P.O. b.i.d., increased to 0.5 mg/kg P.O. three or four times daily. Then increase by 0.5 mg/kg P.O. daily, as needed, to 3 mg/kg two or three times daily. Maximum dosage is 100 mg q.i.d.

➢ Malignant hyperthermic crisis
Adults and children: Initially, 1 mg/kg by I.V. push, repeated as needed up to a cumulative dosage of 10 mg/kg/day

➢ To prevent or minimize malignant hyperthermia in patients who require surgery
Adults and children: 4 to 8 mg/kg P.O. daily in three or four divided doses for 1 to 2 days before surgery; give last dose 3 to 4 hours before surgery. Or 2.5 mg/kg I.V. infused over 1 hour before anesthetics are given.

➢ To prevent recurrence of malignant hyperthermic crisis
Adults: 4 to 8 mg/kg daily P.O. in four divided doses for up to 3 days after initial hyperthermic crisis

Off-label uses

- Heat stroke
- Neuroleptic malignant syndrome

Contraindications

- Active hepatic disease (oral form)
- Patients who use spasticity to maintain posture or balance (oral form)
- Breastfeeding

Precautions

Use cautiously in:

- cardiac, hepatic, renal, or respiratory dysfunction or impairment
- women (especially pregnant women)
- adults older than age 35
- children younger than age 5.

Administration

- For I.V. use, add 60 ml of sterile water for injection to each vial; shake until solution is clear. Protect from direct light and use within 6 hours.
- Give therapeutic or emergency dose by rapid I.V. push. Administer follow-up dose over 2 to 3 minutes.
- Prevent extravasation when giving I.V. Drug has high pH and causes tissue irritation.

Route	Onset	Peak	Duration
P.O.	Slow	Unknown	6-12 hr
I.V.	Rapid	Unknown	Unknown

Adverse reactions

CNS: dizziness, drowsiness, fatigue, malaise, weakness, confusion, depression, insomnia, nervousness, headache, light-headedness, speech disturbances, **seizures**
CV: tachycardia, blood pressure fluctuations, phlebitis, **heart failure**
EENT: double vision, excessive tearing
GI: nausea, vomiting, diarrhea, constipation, abdominal cramps, GI reflux and irritation, hematemesis, difficulty swallowing, anorexia, **GI bleeding**
GU: urinary frequency, dysuria, nocturia, urinary incontinence, hematuria, crystalluria, prostatitis
Hematologic: aplastic anemia, leukopenia, thrombocytopenia, lymphocytic lymphoma
Hepatic: hepatitis
Musculoskeletal: myalgia, backache
Respiratory: suffocating sensation, **respiratory depression, pleural effusion with pericarditis**
Skin: rash, urticaria, pruritus, eczema-like eruptions, sweating, photosensitivity, abnormal hair growth
Other: altered taste, chills, fever, edema

Interactions

Drug-drug. *CNS depressants:* increased CNS depression

Estrogen: increased risk of hepatotoxicity
Verapamil (I.V.): cardiovascular collapse (when given with I.V. dantrolene)
Drug-diagnostic tests. *Alanine aminotransferase, alkaline phosphatase, aspartate aminotransferase, bilirubin, blood urea nitrogen:* increased values
Drug-behaviors. *Alcohol use:* increased CNS depression
Sun exposure: phototoxicity

Patient monitoring

- Obtain baseline liver function test results; monitor periodically during therapy.
- Monitor ECG, serum electrolytes, and urine output regularly.

🔊 With long-term oral therapy, monitor patient for signs and symptoms of hepatotoxicity. Be prepared to discontinue drug if these occur.

- Assess for muscle weakness, poor coordination, and reduced reflexes before and during therapy. Drug may weaken muscles and impair ambulation.

Patient teaching

🔊 Instruct patient receiving prolonged oral therapy to immediately report weakness, malaise, fatigue, nausea, rash, itching, severe diarrhea, bloody or black tarry stools, or yellowing of skin or eyes.

- Inform patient that drug may cause drowsiness, dizziness, or light-headedness.
- Caution patient to avoid driving and other hazardous activities until he knows how drug affects concentration and alertness.
- As appropriate, review all other significant and life-threatening adverse reactions and interactions, especially those related to the drugs, tests, and behaviors mentioned above.

dapsone (DDS)

Avlosulfon✱, Dapsone

Pharmacologic class: Synthetic sulfone
Therapeutic class: Antileprotic, antimalarial
Pregnancy risk category C

Action

Unknown. Bactericidal and bacteriostatic against *Mycobacterium leprae.* Action in dermatitis herpetiformis not established.

Availability

Tablets: 25 mg, 100 mg

Indications and dosages

➢ Leprosy
Adults: 100 mg/day P.O. (given with one or more antileprotics) for 6 to 12 months, depending on disease course
Children ages 10 to 14 years: 50 mg daily for 6 to 12 months, depending on disease course
Children under age 10: As appropriate
➢ Dermatitis herpetiformis
Adults: Initially, 50 mg/day P.O., increased as needed to a maximum of 300 mg/day, then reduced to minimum maintenance level as soon as possible

Off-label uses

- Inflammatory bowel disorders
- Malaria prophylaxis
- *Pneumocystis jiroveci* pneumonia
- Rheumatic and connective tissue disorders

Contraindications

- Hypersensitivity to drug or its derivatives

Precautions

Use cautiously in:

- renal or hepatic impairment, cardio-

pulmonary disease, refractory anemia, glucose-6-phosphate dehydrogenase deficiency
• pregnant or breastfeeding patients.

Administration
• Give with meals if GI upset occurs.

Route	Onset	Peak	Duration
P.O.	Unknown	4-8 hr	Unknown

Adverse reactions
CNS: headache, vertigo, insomnia, paresthesia, peripheral neuropathy, psychosis
CV: tachycardia
EENT: blurred vision, retinal and optic nerve damage, tinnitus
GI: nausea, vomiting, abdominal pain, anorexia, **pancreatitis**
GU: albuminuria, male infertility, **nephrotic syndrome, renal papillary necrosis**
Hematologic: hemolytic anemia, agranulocytosis, aplastic anemia, hypoalbuminemia
Respiratory: pulmonary eosinophilia
Skin: photosensitivity, exfoliative dermatitis, **lupus erythematosus**
Other: fever, hypersensitivity reaction, infectious mononucleosis–like syndrome, **sulfone syndrome**

Interactions
Drug-drug. *Activated charcoal:* decreased dapsone absorption
Didanosine: therapeutic failure of dapsone
Folic acid antagonists (such as methotrexate): increased risk of adverse reactions to dapsone
Para-aminobenzoic acid: antagonistic effect
Probenecid: reduced urinary excretion of dapsone metabolites
Rifampin: increased hepatic metabolism of dapsone, causing reduced blood level
Trimethoprim: increased blood levels of both drugs
Drug-diagnostic tests. *Albumin, granulocytes, hemoglobin:* decreased values
Methemoglobin, reticulocytes: increased values
Drug-behaviors. *Sun exposure:* photosensitivity

d

Patient monitoring
🔊 Monitor patient for sulfone syndrome, a potentially fatal reaction that causes fever, malaise, jaundice with hepatic necrosis, exfoliative dermatitis, lymphadenopathy, methemoglobinemia, and hemolytic anemia.
• Evaluate CBC weekly for first month of therapy, monthly for next 6 months, and then every 6 months. Discontinue drug if tests show decreased white blood cell or platelet count or reduction in hematopoiesis.
• Monitor liver function test results.

Patient teaching
🔊 Instruct patient to immediately report persistent sore throat, fever, chills, malaise, fatigue, swollen lymph nodes, yellowing of skin or eyes, or easy bruising or bleeding.
• Caution patient to avoid driving and other hazardous activities until he knows whether drug affects vision or balance.
• Tell patient drug is intended for long-term use.
• Advise patient to minimize GI upset by eating small, frequent servings of healthy food and drinking plenty of fluids.
• As appropriate, review all other significant and life-threatening adverse reactions and interactions, especially those related to the drugs, tests, and behaviors mentioned above.

darbepoetin alfa

Aranesp

Pharmacologic class: Recombinant human erythropoietin

Therapeutic class: Hematopoietic

Pregnancy risk category C

Action

Stimulates erythropoiesis in bone marrow, increasing red blood cell production

Availability

Albumin solution for injection: 25 mcg/ml, 40 mcg/ml, 60 mcg/ml, 100 mcg/ml, 150 mcg/ml, 200 mcg/ml, 300 mcg/ml, 500 mcg/ml

Polysorbate solution for injection: 25 mcg/ml, 40 mcg/ml, 60 mcg/ml, 100 mcg/ml, 150 mcg/ml, 200 mcg/ml, 300 mcg/ml

Indications and dosages

➢ Anemia caused by chronic renal failure

Adults: Initially, 0.45 mcg/kg I.V. or subcutaneously as a single dose once weekly. Titrate dosage to maintain target hemoglobin concentration no higher than 12 g/dl. Adjust dosage no more often than once monthly.

➢ Chemotherapy-induced anemia

Adults: 2.25 mcg/kg I.V. or subcutaneously q week. Titrate dosage to maintain target hemoglobin concentration no higher than 12 g/dl.

Dosage adjustment

- Conversion from epoetin therapy

Contraindications

- Hypersensitivity to drug
- Uncontrolled hypertension

Precautions

Use cautiously in:

- anemia; thalassemia; porphyria; seizures; underlying hematologic disease, including hemolytic and sickle cell anemia
- pregnant or breastfeeding patients
- children.

Administration

- Give by subcutaneous or I.V. injection only.
- Don't dilute or give with other drug solutions.

Clinical alert: Don't shake. Vigorous shaking may denature drug, making it biologically inactive.

- Give single I.V. dose over 1 minute.
- Discard unused portion. (Drug contains no preservative.)

Route	Onset	Peak	Duration
I.V., subcut.	2-6 wk	Unknown	Unknown

Adverse reactions

CNS: dizziness, headache, fatigue, weakness, **seizures, transient ischemic attack, cerebrovascular accident**

CV: hypertension, hypotension, chest pain, peripheral edema, **arrhythmias, heart failure, cardiac arrest, myocardial infarction, vascular access thrombosis**

GI: nausea, vomiting, diarrhea, constipation, abdominal pain

Metabolic: fluid overload

Musculoskeletal: myalgia; joint, back, and limb pain

Respiratory: cough, upper respiratory tract infection, dyspnea, bronchitis

Skin: pruritus

Other: fever, flulike symptoms, infection, pain at injection site

Interactions

None significant

Patient monitoring

- Assess hemoglobin concentration before starting therapy and then weekly during therapy.
- Observe closely for serious CNS and cardiovascular adverse reactions.
- Know that supplemental iron is recommended for patients with serum ferritin level below 100 mcg/ml or serum transferrin saturation below 20%.

Patient teaching

- Tell patient to report chest pain or other pain, muscle tremors, weakness, and cough or other respiratory symptoms.
- If patient will self-administer drug, tell him to follow exact directions for injection and needle disposal.
- Caution patient to avoid driving and other hazardous activities until he knows how drug affects concentration and alertness.
- Advise patient to minimize GI upset by eating small, frequent servings of healthy food and drinking plenty of fluids.
- Tell patient he'll undergo frequent blood testing during therapy to help determine correct dosage.
- As appropriate, review all other significant and life-threatening adverse reactions.

daunorubicin citrate liposome

DaunoXome

Pharmacologic class: Anthracycline glycoside
Therapeutic class: Antibiotic antineoplastic
Pregnancy risk category D

Action

Inhibits DNA synthesis and DNA-dependent RNA synthesis through intercalation. Formulation increases selectivity of daunorubicin for solid tumors; may increase permeability of tumor neovasculature to some particles in drug's size range.

Availability

Injection: 2 mg/ml

Indications and dosages

➤ First-line cytotoxic therapy for advanced Kaposi's sarcoma associated with human immunodeficiency virus (HIV)
Adults: 40 mg/m^2 I.V. over 1 hour. Repeat q 2 weeks until evidence of disease progression or other complications occur.

Dosage adjustment

- Renal or hepatic impairment

Contraindications

- Hypersensitivity to drug

Precautions

Use cautiously in:
- renal or hepatic impairment, bone marrow depression, cardiac disease, gout, infections
- pregnant or breastfeeding patients.

Administration

- Follow facility policy for preparing and handling antineoplastics.
- Dilute 1:1 with 5% dextrose injection.
- Don't use in-line filter for I.V. infusion.
- If prescribed, premedicate with allopurinol to help prevent hyperuricemia.
- Take steps to prevent extravasation.
- Protect solution from light.

Route	Onset	Peak	Duration
I.V.	Unknown	Unknown	Unknown

Adverse reactions

CNS: headache, fatigue, malaise, confusion, depression, dizziness, drowsiness, emotional lability, anxiety, hallucinations, syncope, tremors, rigors, insomnia, neuropathy, amnesia, hyperactivity, abnormal thinking, **meningitis, seizures**
CV: hypertension, chest pain, palpitations, **myocardial infarction, cardiac arrest**
EENT: abnormal vision, conjunctivitis, eye pain, hearing loss, earache, tinnitus, rhinitis, sinusitis
GI: nausea, vomiting, diarrhea, constipation, abdominal pain, dyspepsia, gastritis, enlarged spleen, fecal incontinence, hemorrhoids, tenesmus, melena, difficulty swallowing, dry mouth, mouth inflammation, **GI hemorrhage**
GU: dysuria, nocturia, polyuria
Hematologic: thrombocytopenia, neutropenia
Hepatic: hepatomegaly
Metabolic: hyperuricemia, dehydration
Musculoskeletal: joint pain, myalgia, muscle rigidity, back pain, abnormal gait
Respiratory: dyspnea, cough, hemoptysis, increased sputum, **pulmonary infiltrations, pulmonary hypertension**
Skin: pruritus, dry skin, seborrhea, folliculitis, alopecia, sweating
Other: bleeding gums, dental caries, altered taste, lymphadenopathy, opportunistic infections, fever, hot flashes, hiccups, thirst, infusion site inflammation, edema, allergic reactions

Interactions

Drug-diagnostic tests. *Granulocytes:* decreased count
Uric acid: increased level

Patient monitoring

- Assess cardiac, renal, and hepatic function before each course of treatment.
- Evaluate CBC with white cell differential before each dose. Withhold dose if granulocyte count is below 750 cells/mm^3.
- Monitor serum uric acid level.

Patient teaching

[Clinical alert] Instruct patient to immediately report swelling, pain, burning, or redness at infusion site, as well as persistent nausea, vomiting, diarrhea, chest pain, arm or leg swelling, difficulty breathing, palpitations, rapid heartbeat, yellowing of skin or eyes, abdominal pain, or bloody stools.

- Tell patient drug makes him more susceptible to infection. Advise him to avoid crowds and exposure to illness.
- Advise patient to minimize GI upset by eating small, frequent servings of healthy foods, drinking plenty of fluids, and chewing gum.
- As appropriate, review all other significant and life-threatening adverse reactions and interactions, especially those related to the tests mentioned above.

daunorubicin hydrochloride

Cerubidine

Pharmacologic class: Anthracycline glycoside
Therapeutic class: Antibiotic antineoplastic
Pregnancy risk category D

Action

Antimitotic and cytotoxic. Forms complexes with DNA by intercalation between base pairs. Inhibits topoisomerase II activity by stabilizing topoisomerase II complex; causes breaks in single- and double-stranded DNA. May also inhibit polymerase activity, influence regulation of gene expression, and cause free radical damage to DNA.

Availability

Injection: 5 mg/ml
Lyophilized powder for injection: 21.4 mg, 53.5 mg

Indications and dosages

➢ Acute nonlymphocytic leukemia
Adults older than age 60: 30 mg/m²/day I.V. on days 1, 2, and 3 of first course and on days 1 and 2 of subsequent courses; given with cytarabine I.V. infusion (7 days for first course, 5 days for subsequent courses)
Adults younger than age 60: 45 mg/m²/day I.V. on days 1, 2, and 3 of first course and on days 1 and 2 of subsequent courses; given with cytarabine I.V. infusion (7 days for first course, 5 days for subsequent courses)
➢ Acute lymphocytic leukemia
Adults: 45 mg/m²/day I.V. on days 1, 2, and 3; vincristine I.V. on days 1, 8, and 15; prednisone P.O. on days 1 through 22, then tapered between days 22 and 29; then asparaginase I.V. on days 22 to 32
Children ages 2 and older: 25 mg/m²/day I.V. on first day every week; may be given in combination with vincristine I.V. on first day every week and prednisone P.O. daily

Dosage adjustment

- Renal or hepatic impairment

Contraindications

- Hypersensitivity to drug

Precautions

Use cautiously in:
- renal or hepatic impairment, bone marrow depression, cardiac disease, gout, infections
- elderly patients
- pregnant or breastfeeding patients.

Administration

- Follow facility policy for preparing and handling antineoplastics.
- If prescribed, premedicate with allopurinol to help prevent hyperuricemia.

Give by I.V. route only.
- Reconstitute vial contents with 4 ml of sterile water for injection to yield 5 mg/ml solution.
- Don't mix with other drugs or heparin.
- Withdraw desired dosage into syringe containing 10 to 15 ml of normal saline solution; then inject into tubing or sidearm of compatible, rapidly flowing I.V. solution over 3 to 5 minutes. For intermittent infusion, mix with 100 ml of normal saline solution and infuse over 30 to 45 minutes.

Take care to prevent extravasation, because drug causes severe local tissue necrosis. If extravasation occurs, stop infusion immediately; according to facility policy, intervene to avoid severe tissue necrolysis, severe cellulitis, thrombophlebitis, and painful induration.

Route	Onset	Peak	Duration
I.V.	Unknown	Unknown	Unknown

Adverse reactions

CV: cardiotoxicity
GI: acute nausea, vomiting, GI mucosal inflammation
GU: urine discoloration
Hematologic: bone marrow depression
Metabolic: hyperuricemia
Skin: rash, contact dermatitis, urticaria, reversible alopecia

Interactions

Drug-drug. *Other antineoplastic, hepatotoxic, or myelosuppressive drugs:* increased risk of toxicity
Drug diagnostic tests. *Granulocytes:* decreased count
Uric acid: increased level

Patient monitoring

🔊 Observe I.V. site closely for extravasation.

- Monitor cardiac, renal, and hepatic function before each course of treatment.
- Evaluate CBC with white cell differential before each dose. Withhold dose if granulocyte count is below 750 cells/mm³.
- Monitor serum uric acid level.

Patient teaching

🔊 Instruct patient to immediately report swelling, pain, burning, or redness at infusion site, as well as persistent nausea, vomiting, diarrhea, bloody stools, abdominal or chest pain, swollen arm or leg, difficulty breathing, palpitations, rapid heartbeat, or yellowing of skin or eyes.

- Inform patient that drug makes him more susceptible to infection. Caution him to avoid crowds and exposure to illness.
- Advise patient to minimize GI upset by eating small, frequent servings of healthy food, drinking plenty of fluids, and chewing gum.
- Tell patient that drug may redden his urine.
- As appropriate, review all other significant and life-threatening adverse reactions and interactions, especially those related to the drugs and tests mentioned above.

delavirdine mesylate

Rescriptor

Pharmacologic class: Nonnucleoside reverse transcriptase inhibitor

Therapeutic class: Antiretroviral

Pregnancy risk category C

Action

Binds to reverse transcriptase enzyme, blocking RNA-dependent and DNA-dependent DNA polymerase synthesis

Availability

Tablets: 100 mg, 200 mg

Indications and dosages

➢ Human immunodeficiency virus (HIV)–1 infection

Adults: 400 mg P.O. t.i.d.

Contraindications

- Hypersensitivity to drug
- Concurrent use of alprazolam, astemizole, ergot derivatives, midazolam, pimozide, terfenadine, or triazolam

Precautions

Use cautiously in:

- hepatic impairment
- pregnant or breastfeeding patients.

Administration

- Know that drug is usually given with at least two other antiretrovirals.
- If patient can't swallow tablets, dissolve 100-mg tablets in water by adding four tablets to at least 3 oz of water; let stand for a few minutes and then stir until completely dissolved. Have patient swallow entire mixture immediately. Then add small amount of water to glass and have him swallow this mixture to ensure that he consumes entire dose.
- Give 200-mg tablets intact; don't dissolve in water.
- If patient has achlorhydria, give drug with acidic beverage, such as orange juice.

🔊 Don't give concurrently with alprazolam, astemizole or terfenadine (no longer available in U.S.), ergot derivatives, midazolam, pimozide, or triazolam.

Route	Onset	Peak	Duration
P.O.	Unknown	1 hr	Unknown

Adverse reactions

CNS: confusion, disorientation, dizziness, drowsiness, agitation, amnesia, changes in dreams, hallucinations, hyperesthesia, poor concentration, mania, nervousness, restlessness, paranoia, paresthesia, tremor, migraine, neuropathy, paralysis, **seizures**
CV: abnormal heart rate and rhythm, peripheral vascular disorder, peripheral edema, hypertension, orthostatic hypotension, cardiac insufficiency, **cardiomyopathy**
EENT: blurred or double vision, nystagmus, conjunctivitis, dry eyes, scleral yellowing, ear pain, otitis media, tinnitus, epistaxis, rhinitis
GI: nausea, diarrhea, constipation, abdominal pain or cramps, dyspepsia, abdominal distention, bloody stools, colitis, diverticulitis, enteritis, gastroenteritis, gastroesophageal reflux, mouth and tongue irritation and ulcers, increased saliva, difficulty swallowing, **GI bleeding, pancreatitis**
GU: hematuria, polyuria, chromaturia, proteinuria, nocturia, urinary tract infection, renal calculi, kidney pain, gynecomastia, erectile dysfunction, epididymitis, hemospermia, testicular pain, vaginal candidiasis, amenorrhea, irregular uterine bleeding
Hematologic: purpura, spleen disorders, eosinophilia, **granulocytosis, disseminated intravascular coagulation, leukopenia, neutropenia, pancytopenia, hemolytic anemia**
Hepatic: hepatotoxicity, hepatic failure, hepatomegaly
Metabolic: hypomagnesemia, hyper glycemia, hyperuricemia, hypocalcemia, hyponatremia, **hypoglycemia, hyperkalemia, metabolic acidosis**
Musculoskeletal: joint pain, arthritis, bone disorders, myalgia, muscle cramps, muscle weakness, bone pain, bone disorders, tendon disorders, tenosynovitis, neck pain and rigidity, limb pain, **tetany, rhabdomyolysis**
Respiratory: pulmonary congestion, dyspnea, pneumonia
Skin: pallor, bruising, yellowing of skin, dermal leukocytoblastic vasculitis, dermatitis, skin dryness and discoloration, erythema, folliculitis, herpes zoster or herpes simplex infection, petechiae, petechial or pruritic rash, seborrhea, alopecia, skin nodules, urticaria, sebaceous or epidermal cyst, angioedema, **erythema multiforme**
Other: tooth abscess, toothache, gingivitis, gum hemorrhage, weight gain or loss, fever, lymphadenopathy, adenopathy, increased thirst, hiccups, facial edema, pain, abscess, bacterial infection, *Mycobacterium tuberculosis* infection, body fat redistribution, hypersensitivity reaction, **sepsis**, **Stevens-Johnson syndrome**

Interactions

Drug-drug. *Alprazolam, astemizole, ergot derivatives, midazolam, pimozide, terfenadine:* increased risk of serious or life-threatening adverse reactions
Antacids, histamine$_2$-receptor antagonists: reduced delavirdine absorption
Bepridil, clarithromycin, estrogen, hormonal contraceptives, indinavir, lopinavir-ritonavir, saquinavir, sildenafil, warfarin: increased blood levels of these drugs
Carbamazepine, phenobarbital, phenytoin, rifabutin, rifampin: loss of virologic response, resistance to delavirdine
Dexamethasone: decreased delavirdine blood level
Didanosine: decreased blood levels of both drugs
Fluoxetine, ketoconazole: 50% increase in delavirdine blood level
Drug-diagnostic tests. *Alanine aminotransferase, alkaline phosphatase, aspartate aminotransferase, bilirubin, creati*

nine, lipase, gamma-glutamyl transpeptidase, triglycerides: increased levels
Granulocytes, hemoglobin, neutrophils, platelets, red blood cells, white blood cells: decreased values
Partial thromboplastin time, prothrombin time: increased
Drug-herbs. *St. John's wort:* loss of virologic response or resistance to delavirdine

Patient monitoring

- Monitor liver function test results frequently when giving drug concurrently with saquinavir.
- Check electrolyte and uric acid levels regularly.

🔊 Monitor patient for serious hepatic, cardiovascular, and CNS problems and hypersensitivity reactions.

Patient teaching

- Tell patient he can take drug with or without food.
- If patient can't swallow tablets, teach him how to dissolve 100-mg tablets in water.

🔊 Tell patient to discontinue drug and consult prescriber immediately if he develops severe rash accompanied by fever, blistering, oral lesions, conjunctivitis, swelling, or muscle aches.

🔊 Tell patient to promptly report unusual fatigue, yellowing of skin or eyes, unusual bruising or bleeding, muscle weakness, or signs and symptoms of infection.

🔊 Advise patient that rash is a major adverse effect, usually occurring 1 to 3 weeks after therapy starts and resolving in 3 to 14 days. Instruct him to report rash promptly.

- Inform patient that drug doesn't cure HIV or reduce its transmission.
- As appropriate, review all other significant and life-threatening adverse reactions and interactions, especially those related to the drugs, tests, and herbs mentioned above.

demeclocycline hydrochloride

Declomycin

Pharmacologic class: Tetracycline
Therapeutic class: Antibiotic
Pregnancy risk category D

Action

Binds with bacterial cell, inhibiting its reproduction and protein synthesis

Availability

Tablets: 150 mg, 300 mg

Indications and dosages

➤ Infections caused by susceptible organisms and when penicillin is contraindicated *(Neisseria gonorrhoeae, Treponema pallidum, Treponema pertenue, Listeria monocytogenes, Clostridium* species; *Bacillus anthracis, Fusobacterium fusiforme, Actinomyces israelii, Neisseria meningitides).* Also, adjunct to amebicides in acute intestinal amebiasis, treatment of severe acne and nongonococcal urethritis, and trachoma and inclusion conjunctivitis caused by *Chlamydia trachomatis*
Adults: 150 mg P.O. q.i.d. or 300 mg P.O. b.i.d. For gonococcal infections, initially 600 mg P.O., followed by 300 mg q 12 hours for 4 days, to a maximum dosage of 3 g.
Children older than age 8: 6.6 to 13.2 mg/kg/day P.O. in two to four divided doses

Off-label uses

- Syndrome of inappropriate antidiuretic hormone secretion (limited use)

Contraindications

- Hypersensitivity to tetracyclines
- Children younger than age 8

Precautions

Use cautiously in:
- marked renal impairment
- significant exposure to sun or ultraviolet light
- pregnant patients.

Administration

- Obtain specimens for culture and sensitivity testing as appropriate before starting therapy.
- Give with full glass of water 1 hour before or 2 hours after meals.
- If patient is receiving antacids, give these at least 2 hours after demeclocycline.

Route	Onset	Peak	Duration
P.O.	Variable	3-4 hr	18-20 hr

Adverse reactions

CNS: dizziness, light-headedness, headache, vertigo, **pseudotumor cerebri**
EENT: blurred vision, tinnitus
GI: nausea, vomiting, diarrhea, tongue inflammation, difficulty swallowing, anorexia, enterocolitis, **pancreatitis, esophageal ulcers**
GU: nephrogenic diabetes insipidus, **acute renal failure**
Hematologic: eosinophilia, **leukocytosis, hemolytic anemia, thrombocytopenia, neutropenia, leukopenia**
Hepatic: hepatic failure, hepatitis
Skin: phototoxicity, rash, urticaria, changes in skin and mucous membrane pigmentation, exfoliative dermatitis, **erythema multiforme**
Other: discolored and poorly calcified permanent teeth (when used during dental development period in children), discolored and poorly calcified primary teeth of fetus (when used by pregnant patient), superinfection, **Stevens-Johnson syndrome**

Interactions

Drug-drug. *Aluminum- or magnesium-containing preparations, antacids, calcium, iron preparations:* decreased demeclocycline absorption
Hormonal contraceptives: decreased contraceptive efficacy
Methoxyflurane: increased risk of nephrotoxicity
Penicillin: decreased demeclocycline activity
Drug-diagnostic tests. *Blood urea nitrogen, hepatic enzymes:* increased levels
Drug-food. *Any food (especially dairy products):* decreased drug absorption

Patient monitoring

- Stay alert for serious GI, hepatic, and skin reactions.
- Monitor hepatic enzyme levels and CBC with white cell differential.

Patient teaching

- Tell patient to take drug on empty stomach with a full glass of water at least 1 hour before or 2 hours after meals.
- Advise patient to avoid dairy products, laxatives, and iron preparations.

[Clinical alert] Instruct patient to promptly report abdominal pain, change in urination pattern, unusual fatigue, yellowing of skin or eyes, rash, or unusual bleeding or bruising.

- Caution patient to avoid driving and other hazardous activities until he knows if drug causes dizziness.
- Tell patient to discard outdated drug products, because these may be toxic.
- Advise patient to minimize GI upset by eating small, frequent servings of healthy food and drinking plenty of fluids.
- As appropriate, review all other significant and life-threatening adverse reactions and interactions, especially those related to the drugs, tests, and foods mentioned above.

denileukin diftitox
Ontak

Pharmacologic class: Biological response modifier
Therapeutic class: Antineoplastic
Pregnancy risk category C

Action
Recombinant DNA–derived cytotoxic protein. Interacts with interleukin-2 (IL-2) receptors on cell surface and inhibits cellular protein synthesis, causing cell death.

Availability
Frozen solution for injection: 150 mcg/ml

Indications and dosages
➤ Persistent or recurrent cutaneous T-cell lymphoma that expresses CD25 component of IL-2 receptor
Adults: 9 or 18 mcg/kg/day I.V. infused over 15 minutes for 5 consecutive days q 21 days

Contraindications
- Hypersensitivity to drug, its components, diphtheria toxin, or IL-2

Precautions
Use cautiously in:
- cardiovascular disease
- elderly patients
- pregnant or breastfeeding patients
- children (safety and efficacy not established).

Administration
- Follow facility procedures for safe handling, administration, and disposal of chemotherapeutic agents.

🔊 Administer by I.V. infusion only. Don't give by I.V. bolus.
- Premedicate with acetaminophen, nonsteroidal anti-inflammatory drugs, and antihistamines, as ordered, to minimize infusion-related events.
- Gently swirl vial to mix, but avoid vigorous agitation.
- Don't mix with other drugs.
- Don't deliver through in-line filter.
- Infuse over at least 15 minutes.

🔊 During infusion, observe closely for signs and symptoms of hypersensitivity reaction.

Route	Onset	Peak	Duration
I.V.	Variable	Variable	Variable

Adverse reactions
CNS: dizziness, paresthesia, nervousness, confusion, insomnia, syncope, headache
CV: hypotension, hypertension, vasodilation, tachycardia, chest pain, **capillary leak syndrome** (with extravasation), **thrombosis, arrhythmias**
EENT: rhinitis, pharyngitis, **laryngospasm**
GI: nausea, vomiting, diarrhea, constipation, flatulence, dyspepsia, difficulty swallowing, anorexia
GU: hematuria, albuminuria, pyuria
Hematologic: anemia, **thrombocytopenia, leukopenia**
Musculoskeletal: myalgia, back or joint pain
Metabolic: hypoalbuminemia, hypocalcemia, hypokalemia, dehydration
Respiratory: dyspnea, cough, lung disorder
Skin: rash, pruritus, sweating
Other: weight loss, edema, flulike symptoms, injection site reaction, **hypersensitivity reactions** including **anaphylaxis**

Interactions
Drug-drug. *Live-virus vaccines:* decreased antibody reaction
Drug-diagnostic tests. *Albumin, calcium, potassium:* decreased levels
Urine creatinine: increased level

Patient monitoring
- Monitor patient closely during first infusion and for 24 hours afterward.
- Evaluate patient for vascular leak syndrome (marked by at least two of the following: edema, hypotension, hypoalbuminemia).
- Monitor CBC, blood chemistry panel, renal and hepatic function, and albumin level. Repeat all tests weekly during therapy.

Patient teaching
Instruct patient to immediately report chest pain, difficulty breathing, chills, burning at infusion site, or throat tightness, redness, swelling, or pain.
- Caution patient to avoid driving and other hazardous activities until he knows how drug affects concentration and alertness.
- Inform patient that drug makes him more susceptible to infection. Advise him to avoid crowds and exposure to illness.
- As appropriate, review all other significant and life-threatening adverse reactions and interactions, especially those related to the drugs and tests mentioned above.

desipramine hydrochloride
Norpramin

Pharmacologic class: Tricyclic antidepressant
Therapeutic class: Antidepressant
Pregnancy risk category NR

Action
Inhibits norepinephrine or serotonin reuptake at presynaptic neuron

Availability
Tablets: 10 mg, 25 mg, 50 mg, 75 mg, 100 mg, 150 mg

Indications and dosages
➢ Depression
Adults: Initially, 100 to 200 mg/day P.O. Increase gradually if needed to a maximum dosage of 300 mg/day.
Adolescents and elderly adults: 25 to 100 mg/day P.O. as a single dose or in divided doses. Increase gradually if needed to a maximum dosage of 150 mg/day.

Off-label uses
- Arthritis pain
- Cancer pain
- Diabetic or peripheral neuropathy
- Tic douloureux

Contraindications
- Hypersensitivity to drug
- Recovery phase of myocardial infarction (MI)
- MAO inhibitor use within past 14 days

Precautions
Use cautiously in:
- cardiovascular disorders, glaucoma, thyroid disorders
- urinary retention
- adolescents and children younger than age 12.

Administration
- Before giving drug, measure patient's sitting and supine blood pressure to assess for orthostasis.
- Give full dose at bedtime to avoid daytime drowsiness.
- Discontinue drug 2 days before surgery.

Don't give within 14 days of MAO inhibitor, because potentially fatal reaction may occur.

Route	Onset	Peak	Duration
P.O.	Unknown	4-6 hr	Unknown

Adverse reactions
CNS: sedation, weakness, anxiety, restlessness, insomnia, delusions, confu-

sion, agitation, hallucinations, disorientation, extrapyramidal reactions, EEG changes, **neuroleptic malignant syndrome, seizures, suicidal behavior or ideation (especially in child or adolescent)**
CV: hypotension, hypertension, tachycardia, palpitations, **arrhythmias, MI, heart block**
EENT: blurred vision, dry eyes, laryngitis
GI: nausea, vomiting, constipation, abdominal cramps, epigastric distress, difficulty swallowing, parotid gland swelling, mouth inflammation, dry mouth, black tongue
GU: urinary retention, delayed voiding, urinary tract dilation, testicular swelling, erectile or other male sexual dysfunction, gynecomastia, menstrual irregularities, galactorrhea, increased or decreased libido
Hematologic: purpura, eosinophilia, **bone marrow depression, agranulocytosis, thrombocytopenia**
Metabolic: syndrome of inappropriate antidiuretic hormone secretion
Musculoskeletal: muscle weakness
Skin: dry skin, photosensitivity, rash, pruritus, petechiae, sweating
Other: peculiar taste, weight gain, edema, hypothermia, flushing, withdrawal symptoms with abrupt drug cessation (dizziness, nausea, vomiting, headache, malaise, sleep disturbances, hyperthermia, irritability, worsening of depression), **sudden death (in children)**

Interactions

Drug-drug. *Adrenergics, anticholinergics:* additive adrenergic or anticholinergic effects
Cimetidine, phenothiazines, quinidine, selective serotonin reuptake inhibitors: increased desipramine effects, possible toxicity
Clonidine: hypertensive crisis
CNS depressants (antihistamines, opioid analgesics, sedative-hypnotics): additive CNS depression
MAO inhibitors: hyperpyretic crisis, severe seizures, death
Sparfloxacin: increased risk of adverse cardiovascular reactions
Drug-diagnostic tests. *Glucose:* increased or decreased level
Drug-food. *Grapefruit juice:* increased drug blood level and effects
Drug-herbs. *Chamomile, hops, kava, skullcap, valerian:* increased CNS depression
S-adenosylmethionine (SAM-e), St. John's wort: adverse serotonergic effects, including serotonin syndrome
Drug-behaviors. *Alcohol use:* increased response to alcohol
Smoking: increased metabolism and decreased efficacy of desipramine

Patient monitoring

🔊 Assess for suicidal tendencies before starting therapy.
- Monitor blood glucose level and CBC with white cell differential during therapy.
- Watch for severe CNS, cardiovascular, and hematologic adverse reactions.

Patient teaching

- Tell patient to take full dose at bedtime to avoid daytime drowsiness.

🔊 Urge patient to promptly report chest pain or easy bruising or bleeding.
- Inform patient that desired therapeutic effect may take 2 to 3 weeks.
- Caution patient that drug may cause physical or psychological dependence.

🔊 Instruct patient or parent to immediately report increasing depression or suicidal ideation (especially in child or adolescent).
- Caution patient to avoid driving and other hazardous activities until he knows how drug affects alertness, vision, and coordination.
- As appropriate, review all other significant and life-threatening adverse reactions and interactions, especially those related to the drugs, tests, foods, herbs, and behaviors mentioned above.

desloratadine

Clarinex, Clarinex Reditabs

Pharmacologic class: Peripherally selective piperidine, selective histamine$_1$-receptor antagonist
Therapeutic class: Antihistamine (nonsedating, second generation)
Pregnancy risk category C

Action

Suppresses histamine release at peripheral histamine$_1$-receptor sites

Availability

Syrup: 2.5 mg/5 ml
Tablets: 5 mg

Indications and dosages

➢ Seasonal and perennial allergic rhinitis; chronic idiopathic urticaria and allergies caused by indoor and outdoor allergens; pruritus; to reduce number and size of hives
Adults and children ages 12 and older: 5 mg/day P.O.
Children ages 6 to 11: 1 tsp (2.5 mg/5 ml syrup) P.O. once daily
Children ages 12 months to 5 years: ½ tsp (1.25 mg in 2.5 ml syrup) P.O. once daily
Children ages 6 to 11 months: 2 ml (1 mg syrup) P.O. once daily

Dosage adjustment

- Hepatic or renal impairment

Contraindications

- Hypersensitivity to drug, its components, or loratadine

Precautions

Use cautiously in:

- renal or hepatic impairment
- elderly patients
- pregnant or breastfeeding patients
- children younger than age 12 (safety and efficacy not established, except syrup).

Administration

- Give with or without food.

Route	Onset	Peak	Duration
P.O.	1 hr	3 hr	24 hr

Adverse reactions

CNS: dizziness, drowsiness, fatigue, headache
CV: tachycardia, palpitations
EENT: pharyngitis, dry throat
GI: nausea, dyspepsia, dry mouth
GU: dysmenorrhea
Musculoskeletal: myalgia
Other: flulike symptoms, hypersensitivity reaction

Interactions

Drug-diagnostic tests. *Bilirubin, hepatic enzymes:* increased values
Skin tests: interference with positive reaction to dermal reactivity indicators

Patient monitoring

- Monitor hepatic and renal function test results.

Patient teaching

- Tell patient he may take drug with or without food.
- Instruct patient to report rapid heartbeat, shortness of breath, rash, persistent flulike symptoms, or muscle ache.
- Caution patient to avoid driving and other hazardous activities until he knows how drug affects concentration and alertness.
- As appropriate, review all other significant adverse reactions and interactions, especially those related to the tests mentioned above.

desmopressin acetate (1-deamino-8-D-arginine vasopressin)

DDAVP, Desmospray, Minirin, Stimate

Pharmacologic class: Posterior pituitary hormone
Therapeutic class: Antidiuretic hormone
Pregnancy risk category B

Action

Enhances water reabsorption by increasing permeability of renal collecting ducts to adenosine monophosphate and water, thereby reducing urinary output and increasing urine osmolality. Also increases factor VIII (antihemophilic factor) activity.

Availability

Injection: 4 mcg/ml in single-dose 1-ml ampules and multidose 10-ml vials
Intranasal solution: 0.1 mg/ml, 1.5 mg/ ml
Intranasal spray (DDAVP): 0.1 mg/ml (10 mcg/spray) in 5-ml spray pump bottle
Tablets: 0.1 mg, 0.2 mg

Indications and dosages

➤ Diabetes insipidus
Adults and children older than age 12: 0.05 mg P.O. b.i.d.; adjust dosage based on patient response. Or 0.1 to 0.4 ml (10 to 40 mcg) daily intranasally as a single dose or in two or three divided doses. Or 0.5 ml (2 mcg) to 1 ml (4 mcg) daily I.V. or subcutaneously, usually in two divided doses.
Children ages 3 months to 12 years: 0.05 to 0.3 ml/day intranasally in one or two divided doses

➤ Hemophilia A; von Willebrand's disease type I
Adults and children: 0.3 mcg/kg I.V.; may repeat dose if needed. Or 300 mcg of intranasal solution containing 1.5 mcg/ml; for patients weighing less than 50 kg (110 lb), total dosage of 150 mcg (one spray of solution containing 1.5 mg/ml into a single nostril) is usually sufficient. If needed to maintain hemostasis during surgery, give intranasal dose 2 hours before surgery or give I.V. dose 30 minutes before surgery.

➤ Primary nocturnal enuresis
Children ages 6 and older: Initially, 20 mcg intranasally at bedtime. Maximum dosage is 40 mcg/day.

Off-label uses

- Chronic autonomic failure (such as nocturnal polyuria, overnight weight loss, morning orthostatic hypotension)

Contraindications

- Hypersensitivity to drug
- Hemophilia A with factor VIII levels less than or equal to 5%
- Von Willebrand's disease type IIB
- Impaired level of consciousness (intranasal form)

Precautions

Use cautiously in:
- coronary artery disease, hypertensive cardiovascular disease, fluid and electrolyte imbalances
- breastfeeding patients.

Administration

- Adjust morning and evening dosages as appropriate to minimize frequent urination and risk of water intoxication.
- Give I.V. dose (diluted in normal saline solution) by infusion over 15 to 30 minutes.

◀ When giving to child with diabetes insipidus, carefully restrict fluid intake to prevent hyponatremia and water intoxication.

Route	Onset	Peak	Duration
P.O.	1 hr	1-5 hr	8-12 hr
I.V.	15-30 min	Unknown	4-12 hr
Intranasal	1 hr	1-1.5 hr	8-12 hr

Adverse reactions

CNS: headache, dizziness, insomnia
CV: slight blood pressure increase, chest pain, palpitations
EENT: rhinitis, epistaxis, sore throat
GI: nausea, abdominal pain
GU: vulvar pain
Respiratory: cough
Other: local erythema, flushing, swelling or burning after injection

Interactions

Drug-drug. *Carbamazepine, chlorpropamide, pressor drugs:* potentiation of desmopressin effects

Patient monitoring

- Monitor urine volume and specific gravity, plasma and urine osmolality, and electrolyte levels in patients with diabetes insipidus.
- Monitor factor VIII antigen levels, activated partial thromboplastin time, and bleeding time in patients with hemophilia.

◀ When giving to child with diabetes insipidus, carefully monitor fluid intake and output.

Patient teaching

- Instruct patient to take drug exactly as prescribed and not to interchange strengths or delivery systems.
- Teach patient how to use prescribed delivery system if taking drug by other than oral route.
- Instruct patient with diabetes insipidus to avoid overhydration and to weigh himself daily. Tell him to report weight gain or swelling of arms or legs. If he's using nasal spray, teach him to inspect nasal membranes regularly and to report increased nasal congestion or swelling.
- Caution elderly patient not to increase fluid intake beyond that sufficient to satisfy thirst.
- As appropriate, review all significant adverse reactions and interactions, especially those related to the drugs mentioned above.

d

dexamethasone

Alti-Dexamethasone♣, Decadron, Dexameth, Dexone, Hexadrol

dexamethasone acetate

Dalalone D.P.

dexamethasone sodium phosphate

Dalalone, Decadron Phosphate

Pharmacologic class: Glucocorticoid
Therapeutic class: Anti-inflammatory
Pregnancy risk category C

Action

Unclear. Reduces inflammation by suppressing polymorphonuclear leukocyte migration, reversing increased capillary permeability, and stabilizing leukocyte lysosomal membranes. Also suppresses immune response (by reducing lymphatic activity), stimulates bone marrow, and promotes protein, fat, and carbohydrate metabolism.

Availability

Elixir: 0.5 mg/5 ml
Oral solution: 0.5 mg/5 ml, 1 mg/ml
Solution for injection (sodium phosphate): 4 mg/ml, 10 mg/ml, 20 mg/ml, 24 mg/ml
Suspension for injection (acetate): 8 mg/ml, 16 mg/ml
Tablets: 0.25 mg, 0.5 mg, 0.75 mg, 1 mg, 1.5 mg, 2 mg, 4 mg, 6 mg

 Indications and dosages

➢ Allergic and inflammatory conditions

Adults: 0.75 to 9 mg/day (dexamethasone) P.O. as a single dose or in divided doses; in severe cases, much higher dosages may be needed. Or 8 to 16 mg (acetate) I.M. q 1 to 3 weeks. Dosage requirements vary and must be individualized based on disease and patient response.

➢ Cerebral edema

Adults: Initially, 10 mg (sodium phosphate) I.V., followed by 4 mg I.M. q 6 hours. Then reduce dosage gradually over 5 to 7 days.

➢ Suppression test for Cushing's syndrome

Adults: 1 mg P.O. at 11 P.M. or 0.5 mg P.O. q 6 hours for 48 hours (with urine collection testing, as ordered)

Off-label uses

- Acute altitude sickness
- Bacterial meningitis
- Bronchopulmonary dysplasia in preterm infants
- Hirsutism
- Suppression test for detection, diagnosis, or management of depression

Contraindications

- Hypersensitivity to drug, benzyl alcohol, bisulfites, EDTA, creatinine, polysorbate 80, or methylparaben
- Systemic fungal infections

Precautions

Use cautiously in:

- renal insufficiency, cirrhosis, diabetes mellitus, diverticulitis, GI disease, cardiovascular disease, hypoprothrombinemia, hypothyroidism, myasthenia gravis, glaucoma, osteoporosis, infections, underlying immunosuppression, psychotic tendencies
- pregnant or breastfeeding patients
- children.

Administration

- Give P.O. dose with food or milk.
- When giving I.M., inject deep into gluteal muscle; rotate sites as needed.
- For I.V. use, drug may be given undiluted as a single dose over 1 minute or added to dextrose or I.V. saline solutions and given as an intermittent infusion at prescribed rate.

Route	Onset	Peak	Duration
P.O.	Unknown	1-2 hr	2.75 days
I.V.	1 hr	1 hr	Variable
I.M. (acetate)	Unknown	8 hr	6 days
I.M. (sodium phosphate)	1 hr	1 hr	6 days

Adverse reactions

CNS: headache, malaise, vertigo, psychiatric disturbances, **increased intracranial pressure, seizures**

CV: hypotension, **thrombophlebitis, myocardial rupture after recent myocardial infarction, thromboembolism**

EENT: cataracts

GI: nausea, vomiting, abdominal distention, dry mouth, anorexia, **peptic ulcer, bowel perforation, pancreatitis, ulcerative esophagitis**

Metabolic: decreased carbohydrate tolerance, hyperglycemia, cushingoid appearance (moon face, buffalo hump), decreased growth (in children), latent diabetes mellitus, sodium and fluid retention, negative nitrogen balance, **adrenal suppression, hypokalemic alkalosis**

Musculoskeletal: muscle wasting, muscle pain, osteoporosis, aseptic joint necrosis, tendon rupture, long bone fractures

Skin: diaphoresis, angioedema, erythema, rash, pruritus, urticaria, contact dermatitis, acne, decreased wound healing, bruising, skin fragility, petechiae

Other: facial edema, weight gain or loss, increased susceptibility to infection, hypersensitivity reactions

Interactions

Drug-drug. *Barbiturates, phenytoin, rifampin:* decreased dexamethasone effects
Digoxin: increased risk of digoxin toxicity
Ephedrine: increased dexamethasone clearance
Estrogen, hormonal contraceptives: blocking of dexamethasone metabolism
Fluoroquinolones: increased risk of tendon rupture
Itraconazole, ketoconazole: increased dexamethasone blood level and effects
Live-virus vaccines: decreased antibody response to vaccine, increased risk of adverse reactions
Loop and thiazide diuretics: additive hypokalemia
Somatrem, somatropin: decreased response to these drugs
Drug-diagnostic tests. *Calcium, potassium:* decreased levels
Cholesterol, glucose: increased levels
Nitroblue tetrazolium test: false-negative result
Drug-herbs. *Echinacea:* increased immune-stimulating effect
Ginseng: potentiation of immune-modulating response
Drug-behaviors. *Alcohol use:* increased risk of gastric irritation and GI ulcers

Patient monitoring

- Monitor blood glucose level closely in diabetic patients receiving drug orally.
- Monitor hemoglobin and potassium levels.
- Assess for occult blood loss.

🔊 In long-term therapy, never discontinue drug abruptly. Dosage must be tapered gradually.

Patient teaching

🔊 Instruct patient to immediately report sudden weight gain, swelling of face or limbs, excessive nervousness or sleep disturbances, excessive body hair growth, vision changes, difficulty breathing, muscle weakness, persistent abdominal pain, or change in stool color.

- Tell patient to take oral drug with or after meals.
- Advise patient to report vision changes.
- Inform patient that drug makes him more susceptible to infection. Advise him to avoid crowds and exposure to illness.

🔊 Caution patient not to stop taking drug abruptly.

- As appropriate, review all other significant and life-threatening adverse reactions and interactions, especially those related to the drugs, tests, herbs, and behaviors mentioned above.

dexmedetomidine hydrochloride

Precedex

Pharmacologic class: Alpha$_2$-adrenoceptor agonist

Therapeutic class: Nonbarbiturate sedative-hypnotic

Pregnancy risk category C

Action

Produces sedation through alpha$_1$ and alpha$_2$ stimulation

Availability

Injection: 100 mcg/ml

Indications and dosages

➢ Sedation of intubated and mechanically ventilated patients
Adults: 1 mcg/kg I.V. as a loading dose

given over 10 minutes, then 0.2 to 0.7 mcg/kg/hour. Don't infuse longer than 24 hours.

Dosage adjustment

- Hepatic or renal impairment
- Elderly patients

Contraindications

- Hypersensitivity to drug
- Complete heart block

Precautions

Use cautiously in:

- renal or hepatic impairment, respiratory depression, arrhythmias
- elderly patients
- pregnant or breastfeeding patients
- children.

Administration

- Infuse I.V. loading dose over 10 minutes.
- Watch for hypertension when giving loading dose.

Clinical alert: Use controlled infusion device for continuous infusion. Calculate infusion rate according to patient's weight and desired sedation level.

- To prepare infusion, add 2 ml of drug to 48 ml of normal saline solution, for a total volume of 50 ml.
- Don't infuse through same I.V. line with plasma or blood.
- Administer only in continually monitored setting.

Route	Onset	Peak	Duration
I.V.	Unknown	Unknown	Unknown

Adverse reactions

CV: bradycardia, hypotension, hypertension, **atrial fibrillation, myocardial infarction**
GI: nausea
GU: oliguria
Hematologic: anemia, **leukocytosis**
Respiratory: hypoxia, **pulmonary edema, pleural effusion**
Other: thirst

Interactions

Drug-drug. *Antipsychotics, inhalation anesthetics, opioids, sedative-hypnotics, skeletal muscle relaxants:* increased CNS depression
Drug-behaviors. *Alcohol use:* increased CNS depression

Patient monitoring

- Assess renal and hepatic function before starting therapy.
- Monitor cardiovascular status continuously.
- Evaluate infusion site for burning and irritation.

Patient teaching

- Tell patient he'll be closely supervised during period of sedation and on arousal.
- As appropriate, review all other significant and life-threatening adverse reactions and interactions, especially those related to the drugs and behaviors mentioned above.

dexmethylphenidate hydrochloride

Focalin

Pharmacologic class: Methylphenidate derivative
Therapeutic class: CNS stimulant
Controlled substance schedule II
Pregnancy risk category C

Action

Thought to block norepinephrine and dopamine reuptake, increasing the concentration of these neurotransmitters in extraneuronal space

Availability

Tablets: 2.5 mg, 5 mg, 10 mg

Indications and dosages

➤ Attention deficit hyperactivity disorder

Adults and children over age 6: In patients not receiving methylphenidate concurrently, 2.5 mg P.O. b.i.d. at least 4 hours apart; increase as needed in 2.5- to 5-mg increments to a maximum of 10 mg b.i.d. (Individualize dosage according to patient needs and response.) In patients receiving methylphenidate concurrently, start with half of methylphenidate dosage; maximum dosage is 10 mg P.O. b.i.d.

Contraindications

- Hypersensitivity to drug
- Glaucoma
- Anxiety, agitation, tension
- Family history or diagnosis of Tourette syndrome
- MAO inhibitor use within past 14 days

Precautions

Use cautiously in:
- hypertension, depression, seizures, cardiovascular disorders, psychosis, drug abuse
- pregnant or breastfeeding patients
- children under age 6 (safety and efficacy not established).

Administration

- Administer at same time each day without regard to meals.
- Don't give within 14 days of MAO inhibitor use.

Route	Onset	Peak	Duration
P.O.	Variable	1-1.5 hr	Unknown

Adverse reactions

CNS: nervousness, insomnia, dizziness, drowsiness, headache, dyskinesia, chorea, Tourette syndrome, **toxic psychosis**

CV: increased or decreased heart rate and blood pressure, tachycardia, angina, palpitations, **arrhythmias**

EENT: blurred vision, visual accommodation problems

GI: nausea, abdominal pain

Hematologic: anemia, **leukopenia, thrombocytopenia**

Hepatic: hepatic dysfunction, hepatic coma

Skin: rash, alopecia

Other: fever, decreased appetite, weight loss, psychological drug dependence, drug tolerance, growth suppression in children (with long-term use)

Interactions

Drug-drug. *Anticoagulants, phenobarbital, phenytoin, primidone, selective serotonin reuptake inhibitors, tricyclic antidepressants:* inhibited metabolism and additive effects of these drugs

Antihypertensives, pressor agents (dopamine, epinephrine): decreased efficacy of these drugs

MAO inhibitors: severe hypertensive crisis

Patient monitoring

- Monitor blood pressure closely, especially in patients receiving antihypertensives concurrently.
- Evaluate cardiac status. Report palpitations and other signs and symptoms of arrhythmias.
- During prolonged therapy, regularly monitor CBC with white cell differential and platelet count.

Patient teaching

- Advise patient or parents that drug should be taken at same time each day.
- Tell patient or parents that drug usually is discontinued if symptoms don't improve within 1 month.
- Instruct parents to monitor child's height and weight, because CNS stimulants have been associated with growth suppression.
- As appropriate, review all other significant and life-threatening adverse

reactions and interactions, especially those related to the drugs mentioned above.

dextran, high-molecular-weight (dextran 70, dextran 75)

Gendex 75, Gentran 70, Gentran 75, Macrodex

dextran, low-molecular-weight (dextran 40)

Gentran 40, Rheomacrodex

Pharmacologic class: Polysaccharide
Therapeutic class: Plasma volume expander
Pregnancy risk category C

Action

Expands plasma volume through colloidal osmotic effects during hypovolemic shock; pulls fluid from interstitial space, moving it into intravascular space

Availability

Injection: 6% dextran 70 in dextrose 5% in water (D_5W) or normal saline solution; 6% dextran 75 in D_5W or normal saline solution; 10% dextran 40 in D_5W or normal saline solution

Indications and dosages

➢ Plasma volume expansion

Adults: Dosage and infusion rate based on amount of fluid lost and hemoconcentration. Usual initial dosage of dextran 70 or 75 is 500 ml of 6% solution I.V., not to exceed 20 ml/kg during first 24 hours. Usual initial dosage of dextran 40 is 500 ml of 10% solution I.V., not to exceed 20 ml/kg during first 24 hours. Beyond 24 hours, usual total daily dosage should not exceed 10 ml/kg and therapy should not exceed 5 days.

Children: Dosage based on weight or body surface area, not to exceed 20 ml/kg I.V. daily

Contraindications

- Hypersensitivity to drug
- Pulmonary edema, cardiac decompensation, severe heart failure
- Thrombocytopenia
- Renal disease with severe oliguria or anuria
- Hypovolemic conditions

Precautions

Use cautiously in:

- active hemorrhage, diabetes mellitus, chronic hepatic disease, abdominal conditions
- pregnant or breastfeeding patients.

Administration

- Give by I.V. infusion only.
- In normovolemic patients, infuse no faster than 4 ml/minute.

Route	Onset	Peak	Duration
I.V.	Immediate	Immediate	Unknown

Adverse reactions

CV: hypotension, **thrombophlebitis, cardiac arrest**
GI: nausea, vomiting
GU: increased urine viscosity, **osmotic nephrosis, renal failure**
Hematologic: reduced platelet function, **prolonged bleeding time, decreased coagulation times**
Metabolic: hyponatremia
Respiratory: wheezing, dyspnea, **bronchospasm, pulmonary edema**
Skin: urticaria, rash, flushing, pruritus, angioedema
Other: chills, infection at injection site, **anaphylaxis**

Interactions

Drug-drug. *Abciximab, aspirin, heparin, thrombolytics, warfarin:* increased bleeding

Drug-diagnostic tests. *Alanine aminotransferase, aspartate aminotransferase:* increased levels

Bilirubin, glucose, hematocrit, hemoglobin, total protein, urine protein: falsely increased levels

Bleeding time: prolonged

Blood typing and cross-matching, Rh typing: test interference

Hematocrit: decreased

Patient monitoring

- Observe patient closely for signs and symptoms of anaphylaxis during first 30 minutes of infusion.
- Evaluate for dehydration after infusion.
- Know that bleeding time may be prolonged temporarily in patients receiving more than 1,000 ml of drug.
- Monitor amount and pattern of fluid intake and output.
- Assess patient's vital signs frequently. Suspect circulatory overload if patient has increased heart and respiratory rates, shortness of breath, and wheezing.

Patient teaching

- As appropriate, review all other significant and life-threatening adverse reactions and interactions, especially those related to the drugs and tests mentioned above.

dextroamphetamine sulfate

Dexedrine, Dexedrine Spansule, DextroStat

Pharmacologic class: Amphetamine

Therapeutic class: Sympathomimetic amine, CNS stimulant

Controlled substance schedule II

Pregnancy risk category C

Action

Produces CNS and respiratory stimulation by promoting release of norepinephrine from nerve terminals

Availability

Capsules (sustained-release): 5 mg, 10 mg, 15 mg

Tablets: 5 mg, 10 mg

Indications and dosages

➢ Attention deficit hyperactivity disorder

Adults: 5 to 60 mg P.O. daily in divided doses

Children ages 6 and older: 5 mg P.O. once or twice daily, increased by 5 mg at weekly intervals

Children ages 3 to 5: 2.5 mg P.O. daily, increased by 2.5 mg at weekly intervals

➢ Narcolepsy

Adults: 5 to 60 mg P.O. daily as a single dose or in divided doses

Children ages 12 and older: 10 mg P.O. daily, increased by 10 mg at weekly intervals until desired response occurs or adult dosage is reached

Children ages 6 to 11: 5 mg P.O. daily, increased by 5 mg at weekly intervals until desired response occurs or adult dosage is reached

Contraindications

- Hypersensitivity to drug or tartrazine
- Glaucoma

- Psychotic disorders
- MAO inhibitor use within past 14 days
- Pregnancy or breastfeeding

Precautions
Use cautiously in:
- cardiovascular disease, hypertension, diabetes mellitus
- history of substance abuse
- elderly patients.

Administration
- Make sure patient swallows sustained-release capsules whole without chewing or crushing.
- Give last daily dose at least 6 hours before patient's bedtime.

Don't give within 14 days of MAO inhibitor, because potentially fatal reaction may occur.

Route	Onset	Peak	Duration
P.O.	1-2 hr	Unknown	2-10 hr
P.O. (sustained)	Unknown	Unknown	Up to 24 hr

Adverse reactions
CNS: hyperactivity, insomnia, restlessness, tremor, depression, dizziness, headache, irritability
CV: palpitations, tachycardia, hypertension, hypotension, **arrhythmias**
GI: nausea, vomiting, constipation, diarrhea, abdominal cramps, dry mouth
GU: erectile dysfunction, increased libido
Skin: urticaria
Other: metallic taste, decreased appetite, physical or psychological drug dependence

Interactions
Drug-drug. *Acetazolamide, sodium bicarbonate:* urine alkalization, leading to increased dextroamphetamine effects
Adrenergic blockers: additive effects
Ammonium chloride, ascorbic acid (large doses): urine acidification, leading to decreased dextroamphetamine effects
Beta-adrenergic blockers, tricyclic antidepressants: increased risk of adverse cardiovascular effects
Guanethidine: reversal of hypotensive effect
MAO inhibitors: hypertensive crisis
Phenothiazines: decreased dextroamphetamine effects
Selective serotonin reuptake inhibitors: increased risk of serotonin syndrome
Drug-diagnostic tests. *Plasma corticosteroids:* increased levels
Drug-food. *Caffeine:* increased stimulant effect
Drug-herbs. *Caffeine-containing herbs, ephedra (ma huang):* increased stimulant effect

Patient monitoring
- Interrupt therapy or reduce dosage periodically to assess drug efficacy in patients with behavior disorders.
- Monitor blood and urine glucose levels carefully in diabetic patient. Drug may alter regular insulin requirements.

Patient teaching
- Tell patient to swallow sustained-release capsules whole with liquid without chewing or crushing.
- Advise patient to take drug early in day to avoid insomnia.
- Instruct patient to avoid driving and other hazardous activities until he knows how drug affects him.
- Caution patient not to stop therapy abruptly but to taper dosage gradually.
- As appropriate, review all other significant and life-threatening adverse reactions and interactions, especially those related to the drugs, tests, foods, and herbs mentioned above.

dextromethorphan hydrobromide

Balminil DM✱, Benylin Adult Formula Cough Syrup, Benylin Pediatric, Broncho-Grippol-DM✱, Calmylin #1✱, Children's Hold, Creo-Terpin, Delsym, DexAlone, DM Syrup, Drixoral Cough and Congestion Liquid Caps, Hold, Koffex-DM✱, Mediquell, Neo-DM✱, Ornex DM, Pertussin Cough Suppressant, Pertussin CS, Pertussin ES, Robidex, Robitussin Cough Calmers, Robitussin Maximum Strength Cough Suppressant, Robitussin Pediatric Cough and Cold, Sedatuss✱, Sucrets Cough Control Formula, Vicks Pediatric Formula 44D

Pharmacologic class: Levorphanol derivative

Therapeutic class: Antitussive (nonnarcotic)

Pregnancy risk category C

Action

Depresses cough reflex through direct effect on cough center in medulla. Has no expectorant action and does not inhibit ciliary action. Although related to opioids structurally, lacks analgesic and addictive properties.

Availability

Gelcaps: 15 mg, 30 mg
Liquid: 3.5 mg/5 ml, 5 mg/5 ml, 7.5 mg/5 ml, 15 mg/5 ml
Lozenges: 5 mg, 7.5 mg
Oral suspension (extended-release): 30 mg/5 ml
Syrup: 7.5 mg/5 ml, 10 mg/15 ml

Indications and dosages

➢ Cough caused by minor viral upper respiratory tract infections or inhaled irritants

Adults and children over age 12: 10 to 20 mg P.O. q 4 hours, or 30 mg P.O. q 6 to 8 hours, or 60 mg of extended-release form P.O. b.i.d. (not to exceed 120 mg/day)

Children ages 6 to 12: 5 to 10 mg P.O. q 4 hours, or 15 mg P.O. q 6 to 8 hours, or 30 mg of extended-release form P.O. q 12 hours (not to exceed 60 mg/day)

Children ages 2 to 6: 2.5 to 5 mg P.O. q 4 hours, or 7.5 mg q 6 to 8 hours, or 15 mg of extended-release form P.O. q 12 hours (not to exceed 30 mg/day)

Dosage adjustment

- Elderly patients

Contraindications

- Hypersensitivity to drug
- Chronic productive cough
- MAO inhibitor use within past 14 days

Precautions

Use cautiously in:

- tartrazine sensitivity
- diabetes mellitus (with sucrose-containing drug products)
- pregnant or breastfeeding patients
- children younger than age 2 (safety not established).

Administration

- Don't administer lozenges to children younger than age 6.

◀ Don't give within 14 days of MAO inhibitors.

Route	Onset	Peak	Duration
P.O.	15-30 min	Unknown	3-6 hr
P.O. (extended)	Unknown	Unknown	9-12 hr

Adverse reactions

CNS: dizziness and sedation
GI: nausea, vomiting, stomach pain

Interactions

Drug-drug. *Amiodarone, fluoxetine, quinidine:* increased dextromethorphan blood level, greater risk of adverse reactions
Antidepressants, antihistamines, opioids, sedative-hypnotics: additive CNS depression
MAO inhibitors, sibutramine: serotonin syndrome (nausea, confusion, blood pressure changes)
Drug-behaviors. *Alcohol use:* additive CNS depression

Patient monitoring

- Monitor cough frequency and type, and assess sputum characteristics.
- Assess hydration status. Increase patient's fluid input to help moisten secretions.

Patient teaching

- Advise patient to avoid irritants, such as smoking, dust, and fumes. Suggest use of humidifier to filter air pollutants.
- Inform patient that treatment aims to decrease coughing frequency and intensity without completely eliminating protective cough reflex.
- Instruct patient to contact health care provider if cough lasts more than 7 days.
- As appropriate, review all other significant adverse reactions and interactions, especially those related to the drugs and behaviors mentioned above.

dextrose (d-glucose)

B-D Glucose, Glutose, Insta-Glucose

Pharmacologic class: Monosaccharide
Therapeutic class: Carbohydrate caloric nutritional supplement
Pregnancy risk category C

Action

Prevents protein and nitrogen loss; promotes glycogen deposition and ketone accumulation (through osmotic diuretic action)

Availability

Injection: 2.5%, 5%, 10%, 20%, 25%, 30%, 40%, 50%, 60%, 70%
Oral gel: 40%
Tablets (chewable): 5 g

Indications and dosages

➢ Insulin-dependent hypoglycemia
Adults and children: Initially, 10 to 20 g P.O., repeated in 10 to 20 minutes if needed based on blood glucose level; or 20 to 50 ml by I.V. infusion or injection of 50% solution given at 3 ml/ minute. Maintenance dosage is 10% to 15% solution by continuous I.V. infusion until blood glucose level reaches therapeutic range.
Infants and neonates: 2 ml/kg of 10% to 25% solution by slow I.V. infusion until blood glucose level reaches therapeutic range
➢ Calorie replacement
Adults and children: 2.5%, 5%, or 10% solution given through peripheral I.V. line, with dosage tailored to patient's need for fluid or calories; or 10% to 70% solution given through large central vein if needed (typically mixed with amino acids or other solution)

Off-label uses

- Varicose veins
- Insulin-secreting islet-cell adenoma

Contraindications

- Hypersensitivity to drug
- Hyperglycemia, diabetic coma
- Hemorrhage
- Heart failure

Precautions

Use cautiously in:
- renal, cardiac, or hepatic impairment; diabetes mellitus.

Administration
- Use aseptic technique when preparing solution. Bacteria thrive in high-glucose environments.

Clinical alert: Infuse concentrations above 10% through central vein.
- Don't infuse concentrated solution rapidly, because doing so may cause hyperglycemia and fluid shifts.

Clinical alert: Never stop infusion abruptly.

Route	Onset	Peak	Duration
P.O.	10-20 min	40 min	Unknown
I.V.	2-3 min	Unknown	Unknown

Adverse reactions
CNS: confusion, loss of consciousness
CV: hypertension, phlebitis, **venous thrombosis, heart failure**
GU: glycosuria, osmotic diuresis
Metabolic: hyperglycemia, hypervolemia, hypovolemia, electrolyte imbalances, **hyperosmolar coma**
Respiratory: pulmonary edema
Skin: flushing, urticaria
Other: chills, fever, dehydration, injection site reaction, infection

Interactions
Drug-drug. *Corticosteroids, corticotropin:* increased risk of fluid and electrolyte imbalances
Drug-diagnostic tests. *Glucose:* increased level

Patient monitoring
Clinical alert: Monitor infusion site frequently to prevent irritation, tissue sloughing, necrosis, and phlebitis.
- Check blood glucose level at regular intervals.
- Monitor fluid intake and output.
- Weigh patient regularly.
- Assess patient for confusion.

Patient teaching
- Teach patient how to recognize signs and symptoms of hypoglycemia and hyperglycemia.
- Provide instructions on glucose self-monitoring.
- As appropriate, review all other significant and life-threatening adverse reactions and interactions, especially those related to the drugs and tests mentioned above.

d

diazepam
Apo-Diazepam*, Diastat, Diazemuls*, Diazepam Intensol, Dizac, Novo-Dipam*, PMS-Diazepam*, Valium, Vivol*

Pharmacologic class: Benzodiazepine
Therapeutic class: Anxiolytic, anticonvulsant, sedative-hypnotic, skeletal muscle relaxant (centrally acting)
Controlled substance schedule IV
Pregnancy risk category D

Action
Produces anxiolytic effect and CNS depression by stimulating gamma-aminobutyric acid receptors. Relaxes skeletal muscles of spine by inhibiting polysynaptic afferent pathways. Controls seizures by enhancing presynaptic inhibition.

Availability
Injection: 5 mg/ml
Oral solution: 1 mg/ml, 5 mg/5 ml
Rectal gel delivery system: 2.5 mg, 10 mg, 15 mg, 20 mg
Sterile emulsion for injection: 5 mg/ml
Tablets: 2 mg, 5 mg, 10 mg

Indications and dosages
➢ Anxiety disorders
Adults: 2 to 10 mg P.O. two to four times daily, depending on symptom severity. Alternatively, for moderate anxiety, 2 to 5 mg I.V., repeated in 3 to 4 hours if needed. For severe anxiety, 5

to 10 mg I.V., repeated in 3 to 4 hours if needed.
Children age 6 months and older: 1 to 2.5 mg P.O. three to four times daily; may increase gradually as needed
➢ Before cardioversion
Adults: 5 to 15 mg I.V. 5 to 10 minutes before cardioversion
➢ Before endoscopy
Adults: Usually, 10 mg I.V. is sufficient; may be increased to 20 mg I.V. Alternatively, 5 to 10 mg I.M. 30 minutes before endoscopy.
➢ Status epilepticus and severe recurrent convulsive seizures
Adults: 5 to 10 mg I.V. slowly, repeated as needed q 10 to 15 minutes, to a maximum of 30 mg; may repeat regimen if needed in 2 to 4 hours. May give I.M. if I.V. delivery is impossible.
Children ages 5 and older: 1 mg I.V. slowly q 2 to 5 minutes, to a maximum of 10 mg; repeat in 2 to 4 hours if needed. May give I.M. if I.V. delivery is impossible.
Children over 1 month to 5 years: 0.2 to 0.5 mg I.V. slowly q 2 to 5 minutes, to a maximum of 5 mg I.V. May give I.M. if I.V. delivery is impossible.
➢ Adjunctive use in selected refractory patients with epilepsy
Adults and children ages 12 and older: 0.2 mg/kg P.R. May repeat 4 to 12 hours later.
Children ages 6 to 11: 0.3 mg/kg P.R. May repeat 4 to 12 hours later.
Children ages 2 to 5: 0.5 mg/kg P.R. May repeat 4 to 12 hours later.
➢ Muscle spasm associated with local pathology, cerebral palsy, athetosis, "stiff-man" syndrome, or tetanus
Adults: 2 to 10 mg P.O. three to four times daily. Or initially, 5 to 10 mg I.V. or I.M., repeated in 3 to 4 hours if needed. Tetanus may necessitate higher dosages.
Elderly or debilitated patients: Initially, 2 to 2.5 mg P.O. once or twice daily, increased gradually as needed and tolerated
Children: 1 to 2.5 mg P.O. three to four times daily
Children ages 5 and older: 5 to 10 mg I.M. or I.V., repeated q 3 to 4 hours as needed to control tetanus spasm
Children over 1 month to 5 years: 1 to 2 mg I.M. or I.V. slowly, repeated q 3 to 4 hours as needed to control tetanus spasm
➢ Acute alcohol withdrawal
Adults: Initially, 10 mg P.O. three to four times during first 24 hours, decreased to 5 mg P.O. three to four times daily p.r.n. Or initially, 10 mg I.M. or I.V.; then 5 to 10 mg I.M. or I.V. in 3 to 4 hours p.r.n.

Off-label uses
• Panic attacks
• Adjunct to general anesthesia

Contraindications
• Hypersensitivity to drug, other benzodiazepines, alcohol, or tartrazine
• Coma or CNS depression
• Narrow-angle glaucoma

Precautions
Use cautiously in:
• hepatic dysfunction, severe renal impairment
• elderly patients
• pregnant or breastfeeding patients (use not recommended)
• children.

Administration
🔊 Administer I.V. infusion slowly into large vein, taking at least 1 minute for each 5 mg in adults or at least 3 minutes for each 0.25 mg/kg in children.
• Know that I.V. route is preferred over I.M. route because of slow or erratic I.M. absorption.
• Don't mix with other drugs or solutions in syringe or container.
• Enforce bed rest for at least 3 hours after I.V. injection.

• Give I.M. injection deeply and slowly into large muscle mass.
• If desired, mix oral solution with liquid or soft food.

Route	Onset	Peak	Duration
P.O.	30-60 min	1-2 hr	Up to 24 hr
I.V.	1-5 min	15-30 min	15-60 min
I.M.	Within 20 min	0.5-1.5 hr	Unknown
P.R.	Unknown	1-2 hr	4-12 hr

Adverse reactions

CNS: dizziness, drowsiness, lethargy, depression, light-headedness, disorientation, anger, manic or hypomanic episodes, restlessness, paresthesia, headache, slurred speech, dysarthria, stupor, tremor, dystonia, vivid dreams, extrapyramidal reactions, mild paradoxical excitation
CV: bradycardia, tachycardia, hypertension, hypotension, palpitations, **cardiovascular collapse**
EENT: blurred vision, diplopia, nystagmus, nasal congestion
GI: nausea, vomiting, diarrhea, constipation, gastric disorders, difficulty swallowing, increased salivation
GU: urinary retention or incontinence, menstrual irregularities, gynecomastia, libido changes
Hematologic: blood dyscrasias including eosinophilia, **leukopenia**, **agranulocytosis,** and **thrombocytopenia**
Hepatic: hepatic dysfunction
Musculoskeletal: muscle rigidity, muscular disturbances
Respiratory: respiratory depression
Skin: dermatitis, rash, pruritus, urticaria, diaphoresis
Other: weight gain or loss, decreased appetite, edema, hiccups, fever, physical or psychological drug dependence or tolerance

Interactions

Drug-drug. *Antidepressants, antihistamines, barbiturates, opioids:* additive CNS depression
Cimetidine, disulfiram, fluoxetine, hormonal contraceptives, isoniazid, ketoconazole, metoprolol, propoxyphene, propranolol, valproic acid: decreased metabolism and enhanced action of diazepam
Digoxin: increased digoxin blood level, possible toxicity
Levodopa: decreased levodopa efficacy
Rifampin: increased metabolism and decreased efficacy of diazepam
Theophylline: decreased sedative effect of diazepam
Drug-diagnostic tests. *Alanine aminotransferase, alkaline phosphatase, aspartate aminotransferase, lactate dehydrogenase:* increased levels
Neutrophils, platelets: decreased counts
Drug-herbs. *Chamomile, hops, kava, skullcap, valerian:* increased CNS depression
Drug-behaviors. *Alcohol use:* increased CNS depression

Patient monitoring

• Supervise ambulation, especially in elderly patients.
• Monitor CBC and kidney and liver function test results.
Avoid sudden drug withdrawal. Taper dosage gradually to termination of therapy.

Patient teaching

• Inform patient he may take drug with or without food; recommend taking it with food if it causes stomach upset.
• Teach caregiver how to administer rectal gel system, if prescribed.
• Caution patient to avoid driving and other hazardous activities until he knows how drug affects concentration and alertness.

- Tell patient to notify prescriber immediately if easy bruising or bleeding occurs.
- Instruct patient to move slowly when sitting up or standing, to avoid dizziness from blood pressure decrease. Advise him to dangle legs briefly before getting out of bed.
- Advise patient not to stop taking drug abruptly.
- Tell female patient not to take drug if she is pregnant or plans to breastfeed.
- As appropriate, review all other significant and life-threatening adverse reactions and interactions, especially those related to the drugs, tests, herbs, and behaviors mentioned above.

diazoxide

Hyperstat IV, Proglycem✱

Pharmacologic class: Vasodilator

Therapeutic class: Antihypertensive (nondiuretic), antihypoglycemic

Pregnancy risk category C

Action

Unclear. Relaxes peripheral arterioles of smooth-muscle cells and reduces peripheral vascular resistance as a result of vasodilation.

Availability

Capsules: 50 mg

Injection: 15 mg/ml in 20-ml ampules

Oral suspension: 50 mg/ml

Indications and dosages

➢ Hypertensive crisis

Adults and children: 1 to 3 mg/kg I.V. bolus, to a maximum dosage of 150 mg q 5 to 15 minutes until adequate response occurs. Repeat as needed q 4 hours or more.

➢ Hypoglycemia secondary to hyperinsulinism

Adults and children: 3 to 8 mg/kg P.O. daily in two to three divided doses q 8 to 12 hours

Newborn and infants: 3.3 mg/kg P.O. q 8 hours

Off-label uses

- Pregnancy-induced hypertension
- Obesity

Contraindications

- Hypersensitivity to drug, thiazides, or sulfonamides
- Compensatory hypertension
- Pheochromocytoma
- Dissecting aortic aneurysm

Precautions

Use cautiously in:

- fluid and electrolyte imbalances; impaired renal, hepatic, cerebral, or cardiac circulation
- pregnant or breastfeeding patients
- children.

Administration

- Keep patient recumbent during I.V. administration and for at least 30 minutes afterward.
- Give single I.V. doses over 10 to 30 seconds. Continuous I.V. infusion can be given at a constant rate (7.5 to 30 mg/minute) until adequate response occurs.

Route	Onset	Peak	Duration
P.O.	1 hr	Unknown	8 hr
I.V.	1 min	2-5 min	2-12 hr

Adverse reactions

CNS: headache, light-headedness, dizziness, weakness, euphoria, **seizures, paralysis, cerebral ischemia**

CV: ECG changes, orthostatic hypotension, angina pectoris, **myocardial ischemia, myocardial infarction, arrhythmias, shock, supraventricular tachycardia, heart failure**

EENT: optic nerve damage

GI: nausea, vomiting, diarrhea, constipation, abdominal discomfort, dry mouth
GU: breast tenderness
Metabolic: hyperglycemia, hyperuricemia, fluid and electrolyte imbalances, sodium and water retention
Skin: inflammation (with extravasation), diaphoresis, flushing
Other: sensation of warmth, edema, pain (with extravasation)

Interactions

Drug-drug. *Antihypertensives (such as beta-adrenergic blockers, hydralazine, methyldopa, minoxidil, nitrates, prazosin, reserpine):* additive hypotension
Hydantoins: decreased hydantoin blood level
Sulfonylureas: hyperglycemia
Thiazide diuretics: increased diazoxide effects
Drug-diagnostic tests. *Blood urea nitrogen, glucose, serum sodium, uric acid:* increased levels
Eosinophils, hematocrit, hemoglobin, platelets, white blood cells: decreased values

Patient monitoring

◀ Measure blood pressure every 5 minutes for first 15 to 30 minutes of infusion or until patient stabilizes.
- Monitor ECG and pulse continuously during and after infusion. Be aware that tachycardia may immediately follow I.V. infusion.
- Assess fluid status; promptly report intake and output changes. If fluid retention occurs, give diuretic, as prescribed.
- Inspect I.V. site regularly for infiltration or extravasation.
- Observe closely for signs and symptoms of heart failure.
- Monitor diabetic patient for loss of glycemic control.

Patient teaching

◀ Instruct patient to immediately report chest pain, dizziness, and severe headache.
- Tell patient to weigh himself daily and report significant gains.
- As appropriate, review all other significant and life-threatening adverse reactions and interactions, especially those related to the drugs and tests mentioned above.

diclofenac potassium

Cataflam, Novo-Difenac-K✤, Novo-Difenac-SR✤

diclofenac sodium

Voltaren, Voltaren SR

Pharmacologic class: Cyclooxygenase inhibitor, nonsteroidal anti-inflammatory drug (NSAID)
Therapeutic class: Nonopioid analgesic, antiarthritic
Pregnancy risk category B (third trimester: ***D***)

Action

Unclear. Thought to block activity of cyclooxygenase, thereby inhibiting inflammatory responses of vasodilation and swelling and blocking transmission of painful stimuli.

Availability

Tablets: 50 mg, 75 mg
Tablets (delayed-release): 25 mg, 50 mg, 75 mg
Tablets (extended-release): 100 mg

Indications and dosages

➢ Analgesia; dysmenorrhea
Adults: Initially, 100 mg P.O., then 50 mg t.i.d. as needed

➢ Rheumatoid arthritis
Adults: Initially, 50 mg P.O. three to four times daily. After initial response, reduce to lowest dosage that controls symptoms. Usual maintenance dosage is 25 mg t.i.d.
➢ Osteoarthritis
Adults: Initially, 50 mg P.O. two to three times daily. After initial response, reduce to lowest dosage that controls symptoms.
➢ Ankylosing spondylitis
Adults: 25 mg P.O. four to five times daily. After initial response, reduce to lowest dosage that controls symptoms.

Dosage adjustment
• Renal impairment
• Elderly patients

Off-label uses
• Post-radial keratotomy symptoms
• Dental pain

Contraindications
• Hypersensitivity to drug or its components, other NSAIDs, or aspirin
• Active GI bleeding or ulcer disease

Precautions
Use cautiously in:
• severe cardiovascular, renal, or hepatic disease; bleeding tendency
• history of porphyria or ulcer disease
• concurrent anticoagulant use
• elderly patients
• pregnant or breastfeeding patients
• children.

Administration
• Give on empty stomach 1 hour before or after a meal.
• If drug causes GI upset, give with milk or meals.
• Make sure patient swallows extended-release form whole without chewing or crushing.

Route	Onset	Peak	Duration
P.O.	10 min	1 hr	8 hr
P.O. (delayed)	30 min	2-3 hr	8 hr
P.O. (extended)	Unknown	5-6 hr	Unknown

Adverse reactions
CNS: dizziness, drowsiness, headache
CV: hypertension
EENT: tinnitus
GI: diarrhea, abdominal pain, dyspepsia, heartburn, peptic ulcer, **GI bleeding, GI perforation**
GU: dysuria, frequent urination, hematuria, proteinuria, nephritis, **acute renal failure**
Hematologic: prolonged bleeding time
Hepatic: hepatotoxicity
Skin: eczema, photosensitivity, rash, contact dermatitis, dry skin, exfoliation
Other: allergic reactions (including edema), **anaphylaxis**

Interactions
Drug-drug. *Anticoagulants, antiplatelet agents, cephalosporins, plicamycin, thrombolytics:* increased risk of bleeding
Antihypertensives, diuretics: decreased efficacy of these drugs
Antineoplastics: increased risk of hematologic adverse reactions
Colchicine, corticosteroids, other NSAIDs: additive adverse GI effects
Cyclosporine, probenecid: increased risk of diclofenac toxicity
Digoxin, lithium, methotrexate, phenytoin, theophylline: increased levels of these drugs, greater risk of toxicity
Potassium-sparing diuretics: increased risk of hyperkalemia
Drug-diagnostic tests. *Alanine aminotransferase, alkaline phosphatase, aspartate aminotransferase, blood urea nitrogen, creatinine, electrolytes, lactate dehydrogenase, urine uric acid:* increased values

Bleeding time: prolonged
Hematocrit, hemoglobin, platelets, serum uric acid, urine electrolytes, white blood cells: decreased values
Drug-herbs. *Anise, arnica, chamomile, clove, dong quai, fenugreek, feverfew, garlic, ginger, ginkgo, ginseng, and others:* increased risk of bleeding
Drug-behaviors. *Alcohol use:* increased risk of adverse GI effects

Patient monitoring

- Monitor hepatic and renal function.
- Observe for and report signs and symptoms of bleeding.
- Assess for hypertension.
- Monitor sodium and potassium levels in patients receiving potassium-sparing diuretics.
- Weigh patient to detect fluid retention. Report gain of more than 2 lb in 24 hours.

Patient teaching

- Instruct patient to take drug on empty stomach 1 hour before or after a meal.
- Advise patient not to lie down for 15 to 30 minutes after taking drug, to minimize esophageal irritation.
- Instruct patient to stop taking drug and contact prescriber promptly if he experiences ringing or buzzing in ears, dizziness, GI discomfort, or bleeding.
- Caution patient not to take over-the-counter analgesics during diclofenac therapy.
- As appropriate, review all other significant and life-threatening adverse reactions and interactions, especially those related to the drugs, tests, herbs, and behaviors mentioned above.

dicloxacillin sodium

Pharmacologic class: Penicillinase-resistant penicillin
Therapeutic class: Anti-infective
Pregnancy risk category B

Action

Inhibits cell-wall synthesis during bacterial cell division and multiplication; resists penicillinase enzymes produced by bacteria

Availability

Capsules: 125 mg, 250 mg, 500 mg
Oral solution: 62.5 mg/5 ml

Indications and dosages

➤ Systemic infections caused by penicillinase-producing staphylococci
Adults and children weighing 40 kg (88 lb) or more: 125 to 250 mg P.O. q 6 hours. More severe infection may require higher dosage.
Children weighing less than 40 kg (88 lb): 12.5 to 25 mg/kg P.O. daily in divided doses q 6 hours, depending on severity of infection

Contraindications

- Hypersensitivity to drug, other penicillins, or cephalosporins

Precautions

Use cautiously in:
- severe renal insufficiency, infectious mononucleosis
- pregnant or breastfeeding patients.

Administration

- Ask patient about history of allergy to penicillin or cephalosporins before giving.
- Give on empty stomach at least 1 hour before or 2 hours after meals.
- Administer with water only. Don't give with acidic juices or carbonated

beverages, which may inactivate drug effects.

Route	Onset	Peak	Duration
P.O.	Unknown	2 hr	6 hr

Adverse reactions

CNS: lethargy, hallucinations, anxiety, confusion, agitation, depression, fatigue, dizziness, **seizures**
CV: vein irritation, **thrombophlebitis, heart failure**
GI: nausea, vomiting, diarrhea, bloody diarrhea, abdominal pain, gastritis, enterocolitis, oral and rectal candidiasis, stomatitis, glossitis, sore mouth, **pseudomembranous colitis**
GU: vaginitis, nephropathy, **interstitial nephritis**
Hematologic: eosinophilia, anemia, **neutropenia, hemolytic anemia, agranulocytosis, leukopenia, thrombocytopenic purpura, thrombocytopenia**
Hepatic: hepatitis
Respiratory: wheezing
Skin: rash, urticaria
Other: overgrowth of nonsusceptible organisms, superinfection, fever, hypersensitivity reactions, **serum sickness, anaphylaxis**

Interactions

Drug-drug. *Aminoglycosides:* decreased drug blood levels
Chloramphenicol, tetracycline: decreased efficacy of both drugs
Hormonal contraceptives: decreased contraceptive efficacy
Drug-diagnostic tests. *Conjugated estrone or estriol-glucuronide (in pregnant women), estradiol, granulocytes, hemoglobin, platelets, total conjugated estriol, white blood cells:* decreased levels
Coombs' test, urine glucose: false-positive results
Eosinophils: increased count
Drug-food. *Any food:* interference with drug absorption and efficacy
Carbonated beverages, juices: drug inactivation

Patient monitoring

- In long-term therapy, monitor renal, hepatic, and hematopoietic functions and evaluate blood cultures weekly.

Patient teaching

- Advise patient to contact prescriber if nausea, diarrhea, or other GI effects occur.
- Instruct patient to complete entire course of therapy, even if he feels better.

Clinical alert: Tell patient to report rash immediately.

- As appropriate, review all other significant and life-threatening adverse reactions and interactions, especially those related to the drugs, tests, and foods mentioned above.

dicyclomine

Bentyl, Bentylol✱, Formulex✱, Spasmoban

Pharmacologic class: Anticholinergic
Therapeutic class: Antispasmodic
Pregnancy risk category B

Action

Thought to exert direct effect on GI smooth muscle by inhibiting acetylcholine at receptor sites, thereby reducing GI tract motility and tone

Availability

Capsules: 10 mg, 20 mg
Solution for injection: 10 mg/ml
Syrup: 10 mg/5 ml
Tablets: 10 mg, 20 mg

Indications and dosages

➢ Irritable bowel syndrome in patients unresponsive to usual interventions

Adults: 20 mg P.O. or I.M. q.i.d.; may increase up to 160 mg/day

Contraindications

- Hypersensitivity to drug
- GI or genitourinary tract obstruction
- Severe ulcerative colitis
- Reflux esophagitis
- Unstable cardiovascular status
- Glaucoma
- Myasthenia gravis
- Breastfeeding
- Infants younger than 6 months

Precautions

Use cautiously in:
- hepatic or renal impairment, autonomic neuropathy, cardiovascular disease, prostatic hypertrophy
- elderly patients
- pregnant patients (safety not established).

Administration

- Give 30 to 60 minutes before meals; give bedtime dose at least 2 hours after evening meal.

Don't administer by I.V. route.

- Don't give by I.M. route for more than 2 days.

Route	Onset	Peak	Duration
P.O., I.M.	Unknown	Unknown	Unknown

Adverse reactions

CNS: confusion, drowsiness, light-headedness (with I.M. use), psychosis
CV: palpitations, tachycardia
EENT: blurred vision, increased intraocular pressure
GI: nausea, vomiting, constipation, heartburn, decreased salivation, dry mouth, **paralytic ileus**
GU: urinary hesitancy or retention, erectile dysfunction, decreased lactation
Skin: decreased sweating, rash, itching, urticaria
Other: pain and redness at I.M. site, allergic reactions including **anaphylaxis**

Interactions

Drug-drug. *Adsorbent antidiarrheals, antacids:* decreased dicyclomine absorption
Cyclopropane anesthetics: increased risk of cardiovascular adverse reactions
Oral drugs: altered absorption of these drugs
Potassium (oral): increased GI mucosal lesions
Other anticholinergics (including antihistamines, disopyramide, quinidine): additive anticholinergic effects
Drug-diagnostic tests. *Gastric acid secretion test:* antagonism of pentagastrin and histamine (testing agents)

Patient monitoring

Stay alert for anaphylaxis.

- Monitor vital signs and fluid intake and output. Ask patient about palpitations.

Assess for light-headedness, confusion, and rash after I.M. injection.

- Evaluate patient's vision, particularly for blurring and other signs and symptoms of increasing intraocular pressure.
- Assess bowel pattern, particularly for signs and symptoms of paralytic ileus.

Patient teaching

- Instruct patient to take drug 30 to 60 minutes before meals and to take bedtime dose at least 2 hours after evening meal.
- Advise patient not to take antacids or adsorbent antidiarrheals within 2 hours of dicyclomine.

Urge patient to promptly report rash, abdominal pain, decreased urinary output, or absence of bowel movements.

- Caution patient to avoid driving or other hazardous activities until he knows how drug affects concentration, vision, and alertness.
- Advise patient to minimize GI upset by eating small, frequent servings of healthy food and drinking plenty of fluids.

• As appropriate, review all other significant and life-threatening adverse reactions and interactions, especially those related to the drugs and tests mentioned above.

didanosine (ddI, 2,3-dideoxyinosine)

Videx, Videx EC

Pharmacologic class: Nucleoside reverse transcriptase inhibitor
Therapeutic class: Antiretroviral, antiviral
Pregnancy risk category B

Action

Inhibits replication of human immunodeficiency virus (HIV) by disrupting synthesis of DNA polymerase, an enzyme crucial to DNA and RNA formation

Availability

Capsules (delayed-release): 125 mg, 200 mg, 250 mg, 400 mg
Powder for oral solution (buffered): 100 mg/packet, 167 mg/packet, 250 mg/packet
Powder for oral solution (pediatric): 2 g in 4-oz glass bottle, 4 g in 8-oz glass bottle
Tablets (buffered, chewable): 25 mg, 50 mg, 100 mg, 150 mg, 200 mg

Indications and dosages

➤ HIV infection

Adults weighing 60 kg (132 lb) or more: 200 mg (tablets) P.O. q 12 hours, or 400 mg (capsules) P.O. once daily, or 250 mg (buffered powder) P.O. q 12 hours
Adults weighing less than 60 kg (132 lb): 125 mg (tablets) P.O. q 12 hours, or 250 mg (capsules) P.O. once daily, or 167 mg (buffered powder) P.O. q 12 hours
Children: 120 mg/m^2 (tablets or powder for oral solution, pediatric) P.O. q 12 hours

Dosage adjustment

• Renal impairment

Contraindications

• Hypersensitivity to drug

Precautions

Use cautiously in:
• renal or hepatic impairment, peripheral neuropathy, phenylketonuria, hyperuricemia
• elderly patients
• pregnant or breastfeeding patients
• children.

Administration

• Know that drug is usually given in conjunction with other antiretrovirals.
• Give on empty stomach 30 minutes before or 2 hours after a meal.
• Don't administer with fruit juice.
• Know that pharmacist must prepare pediatric powder for oral solution by diluting with water and antacid to a concentration of 10 mg/ml.
• Be aware that delayed-release capsules aren't intended for use in children.

Route	Onset	Peak	Duration
P.O.	Unknown	0.5-1 hr	Unknown

Adverse reactions

CNS: dizziness, anxiety, abnormal thinking, hypoesthesia, agitation, confusion, hypertonia, asthenia, peripheral neuropathy, **seizures, coma**
CV: peripheral coldness, palpitations, hypotension, bradycardia, weak pulse, pseudoaneurysm, incomplete atrioventricular (AV) block, **complete AV block, nodal arrhythmias, ventricular tachycardia, thrombophlebitis, embolism**

EENT: diplopia, abnormal vision, ocular hypotony, iritis, retinal detachment
GI: nausea, vomiting, diarrhea, abdominal enlargement, dyspepsia, ileus, GI reflux, hematemesis, dysphagia, dry mouth, **pancreatitis**
GU: urinary retention, frequency, or incontinence; dysuria; cystalgia; prostatitis; **renal dysfunction; nephrotoxicity**
Hematologic: anemia, **leukocytosis, thrombocytopenia, bleeding, neutropenia**
Hepatic: hepatomegaly with steatosis
Metabolic: diabetes mellitus, **hyperkalemia, lactic acidosis**
Musculoskeletal: muscle contractions
Respiratory: pneumonia, crackles, rhonchi, bronchitis, pleurisy, dyspnea, wheezing, **pleural effusion, pulmonary edema, pulmonary embolism, bronchospasm**
Skin: diaphoresis, pallor, rash, urticaria, pruritus, bullous eruption, petechiae, cellulitis, abscess
Other: edema, development of human antichimeric antibodies

Interactions

Drug-drug. *Allopurinol, ganciclovir (oral):* increased didanosine blood level
Amprenavir, delavirdine, indinavir, ritonavir, saquinavir: altered didanosine pharmacokinetics
Antacids, other drugs that increase gastric pH: increased risk of didanosine toxicity
Co-trimoxazole, pentamidine: increased risk of pancreatic toxicity
Dapsone, fluoroquinolones, ketoconazole: decreased blood levels of these drugs
Itraconazole: decreased itraconazole blood level
Methadone: 50% decrease in didanosine blood level
Drug-diagnostic tests. *Alanine aminotransferase, alkaline phosphatase, aspartate aminotransferase, bilirubin, uric acid:* increased levels
Granulocytes, hemoglobin, platelets, white blood cells: decreased values
Drug-food. *Any food:* decreased rate and extent of drug absorption

Patient monitoring

- [Clinical alert] Monitor for signs and symptoms of pancreatitis. Report these to prescriber immediately.
- [Clinical alert] Assess carefully for signs and symptoms of lactic acidosis, such as dizziness, light-headedness, and bradycardia.
- Monitor for signs and symptoms of peripheral neuropathy.
- In patients with renal impairment, watch for drug toxicity and hypermagnesemia (suggested by muscle weakness and confusion).

Patient teaching

- Tell patient to take drug on empty stomach and to chew tablets without crushing or breaking.
- Advise patient using buffered powder to mix it with water, not juice, and to let powder dissolve for several minutes before taking.
- [Clinical alert] Instruct patient to immediately report abdominal pain, nausea, or vomiting.
- As appropriate, review all other significant and life-threatening adverse reactions and interactions, especially those related to the drugs, tests, and foods mentioned above.

diflunisal

Dolobid

Pharmacologic class: Nonsteroidal anti-inflammatory drug
Therapeutic class: Nonopioid analgesic, anti-inflammatory
Pregnancy risk category C

Action
Unclear. Thought to act by inhibiting prostaglandin synthesis.

Availability
Tablets: 250 mg, 500 mg

Indications and dosages
➢ Osteoarthritis; rheumatoid arthritis
Adults: 500 to 1,000 mg P.O. daily in two divided doses, usually given q 12 hours, to a maximum of 1,500 mg/day
➢ Mild to moderate pain
Adults: 1 g P.O., followed by 500 mg q 8 to 12 hours; or 500 mg P.O., followed by 250 mg q 8 to 12 hours (depending on severity of pain and patient's age, weight, and response)

Dosage adjustment
- Elderly patients

Contraindications
- Hypersensitivity to drug
- Acute asthmatic attacks
- Bleeding disorders
- Vitamin K deficiency
- Children younger than age 12

Precautions
Use cautiously in:
- renal impairment, compromised cardiac function, hypertension, peptic ulcer
- elderly patients.

Administration
- Give tablets whole with food or milk.

Route	Onset	Peak	Duration
P.O.	1 hr	2-3 hr	8-12 hr

Adverse reactions
CNS: dizziness, insomnia, drowsiness, headache, fatigue
EENT: tinnitus
GI: nausea, vomiting, diarrhea, constipation, flatulence, stomatitis
GU: hematuria, **renal impairment, interstitial nephritis**
Skin: rash, pruritus, sweating, **erythema multiforme**
Other: Stevens-Johnson syndrome

Interactions
Drug-drug. *Acetaminophen, hydrochlorothiazide, indomethacin:* increased levels of these drugs
Antacids, aspirin: decreased diflunisal blood level
Anticoagulants, thrombolytics: enhanced anticoagulant effect
Cyclosporine: increased risk of nephrotoxicity
Methotrexate: increased risk of methotrexate toxicity

Patient monitoring
- Monitor fluid intake and output for signs of renal impairment. Assess for dysuria and hematuria.

🔊 Watch for signs and symptoms of erythema multiforme (sore throat, fever, rash, cough, iris lesions, mouth sores). Report early signs before condition can progress to Stevens-Johnson syndrome.
- Assess nutritional and hydration status.
- Monitor neurologic status.

Patient teaching
- Instruct patient to swallow tablets whole with food or milk.
- If patient needs antacids, advise him not to take them within 2 hours of diflunisal.
- Caution patient to avoid driving and other hazardous activities until he knows how drug affects concentration, balance, hearing, and alertness.
- Advise patient to minimize GI upset by eating small, frequent servings of healthy food and ensuring adequate fluid intake.

🔊 Tell patient to promptly report rash and other signs and symptoms of erythema multiforme.
- As appropriate, review all other significant and life-threatening adverse

reactions and interactions, especially those related to the drugs mentioned above.

digoxin

Digitek, Lanoxicaps, Lanoxin, Novo-Digoxin ✦

Pharmacologic class: Cardiac glycoside
Therapeutic class: Inotropic, antiarrhythmic
Pregnancy risk category C

Action

Increases force and velocity of myocardial contraction and prolongs refractory period of atrioventricular (AV) node by increasing calcium entry into myocardial cells. Slows conduction through sinoatrial and AV nodes and produces antiarrhythmic effect.

Availability

Capsules: 0.05 mg, 0.1 mg, 0.2 mg
Elixir (pediatric): 0.05 mg/ml
Injection: 0.05 mg/ml, 0.1 mg/ml, 0.25 mg/ml
Tablets: 0.125 mg, 0.25 mg, 0.5 mg

Indications and dosages

➤ Heart failure; tachyarrhythmias; atrial fibrillation and flutter; paroxysmal atrial tachycardia

Adults: For rapid digitalizing, 0.6 to 1 mg I.V. over 24 hours, with 50% of total dosage given initially and additional fractions given at 4- to 8-hour intervals; or digitalizing dose of 0.75 to 1.25 mg P.O. over 24 hours, with 50% of total dosage given initially and additional fractions given at 4- to 8-hour intervals. Maintenance dosage is 0.063 to 0.5 mg/day (tablets) or 0.35 to 0.5 mg/day (gelatin capsules), depending on lean body weight, renal function, and drug blood level.

Children older than age 10: For rapid digitalizing, 8 to 12 mcg/kg I.V. over 24 hours, with 50% of total dosage given initially and additional fractions given at 4- to 8-hour intervals; or digitalizing dose of 10 to 15 mcg/kg P.O. over 24 hours, with 50% of total dosage given initially and additional fractions given at 6- to 8-hour intervals. Maintenance dosage is 25% to 35% of loading dosage, given daily as a single dose (determined by renal function).

Children ages 5 to 10: For rapid digitalizing, 15 to 30 mcg/kg I.V. over 24 hours, with 50% of total dosage given initially and additional fractions given at 4- to 8-hour intervals; or digitalizing dose of 20 to 35 mcg/kg P.O. over 24 hours, with 50% of total dosage given initially and additional fractions given at 6- to 8-hour intervals. Maintenance dosage is 25% to 35% of loading dosage, given daily in two divided doses (determined by renal function).

Children ages 2 to 5: For rapid digitalizing, 25 to 35 mcg/kg I.V. over 24 hours, with 50% of total dosage given initially and additional fractions given at 4- to 8-hour intervals; or digitalizing dose of 30 to 40 mcg/kg P.O. over 24 hours, with 50% of total dosage given initially and additional fractions given at 6- to 8-hour intervals. Maintenance dosage is 25% to 35% of loading dosage, given daily in two divided doses (determined by renal function).

Children ages 1 to 2: For rapid digitalizing, 30 to 50 mcg/kg I.V. over 24 hours, with 50% of total dosage given initially and additional fractions given at 4- to 8-hour intervals; or digitalizing dose of 35 to 60 mcg/kg P.O. over 24 hours, with 50% of total dosage given initially and additional fractions given at 6- to 8-hour intervals. Maintenance dosage is 25% to 35% of loading dosage, given daily in two divided doses (determined by renal function).

Infants (full-term): For rapid digitalizing, 20 to 30 mcg/kg I.V. over 24 hours,

with 50% of total dosage given initially and additional fractions given at 4- to 8-hour intervals; or digitalizing dose of 25 to 35 mcg/kg P.O. over 24 hours, with 50% of total dosage given initially and additional fractions given at 6- to 8-hour intervals. Maintenance dosage is 25% to 35% of loading dosage, given daily in two divided doses (determined by renal function).
Infants (premature): For rapid digitalizing, 15 to 25 mcg/kg I.V. over 24 hours, with 50% of total dosage given initially and additional fractions given at 4- to 8-hour intervals; or digitalizing dose of 20 to 30 mcg/kg P.O. over 24 hours, with 50% of total dosage given initially and additional fractions given at 6- to 8-hour intervals. Maintenance dosage is 20% to 30% of loading dosage, given daily in two divided doses (determined by renal function).

Dosage adjustment

- Renal impairment
- Hyperthyroidism
- Elderly patients

Off-label uses

- Supraventricular tachyarrhythmias
- Intrauterine tachyarrhythmias

Contraindications

- Hypersensitivity to drug
- Uncontrolled ventricular arrhythmias
- AV block
- Idiopathic hypertrophic subaortic stenosis
- Constrictive pericarditis

Precautions

Use cautiously in:
- renal or hepatic impairment, electrolyte imbalances, myocardial infarction, thyroid disorders
- obesity
- elderly patients
- pregnant or breastfeeding patients.

Administration

- Measure apical pulse for 1 full minute before administering. If rate is below 60 beats/minute, withhold dose, notify prescriber, and check drug blood level for toxicity.
- Administer I.V. drug undiluted, or dilute with sterile water for injection, normal saline solution, or dextrose 5% in water as directed.

Clinical alert: Know that drug has narrow therapeutic index, so dosage must be monitored regularly and patient must be monitored for signs and symptoms of toxicity.

- Know that for rapid effect, initial digitalizing dose generally is given in several divided doses over 12 to 24 hours.
- Be aware that dosages used for atrial arrhythmias generally are higher than those used for inotropic effect.

Route	Onset	Peak	Duration
P.O.	0.5-2 hr	2-6 hr	2-4 days
I.V.	5-30 min	1-5 hr	2-4 days

Adverse reactions

CNS: fatigue, headache, asthenia
CV: bradycardia, ECG changes, **arrhythmias**
EENT: blurred or yellow vision
GI: nausea, vomiting, diarrhea
GU: gynecomastia
Hematologic: thrombocytopenia
Other: decreased appetite

Interactions

Drug-drug. *Amiodarone, cyclosporine, diclofenac, diltiazem, propafenone, quinidine, quinine, verapamil:* increased digoxin blood level, possibly leading to toxicity
Amphotericin B, corticosteroids, mezlocillin, piperacillin, thiazide and loop diuretics, ticarcillin: hypokalemia, increased risk of digoxin toxicity

Antacids, cholestyramine, colestipol, kaolin/pectin: decreased digoxin absorption
Beta-adrenergic blockers, other antiarrhythmics (including disopyramide, quinidine): additive bradycardia
Laxatives (excessive use): hypokalemia, increased risk of digoxin toxicity
Spironolactone: reduced digoxin clearance, increased risk of digoxin toxicity
Thyroid hormones: decreased digoxin efficacy
Drug-diagnostic tests. *Creatine kinase:* increased level
Drug-food. *High-fiber meal:* decreased digoxin absorption
Drug-herbs. *Coca seed, coffee seed, cola seed, guarana seed, horsetail, licorice, natural stimulants (such as aloe), yerba maté:* increased risk of digoxin toxicity and hypokalemia
Ephedra (ma huang): arrhythmias
Hawthorn: increased risk of adverse cardiovascular effects
Indian snakeroot: bradycardia
Psyllium: decreased digoxin absorption
St. John's wort: decreased blood level and effects of digoxin

Patient monitoring

- Assess apical pulse regularly for 1 full minute. If rate is less than 60 beats/minute, withhold dose and notify prescriber.

[Clinical alert] Monitor for signs and symptoms of drug toxicity (such as nausea, vomiting, visual disturbances, arrhythmias, and altered mental status). Be aware that therapeutic digoxin levels range from 0.5 to 2 ng/ml.

- Monitor ECG and blood levels of digoxin, potassium, magnesium, calcium, and creatinine.
- Stay alert for hypocalcemia. Know that this condition may predispose patient to digoxin toxicity and may decrease digoxin efficacy.

[Clinical alert] Watch closely for hypokalemia and hypomagnesemia. Know that digoxin toxicity may occur with these conditions despite digoxin blood levels below 2 ng/ml.

Patient teaching

- Advise patient to check pulse rate regularly. If it's below 60 or above 110 beats/minute, tell him to withhold dose and notify prescriber.
- Instruct patient not to take over-the-counter drugs without prescriber's approval.

[Clinical alert] Teach patient how to recognize and report signs and symptoms of digoxin toxicity.

- Stress importance of follow-up testing as directed by prescriber.
- As appropriate, review all other significant and life-threatening adverse reactions and interactions, especially those related to the drugs, tests, foods, and herbs mentioned above.

dihydroergotamine mesylate

D.H.E. 45, Dihydroergotamine-Sandoz✤, Migranal

Pharmacologic class: Alpha-adrenergic blocker
Therapeutic class: Vasoconstrictor, vascular headache suppressant
Pregnancy risk category X

Action

Stimulates alpha-adrenergic receptors, causing intracranial and peripheral vasoconstriction. Also activates 5-hydroxytryptamine-1D receptors to inhibit release of proinflammatory neuropeptides.

Availability

Injection: 1 mg/ml
Nasal spray: 4 mg/ml in ampule with applicator

Indications and dosages

➤ Vascular headaches, including migraine and cluster headaches

Adults: 1 mg I.M. or subcutaneously; may repeat in 1 hour to a total dosage of 3 mg (not to exceed 3 mg/day or 6 mg/week). Or 1 mg I.V.; may repeat in 1 hour (not to exceed 2 mg/day or 6 mg/week). Or one spray (0.5 mg) in each nostril, repeated after 15 minutes to a total dosage of 2 mg (not to exceed 3 mg/24 hours or 4 mg/week).

Off-label uses

- Intracranial hypertension
- Prevention of orthostatic hypotension
- Deep-vein thrombosis, pulmonary embolism

Contraindications

- Hypersensitivity to drug
- Cardiovascular disease, hypertension, peripheral vascular disease
- Severe renal or hepatic disease
- Concurrent use of potent vasoconstrictors
- Pregnancy or breastfeeding

Precautions

Use cautiously in:

- diabetes mellitus
- concurrent use of beta-adrenergic blockers, macrolide antibiotics, or nitrates
- children younger than age 6.

Administration

- Give at first sign of migraine or as soon as possible after symptom onset.
- For I.V. use, drug may be given undiluted over 1 minute.

Route	Onset	Peak	Duration
I.V.	<5 min	15 min-2 hr	8 hr
I.M., subcut.	15-30 min	15 min-2 hr	8 hr
Nasal	Within 30 min	Unknown	Unknown

Adverse reactions

CNS: dizziness, fatigue, numbness or tingling in fingers or toes

CV: angina pectoris, intermittent claudication, sinus tachycardia, sinus bradycardia, **myocardial infarction**

EENT: rhinitis, throat irritation

GI: nausea, vomiting, diarrhea, abdominal pain

Musculoskeletal: stiffness or weakness of arms, legs, neck, or shoulders; muscle pain

Other: altered taste, polydipsia

Interactions

Drug-drug. *Beta-adrenergic blockers, macrolides, vasoconstrictors:* increased risk of peripheral vasoconstriction

Nitrates: antagonism of antianginal effects

Drug-behaviors. *Smoking:* increased risk of peripheral vasoconstriction

Patient monitoring

- Monitor cardiac status, especially when giving large doses.
- Assess for and report numbness and tingling of fingers and toes, arm or leg weakness, muscle pain, and intermittent claudication.

Patient teaching

- Advise patient to take drug at first sign of migraine.
- Instruct patient to lie down in dark, quiet room for several hours after taking dose.
- [Clinical alert] Tell patient to immediately report chest pain, nausea, vomiting, change in heartbeat, numbness, tingling, or pain or weakness in arms or legs.
- As appropriate, review all other significant and life-threatening adverse reactions and interactions, especially those related to the drugs and behaviors mentioned above.

diltiazem hydrochloride

Apo-Diltiaz♣, Apo-Diltiazem♣, Cardizem, Cardizem CD, Cardizem LA, Cartia XT, Dilacor-XR, Diltia XT, Gen-Diltiazem♣, Novo-Diltazem♣, Nu-Diltiaz♣, Syn-Diltiazem, Tiazac

Pharmacologic class: Calcium channel blocker

Therapeutic class: Antianginal, antiarrhythmic (class IV), antihypertensive

Pregnancy risk category C

Action

Inhibits calcium from entering myocardial and vascular smooth-muscle cells, thereby depressing myocardial and smooth-muscle contraction and decreasing impulse formation and conduction velocity. As a result, systolic and diastolic pressures decrease.

Availability

Capsules (extended-release, sustained-release): 60 mg, 90 mg, 120 mg, 180 mg, 240 mg, 300 mg, 360 mg, 420 mg
Injection: 5 mg/ml in 10-ml vials, 25-mg ready-to-use syringes, 100-mg Monovial
Tablets: 30 mg, 60 mg, 90 mg, 120 mg

Indications and dosages

➢ Angina pectoris and vasospastic (Prinzmetal's) angina; hypertension; supraventricular tachyarrhythmias; atrial flutter or fibrillation

Adults: 30 to 90 mg P.O. three to four times daily (tablets), or 60 to 120 mg P.O. b.i.d. (sustained-release), or 180 to 240 mg P.O. once daily (extended-release), adjusted after 14 days as needed, up to a total daily dosage of 360 mg. Or 0.25 mg/kg by I.V. bolus over 2 minutes; if response is inadequate after 15 minutes, may give 0.35 mg/kg over 2 minutes; may follow with continuous I.V. infusion at 10 mg/hour (at a range of 5 to 15 mg/hour) for up to 24 hours.

Dosage adjustment

- Severe hepatic or renal impairment
- Elderly patients

Off-label uses

- Unstable angina, coronary artery bypass graft surgery
- Tardive dyskinesia
- Migraine
- Hyperthyroidism
- Raynaud's phenomenon

Contraindications

- Hypersensitivity to drug
- Atrial flutter or fibrillation associated with shortened refractory period (Wolff-Parkinson-White syndrome, with I.V. use)
- Recent myocardial infarction or pulmonary congestion
- Cardiogenic shock, concurrent I.V. beta-blocker therapy, ventricular tachycardia, neonates (with I.V. use, because of benzyl alcohol in syringe formulation)
- Sick sinus syndrome, second- or third-degree atrioventricular block (except in patients with ventricular pacemakers)
- Hypotension (systolic pressure below 90 mm Hg)

Precautions

Use cautiously in:
- severe hepatic or renal impairment, heart failure
- history of serious ventricular arrhythmias
- elderly patients
- pregnant or breastfeeding patients
- children (safety not established).

Administration

- When giving I.V., dilute in dextrose 5% in water or normal saline solution.

• Give I.V. bolus dose over 2 minutes; a second bolus may be given after 15 minutes.
• Administer continuous I.V. infusion at a rate of 5 to 15 mg/hour.
🔊 When giving by continuous I.V. infusion, make sure emergency equipment is available and that patient has continuous ECG monitoring with frequent blood pressure monitoring.
• Don't crush tablets or sustained-release capsules; they must be swallowed whole.
• Withhold dose if systolic blood pressure falls below 90 mm Hg, diastolic pressure is below 60 mm Hg, or apical pulse is slower than 60 beats/minute.

Route	Onset	Peak	Duration
P.O.	30 min	2-3 hr	6-8 hr
P.O. (sustained)	Unknown	Unknown	12 hr
P.O. (extended)	Unknown	14 hr	Up to 24 hr
I.V.	2-5 min	2-4 hr	Unknown

Adverse reactions

CNS: headache, abnormal dreams, anxiety, confusion, dizziness, drowsiness, nervousness, psychiatric disturbances, asthenia, paresthesia, syncope, tremor
CV: peripheral edema, bradycardia, chest pain, hypotension, palpitations, tachycardia, **arrhythmias, heart failure**
EENT: blurred vision, tinnitus, epistaxis
GI: nausea, vomiting, diarrhea, constipation, dyspepsia, dry mouth
GU: urinary frequency, dysuria, nocturia, polyuria, gynecomastia, sexual dysfunction
Hematologic: anemia, **leukopenia, thrombocytopenia**
Metabolic: hyperglycemia
Musculoskeletal: joint stiffness, muscle cramps
Respiratory: cough, dyspnea
Skin: rash, dermatitis, flushing, diaphoresis, photosensitivity, pruritus, urticaria, **erythema multiforme**
Other: unpleasant taste, gingival hyperplasia, weight gain, decreased appetite, **Stevens-Johnson syndrome**

Interactions

Drug-drug. *Beta-adrenergic blockers, digoxin, disopyramide, phenytoin:* bradycardia, conduction defects, heart failure
Carbamazepine, cyclosporine, quinidine: decreased diltiazem metabolism, increased risk of toxicity
Cimetidine, ranitidine: increased blood level and effects of diltiazem
Fentanyl, nitrates, other antihypertensives, quinidine: additive hypotension
HMG-CoA reductase inhibitors, imipramine, sirolimus, tacrolimus: increased blood levels of these drugs
Lithium: decreased lithium blood level, reduced antimanic control
Nonsteroidal anti-inflammatory drugs: decreased antihypertensive effect of diltiazem
Theophylline: increased theophylline effects
Drug-diagnostic tests. *Hepatic enzymes:* increased levels
Drug-food. *Grapefruit juice:* increased blood level and effects of diltiazem
Drug-behaviors. *Acute alcohol ingestion:* additive hypotension

Patient monitoring

• Check blood pressure and ECG before starting therapy, and monitor closely during dosage adjustment period. Withhold dose if systolic pressure is below 90 mm Hg.
🔊 Monitor for signs and symptoms of heart failure and worsening arrhythmias.
• Supervise patient during ambulation.

Patient teaching

- Advise patient to change position slowly to minimize light-headedness and dizziness.
- Caution patient to avoid driving and other hazardous activities until he knows how drug affects concentration and alertness.
- As appropriate, review all other significant and life-threatening adverse reactions and interactions, especially those related to the drugs, tests, foods, and behaviors mentioned above.

dimenhydrinate

Apo-Dimenhydrinate♣, Calm X, Dimetabs, Dinate, Dramamine, Dramanate♣, Gravol♣, Hydrate, PMS-Dimenhydrinate♣, Travamine♣, Triptone Caplets

Pharmacologic class: Anticholinergic
Therapeutic class: Antiemetic, antivertigo agent
Pregnancy risk category B

Action

Prevents nausea and vomiting by inhibiting vestibular stimulation of chemoreceptor trigger zone and inhibiting stimulation of vomiting center in brain

Availability

Capsules: 50 mg
Capsules (extended-release): 25 mg
Elixir: 12.5 mg/5 ml, 15 mg/5 ml
Injection: 50 mg/ml
Liquid: 12.5 mg/4 ml, 15.62 mg/5 ml
Suppositories: 50 mg, 100 mg
Tablets: 50 mg
Tablets (chewable): 50 mg

Indications and dosages

➢ Prevention and treatment of nausea, vomiting, dizziness, and vertigo

Adults and children ages 12 and older: 50 to 100 mg P.O. q 4 hours (not to exceed 400 mg/day), or 50 to 100 mg P.R. q 6 to 8 hours, or 50 mg I.M. or I.V. q 4 hours p.r.n.
Children ages 6 to 12: 25 to 50 mg P.O. q 6 to 8 hours (not to exceed 150 mg/day), or 25 to 50 mg P.R. q 8 to 12 hours, or 1.25 mg/kg I.M. (37.5 mg/m^2) q 6 hours p.r.n.
Children ages 2 to 6: 12.5 to 25 mg P.O. q 6 to 8 hours (not to exceed 75 mg/day)

Contraindications

- Hypersensitivity to drug or tartrazine
- Alcohol intolerance

Precautions

Use cautiously in:
- angle-closure glaucoma, seizure disorders, prostatic hypertrophy.

Administration

- For I.V. use, dilute with dextrose 5% in water or normal saline solution.
- Give each 50-mg I.V. dose over 2 minutes.

Clinical alert: Don't administer by I.V. route to premature or low-birth-weight infants. Solution contains benzyl alcohol, which can cause fatal "gasping" syndrome.

Route	Onset	Peak	Duration
P.O.	15-60 min	1-2 hr	3-6 hr
I.V.	Rapid	Unknown	3-6 hr
I.M.	20-30 min	1-2 hr	3-6 hr
P.R.	30-45 min	Unknown	6-12 hr

Adverse reactions

CNS: drowsiness, dizziness, headache, paradoxical stimulation (in children)
CV: hypotension, palpitations
EENT: blurred vision, tinnitus
GI: diarrhea, constipation, dry mouth
GU: dysuria, urinary frequency
Skin: photosensitivity
Other: decreased appetite, pain at I.M. site

Interactions

Drug-drug. *Disopyramide, quinidine, tricyclic antidepressants:* increased anticholinergic effects
MAO inhibitors: intensified and prolonged anticholinergic effects
Other CNS depressants (such as antihistamines, opioids, sedative-hypnotics): additive CNS depression
Ototoxic drugs (such as aminoglycosides, ethacrynic acid): masking of signs or symptoms of ototoxicity
Drug-diagnostic tests. *Allergy skin tests:* false-negative results
Drug-behaviors. *Alcohol use:* increased CNS depression

Patient monitoring

- Assess for lethargy and drowsiness.
- Monitor for dizziness, nausea, and vomiting (possible indicators of drug toxicity).

Patient teaching

- To prevent motion sickness, advise patient to take drug 30 minutes before traveling and to repeat dose before meals and at bedtime.
- Instruct patient to avoid driving and other hazardous activities until he knows how drug affects concentration and alertness.
- Caution patient to avoid alcohol and sedative-hypnotics during therapy.
- As appropriate, review all other significant adverse reactions and interactions, especially those related to the drugs, tests, and behaviors mentioned above.

dinoprostone (prostaglandin E_2, PGE_2)

Cervidil Vaginal Insert, Prepidil Endocervical Gel, Prostin E2 Vaginal Suppository

Pharmacologic class: Oxytocic, prostaglandin
Therapeutic class: Abortifacient, cervical ripening agent
Pregnancy risk category C

Action

Initiates strong contractions of uterine smooth muscle by stimulating myometrium and promoting cervical softening, effacement, and dilation

Availability

Endocervical gel: 0.5 mg in 3-g gel vehicle in prefilled syringe with catheter
Vaginal insert: 10 mg
Vaginal suppositories: 20 mg

Indications and dosages

➢ Cervical ripening
Adults: 0.5 mg endocervical gel vaginally; if response is poor, may repeat in 6 hours (not to exceed 1.5 mg in 24 hours). Or one 10-mg vaginal insert.
➢ To induce abortion
Adults: One 20-mg vaginal suppository; repeat q 3 to 5 hours (not to exceed total dosage of 240 mg or duration of 48 hours).

Off-label uses

- Drug-induced GI bleeding

Contraindications

- Hypersensitivity to prostaglandins or additives in gel or suppository
- Active genital herpes infection
- Acute pelvic inflammatory disease

• Ruptured membranes, placenta previa, or unexplained vaginal bleeding during pregnancy

Precautions

Use cautiously in:
• pulmonary, cardiac, renal, or hepatic disease; asthma; hypotension; adrenal disorders; diabetes mellitus; epilepsy; glaucoma
• multiparity.

Administration

• Keep patient prone for 10 minutes after administration to prevent drug expulsion and enhance absorption.
• Store suppositories in freezer; bring to room temperature before using.

Route	Onset	Peak	Duration
Vaginal (gel)	Rapid	30-45 min	Unknown
Vaginal (insert)	Rapid	Unknown	12 hr
Vaginal (suppository)	10 min	Unknown	2-3 hr

Adverse reactions

CNS: headache, drowsiness, syncope
CV: hypotension, hypertension
GI: nausea, vomiting, diarrhea
GU: urinary tract infection, vaginal or uterine pain, uterine contractile abnormalities, warm vaginal sensation, **uterine hypertonicity, uterine rupture**
Musculoskeletal: back pain
Respiratory: cough, dyspnea, wheezing
Other: allergic reactions including chills, fever, and **anaphylaxis**

Interactions

Drug-drug. *Other oxytocics:* increased oxytocic effects

Patient monitoring

◀⁝ Monitor uterine contractions and observe for excessive vaginal bleeding and cramping. Record sanitary pad count.
• Monitor vital signs and assess for drug-induced fever. Report significant blood pressure and pulse changes.
• Assess for wheezing, chest pain, and dyspnea.
• Evaluate for GI upset. To minimize, give antiemetic before dinoprostone therapy.

Patient teaching

• Advise patient to stay in prone position for 10 minutes after administration.
• Instruct patient to report fever, bleeding, or abdominal cramps.
• Tell patient to avoid douches, tampons, tub baths, and sexual intercourse for at least 2 weeks after receiving drug.
• As appropriate, review all other significant and life-threatening adverse reactions and interactions, especially those related to the drugs mentioned above.

diphenhydramine hydrochloride

Allerdryl✱, AllerMax, Banophen, Benadryl, Benadryl Allergy, Benadryl Dye-Free Allergy, Compoz, Compoz Nighttime Sleep Aid, Diphen AF, Diphen Cough, Diphenhist, Genahist, Hyrexin, Maximum Strength Nytol, Maximum Strength Sleepinal, Midol PM, Nervine Nighttime Sleep Aid, Nytol, Siladryl, Sleep-Eze D, Sominex, Twilite, Unisom Nighttime Sleep-Aid

Pharmacologic class: Ethanolamine derivative, nonselective histamine$_1$-receptor antagonist

Therapeutic class: Antihistamine, antitussive, antiemetic, antivertigo agent, antidyskinetic

Pregnancy risk category B

Action

Interferes with histamine effects at histamine$_1$-receptor sites; prevents but doesn't reverse histamine-mediated response. Also possesses CNS depressant and anticholinergic properties.

Availability

Capsules: 25 mg, 50 mg
Elixir: 12.5 mg/5 ml
Injection: 10 mg/ml, 50 mg/ml
Syrup: 12.5 mg/5 ml
Tablets: 25 mg, 50 mg
Tablets (chewable): 12.5 mg, 25 mg

Indications and dosages

➢ Allergy symptoms caused by histamine release (including anaphylaxis, seasonal and perennial allergic rhinitis, and allergic dermatoses); nausea; vertigo

Adults and children over age 12: 25 to 50 mg P.O. q 4 to 6 hours, or 10 to 50 mg I.V. or I.M. q 2 to 3 hours p.r.n. (Some patients may need up to 100 mg.) Don't exceed 400 mg/day.

Children ages 6 to 12: 12.5 to 25 mg P.O. q 4 to 6 hours, or 1.25 mg/kg (37.5 mg/m^2) I.M. or I.V. q.i.d. Don't exceed 150 mg/day.

Children ages 2 to 5: 6.25 mg P.O. q 4 to 6 hours. Don't exceed 37.5 mg/day.

➢ Cough

Adults: 25 mg P.O. q 4 hours p.r.n. Don't exceed 150 mg/day.

Children ages 6 to 12: 12.5 mg P.O. q 4 hours. Don't exceed 75 mg/day.

Children ages 2 to 5: 6.25 mg P.O. q 4 hours. Don't exceed 37.5 mg/24 hours.

➢ Dyskinesia; Parkinson's disease

Adults: Initially, 25 mg P.O. t.i.d.; may be increased to a maximum of 50 mg q.i.d.

➢ Mild nighttime sedation

Adults: 50 mg P.O. 20 to 30 minutes before bedtime

Dosage adjustment

- Elderly patients

Off-label uses

- Drug-induced extrapyramidal reactions

Contraindications

- Hypersensitivity to drug
- Alcohol intolerance
- Acute asthma attacks
- MAO inhibitor use within past 14 days
- Breastfeeding

Precautions

Use cautiously in:

- severe hepatic disease, angle-closure glaucoma, seizure disorders, prostatic hypertrophy
- elderly patients
- pregnant patients (safety not established).

Administration

- For motion sickness, administer 30 minutes before activity.
- Give oral doses with food or milk to minimize adverse GI effects.
- For I.V. use, check compatibility before mixing with other drugs.
- Inject I.M. dose deep into large muscle mass; rotate sites.
- Discontinue drug 4 days before allergy skin testing to avoid misleading results.

Clinical alert: Don't give within 14 days of MAO inhibitors.

Route	Onset	Peak	Duration
P.O.	15-60 min	1-4 hr	4-8 hr
I.V.	Rapid	Unknown	4-8 hr
I.M.	20-30 min	1-4 hr	4-8 hr

Adverse reactions

CNS: drowsiness, dizziness, headache, paradoxical stimulation (especially in children)
CV: hypotension, palpitations
EENT: blurred vision, tinnitus
GI: diarrhea, constipation, dry mouth

GU: dysuria, urinary frequency or retention
Skin: photosensitivity
Other: decreased appetite, pain at I.M. injection site

Interactions

Drug-drug. *Antihistamines, opioids, sedative-hypnotics:* additive CNS depression
Disopyramide, quinidine, tricyclic antidepressants: increased anticholinergic effects
MAO inhibitors: intensified and prolonged anticholinergic effects
Drug-diagnostic tests. *Skin allergy tests:* false-negative results
Hemoglobin, platelets: decreased values
Drug-herbs. *Angel's trumpet, jimson weed, scopolia:* increased anticholinergic effects
Chamomile, hops, kava, skullcap, valerian: increased CNS depression
Drug-behaviors. *Alcohol use:* increased CNS depression

Patient monitoring

- Monitor cardiovascular status, especially in patients with cardiovascular disease.
- Supervise patient during ambulation. Use side rails as necessary.

Patient teaching

- Advise patient to take drug with food if it causes GI upset.
- Caution patient to avoid driving and other hazardous activities until he knows how drug affects concentration and alertness.
- As appropriate, review all other significant adverse reactions and interactions, especially those related to the drugs, tests, herbs, and behaviors mentioned above.

diphenoxylate hydrochloride and atropine sulfate

Logen, Lomanate, Lomotil, Lonox

Pharmacologic class: Anticholinergic, meperidine congener
Therapeutic class: Antidiarrheal
Controlled substance schedule V
Pregnancy risk category C

Action

Acts on smooth muscle of GI tract by decreasing peristalsis, which inhibits motility. (Small amount of atropine is added to reduce abuse potential.)

Availability

Liquid: 2.5 mg diphenoxylate and 0.025 mg atropine/5 ml
Tablets: 2.5 mg diphenoxylate and 0.025 mg atropine

Indications and dosages

➢ Diarrhea
Adults: Initially, 5 mg P.O. three to four times daily, then 5 mg/day as needed (not to exceed 20 mg/day). Decrease dosage when desired response occurs.
Children: Initially, 0.3 to 0.4 mg/kg P.O. (liquid only) daily in four divided doses. Decrease dosage when desired response occurs.

Dosage adjustment

- Respiratory disease
- Elderly patients

Contraindications

- Hypersensitivity to drug
- Obstructive jaundice
- Diarrhea associated with pseudomembranous colitis or enterotoxin-producing bacteria
- Angle-closure glaucoma

- Concurrent MAO inhibitor use
- Children younger than age 2

Precautions

Use cautiously in:

- inflammatory bowel disease; prostatic hypertrophy; severe hepatic disease (use with extreme caution)
- concurrent use of drugs that cause physical dependence; history of physical drug dependence
- elderly patients
- pregnant or breastfeeding patients
- children (safety not established in children younger than age 12).

Administration

◀ Don't confuse brand name Lomotil with Lamictal (an anticonvulsant). Serious errors have been reported.

- Withhold drug if patient has severe fluid or electrolyte imbalance.
- Administer with food if GI upset occurs.

◀ Don't give within 14 days of MAO inhibitors.

Route	Onset	Peak	Duration
P.O.	45-60 min	2 hr	3-4 hr

Adverse reactions

CNS: dizziness, confusion, drowsiness, headache, insomnia, nervousness
CV: tachycardia
EENT: blurred vision, dry eyes
GI: nausea, vomiting, constipation, epigastric distress, ileus, dry mouth
GU: urinary retention
Skin: flushing

Interactions

Drug-drug. *CNS depressants (including antihistamines, sedative-hypnotics, opioids):* increased CNS depression
Anticholinergic-like drugs (including tricyclic antidepressants, disopyramide): increased anticholinergic effects
MAO inhibitors: hypertensive crisis
Drug-diagnostic tests. *Amylase:* increased level
Drug-herbs. *Angel's trumpet, jimsonweed, scopolia:* increased anticholinergic effects
Drug-behaviors. *Alcohol use:* increased CNS depression

Patient monitoring

◀ Assess for and report abdominal distention and signs or symptoms of decreased peristalsis.

- Watch for signs and symptoms of dehydration.
- Assess frequency and consistency of bowel movements.

Patient teaching

- Instruct patient to report persistent diarrhea.
- Caution patient to avoid driving and other hazardous activities until he knows how drug affects concentration and alertness.
- Tell patient that prolonged use may lead to dependence.
- As appropriate, review all other significant adverse reactions and interactions, especially those related to the drugs, tests, herbs, and behaviors mentioned above.

dipyridamole

Apo-Dipyridamole FC✦, Apo-Dipyridamole SC✦, Novo-Dipiradol✦, Persantine

Pharmacologic class: Platelet adhesion inhibitor

Therapeutic class: Antiplatelet agent, diagnostic agent (coronary vasodilator)

Pregnancy risk category B

Action

Unclear. May reduce platelet aggregation by inhibiting phosphodiesterase, adenosine uptake, or formation of thromboxane A_2. Produces vasodilation, thereby increasing coronary blood flow.

Availability

Injection: 10 mg/2 ml
Tablets: 25 mg, 50 mg, 75 mg, 100 mg

Indications and dosages

➢ To prevent thromboembolism in patients with prosthetic heart valves
Adults: 75 to 100 mg P.O. q.i.d.
➢ Alternative to exercise in thallium myocardial perfusion imaging
Adults: 0.57 mg/kg I.V. infused over 4 minutes (0.142 mg/kg/minute). Maximum I.V. dosage is 60 mg.

Off-label uses

- Prevention of myocardial reinfarction (given with aspirin)
- Thrombotic thrombocytopenia purpura

Contraindications

- Hypersensitivity to drug

Precautions

Use cautiously in:
- hypotension, platelet defects
- pregnant or breastfeeding patients (safety not established)
- children younger than age 12 (safety not established).

Administration

- Know that drug is usually given with warfarin when used to prevent thromboembolism.
- Dilute I.V. solution with dextrose 5% in water or normal or half-normal saline solution, as directed.
- Give single I.V. dose over 4 minutes.
- When used as diagnostic agent, administer within 5 minutes of thallium injection.
- Give oral form with a full glass of water at least 1 hour before or 2 hours after meals. If gastric distress occurs, give with food.

Route	Onset	Peak	Duration
P.O.	Unknown	Unknown	Unknown
I.V.	Unknown	6.5 min	30 min

Adverse reactions

CNS: dizziness, headache, syncope; transient cerebral ischemia or weakness (with I.V. use)
CV: hypotension, **arrhythmias, myocardial infarction** (all with I.V. use)
GI: nausea, vomiting diarrhea, dyspepsia
Hematologic: prolonged bleeding time
Respiratory: bronchospasm (with I.V. use)
Skin: rash, flushing (with I.V. use)

Interactions

Drug-drug. *Anticoagulants, cefamandole, cefoperazone, cefotetan, nonsteroidal anti-inflammatory drugs, plicamycin, sulfinpyrazone, thrombolytics, valproic acid:* increased risk of bleeding
Aspirin: increased effect on platelet aggregation
Theophylline: negation of dipyridamole effects during thallium imaging
Drug-behaviors. *Alcohol use:* increased risk of hypotension

Patient monitoring

- Monitor for therapeutic efficacy, including improved exercise tolerance and decreased need for nitrates.
- Assess platelet and coagulation studies regularly.
- Monitor ECG and vital signs, especially blood pressure.

Patient teaching

- Advise patient to take drug 1 hour before or 2 hours after meals for best absorption.
- As appropriate, review all other significant and life-threatening adverse reactions and interactions, especially those related to the drugs and behaviors mentioned above.

dirithromycin

Dynabac

Pharmacologic class: Macrolide
Therapeutic class: Anti-infective
Pregnancy risk category C

Action

Binds to 50S ribosomal subunit of susceptible bacteria, inhibiting protein synthesis

Availability

Tablets: 250 mg

Indications and dosages

➢ Acute and chronic bronchitis or other respiratory infections
Adults and children ages 12 and older: 500 mg P.O. daily for 5 to 7 days
➢ Community-acquired pneumonia caused by *Legionella pneumophila, Mycoplasma pneumoniae,* or *Streptococcus pneumoniae*
Adults and children ages 12 and older: 500 mg P.O. daily for 14 days
➢ Pharyngitis or tonsillitis caused by *Streptococcus pyogenes*
Adults and children ages 12 and older: 500 mg P.O. daily for 10 days

Contraindications

- Hypersensitivity to drug or other macrolides
- Known, suspected, or potential bacteremia
- Concurrent use of astemizole, cisapride, pimozide, or terfenadine

Precautions

Use cautiously in:
- renal or hepatic impairment, colitis
- pregnant or breastfeeding patients.

Administration

- Obtain specimens for culture and sensitivity testing as necessary before starting therapy.
- Give with food or within 1 hour of a meal.
- Make sure patient swallows tablets whole without cutting, crushing, or chewing.

Don't give concurrently with astemizole or terfenadine (no longer available in U.S.), cisapride, or pimozide.

Route	Onset	Peak	Duration
P.O.	Unknown	4 hr	Unknown

Adverse reactions

CNS: headache, dizziness, vertigo, asthenia, insomnia
GI: nausea, diarrhea, vomiting, abdominal pain, dyspepsia, flatulence, **pseudomembranous colitis**
Metabolic: hyperkalemia
Respiratory: increased cough, dyspnea
Other: nonspecific pain, superinfection

Interactions

Drug-drug. *Antacids, histamine$_2$-receptor antagonists:* increased absorption of dirithromycin
Astemizole, cisapride, pimozide, terfenadine: increased risk of arrhythmias and sudden death
Digoxin: increased digoxin blood level
Drug-diagnostic tests. *Alanine aminotransferase, alkaline phosphatase, aspartate aminotransferase, bilirubin, creatine kinase, eosinophils, gamma-glutamyltransferase, lactate dehydrogenase, neutrophils, platelets, potassium:* increased levels
Drug-food. *Any food:* increased absorption of dirithromycin

Patient monitoring

- Monitor for signs and symptoms of superinfection.

Patient teaching

• Instruct patient to take tablets whole, within 1 hour of a meal.

Tell patient to report signs and symptoms of worsening infection, superinfection (such as loose, foul-smelling stools, vaginal itching, sudden fever, cough), or pseudomembranous enterocolitis (such as severe diarrhea or vomiting).

• As appropriate, review all other significant and life-threatening adverse reactions and interactions, especially those related to the drugs, tests, and foods mentioned above.

disopyramide

Rythmodan✱, Rythmodan-LA✱

disopyramide phosphate

Norpace, Norpace CR

Pharmacologic class: Pyridine derivative

Therapeutic class: Ventricular and supraventricular antiarrhythmic (class IA), antitachyarrhythmic

Pregnancy risk category C

Action

Slows diastolic depolarization rate, reduces upstroke velocity, and prolongs duration of action potential and refractory period. Also decreases disparity in refractoriness between infarcted and adjacent normally perfused myocardium.

Availability

Capsules: 100 mg, 150 mg
Capsules (extended release): 100 mg, 150 mg
Tablets (extended-release): 150 mg

Indications and dosages

➤ Ventricular tachycardia and other ventricular arrhythmias not severe enough to require cardioversion

Adults weighing more than 50 kg (110 lb): Initially, 200 to 300 mg P.O. as a loading dose, then 150 mg P.O. q 6 hours (conventional capsules) or 300 mg P.O. q 12 hours (extended-release forms)

Adults weighing 50 kg (110 lb) or less: 100 mg P.O. q 6 hours (conventional capsules) or 200 mg P.O. q 12 hours (extended-release capsules)

Children ages 12 to 18: 6 to 15 mg/kg P.O. daily in four divided doses given q 6 hours

Children ages 4 to 11: 10 to 15 mg/kg P.O. daily in four divided doses given q 6 hours

Children ages 1 to 3: 10 to 20 mg/kg P.O. daily in four divided doses given q 6 hours

Children younger than age 1: 10 to 30 mg/kg P.O. daily in four divided doses given q 6 hours

Dosage adjustment

• Renal or hepatic insufficiency
• Acute myocardial infarction

Off-label uses

• Paroxysmal supraventricular tachycardia

Contraindications

• Hypersensitivity to drug
• Cardiogenic shock
• Second- or third-degree heart block
• Sick sinus syndrome
• Congenital QT prolongation

Precautions

Use cautiously in:

• heart failure, left ventricular dysfunction, conduction abnormalities, hepatic or renal insufficiency, prostate enlargement, myasthenia gravis, glaucoma, diabetes mellitus

- pregnant or breastfeeding patients
- children.

Administration

- Start therapy 6 to 12 hours after last quinidine dose or 3 to 6 hours after last procainamide dose.

🔊 Know that patient with atrial flutter or fibrillation should receive digitalis before starting disopyramide therapy to ensure that drug doesn't increase ventricular rate.

Route	Onset	Peak	Duration
P.O.	Rapid	2 hr	Unknown
P.O. (extended)	Unknown	4.9 ± 1.4 hr	Unknown
I.V.	Unknown	Unknown	Unknown

Adverse reactions

CNS: dizziness, agitation, depression, fatigue, headache, nervousness, acute psychosis, syncope
CV: chest pain, orthostatic hypotension, **heart failure, heart block, arrhythmias**
EENT: blurred vision, angle-closure glaucoma, dry eyes, dry nose
GI: nausea, vomiting, diarrhea, constipation, abdominal pain, bloating, flatulence, dry mouth
GU: urinary hesitancy or retention, erectile dysfunction
Hematologic: anemia, **thrombocytopenia, agranulocytosis**
Hepatic: jaundice
Metabolic: hypokalemia, **hypoglycemia**
Musculoskeletal: muscle weakness, myalgia
Respiratory: dyspnea
Skin: rash, pruritus, dermatoses
Other: edema, decreased appetite, weight gain

Interactions

Drug-drug. *Antiarrhythmics, fluoroquinolones:* widened QRS complex or QT interval
Anticholinergics: increased risk of adverse effects
Clarithromycin, erythromycin: increased disopyramide blood level
Phenytoin: increased disopyramide metabolism and blood level
Rifampin: decreased disopyramide blood level
Drug-diagnostic tests. *Blood urea nitrogen, creatinine, hepatic enzymes, lipids:* increased levels
Glucose, hematocrit, hemoglobin: decreased levels
Drug-herbs. *Aloe, buckthorn bark or berry, cascara sagrada bark, senna pod or leaf:* increased drug action
Jimsonweed: increased risk of adverse cardiovascular effects

Patient monitoring

- Check apical pulse before administering. Withhold dose if rate is below 60 or above 120 beats/minute.
- Monitor ECG for complete heart block.

🔊 Assess closely for signs and symptoms of heart failure.

- Evaluate for signs and symptoms of fluid retention, such as rapid weight gain.
- Monitor electrolyte levels regularly, checking especially for hypokalemia.

Patient teaching

- Tell patient to weigh himself daily and report weekly gain of more than 2 lb (1 kg).

🔊 Instruct patient to watch for and promptly report ankle swelling.

- Advise patient to move slowly when sitting up or standing, to avoid dizziness or light-headedness from sudden blood pressure decrease.
- Caution patient to avoid driving and other hazardous activities until he knows how drug affects concentration and alertness.
- As appropriate, review all other significant and life-threatening adverse

reactions and interactions, especially those related to the drugs, tests, and herbs mentioned above.

dobutamine hydrochloride

Dobutrex

Pharmacologic class: Sympathomimetic, adrenergic
Therapeutic class: Inotropic
Pregnancy risk category B

Action

Stimulates beta$_1$-adrenergic receptors of heart, causing a positive inotropic effect that increases myocardial contractility and stroke volume. Also reduces peripheral vascular resistance, decreases ventricular filling pressure, and promotes atrioventricular conduction.

Availability

Injection: 12.5 mg/ml in 20-ml vials

Indications and dosages

➢ Short-term treatment of cardiac decompensation caused by depressed contractility (such as during refractory heart failure); adjunct in cardiac surgery
Adults: 2.5 to 10 mcg/kg/minute I.V. as a continuous infusion, adjusted to hemodynamic response

Dosage adjustment

- Elderly patients

Off-label uses

- Adjunct in myocardial infarction (MI) and septic shock
- Diagnosis of coronary artery disease (echocardiography stress test, ventriculography, computed tomography)

Contraindications

- Hypersensitivity to drug
- Idiopathic hypertrophic subaortic stenosis

Precautions

Use cautiously in:
- hypertension, MI, atrial fibrillation, hypovolemia
- pregnant or breastfeeding patients
- children.

Administration

- Use infusion pump or microdrip I.V. infusion set.
- Dilute with dextrose 5% in water or normal saline solution to at least 50 ml of solution. Know that drug is incompatible with alkaline solutions, such as sodium bicarbonate injection.

Route	Onset	Peak	Duration
I.V.	1-2 min	10 min	Brief

Adverse reactions

CNS: headache
CV: hypertension, hypotension, tachycardia, premature ventricular contractions, angina, palpitations, nonspecific chest pain, phlebitis
GI: nausea, vomiting
Metabolic: hypokalemia
Respiratory: dyspnea, **asthma attacks**
Skin: extravasation with tissue necrosis
Other: hypersensitivity reactions including **anaphylaxis**

Interactions

Drug-drug. *Beta-adrenergic blockers:* increased alpha-adrenergic effects
Bretylium: potentiation of vasopressor activity
Cyclopropane, halothane: serious arrhythmias
Guanethidine: decreased hypotensive effects
Thyroid hormone: increased cardiovascular effects
Tricyclic antidepressants: potentiation of cardiovascular and vasopressor effects

Drug-herbs. *Rue:* increased inotropic potential

Patient monitoring

- As needed, correct hypovolemia before starting therapy by giving volume expanders, as prescribed.
- Monitor ECG and blood pressure continuously during administration.
- Monitor fluid intake and output.

Clinical alert: Assess electrolyte levels. Stay especially alert for hypokalemia.

Patient teaching

- Instruct patient to report anginal pain, headache, leg cramps, and shortness of breath.
- Explain need for close observation and monitoring.
- As appropriate, review all other significant and life-threatening adverse reactions and interactions, especially those related to the drugs and herbs mentioned above.

docetaxel

Taxotere

Pharmacologic class: Mitosis inhibitor
Therapeutic class: Antineoplastic
Pregnancy risk category D

Action

Inhibits cellular mitosis by disrupting microtubular network

Availability

Injection concentrate: 20 mg, 80 mg

Indications and dosages

➢ Metastatic breast cancer unresponsive to previous regimens
Adults: 60 to 100 mg/m² I.V. over 1 hour q 3 weeks

➢ Metastatic non-small-cell lung cancer; androgen-independent (hormone refractory) metastatic prostate cancer
Adults: 75 mg/m² I.V. over 1 hour q 3 weeks

Dosage adjustment

- Febrile neutropenia

Contraindications

- Hypersensitivity to drug or polysorbate 80
- Hepatic impairment
- Neutrophil count below 1,500 cells/mm³

Precautions

Use cautiously in:
- females of childbearing age
- pregnant or breastfeeding patients.

Administration

Clinical alert: Don't let drug concentrate contact plasticized polyvinyl chloride equipment or devices.

- Know that when used for prostate cancer, drug must be given with prednisone, as prescribed.
- Dilute with accompanying diluent solution; rotate vial gently to mix. Once foam has largely dissipated, withdraw prescribed amount of drug and mix in glass or polypropylene bottle or in plastic bag with 250 ml of normal saline solution or dextrose 5% in water.
- Mix solution thoroughly and infuse over 1 hour, using polyethylene-lined infusion set.

Route	Onset	Peak	Duration
I.V.	Rapid	Unknown	7 days

Adverse reactions

CNS: fatigue, asthenia, neurosensory deficits, peripheral neuropathy
CV: peripheral edema, **cardiac tamponade, pericardial effusion**
GI: nausea, vomiting, diarrhea, stomatitis, ascites
Hematologic: anemia, **thrombocytopenia, leukopenia**

Musculoskeletal: myalgia, joint pain
Respiratory: bronchospasm, pulmonary edema
Skin: alopecia, rash, dermatitis, desquamation, erythema, nail disorders
Other: edema, hypersensitivity reactions including **anaphylaxis**

Interactions

Drug-drug. *Antineoplastics:* additive bone marrow depression
Cyclosporine, erythromycin, ketoconazole, troleandomycin: significant change in docetaxel effects
Live-virus vaccines: increased risk of infection

Patient monitoring

🔈 Watch for signs and symptoms of anaphylaxis or other hypersensitivity reactions, especially with first two doses.
• Monitor vital signs and fluid intake and output. Watch for signs and symptoms of fluid overload and bronchospasm.
• Monitor CBC, and assess for signs and symptoms of blood dyscrasias.
• Observe I.V. site frequently for extravasation.
• Assess neurologic status to detect neurosensory deficits and peripheral neuropathy.

Patient teaching

• Instruct patient to weigh himself daily and to immediately report sudden weight gain or difficulty breathing.
🔈 Tell patient to report signs and symptoms of blood dyscrasias. Inform him that he'll undergo frequent blood testing to monitor these effects.
🔈 Advise patient to immediately report rash or difficulty breathing.
• Inform patient that hair loss is common with docetaxel use, but that hair will grow back after therapy ends.
• Advise female patient of childbearing age to use effective contraception during therapy and to notify prescriber if she suspects pregnancy.
• As appropriate, review all other significant and life-threatening adverse reactions and interactions, especially those related to the drugs mentioned above.

docusate calcium

DC Softgels, Pro-Cal-Sof, Stool Softener DC, Sulfolax, Surfak Liquigels

docusate sodium

Colace, Diocto, D.O.S. Softgels, D-S-S, Genasoft Softgels, Modane Soft, Regulax SS, Silace

Pharmacologic class: Emollient
Therapeutic class: Stool softener, surfactant
Pregnancy risk category C

Action

Increases absorption of liquid into stool, resulting in softening of fecal mass. Also promotes electrolyte and water secretion into colon.

Availability

docusate calcium
Capsules: 240 mg
Capsules (soft gels): 240 mg
docusate sodium
Capsules: 50 mg, 100 mg, 250 mg
Capsules (soft gels): 100 mg, 250 mg
Liquid: 150 mg/15 ml
Syrup: 50 mg/15 ml, 60 mg/15 ml, 20 mg/5 ml, 100 mg/30 ml, 150 mg/15 ml
Tablets: 100 mg

Indications and dosages

➢ Stool softener
Adults and children older than age 12: 240 mg (docusate calcium) or 50 to

200 mg (docusate sodium) P.O. daily until bowel movements are normal
Children ages 6 to 12: 40 to 120 mg (docusate sodium) P.O. daily
Children ages 3 to 6: 20 to 60 mg (docusate sodium) P.O. daily

Contraindications
- Hypersensitivity to drug
- Abdominal pain, nausea, or vomiting
- Intestinal obstruction

Precautions
Use cautiously in:
- pregnant or breastfeeding patients.

Administration
- Give tablets and capsules with full glass of water.
- Give liquid solution with milk or fruit juice.
- Be aware that excessive or long-term use may lead to laxative dependence.

Route	Onset	Peak	Duration
P.O.	24-48 hr (up to 5 days)	Unknown	Unknown

Adverse reactions
EENT: throat irritation
GI: nausea, diarrhea, mild cramps
Skin: rash
Other: bitter taste, decreased appetite, laxative dependence

Interactions
Drug-drug. *Mineral oil:* increased mineral oil absorption, causing toxicity
Warfarin: decreased warfarin effects (with high doses)

Patient monitoring
- If diarrhea occurs, withhold drug and notify prescriber.
- Know that therapeutic efficacy usually becomes apparent 1 to 3 days after first dose.

Patient teaching
- Instruct patient to drink sufficient fluids with each dose and to increase fluid intake during the day.
- Advise patient to prevent constipation by increasing fluids and consuming more dietary fiber (as in fruits and bran).
- Inform patient that excessive or prolonged use may lead to laxative dependence.
- As appropriate, review all other significant adverse reactions and interactions, especially those related to the drugs mentioned above.

dofetilide
Tikosyn

Pharmacologic class: Methanesulfonamide derivative
Therapeutic class: Antiarrhythmic (class III)
Pregnancy risk category C

Action
Selectively blocks potassium channels, prolonging ventricular refractory period and action potential. Has no effect on sodium channels.

Availability
Capsules: 125 mcg, 250 mcg, 500 mcg

Indications and dosages
➢ To convert atrial fibrillation and atrial flutter to normal sinus rhythm; to maintain normal sinus rhythm
Adults: 500 mcg P.O. b.i.d. if creatinine clearance exceeds 60 ml/minute

Dosage adjustment
- Renal impairment

Off-label uses
- Ventricular arrhythmias

Contraindications

- Hypersensitivity to drug
- Arrhythmias
- Severe renal impairment
- Concurrent use of cimetidine, ketoconazole, megestrol, prochlorperazine, trimethoprim, sulfamethoxazole, or verapamil

Precautions

Use cautiously in:
- mild to moderate renal or hepatic impairment, ventricular arrhythmias
- pregnant or breastfeeding patients
- children younger than age 18.

Administration

Be aware that therapy must be initiated in setting that allows continuous ECG monitoring by trained personnel for at least 3 days. Such monitoring must be repeated with dosage changes.
- Know that patients with atrial fibrillation require anticoagulation before and during therapy.
- Dosage must be individualized according to creatinine clearance and QTc interval (or QT interval if heart rate is below 60 beats/minute), as determined before first dose.
- Know that patient shouldn't be discharged for at least 12 hours after conversion to normal sinus rhythm.

Route	Onset	Peak	Duration
P.O.	Unknown	2-3 hr	Unknown

Adverse reactions

CNS: headache, dizziness, insomnia, anxiety, migraine, asthenia, paresthesia, syncope, **cerebral ischemia, cerebrovascular accident**
CV: chest pain, angina, hypertension, palpitations, bradycardia, peripheral edema, **atrial or ventricular fibrillation, ventricular tachycardia, cardiac arrest, myocardial infarction, torsades de pointes, AV block, bundle-branch block**
GI: nausea, diarrhea, abdominal pain
GU: urinary tract infection
Hepatic: hepatic damage
Musculoskeletal: back pain, joint pain, facial paralysis
Respiratory: respiratory tract infection, dyspnea, increased cough
Skin: rash, diaphoresis, angioedema
Other: flulike symptoms

Interactions

Drug-drug. *Amiloride, amiodarone, azole antifungals, cannabinoids, cimetidine, diltiazem, ketoconazole, macrolides, megestrol, metformin, nefazodone, norfloxacin, prochlorperazine, protease inhibitors, quinine, selective serotonin reuptake inhibitors, sulfamethoxazole, triamterene, trimethoprim, verapamil, zafirlukast:* increased dofetilide blood level
Drug-food. *Grapefruit juice:* decreased metabolism and increased blood level of dofetilide

Patient monitoring

- Monitor ECG regularly during first 3 months of therapy, then periodically.
- Monitor electrolyte levels, QTc interval, renal function, and creatinine clearance.
- Assess patient for signs and symptoms of electrolyte imbalances, such as nausea, vomiting, diaphoresis, and diarrhea.

Patient teaching

- Explain reason for initial monitoring and follow-up.

Instruct patient to immediately report prolonged vomiting, diarrhea, or excessive sweating.
- As appropriate, review all other significant and life-threatening adverse reactions and interactions, especially those related to the drugs and foods mentioned above.

dolasetron mesylate
Anzemet

Pharmacologic class: Selective serotonin subtype 3 (5-HT_3) receptor antagonist
Therapeutic class: Antiemetic
Pregnancy risk category B

Action
Blocks serotonin activation at receptor sites in vagal nerve terminals and in chemoreceptor trigger zone in CNS, decreasing the vomiting reflex

Availability
Injection: 12.5 mg/0.625-ml ampules, 20 mg/ml in 5-ml vials
Tablets: 50 mg, 100 mg

Indications and dosages
➢ Chemotherapy-induced nausea and vomiting
Adults: 100 mg P.O. 1 hour before chemotherapy or 1.8 mg/kg I.V. 30 minutes before chemotherapy
Children ages 2 to 16: 1.8 mg/kg P.O. within 1 hour before chemotherapy or 1.8 mg/kg I.V. (not to exceed 100 mg) 30 minutes before chemotherapy
➢ Prevention or treatment of postoperative nausea and vomiting
Adults: 100 mg P.O. within 2 hours before surgery or 12.5 mg I.V. 15 minutes before cessation of anesthesia (for prevention) or as soon as nausea or vomiting begins (for treatment)
Children ages 2 to 16: 1.2 mg/kg P.O. (up to 100 mg/dose) within 2 hours before surgery or 0.35 mg/kg I.V. (up to 12.5 mg) 15 minutes before cessation of anesthesia (for prevention) or as soon as nausea or vomiting begins (for treatment)

Contraindications
- Hypersensitivity to drug
- Arrhythmias

Precautions
Use cautiously in:
- risk factors for prolonged cardiac conduction intervals
- pregnant or breastfeeding patients (safety not established).

Administration
- Give oral dose at least 1 hour before chemotherapy for best results.
- To prevent postoperative nausea, give oral dose within 2 hours before surgery.
- If patient has difficulty swallowing tablet, injection solution may be mixed with apple or apple-grape juice and given orally.
- For I.V. use, single dose may be given undiluted over 30 seconds. For I.V. infusion, dilute in normal saline solution, dextrose 5% in water, or lactated Ringer's solution, and give single dose over at least 15 minutes. Don't mix with other drugs.
- Flush I.V. line before and after infusion.

Route	Onset	Peak	Duration
P.O.	Unknown	1-2 hr	Up to 24 hr
I.V.	Unknown	15-30 min	Up to 24 hr

Adverse reactions
CNS: headache (increased in cancer patients), dizziness, fatigue, syncope
CV: bradycardia, tachycardia, ECG changes, hypertension, hypotension
GI: diarrhea, constipation, dyspepsia, abdominal pain
GU: urinary retention, **oliguria**
Skin: pruritus, rash
Other: chills, fever, decreased appetite

Interactions
Drug-drug. *Antiarrhythmics, anthracycline (high cumulative doses), diuretics:* increased risk of conduction abnormalities

Drugs that affect hepatic microsomal enzymes: altered dolasetron blood level
Drug-diagnostic tests. *Alanine aminotransferase, aspartate aminotransferase:* increased levels

Patient monitoring

• Monitor closely for excessive diuresis.
🔊 Watch for ECG changes, including prolonged PR interval and widened QRS complex, especially in patients receiving antiarrhythmics concurrently.

Patient teaching

• Instruct patient to take drug 1 to 2 hours before chemotherapy.
• Inform patient that drug commonly causes headache.
• As appropriate, review all other significant and life-threatening adverse reactions and interactions, especially those related to the drugs and tests mentioned above.

donepezil hydrochloride

Aricept

Pharmacologic class: Acetylcholinesterase inhibitor
Therapeutic class: Anti-Alzheimer's agent
Pregnancy risk category C

Action

Reversibly inhibits acetylcholinesterase hydrolysis in CNS, leading to increased acetylcholine level and temporary cognitive improvement in patients with Alzheimer's disease

Availability

Tablets: 5 mg, 10 mg

Indications and dosages

➤ Mild to moderate Alzheimer's disease
Adults: Initially, 5 mg P.O. daily at bedtime. After 4 to 6 weeks, may increase dosage to 10 mg.

Contraindications

• Hypersensitivity to drug or piperidine derivatives
• Pregnancy or breastfeeding

Precautions

Use cautiously in:
• cardiovascular disease, chronic obstructive pulmonary disease (COPD)
• history of ulcers, GI bleeding, or sick sinus syndrome
• concurrent use of nonsteroidal anti-inflammatory drugs (NSAIDs).

Administration

• Give with or without food.
• For best response, give at bedtime.

Route	Onset	Peak	Duration
P.O.	Unknown	3-4 hr	Unknown

Adverse reactions

CNS: headache, dizziness, vertigo, fatigue, depression, aggression, irritability, restlessness, nervousness, paresthesia, insomnia, abnormal dreams, tremor, aphasia, **seizures**
CV: chest pain, bradycardia, hypertension, hypotension, vasodilation, **atrial fibrillation**
EENT: cataracts, blurred vision, eye irritation, sore throat
GI: nausea, vomiting, diarrhea, bloating, epigastric pain, fecal incontinence, **GI bleeding**
GU: urinary frequency, increased libido
Hepatic: hepatotoxicity
Metabolic: dehydration
Musculoskeletal: muscle cramps, arthritis, bone fracture

Respiratory: dyspnea, bronchitis
Skin: pruritus, urticaria, bruising, diaphoresis, rash, flushing
Other: toothache, decreased appetite, weight loss, hot flashes, influenza

Interactions

Drug-drug. *Anticholinergics:* reduced donepezil effects
Anticholinesterases, cholinomimetics: synergistic effects
Carbamazepine, dexamethasone, phenobarbital, phenytoin, rifampin: accelerated donepezil elimination
NSAIDs: increased risk of GI bleeding
Drug-herbs. *Jaborandi tree, pill-bearing spurge:* increased risk of drug toxicity

Patient monitoring

Watch closely for increased bronchoconstriction in patients with history of asthma or COPD.
- Assess cardiovascular status. Drug may cause bradycardia from increased vagal tone.
- Monitor closely for signs and symptoms of GI ulcers and bleeding, especially if patient takes NSAIDs concurrently.

Patient teaching

- Advise patient to take drug at bedtime.
- Inform patient that drug may slow the heart rate, leading to fainting episodes.

Instruct patient to immediately report signs or symptoms of GI ulcers ("coffee-ground" vomitus, black tarry stools, and abdominal pain), irregular heart beat, unusual tiredness, or yellowing of skin or eyes.
- As appropriate, review all other significant and life-threatening adverse reactions and interactions, especially those related to the drugs and herbs mentioned above.

dopamine hydrochloride

Intropin, Revimine✱

Pharmacologic class: Catecholamine, adrenergic
Therapeutic class: Inotropic, vasopressor
Pregnancy risk category C

Action

Causes norepinephrine release (mainly on dopaminergic receptors), leading to vasodilation of renal and mesenteric arteries. Also exerts inotropic effects on heart, which increases the heart rate, blood flow, myocardial contractility, and stroke volume.

Availability

Injection for dilution: 40 mg/ml, 80 mg/ml, 160 mg/ml
Premixed injection: 0.8 mg/ml, 1.6 mg/ml, 3.2 mg/ml in 250 ml and 500 ml of dextrose 5% in water

Indications and dosages

➢ Shock; hemodynamic imbalance; hypotension
Adults and children: 2 to 5 mcg/kg/minute by I.V. infusion. Titrate dosage to desired response; may increase infusion by 1 to 4 mcg/kg/minute at 10- to 30-minute intervals.

Off-label uses

- Chronic obstructive pulmonary disease
- Heart failure

Contraindications

- Hypersensitivity to drug or bisulfites
- Tachyarrhythmias, ventricular fibrillation
- Pheochromocytoma

Precautions

Use cautiously in:
- hypovolemia, myocardial infarction, occlusive vascular disease, diabetic endarteritis, atrial embolism
- concurrent MAO inhibitor use
- pregnant or breastfeeding patients
- children.

Administration

- Give I.V. infusion using metered pump or other device that controls flow.
- Add 200 to 400 mg of dopamine to 250 to 500 ml of normal saline solution, 5% dextrose injection, 5% dextrose and half-normal saline solution, or 5% dextrose in lactated Ringer's solution.
- Infuse into large (preferably central) vein to avoid extravasation.

🔊 Don't give concurrently with MAO inhibitors. Reduce dosage if patient has received MAO inhibitor recently.

Route	Onset	Peak	Duration
I.V.	1-2 min	Unknown	<10 min

Adverse reactions

CNS: headache
CV: palpitations, hypotension, angina, ECG changes, tachycardia, vasoconstriction, **arrhythmias**
EENT: mydriasis
GI: nausea, vomiting
Metabolic: azotemia, hyperglycemia
Respiratory: dyspnea, asthma attacks
Skin: piloerection
Other: irritation at injection site, **gangrene of extremities** (with high doses for prolonged periods or in occlusive vascular disease)

Interactions

Drug-drug. *Alpha- or beta-adrenergic blockers:* antagonism of dopamine effects
Ergot alkaloids: extreme blood pressure increase
Guanethidine: decreased cardiostimulatory effects
Inhalation anesthetics: increased risk of hypertension, arrhythmias
MAO inhibitors: hypertensive crisis
Oxytocics: severe, persistent hypotension
Phenytoin: seizures, severe hypotension, bradycardia
Tricyclic antidepressants: decreased pressor response
Drug-diagnostic tests. *Glucose, nitrogenous compounds, urine catecholamines:* increased levels

Patient monitoring

- Monitor blood pressure, pulse, urinary output, and pulmonary artery wedge pressure during infusion.

🔊 Inspect I.V. site regularly for irritation. Avoid extravasation.

🔊 Monitor color and temperature of extremities.

🔊 Never stop infusion abruptly, because this may cause severe hypotension. Instead, taper gradually.

Patient teaching

- Explain the need for close observation during infusion.
- Instruct patient to report adverse reactions and I.V. site discomfort.
- As appropriate, review all other significant and life-threatening adverse reactions and interactions, especially those related to the drugs and tests mentioned above.

dornase alfa

Pulmozyme

Pharmacologic class: Recombinant human deoxyribonuclease I

Therapeutic class: Cystic fibrosis agent, mucolytic enzyme, respiratory inhalant

Pregnancy risk category B

Action

Selectively cleaves to DNA in sputum, decreasing viscosity of pulmonary secretions

Availability

Inhalation solution: 2.5-mg ampule (1 mg/ml)

Indications and dosages

➢ To reduce respiratory tract infections and improve pulmonary function

Adults and children older than age 5: One ampule (2.5 mg) inhaled once daily

Contraindications

- Hypersensitivity to drug, its components, or products derived from Chinese hamster ovary cells
- Status asthmaticus
- Respiratory tract infection

Precautions

Use cautiously in:

- nonasthmatic bronchial disease, asthma controlled by bronchodilators
- pregnant or breastfeeding patients.

Administration

- Don't shake or dilute drug.
- Use only with approved nebulizer.
- Discard cloudy or discolored solution.

Route	Onset	Peak	Duration
Inhalation	3-7 days	9 days	Unknown

Adverse reactions

CV: chest pain

EENT: conjunctivitis, rhinitis, pharyngitis, hemoptysis, voice changes

Respiratory: dyspnea, increased sputum, wheezing

Skin: rash, urticaria, pruritus

Other: hypersensitivity reactions

Interactions

None known

Patient monitoring

- Assess patient periodically. Report improvement in dyspnea and sputum clearance.
- Monitor for signs and symptoms of hypersensitivity reaction.

Patient teaching

- Teach patient how to use nebulizer.
- Instruct patient to report rash, hives, and itching.
- As appropriate, review all other significant adverse reactions mentioned above.

doxapram hydrochloride

Dopram

Pharmacologic class: CNS and respiratory stimulant

Therapeutic class: Analeptic

Pregnancy risk category B

Action

Activates peripheral carotid, aortic, and other chemoreceptors to stimulate respiration. Increases tidal volume and respiratory rate by directly stimulating respiratory center in medulla oblongata.

Availability

Injection: 20 mg/ml

Indications and dosages

➢ Respiratory depression after anesthesia

Adults and adolescents: 5 mg/minute by I.V. infusion until desired response occurs; then reduce to 1 to 3 mg/minute, to a maximum cumulative dosage of 4 mg/kg (or 300 mg). Or 0.5 to 1 mg/kg I.V. injection, repeated q 5 minutes, if needed, to a maximum total dosage of 1.5 mg/kg.

➢ Chronic pulmonary disease related to acute hypercapnia

Adults: 1 to 2 mg/minute by I.V. infusion, using a concentration of 2 mg/ml, to a maximum of 3 mg/minute. Infusion shouldn't exceed 2 hours.

➢ Drug-induced CNS depression

Adults: Initially, 2 mg/kg I.V., repeated in 5 minutes and then q 1 to 2 hours until patient awakens, to a maximum daily dosage of 3 g. For infusion, priming dose of 2 mg/kg I.V.; if no response occurs, continue for 1 to 2 hours as needed; if some response occurs, give I.V. infusion of 250 mg in 250 ml of saline solution or dextrose 5% in water at 1 to 3 mg/minute until patient awakens. Don't infuse longer than 2 hours or give more than 3 g/day.

Off-label uses

- Laryngospasm secondary to postoperative tracheal extubation

Contraindications

- Hypersensitivity to drug
- Cardiovascular disorders
- Cerebrovascular accident
- Head injury, seizures
- Respiratory failure, restrictive respiratory disease
- Neonates

Precautions

Use cautiously in:

- bronchial asthma, arrhythmias, increased intracranial pressure, hyperthyroidism, pheochromocytoma, metabolic disorders
- pregnant or breastfeeding patients.

Administration

- Ensure adequate airway and oxygenation before administering.
- Give I.V. slowly to avoid hemolysis.
- Know that doxapram is compatible with 5% and 10% dextrose in water and with normal saline solution.

Don't mix with thiopental sodium, bicarbonate, or aminophylline, because precipitates or gas may form.

Route	Onset	Peak	Duration
I.V.	20-40 sec	1-2 min	5-12 min

Adverse reactions

CNS: weakness, dizziness, drowsiness, headache, dysarthria, dysphonia, disorientation, hyperactivity, paresthesia, **loss of consciousness, seizures**

CV: hypotension, bradycardia, chest pain or tightness, heart rate changes, **thrombophlebitis, atrioventricular block, arrhythmias, cardiac arrest**

EENT: lacrimation, diplopia, miosis, conjunctival hyperemia, sneezing, **laryngospasm**

GI: nausea, vomiting, diarrhea, abdominal cramps, increased salivation, dysphagia

GU: urinary frequency or incontinence, albuminuria

Musculoskeletal: muscle cramps, fasciculations

Respiratory: dyspnea, increased secretions, **respiratory muscle paralysis, central respiratory paralysis, bronchospasm, respiratory depression, respiratory arrest**

Skin: rash, diaphoresis, flushing

Other: burning or hot sensation in genitalia and perineal areas

Interactions

Drug-drug. *General anesthetics:* increased risk of self-limiting arrhythmias

MAO inhibitors, sympathomimetics: potentiation of adverse cardiovascular effects
Skeletal muscle relaxants: masking of residual effects of these drugs
Drug-diagnostic tests. *Blood urea nitrogen:* increased level
Erythrocytes, hematocrit, hemoglobin, red blood cells, white blood cells: decreased levels

Patient monitoring

- Assess blood pressure, pulse, deep tendon reflexes, airway, and arterial blood gas values before starting therapy and frequently during infusion.
- Monitor I.V. site frequently for irritation and thrombophlebitis.

Discontinue infusion immediately if hypotension or dyspnea suddenly develops.

Patient teaching

- Instruct patient to report adverse reactions promptly.
- As appropriate, review all other significant and life-threatening adverse reactions and interactions, especially those related to the drugs and tests mentioned above.

doxazosin mesylate

Cardura

Pharmacologic class: Sympatholytic, peripherally acting antiadrenergic
Therapeutic class: Antihypertensive
Pregnancy risk category C

Action

Blocks $alpha_1$-adrenergic receptors, promoting vasodilation. Also reduces urethral resistance, relieving obstruction and improving urine flow and other symptoms of benign prostatic hypertrophy (BPH).

Availability

Tablets: 1 mg, 2 mg, 4 mg, 8 mg

Indications and dosages

➢ Hypertension

Adults: 1 mg P.O. once daily. May increase dosage gradually q 2 weeks, up to 2 to 16 mg daily, as needed.

➢ BPH

Adults: 1 mg P.O. once daily. May increase dosage gradually, up to 8 mg daily, as needed.

Off-label uses

- Pheochromocytoma
- Syndrome X

Contraindications

- Hypersensitivity to drug or quinazoline derivatives

Precautions

Use cautiously in:

- renal or hepatic impairment, heart failure
- elderly patients
- pregnant or breastfeeding patients
- children (safety not established).

Administration

- Give initial dose at bedtime to minimize orthostatic hypotension and syncope.
- Know that incidence of orthostatic hypotension increases greatly when daily dosage exceeds 4 mg and that it usually occurs within 6 hours of administration.

Route	Onset	Peak	Duration
P.O.	1-2 hr	2-6 hr	24 hr

Adverse reactions

CNS: dizziness, vertigo, headache, depression, drowsiness, fatigue, nervousness, weakness, asthenia
CV: orthostatic hypotension, chest pain, palpitations, tachycardia, **arrhythmias**

EENT: abnormal or blurred vision, conjunctivitis, epistaxis, rhinitis, pharyngitis
GI: nausea, vomiting, diarrhea, constipation, abdominal discomfort, flatulence, dry mouth
GU: decreased libido, sexual dysfunction
Respiratory: dyspnea
Musculoskeletal: joint pain, arthritis, gout, myalgia
Skin: flushing, rash, pruritus
Other: edema

Interactions

Drug-drug. *Clonidine, nitrates, other antihypertensives:* decreased antihypertensive effect
Drug-diagnostic tests. *Neutrophils, white blood cells:* decreased counts
Drug-herbs. *Butcher's broom:* decreased doxazosin effects
Drug-behaviors. *Alcohol use:* additive hypotension

Patient monitoring

- Monitor blood pressure with patient lying down and standing up every 2 to 6 hours after initial dose or after a dosage increase (when orthostatic hypotension is most likely to occur).

Patient teaching

- Caution patient not to drive or perform other activities requiring alertness for 12 to 24 hours after first dose.
- Tell patient to move slowly when sitting up or standing, to avoid dizziness or light-headedness from sudden blood pressure decrease.
- Advise patient to report episodes of dizziness or palpitations.
- As appropriate, review all other significant and life-threatening adverse reactions and interactions, especially those related to the drugs, tests, herbs, and behaviors mentioned above.

d

doxepin hydrochloride

Apo-Doxepin✱, Novo-Doxepin✱, Sinequan, Xepin, Zonalon

Pharmacologic class: Tricyclic antidepressant
Therapeutic class: Antidepressant, anxiolytic, antipruritic
Pregnancy risk category C

Action

Unknown. May prevent reuptake of norepinephrine, serotonin, or both at presynaptic neurons, increasing levels of these neurotransmitters in CNS. Exact mechanism in pruritus also unknown, but drug is a potent histamine$_1$- and histamine$_2$-blocker.

Availability

Capsules: 10 mg, 25 mg, 50 mg, 75 mg, 100 mg, 150 mg
Cream (topical): 5% in 30-g tube
Oral concentrate: 10 mg/ml

Indications and dosages

➢ Endogenous depression; anxiety
Adults: Initially, 25 mg P.O. t.i.d., increased as needed up to 150 mg daily in outpatients and 300 mg daily in hospitalized patients.
Elderly adults: Initially, 25 to 50 mg P.O. daily; may be increased as needed
➢ Short-term relief of histamine-mediated pruritus of moderate severity accompanying such conditions as eczematous dermatitis
Adults: Apply a thin film of cream to skin q.i.d., with 3 to 4 hours between applications, for a maximum of 8 days.

Off-label uses

- Adjunct in peptic ulcer disease

Contraindications
- Hypersensitivity to drug or other dibenzoxepins
- Glaucoma
- Predisposition to urinary retention
- MAO inhibitor use within past 14 days

Precautions
Use cautiously in:
- cardiovascular disease, prostatic enlargement, seizures
- elderly patients
- pregnant or breastfeeding patients.

Administration
- If desired, mix contents of capsule with food.
- Dilute oral concentrate with 120 ml of water, milk, or juice. Be aware that drug is incompatible with carbonated beverages.
- Know that drug may be given at bedtime to prevent daytime sleepiness.

◀ Don't give within 14 days of MAO inhibitor, because drug interaction may cause cardiovascular instability.

◀ Avoid concurrent use of other CNS depressants, because inadvertent overdose may occur.

- With topical cream, don't apply to broken skin or use occlusive dressings, because doing so increases dermal absorption.
- Be aware that drug is usually given in conjunction with psychotherapy when used for depression.

Route	Onset	Peak	Duration
P.O.	Unknown	2 hr	Unknown
Topical	Unknown	Unknown	Unknown

Adverse reactions
CNS: fatigue, sedation, agitation, confusion, hallucinations, drowsiness, dizziness, extrapyramidal reactions, poor concentration, syncope, **seizures, cerebrovascular accident, increased risk of suicide or suicidal ideation** (especially in child or adolescent)
CV: hypotension, orthostatic hypotension, hypertension, vasculitis, ECG changes, tachycardia, palpitations, **arrhythmias, myocardial infarction, heart block**
EENT: blurred vision, increased intraocular pressure, lacrimation, tinnitus, nasal congestion
GI: nausea, constipation, dry mouth, **paralytic ileus**
GU: urinary retention, delayed voiding, urinary tract dilation, gynecomastia, galactorrhea, menstrual irregularities, testicular swelling, libido changes
Hematologic: purpura, **bone marrow depression, eosinophilia, agranulocytosis, thrombocytopenia, leukopenia**
Metabolic: hyperglycemia, **hypoglycemia**
Skin: photosensitivity; rash; urticaria; pruritus; diaphoresis; flushing; petechiae; alopecia; local burning, stinging, tingling, irritation, or rash (with topical use)
Other: increased appetite, weight gain or loss, hyperthermia, chills, edema, drug-induced fever, hypersensitivity reactions

Interactions
Drug-drug. *Barbiturates, CNS depressants (including antihistamines, clonidine, opioids, sedative-hypnotics):* additive CNS depression
Carbamazepine, class IC antiarrhythmics (flecainide, propafenone), other antidepressants, other CYP450-2D6 inhibitors (amiodarone, cimetidine, quinidine, ritonavir), phenothiazines: increased doxepin blood level and effects
Clonidine: hypertensive crisis
Guanethidine: antagonism of antihypertensive effects
Levodopa: delayed or decreased levodopa absorption, hypertension
MAO inhibitors: tachycardia, seizures, potentially fatal reactions
Rifamycin: decreased doxepin effects

Selective serotonin reuptake inhibitors: increased risk of toxicity
Sparfloxacin: increased risk of adverse cardiovascular effects
Drug-diagnostic tests. *Bilirubin, hepatic enzymes:* increased levels
Glucose: increased or decreased level
Liver function tests: altered results
Drug-herbs. *Angel's trumpet, jimsonweed, scopolia:* increased anticholinergic effects
Chamomile, hops, kava, skullcap, valerian: increased CNS depression
Evening primrose oil: additive or synergistic effects
S-adenosylmethionine (SAM-e), St. John's wort, yohimbe: serotonin syndrome
Drug-behaviors. *Alcohol use:* increased CNS depression
Smoking: increased drug metabolism and altered effects
Sun exposure: increased risk of photosensitivity reactions

Patient monitoring

Record mood changes and watch for suicidal tendencies, especially in child or adolescent.
• Assess bowel elimination pattern. Increase fluids and administer stool softeners as ordered to ease constipation.
• Monitor fluid intake and output. Report changes in voiding pattern.
• Monitor liver function test results, CBC with white cell differential, and glucose level.

Patient teaching

• Advise patient on long-term therapy not to stop taking drug abruptly because this may lead to nausea, headache, and malaise.
Instruct patient and significant other, as appropriate, to monitor mental status carefully and to immediately report increased depression or suicidal thoughts or behavior (especially when used in child or adolescent).
Tell patient to promptly report easy bruising or bleeding.
• Caution patient to avoid driving and other hazardous activities until he knows how drug affects concentration and alertness.
• Instruct patient to move slowly when sitting up or standing, to avoid dizziness or light-headedness from sudden blood pressure decrease.
• Explain that drowsiness and dizziness usually subside after several weeks.
• Tell patient that using topical cream on more than 10% of body surface area may cause drowsiness.
• Caution patient using topical cream not to apply it to broken skin and not to use occlusive dressings. Also tell him to avoid contact with eyes and to rinse eyes thoroughly with warm water if contact occurs.
• As appropriate, review all other significant and life-threatening adverse reactions and interactions, especially those related to the drugs, tests, herbs, and behaviors mentioned above.

doxorubicin hydrochloride

Adriamycin PFS, Adriamycin RDF, Rubex

Pharmacologic class: Anthracycline
Therapeutic class: Antibiotic antineoplastic
Pregnancy risk category D

Action

Unclear. Thought to inhibit DNA and RNA synthesis by forming complex with DNA. Also exerts immunosuppressive activity. Cell-cycle–S-phase specific.

Availability

Injection (preservative-free): 2 mg/ml

Powder for injection: 10 mg, 20 mg, 50 mg, 100 mg, 150 mg

Indications and dosages

➢ Solid tumors, including bladder, breast, lung, stomach, and thyroid cancers; malignant lymphomas, including Hodgkin's disease; acute leukemia; Wilms' tumor; neuroblastoma

Adults: 60 to 75 mg/m² I.V. as a single dose at 21-day cycles, or 30 mg/m² I.V. as a single daily dose on first to third days of 4-week cycle, or 20 mg/m² I.V. once weekly. Maximum cumulative dosage is 550 mg/m².

Dosage adjustment

- Bone marrow depression
- Impaired cardiac or hepatic function

Off-label uses

- Endometrial carcinoma, islet cell carcinoma
- Chronic lymphocytic leukemia
- Multiple myeloma

Contraindications

- Hypersensitivity to drug
- Severe bone marrow depression
- Previous treatment with maximum cumulative doses of doxorubicin, other anthracyclines, or anthracenes

Precautions

Use cautiously in:

- cardiac disease, hepatic impairment, depressed bone marrow reserve, CNS metastases, brain tumor, malignant melanoma, renal carcinoma
- elderly patients
- females of childbearing age
- pregnant or breastfeeding patients
- children.

Administration

- Follow facility policy for handling and preparing antineoplastics.

Don't dilute solution with bacteriostatic diluent. Don't mix with other drugs.

- Dilute as directed with normal saline solution to a final concentration of 2 mg/ml.
- Administer slowly over 3 to 5 minutes into tubing of free-flowing I.V. infusion of normal saline solution or dextrose 5% in water.
- Deliver into large vein using butterfly needle. Avoid veins over joints or extremities with compromised venous or lymphatic drainage.

Avoid rapid infusion, because this may increase risk of acute infusion-related reactions (back pain, chest tightness, flushing).

If extravasation occurs, stop infusion immediately, apply ice, and notify prescriber.

Route	Onset	Peak	Duration
I.V.	Rapid	2 hr	24-36 days

Adverse reactions

CNS: drowsiness, dizziness, asthenia, fatigue, malaise, paresthesia, headache, depression, insomnia, anxiety, emotional lability

CV: chest pain, hypotension, tachycardia, peripheral edema, **cardiomyopathy, heart failure, arrhythmias, pericardial effusion**

GI: nausea, vomiting, diarrhea, constipation, enlarged abdomen, abdominal pain, dyspepsia, oral candidiasis, moniliasis, stomatitis, glossitis, esophagitis, dysphagia

GU: albuminuria, hyperuricosuria, red urine

Hematologic: anemia, **leukopenia, thrombocytopenia, neutropenia, bone marrow depression**

Metabolic: hyperglycemia, hypocalcemia

Musculoskeletal: myalgia, back pain

Respiratory: dyspnea, increased cough, pneumonia

Skin: rash, dry skin, pruritus, skin discoloration, alopecia, diaphoresis, exfoliative dermatitis, palmar-plantar erythrodysesthesia

Other: abnormal taste, infection, chills, fever, herpes zoster, injection site reactions, allergic reactions including **anaphylaxis, acute infusion-associated reactions**

Interactions

Drug-drug. *Antineoplastics:* additive bone marrow depression
Cyclophosphamide: increased risk of hemorrhagic cystitis, increased cardiotoxicity
Cyclosporine: profound and prolonged hematologic toxicity, increased risk of coma and seizures
Dactinomycin (in children): increased risk of pneumonitis
Live-virus vaccines: decreased antibody response to vaccine, increased risk of adverse reactions
Mercaptopurine: hepatitis
Paclitaxel (if given first): reduced doxorubicin clearance, increased incidence and severity of neutropenia and stomatitis
Phenobarbital: increased clearance and decreased effects of doxorubicin
Phenytoin: decreased phenytoin blood level
Progesterone: increased incidence and severity of neutropenia and thrombocytopenia
Streptozocin: increased doxorubicin half-life
Verapamil: increased doxorubicin blood level
Drug-diagnostic tests. *Alkaline phosphatase, bilirubin, glucose, prothrombin time, serum and urine uric acid:* increased levels
Calcium, hemoglobin, neutrophils, platelets, white blood cells (WBCs): decreased levels

Patient monitoring

🔈 Watch for acute life-threatening arrhythmias, which may occur during or within a few hours after administration.
🔈 Monitor for cardiomyopathy and subsequent heart failure with chronic overdose (more common in children).
• Stay alert for erythematous streaking along vein next to injection site, which may indicate too-rapid infusion.
• Watch for nausea and vomiting. Administer antiemetics as needed.
🔈 Check for superinfection or hemorrhage caused by persistent bone marrow depression (but expect WBC counts as low as 1,000/mm^3 during therapy).
🔈 Watch closely for infusion-related reactions and anaphylaxis.
• Monitor CBC, hepatic profile, coagulation tests, ejection fraction, and glucose, uric acid, and calcium blood levels.

Patient teaching

🔈 Advise patient to promptly report irregular heartbeats, easy bruising or bleeding, or signs of hypersensitivity reaction, such as a rash.
• Caution patient to avoid people with colds, flu, or other contagious illnesses.
• Explain that drug may cause complete but reversible hair loss.
• Inform patient that drug may turn urine red for 1 or 2 days.
• As appropriate, review all other significant and life-threatening adverse reactions and interactions, especially those related to the drugs and tests mentioned above.

doxorubicin hydrochloride, liposomal

Caelyx✤, Doxil

Pharmacologic class: Anthracycline
Therapeutic class: Antibiotic antineoplastic
Pregnancy risk category D

Action
Unclear. Thought to inhibit DNA and RNA synthesis by forming complex with DNA. Also exerts immunosuppressive activity. Liposomal encapsulation increases uptake by tumors, prolongs drug action, and may decrease toxicity. Cell-cycle–S-phase specific.

Availability
Liposomal dispersion for injection: 20 mg/10 ml in 10-ml vials

Indications and dosages
➢ AIDS-related Kaposi's sarcoma
Adults: 20 mg/m² I.V. over 30 minutes once q 3 weeks
➢ Metastatic ovarian carcinoma
Adults: Initially, 50 mg/m² I.V. at a rate of 1 mg/minute q 4 weeks for at least four courses. If no adverse reactions occur, increase infusion rate to complete the infusion over 1 hour.

Dosage adjustment
- Hepatic impairment

Contraindications
- Hypersensitivity to drug
- Malignant melanoma
- CNS metastases
- Bone marrow depression
- Cardiac disease
- Breastfeeding

Precautions
Use cautiously in:
- hepatic impairment, brain tumor, renal carcinoma
- elderly patients
- females of childbearing age
- pregnant patients
- children.

Administration
- Follow facility policy for handling and preparing antineoplastics.
- Dilute dose (up to 90 mg) in 250 ml of dextrose 5% in water. Don't use any other diluent.

[Clinical alert] Don't dilute solution with bacteriostatic diluent. Don't mix with other drugs.
- Don't use in-line filter.
- Administer slowly by I.V. infusion. Don't give as I.V. bolus.

[Clinical alert] Avoid rapid infusion, which may increase the risk of infusion-related reactions (back pain, chest tightness, flushing).

[Clinical alert] If extravasation occurs, stop infusion immediately, apply ice, and notify prescriber.
- Don't give I.M. or subcutaneously.
- Know that drug is a translucent red dispersion, not a clear solution.

Route	Onset	Peak	Duration
I.V.	10 days	14 days	21-24 days

Adverse reactions
CNS: drowsiness, dizziness, asthenia, fatigue, malaise, paresthesia, headache, depression, insomnia, anxiety, emotional lability
CV: chest pain, hypotension, tachycardia, peripheral edema, **cardiomyopathy, heart failure, arrhythmias, pericardial effusion**
GI: nausea, vomiting, diarrhea, constipation, abdominal pain, enlarged abdomen, dyspepsia, moniliasis, stomatitis, glossitis, oral candidiasis, esophagitis, dysphagia
GU: albuminuria, red urine
Hematologic: anemia, **leukopenia, thrombocytopenia, neutropenia, bone marrow depression**
Hepatic: jaundice
Metabolic: hypocalcemia, hyperglycemia
Musculoskeletal: myalgia, back pain
Respiratory: dyspnea, increased cough, pneumonia
Skin: rash, dry skin, pruritus, skin discoloration, alopecia, diaphoresis, exfoliative dermatitis, palmar-plantar erythrodysesthesia
Other: altered taste, fever, chills, infection, herpes zoster, injection site reac-

tions, allergic reactions including **anaphylaxis, acute infusion reaction**

Interactions

Drug-drug. *Antineoplastics:* additive bone marrow depression
Cyclophosphamide: increased risk of hemorrhagic cystitis
Cyclosporine: profound and prolonged hematologic toxicity, increased risk of coma and seizures, increased cardiotoxicity
Dactinomycin (in children): increased risk of pneumonitis
Live-virus vaccines: decreased antibody response to vaccine, increased risk of adverse reactions
Mercaptopurine: hepatitis
Paclitaxel (if administered first): reduced doxorubicin clearance, increased incidence and severity of neutropenia and stomatitis
Phenobarbital: increased clearance and decreased effects of doxorubicin
Phenytoin: decreased phenytoin blood level
Progesterone: increased risk and severity of neutropenia and thrombocytopenia
Streptozocin: prolonged doxorubicin half-life
Verapamil: increased doxorubicin blood level
Drug-diagnostic tests. *Alkaline phosphatase, bilirubin, glucose, prothrombin time, serum and urine uric acid:* increased levels
Calcium, hemoglobin, neutrophils, platelets, white blood cells: decreased levels

Patient monitoring

◀ Observe patient closely for anaphylaxis and bleeding problems.
◀ Stay alert for acute life-threatening arrhythmias, which may occur during or within a few hours after administration.
◀ Assess for cardiomyopathy and subsequent heart failure with chronic overdose (more common in children).
◀ Monitor closely for acute infusion reaction.
- Assess for and report liver engorgement and yellowing of skin or eyes.
- Check CBC, coagulation tests, hepatic profile, and bilirubin, glucose, calcium and uric acid levels.
- Watch for nausea and vomiting. Give antiemetics, as needed and prescribed.
- Assess for constipation and give fluids and stool softeners, as needed and prescribed.

Patient teaching

◀ Instruct patient to immediately report shortness of breath, rash, chest pain, or palpitations.
- Advise patient to avoid people with colds, flu, or other contagious illnesses.
- As appropriate, review all other significant and life-threatening adverse reactions and interactions, especially those related to the drugs and tests mentioned above.

doxycycline

Vibramycin

doxycycline calcium

Vibramycin

doxycycline hyclate

Apo-Doxy✤, Doryx, Doxy-Caps, Doxy 100, Doxy 200, Doxycin✤, Periostat, Vibramycin, Vibra-Tabs

doxycycline monohydrate

Monodox

Pharmacologic class: Tetracycline
Therapeutic class: Anti-infective
Pregnancy risk category D

Action

Unclear. Thought to inhibit bacterial protein synthesis at 30S and 50S ribosomal subunit and to alter cytoplasmic membrane of susceptible organisms.

Availability

Capsules: 20 mg, 50 mg, 100 mg
Capsules (coated pellets): 75 mg, 100 mg
Powder for injection: 100 mg, 200 mg
Powder for oral suspension: 25 mg/5 ml
Syrup: 50 mg
Tablets: 20 mg, 50 mg, 75 mg, 100 mg

Indications and dosages

➢ Infections caused by unusual organisms, including *Mycoplasma, Chlamydia,* and *Rickettsia* organisms
Adults and children weighing more than 45 kg (99 lb): 100 mg P.O. q 12 hours on first day, followed by 100 to 200 mg P.O. once daily; or 50 to 100 mg P.O. q 12 hours; or 200 mg I.V. once daily; or 100 mg I.V. q 12 hours on first day, followed by 100 to 200 mg I.V. once daily; or 50 to 100 mg I.V. q 12 hours
Children weighing 45 kg (99 lb) or less: 2.2 mg/kg P.O. q 12 hours on first day, followed by 2.2 to 4.4 mg/kg/day P.O. once daily; or 1.1 to 2.2 mg/kg P.O. q 12 hours; or 4.4 mg/kg I.V. once daily; or 2.2 mg/kg I.V. q 12 hours on first day, followed by 2.2 to 4.4 mg/kg I.V. once daily; or 1.1 to 2.2 mg/kg I.V. q 12 hours
➢ Gonorrhea in penicillin-allergic patients
Adults and children weighing more than 45 kg (99 lb): 100 mg P.O. q 12 hours for 7 days; or 300 mg P.O. initially, followed by another 300 mg P.O. 1 hour later
➢ Lyme disease
Adults and children weighing more than 45 kg (99 lb): 100 mg P.O. b.i.d. for 10 to 30 days
➢ Periodontitis
Adults and children weighing more than 45 kg (99 lb): 20 mg P.O. b.i.d. for up to 9 months
➢ Anthrax
Adults and children weighing more than 45 kg (99 lb): 100 mg P.O. b.i.d. for 60 days; or 100 mg I.V. q 12 hours for 60 days, changing to oral route when appropriate
Children weighing 45 kg (99 lb) or less: 2.2 mg/kg P.O. b.i.d. for 60 days; or 100 mg I.V. q 12 hours for 60 days, changing to oral route when appropriate
➢ Prevention of malaria caused by *Plasmodium falciparum* in short-term travelers (less than 4 months)
Adults: 100 mg/day P.O. starting 1 to 2 days before travel begins and continuing during and for 4 weeks after travel
Children: 2 mg/kg/day P.O., up to adult dosage of 100 mg/day, starting 1 to 2 days before travel begins and continuing during and for 4 weeks after travel

Off-label uses

- Traveller's diarrhea
- Pleural effusion

Contraindications

- Hypersensitivity to drug, other tetracyclines, or bisulfites (with some drug products)

Precautions

Use cautiously in:
- renal disease, hepatic impairment, nephrogenic diabetes insipidus, cachexia
- pregnant or breastfeeding patients
- children younger than age 8.

Administration

- Obtain specimens for culture and sensitivity testing, as ordered, before first dose.

◀ Don't give in conjunction with methoxyflurane anesthetic. Severe or fatal kidney damage may result.

• Reconstitute powder for injection with dextrose 5% in water, normal saline solution, lactated Ringer's solution, or dextrose 5% in lactated Ringer's solution.
• Don't infuse solutions with concentrations above 1 mg/ml.
• Infuse 100-mg dose over at least 1 hour.
• Complete infusion within 12 hours of dilution, unless diluted with lactated Ringer's solution or dextrose 5% in lactated Ringer's solution; in this case, complete infusion within 6 hours.
Clinical alert: Don't give during last half of pregnancy or to children under age 8 unless other drugs are likely to be ineffective or are contraindicated. Drug may retard bone growth and cause tooth discoloration and malformation.

Route	Onset	Peak	Duration
P.O.	1-2 hr	1.5-4 hr	12 hr
I.V.	Rapid	End of infusion	12 hr

Adverse reactions

CNS: paresthesia, **pseudotumor cerebri**
CV: phlebitis, **thrombophlebitis, pericarditis**
EENT: vestibular reactions, hoarseness, pharyngitis
GI: nausea, vomiting, diarrhea, esophagitis, epigastric distress, enterocolitis, anogenital lesions or inflammation, glossitis, oral candidiasis, black hairy tongue, **pancreatitis**
GU: dark yellow or brown urine, vaginal candidiasis
Hematologic: hemolytic anemia, neutropenia, thrombocytopenia
Hepatic: hepatotoxicity
Musculoskeletal: bone growth retardation (in children younger than age 8)
Skin: photosensitivity, maculopapular or erythematous rash, hyperpigmentation, urticaria
Other: tooth enamel defects, increased appetite, phlebitis at I.V. site, superinfection, hypersensitivity reactions including **anaphylaxis**

Interactions

Drug-drug. *Adsorbent antidiarrheals; antacids; calcium, iron, and magnesium preparations:* decreased doxycycline absorption
Barbiturates, carbamazepine, hormonal contraceptives containing estrogen, phenytoin, rifamycin: decreased doxycycline efficacy
Cholestyramine, colestipol: decreased oral absorption of doxycycline
Methoxyflurane: increased nephrotoxicity
Penicillin: decreased penicillin activity
Sucralfate: prevention of doxycycline absorption from GI tract
Warfarin: enhanced warfarin effects
Drug-diagnostic tests. *Alkaline phosphatase, alanine aminotransferase, amylase, aspartate aminotransferase, bilirubin, blood urea nitrogen (BUN), eosinophils:* increased levels
Hemoglobin, neutrophils, platelets, white blood cells: decreased levels
Urine catecholamines: false elevations
Drug-food. *Calcium-containing foods:* decreased drug absorption
Drug-behaviors. *Alcohol use:* decreased anti-infective effect of doxycycline
Sun exposure: increased risk of photosensitivity

Patient monitoring

• Evaluate I.V. site regularly. Apply cool compresses as needed.
Clinical alert: Monitor for hypersensitivity reactions, including anaphylaxis.
• Monitor hepatic profile, CBC, BUN, and creatinine levels.
• Assess for hypercoagulability in patients taking warfarin concurrently.
• Monitor for digoxin toxicity in patients taking digoxin concurrently.

Patient teaching

• Advise patient to take with 8 oz of water to ensure passage into stomach.

• Tell patient to take on empty stomach at least 1 hour before meals or 2 hours afterwards.
• Instruct patient to take at least 1 hour before bedtime to prevent esophagitis.
🔊 Tell patient to immediately report painful swallowing, abdominal pain, easy bruising or bleeding, or signs of hypersensitivity (such as rash).
• Advise female patient to tell prescriber if she is pregnant.
• Instruct patient to avoid alcohol use and large amounts of calcium-containing foods (such as dairy products and some green leafy vegetables, such as spinach).
• Stress importance of good oral hygiene.
• As appropriate, review all other significant and life-threatening adverse reactions and interactions, especially those related to the drugs, tests, foods, and behaviors mentioned above.

dronabinol

Marinol

Pharmacologic class: Cannabinoid
Therapeutic class: Antiemetic
Controlled substance IV
Pregnancy risk category B

Action

Unknown. May exert antiemetic effect by inhibiting vomiting control mechanism in medulla oblongata.

Availability

Capsules: 2.5 mg, 5 mg, 10 mg

Indications and dosages

➢ Prevention of nausea and vomiting caused by chemotherapy
Adults and children: Initially, 5 mg/m² P.O. 1 to 3 hours before chemotherapy. Repeat dose q 2 to 4 hours after chemotherapy, up to four to six doses per day. If 5-mg/m² dose is ineffective and patient has no significant adverse reactions, dosage may be increased in increments of 2.5 mg/m² to a maximum dosage of 15 mg/m².
➢ Appetite stimulant
Adults and children: Initially, 2.5 mg P.O. b.i.d. May reduce dosage to 2.5 mg/day given as a single evening or bedtime dose. Maximum dosage is 10 mg P.O. b.i.d.

Contraindications

• Hypersensitivity to cannabinoids or sesame oil
• Breastfeeding

Precautions

Use cautiously in:
• hypertension, heart disease, bipolar disorder, schizophrenia, drug abuse
• pregnant patients.

Administration

• When used to stimulate appetite, give before lunch and dinner.

Route	Onset	Peak	Duration
P.O.	30-60 min	2-4 hr	4-6 hr

Adverse reactions

CNS: drowsiness, anxiety, impaired coordination, irritability, depression, headache, hallucinations, memory loss, paresthesia, ataxia, paranoia, disorientation, nightmares, speech difficulties, syncope, **suicidal ideation**
CV: tachycardia, hypotension, hypertension
EENT: visual disturbances, tinnitus
GI: dry mouth
Skin: facial flushing, diaphoresis

Interactions

Drug-drug. *Anticholinergics, antihistamines, tricyclic antidepressants:* increased tachycardia and hypertension
CNS depressants: increased CNS depression

Ritonavir: increased dronabinol blood level and risk of toxicity
Drug-behaviors. *Alcohol use:* increased CNS depression

Patient monitoring
- Monitor vital signs for hypotension and tachycardia.

Check for adverse CNS reactions. Report significant depression, paranoid reaction, or emotional lability.
- Monitor nutritional status and hydration.

Patient teaching
- Teach patient about drug's significant adverse CNS and cardiovascular effects. Emphasize that he should take it only as prescribed and needed.

Advise patient (and significant other) to immediately report depression, suicidal thoughts, paranoid reactions, and other serious CNS reactions.
- Caution patient to avoid driving and other hazardous activities until he knows how drug affects concentration and alertness.
- As appropriate, review all other significant and life-threatening adverse reactions and interactions, especially those related to the drugs and behaviors mentioned above.

droperidol
Inapsine

Pharmacologic class: Butyrophenone
Therapeutic class: General anesthetic, antiemetic
Pregnancy risk category C

Action
Produces marked sedation by directly blocking subcortical receptors. Produces antiemetic effect by blocking CNS receptors in chemoreceptor trigger zone.

Availability
Injection: 2.5 mg/ml in 1-ml, 2-ml, and 5-ml ampules and in 2-ml, 5-ml, and 10-ml vials

Indications and dosages
➢ Perioperative nausea and vomiting
Adults: Initially, 2.5 mg I.M. or I.V. Additional doses of 1.25 mg may be given. Dosages are highly individualized according to patient's age, weight, physical status, and underlying pathologic condition.
Children ages 2 to 12: Initially, 0.1 mg/kg I.M. or I.V. Additional doses up to a total of 2.5 mg may be given. Dosages are highly individualized according to patient's age, weight, physical status, and underlying clinical condition.

Dosage adjustment
- Elderly or debilitated patients
- High-risk patients (such as patients over age 65 and those with heart failure, alcohol abuse, or other factors that predispose to prolonged QT interval)
- Patients who have received other CNS depressants (such as analgesics or anesthetics)

Off-label uses
- Chemotherapy-induced nausea and vomiting (principally with cisplatin)

Contraindications
- Hypersensitivity to drug
- Known or suspected QT-interval prolongation (more than 440 millisec in males or 450 millisec in females)

Precautions
Use cautiously in:
- severe cardiac or renal disease, diabetes mellitus, respiratory insufficiency, prostatic hypertrophy, angle-closure glaucoma, CNS depression, CNS tumors, intestinal obstruction, bone marrow depression
- elderly patients

• pregnant or breastfeeding patients
• children younger than age 2.

Administration

• Know that drug is indicated to ease perioperative nausea and vomiting only in patients who don't respond adequately to other treatment.
• Be aware that drug doesn't need to be diluted for I.V. or I.M. use.
• Give by slow I.V. injection, or inject I.M. into large muscle.

Route	Onset	Peak	Duration
I.V., I.M.	3-10 min	30 min	2-4 hr

Adverse reactions

CNS: weakness, dysarthria, dysphonia, dizziness, extrapyramidal reactions, headache, postoperative hallucinatory episodes with transient depression, tremor, irritability, paresthesia, aggression, vertigo, ataxia, **loss of consciousness, seizures, neuroleptic malignant syndrome**
CV: chest pain, hypertension, hypotension, vasodilation, **arrhythmias, atrial fibrillation**
EENT: cataracts, blurred vision, eye irritation, sore throat
GI: nausea, vomiting, diarrhea, abdominal cramps, bloating, epigastric pain, fecal incontinence, increased salivation, dysphagia
GU: urinary frequency, increased libido
Hepatic: cholestatic jaundice
Metabolic: dehydration
Musculoskeletal: muscle cramps, arthritis, bone fractures
Respiratory: bronchitis, dyspnea
Skin: bruising, rash, urticaria, facial sweating, diaphoresis, pruritus, flushing
Other: toothache, weight loss, hot flashes, influenza, chills

Interactions

Drug-drug. *Antihypertensives, nitrates:* additive hypertension
CNS depressants (including antidepressants, antihistamines, opioids): additive CNS depression
Drug-herbs. *Chamomile, hops, kava, skullcap, valerian:* increased CNS depression
Drug-behaviors. *Alcohol use:* additive CNS depression

Patient monitoring

🔊 Monitor QT interval; report prolongation. Also watch for torsades de pointes.
🔊 Know that drug may cause sudden death at high doses (above 25 mg) in patients at risk for arrhythmias.
🔊 Monitor for signs and symptoms of neuroleptic malignant syndrome, such as hyperthermia, severe extrapyramidal symptoms, altered mental status, stupor, coma, hypertension, tachycardia, pallor, or diaphoresis. (However, this syndrome is rare.)
• Assess vital signs frequently. Stay alert for orthostatic hypotension and tachycardia. Keep I.V. fluids and vasopressors on hand to treat pronounced hypotension.
🔊 Don't place hypotensive patient in Trendelenburg position because this may deepen anesthesia, precipitating respiratory arrest.
• Avoid abrupt position changes.
• Observe for signs and symptoms of respiratory compromise if drug is used concurrently with narcotics.

Patient teaching

• Advise patient not to drink alcohol or take CNS depressants for 24 hours after receiving drug.
• Tell patient drug may cause extreme drowsiness for several days after administration.
• Caution patient not to drive or perform other activities requiring mental alertness.
• Instruct patient to change positions slowly.

• As appropriate, review all other significant and life-threatening adverse reactions and interactions, especially those related to the drugs, herbs, and behaviors mentioned above.

drotrecogin alfa (activated)
Xigris

Pharmacologic class: Activated protein C (recombinant)
Therapeutic class: Antisepsis drug
Pregnancy risk category C

Action
Antisepsis action unknown. May produce indirect profibrinolytic activity by hindering plasminogen activator inhibitor-1 and limiting generation of activated thrombin-activatable fibrinolysis inhibitor. Produces anti-inflammatory effect by inhibiting human tumor necrosis factor production and suppressing thrombin-induced inflammatory responses.

Availability
Powder for injection (lyophilized): 5 mg, 20 mg

Indications and dosages
➤ Severe sepsis
Adults: 24 mcg/kg/hour I.V. for a total duration of 96 hours

Contraindications
• Hypersensitivity to drug or its components
• Intracranial neoplasm or lesion or evidence of cerebral herniation
• Intracranial or intraspinal surgery within past 2 months
• Hemorrhagic stroke within past 3 months
• Severe head trauma or trauma with increased risk of bleeding
• Active bleeding or high risk of bleeding
• Patients undergoing bone marrow therapy
• Current use of epidural catheter

Precautions
Use cautiously in:
• intracranial arteriovenous malformation, chronic severe hepatic disease, recent GI bleeding
• concurrent use of heparin, thrombolytics, oral anticoagulants, or aspirin
• pregnant patients
• children (safety and efficacy not established).

Administration
• Mix with normal saline solution, lactated Ringer's solution, or dextrose 5% in water.
• Prepare immediately before use. Hang infusion bag within 3 hours of reconstitution; complete infusion within 12 hours after preparation.
• Administer only through infusion pump.
• Don't infuse with any other drug.
• Give entire regimen over 96 hours.
Clinical alert: Discontinue drug 2 hours before invasive procedures.
• Be aware that once hemostasis occurs, drug therapy may resume immediately after uncomplicated invasive procedures or 12 hours after major invasive procedures (such as surgery).

Route	Onset	Peak	Duration
I.V.	Rapid	Unknown	Unknown

Adverse reactions
CNS: intracranial hemorrhage
GI: intra-abdominal, retroperitoneal, or other GI tract bleeding
GU: bleeding
Hematologic: bleeding
Skin: bruising
Other: skin and soft-tissue bleeding, **intrathoracic bleeding**

Interactions

Drug-drug. *Anticoagulants, aspirin, glycoprotein IIb/IIIa inhibitors, indomethacin, phenylbutazone, thrombolytics:* increased risk of bleeding
Drug-diagnostic tests. *Activated partial thromboplastin time (APTT), prothrombin time (PT):* prolonged
Hematocrit: decreased

Patient monitoring

🔊 Know that no antidote exists. Monitor closely for signs and symptoms of hemorrhage. Stop infusion if clinically significant bleeding occurs.
- Monitor PT and CBC (especially platelet count).
- Realize that drug may variably prolong APTT and thus doesn't reliably indicate coagulopathy.

Patient teaching

- As appropriate, review all other significant and life-threatening adverse reactions and interactions, especially those related to the drugs and tests mentioned above.

duloxetine hydrochloride

Cymbalta

Pharmacologic class: Selective serotonin and norepinephrine reuptake inhibitor
Therapeutic class: Antidepressant
Pregnancy risk category C

Action

Unknown. May potentiate serotonergic and noradrenergic activity in CNS.

Availability

Capsules: 20 mg, 30 mg, 60 mg

Indications and dosages

➢ Major depressive disorder
Adults: 20 to 30 mg P.O. b.i.d.
➢ Neuropathic pain associated with peripheral neuropathy
Adults: 60 mg P.O. once daily

Contraindications

- Hypersensitivity to drug or its components
- MAO inhibitor use within past 14 days
- Uncontrolled angle-closure glaucoma

Precautions

Use cautiously in:
- hepatotoxicity, severe renal impairment, seizure disorder, activation of mania or hypomania, controlled angle-closure glaucoma
- heavy alcohol use
- pregnant or breastfeeding patients
- children.

Administration

- Give without regard to meals.
- Make sure patient swallows capsules whole without chewing or crushing. Don't sprinkle contents onto food or mix with liquids.

🔊 Don't give within 14 days of MAO inhibitors. Don't give MAO inhibitors within 5 days of duloxetine withdrawal.

Route	Onset	Peak	Duration
P.O.	Unknown	6 hr	Unknown

Adverse reactions

CNS: fatigue, somnolence, dizziness, tremor, insomnia, anxiety, worsening of depression, increased risk of suicide or suicidal ideation (especially in child or adolescent)
EENT: blurred vision
GI: nausea, vomiting, diarrhea, constipation, dry mouth
GU: abnormal orgasm, erectile or ejaculatory dysfunction, delayed ejaculation, decreased libido
Skin: increased sweating, hot flashes
Other: decreased appetite, weight loss

Interactions

Drug-drug. *Cimetidine, quinolone antibiotics:* decreased duloxetine half-life
Desipramine, flecainide, phenothiazines, propafenone, tricyclic antidepressants: increased blood levels of these drugs
Fluoxetine, paroxetine, quinidine: increased duloxetine blood level
Fluvoxamine: increased duloxetine half-life
Drug-diagnostic tests. *Alanine aminotransferase, alkaline phosphatase, aspartate aminotransferase, creatine kinase:* increased levels
Drug-behaviors. *Alcohol use:* increased risk of hepatic damage
Smoking: decreased duloxetine bioavailability

Patient monitoring

Monitor patient's mental status carefully. Stay alert for mood changes and signs of suicidal ideation, especially in child or adolescent
- Monitor liver function test results and creatinine level for evidence of hepatic impairment.

Don't stop drug therapy abruptly. Dosage must be tapered gradually.

Patient teaching

- Tell patient he can take drug without regard to meals.
- Instruct patient to swallow capsules whole without chewing or crushing. Tell him not to sprinkle contents onto food or mix with liquids.

Advise patient (and parent or significant other as appropriate) to monitor mental status carefully and to immediately report increased depression or suicidal thoughts or behavior (especially in child or adolescent).

Tell patient not to stop taking drug abruptly. Dosage must be tapered gradually.
- Caution patient to avoid driving and other hazardous activities until he knows how drug affects concentration and alertness.
- Instruct patient to avoid heavy alcohol use while taking drug because of increased risk of hepatic damage.
- Tell female patient to notify prescriber if she is pregnant or breastfeeding or plans to become pregnant or to breastfeed.
- As appropriate, review all other significant adverse reactions and interactions, especially those related to the drugs, tests, and behaviors mentioned above.

dutasteride

Avodart

Pharmacologic class: Synthetic 4-azasteroid compound
Therapeutic class: 5-alpha-reductase inhibitor, sex hormone
Pregnancy risk category X

Action

Inhibits 5-alpha-reductase, an intracellular enzyme present in liver, skin, and prostate that's required for conversion of testosterone to 5-alpha-dihydrotestosterone (DHT). DHT appears to be the principal androgen responsible for stimulating prostatic growth.

Availability

Capsules: 0.5 mg

Indications and dosages

➤ Symptomatic benign prostatic hypertrophy
Adults: 0.5 mg P.O. daily

Contraindications

- Hypersensitivity to drug, its components, other 5-alpha-reductase inhibitors, xanthines (such as coffee, theobromine), or ethylenediamine
- Women
- Children

Precautions
Use cautiously in:
- hepatic impairment
- elderly patients.

Administration
Clinical alert: Wear gloves when handling and administering, because drug may be absorbed through skin.
- Don't handle drug if you're pregnant or plan to become pregnant.
- Don't open or crush capsule.
- Give without regard to food.

Route	Onset	Peak	Duration
P.O.	Rapid	2-3 hr	Unknown

Adverse reactions
GI: dyspepsia
GU: decreased libido, decreased ejaculatory volume, erectile dysfunction, gynecomastia

Interactions
Drug-drug. *Cimetidine, ciprofloxacin, diltiazem, ketoconazole, other drugs metabolized by CYP450-3A4 pathway, ritonavir, verapamil:* increased dutasteride blood level
Drug-diagnostic tests. *Prostate-specific antigen (PSA):* decreased level
Thyroid-stimulating hormone: increased level

Patient monitoring
- Monitor fluid intake and output. Assess for ease of starting urine stream and for urinary urgency or frequency.
- Check baseline PSA level; reevaluate at 3 to 6 months.

Patient teaching
- Tell patient to take drug with full glass of water without crushing or opening capsule.
- Instruct patient not to take capsule if it's cracked or leaking.
- Inform patient that drug decreases testosterone production in prostate.
- Tell patient to report dysuria and urinary urgency.

Clinical alert: Advise patient not to donate blood for at least 6 months after final dose.
- Inform patient that drug may decrease ejaculatory volume.
- Explain that sexual side effects eventually will subside.
- As appropriate, review all other significant adverse reactions and interactions, especially those related to the drugs and tests mentioned above.

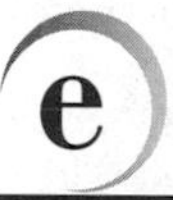

edrophonium chloride
Enlon, Reversol, Tensilon

Pharmacologic class: Anticholinesterase
Therapeutic class: Diagnostic drug, muscle stimulant, antidote
Pregnancy risk category C

Action
Reversibly inhibits cholinesterase, blocking acetylcholine from its release sites in parasympathetic and somatic efferent nerves and increasing acetylcholine concentration in synapses

Availability
Injection: 10 mg/ml in 1-ml ampules and in 10-ml and 15-ml vials

Indications and dosages
➢ Diagnostic aid in myasthenia gravis (Tensilon test)
Adults: 1 to 2 mg I.V. over 15 to 30 seconds; if no response occurs within 45 seconds, give 8 mg. Alternatively, 10 mg I.M.

Children weighing more than 34 kg (75 lb): 2 mg I.V.; if no response occurs within 45 seconds, give 1 mg q 45 seconds, to a maximum of 10 mg. Alternatively, 5 mg I.M.
Children weighing 34 kg (75 lb) or less: 1 mg I.V.; if no response occurs within 45 seconds, give 1 mg q 45 seconds, to a maximum of 5 mg. Alternatively, 2 mg I.M.
➢ To differentiate myasthenic crisis from cholinergic crisis
Adults: 1 mg I.V.; if no response occurs in 1 minute, repeat dose once. Increased muscle strength confirms myasthenic crisis; weakness or no increase in muscle strength confirms cholinergic crisis.
➢ Antidote for curare to reverse nondepolarizing neuromuscular blocking action
Adults: 10 mg I.V. given over 30 to 45 seconds. Repeat dose q 5 to 10 minutes p.r.n. to a maximum of 40 mg.

Contraindications

- Hypersensitivity to drug or sulfites
- Mechanical GI or urinary tract obstruction
- Peritonitis
- Breastfeeding

Precautions

Use cautiously in:
- bronchial asthma, peptic ulcer, bradycardia, arrhythmias, vagotonia, hyperthyroidism, epilepsy, recent coronary occlusion
- pregnant patients.

Administration

- Withdraw anticholinesterase drugs at least 8 hours before test.

[Clinical alert] Keep atropine (edrophonium antidote) readily available.
[Clinical alert] Keep advanced life-saving equipment on hand during administration, because drug may cause respiratory distress.
[Clinical alert] Administer only when continuous ECG monitoring is available.

- Know that drug may be given undiluted and that maximum concentration is 10 mg/ml.
- Frequently assess muscle strength when giving drug for diagnostic or differentiating indications.

Route	Onset	Peak	Duration
I.V.	<1 min	Unknown	5-20 min
I.M.	2-10 min	Unknown	10-40 min

Adverse reactions

CNS: asthenia, dysarthria, dysphonia, dizziness, drowsiness, headache, syncope, **loss of consciousness, seizures**
CV: hypotension, **thrombophlebitis** (with I.V. use), **atrioventricular block, cardiac arrest, bradycardia**
EENT: lacrimation, diplopia, miosis, conjunctival hyperemia
GI: nausea, vomiting, diarrhea, abdominal cramps, increased salivation, dysphagia
GU: urinary frequency or incontinence
Musculoskeletal: muscle cramps, fasciculations
Respiratory: increased secretions, dyspnea, **respiratory muscle paralysis, respiratory depression, central respiratory paralysis, respiratory arrest, bronchospasm, laryngospasm**
Skin: rash, diaphoresis, flushing
Other: anaphylaxis

Interactions

Drug-drug. *Aminoglycosides:* prolonged or increased muscle weakness
Cholinergics: increased cholinergic effects that mimic myasthenia weakness
Corticosteroids, magnesium, procainamide, quinidine: antagonism of cholinergic effects
Depolarizing neuromuscular blockers: increased neuromuscular blockade, prolonged respiratory depression
Local and general anesthetics: antagonism of cholinergic effects

Drug-diagnostic tests. *Urine cannabinoid test:* false-positive result
Drug-food. *High-fat meals:* decreased drug absorption
Drug-herbs. *Jaborandi, pill-bearing spurge:* additive effects

Patient monitoring

◀ When giving as diagnostic test for myasthenia gravis, monitor closely for cholinergic crisis (skeletal muscle fasciculations and increased muscle weakness, especially in respiratory muscles) after 2-mg dose. If cholinergic crisis occurs, discontinue drug and give atropine I.V. as prescribed.
◀ Assess for bradycardia, hypotension, and cardiac arrest.
• Monitor I.V. site closely.
• Observe for nausea and vomiting. Give antiemetics, as prescribed.

Patient teaching

• Tell patient that increased muscle strength is a positive response to drug.
• Advise patient to report vision changes.
• Caution patient to avoid driving and other hazardous activities until he knows how drug affects concentration and alertness.
• As appropriate, review all other significant and life-threatening adverse reactions and interactions, especially those related to the drugs, tests, foods, and herbs mentioned above.

efavirenz

Sustiva

Pharmacologic class: Nonnucleoside reverse transcriptase inhibitor
Therapeutic class: Antiretroviral
Pregnancy risk category C

Action

Inhibits human immunodeficiency virus (HIV) reverse transcriptase (required for transcription of HIV-1 RNA to DNA), leading to viral cell death

Availability

Capsules: 50 mg, 100 mg, 200 mg
Tablets: 600 mg

Indications and dosages

➢ HIV infection (given with one or more additional antiretrovirals)
Adults and children older than age 3 and weighing more than 40 kg (88 lb): 600 mg P.O. once daily
Children weighing 32.5 to 40 kg (71.5 to 88 lb): 400 mg P.O. once daily
Children weighing 25 to 32.5 kg (55 to 71.5 lb): 350 mg P.O. once daily
Children weighing 20 to 25 kg (44 to 55 lb): 300 mg P.O. once daily
Children weighing 15 to 20 kg (33 to 44 lb): 250 mg P.O. once daily
Children weighing 10 to 15 kg (22 to 33 lb): 200 mg P.O. once daily

Contraindications

• Hypersensitivity to drug
• Concurrent use of astemizole, cisapride, midazolam, triazolam, or ergot derivatives

Precautions

Use cautiously in:
• hypercholesterolemia, hepatic impairment, concurrent use of hepatotoxic drugs, mental illness, or substance abuse
• pregnant or breastfeeding patients
• children.

Administration

• Give on empty stomach.
• Know that drug is given with other antiretrovirals.

Route	Onset	Peak	Duration
P.O.	Rapid	3-5 hr	24 hr

Adverse reactions

CNS: dizziness, drowsiness, fatigue, insomnia, abnormal dreams, hypoesthesia, depression, headache, poor concentration, nervousness, anxiety, CNS depression, **suicidal ideation**
CV: arrhythmias
GI: nausea, diarrhea, flatulence, abdominal pain, dyspepsia
GU: hematuria, renal calculi
Hepatic: hepatotoxicity
Respiratory: respiratory depression
Skin: rash, diaphoresis, pruritus, **erythema multiforme, toxic epidermal necrolysis, Stevens-Johnson syndrome**
Other: increased appetite

Interactions

Drug-drug. *Clarithromycin, indinavir:* reduced blood levels of these drugs
CNS depressants (including antidepressants, antihistamines, opioids): increased CNS depression
CYP450 inducers (including phenobarbital, rifabutin, rifampin): increased clearance and decreased blood level of efavirenz
Ergot alkaloids, estrogen, midazolam, ritonavir, triazolam: increased blood levels of these drugs, greater risk of serious adverse reactions (including arrhythmias, CNS and respiratory depression, and hepatotoxicity)
Hormonal contraceptives: increased ethinyl estradiol blood level
Saquinavir: decreased saquinavir blood level
Warfarin: increased or decreased warfarin effects
Drug-diagnostic tests. *Alanine aminotransferase, aspartate aminotransferase, gamma-glutamyltransferase, total cholesterol, triglycerides:* increased levels
Urine cannabinoid test: false-positive result
Drug-food. *High-fat meal:* increased drug absorption
Drug-herbs. *St. John's wort:* decreased efavirenz blood level and efficacy, drug resistance
Drug-behaviors. *Alcohol use:* increased CNS depression

Patient monitoring

- Monitor dietary intake and hepatic and lipid profile.
- Closely monitor patients with hepatic failure.
- [Clinical alert] Record mood changes and stay alert for suicidal ideation or behavior.
- Be aware that drug may cause hypercholesterolemia.
- Know that amount of HIV in blood may increase if patient stops drug therapy even briefly.

Patient teaching

- Instruct patient to take with full glass of water, preferably at bedtime to improve tolerance of CNS effects. Also tell him to avoid taking drug with high-fat meals.
- Inform patient that drug must be taken in combination with other antiretrovirals.
- Tell patient that drug doesn't cure HIV or AIDS and that he can still transmit virus to others.
- [Clinical alert] Advise patient to report suicidal thoughts and other psychiatric symptoms.
- Caution patient to avoid driving and other hazardous activities until he knows how drug affects concentration and alertness.
- [Clinical alert] Tell female patient to immediately inform prescriber if she becomes pregnant.
- As appropriate, review all other significant and life-threatening adverse reactions and interactions, especially those related to the drugs, tests, foods, herbs, and behaviors mentioned above.

eletriptan hydrobromide
Relpax

Pharmacologic class: 5-hydroxytryptamine-1 (5-HT_1) receptor agonist
Therapeutic class: Antimigraine agent
Pregnancy risk category C

Action
Binds with serotonin 5-HT_{1B} receptors on intracranial blood vessels and serotonin 5-HT_{1D} receptors on sensory nerve endings, constricting cranial arteries and thereby relieving migraine

Availability
Tablets: 20 mg, 40 mg

Indications and dosages
➢ Migraine with or without aura
Adults: Initially, 20 to 40 mg P.O.; may repeat in 2 hours if headache returns after initial improvement. Maximum dosage is 80 mg/day.

Contraindications
- Hypersensitivity to drug
- Basilar and hemiplegic migraine
- Severe hepatic disease
- Ischemic heart disease
- Peripheral vascular disease
- Cerebrovascular syndromes
- Uncontrolled hypertension
- Within 24 hours of another serotonin agonist or ergot-type drug

Precautions
Use cautiously in:
- hepatic or renal impairment, diabetes mellitus, hypercholesterolemia, cardiac disorders
- elderly patients
- pregnant or breastfeeding patients
- children.

Administration
- Give first dose as soon as migraine symptoms arise.

Clinical alert: Be aware that first dose should be given under close supervision to patients with coronary artery disease.
- If headache improves but then recurs, give second dose at least 2 hours after first.
- Be aware that drug's safety in treating an average of more than three headaches within a 30-day period has not been established.

Route	Onset	Peak	Duration
P.O.	2 hr	2-3 hr	Unknown

Adverse reactions
CNS: dizziness, insomnia, drowsiness, headache, fatigue, anxiety, paresthesia, asthenia, **cerebrovascular ischemia**
CV: chest pain, palpitations, hypertension, **cardiovascular ischemia**
GI: nausea, vomiting, diarrhea, dry mouth
Musculoskeletal: muscle weakness
Respiratory: chest tightness or pressure
Skin: flushing
Other: hot or cold sensation

Interactions
Drug-drug. *Antihistamines, ergotamine, ergot derivatives:* increased vasospastic effects
CYP450-3A4 inhibitors (such as clarithromycin, ketoconazole, propranolol): increased eletriptan blood level
MAO inhibitors: increased eletriptan effects

Patient monitoring
- Monitor vital signs and assess for chest pain, tightness, or pressure.

Patient teaching
- Instruct patient to take first dose as soon as migraine symptoms occur. If headache improves but then recurs,

advise him to take second dose at least 2 hours after first.
• Caution patient to avoid driving and other hazardous activities until drug no longer affects concentration and alertness.
• Tell patient to report chest pain, pressure, or tightness.
• Inform patient that drug won't prevent migraines and isn't effective against other headache types.
• As appropriate, review all other significant and life-threatening adverse reactions and interactions, especially those related to the drugs mentioned above.

emtricitabine

Emtriva

Pharmacologic class: Nucleoside reverse transcriptase inhibitor
Therapeutic class: Antiretroviral
Pregnancy risk category B

Action

Inhibits activity of human immunodeficiency virus-1 (HIV-1) reverse transcriptase by competing with natural substrate and by its incorporation into nascent viral DNA, thereby halting viral replication

Availability

Capsules: 200 mg

Indications and dosages

➢ HIV-1 infection
Adults: 200 mg P.O. once daily

Dosage adjustment

• Renal impairment

Contraindications

• Hypersensitivity to drug or its components

Precautions

Use cautiously in:
• renal impairment
• increased risk for lactic acidosis or hepatic impairment
• obese patients
• elderly patients
• children (safety and efficacy not established).

Administration

• Give with or without food.
• Know that drug is given with other antiretrovirals.

Route	Onset	Peak	Duration
P.O.	Rapid	1-2 hr	Unknown

Adverse reactions

CNS: dizziness, headache, insomnia, abnormal dreams, depression, peripheral neuritis or neuropathy, paresthesia
EENT: rhinitis
GI: nausea, vomiting, diarrhea, abdominal pain, dyspepsia
Hepatic: hepatotoxicity
Metabolic: cushingoid appearance (buffalo hump, moon face), **lactic acidosis**
Musculoskeletal: joint pain, myalgia
Respiratory: increased cough
Skin: rash, skin discoloration (hyperpigmentation on palms and soles)
Other: body fat redistribution

Interactions

Drug-drug. *Tenofovir disoproxil fumarate:* increased emtricitabine effect
Drug-diagnostic tests. *Alanine aminotransferase, amylase, aspartate aminotransferase, bilirubin, creatine kinase, lipase, triglycerides:* increased levels
Glucose: increased or decreased level
Neutrophils: decreased count

Patient monitoring

🔈 Monitor closely (especially in females and obese patients) for signs and symptoms of lactic acidosis and hepa-

totoxicity, even if patient doesn't have marked transaminase elevations.
• Assess neurologic status, checking especially for depression, peripheral neuropathy, and paresthesia.
• Monitor neutrophil count, lipid panel, liver function tests, and blood glucose level.
Clinical alert: Monitor patient closely for several months after drug withdrawal. Severe, acute exacerbations of hepatitis B virus (HBV) have been reported after discontinuation in patients co-infected with HBV and HIV.
• Monitor nutritional and hydration status in light of GI adverse effects and underlying disease.
• Watch for cushingoid appearance and body fat redistribution.

Patient teaching

• Tell patient to take a missed dose as soon as he remembers. However, if it's almost time for next dose, tell him to skip the missed dose and take next dose as scheduled.
Clinical alert: Instruct patient not to change dosage or stop taking drug unless prescriber approves.
Clinical alert: Tell patient to immediately report signs or symptoms of lactic acidosis—unusual tiredness or muscle pain, difficulty breathing, stomach pain with nausea and vomiting, coldness, dizziness or light-headedness, or fast or irregular heartbeat.
Clinical alert: Instruct patient to immediately report signs or symptoms of liver problems—unusual tiredness, yellowing of skin or eyes, dark urine, light-colored feces, appetite loss, nausea, or pain in lower abdominal area.
• Advise patient to report adverse CNS reactions and to use good judgment about driving and other hazardous activities.
• Caution patient that drug may cause depression. Tell him to notify prescriber if he develops symptoms.
• Inform patient that drug may cause body fat redistribution, dark areas on palms and soles, and rash.
• Tell female patient to inform prescriber if she is pregnant or plans to become pregnant.
• Caution HIV-positive patient not to breastfeed.
• As appropriate, review all other significant and life-threatening adverse reactions and interactions, especially those related to the drugs and tests mentioned above.

emtricitabine and tenofovir disoproxil fumarate

Truvada

Pharmacologic class: Nucleoside/nucleotide reverse-transcriptase inhibitor combination
Therapeutic class: Antiretroviral
Pregnancy risk category B

Action

Inhibits activity of human immunodeficiency virus-1 (HIV-1) reverse transcriptase by competing with natural substrate and by its incorporation into nascent viral DNA, thereby halting viral replication. Tenofovir disoproxil fumarate inhibits activity of HIV-1 reverse transcriptase by competing with the natural substrate deoxyadenosine 5′-triphosphate and by its incorporation into viral DNA, resulting in chain termination.

Availability

Tablets: 200 mg emtricitabine/300 mg tenofovir disoproxil fumarate

Indications and dosages

➢ HIV-1 infection in adults
Adults: 1 tablet P.O. daily

Dosage adjustment
- Renal impairment

Contraindications
- Hypersensitivity to drug or its components

Precautions
Use cautiously in:
- renal impairment
- increased risk of lactic acidosis or hepatic impairment
- decreased bone density
- obese patients
- elderly patients
- children (safety and efficacy not established).

Administration
- Give with or without food.
- Don't give with drug products containing lamivudine.
- Know that drug is usually given with other antiretrovirals.

Route	Onset	Peak	Duration
P.O.	Rapid	1-2 hr	Unknown

Adverse reactions
CNS: headache, insomnia, abnormal dreams, asthenia, dizziness, depressive disorder, neuropathy, peripheral neuropathy, peripheral neuritis, paresthesia
CV: chest pain
EENT: rhinitis
GI: nausea, vomiting, diarrhea, abdominal pain, anorexia, dyspepsia, flatulence, **pancreatitis**
GU: hematuria, glycosuria, proteinuria, proximal tubulopathy, **renal insufficiency, acute tubular necrosis, renal failure, acute renal failure, Fanconi syndrome**
Hepatic: hepatotoxicity
Metabolic: cushingoid appearance (buffalo hump, moon face), hypophosphatemia, **lactic acidosis**
Musculoskeletal: arthralgia, myalgia, back pain
Respiratory: dyspnea, increased cough, pneumonia
Skin: sweating, rash, pruritus, urticaria, skin discoloration (hyperpigmentation of palms and soles)
Other: weight loss, fever, allergic reaction, body fat redistribution

Interactions
Drug-drug. *Acyclovir, adefovir dipivoxil, cidofovir, ganciclovir, valacyclovir, valganciclovir:* increased concentration of emtricitabine/tenofovir
Atazanavir, lopinavir/ritonavir: increased tenofovir concentration
Didanosine: increased didanosine concentration
Drug-diagnostic tests. *Alanine phosphatase, amylase, aspartate aminotransferase, bilirubin, creatine kinase, creatinine, lipase, urine and serum glucose:* increased levels
Neutrophils: decreased count

Patient monitoring
[Clinical alert] Monitor patient closely (especially female or obese patient) for signs and symptoms of lactic acidosis and hepatotoxicity, even if patient doesn't have marked transaminase elevations.
- Assess neurologic status, especially for depression, peripheral neuropathy, and paresthesia.
- Monitor neutrophil count, lipid panel, liver function test results, and blood glucose level.
- Monitor renal function closely, especially if patient is receiving nephrotoxic agents.

[Clinical alert] Monitor patient closely for several months after drug withdrawal. Severe, acute exacerbations of hepatitis B virus (HBV) have been reported after discontinuation in patients co-infected with HBV and HIV.
- Monitor nutritional and hydration status in light of GI adverse effects and underlying disease.
- Watch for cushingoid appearance and body fat redistribution.

Patient teaching

Clinical alert: Instruct patient not to change dosage or stop taking drug unless prescriber approves.

Clinical alert: Advise patient to immediately report signs or symptoms of lactic acidosis—unusual tiredness or muscle pain, difficulty breathing, stomach pain with nausea and vomiting, coldness, dizziness or light-headedness, and fast or irregular heartbeat.

Clinical alert: Instruct patient to immediately report signs and symptoms of liver problems—unusual tiredness, yellowing of skin or eyes, dark urine, light-colored feces, appetite loss, nausea, and lower abdominal pain.

- Advise patient to notify prescriber of adverse CNS reactions and to use good judgment about driving and other hazardous activities.
- Inform patient that drug may cause depression. Tell him to notify prescriber if he develops symptoms.
- Inform patient that drug may cause body fat redistribution, rash, and dark areas on palms and soles.
- Advise patient to tell prescriber if he has bone problems before taking drug.
- Tell female patient to inform prescriber if she is pregnant or plans to become pregnant.
- Caution HIV-positive patient not to breastfeed.
- If patient misses a dose, instruct him to take it as soon as he remembers. However, if it's almost time for next dose, tell him to skip the missed dose and take next dose as scheduled.
- As appropriate, review all other significant and life-threatening adverse reactions and interactions, especially those related to the drugs and tests mentioned above.

enalapril maleate
Vasotec

enalaprilat
Vasotec IV

Pharmacologic class: Angiotensin-converting enzyme (ACE) inhibitor
Therapeutic class: Antihypertensive
Pregnancy risk category C (first trimester), ***D*** (second and third trimesters)

Action

Inhibits conversion of angiotensin I to angiotensin II, a potent vasoconstrictor; inactivates bradykinin and prostaglandins. Also increases plasma renin and potassium levels and reduces aldosterone levels, resulting in systemic vasodilation.

Availability

Injection: 1.25 mg/ml
Tablets: 2.5 mg, 5 mg, 10 mg, 20 mg

Indications and dosages

➢ Hypertension

Adults: For patients not taking concomitant diuretics—initially, 5 mg P.O. once daily, increased after 1 to 2 weeks as needed to a maintenance dosage of 10 to 40 mg P.O. daily given as a single dose or in two divided doses; or 1.25 mg I.V. q 6 hours. For patients taking diuretics—initially, 2.5 mg P.O. or 0.625 mg I.V.

Children: 0.08 mg/kg P.O. once daily; may be increased based on blood pressure response up to 5 mg daily. Maximum dosage is 0.58 mg/kg/dose.

➢ Heart failure

Adults: Initially, 2.5 mg P.O. once or twice daily, increased after 1 to 2 weeks as needed to maintenance dosage of 5 to 40 mg P.O. daily given as a single dose or in two divided doses

➢ Asymptomatic left ventricular dysfunction

Adults: Initially, 2.5 mg P.O. once or twice daily, increased after 1 to 2 weeks as needed to a maximum of 20 mg/day in divided doses

Dosage adjustment

- Renal impairment

Off-label uses

- Diabetic nephropathy
- Hypertensive emergency

Contraindications

- Hypersensitivity to drug or other ACE inhibitors
- Angioedema
- Pregnancy

Precautions

Use cautiously in:

- renal or hepatic impairment, hypovolemia, hyponatremia, aortic stenosis, hypertrophic cardiomyopathy, cerebrovascular or cardiac insufficiency
- black patients with hypertension
- concurrent diuretic use
- elderly patients
- breastfeeding patients
- children.

Administration

- Give oral doses with food or beverage.
- Discontinue diuretics for 2 to 3 days before starting drug, if possible.
- Know that I.V. administration is usually reserved for patients who cannot take P.O. form.
- Be aware that I.V. administration isn't recommended for pediatric patients.
- Administer I.V. dose either undiluted or diluted in 50 ml of dextrose 5% in water, normal saline solution, dextrose 5% in normal saline solution, or dextrose 5% in lactated Ringer's solution.
- Give single I.V. dose by push or piggyback over 5 minutes. If patient's at risk for hypotension, infusion may be given over 1 hour.

Route	Onset	Peak	Duration
P.O.	1 hr	4-6 hr	24 hr
I.V.	15 min	3-4 hr	6 hr

e

Adverse reactions

CNS: dizziness, fatigue, headache, insomnia, drowsiness, vertigo, asthenia, paresthesia, ataxia, confusion, depression, nervousness, **cerebrovascular accident**

CV: orthostatic hypotension, palpitations, angina pectoris, tachycardia, peripheral edema, **arrhythmias, cardiac arrest**

EENT: sinusitis

GI: nausea, vomiting, constipation, dyspepsia, abdominal pain, dry mouth, **pancreatitis**

GU: proteinuria, urinary tract infection, erectile dysfunction, decreased libido, **oliguria**

Hematologic: agranulocytosis, bone marrow depression

Hepatic: hepatitis

Metabolic: hyponatremia, **hyperkalemia**

Respiratory: cough, upper respiratory tract infection, asthma, bronchitis, dyspnea, **eosinophilic pneumonitis**

Skin: rash, alopecia, photosensitivity, diaphoresis, exfoliative dermatitis, angioedema, **erythema multiforme**

Other: altered taste, fever, increased appetite, anaphylactoid reactions

Interactions

Drug-drug. *Allopurinol:* increased risk of hypersensitivity reaction

Antacids: decreased enalapril absorption

Cyclosporine, indomethacin, potassium-sparing diuretics, potassium supplements: hyperkalemia

Digoxin, lithium: increased blood levels of these drugs, possible toxicity
Diuretics, nitrates, other antihypertensives, phenothiazines: additive hypotension
Nonsteroidal anti-inflammatory drugs: decreased antihypertensive response
Rifampin: decreased enalapril efficacy
Drug-diagnostic tests. *Alanine aminotransferase, alkaline phosphatase, aspartate aminotransferase, bilirubin, blood urea nitrogen (BUN), creatinine, potassium:* increased levels
Antinuclear antibodies: positive titer
Sodium: decreased level
Drug-food. *Salt substitutes containing potassium:* hyperkalemia
Drug-herbs. *Capsaicin:* increased incidence of cough
Drug-behaviors. *Acute alcohol ingestion:* additive hypotension
Sun exposure: photosensitivity reaction

Patient monitoring

🔈 Assess for rapid blood pressure drop leading to cardiovascular collapse, especially when giving with diuretics.
🔈 In patient with renal insufficiency or renal artery stenosis, monitor for worsening renal function.
- After initial dose, observe patient closely for at least 2 hours until blood pressure has stabilized. Then continue to observe for additional hour.
- Monitor vital signs, fluid intake and output, and daily weight.
- Supervise patient during ambulation until effects of drug are known.
- Monitor liver function tests, BUN, and creatinine and electrolyte levels.

Patient teaching

- Inform patient that drug's full effect may not occur for several weeks.
- Advise patient to report persistent dry cough with nasal congestion.

🔈 Tell patient to immediately report swelling of face, eye area, tongue, lips, hands, or feet; rash, hives, or severe itching; unexplained fever; unusual tiredness; yellowing of skin or eyes; abdominal pain; or easy bruising.
- Instruct patient to move slowly when sitting up or standing, to avoid dizziness or light-headedness from sudden blood pressure decrease.
- As appropriate, review all other significant and life-threatening adverse reactions and interactions, especially those related to the drugs, tests, foods, herbs, and behaviors mentioned above.

enfuvirtide

Fuzeon

Pharmacologic class: Human immunodeficiency-1 (HIV-1) fusion inhibitor
Therapeutic class: Antiretroviral
Pregnancy risk category B

Action

Interferes with entry of HIV-1 into cells by inhibiting fusion of viral and cellular membranes

Availability

Powder for injection: 90 mg/1-ml vial

Indications and dosages

➢ HIV-1 infection
Adults: 90 mg subcutaneously b.i.d. in upper arm, anterior thigh, or abdomen
Children ages 6 to 16: 2 mg/kg subcutaneously b.i.d. in upper arm, anterior thigh, or abdomen. Maximum dosage is 90 mg b.i.d.

Contraindications

- Hypersensitivity to drug or its components

Precautions

Use cautiously in:
- increased risk of pneumonia

- injection site reaction
- elderly patients
- children younger than age 6 (safety and efficacy not established).

Administration

- Rotate injection sites.
- Be aware that preferred injection sites are upper arm, anterior thigh, and abdomen.
- Reconstitute with 1.1 ml of sterile water for injection, and gently tap vial for 10 seconds. Then gently roll vial between hands or allow vial to stand until product dissolves completely (could take up to 45 minutes).
- Know that drug is usually given with other antiretrovirals.
- Use reconstituted solution immediately.

Route	Onset	Peak	Duration
Subcut.	Unknown	4 hr	Unknown

Adverse reactions

CNS: fatigue, asthenia, insomnia, depression, anxiety, peripheral neuropathy
EENT: conjunctivitis, sinusitis
GI: nausea, diarrhea, upper abdominal pain, dry mouth, anorexia, pancreatitis
Hematologic: lymphadenopathy
Musculoskeletal: limb pain, myalgia
Respiratory: cough, pneumonia
Skin: folliculitis
Other: taste disturbance, decreased appetite, weight loss, herpes simplex infection, injection site reactions (erythema, induration, nodules, cysts, mild to moderate pain, infection), flulike illness, hypersensitivity reactions

Interactions

Drug-diagnostic tests. *Alanine aminotransferase, amylase, aspartate aminotransferase, creatine kinase, eosinophils, gamma-glutamyltransferase, lipase, triglycerides:* increased levels
Hemoglobin: decreased level

Patient monitoring

- Inspect injection sites frequently for adverse reactions.
- Monitor CBC with white cell differential, lipid panel, liver function test results, and gastric enzymes levels.
- Watch for hypersensitivity reactions.
- Monitor nutritional and hydration status in light of GI adverse effects and underlying disease.

Patient teaching

- Teach patient (or caregiver) how to reconstitute and self-administer drug, as appropriate.
- [Clinical alert] Instruct patient not to change dosage or stop taking drug unless prescriber approves.
- [Clinical alert] Tell patient to immediately report signs or symptoms of hypersensitivity reaction (such as rash, fever, nausea and vomiting, and chills).
- Teach patient how to recognize signs and symptoms of injection site reaction. Tell him to contact prescriber if these occur, especially if they last more than 7 days.
- Advise female patient to notify prescriber if she is pregnant or plans to become pregnant.
- Tell HIV-infected patient not to breastfeed.
- If patient misses a dose, instruct him to take it as soon as he remembers. However, if it's almost time for next dose, tell him to skip the missed dose and take next dose on schedule.
- As appropriate, review all other significant adverse reactions and interactions, especially those related to the tests mentioned above.

enoxaparin sodium

Lovenox

Pharmacologic class: Low-molecular-weight heparin
Therapeutic class: Anticoagulant
Pregnancy risk category B

Action

Inhibits thrombus and clot formation by blocking factor Xa and factor IIa. This inhibition accelerates formation of antithrombin III-thrombin complex (a coagulation inhibitor), thereby deactivating thrombin and preventing conversion of fibrinogen to fibrin.

Availability

Solution for injection: 30 mg/0.3 ml, 40 mg/0.4 ml, 60 mg/0.6 ml, 80 mg/0.8 ml, 100 mg/1 ml (all in prefilled syringes); 300 mg/3 ml (in multidose vials)

Indications and dosages

➢ Prevention of pulmonary embolism and deep-vein thrombosis (DVT) after abdominal surgery

Adults: 40 mg subcutaneously 2 hours before surgery, repeated 24 hours after initial dose (provided hemostasis has been established) and continued once daily for 7 to 10 days until risk of DVT has diminished

➢ Prevention of pulmonary embolism and DVT after hip or knee replacement surgery

Adults: 30 mg subcutaneously 12 to 24 hours after surgery (provided hemostasis has been established), repeated q 12 hours for 7 to 10 days until risk of DVT has diminished. Alternatively, hip-replacement patient may receive 40 mg subcutaneously 12 hours before surgery and then once daily for 3 weeks, for a total of 4 weeks of therapy.

➢ Prevention of ischemic complications of unstable angina or non-Q-wave myocardial infarction

Adults: 1 mg/kg subcutaneously q 12 hours, given with aspirin 100 to 325 mg P.O. once daily until patient is clinically stable

➢ Hospitalized patients with acute DVT with or without pulmonary embolism (PE) (given with warfarin sodium)

Adults: 1 mg/kg subcutaneously q 12 hours or 1.5 mg/kg subcutaneously once daily for 5 to 7 days until therapeutic effect is established. Warfarin therapy usually begins within 72 hours of enoxaparin injection.

➢ Outpatients with acute DVT without PE (given with warfarin sodium)

Adults: 1 mg/kg subcutaneously q 12 hours for 5 to 7 days until therapeutic effect is established. Warfarin therapy usually begins within 72 hours of enoxaparin injection.

Dosage adjustment

- Patients weighing less than 45 kg (99 lb)
- Creatinine clearance below 30 ml/minute

Off-label uses

- Prevention of clots associated with hemodialysis
- Prevention of thrombosis during pregnancy

Contraindications

- Hypersensitivity to drug, heparin, sulfites, benzyl alcohol, or pork products
- Thrombocytopenia
- Active major bleeding

Precautions

Use cautiously in:

- severe hepatic or renal disease, retinopathy (hypertensive or diabetic), uncontrolled hypertension, hemor-

rhagic stroke, bacterial endocarditis, GI bleeding or other bleeding disorders
• recent history of ulcer disease, history of congenital or acquired bleeding disorder, history of thrombocytopenia related to heparin use
• recent CNS surgery
• pregnant or breastfeeding patients
• children.

Administration

🔊 Be aware that enoxaparin is a high-alert drug.
• Use tuberculin syringe with multidose vial to ensure accurate dosage.
• Don't expel air bubble from syringe before administering.
• Inject drug deep subcutaneously with patient in supine position. Alternate left and right anterolateral and posterolateral abdominal wall sites.
• Don't rub injection site.
🔊 Don't give by I.M. or I.V. route.

Route	Onset	Peak	Duration
Subcut.	Unknown	3-5 hr	24 hr

Adverse reactions

CNS: dizziness, headache, insomnia, confusion, **cerebrovascular accident**
CV: edema, chest pain, **atrial fibrillation, heart failure**
GI: nausea, vomiting, constipation
GU: urinary retention
Hematologic: anemia, **bleeding tendency, thrombocytopenia, hemorrhage**
Metabolic: hyperkalemia
Skin: bruising, pruritus, rash, urticaria
Other: fever; pain, irritation, or erythema at injection site

Interactions

Drug-drug. *Warfarin, other drugs that affect platelet function (including abciximab, aspirin, clopidogrel, dextran, dipyridamole, eptifibatide, nonsteroidal anti-inflammatory drugs [NSAIDs], some penicillins, ticlopidine, tirofiban):* increased risk of bleeding
Drug-diagnostic tests. *Hepatic enzymes:* reversible increases
Hemoglobin, platelets: decreased levels
Drug-herbs. *Anise, arnica, chamomile, clove, feverfew, garlic, ginger, ginkgo, ginseng:* increased risk of bleeding

Patient monitoring

• Monitor CBC and platelet counts. Watch for signs and symptoms of bleeding or bruising.
• Monitor fluid intake and output. Watch for fluid retention and edema.

Patient teaching

• If patient will self-administer drug, teach proper injection technique.
🔊 Instruct patient to promptly report irregular heart beat, unusual bleeding or bruising, rash, or hives.
• Teach patient safety measures to avoid bruising or bleeding.
• Advise patient to weigh himself regularly and to report gains.
• As appropriate, review all other significant and life-threatening adverse reactions and interactions, especially those related to the drugs, tests, and herbs mentioned above.

entacapone

Comtan

Pharmacologic class: Catechol O-methyltransferase (COMT) inhibitor
Therapeutic class: Antidyskinetic
Pregnancy risk category C

Action

Inhibits COMT, the primary enzyme involved in metabolizing levodopa. This inhibition increases levodopa blood level and duration of action, easing symptoms of Parkinson's disease.

Availability

Tablets: 200 mg

Indications and dosages

➢ Adjunctive treatment of idiopathic Parkinson's disease in patients experiencing wearing off of carbidopa-levodopa effects
Adults: 200 mg P.O. with each carbidopa-levodopa dose, to a maximum of eight times daily (1,600 mg)

Contraindications

- Hypersensitivity to drug
- Pregnancy or breastfeeding

Precautions

Use cautiously in:
- hepatic or renal dysfunction, hypertension, heart disease.

Administration

- Give without regard to food.
- Administer at same time as carbidopa-levodopa. Make sure patient swallows tablet whole.

Don't withdraw drug abruptly.

Route	Onset	Peak	Duration
P.O.	Variable	1 hr	Unknown

Adverse reactions

CNS: dizziness, depression, drowsiness, disorientation, memory loss, agitation, delusions, hallucinations, paranoia, euphoria, dyskinesia, hyperkinesia, light-headedness, paresthesia, heaviness of limbs, numbness of fingers
CV: tachycardia, orthostatic hypotension, hypertension
GI: nausea, vomiting, epigastric pain, flatulence
GU: urine discoloration
Respiratory: upper respiratory tract infection, dyspnea, sinus congestion
Other: fever

Interactions

Drug-drug. *Ampicillin, chloramphenicol, cholestyramine, erythromycin, probenecid, rifampin:* decreased entacapone excretion
Bitolterol, dobutamine, dopamine, epinephrine, isoetherine, methyldopa, norepinephrine: increased heart rate, increased risk of arrhythmias, excessive blood pressure changes
MAO inhibitors: increased risk of toxicity
Drug-behaviors. *Alcohol use:* increased risk of adverse reactions

Patient monitoring

- Monitor vital signs, watching especially for orthostatic hypotension.
- Evaluate neurologic status closely. Check for hallucinations and new onset or exacerbation of dyskinesia.
- Assess respiratory status, particularly for dyspnea and signs and symptoms of upper respiratory tract infection.
- Monitor nutritional and hydration status if patient experiences vomiting.

Patient teaching

- Instruct patient to swallow tablet whole and to take it at same time as carbidopa-levodopa.

Caution patient not to stop taking drug abruptly.

- Advise patient to move slowly when sitting up or standing, to avoid dizziness or light-headedness from sudden blood pressure decrease.
- Caution patient to avoid driving and other hazardous activities until drug no longer affects concentration and alertness.

Instruct patient (and caregiver) to institute safety measures at home to prevent injury related to disease or drug's adverse CNS effects.

- As appropriate, review all other significant adverse reactions and interactions, especially those related to the drugs and behaviors mentioned above.

ephedrine

ephedrine sulfate

Pharmacologic class: Sympathomimetic
Therapeutic class: Bronchodilator, vasopressor, nasal decongestant
Pregnancy risk category C

Action

Stimulates $beta_2$-adrenergic receptors, relaxing bronchial smooth muscle and relieving bronchospasm. Also stimulates alpha-adrenergic receptors and promotes norepinephrine release from sympathetic neurons, which increases blood pressure and cardiac output.

Availability

Capsules: 25 mg, 50 mg
Injection: 25 mg/ml, 30 mg/ml, 50 mg/ml
Nasal jelly: 0.6%
Nasal spray: 0.25%

Indications and dosages

➤ Hypotension
Adults: 25 mg P.O. one to four times daily, or 25 to 50 mg I.M. or subcutaneously, or 10 to 25 mg I.V. p.r.n. Maximum dosage is 150 mg daily.
Children: 3 mg/kg or 25 to 100 mg/m² subcutaneously or I.V. daily in four to six divided doses
➤ Bronchodilation; nasal decongestion
Adults and children older than age 12: 12.5 to 50 mg P.O. q 3 to 4 hours p.r.n; maximum dosage is 150 mg daily. As a decongestant, two or three sprays in each nostril, or nasal jelly applied in each nostril q 4 hours.
Children ages 6 to 12: 6.25 to 12.5 mg P.O. q 4 hours; maximum dosage is 75 mg daily. As a decongestant, one or two sprays in each nostril q 4 hours.
Children older than age 2: 2 to 3 mg/kg or 100 mg/m² P.O. daily in four to six divided doses. As a decongestant, one or two sprays in each nostril q 4 hours.

Contraindications

- Hypersensitivity to drug
- Severe coronary artery disease
- Angina pectoris
- Angle-closure glaucoma
- MAO inhibitor use within past 14 days

Precautions

Use cautiously in:
- hypertension, heart disease, hepatic or renal dysfunction, hyperthyroidism, diabetes mellitus, prostatic hypertrophy
- elderly patients
- breastfeeding patients.

Administration

- Give direct I.V. injection slowly, giving each 10 mg-dose over 1 minute.

Route	Onset	Peak	Duration
P.O.	15-60 min	Unknown	3-5 hr
I.V.	5 min	Unknown	1 hr
I.M., subcut.	10-20 min	Unknown	0.5-1 hr
Intranasal	Unknown	Unknown	Unknown

Adverse reactions

CNS: dizziness, headache, euphoria, insomnia, nervousness, confusion, delirium, tremor, **cerebral hemorrhage**
CV: palpitations, tachycardia, hypertension, precordial pain, **arrhythmias**
EENT: dry nose or throat
GI: nausea, vomiting, epigastric pain, flatulence
GU: urinary retention, dysuria
Musculoskeletal: muscle weakness
Skin: diaphoresis

Interactions

Drug-drug. *Acetazolamide:* increased ephedrine blood level
Alpha-adrenergic blockers: unopposed beta-adrenergic effects, resulting in hypotension
Antihypertensives: decreased antihypertensive effects
Beta-adrenergic blockers: unopposed alpha-adrenergic effects, resulting in hypertension
Cardiac glycosides, general anesthetics: increased risk of ventricular arrhythmias
Ergot alkaloids: enhanced vasoconstrictor and pressor effects
Guanadrel, guanethidine: potentiation of pressor response
MAO inhibitors, tricyclic antidepressants: severe hypertension
Methyldopa, reserpine: inhibition of ephedrine's effects

Patient monitoring

- 🔈 Monitor vital signs and ECG, staying alert for tachycardia, arrhythmia, and hypertension.
- Assess cardiovascular status closely. Ask patient about precordial pain.
- 🔈 Monitor neurologic status, particularly for signs and symptoms of cerebral hemorrhage.
- Measure fluid intake and output, and watch for urinary retention.

Patient teaching

- Tell patient taking drug orally that insomnia may occur. Encourage him to take dose at least 2 hours before bedtime.
- Inform patient that drug may cause abnormal heartbeats. Assure him that he'll be closely monitored, and instruct him to report chest pain.
- 🔈 Urge patient to promptly report severe headache or significant CNS changes.
- Caution patient to avoid driving and other hazardous activities until he knows how drug affects concentration and alertness.
- As appropriate, review all other significant and life-threatening adverse reactions and interactions, especially those related to the drugs mentioned above.

epinephrine

Bronkaid Mistometer✱, Primatene Mist, Twinject

epinephrine bitartrate

Bronitin Mist

epinephrine hydrochloride

EpiPen, EpiPen Jr.

Pharmacologic class: Sympathomimetic (direct acting)
Therapeutic class: Bronchodilator, mydriatic
Pregnancy risk category C

Action

Stimulates alpha- and beta-adrenergic receptors, causing relaxation of cardiac and bronchial smooth muscle and dilation of skeletal muscles. Also decreases aqueous humor production, increases aqueous outflow, and dilates pupils by contracting dilator muscle.

Availability

Aerosol inhaler: 160 mcg, 200 mcg, 220 mcg, 250 mcg
Auto-injector for I.M. injection: 1:2,000 (0.5 mg/ml)
Injection: 0.01 mg/ml, 0.1 mg/ml, 0.5 mg/ml, 1 mg/ml, 5 mg/ml parenteral suspension
Nebulizer inhaler: 1%, 1.25%, 2.25%
Ophthalmic drops: 0.5%, 1%, 2%
Solution: 1:200,000

Indications and dosages

➢ Bronchodilation; anaphylaxis; hypersensitivity reaction

Adults: 0.1 to 0.5 ml of 1:1,000 solution subcutaneously or I.M., repeated q 10 to 15 minutes p.r.n. Or 0.1 to 0.25 ml of 1:10,000 solution I.V. slowly over 5 to 10 minutes; may repeat q 5 to 15 minutes p.r.n. or follow with a continuous infusion of 1 mcg/minute, increased to 4 mcg/minute p.r.n. For emergency treatment, EpiPen delivers 0.3 mg I.M. of 1:1,000 epinephrine.

Children: For emergency treatment, EpiPen Jr. delivers 0.15 mg I.M. of 1:2,000 epinephrine.

➢ Acute asthma attack

Adults and children ages 4 and older: 160 to 250 mcg metered aerosol (equivalent to one inhalation); repeat once after 1 minute, if needed. Don't give subsequent doses for at least 3 hours. Or one to three deep inhalations of 1% solution with hand-held nebulizer, repeated q 3 hours p.r.n.

➢ To restore cardiac rhythm in cardiac arrest

Adults: 0.5 to 1 mg I.V., repeated q 3 to 5 minutes, if needed. If no response, may give 3 to 5 mg I.V. q 3 to 5 minutes.

➢ Chronic simple glaucoma

Adults: One drop in affected eye once or twice daily. Adjust dosage to meet patient's needs.

➢ To prolong local anesthetic effects

Adults and children: 1:200,000 concentration with local anesthetic

Contraindications

- Hypersensitivity to drug, its components, or sulfites
- Angle-closure glaucoma
- Cardiac disease
- Cerebral arteriosclerosis
- MAO inhibitor use within past 14 days
- Labor
- Breastfeeding

Precautions

Use cautiously in:

- hypertension, hyperthyroidism, diabetes, prostatic hypertrophy
- elderly patients
- pregnant patients
- children.

Administration

- In anaphylaxis, use I.M. route, not subcutaneous route, if possible.

🔊 Inject EpiPen and EpiPen Jr. only into anterolateral aspect of thigh. Don't inject into buttocks or give I.V.

🔊 Be aware that not all epinephrine solutions can be given I.V. Check manufacturer's label.

- For I.V. injection, give each 1-mg dose over at least 1 minute. For continuous infusion, use rate of 1 to 10 mcg/minute, adjusting to desired response.
- Use Epi-Pen Jr. for patients weighing less than 30 kg (66 lb).

🔊 Don't give within 14 days of MAO inhibitors.

Route	Onset	Peak	Duration
I.V.	Immediate	5 min	Short
I.M.	Variable	Unknown	1-4 hr
Subcut.	5-15 min	0.5 hr	1-4 hr
Inhalation	1-5 min	Unknown	1-3 hr

Adverse reactions

CNS: nervousness, anxiety, tremor, vertigo, headache, disorientation, agitation, drowsiness, fear, dizziness, asthenia, **cerebral hemorrhage, cerebrovascular accident** (CVA)

CV: palpitations, widened pulse pressure, hypertension, tachycardia, angina, ECG changes, **ventricular fibrillation, shock**

GI: nausea, vomiting

GU: decreased urinary output, urinary retention, dysuria

Respiratory: dyspnea, **pulmonary edema**

Skin: urticaria, pallor, diaphoresis, necrosis
Other: hemorrhage at injection site

Interactions

Drug-drug. *Alpha-adrenergic blockers:* hypotension from unopposed beta-adrenergic effects
Antihistamines, thyroid hormone, tricyclic antidepressants: severe sympathomimetic effects
Beta-adrenergic blockers (such as propranolol): vasodilation and reflex tachycardia
Cardiac glycosides, general anesthetics: increased risk of ventricular arrhythmias
Diuretics: decreased vascular response
Doxapram, mazindol, methylphenidate: enhanced CNS stimulation or pressor effects
Ergot alkaloids: decreased vasoconstriction
Guanadrel, guanethidine: enhanced pressor effects of epinephrine
Levodopa: increased risk of arrhythmias
Levothyroxine: potentiation of epinephrine effects
MAO inhibitors: increased risk of hypertensive crisis
Drug-diagnostic tests. *Glucose:* transient elevation
Lactic acid: elevated level (with prolonged use)

Patient monitoring

🔊 Monitor vital signs, ECG, and cardiovascular and respiratory status. Watch for ventricular fibrillation, tachycardia, arrhythmias, and signs and symptoms of shock. Ask patient about anginal pain.
- Assess drug's effect on underlying problem (such as anaphylaxis or asthma attack), and repeat dose as needed.

🔊 Monitor neurologic status, particularly for decreased level of consciousness and other signs and symptoms of cerebral hemorrhage or CVA.
- Monitor fluid intake and output, watching for urinary retention or decreased urinary output.
- Inspect injection site for hemorrhage or skin necrosis.

Patient teaching

- Teach patient who uses auto-injector how to use syringe correctly, when to inject drug, and when to repeat doses.
- Teach patient who uses hand-held nebulizer correct use of equipment and drug. Explain indications for both initial dose and repeat doses.

🔊 Inform patient that drug may cause serious adverse effects. Tell him which symptoms to report.
- If patient will self-administer drug outside of health care setting, explain need for prompt evaluation by a health care provider to ensure that underlying disorder has been corrected.
- As appropriate, review all other significant and life-threatening adverse reactions and interactions, especially those related to the drugs and tests mentioned above.

epirubicin hydrochloride

Ellence, Pharmorubicin RDF

Pharmacologic class: Anthracycline
Therapeutic class: Antibiotic antineoplastic
Pregnancy risk category D

Action

Unknown. Forms complex with DNA by intercalation with nucleotide base pairs, causing inhibition of DNA, RNA, and protein synthesis.

Availability

Injection: 2 mg/ml, 50 mg/25 ml, 200 mg/dl

Indications and dosages

➤ Adjunctive therapy in patients with axillary-node tumor involvement after resection of primary breast cancer

Adults: 100 to 120 mg/m² by I.V. infusion over 3 to 5 minutes on first day of each cycle or divided equally in two doses on days 1 and 8 of each cycle; repeat cycle q 3 to 4 weeks for six cycles in conjunction with cyclophosphamide and fluorouracil. After first cycle, dosage adjustments are based on toxicity. For patients with platelet count below 50,000/mm³, absolute neutrophil count (ANC) below 250/mm³, neutropenic fever, or grade 3 or 4 nonhematologic toxicity, reduce first day's dosage in subsequent cycles to 75% and delay subsequent cycles until platelet count is at least 100,000/mm³, ANC is at least 1,500/mm³, and nonhematologic toxicity recovers to grade 1 or better.

Off-label uses

- Cancer of bladder, lung, nasopharynx, endometrium, and ovaries

Contraindications

- Hypersensitivity to drug
- Myocardial insufficiency
- Severe hepatic dysfunction
- Baseline neutrophil count below 1,500/mm³
- Cumulative doses above 900 mg/m²

Precautions

Use cautiously in:

- heart disease, hepatic disease
- previous or recent radiation therapy
- pregnant or breastfeeding patients
- children.

Administration

- Be aware that drug may be given with antibiotics.
- Know that previous anthracycline use must be considered when determining dosage because of increased risk of heart failure.
- Follow facility policy for administration and disposal of carcinogenic drugs.

Clinical alert: Avoid extravasation. If patient complains of burning or stinging, switch infusion to a different vein.

- Administer premixed solution over 3 to 5 minutes into tubing of free-flowing I.V. line containing dextrose 5% in water or normal saline solution.
- Direct I.V. push is not recommended because of extravasation risk.
- If patient develops facial flushing or red streak in the vein being infused, slow infusion rate.

Route	Onset	Peak	Duration
I.V.	Unknown	Unknown	Unknown

Adverse reactions

CNS: lethargy
CV: **cardiomyopathy, heart failure**
EENT: conjunctivitis, keratitis
GI: nausea, vomiting, diarrhea, mucositis
GU: reddish urine, amenorrhea
Hematologic: anemia, **leukopenia, neutropenia, thrombocytopenia**
Skin: alopecia; rash; pruritus; darkening of soles, palms, or nails
Other: increased appetite, infection, fever, hot flashes, tissue necrosis

Interactions

Drug-drug. *Calcium channel blockers:* increased risk of heart failure
Cimetidine: increased epirubicin blood level
Cytotoxic drugs: additive toxicity
Live-virus vaccines: increased risk of infection
Trastuzumab: increased risk of cardiac dysfunction
Drug-diagnostic tests. *Hemoglobin, neutrophils, platelets, white blood cells:* decreased values

Patient monitoring

🔈 Monitor vital signs, left ventricular ejection fraction, and cardiovascular status carefully. Watch for signs and symptoms of cardiomyopathy and heart failure.
- Assess nutritional status and hydration in light of GI adverse effects.

🔈 Monitor CBC with white cell differential and watch for signs and symptoms of blood dyscrasias.
- Check temperature. Stay alert for fever and other signs or symptoms of infection.

Patient teaching

- Inform patient that drug may cause tissue damage at injection site. Tell him to report pain, burning, or swelling.

🔈 Instruct patient to immediately report sudden weight gain, swelling, or shortness of breath.

🔈 Tell patient to promptly report unusual bruising or bleeding, fever, or signs and symptoms of infection.
- Explain that drug will cause hair loss but that hair should grow back within a few months after therapy.
- Advise female patient that drug may cause premature menopause or permanent cessation of menses.
- As appropriate, review all other significant and life-threatening adverse reactions and interactions, especially those related to the drugs and tests mentioned above.

eplerenone

Inspra

Pharmacologic class: Aldosterone receptor blocker
Therapeutic class: Antihypertensive
Pregnancy risk category B

Action

Binds to and blocks aldosterone receptors, disrupting normal sodium and water reabsorption and causing sodium and water excretion to increase. These actions reduce blood volume and blood pressure.

Availability

Tablets: 25 mg, 50 mg, 100 mg

Indications and dosages

➢ Hypertension
Adults: 50 mg/day P.O. as a single dose. After 4-week trial, may increase to 50 mg P.O. b.i.d. if necessary.
➢ Heart failure; postmyocardial infarction (MI)
Adults: Initially, 25 mg P.O. once daily. After 1 month, may increase to maximum dosage of 50 mg P.O. once daily.

Contraindications

- Hypersensitivity to drug
- Hyperkalemia
- Type 2 diabetes mellitus with microalbuminuria
- Severe renal impairment

Precautions

Use cautiously in:
- hepatic impairment
- pregnant or breastfeeding patients
- children (safety and efficacy not established).

Administration

- Give with or without food.
- Know that drug may be given alone or with other antihypertensives.

Route	Onset	Peak	Duration
P.O.	Slow	1.5 hr	Unknown

Adverse reactions

CNS: headache, dizziness, fatigue
CV: angina, **MI**
GI: diarrhea, abdominal pin
GU: albuminuria, vaginal bleeding,

changes in sexual function, gynecomastia and breast pain (in men)
Metabolic: hypercholesterolemia, **hyperkalemia**
Respiratory: cough
Other: flulike symptoms

Interactions

Drug-drug. *Angiotensin-converting enzyme inhibitors:* increased risk of hyperkalemia
CYP450-3A4 inhibitors: serious toxic effects
Lithium: increased risk of toxicity
Nonsteroidal anti-inflammatory drugs: decreased hypertensive effect of eplerenone

Patient monitoring

- Monitor electrolyte levels, and watch for signs and symptoms of hyperkalemia.
- Check vital signs, and ask patient about chest pain.
- Monitor lipid panel.
- Assess for new onset of persistent dry cough or flulike symptoms.

Patient teaching

Advise patient to immediately report chest pain, flulike symptoms, or persistent dry cough.
- Caution patient to avoid driving and other hazardous activities until he knows how drug affects concentration and alertness.
- Inform patient that drug may affect sexual function. Encourage him to discuss this issue with prescriber.
- Advise female patient to discuss pregnancy or breastfeeding with prescriber before starting drug.
- As appropriate, review all other significant and life-threatening adverse reactions and interactions, especially those related to the drugs mentioned above.

epoetin alfa

Epogen, Eprex, Procrit

Pharmacologic class: Recombinant human erythropoietin
Therapeutic class: Biological response modifier
Pregnancy risk category C

Action

Binds to erythropoietin, stimulating mitotic activity of erythroid progenitor cells in bone marrow and causing release of reticulocytes from bone marrow into bloodstream, where they become mature red blood cells

Availability

Injection: 2,000 units/ml, 3,000 units/ml, 4,000 units/ml, 10,000 units/ml; 10,000 units/ml and 20,000 units/ml in multidose vials

Indications and dosages

➢ Anemia associated with chronic renal failure
Adults: Initially, 50 to 100 units/kg I.V. or subcutaneously three times weekly. May be increased after 8 weeks if hematocrit is still below target range.
➢ Anemia caused by zidovudine therapy in patients with human immunodeficiency virus infection
Adults: 100 units/kg I.V. or subcutaneously three times weekly for 8 weeks or until hematocrit level is adequate. If desired response isn't reached after 8 weeks, dosage may be increased by 50 to 100 units/kg I.V. or subcutaneously three times weekly; after 4 to 8 weeks, dosage may be further increased, as prescribed, to a maximum dosage of 300 units/kg I.V. or subcutaneously three times weekly.
➢ Anemia associated with cancer chemotherapy
Adults: 150 units/kg subcutaneously

three times weekly for 8 weeks or until hematocrit level is adequate. If desired response isn't reached after 8 weeks, dosage may be increased to a maximum of 300 units/kg subcutaneously three times weekly.

➢ To reduce need for blood transfusion in surgical patients
Adults: 300 units/kg subcutaneously daily for 10 days before surgery, on day of surgery, and for 4 days after surgery; or 600 units/kg subcutaneously weekly starting 3 weeks before surgery, followed by additional dose on day of surgery

➢ Anemia in children with chronic renal failure who are on dialysis
Children ages 1 month to 16 years: 50 units/kg I.V. or subcutaneously three times weekly. Maintenance dosage is individualized to maintain hematocrit within target range.

Contraindications

- Hypersensitivity to drug, human albumin, or products derived from mammal cells
- Uncontrolled hypertension

Precautions

Use cautiously in:

- renal insufficiency
- pregnant or breastfeeding patients
- children.

Administration

- For I.V. use, give single dose by direct I.V. injection over at least 1 minute, and follow with saline flush.
- If patient is on hemodialysis, administer drug into venous return line of dialysis tubing after patient completes dialysis session.
- Know that supplemental iron may be needed to support erythropoiesis and avoid iron depletion.

◀ Avoid using multidose vials in premature infants because of benzyl alcohol content.

Route	Onset	Peak	Duration
I.V.	Immediate	Immediate	Unknown
Subcut.	Unknown	5-24 hr	Unknown

Adverse reactions

CNS: headache, paresthesia, fatigue, dizziness, asthenia, **seizures**
CV: hypertension, increased clotting of arteriovenous grafts
GI: nausea, vomiting, diarrhea
Metabolic: hyperuricemia, hyperphosphatemia, **hyperkalemia**
Musculoskeletal: joint pain
Respiratory: cough, dyspnea
Skin: rash, urticaria
Other: fever, edema, injection site pain

Interactions

Drug-diagnostic tests. *Blood urea nitrogen, creatinine, phosphate, potassium, uric acid:* increased levels

Patient monitoring

- Monitor vital signs and cardiovascular status, especially for hypertension and edema.
- Assess arteriovenous graft for patency, because drug may increase clotting at graft.
- Monitor electrolyte and uric acid levels. Watch closely for hyperuricemia, hyperkalemia, and hyperphosphatemia.
- Check temperature for fever.
- Monitor neurologic status for signs and symptoms of impending seizure.
- Evaluate nutritional status and hydration in light of GI adverse effects.

Patient teaching

◀ Instruct patient to monitor weight and blood pressure regularly and to immediately report hypertension, sudden weight gain, or swelling.

- Caution patient to avoid driving and other hazardous activities until he knows how drug affects concentration, motor skills, and alertness.

• Tell patient to minimize GI upset by eating small, frequent servings of food and drinking plenty of fluids.
• Advise female patient to discuss pregnancy or breastfeeding with prescriber before starting drug.
• As appropriate, review all other significant and life-threatening adverse reactions and interactions, especially those related to the tests mentioned above.

eprosartan mesylate

Teveten

Pharmacologic class: Angiotensin II receptor antagonist

Therapeutic class: Antihypertensive

Pregnancy risk category C (first trimester), ***D*** (second and third trimesters)

Action

Blocks aldosterone-stimulating and vasoconstrictive effects of angiotensin II at receptor sites in vascular smooth muscles and adrenal glands, decreasing vascular resistance

Availability

Tablets: 400 mg, 600 mg

Indications and dosages

➢ Hypertension

Adults: 600 mg P.O. once daily or in divided doses b.i.d.

Contraindications

• Hypersensitivity to drug
• Hypotension
• Pregnancy or breastfeeding

Precautions

Use cautiously in:
• heart failure, renal or hepatic impairment, obstructive biliary disorders, volume or sodium depletion
• concurrent high-dose diuretic therapy
• black patients
• females of childbearing age
• children younger than age 18 (safety not established).

Administration

• Give initial dose in supervised medical setting, and monitor blood pressure for 2 hours after administration.
• Know that drug may be given alone or with other antihypertensives.
• Be prepared to treat transient hypotension by placing patient in supine position and giving I.V. normal saline infusion as needed.

Route	Onset	Peak	Duration
P.O.	Unknown	6 hr	24 hr

Adverse reactions

CNS: dizziness, fatigue, headache, syncope

CV: hypotension, chest pain, peripheral edema

EENT: sinus disorders

GI: nausea, diarrhea, constipation, abdominal pain, dry mouth

GU: albuminuria, **renal failure**

Hepatic: hepatitis

Metabolic: gout, **hyperkalemia**

Musculoskeletal: joint pain, back pain, muscle weakness

Respiratory: upper respiratory tract infection, cough, bronchitis

Skin: angioedema

Other: dental pain, fever, facial edema

Interactions

Drug-drug. *Antihypertensives, diuretics:* increased risk of hypotension

Nonsteroidal anti-inflammatory drugs: decreased antihypertensive effect of eprosartan

Potassium-sparing diuretics, potassium supplements: increased risk of hyperkalemia

Drug-diagnostic tests. *Albumin:* elevated level

Drug-food. *Salt substitutes containing potassium:* increased risk of hyperkalemia
Drug-herbs. *Ephedra (ma huang):* antagonism of eprosartan action
Drug-behaviors. *Alcohol use:* increased CNS depression

Patient monitoring
- Monitor vital signs, particularly for hypotension after administration.
- Assess cardiovascular status, especially for chest pain, syncope, and edema.
- Monitor liver and kidney function test results, watching for drug-induced hepatitis or renal failure.
- Assess respiratory status. Stay alert for dry, persistent cough and signs and symptoms of respiratory infections.
- Monitor electrolyte levels, and watch for signs and symptoms of hyperkalemia.

Patient teaching
- Instruct patient to take drug at same time each day, with or without food.

◀ Inform patient that drug may cause angioedema. Instruct him to immediately report facial or lip swelling, fever, or sore throat.

◀ Advise patient to immediately report chest pain, fainting, decreased urine output, unusual tiredness, yellowing of skin or eyes, or swelling.

◀ Tell female patient to contact prescriber right away if she suspects she's pregnant.

- Caution female not to breastfeed while taking drug.
- As appropriate, review all other significant and life-threatening adverse reactions and interactions, especially those related to the drugs, tests, foods, herbs, and behaviors mentioned above.

eptifibatide
Integrilin

Pharmacologic class: Platelet aggregation inhibitor
Therapeutic class: Antiplatelet agent
Pregnancy risk category B

Action
Decreases platelet aggregation by binding to platelet-receptor glycoprotein, preventing binding of fibrinogen to platelets, which causes thrombus formation

Availability
Injection: 10-ml vial (2 mg/ml), 100-ml vial (0.75 mg/ml)

Indications and dosages
➢ Acute coronary syndrome (unstable angina or non-Q-wave myocardial infarction)
Adults: 180 mcg/kg I.V. bolus (to maximum of 22.6 mg) over 1 to 2 minutes, followed by a continuous infusion of 2 mcg/kg/minute (to a maximum of 15 mg/hour) for up to 72 hours
➢ Prevention of thrombosis related to percutaneous coronary intervention (PCI)
Adults: 180 mcg/kg (to a maximum of 22.6 mg) I.V. bolus immediately before PCI, then a continuous infusion of 2 mcg/kg/minute (to a maximum of 15 mg/hour), followed by a second 180-mcg/kg bolus 10 minutes after first bolus. Continue infusion until discharge or for up to 24 hours.

Dosage adjustment
- Renal impairment

Contraindications
- Hypersensitivity to drug or its components

- Severe hypertension
- Bleeding disorders
- Renal dialysis or creatinine level of at least 4 mg/dl
- Recent cerebrovascular accident
- Recent surgery

Precautions

Use cautiously in:

- renal insufficiency
- elderly patients
- pregnant or breastfeeding patients
- children (safety and efficacy not established).

Administration

- Withdraw single bolus dose from 10-ml vial into syringe, and give by I.V. push over 1 to 2 minutes. Follow single I.V. bolus dose with continuous I.V. infusion given undiluted from 100-ml vial spiked with infusion set connected to infusion control device.
- Don't administer through same I.V. line as furosemide.

Route	Onset	Peak	Duration
I.V.	Immediate	Immediate	4-6 hr

Adverse reactions

CNS: headache, dizziness, asthenia, syncope
CV: hypotension
GI: nausea, diarrhea, constipation
GU: hematuria
Hematologic: bleeding tendency, thrombocytopenia
Skin: flushing
Other: bleeding at femoral access site

Interactions

Drug-drug. *Clopidogrel, dipyridamole, nonsteroidal anti-inflammatory drugs, oral anticoagulants, thrombolytics, ticlopidine:* increased risk of bleeding
Other platelet aggregation inhibitors: serious bleeding
Drug-diagnostic tests. *Platelets:* decreased count
Drug-herbs. *Most commonly used herbs:* increased anticoagulant effect of eptifibatide

Patient monitoring

- Monitor vital signs and assess cardiovascular status, especially for syncope and hypotension.
- Monitor coagulation studies, CBC, and platelet count. Watch for signs and symptoms of abnormal bleeding or bruising and hematuria.
- Check carefully for bleeding at all sites of invasive procedures, particularly femoral access site.

Patient teaching

- Tell patient drug may cause serious adverse effects but can help prevent a heart attack. Reassure him that he'll be closely monitored during therapy.
- Instruct patient to immediately report fainting or abnormal bruising or bleeding.
- Teach patient safety measures to avoid bruising or bleeding.
- As appropriate, review all other significant and life-threatening adverse reactions and interactions, especially those related to the drugs, tests, and herbs mentioned above.

ertapenem sodium

Invanz

Pharmacologic class: Carbapenem
Therapeutic class: Anti-infective
Pregnancy risk category B

Action

Inhibits cell-wall synthesis in bacteria, causing cell death

Availability

Powder for infusion (lyophilized): 1 g/vial

Indications and dosages

➤ Community-acquired pneumonia; skin infections; complicated genitourinary (GU) infections; complicated intra-abdominal infections; acute pelvic infections
Adults: 1 g I.M. or I.V. daily. Length of treatment varies with type of infection: community-acquired pneumonia, 10 to 14 days; skin and skin structures, 7 to 14 days; GU, 10 to 14 days; intra-abdominal, 5 to 14 days; acute pelvic, 3 to 10 days.

Dosage adjustment

- Renal impairment

Contraindications

- Hypersensitivity to drug, its components, other carbapenems, or beta-lactams
- I.M. injection in patients allergic to lidocaine or other amide local anesthetics

Precautions

Use cautiously in:
- seizure disorder
- pregnant or breastfeeding patients
- children (safety and efficacy not established).

Administration

- Reconstitute for I.V. use by adding to vial 10 ml of sterile or bacteriostatic water or normal saline for injection. Don't use diluents containing dextrose.
- Further dilute reconstituted drug in 50 ml of normal saline solution; infuse over 30 minutes. Don't mix or infuse with other drugs.
- Reconstitute for I.M. use by adding 3.2 ml of 1% lidocaine to vial and shaking well.
- Inject I.M. dose deep into large muscle mass, such as gluteus maximus or lateral thigh.

Route	Onset	Peak	Duration
I.V.	Rapid	30 min	Unknown
I.M.	10 min	2.3 hr	Unknown

Adverse reactions

CNS: headache, dizziness, asthenia, fatigue, insomnia, altered mental status, anxiety, **seizures**
CV: hypotension, hypertension, chest pain, phlebitis, **thrombophlebitis, arrhythmias, heart failure**
EENT: pharyngitis
GI: nausea, vomiting, diarrhea, constipation, abdominal pain, dyspepsia, gastroesophageal reflux disease, **pseudomembranous colitis**
GU: vaginitis
Hepatic: hepatotoxicity
Respiratory: crackles, cough, dyspnea, wheezing, **respiratory distress**
Skin: rash, **erythema multiforme, Stevens-Johnson syndrome, toxic epidermal necrolysis**
Other: fever, pain, induration, and inflammation at I.V. site; edema; hypersensitivity reactions including **anaphylaxis**

Interactions

Drug-drug. *Probenecid:* increased blood level and half-life of ertapenem

Patient monitoring

- [Clinical alert] Monitor vital signs, ECG, and cardiovascular status closely. Stay alert for arrhythmias, edema, respiratory distress, and other signs and symptoms of heart failure.
- [Clinical alert] Assess neurologic status, and watch for signs of impending seizure.
- [Clinical alert] Monitor bowel pattern, and stay alert for signs and symptoms of pseudomembranous colitis.
- Inspect injection site for evidence of thrombophlebitis and induration.
- [Clinical alert] Watch for indications of erythema multiforme (sore throat, rash, cough, iris lesions, mouth sores, fever). Report

early signs before condition progresses to Stevens-Johnson syndrome, and stay alert for other hypersensitivity reactions (including anaphylaxis).

Patient teaching

- Tell patient to notify nurse right away if drug causes pain or swelling at injection site.
- Inform patient that drug can be toxic to many organ systems. Tell him to promptly report significant adverse reactions.
- Tell female patient to inform prescriber of pregnancy or breastfeeding before taking drug.
- As appropriate, review all other significant and life-threatening adverse reactions and interactions, especially those related to the drugs mentioned above.

erythromycin

Apo-Erythro✦, Apo-Erythro-EC, Diomycin✦, E-Base, E-Mycin, Erybid✦, ERYC, Ery-Tab, Erythromid✦, PCE✦

erythromycin estolate

Ilosone, Novo-rythro✦

erythromycin ethylsuccinate

Apo-Erythro-ES✦, E.E.S., EryPed

erythromycin gluceptate

Ilotycin Gluceptate

erythromycin lactobionate

Erythrocin

erythromycin stearate

Erythrocin Stearate, Erythrocot, My-E

erythromycin (topical)

Akne-Mycin, A/T/S, Emgel, Erycette, Erygel, EryMax, Ery-Sol, Erythra-Derm, Erythro-Statin, ETS, Sans-Acne✦, Staticin, Theramycin Z, T-Stat

Pharmacologic class: Macrolide
Therapeutic class: Anti-infective
Pregnancy risk category B

Action

Binds with 50S subunit of susceptible bacterial ribosomes, suppressing protein synthesis in bacterial cells and causing cell death

Availability

erythromycin base
Capsules (delayed-release): 250 mg
Tablets (enteric-coated): 250 mg, 333 mg
Tablets (film-coated): 500 mg
Tablets (with polymer-coated particles): 333 mg, 500 mg
erythromycin estolate
Capsules: 250 mg
Oral suspension: 125 mg/5 ml, 250 mg/5 ml
Tablets: 500 mg
erythromycin ethylsuccinate
Drops: 100 mg/2.5 ml
Oral suspension: 200 mg/5 ml, 400 mg/5 ml
Tablets: 400 mg
Tablets (chewable): 200 mg
erythromycin gluceptate
Powder for injection: 500 mg, 1 g
erythromycin lactobionate
Powder for injection: 500 mg, 1 g
erythromycin stearate
Tablets (film-coated): 250 mg
erythromycin (topical)
Gel, ointment, solution: 2%

Indications and dosages

➢ Pelvic inflammatory disease
Adults: 500 mg (base) I.V. q 6 hours for 3 days, then 250 mg (base, estolate,

or stearate) or 400 mg (ethylsuccinate) q 6 hours for 7 days

➢ Syphilis
Adults: 500 mg (base, estolate, or stearate) P.O. q.i.d. for 14 days

➢ Most upper and lower respiratory tract infections; otitis media; skin infections; legionnaires' disease
Adults: 250 mg P.O. q 6 hours, or 333 mg P.O. q 8 hours, or 500 mg P.O. q 12 hours (base, estolate, or stearate); or 400 mg P.O. q 6 hours or 800 mg P.O. q 12 hours (ethylsuccinate); or 250 to 500 mg I.V. (up to 1 g) q 6 hours (gluceptate or lactobionate)
Children: 30 to 50 mg/kg/day (base, estolate, ethylsuccinate, or lactobionate) I.V. or P.O., in divided doses q 6 hours when giving I.V. and q 6 to 8 hours when giving P.O. Maximum dosage is 2 g/day for base or estolate, 3.2 g/day for ethylsuccinate, and 4 g/day for lactobionate.

➢ Intestinal amebiasis
Adults: 250 mg (base, estolate, or stearate) or 400 mg (ethylsuccinate) P.O. q 6 hours for 10 to 14 days
Children: 30 to 50 mg/kg/day (base, estolate, ethylsuccinate, or stearate) P.O. in divided doses over 10 to 14 days

➢ Conjunctivitis of the newborn
Neonates: 50 mg/kg/day (estolate or ethylsuccinate) P.O. in four divided doses for at least 14 days

➢ Pertussis
Children: 40 to 50 mg/kg/day (estolate preferred) P.O. in four divided doses for 14 days

➢ Pneumonia of infancy
Infants: 50 mg/kg/day (estolate or ethylsuccinate) P.O. in four divided doses for at least 3 weeks

➢ Acne
Adults and children older than age 12: 2% ointment, gel, or solution applied topically b.i.d.

Dosage adjustment
• Hepatic impairment

Off-label uses
• Chancroid

Contraindications
• Hypersensitivity to drug or tartrazine
• Hepatic impairment (with estolate)
• Pregnancy (with estolate)

Precautions
Use cautiously in:
• myasthenia gravis
• hepatic disease.

Administration
🔊 Be aware that ventricular arrhythmias and sudden death may occur if drug is given concurrently with potent CYP3A inhibitors (such as clarithromycin, diltiazem, nitroimidazole antifungal agents, protease inhibitors, verapamil, and troleandomycin).
• Give erythromycin ethylsuccinate and delayed-release products without regard to meals, but avoid giving with grapefruit juice.
• Give erythromycin base or stearate 1 hour before or 2 hours after meals for optimal absorption.
• Follow label directions to reconstitute drug for I.V. use. For intermittent infusion, infuse each 250 mg in at least 100 ml of normal saline solution over 20 to 60 minutes. Continuous infusion may be given over 6 to 24 hours as directed.

Route	Onset	Peak	Duration
P.O.	1 hr	1-4 hr	6-12 hr
I.V.	Rapid	End of infusion	6-12 hr

Adverse reactions
CV: torsades de pointes, arrhythmias
EENT: ototoxicity
GI: nausea, vomiting, diarrhea, abdominal pain or cramps
Hepatic: hepatic dysfunction, hepatitis
Skin: rash

Other: increased appetite, aggravation of weakness in myasthenia gravis, allergic reactions, superinfection, phlebitis at I.V. site

Interactions

Drug-drug. *Alfentanil, alprazolam, bromocriptine, buspirone, carbamazepine, clozapine, cyclosporine, diazepam, disopyramide, ergot alkaloids, felodipine, methylprednisolone, midazolam, tacrolimus, theophylline, triazolam, vinblastine, warfarin:* increased blood levels and risk of toxicity from these drugs
Clindamycin, lincomycin: antagonism of erythromycin's effects
CYP3A inhibitors: increased erythromycin blood level, with risk of ventricular arrhythmias and sudden death
Digoxin: increased digoxin blood level
HMG-CoA reductase inhibitors: increased risk of myopathy and rhabdomyolysis
Hormonal contraceptives: decreased contraceptive efficacy
Pimozide, sparfloxacin: increased risk of serious arrhythmias
Rifabutin, rifampin: decreased erythromycin effects, increased risk of adverse GI reactions
Theophylline: increased theophylline blood level, decreased erythromycin blood level
Drug-diagnostic tests. *Alanine aminotransferase, alkaline phosphatase, aspartate aminotransferase, bilirubin:* increased levels
Urine catecholamines: false elevations
Drug-food. *Grapefruit juice:* increased erythromycin blood level

Patient monitoring

- Check temperature, and watch for signs and symptoms of superinfection.
- Monitor liver function tests. Watch for signs and symptoms of hepatotoxicity.
- Assess patient's hearing for signs of ototoxicity.

Patient teaching

- Instruct patient to take with 8 oz of water 1 hour before or 2 hours after meals, and to avoid grapefruit juice.
- If drug causes GI upset, encourage patient to take it with food.
- Tell patient not to swallow chewable tablets whole and not to chew or crush enteric-coated tablets.
- 🔊 Advise patient to immediately report irregular heart beats, unusual tiredness, yellowing of skin or eyes, or signs and symptoms of new infection.
- Tell patient he'll undergo periodic blood tests to monitor liver function.
- As appropriate, review all other significant and life-threatening adverse reactions and interactions, especially those related to the drugs, tests, and foods mentioned above.

escitalopram oxalate

Lexapro

Pharmacologic class: Selective serotonin reuptake inhibitor
Therapeutic class: Antidepressant
Pregnancy risk category C

Action

Prevents serotonin reuptake by CNS neurons, making more serotonin available in brain and thereby relieving depression

Availability

Oral solution: 5 mg/5 ml
Tablets: 10 mg, 20 mg

Indications and dosages

➤ Major depression
Adults: Initially, 10 mg P.O. daily as a single dose. After at least 1 week, may increase to 20 mg P.O. daily, as needed.

Elderly adults and patients with hepatic impairment: Maximum dosage of 10 mg P.O. daily as a single dose
➢ Generalized anxiety disorder
Adults: 10 mg/day P.O as a single dose in the morning or evening, increased to 20 mg/day P.O. as needed

Contraindications

• Hypersensitivity to drug
• MAO inhibitor use within past 14 days

Precautions

Use cautiously in:
• renal or hepatic impairment, suicidal tendency
• elderly patients
• pregnant or breastfeeding patients.

Administration

• Give with or without food.
Don't give within 14 days of MAO inhibitor.

Route	Onset	Peak	Duration
P.O.	Slow	3.5-6.5 hr	Unknown

Adverse reactions

CNS: drowsiness, dizziness, insomnia, fatigue, **increased risk of suicide or suicidal ideation** (especially in child or adolescent)
EENT: rhinitis, sinusitis
GI: nausea, vomiting, diarrhea, constipation, dyspepsia, abdominal pain, dry mouth
GU: ejaculatory disorders, erectile dysfunction, anorgasmia (in females), decreased libido
Other: increased appetite, flulike symptoms, **serotonin syndrome**

Interactions

Drug-drug. *Carbamazepine, lithium:* decreased effects of escitalopram
Citalopram: increased risk of serious toxic effects
MAO inhibitors: increased escitalopram blood level and risk of toxicity
Triptans: weakness, hyperreflexia, incoordination
Drug-herbs. *Ginkgo, St. John's wort:* increased risk of adverse effects
Drug-behaviors. *Alcohol use:* increased motor impairment

Patient monitoring

Assess patient's mood closely. Watch for signs and symptoms of increased depression or suicidal ideation (especially in child or adolescent).
• Monitor patient's prescription refills to help detect drug hoarding or overuse.
• Check nutritional and hydration status in light of GI adverse effects.

Patient teaching

• Advise patient to minimize GI upset by eating small, frequent servings of food and drinking plenty of fluids.
• Inform patient that full drug effect may take up to 4 weeks. Caution him not to overuse drug.
Tell patient (and parent or significant other as appropriate) to contact prescriber immediately if depression worsens or suicidal thoughts develop (especially in child or adolescent).
• Caution patient to avoid driving and other hazardous activities until he knows how drug affects concentration and alertness.
• As appropriate, review all other significant and life-threatening adverse reactions and interactions, especially those related to the drugs, herbs, and behaviors mentioned above.

esmolol hydrochloride
Brevibloc

Pharmacologic class: Beta-adrenergic blocker (cardioselective)
Therapeutic class: Antiarrhythmic, antihypertensive
Pregnancy risk category C

Action
Blocks stimulation of beta-adrenergic receptors (primarily $beta_1$ receptors), thereby reducing atrioventricular conduction and cardiac output and decreasing blood pressure

Availability
Injection: 10 mg/ml, 250 mg/ml

Indications and dosages
➢ Supraventricular tachycardia
Adults: Initially, a loading dose of 500 mcg/kg/minute by I.V. infusion over 1 minute, followed by a maintenance infusion of 50 mcg/kg/minute over 4 minutes. If desired response doesn't occur after 5 minutes, repeat loading dose and increase maintenance infusion to 100 mcg/kg/minute for 4 minutes. Repeat sequence as needed, with maintenance dosage increased in increments of 50 mcg/kg/minute, to a maximum maintenance infusion of 200 mcg/kg/minute for 48 hours.
➢ Sinus tachycardia or hypertension
Adults: Initially, 80 mg (1 mg/kg) by I.V. bolus over 30 seconds; then, if needed, 150 mcg/kg/minute by I.V. infusion, to a maximum of 300 mcg/kg/minute

Off-label uses
- Acute myocardial ischemia

Contraindications
- Hypersensitivity to drug
- Heart failure
- Heart block greater than third degree
- Sinus bradycardia
- Cardiogenic shock

Precautions
Use cautiously in:
- renal impairment, diabetes, bronchospasm, cardiac disease, cerebrovascular insufficiency, peripheral vascular disease, hyperthyroidism, myasthenic conditions
- pregnant or breastfeeding patients.

Administration
- Be aware that compatible solutions include 5% dextrose for injection, 5% dextrose in lactated Ringer's injection, 5% dextrose in Ringer's injection, 5% dextrose in 0.45% or 0.9% sodium chloride injection, and lactated Ringer's injection.
- Don't mix with 5% sodium bicarbonate injection.
- Dilute 250-mg/ml dose to a concentration of 10 mg/ml, and administer by infusion control device.
- Know that maximum I.V. solution concentration is 10 mg/ml.
- Large fluid volumes may be needed to infuse drug. Use caution when excessive fluids could be harmful.

Route	Onset	Peak	Duration
I.V.	Immediate	30 min	30 min after infusion

Adverse reactions
CNS: anxiety, depression, dizziness, drowsiness, headache, agitation, fatigue, confusion, speech disorders, asthenia
CV: peripheral ischemia, chest pain, bradycardia, hypotension
GI: nausea, vomiting, heartburn
GU: urinary retention
Respiratory: wheezing, dyspnea
Skin: flushing, pallor, erythema
Other: altered taste, fever, chills, ede-

ma, midscapular pain, inflammation or induration at infusion site

Interactions

Drug-drug. *Alpha$_1$-adrenergic blockers:* exaggerated antihypertensive effect
Catecholamines, reserpine: increased bradycardia and hypotension
Digoxin: increased digoxin blood level
Morphine: increased esmolol blood level
Succinylcholine: prolonged neuromuscular blockade
Drug-herbs. *Ephedra (ma huang), St. John's wort, yohimbe:* decreased antihypertensive effect

Patient monitoring

- Monitor vital signs and ECG, particularly for hypotension.
- Assess neurologic status, and institute safety measures as needed.
- Monitor fluid intake and output, watching for urinary retention.
- Check I.V. site regularly.

Patient teaching

- Explain to patient that drug is an emergency measure to control blood pressure, arrhythmias, or heart rate.
- Ensure patient he'll be closely monitored throughout drug therapy.
- Tell patient to report pain or redness at I.V. site.
- As appropriate, review all other significant adverse reactions and interactions, especially those related to the drugs and herbs mentioned above.

esomeprazole magnesium

Nexium

Pharmacologic class: Proton pump inhibitor
Therapeutic class: Antiulcer agent
Pregnancy risk category C

Action

Reduces gastric acid production by inhibiting enzyme activity in gastric parietal cells, preventing transport of hydrogen ions into gastric lumen

Availability

Capsules (delayed-release): 20 mg, 40 mg

Indications and dosages

➣ Gastroesophageal reflux disease (GERD)
Adults: 20 to 40 mg P.O. once daily for 4 to 8 weeks
➣ Symptomatic GERD
Adults: 20 mg P.O. once daily for 4 to 8 weeks p.r.n.
➣ Prevention of erosive esophagitis
Adults: 20 mg P.O. once daily
➣ Duodenal ulcer associated with *Helicobacter pylori* infection (as part of triple therapy)
Adults: 40 mg P.O. once daily for 10 days, given in combination with amoxicillin 1,000 mg b.i.d. for 10 days and with clarithromycin 500 mg b.i.d. for 10 days

Contraindications

- Hypersensitivity to drug or its components

Precautions

Use cautiously in:
- severe hepatic impairment
- pregnant or breastfeeding patients
- children younger than age 18 (safety not established).

Administration

- Give 1 hour before or 2 hours after a meal.
- Know that contents of capsules may be mixed with applesauce.
- Don't crush capsules or pellets.

Route	Onset	Peak	Duration
P.O.	Rapid	1.6 hr	24 hr

Adverse reactions

CNS: headache, dizziness, asthenia, vertigo, apathy, anxiety, paresthesia, insomnia, abnormal dreams
EENT: sinusitis, epistaxis
GI: nausea, vomiting, diarrhea, constipation, abdominal pain, flatulence, dry mouth
Respiratory: upper respiratory tract infection, cough
Skin: rash, inflammation, urticaria, pruritus, alopecia, dry skin

Interactions

Drug-drug. *Digoxin, iron salts, ketoconazole:* altered absorption and effects of these drugs
Drug-diagnostic tests. *Alanine aminotransferase, alkaline phosphatase, aspartate aminotransferase, bilirubin, creatinine, uric acid:* increased levels
Hemoglobin, platelets, potassium, sodium, thyroxine, white blood cells: altered levels

Patient monitoring

- Monitor neurologic status, especially for dizziness, headache, paresthesia, and asthenia.
- Watch for signs and symptoms of EENT and respiratory infections.
- Assess nutritional and hydration status in light of adverse GI effects.
- Check for rash and other signs of hypersensitivity.
- Monitor liver function test results if patient is on long-term therapy.

Patient teaching

- Instruct patient to take drug 1 hour before or 2 hours after a meal.
- If patient has trouble swallowing capsule, tell him to open it, sprinkle pellets into soft food (such as applesauce), and take right away.
- Caution patient to avoid driving and other hazardous activities until he knows how drug affects concentration and alertness.
- Advise female patient to tell prescriber if she's pregnant or breastfeeding.
- As appropriate, review all other significant adverse reactions and interactions, especially those related to the drugs and tests mentioned above.

e

estradiol
Estrace, Estring, Estrogel, Gynodiol, Innofem

estradiol acetate
Femring

estradiol cypionate
Depo-Estradiol

estradiol hemihydrate
Estrasorb

estradiol transdermal system
Alora, Climara, Esclim, Estraderm, FemPatch, Menostar, Vivelle

estradiol valerate
Clinagen LA 40, Delestrogen, Femogex✤

Pharmacologic class: Estrogen
Therapeutic class: Hormone
Pregnancy risk category X

Action

Binds to nuclear receptors in responsive tissues (such as female genital organs, breasts, and pituitary gland), enhancing DNA, RNA, and protein synthesis. In androgen-dependent prostate cancer, competes for androgen receptor sites, inhibiting androgen activity. Also decreases pituitary release of follicle-stimulating hormone and luteinizing hormone.

Availability

Injection (cypionate in oil): 5 mg/ml
Injection (valerate in oil): 10 mg/ml, 20 mg/ml, 40 mg/ml
Tablets: 0.5 mg, 1 mg, 1.5 mg, 2 mg
Tablets (film-coated): 25.8 mcg estradiol hemidrate (equivalent to 25 mcg estradiol)
Transdermal system: 25 mcg/24-hour release rate, 37.5 mcg/24-hour release rate, 50 mcg/24-hour release rate, 75 mcg/24-hour release rate, 100 mcg/24-hour release rate
Vaginal cream: 100 mcg/g
Vaginal ring: 2 mg released over 90 days
Vaginal tablets: 25 mcg

Indications and dosages

➢ Symptoms of menopause, atrophic vaginitis, female hypogonadism, ovarian failure, and osteoporosis
Adults: 0.5 to 2 mg (estradiol) P.O. daily continuously or cyclically. Or 1 to 5 mg (cypionate) or 10 to 20 mg (valerate) I.M. monthly. Or 50- or 100-mcg/24-hour transdermal patch applied twice weekly (Alora, Estraderm) or weekly (Climara). Or 25-mcg/24-hour patch applied q 7 days (FemPatch) or 37.5- to 100-mcg transdermal patch applied twice weekly (Vivelle). Or 2 to 4 g (0.2 to 0.4 mg) vaginal cream (estradiol) applied daily for 1 to 2 weeks, then decreased to 1 to 2 g/day for 1 to 2 weeks, then a maintenance dose of 1 g one to three times weekly for 3 weeks, then off for 1 week; repeat cycle once vaginal mucosa has been restored. Or 2-mg vaginal ring q 3 months or 25-mcg vaginal tablet once daily for 2 weeks, then twice weekly.
➢ Postmenopausal breast cancer
Adults: 10 mg P.O. t.i.d. (estradiol)
➢ Prostate cancer
Adults: 1 to 2 mg P.O. t.i.d. (estradiol) or 30 mg I.M. q 1 to 2 weeks (valerate)

Contraindications

- Hypersensitivity to drug or its components
- Thromboembolic disease (current or previous)
- Undiagnosed vaginal bleeding
- Breast or reproductive system cancer (except in metastatic disease)
- Estrogen-dependent neoplasms
- Pregnancy

Precautions

Use cautiously in:
- cardiovascular, hepatic, or renal disease
- breastfeeding patients.

Administration

- Inject I.M. dose deep into large muscle mass; rotate injection sites.
- If switching from oral to transdermal estrogen, apply patch 1 week after withdrawal of oral therapy.

Route	Onset	Peak	Duration
P.O.	Slow	Days	Unknown
I.M.	Unknown	Unknown	Unknown
Transdermal	Unknown	Unknown	3-4 days (Estraderm) 7 days (Climara)
Vaginal ring	Unknown	Unknown	90 days
Vaginal tablet	Unknown	Unknown	3-4 days

Adverse reactions

CNS: headache, dizziness, lethargy, depression
CV: hypertension, **myocardial infarction (MI), thromboembolism**
EENT: contact lens intolerance, worsening of myopia or astigmatism
GI: nausea, vomiting
GU: amenorrhea, dysmenorrhea, breakthrough bleeding, cervical erosions, decreased libido, vaginal candidiasis, erectile dysfunction, testicular

atrophy, gynecomastia, breast pain or tenderness
Hepatic: jaundice
Metabolic: sodium and fluid retention, hypercalcemia, hyperglycemia
Musculoskeletal: leg cramps
Skin: oily skin, acne, pigmentation changes, urticaria
Other: weight loss or gain, edema, increased appetite

Interactions

Drug-drug. *Insulin, oral hypoglycemics, warfarin:* altered requirements for these drugs
Drug-diagnostic tests. *Antithrombin III, folate, low-density lipoproteins, pyridoxine, total cholesterol, urine pregnanediol:* decreased levels
Cortisol; factors VII, VIII, IX, and X; glucose; high-density lipoproteins; phospholipids; prolactin; prothrombin; sodium; triglycerides: increased levels
Metyrapone test: false decrease
Thyroid function tests: false interpretation
Drug-behaviors. *Smoking:* increased risk of adverse CV reactions

Patient monitoring

🔊 Monitor vital signs and cardiovascular status, especially for hypertension, thromboembolism, and MI.
• Assess vision.
• In diabetic patient, monitor blood glucose level and watch for signs and symptoms of hyperglycemia.

Patient teaching

• Instruct patient to place transdermal patch on clean, dry skin area.
• Teach proper technique for use of vaginal tablet, ring, or cream, as appropriate.
• Tell patient drug may cause loss of libido (in women) or erectile dysfunction (in men). Encourage patient to discuss these issues with prescriber.
🔊 Teach patient to recognize and immediately report signs and symptoms of thromboembolism.
🔊 Caution patient not to take drug if she is or plans to become pregnant.
• Advise patient that drug may worsen nearsightedness or astigmatism and make contact lenses uncomfortable.
• As appropriate, review all other significant and life-threatening adverse reactions and interactions, especially those related to the drugs, tests, and behaviors mentioned above.

estrogens, conjugated

C.E.S.✱, Congest✱, Premarin, Premarin Intravenous

Pharmacologic class: Estrogen
Therapeutic class: Replacement hormone, antineoplastic, antiosteoporotic
Pregnancy risk category X

Action

Bind to nuclear receptors in responsive tissues (such as female genital organs, breasts, and pituitary gland), enhancing DNA, RNA, and protein synthesis. In androgen-dependent prostate cancer, compete for androgen receptor sites, inhibiting androgen activity. Also decrease pituitary release of follicle-stimulating and luteinizing hormones.

Availability

Powder for injection: 25 mg/5 ml
Tablets: 0.3 mg, 0.625 mg, 0.9 mg, 1.25 mg, 2.5 mg
Vaginal cream: 0.625 mg/g

Indications and dosages

➢ Ovariectomy; primary ovarian failure
Adults: 1.25 mg P.O. daily continuously or in cycles of 3 weeks on and 1 week off

➢ Osteoporosis and menopausal symptoms
Adults: 0.3 to 1.25 mg P.O. daily continuously or in cycles of 3 weeks on and 1 week off
➢ Female hypogonadism
Adults: 0.3 to 0.625 mg P.O. daily, given in cycles of 3 weeks on and 1 week off
➢ Inoperable breast cancer in men and postmenopausal women
Adults: 10 mg P.O. t.i.d. for 3 months or more
➢ Inoperable prostate carcinoma
Adults: 1.25 to 2.5 mg P.O. t.i.d.
➢ Uterine bleeding caused by hormonal imbalance
Adults: 25 mg I.M. or I.V., repeated in 6 to 12 hours if necessary
➢ Atrophic vaginitis
Adults: 0.5 to 2 g (vaginal cream) intravaginally daily in cycles of 3 weeks on and 1 week off

Contraindications
- Hypersensitivity to drug or its components
- Thromboembolic disease (current or previous)
- Undiagnosed vaginal bleeding
- Breast or reproductive system cancer (except metastatic disease)
- Estrogen-dependent neoplasms
- Pregnancy

Precautions
Use cautiously in:
- cardiovascular disease, severe hepatic or renal disease, asthma, bone disease, migraine, seizures, breast disease
- family history of breast or genital tract cancer
- breastfeeding patients.

Administration
- Know that drug is compatible with dextrose 5% in water and normal saline solution.

Route	Onset	Peak	Duration
P.O., I.M.	Unknown	Unknown	6-12 hr
I.V.	Rapid	Unknown	6-12 hr
Intravaginal	Unknown	Unknown	Unknown

Adverse reactions
CNS: headache, dizziness, lethargy, depression, asthenia, paresthesia, syncope, **cerebrovascular accident** (CVA), **seizures**
CV: hypertension, chest pain, **myocardial infarction (MI), thromboembolism**
EENT: contact lens intolerance, worsening of myopia or astigmatism, otitis media, sinusitis, rhinitis, pharyngitis
GI: nausea, vomiting, diarrhea, abdominal cramps, bloating, enlarged abdomen, dyspepsia, flatulence, gastritis, gastroenteritis, hemorrhoids, colitis, gallbladder disease, anorexia, **pancreatitis**
GU: urinary incontinence, dysuria, urinary tract infection, amenorrhea, dysmenorrhea, endometrial hyperplasia, vaginal candidiasis, leukorrhea, vaginal hemorrhage, genital eruptions, gynecomastia, breast tenderness, breast enlargement or secretion, reduced libido, erectile dysfunction, testicular atrophy, **increased risk of breast cancer, endometrial cancer, hemolytic uremic syndrome**
Hepatic: cholestatic jaundice, **hepatic adenoma**
Metabolic: hyperglycemia, hypercalcemia, sodium and fluid retention, reduced carbohydrate tolerance
Musculoskeletal: leg cramps, back pain, skeletal pain
Respiratory: upper respiratory tract infection, bronchitis, **pulmonary embolism**
Skin: acne, oily skin, pigmentation changes, urticaria, pruritus, erythema nodosum, hemorrhagic eruption, skin hypertrophy, hirsutism, alopecia, **erythema multiforme**

Other: edema, weight changes, increased appetite, hypersensitivity reaction

Interactions

Drug-drug. *Corticosteroids:* enhanced corticosteroid effects
CYP450 inducers (such as barbiturates, rifampin): decreased estrogen efficacy
Hypoglycemics, warfarin: altered requirement for these drugs
Phenytoin: loss of seizure control
Tamoxifen: interference with tamoxifen effects
Tricyclic antidepressants: reduced antidepressant effects
Drug-diagnostic tests. *Antithrombin III, folate, low-density lipoproteins, pyridoxine, total cholesterol, urine pregnanediol:* decreased values
Cortisol; factors VII, VIII, IX, and X; glucose; high-density lipoproteins; phospholipids; prolactin; prothrombin; sodium; triglycerides: increased values
Metyrapone test: false decrease
Thyroid function tests: false interpretation
Drug-food. *Caffeine:* increased caffeine blood level
Drug-herbs. *Black cohosh:* increased risk of adverse reactions
Red clover: interference with estrogen effects
Saw palmetto: antiestrogenic effects
St. John's wort: decreased drug blood level and effects
Drug-behaviors. *Smoking:* increased risk of adverse cardiovascular reactions

Patient monitoring

- Monitor liver function test results and assess abdomen for enlarged liver.
- Evaluate patient for breast tenderness and swelling. As needed, give analgesics and apply cool compresses.
- Monitor fluid intake and output, and weigh patient daily.

🔊 Know that drug increases risk of thromboembolism, CVA, and MI.

- Check serum phosphatase level in patients with prostate cancer.
- Monitor calcium, glucose, and folic acid levels.
- Evaluate bone density annually.

Patient teaching

🔊 Teach patient to recognize and report signs and symptoms of thromboembolism.

🔊 Caution patient not to take drug if she is or plans to become pregnant.

- Tell patient to report breakthrough vaginal bleeding.
- Recommend that patient have routine breast examinations.
- As appropriate, review all other significant and life-threatening adverse reactions and interactions, especially those related to the drugs, tests, foods, herbs, and behaviors mentioned above.

estrogens, esterified

Menest

Pharmacologic class: Estrogen
Therapeutic class: Replacement hormone, antineoplastic, antiosteoporotic
Pregnancy risk category X

Action

Bind to nuclear receptors in responsive tissues (such as female genital organs, breasts, and pituitary gland), enhancing DNA, RNA, and protein synthesis. In androgen-dependent prostate cancer, compete for androgen receptor sites, inhibiting androgen activity. Also decrease pituitary release of follicle-stimulating hormone and luteinizing hormone.

Availability

Tablets: 0.3 mg, 0.625 mg, 1.25 mg, 2.5 mg

Indications and dosages

➢ Moderate to severe vasomotor symptoms or atrophic vaginitis
Adults: 0.3 to 1.25 mg P.O. daily, adjusted to lowest effective dosage; usually given in cycles of 3 weeks on, 1 week off

➢ Female hypogonadism
Adults: 2.5 to 7.5 mg P.O. daily in divided doses for 20 days, followed by 10-day rest period. If no bleeding occurs, repeat same dosing schedule. If bleeding occurs before end of rest period, start 20-day estrogen-progestin cycle, with progestin P.O. given during last 5 days of estrogen therapy.

➢ Inoperable prostate cancer
Adults: 1.25 to 2.5 mg P.O. t.i.d.

➢ Selected breast cancers (inoperable, progressing)
Adults: 10 mg P.O. t.i.d. for at least 3 months

➢ Prevention of osteoporosis
Adults: Initially, 0.3 mg P.O. daily, increased as needed to a maximum of 1.25 mg/day

Contraindications

- Hypersensitivity to drug or its components
- Thromboembolic disease (current or previous)
- Undiagnosed vaginal bleeding
- Breast and reproductive cancers (except metastatic disease)
- Estrogen-dependent neoplasms
- Pregnancy

Precautions

Use cautiously in:
- cardiovascular disease, severe hepatic or renal disease, asthma, bone disease, migraines, seizures, breast nodules, fibrocystic breasts
- family history of breast or genital tract cancer
- breastfeeding patients.

Administration

- Administer with food or fluids.
- Give cyclically as prescribed, except when used palliatively for cancer treatment.

Route	Onset	Peak	Duration
P.O.	Slow	Days	Unknown

Adverse reactions

CNS: headache, dizziness, lethargy, depression, asthenia, paresthesia, syncope, **increased risk of cerebrovascular accident (CVA), seizures**
CV: hypertension, chest pain, **myocardial infarction (MI), thromboembolism**
EENT: contact lens intolerance, worsening of myopia or astigmatism, otitis media, sinusitis, rhinitis, pharyngitis
GI: nausea, vomiting, diarrhea, dyspepsia, flatulence, gastritis, gastroenteritis, enlarged abdomen, hemorrhoids, colitis, gallbladder disease, anorexia, **pancreatitis**
GU: urinary incontinence, dysuria, amenorrhea, dysmenorrhea, endometrial hyperplasia, urinary tract infection, leukorrhea, vaginal discomfort or pain, vaginal hemorrhage, genital eruptions, gynecomastia, breast tenderness, breast enlargement or secretion, reduced libido, erectile dysfunction, testicular atrophy, **increased risk of breast cancer, endometrial cancer, hemolytic uremic syndrome**
Hepatic: cholestatic jaundice, **hepatic adenoma**
Metabolic: hyperglycemia, hypercalcemia, sodium and fluid retention, reduced carbohydrate tolerance
Musculoskeletal: leg cramps, back pain, skeletal pain
Respiratory: upper respiratory tract infection, bronchitis, **pulmonary embolism**
Skin: acne, increased pigmentation, urticaria, pruritus, erythema nodosum, hemorrhagic eruption, alopecia, hirsutism

Other: increased appetite, weight changes, edema, flulike symptoms, hypersensitivity reactions

Interactions

Drug-drug. *Corticosteroids:* enhanced corticosteroid effects
CYP450 inducers (such as barbiturates, rifampin): decreased estrogen efficacy
Hypoglycemics, warfarin: altered requirement for these drugs
Phenytoin: loss of seizure control
Tamoxifen: interference with tamoxifen efficacy
Tricyclic antidepressants: reduced antidepressant effect
Drug-diagnostic tests. *Antithrombin III, folate, low-density lipoproteins, pyridoxine, total cholesterol, urine pregnanediol:* decreased values
Cortisol; factors VII, VIII, IX, and X; glucose; high-density lipoproteins; phospholipids; prolactin; prothrombin; sodium; triglycerides: increased values
Metyrapone test: false decrease
Thyroid function tests: false interpretation
Drug-food. *Caffeine:* increased caffeine blood level
Drug-herbs. *Black cohosh:* increased risk of adverse reactions
Red clover: interference with estrogen therapy
Saw palmetto: antiestrogenic effects
St. John's wort: decreased drug blood level and effects
Drug-behaviors. *Smoking:* increased risk of adverse cardiovascular reactions

Patient monitoring

- Monitor fluid intake and output, and weigh patient daily.
- Evaluate patient for breast tenderness and swelling. As needed, administer analgesics and apply cool compresses.

[Clinical alert] Know that drug increases risk of thromboembolism, CVA, and MI.

- Monitor liver function test results, and assess abdomen for enlarged liver.
- Check serum phosphatase level in patients with prostate cancer, and adjust dosage as appropriate.
- Monitor calcium, glucose, and folic acid levels.

Patient teaching

[Clinical alert] Teach patient to recognize and immediately report signs and symptoms of thromboembolism.

[Clinical alert] Caution patient not to take drug if she is or plans to become pregnant.

- Teach patient how to perform breast self-examination. Emphasize importance of monthly checks.
- Tell patient to report breakthrough vaginal bleeding.
- Mention that drug may cause contact lens intolerance. Advise patient to report vision changes.
- Inform male patient that drug may cause gynecomastia.
- As appropriate, review all other significant and life-threatening adverse reactions and interactions, especially those related to the drugs, tests, foods, herbs, and behaviors mentioned above.

etanercept

Enbrel

Pharmacologic class: Immunomodulator

Therapeutic class: Antiarthritic

Pregnancy risk category B

Action

Reacts with and deactivates free-floating tumor necrosis factor, responsible for inflammation

Availability

Powder for injection: 25 mg in multiple-use vial
Prefilled syringe (single-use): 50 mg/ml

Indications and dosages

➢ Moderately to severely active rheumatoid arthritis; ankylosing spondylitis; psoriatric arthritis

Adults: 50 mg subcutaneously q week given as a single injection. Dosages above 50 mg/week are not recommended.

➢ Chronic moderate to severe plaque psoriasis

Adults ages 18 and older: 50 mg subcutaneously twice weekly (given 3 or 4 days apart) for 3 months, followed by reduction to a maintenance dosage of 50 mg weekly

➢ Polyarticular-course juvenile rheumatoid arthritis

Children ages 4 to 17: 0.8 mg/kg subcutaneously q week, to a maximum of 50 mg weekly

Contraindications

- Hypersensitivity to drug or its components
- Sepsis

Precautions

Use cautiously in:

- immunosuppression, chronic infection, heart failure
- latex allergy (needle cover of diluent syringe contains latex)
- elderly patients
- pregnant or breastfeeding patients
- children younger than age 4.

Administration

- Inject subcutaneously into thigh, abdomen, or upper arm.
- For adult, use single-use, 50 mg/ml prefilled syringe.
- For child weighing 63 kg (138 lb) or more, use single-use, 50 mg/ml prefilled syringe for weekly dose; for child weighing 31 to 62 kg (68 to 137 lb), administer total weekly dose from multiple-use vial as two injections on same day or 3 or 4 days apart; for child weighing less than 31 kg (68 lb), give as a single weekly injection using multiple-use vial.
- Rotate injection sites.

Route	Onset	Peak	Duration
Subcut.	Slow	72 hr	Unknown

Adverse reactions

CNS: asthenia, headache, depression, dizziness, paresthesia, fatigue, demyelinating disorders (such as multiple sclerosis and myelitis), **cerebral hemorrhage, seizures, cerebrovascular accident (CVA)**

CV: hypotension, hypertension, chest pain, **deep-vein thrombosis, thrombophlebitis, myocardial ischemia, myocardial infarction (MI), heart failure**

EENT: ocular inflammation, pharyngitis, rhinitis, sinusitis

GI: nausea, vomiting, diarrhea, abdominal pain, dyspepsia, anorexia, cholecystitis, **abdominal abscess, GI hemorrhage, intestinal perforation, pancreatitis**

GU: pyelonephritis, membranous glomerulonephropathy

Hematologic: anemia, **aplastic anemia, leukopenia, pancytopenia, thrombocytopenia**

Metabolic: hypomagnesemia

Musculoskeletal: bursitis, polymyositis, joint pain

Respiratory: cough, congestion, dyspnea, bronchitis, pneumonia, **pulmonary embolism, interstitial lung disease**

Skin: flushing, cellulitis, pruritus, rash, cutaneous vasculitis, urticaria, alopecia, angioedema

Other: altered taste, weight gain, adenopathy, fever, irritation at injection site, peripheral edema, flulike symptoms, autoantibody formation, **lupus-like syndrome, serious infections**

Interactions
None significant

Patient monitoring
Clinical alert: Watch for signs and symptoms of pancytopenia and infection.
Clinical alert: Monitor for evidence of GI bleeding, lupus-like syndrome, and serious hypersensitivity reactions. Stop therapy immediately if these occur.
• Monitor CBC and coagulation studies.
Clinical alert: Check for signs and symptoms of cardiac compromise and cerebrovascular events.
• Monitor pulmonary function test results periodically to assess lung status.
• Assess patient's ability to self-administer drug.
• Check for irritation at injection site. As needed, apply cool compresses.
• Examine eyes for conjunctival dryness. As needed, apply artificial tears.

Patient teaching
Clinical alert: Tell patient to withhold dose and contact prescriber if he develops signs or symptoms of infection or is exposed to anyone with chickenpox.
Clinical alert: Tell patient to immediately report hypersensitivity reaction, neurologic or respiratory problems, sudden weight gain, chest pain, or easy bruising or bleeding.
• Teach patient or caregiver how to administer drug and handle and dispose of equipment.
• Caution patient not to get live-virus vaccines.
• Tell female to inform prescriber if she is pregnant or breastfeeding.
• Advise patient to expect redness, swelling, and pain at injection site. Assure him that these problems will diminish over time.
• As appropriate, review all other significant and life-threatening adverse reactions mentioned above.

ethambutol hydrochloride
Etibi*, Myambutol

Pharmacologic class: Synthetic antitubercular
Therapeutic class: Antitubercular, antileprotic
Pregnancy risk category B

Action
Unknown. Thought to interfere with RNA synthesis of bacterial metabolites, decreasing mycobacterial replication.

Availability
Tablets: 100 mg, 400 mg

Indications and dosages
➢ Adjunct in tuberculosis and atypical mycobacterial infection caused by *Mycobacterium tuberculosis*
Adults and adolescents: In patients who haven't received previous antitubercular therapy, 15 mg/kg P.O. daily. In patients who have received previous antitubercular therapy, 25 mg/kg P.O. daily, decreased after 60 days to 15 mg/kg daily.

Dosage adjustment
• Renal impairment

Contraindications
• Hypersensitivity to drug

Precautions
Use cautiously in:
• impaired renal or hepatic function, cataracts, optic neuritis, recurrent eye inflammation, diabetic retinopathy, gout
• pregnant patients
• children younger than age 13.

Administration

• Obtain specimens for culture and sensitivity testing, as necessary, before starting therapy and periodically throughout therapy.
• Give with food.

Route	Onset	Peak	Duration
P.O.	Rapid	2-4 hr	24 hr

Adverse reactions

CNS: confusion, disorientation, malaise, dizziness, hallucinations, headache, peripheral neuritis
EENT: optic neuritis, blurred vision, decreased visual acuity, red-green color blindness, eye pain
GI: nausea, vomiting, abdominal pain, GI upset, anorexia
Hematologic: eosinophilia, **thrombocytopenia**
Hepatic: transient hepatic impairment
Metabolic: hyperuricemia, **hypoglycemia**
Musculoskeletal: joint pain, gouty arthritis
Respiratory: bloody sputum, **pulmonary infiltrates**
Skin: rash, pruritus, toxic epidermal necrolysis
Other: fever, **anaphylactoid reactions**

Interactions

Drug-drug. *Aluminum salts:* delayed and reduced ethambutol absorption
Other neurotoxic drugs: increased risk of neurotoxicity
Drug-diagnostic tests. *Alanine aminotransferase, aspartate aminotransferase, bilirubin, uric acid:* increased levels
Glucose: decreased level

Patient monitoring

⚠ Watch for serious adverse reactions, such as thrombocytopenia, respiratory problems, and anaphylactoid reactions.
• Monitor liver function tests, CBC, and blood urea nitrogen, creatinine glucose, and serum uric acid levels.
• Give analgesics for drug-induced pain, as prescribed.
• Observe for signs and symptoms of gout.

Patient teaching

• Instruct patient to take with 8 oz of water. If stomach upset occurs, advise him to take with food.
• If patient must take antacids, advise him to take only aluminum-free antacids.
⚠ Tell patient to immediately report easy bruising or bleeding, respiratory problems, or signs and symptoms of hypersensitivity reactions.
• Advise patient to report vision changes and to have annual eye exams. Reassure him that visual disturbances will subside within several weeks to months after drug is discontinued.
• As appropriate, review all other significant and life-threatening adverse reactions and interactions, especially those related to the drugs and tests mentioned above.

etidronate disodium

Didronel, Didronel IV

Pharmacologic class: Bisphosphonate
Therapeutic class: Bone resorption inhibitor, hypocalcemic agent
Pregnancy risk category B (oral use), *C* (I.V. use)

Action

Blocks calcium absorption, slowing bone metabolism and reducing bone resorption and formation

Availability

Injection: 300 mg/ampule in 6-ml ampules
Tablets: 200 mg, 400 mg

Indications and dosages

➢ Paget's disease
Adults: 5 to 10 mg/kg P.O. daily as a single dose for up to 6 months, or 11 to 20 mg/kg P.O. daily for up to 3 months
➢ Heterotopic ossification after hip replacement
Adults: 20 mg/kg P.O. daily for 1 month before and 3 months after surgery
➢ Heterotopic ossification in spinal cord injury
Adults: Initially, 20 mg/kg P.O. daily for 2 weeks, decreased to 10 mg/kg P.O. daily for 10 weeks
➢ Hypercalcemia related to cancer
Adults: 7.5 mg/kg/day I.V. infused over at least 2 hours for 3 consecutive days; may continue infusion for up to 7 days if necessary. P.O. dosing may begin after last infusion.

Contraindications

- Hypersensitivity to drug or its components
- Severe renal impairment
- Osteomalacia (tablets)

Precautions

Use cautiously in:
- moderate renal impairment, long bone fractures, heart failure, hypocalcemia, hypovitaminosis D
- pregnant or breastfeeding patients
- children (safety not established).

Administration

- For I.V. use, dilute with 250 ml of normal saline solution. Infuse slowly over at least 2 hours.
- Give oral dose with water or juice 2 hours before meals.
- Make sure patient doesn't eat for 2 hours after receiving dose.
- Know that therapy longer than 3 months is not recommended.

Route	Onset	Peak	Duration
P.O. (Paget's)	1 mo	Unknown	1 yr
P.O. (ossif.)	Unknown	Unknown	Several mo
I.V. (hypercalc.)	24 hr	3 days	11 days

e

Adverse reactions

All reactions occur only with I.V. use unless otherwise noted.
CNS: seizures
GI: nausea, constipation, stomatitis
Hematologic: anemia
Metabolic: hypomagnesemia, hypophosphatemia, fluid overload
Musculoskeletal: bone pain and tenderness, fractures (all with oral use)
Respiratory: dyspnea
Skin: rash (with oral use)
Other: taste loss, metallic taste, fever

Interactions

Drug-drug. *Antacids; buffers containing aluminum, calcium, iron, or magnesium; mineral supplements:* decreased etidronate absorption
Calcitonin: additive hypocalcemic effect
Warfarin: increased prothrombin time
Drug-diagnostic tests. *Blood urea nitrogen (BUN), creatinine:* increased levels
Calcium, magnesium: decreased levels
Liver function tests: elevated values
Drug-food. *Foods high in aluminum, calcium, iron, or magnesium:* decreased etidronate absorption

Patient monitoring

- Monitor fluid intake and output.
- Clinical alert: Watch for seizures.
- Monitor patient for GI discomfort. Divide doses as needed to ease symptoms.
- Assess bowel pattern. If constipation occurs, increase fluids and administer stool softeners, as prescribed.

• Monitor calcium, phosphorus, magnesium, creatinine, and BUN levels; liver function tests; and bone scans.

Patient teaching

• Instruct patient not to take drug with food because of decreased drug absorption.
• Tell patient not to consume high-calcium products, such as milk or antacids, within 2 hours of taking dose.
• Stress importance of eating a diet high in vitamin D and calcium.
• Advise patient to report bone pain or decreased range of motion.
• As appropriate, review all other significant adverse and life-threatening reactions and interactions, especially those related to the drugs, tests, and foods mentioned above.

etodolac

Apo-Etodolac♣, Lodine, Lodine XL, Ultradol♣

Pharmacologic class: Pyranocarboxylic acid, nonsteroidal anti-inflammatory drug (NSAID)

Therapeutic class: Nonopioid analgesic

Pregnancy risk category C (first and second trimesters), ***D*** (third trimester)

Action

Blocks activity of cyclooxygenase (which is needed for prostaglandin synthesis), easing pain and reducing inflammation

Availability

Capsules: 200 mg, 300 mg
Tablets: 400 mg, 500 mg
Tablets (extended-release): 400 mg, 500 mg, 600 mg

Indications and dosages

➢ Osteoarthritis; rheumatoid arthritis
Adults: 300 mg P.O. two or three times daily; or 400 mg, 500 mg, or 600 mg P.O. b.i.d.; or 400 to 1,000 mg P.O. (extended-release tablets) once daily
➢ Mild to moderate pain
Adults: 200 to 400 mg P.O. q 6 to 8 hours, not to exceed 1,200 mg/day

Contraindications

• Hypersensitivity to drug or its components
• Concurrent use of other NSAIDs
• Active GI bleeding or ulcer disease

Precautions

Use cautiously in:
• severe cardiovascular, renal, or hepatic disease
• elderly patients
• breastfeeding patients
• children (safety not established).

Administration

• Give with food or antacids to reduce GI upset.
• Make sure patient swallows extended-release tablets whole without crushing or chewing.
• Withhold drug several days before invasive surgery, as ordered.

Route	Onset	Peak	Duration
P.O.	30 min	1-2 hr	4-12 hr
P.O. (extended)	Unknown	3-12 hr	6-12 hr

Adverse reactions

CNS: dizziness, malaise, weakness, depression, nervousness
CV: hypertension
EENT: blurred vision, tinnitus
GI: nausea, vomiting, constipation, diarrhea, flatulence, dyspepsia, peptic ulcer, duodenitis, intestinal ulceration, gastritis, melena
GU: dysuria, urinary frequency, polyuria, **renal failure**
Hematologic: thrombocytopenia
Hepatic: cholestatic jaundice, **cholestatic hepatitis, hepatic necrosis**

Skin: rash, skin peeling, cutaneous vasculitis with purpura, hyperpigmentation
Other: fluid retention, chills, fever, allergic reaction

Interactions

Drug-drug. *Aminoglycosides:* elevated aminoglycoside blood level (in premature infants)
Anticoagulants: prolonged prothrombin time
Beta-adrenergic blockers: reduced antihypertensive effect
Bisphosphonates: increased risk of gastric ulcers
Cholestyramine: decreased etodolac absorption
Cyclosporine: increased risk of nephrotoxicity
Diuretics: decreased diuretic effect
Lithium: increased lithium blood level, greater risk of toxicity
Methotrexate: increased risk of methotrexate toxicity
Phenylbutazone: increased etodolac effects
Phenytoin: increased phenytoin blood level
Salicylates: decreased etodolac blood level
Drug-diagnostic tests. *Bleeding time:* prolonged
Blood urea nitrogen (BUN), creatinine, hepatic enzymes: increased levels
Urine bilirubin, urine ketones: false-positive results
Drug-herbs. *Arnica, chamomile, clove, dong quai, feverfew, garlic, ginkgo, ginseng:* increased risk of bleeding
White willow: increased etodolac effects
Drug-behaviors. *Alcohol use:* increased risk of adverse effects
Sun exposure: phototoxicity

Patient monitoring

- Monitor CBC, liver function tests, BUN, creatinine level, and coagulation studies.
- Assess for GI bleeding and gastric upset. Administer antacids as needed and prescribed.
- Know that drug may cause false-positive urine bilirubin and urine ketone test results.

◀ Monitor patient for signs and symptoms of thrombocytopenia and increased bleeding time.

- Assess for fluid retention and weigh patient daily.
- Watch for decreased blood pressure control in hypertensive patients.

Patient teaching

- Instruct patient to take with meals if possible.
- Tell patient to swallow extended-release tablets whole without crushing or chewing.

◀ Instruct patient to immediately report unusual bleeding or bruising, change in urination pattern, unusual tiredness, or yellowing of skin or eyes.

- Advise patient to avoid activities that can cause injury.
- As appropriate, review all other significant and life-threatening adverse reactions and interactions, especially those related to the drugs, tests, herbs, and behaviors mentioned above.

etonogestrel and ethinyl estradiol vaginal ring

NuvaRing

Pharmacologic class: Sex hormone
Therapeutic class: Contraceptive
Pregnancy risk category X

Action

Inhibits ovulation by altering cervical mucosa and endometrium of uterus. This inhibition prevents sperm from entering the uterus, thereby preventing implantation.

Availability

Vaginal ring: 0.12 mg etonogestrel and 0.015 mg ethinyl estradiol delivered daily over 3 weeks

Indications and dosages

➢ To prevent pregnancy
Adults: Place one ring into vagina and leave in place for 3 weeks, then remove for 1 week. Insert next ring on same day of week as in previous cycle.

Contraindications

- Hypersensitivity to drug or its components
- Breast and uterine cancers or other known or suspected estrogen-dependent neoplasms
- Valvular heart disease with complications
- Thromboembolic disease (current or previous)
- Severe hypertension
- Diabetes with vascular involvement
- Headache with focal neurologic symptoms
- Hepatic tumors, cholestatic jaundice
- Major surgery with prolonged immobilization
- Undiagnosed vaginal bleeding
- Patients older than age 35 who smoke more than 15 cigarettes daily
- Pregnancy or breastfeeding

Precautions

Use cautiously in:
- underlying cardiovascular disease, severe hepatic or renal disease, asthma, bone disease, migraines, breast disease, seizures, sexually transmitted diseases
- family history of breast or genital tract cancers.

Administration

- Be aware that the best way to insert ring is with patient lying down, squatting, or standing and one leg raised.

Route	Onset	Peak	Duration
Vaginal	Rapid	Unknown	Unknown

Adverse reactions

CNS: headache, dizziness, lethargy, depression, **increased risk of cerebrovascular accident, seizures**
CV: hypertension, **myocardial infarction, thromboembolism**
EENT: worsening of myopia or astigmatism
GI: nausea, vomiting, abdominal cramps, bloating, **pancreatitis**
GU: amenorrhea, loss of libido, vaginal candidiasis, breast tenderness, breast enlargement or secretion, **increased risk of endometrial and breast cancer**
Hepatic: cholestatic jaundice, **hepatic adenoma**
Metabolic: sodium and fluid retention
Respiratory: pulmonary embolism
Other: increased appetite, weight changes, edema

Interactions

Drug-drug. *Acetaminophen:* decreased acetaminophen blood level
Anti-infectives, barbiturates, carbamazepine, fosphenytoin, rifampin: decreased contraceptive efficacy
Corticosteroids: increased corticosteroid effects
Cyclosporine: increased risk of cyclosporine toxicity
CYP3A4 inhibitors (such as itraconazole, ketoconazole): increased hormone levels
Dantrolene, other hepatotoxic drugs: increased risk of hepatotoxicity
Hypoglycemics, warfarin: altered requirements for these drugs
Miconazole (vaginal capsules): increased hormone levels
Phenytoin: loss of seizure control
Protease inhibitors: increased contraceptive metabolism
Tamoxifen: interference with tamoxifen efficacy
Tricyclic antidepressants: reduced antidepressant effects
Drug-diagnostic tests. *Antithrombin III, folate, low-density lipoproteins, pyri-*

doxine, total cholesterol: decreased levels
Cortisol; factors VII, VIII, IX, and X; glucose; high-density lipoproteins; phospholipids; prolactin; prothrombin; sodium; triglycerides: increased levels
Drug-food. *Caffeine:* increased caffeine blood level
Drug-herbs. *Black cohosh:* increased risk of adverse reactions
Red clover: interference with contraceptive action
Saw palmetto: antiestrogenic effects
St. John's wort: decreased contraceptive blood level and effects
Drug-behaviors. *Smoking:* increased risk of adverse cardiovascular reactions

Patient monitoring

- Monitor CNS status. Report adverse CNS reactions immediately.
- Assess blood pressure frequently.
- Monitor patient for depression.
- Watch for jaundice and liver engorgement.
- Check for dry eyes. Administer artificial tears as needed.
- Monitor glucose, calcium, and electrolyte levels and lipid profile.

Patient teaching

- Explain that for continued contraception, a new implant must be inserted exactly 1 week after old one is removed, even if patient is menstruating.
- Tell patient to insert and remove ring on same day of week and at same time of day.
- Tell patient that if ring slips out, she should replace it within 3 hours to ensure adequate contraceptive protection.
- Inform patient that smoking during therapy may increase risk of blood clots, phlebitis, and stroke.
- Tell patient to immediately report signs and symptoms of depression, sudden chest pain, difficulty breathing, or yellowing of skin or eyes.
- Teach patient how to perform breast self-examinations. Emphasize importance of monthly checks.
- As appropriate, review all other significant and life-threatening adverse reactions and interactions, especially those related to the drugs, tests, foods, herbs, and behaviors mentioned above.

e

etoposide (VP-16-213)

Toposar, VePesid

etoposide phosphate

Etopophos

Pharmacologic class: Podophyllotoxin derivative
Therapeutic class: Antineoplastic
Pregnancy risk category D

Action

Damages DNA before mitosis by inhibiting topoisomerase II enzyme. This action impairs DNA synthesis and inhibits selected cancer cell growth. Cell-cycle-phase specific.

Availability

Capsules: 50 mg
Injection: 20 mg/ml
Powder for injection (phosphate): 100 mg in single-dose vials

Indications and dosages

➤ Testicular cancer
Adults: 50 to 100 mg/m^2 I.V. daily for 5 days. Or 100 mg/m^2 I.V. on days 1, 3, and 5, with course repeated q 3 to 4 weeks.
➤ Small-cell carcinoma of lung
Adults: 70 mg/m^2 (rounded up or down to nearest 50 mg) P.O. daily for 4 days, then a maximum of 100 mg/m^2 (rounded up or down to nearest 50 mg) P.O. daily for 5 days every 3 to 4 weeks. Alternatively, 35 mg/m^2 I.V. dai-

ly for 4 days, then a maximum of 50 mg/m² I.V. daily for 5 days q 3 to 4 weeks.

Dosage adjustment
- Renal impairment

Off-label uses
- AIDS-related Kaposi's sarcoma
- Wilms' tumor
- Neuroblastoma
- Malignant lymphoma
- Hodgkin's disease
- Ovarian neoplasms

Contraindications
- Hypersensitivity to drug or its components

Precautions
Use cautiously in:
- active infections, decreased bone marrow reserve, renal or hepatic impairment
- pregnant patients and patients with childbearing potential
- breastfeeding patients
- children (safety and efficacy not established).

Administration
- For I.V. concentrations above 0.4 mg/ml, mix each 100 mg with 250 to 500 ml of dextrose 5% in water or normal saline solution, to help prevent crystallization.
- Give I.V. infusion over 30 to 60 minutes. Don't use in-line filter.

🔊 Avoid rapid infusion, which may cause severe hypotension and bronchospasm.
- Administer with antiemetics, as prescribed.
- Wear disposable gloves when handling. If drug comes into contact with skin, wash thoroughly with soap and water.
- Be aware that drug is given with other chemotherapeutic agents.

Route	Onset	Peak	Duration
P.O., I.V.	7-14 days	9-16 days	20 days

Adverse reactions
CNS: drowsiness, fatigue, headache, vertigo, peripheral neuropathy
CV: hypotension (with I.V. use), **heart failure, myocardial infarction**
GI: nausea, vomiting, stomatitis
GU: sterility
Hematologic: anemia, **leukopenia, thrombocytopenia, bone marrow depression**
Hepatic: hepatotoxicity
Metabolic: hyperuricemia
Musculoskeletal: muscle cramps
Respiratory: pulmonary edema, bronchospasm
Other: alopecia, fever, phlebitis at I.V. site, allergic reactions including **anaphylaxis**

Interactions
Drug-drug. *Live-virus vaccines:* increased risk of adverse reactions
Other antineoplastics: additive bone marrow depression
Drug-diagnostic tests. *Hemoglobin, neutrophils, platelets, red blood cells, while blood cells:* decreased values
Uric acid: increased level

Patient monitoring
🔊 Monitor blood pressure during and after infusion. Stop infusion if severe hypotension occurs.
- With I.V. use, monitor infusion rate closely to prevent infusion reactions.
- Throughout infusion, check I.V. site for extravasation, which may cause thrombophlebitis.

🔊 Keep diphenhydramine, hydrocortisone, epinephrine, and artificial airway at hand in case anaphylaxis occurs.
- Assess for CNS adverse effects. Assist patient during ambulation as needed.

🔊 Monitor for signs and symptoms of bone marrow depression.

• Monitor CBC, liver function tests, and blood urea nitrogen and creatinine levels. Report platelet count below 50,000/mm³ or neutrophil count below 500/mm³.

Patient teaching

• Instruct patient to inspect mouth daily for ulcers and bleeding gums.

Tell patient to immediately report difficulty breathing or signs and symptoms of allergic reaction.

Caution female of childbearing age to avoid pregnancy and breastfeeding during drug therapy.

• Instruct patient to move slowly when sitting up or standing, to avoid lightheadedness or dizziness from sudden blood pressure decrease.

• Tell patient drug may cause hair loss.

• As appropriate, review all other significant and life-threatening adverse reactions and interactions, especially those related to the drugs and tests mentioned above.

exemestane

Aromasin

Pharmacologic class: Aromatase inhibitor

Therapeutic class: Hormonal antineoplastic

Pregnancy risk category D

Action

Inhibits conversion of androgens to estrogen, which reduces estrogen concentrations and limits cancer cell growth in estrogen-dependent breast tumors

Availability

Tablets: 25 mg

Indications and dosages

➢ Advanced breast cancer

Adults: 25 mg P.O. once daily after a meal

Contraindications

• Hypersensitivity to drug or its components

Precautions

Use cautiously in:

• moderate to severe hepatic insufficiency or renal impairment
• concurrent use of estrogen-containing drugs
• premenopausal women
• pregnant or breastfeeding patients
• children (safety and efficacy not established).

Administration

• Administer after meals with a full glass of water.

• Know that drug shouldn't be taken by premenopausal women or by patients receiving drugs that contain estrogen.

Route	Onset	Peak	Duration
P.O.	Unknown	1-2 hr	24 hr

Adverse reactions

CNS: headache, dizziness, confusion, asthenia, fatigue, weakness, hypoesthesia, paresthesia, pain, anxiety, insomnia, depression

CV: hypertension, chest pain

EENT: sinusitis

GI: nausea, vomiting, diarrhea, constipation, abdominal pain, dyspepsia, anorexia

GU: urinary tract infection

Musculoskeletal: pathologic fractures, arthritis, back pain, skeletal pain

Respiratory: dyspnea, cough, bronchitis, upper respiratory tract infection

Skin: rash, itching, alopecia, diaphoresis

Other: increased appetite, fever, hot flashes, infection, flulike symptoms, edema, lymphedema

Interactions

Drug-drug. *CYP3A4 inducers:* decreased exemestane blood level

Patient monitoring

- Monitor vital signs, especially blood pressure.
- Check for adverse GI reactions. Give antiemetics, as prescribed, for nausea and vomiting.
- Assess bowel elimination pattern. Increase fluids and administer stool softeners, as needed, to ease constipation.
- Monitor pain level. Administer analgesics, as prescribed, to relieve pain.
- Monitor liver function tests, CBC, and blood urea nitrogen, creatinine, and electrolyte levels.

Patient teaching

- Advise patient to take with full glass of water after a meal.
- Tell patient to report depression, insomnia, or excessive anxiety.
- Instruct patient to wear cotton clothing to let skin breathe if drug causes increased sweating or hot flashes.
- As appropriate, review all other significant adverse reactions and interactions, especially those related to the drugs mentioned above.

ezetimibe

Zetia

Pharmacologic class: Cholesterol absorption inhibitor

Therapeutic class: Antihyperlipidemic

Pregnancy risk category C

Action

Inhibits cholesterol absorption in intestine, decreasing intestinal delivery of cholesterol to liver and increasing systemic cholesterol clearance. Net effect is decreased serum cholesterol level.

Availability

Tablets: 10 mg

Indications and dosages

➢ Adjunct to diet and exercise in primary hypercholesterolemia; adjunct to other lipid-lowering drugs in homozygous familial hypercholesterolemia; adjunct to diet in homozygous sitosterolemia

Adults: 10 mg/day P.O.

Contraindications

- Hypersensitivity to drug or its components
- Active hepatic disease or unexplained, persistent transaminase elevations (when given with HMG-CoA reductase inhibitors)
- Pregnancy (when given with HMG-CoA reductase inhibitors)

Precautions

Use cautiously in:

- renal or hepatic impairment
- elderly patients
- pregnant patients not receiving HMG-CoA reductase inhibitors
- breastfeeding patients
- children younger than age 10.

Administration

- Give with or without food.
- Be aware that drug may be given concurrently with HMG-CoA reductase inhibitor (such as atorvastatin or simvastatin).
- Give at least 2 hours before or 4 hours after bile acid sequestrant (if prescribed).

Route	Onset	Peak	Duration
P.O.	Moderate	4-12 hr	Unknown

Adverse reactions

CNS: headache, dizziness, fatigue
EENT: pharyngitis, sinusitis
GI: nausea, vomiting, diarrhea, abdominal pain, flatulence, dyspepsia, dry mouth, anorexia

Musculoskeletal: back pain, myalgia, joint pain
Respiratory: pneumonia, upper respiratory tract infection
Other: viral infection

Interactions

Drug-drug. *Cholestyramine:* decreased ezetimibe blood level
Cyclosporine, fenofibrate, gemfibrozil: increased ezetimibe blood level
Fibrates: increased risk of cholesterol excretion into gallbladder
Immunosuppressants: increased immunosuppression and bone marrow depression
Drug-diagnostic tests. *Liver function tests:* increased values

Patient monitoring

- Monitor hepatic and lipid profiles.
- Assess for and report unexplained muscle pain.

Patient teaching

- Teach patient about role of diet, exercise, and weight loss in lowering cholesterol levels.
- Instruct patient to report GI upset.
- Caution female patient to avoid pregnancy during therapy.
- Advise patient to use hard candy or gum to relieve dry mouth.
- As appropriate, review all other significant adverse reactions and interactions, especially those related to the drugs and tests mentioned above.

ezetimibe/simvastatin

Vytorin

Pharmacologic class: Combination selective cholesterol absorption inhibitor and HMG-CoA reductase inhibitor
Therapeutic class: Antihyperlipidemic
Pregnancy risk category X

Action

Inhibits cholesterol production in liver and blocks intestinal cholesterol absorption, which decreases intestinal delivery of cholesterol to liver and increases systemic cholesterol clearance. Net effect is reduction in levels of total cholesterol, low-density lipoproteins, apolipoprotein B, triglycerides, and non-high-density-lipoprotein cholesterol (non-HDL-C). Also increases HDL level.

Availability

Tablets: Vytorin 10/10 (10 mg ezetimibe/10 mg simvastatin), Vytorin 10/20 (10 mg ezetimibe/20 mg simvastatin), Vytorin 10/40 (10 mg ezetimibe/40 mg simvastatin), Vytorin 10/ 80 (10 mg ezetimibe/80 mg simvastatin)

Indications and dosages

➢ High LDL levels in primary hypercholesterolemia or mixed hyperlipidemia
Adults: Dosage individualized, usually starting with Vytorin 10/20 P.O. daily. Patients requiring less aggressive LDL reduction may begin with Vytorin 10/10; patients needing LDL reductions of more than 55% may start with Vytorin 10/40.
➢ Elevated total cholesterol and LDL levels in homozygous familial hypercholesterolemia
Adults: Initially, Vytorin 10/40 or Vytorin 10/80 P.O. in evening

Dosage adjustment

- Severe renal insufficiency
- Moderate hepatic insufficiency

Contraindications

- Hypersensitivity to drug or its components
- Active hepatic disease or unexplained, persistent transaminase elevations
- Pregnancy or breastfeeding

Precautions

Use cautiously in:

- severe renal insufficiency
- history of hepatic disease
- substantial alcohol consumption
- concurrent cyclosporine therapy.

Administration

- Know that patient should be placed on standard cholesterol-lowering diet before receiving drug and should continue on this diet throughout therapy.
- Be aware that cholesterol and liver function tests should be done before therapy starts.

🔊 Don't give to patient with severe renal insufficiency unless he has previously tolerated 5 mg or more of simvastatin.

- Give at least 2 hours before or 4 hours after bile acid sequestrant (if prescribed).
- Don't give with grapefruit juice.

Route	Onset	Peak	Duration
P.O.	Unknown	Unknown	Unknown

Adverse reactions

CNS: fatigue, headache
EENT: sinusitis, pharyngitis
GI: nausea, diarrhea, abdominal pain
Hepatic: hepatotoxicity (rare)
Musculoskeletal: arthralgia, myalgia, back pain, pain in extremities, myopathy, **rhabdomyolysis** (rare)
Respiratory: cough, upper respiratory tract infection
Other: influenza, hypersensitivity reactions

Interactions

Drug-drug. *Amiodarone, verapamil:* increased risk of myopathy and rhabdomyolysis
Cholestyramine: decreased ezetimibe blood level with further LDL reduction
Cyclosporine: increased ezetimibe blood level
CYP3A4 inhibitors (clarithromycin, cyclosporine, erythromycin, itraconazole, ketoconazole, nefazodone, protease inhibitors), gemfibrozil and other fibrates, niacin (in doses above 1 g/day): increased risk of myopathy
Digoxin: increased digoxin blood level
Warfarin: modest anticoagulant potentiation
Drug-diagnostic tests. *Creatine kinase (CK), hepatic enzymes:* increased levels
Drug-food. *Grapefruit juice:* increased risk of myopathy
Oat bran: impaired drug absorption
Drug-herbs. *Chaparral, comfrey, eucalyptus, germander, jin bu huan, kava, skullcap, valerian:* possible additive hepatotoxicity
St. John's wort: significant reduction in simvastatin bioavailability

Patient monitoring

- Monitor cholesterol levels and liver function test results before therapy starts and thereafter as indicated.
- Closely monitor patients with complicated medical histories, especially those with renal insufficiency from long-standing diabetes.

🔊 Watch for unexplained muscle pain, tenderness, or weakness. Report this finding promptly and check CK level closely for evidence of myopathy.

🔊 Discontinue drug if myopathy is diagnosed or suspected.

- Be aware that patients taking Vytorin 10/80 should have an additional liver function test before therapy starts, 3 months after titration, and periodically during first year.

Patient monitoring

- Instruct patient to take 2 hours before or 4 hours after bile acid sequestrant (if prescribed).
- Advise patient not to take with large amounts of grapefruit juice.
- Teach patient about role of diet, exercise, and weight loss in lowering cholesterol.

🔊 Tell patient that myopathy can occur when therapy starts or during

dosage titration. Instruct him to immediately report unexplained muscle pain or tenderness or weakness.
- Advise patient to tell all prescribers he's taking this drug before starting any new drug.
- Caution female patient not to become pregnant or breastfeed while taking drug.
- Tell patient to limit or avoid alcohol use during therapy.
- As appropriate, review all other significant and life-threatening adverse reactions and interactions, especially those related to the drugs, tests, foods, and herbs mentioned above.

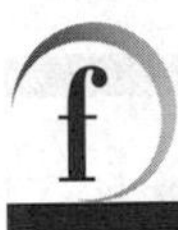

factor IX (human)
AlphaNine SD, Mononine

factor IX (recombinant)
BeneFix

factor IX complex
Bebulin VH, Profilnine SD, Proplex T (heat-treated)

Pharmacologic class: Blood modifier
Therapeutic class: Antihemophilic
Pregnancy risk category C

Action
Converts fibrinogen to fibrin, increasing levels of clotting factors

Availability
Powder for injection: Various strengths; units specified on label

Indications and dosages
➢ Factor IX deficiency (hemophilia B or Christmas disease); anticoagulant overdose
Adults and children: Dosage individualized; drug administered I.V. Use following equations to calculate approximate units needed:
Human product—1 unit/kg times body weight (in kg) times desired increase in factor IX level, expressed as percentage of normal
Recombinant product—1.2 units/kg times body weight (in kg) times desired increase in factor IX level, expressed as percentage of normal
Proplex T—0.5 unit/kg times body weight (in kg) times desired increase in factor IX level, expressed as percentage of normal

Off-label uses
- Hepatic dysfunction
- Esophagitis
- Unspecified GI hemorrhage (human product)

Contraindications
- Hypersensitivity to mouse or hamster protein (with BeneFix)
- Fibrinolysis

Precautions
Use cautiously in:
- recent surgery
- pregnant patients
- children younger than age 6 (safety and efficacy not established).

Administration
- Give by slow I.V. infusion. Average infusion rate is 100 units (2 to 3 ml)/minute; don't exceed 10 ml/minute.
- If prescribed, administer hepatitis B vaccine before giving factor IX.
- Know that dosage is highly individualized according to degree of factor IX deficiency, patient's weight, and bleeding severity.

• Don't use glass syringe. Don't shake reconstituted solution or mix with other I.V. solutions.

Route	Onset	Peak	Duration
I.V.	Immediate	10-30 min	Unknown

Adverse reactions

CNS: light-headedness, paresthesia, headache
CV: blood pressure changes, **thromboembolic reactions, myocardial infarction** (MI)
EENT: allergic rhinitis
GI: nausea, vomiting
Hematologic: disseminated intravascular coagulation (DIC)
Respiratory: pulmonary embolism
Skin: rash, flushing, diaphoresis, pruritus, urticaria
Other: altered taste, fever, chills, burning sensation in jaw and skull, pain at I.V. injection site, hypersensitivity reactions including **anaphylaxis**

Interactions

Drug-drug. *Aminocaproic acid:* increased risk of thrombosis

Patient monitoring

• Be aware that factor IX complex may transmit hepatitis.
• Closely monitor vital signs during infusion.
🔊 Observe for hemolytic reaction. If it occurs, stop infusion, flush line with saline solution, and notify prescriber immediately.
• Monitor I.V. injection site closely.
🔊 Monitor coagulation studies closely. Know that drug may cause thromboembolic disorders, including MI and DIC.

Patient teaching

• Inform patient that drug may transmit diseases.
🔊 Tell patient to immediately report signs and symptoms of hypersensitivity reaction, including rash, hives, tightness in chest, wheezing, shortness of breath, and swelling of throat or lips.
🔊 Advise patient to immediately report unusual bleeding or bruising.
• Caution patient to avoid activities that can cause injury.
• Tell patient to wear medical identification stating that he has a blood-clotting disorder.
• Instruct patient to notify surgeon or dentist of his blood-clotting disorder before surgery or invasive dental procedures.
• As appropriate, review all other significant and life-threatening adverse reactions and interactions, especially those related to the drugs mentioned above.

famciclovir

Famvir

Pharmacologic class: Synthetic nucleoside
Therapeutic class: Antiviral
Pregnancy risk category B

Action

Converts to penciclovir and selectively inhibits DNA polymerase and viral DNA synthesis

Availability

Tablets: 125 mg, 250 mg, 500 mg

Indications and dosages

➢ Acute herpes zoster infection (shingles)
Adults: 500 mg P.O. q 8 hours for 7 days
➢ Recurrent genital herpes
Adults: 125 mg P.O. b.i.d. for 5 days, starting as soon as symptoms appear
➢ Suppression of recurrent genital herpes
Adults: 250 mg P.O. b.i.d. for up to 1 year

➢ Recurrent herpes simplex infection in patients with human immunodeficiency virus
Adults: 500 mg P.O. b.i.d. for 7 days

Dosage adjustment

- Renal impairment

Contraindications

- Hypersensitivity to drug or its components

Precautions

Use cautiously in:

- renal or hepatic impairment
- elderly patients
- pregnant or breastfeeding patients
- children younger than age 18.

Administration

- Know that for best response, therapy should begin within 6 hours of onset of genital herpes symptoms or lesions.
- Give with or without food.

Route	Onset	Peak	Duration
P.O.	Unknown	1 hr	Unknown

Adverse reactions

CNS: headache, fatigue, dizziness, drowsiness, paresthesia, insomnia
EENT: pharyngitis, sinusitis
GI: nausea, vomiting, diarrhea, constipation, abdominal pain, anorexia
Musculoskeletal: back pain, joint pain
Skin: pruritus, rash
Other: fever

Interactions

Drug-drug. *Digoxin:* increased digoxin blood level, increased risk of toxicity
Probenecid: increased blood level of penciclovir (active antiviral compound of famciclovir)

Patient monitoring

- When giving concurrently with digoxin, monitor digoxin blood level and evaluate for digoxin toxicity.
- Monitor CBC, blood urea nitrogen, creatinine, and electrolyte levels.
- Be aware that drug may take several weeks to reach therapeutic level.
- Know that renal failure may raise blood drug level, increasing the risk of adverse reactions.
- Avoid direct contact with infected areas. Wash hands frequently and wear gloves during patient contact.

Patient teaching

- Instruct patient to take with food or milk to avoid upset stomach.
- Inform patient that drug doesn't cure herpes but only decreases pain and itching by allowing sores to heal and preventing new ones from forming.
- Advise patient to wear loose-fitting clothing to avoid irritating lesions.
- Tell patient to report rash or itching.
- Instruct female patient to tell prescriber if she is pregnant or breastfeeding.
- As appropriate, review all other significant adverse reactions and interactions, especially those related to the drugs mentioned above.

famotidine

Apo-Famotidine✤ Gen-Famotidine✤, Mylanta AR, Novo-Famotidine✤, Nu-Famotidine✤, Pepcid, Pepcid AC, Pepcid AC Acid Controller, Pepcid RPD, Rhoxal-Famotidine✤

Pharmacologic class: Histamine$_2$-receptor antagonist
Therapeutic class: Antiulcer drug
Pregnancy risk category B

Action

Blocks action of histamine at histamine$_2$-receptor sites in gastric parietal cells, inhibiting gastric acid secretion and stabilizing pepsin

Availability

Gelcaps: 10 mg
Oral suspension: 40 mg/5 ml
Solution for injection: 10 mg/ml, 20 mg/50 ml of normal saline solution
Tablets: 10 mg, 20 mg, 40 mg
Tablets (chewable): 10 mg
Tablets (orally disintegrating): 20 mg, 40 mg

Indications and dosages

➢ Active duodenal ulcers and benign gastric ulcers
Adults: 40 mg P.O. once daily at bedtime or 20 mg P.O. b.i.d. for up to 8 weeks
➢ Prophylaxis of duodenal ulcers
Adults: 20 mg P.O. once daily at bedtime
➢ Gastroesophageal reflux disease
Adults: 20 mg P.O. b.i.d. for up to 6 weeks. Maximum dosage is 40 mg b.i.d. for up to 12 weeks.
Children ages 1 to 16: 1 mg/kg P.O. daily in two divided doses, to a maximum of 40 mg b.i.d.
➢ Gastric hypersecretory conditions (such as Zollinger-Ellison syndrome)
Adults: Initially, 20 mg P.O. q 6 hours, increased as needed to 160 mg q 6 hours
➢ Hospitalized patients with pathologic hypersecretory conditions or ulcers; patients who can't take oral drugs
Adults: 20 mg I.V. q 12 hours
➢ Prevention or treatment of heartburn, acid indigestion, and sour stomach (Pepcid AC only)
Adults: For prevention, 10 mg P.O. 1 hour before eating, or 10-mg chewable tablet 15 minutes before eating, to a maximum of 20 mg/24 hours for up to 2 weeks. For symptomatic treatment, 10 mg P.O. once or twice daily.

Dosage adjustment

- Renal impairment

Contraindications

- Hypersensitivity to drug or other histamine$_2$-receptor antagonists
- Alcohol intolerance (some oral liquid products)

Precautions

Use cautiously in:
- renal impairment
- elderly patients
- pregnant or breastfeeding patients.

Administration

- Be aware that drug usually is given in one daily dose to patients with renal insufficiency.
- Give P.O. form with foods or liquids.
- Dilute I.V. form with 10 ml dextrose 5% in water or normal saline solution (100 ml) for I.V. piggyback administration.
- Deliver by I.V. push over 2 minutes or intermittent infusion over 30 minutes.
- Know that drug may cause transient irritation at I.V. site.

Route	Onset	Peak	Duration
P.O.	Within 1 hr	1-4 hr	6-12 hr
I.V.	Rapid	0.5-3 hr	8-15 hr

Adverse reactions

CNS: dizziness, headache, paresthesia, asthenia
CV: palpitations
GI: nausea, diarrhea, constipation, dry mouth, anorexia
EENT: orbital edema, conjunctival redness, tinnitus
Musculoskeletal: musculoskeletal pain
Skin: flushing, acne, dry skin
Other: altered taste, fever, pain at injection site, **hypersensitivity reactions**

Interactions

Drug-food. *Caffeine-containing foods:* increased gastric irritation
Drug-herbs. *Yerba maté:* decreased famotidine clearance

Drug-behaviors. *Alcohol use, smoking:* increased gastric irritation

Patient monitoring

- Assess patient for GI signs and symptoms.
- Monitor blood urea nitrogen and creatinine levels in patients with renal impairment.

Patient teaching

- Tell patient that drug is most effective when taken at bedtime.
- Inform patient that pain relief may not begin until several days after therapy starts.
- Caution patient to avoid alcohol, caffeine, and smoking because they may increase gastric irritation.
- Tell female patient to inform prescriber if she is pregnant or breastfeeding.
- As appropriate, review all other significant and life-threatening adverse reactions and interactions, especially those related to the foods, herbs, and behaviors mentioned above.

fat emulsions (I.V.)

Intralipid 10%, Intralipid 20%, Liposyn II 10%, Liposyn II 20%, Liposyn III 10%, Liposyn III 20%

Pharmacologic class: Lipid
Therapeutic class: Nutritional caloric agent and fatty acid
Pregnancy risk category C

Action

Increases plasma triglyceride levels and converts triglycerides to free fatty acids; increases oxygen consumption and heat production and serves as calorie source

Availability

Injection: 50 ml (10%, 20%), 100 ml (10%, 20%), 200 ml (10%, 20%), 250 ml (10%, 20%), 500 ml (10%, 20%)

Indications and dosages

➢ To prevent fatty acid deficiency
Adults: 500 ml (10% of total caloric intake) I.V. twice weekly, initially infused at 1 ml/minute for 30 minutes, not to exceed 500 ml over 4 to 6 hours
➢ Treatment of fatty acid deficiency
Adults and children: 8% to 10% of total caloric intake I.V.
➢ Adjunct to total parenteral nutrition (TPN)
Adults: 1 ml/minute I.V. for 15 to 30 minutes (10% emulsion), or 0.5 ml/minute I.V. for 15 to 30 minutes (20% emulsion). If no adverse effects occur, increase rate to 500 ml over 4 to 8 hours, not to exceed 2.5 g/kg/day.
Children: 0.1 ml/minute I.V. for 10 to 15 minutes (10% emulsion), or 0.05 ml/minute I.V. for 10 to 15 minutes (20% emulsion). If no adverse effects occur, increase rate to 1 g/kg over 4 hours, not to exceed 3 g/kg/day. Fat emulsion provides up to 60% of daily caloric intake; protein-carbohydrate TPN should supply remaining 40%.

Contraindications

- Hypersensitivity to drug
- Allergy to eggs
- Acute pancreatitis, pathologic hyperlipidemia, lipid nephrosis

Precautions

Use cautiously in:
- renal impairment, severe hepatic impairment, pulmonary disease, anemia
- pregnant patients
- premature infants.

Administration

Clinical alert: Ask patient if he's allergic to eggs before starting therapy. If he's allergic, withhold dose.

• Infuse as directed using administration pump. Don't use in-line filter (drug particles are bigger than filter).
• Drug may be piggybacked into TPN infusion proximal to infusion site but past hyperalimentation filter. Hang drug higher than TPN bag, to prevent backup into bag.
• Change I.V. tubing with each new bottle, to prevent bacterial growth.

Route	Onset	Peak	Duration
I.V.	Rapid	Immediate	Unknown

Adverse reactions

GI: splenomegaly (with prolonged use)
Hematologic: leukocytosis, thrombocytopenia, leukopenia (with prolonged use)
Hepatic: jaundice, **hepatomegaly** (with prolonged use)
Metabolic: metabolic acidosis
Respiratory: reduced pulmonary diffusion capacity, **pulmonary edema**
Other: overloading syndrome with prolonged use (causing **focal seizures, fever, leukocytosis, splenomegaly, shock); sepsis; hypersensitivity reaction**

Interactions

Drug-diagnostic tests. *Bilirubin, lipids, hepatic enzymes:* increased levels
Liver function tests: abnormal results
Platelets, white blood cells: decreased counts

Patient monitoring

Clinical alert: Observe closely for serious adverse reactions during first few hours of infusion.
• Monitor I.V. site closely. Change site as needed.
• Assess for hepatomegaly and splenomegaly. Report positive findings.
• Monitor CBC, lipid and hepatic profiles, coagulation studies, and electrolyte and glucose levels.
• Monitor fluid intake and output. Assess for fluid overload (caused by osmotic pull of fat emulsion).

Patient teaching

• Instruct patient to report shortness of breath or injection site reactions.
• Tell female patient to inform prescriber if she is pregnant.
• As appropriate, review all other significant and life-threatening adverse reactions and interactions, especially those related to the tests mentioned above.

felodipine

Plendil, Renedil✤

Pharmacologic class: Calcium channel blocker
Therapeutic class: Antihypertensive, antianginal
Pregnancy risk category C

Action

Impedes extracellular calcium ion movement across membranes of myocardial muscle cells, depressing myocardial contractility and impulse formation; slows impulse conduction velocity and dilates coronary arteries and peripheral arterioles. Net effect is reduced cardiac workload and lower blood pressure.

Availability

Tablets (extended-release): 2.5 mg, 5 mg, 10 mg

Indications and dosages

➢ Hypertension
Adults: Initially, 5 mg P.O. daily. Depending on response, may decrease to 2.5 mg or increase to a maximum of 10 mg P.O. daily at 2-week intervals.

Dosage adjustment
- Hepatic impairment
- Elderly patients

Off-label uses
- Heart failure
- Angina pectoris or vasospastic (Prinzmetal's) angina

Contraindications
- Hypersensitivity to drug

Precautions
Use cautiously in:
- cardiac disease, arrhythmias, severe hepatic or renal impairment
- elderly patients
- pregnant or breastfeeding patients
- children (safety not established).

Administration
- Give without regard to meals.
- Make sure patient swallows tablet whole without crushing or chewing.

Route	Onset	Peak	Duration
P.O.	1 hr	2-4 hr	Up to 24 hr

Adverse reactions
CNS: headache, drowsiness, dizziness, syncope, nervousness, anxiety, psychiatric disturbances, paresthesia, insomnia, asthenia, confusion, irritability
CV: chest pain, peripheral edema, hypotension, palpitations, tachycardia, angina, **arrhythmias, myocardial infarction, atrioventricular block**
EENT: rhinorrhea, sneezing, pharyngitis
GI: nausea, vomiting, diarrhea, constipation, abdominal discomfort, dyspepsia, abdominal cramps, flatulence, dry mouth
Hematologic: anemia
Musculoskeletal: back pain
Respiratory: bronchitis
Skin: dermatitis, rash, pruritus, urticaria, erythema
Other: dysgeusia, gingival hyperplasia, facial edema, thirst, warm sensation

Interactions
Drug-drug. *Antifungals, cimetidine, erythromycin, propranolol, ranitidine:* increased felodipine blood level, increased risk of toxicity
Barbiturates, hydantoins: decreased felodipine blood level
Beta-adrenergic blockers, digoxin, disopyramide, phenytoin: bradycardia, conduction defects, heart failure
Fentanyl, nitrates, other antihypertensives, quinidine: additive hypotension
Nonsteroidal anti-inflammatory drugs: decreased antihypertensive effects
Drug-food. *Grapefruit juice:* increased felodipine blood level and effects
Drug-behaviors. *Acute alcohol ingestion:* additive hypotension

Patient monitoring
[Clinical alert] Don't give to patient with heart block unless he has a pacemaker.
[Clinical alert] Use extreme caution when administering to patients with pulmonary hypertension, renal insufficiency, heart failure, or compromised ventricular function (especially those receiving beta-adrenergic blockers concurrently).
- Monitor fluid intake and output, and weigh patient daily.
- Monitor ECG and vital signs. Assess for signs and symptoms of heart block.
- Assess for reflex tachycardia, angina, and sustained hypotension.
- Check hepatic profile and alkaline phosphatase level in patients with hepatic impairment.

Patient teaching
- Tell patient drug controls but doesn't cure high blood pressure, so he should keep taking it even if he feels well.
- Instruct patient to move slowly when rising, to avoid light-headedness or dizziness from sudden blood pressure decrease.
- Explain that exercise and hot weather may increase drug's hypotensive effects.
- Tell patient to report peripheral edema, persistent headache, or flushing.

• Advise patient to use hard candy or gum if dry mouth or thirst occurs.
• Tell female patient to inform prescriber if she is pregnant or breastfeeding.
• As appropriate, review all other significant and life-threatening adverse reactions and interactions, especially those related to the drugs, foods, and behaviors mentioned above.

fenofibrate

Apo-Fenofibrate✱, Nu-Fenofibrate✱, Tricor

Pharmacologic class: Fibric acid derivative

Therapeutic class: Antihyperlipidemic

Pregnancy risk category C

Action

Inhibits triglyceride synthesis in liver, reducing levels of low- and very-low-density lipoproteins. Also increases uric acid secretion.

Availability

Capsules (micronized): 67 mg, 134 mg, 200 mg
Tablets: 54 mg, 160 mg

Indications and dosages

➢ To decrease levels of low-density lipoproteins, total cholesterol, triglycerides, and apolipoprotein B
Adults: 200-mg capsule or 160-mg tablet P.O. daily
➢ Hypertriglyceridemia
Adults: Initially, 67 to 200 mg/day P.O. (capsules) or 54 to 160 mg/day (tablets); may increase as needed q 4 to 8 weeks up to 200 mg/day (capsules) or 160 mg/day (tablets)

Dosage adjustment

• Renal impairment
• Elderly patients

Off-label uses

• Hyperlipoproteinemia types III, IIa, and IIb (as adjunct to diet)
• Polymetabolic syndrome X

Contraindications

• Hypersensitivity to drug
• Hepatic disease or unexplained, persistent liver function test abnormalities
• Severe renal impairment
• Gallbladder disease
• Breastfeeding

Precautions

Use cautiously in:
• pancreatitis, cholelithiasis
• patients receiving warfarin concurrently
• pregnant patients
• children.

Administration

Before giving, be aware of potentially serious interactions, such as with nephrotoxic drugs.
• Administer with meals.
• Give bile acid sequestrants at least 1 hour before or 4 to 6 hours after fenofibrate.

Route	Onset	Peak	Duration
P.O.	Variable	6-8 hr	Unknown

Adverse reactions

CNS: drowsiness, dizziness, fatigue, headache, migraine, insomnia, depression, vertigo, nervousness, anxiety, paresthesia, hypotonia, neuralgia
CV: tachycardia, varicose veins, phlebitis, angina, hypertension, hypotension, peripheral vascular disease, vasodilation, ECG abnormalities, coronary artery disease, **arrhythmias, ventricular extrasystoles, myocardial infarction, atrial fibrillation**
EENT: conjunctivitis, abnormal vision, cataracts, refraction disorder, otitis media, rhinitis, sinusitis, pharyngitis, laryngitis

GI: nausea, vomiting, diarrhea, constipation, abdominal pain, flatulence, dyspepsia, gastritis, gastroenteritis, esophagitis, duodenal or peptic ulcer, colitis, cholelithiasis, cholecystitis, rectal disorder, **rectal hemorrhage**
GU: urinary frequency, dysuria, cystitis, urolithiasis, prostatic disorder, gynecomastia, vaginal candidiasis, decreased libido, **renal dysfunction**
Hematologic: eosinophilia, anemia, lymphadenopathy, **thrombocytopenia, leukopenia**
Hepatic: fatty liver deposits
Metabolic: hyperuricemia, gout, **hypoglycemia**
Musculoskeletal: back, muscle, or joint pain; myositis; arthritis; tenosynovitis; arthrosis; bursitis
Respiratory: respiratory disorders, bronchitis, increased cough, dyspnea, pneumonia, **asthma**
Skin: rash, pruritus, urticaria, bruising, acne, eczema, diaphoresis, dermatitis, herpes simplex, herpes zoster, alopecia, nail disorder
Other: weight loss or gain, edema, fever, flulike symptoms, hypersensitivity reactions

Interactions

Drug-drug. *Bile acid sequestrants (resins):* decreased absorption and efficacy of fenofibrate
Immunosuppressants, other nephrotoxic drugs: increased risk of renal toxicity
Oral anticoagulants: increased risk of bleeding
Statins (such as simvastatin): rhabdomyolysis, acute renal failure
Drug-diagnostic tests. *Alanine aminotransferase, alkaline phosphatase, aspartate aminotransferase, blood urea nitrogen, creatinine, gamma-glutamyltransferase, uric acid:* increased values
Granulocytes, hemoglobin, neutrophils, platelets, white blood cells (WBCs): decreased values
Liver function tests: abnormal results
Drug-food. *Any food:* increased drug absorption
Drug-behaviors. *Alcohol use:* elevated triglyceride level

Patient monitoring

- Assess creatine kinase and lipid levels and liver function test results.
- Monitor CBC and WBC count. Expect these to decrease at start of therapy, then stabilize.

Patient teaching

- Instruct patient to take with meals for best effect.
- Remind patient that he still needs to follow a triglyceride-lowering diet.
- Caution patient to avoid driving and other hazardous activities until he knows how drug affects concentration and alertness.
- Advise patient to minimize GI upset by eating frequent, small servings of food and drinking plenty of fluids.
- Tell patient that drug may take up to 2 months to alter lipid values.
- Inform breastfeeding patient that she must choose between taking fenofibrate and breastfeeding.
- Tell female patient to inform prescriber if she is pregnant.
- Inform patient that he'll undergo regular blood testing.
- As appropriate, review all other significant and life-threatening adverse reactions and interactions, especially those related to the drugs, tests, foods, and behaviors mentioned above.

fenoldopam mesylate

Corlopam

Pharmacologic class: Dopamine receptor agonist (vasodilator)
Therapeutic class: Emergency antihypertensive
Pregnancy risk category B

Action
Stimulates dopamine$_1$ postsynaptic receptors, causing vasodilation, decreasing blood pressure and total peripheral resistance, and increasing renal blood flow

Availability
Ampules: 10 mg/ml in single-dose, 5-ml ampules

Indications and dosages
➢ Short-term (up to 48 hours) hospital management of severe hypertension when rapid blood pressure reduction is indicated
Hospitalized adults: Dosages highly individualized based on rate and magnitude of desired blood pressure decrease. Dosages of 0.01 to 1.6 mcg/kg/minute I.V. infusion have been studied in clinical trials. Titrate upward or downward no more often than q 15 minutes to achieve desired blood pressure, at recommended increments of 0.05 to 0.1 mcg/kg/minute.
➢ Short-term (up to 4 hours) blood pressure reduction in hospitalized children
Hospitalized children: Dosages highly individualized based on rate and magnitude of desired blood pressure decrease. Dosages of 0.2 mcg/kg/minute I.V. were used initially in clinical trials; dosage increases up to 0.3 to 0.5 mcg/kg/minute q 20 to 30 minutes for up to 4 hours were well tolerated; dosages above 0.8 mcg/kg/minute have produced tachycardia with no additional benefit.

Contraindications
• Hypersensitivity to drug or sulfites

Precautions
Use cautiously in:
• glaucoma, increased intraocular pressure (IOP), tachycardia, hypotension, hypokalemia, hepatic disease
• patients receiving concurrent beta-adrenergic blockers.

Administration
Don't give as I.V. bolus. Give only by slow, continuous I.V. infusion using infusion pump, at a concentration of 40 mcg/ml or less (60 mcg/ml or less for children).
• Be aware that compatible solutions are 0.9% sodium chloride injection and 5% dextrose injection.

Route	Onset	Peak	Duration
I.V.	15 min	20 min	Unknown

Adverse reactions
CNS: anxiety, dizziness, headache, light-headedness, insomnia, nervousness
CV: angina pectoris, nonspecific chest pain, hypotension, palpitations, ST-segment and T-wave changes, tachycardia, bradycardia, **heart failure, ischemic heart disease, myocardial infarction**
EENT: increased IOP, nasal congestion
GI: nausea, vomiting, diarrhea, constipation, abdominal pain and fullness
GU: urinary tract infection, **oliguria**
Hematologic: leukocytosis, bleeding tendency
Metabolic: hypokalemia
Musculoskeletal: leg cramps, back pain
Respiratory: dyspnea, upper respiratory tract infection
Skin: diaphoresis, flushing
Other: injection site pain, fever, hypersensitivity reactions including **anaphylaxis**

Interactions
Drug-drug. *Beta-adrenergic blockers:* increased hypotension
Dopamine antagonists, metoclopramide: decreased fenoldopam effects
Drug-diagnostic tests. *Aminotransferase, blood urea nitrogen, creatinine,*

glucose, lactate dehydrogenase, potassium: decreased levels

Patient monitoring

- Watch closely for signs and symptoms of anaphylaxis or severe asthma.

Check blood pressure carefully at least every 15 minutes to detect hypotension, especially in patient with acute cerebral infarction or hemorrhage.

- When desired blood pressure decrease occurs, discontinue therapy or taper dosage as ordered.
- Know that patients with asthma are at higher risk for sulfite sensitivity.
- Assess respiratory and cardiac status regularly.
- Monitor potassium level closely.
- Evaluate fluid intake and urinary output.

Patient teaching

Tell patient to immediately report signs or symptoms of anaphylaxis or breathing problems.

- Tell patient that drug may cause rapid heart rate and excessively lower blood pressure, possibly resulting in dizziness.

fentanyl citrate

Sublimaze

fentanyl transdermal system

Duragesic, Duragesic 25, Duragesic 50, Duragesic 75, Duragesic 100

fentanyl transmucosal

Actiq, Fentanyl Oralet

Pharmacologic class: Opioid agonist
Therapeutic class: Opioid analgesic, anesthesia adjunct
Controlled substance schedule II
Pregnancy risk category C

Action

Binds to specific opioid receptors in CNS, inhibiting pain pathways, altering pain perception, and increasing the pain threshold

Availability

Injection: 0.05 mg/ml
Transdermal system: 25 mcg/hour, 50 mcg/hour, 75 mcg/hour, 100 mcg/hour
Transmucosal lozenges: 200 mcg, 400 mcg, 600 mcg, 800 mcg, 1,200 mcg, 1,600 mcg

Indications and dosages

➢ Breakthrough pain in opioid-tolerant patients with cancer

Adults: One 200-mcg lozenge dissolved in mouth over 15 minutes; an additional unit may be given 15 minutes later. If patient requires more than 1 unit per episode (as evaluated over several episodes), dosage may be increased; for optimal use or titration, don't exceed 4 units/day.

➢ Management of chronic pain in patients requiring opioid analgesics

Adults: Initially, 25 mcg/hour (transdermal system); no more than 25 mcg/hour in patients who have not been receiving opioids. To calculate dosage for patients already receiving opioids, assess 24-hour requirement for current opioid. Using recommended equianalgesic table, convert to an equivalent amount of morphine/24 hours. Then use recommended fentanyl conversion table to convert to fentanyl transdermal. During dosage titration, keep additional short-acting opioids at hand to treat breakthrough pain; morphine 10 mg I.M. or 60 mg P.O. q 4 hours (60 mg/24 hours I.M. or 360 mg/24 hours P.O.) is roughly equivalent to transdermal fentanyl 100 mcg/hour. Transdermal patch lasts 72 hours in most patients, but some patients require new patch q 48 hours. Titrate upward by 25 mcg/hour q 72 hours.

➢ Short-term analgesia during anesthesia and immediate preoperative and postoperative periods
Adults: 0.05 to 0.1 mg I.M. 30 to 60 minutes before surgery and as adjunct to general anesthesia; total dosage is 0.002 mg/kg. Maintenance dosage during surgery is 0.025 to 0.1 mg I.V. or I.M. Postoperatively, 0.05 to 0.1 mg I.M. to control pain, tachypnea, or emergence delirium; repeat in 1 to 2 hours if needed.
Children ages 2 to 12: 2 to 3 mcg/kg I.V., depending on vital signs; or 5 to 15 mcg/kg transmucosally
➢ General anesthesia (with oxygen only)
Adults: 0.05 to 0.1 mg/kg I.V. for high-dose therapy. Up to 0.12 mg/kg may be necessary.
➢ Adjunct to regional anesthesia
Adults: 0.05 to 0.1 mg I.M. or slow I.V. over 1 to 2 minutes

Dosage adjustment
• Elderly patients

Contraindications
• Hypersensitivity to drug or transdermal adhesive
• Alcohol intolerance
• Acute bronchial asthma
• Pregnancy (transdermal system)
• Breastfeeding
• Children younger than age 18 who weigh less than 50 kg (110 lb)

Precautions
Use cautiously in:
• diabetes mellitus, severe or chronic pulmonary or hepatic disease, cardiovascular disease, CNS tumors, adrenal insufficiency, hypothyroidism, renal impairment
• alcoholism or drug abuse
• elderly patients
• pregnant patients
• children younger than age 2 (safety not established).

Administration
• Before applying transdermal patch, clip hair at site (don't use razor). Wash area with clean water only; dry well.
• Apply transdermal patch to nonirritated, nonirradiated flat surface. Press firmly in place for 30 seconds.
• In elderly patients, don't initiate fentanyl patch at dosages above 25 mcg/hour unless patient is already receiving more than 135 mg/day of oral morphine or equivalent.
• Inject I.V. dose slowly over 3 to 5 minutes.
🔊 Have narcotic antagonist (naloxone) and emergency equipment available when giving drug I.V.
• Be aware that drug isn't recommended to control mild or intermittent pain.

Route	Onset	Peak	Duration
I.V.	1-2 min	3-5 min	0.5-1 hr
I.M.	7-8 min	20-30 min	1-2 hr
Transdermal	6 hr	12-24 hr	72 hr
Transmucosal	Rapid	15-30 min	Several hr

Adverse reactions
CNS: headache, dizziness, vertigo, floating feeling, lethargy, confusion, light-headedness, nervousness, hallucinations, delirium, insomnia, anxiety, fear, mood changes, tremor, sedation, **coma, seizures**
CV: palpitations, hypotension, hypertension, tachycardia, bradycardia, **arrhythmias, circulatory depression, cardiac arrest, shock**
EENT: blurred vision, diplopia, **laryngospasm**
GI: nausea, vomiting, constipation, biliary tract spasm, dry mouth, anorexia
GU: urinary retention or hesitancy, ureteral or vesical sphincter spasm, decreased libido, erectile dysfunction, **oliguria**
Musculoskeletal: skeletal and thoracic muscle rigidity

Respiratory: slow and shallow respirations, suppressed cough reflex, **apnea, bronchospasm**
Skin: local skin irritation (with transdermal system), rash, urticaria, pruritus, diaphoresis, flushing, erythema, cold sensitivity
Other: physical or psychological drug dependence, drug tolerance, pain or phlebitis at injection site

Interactions

Drug-drug. *Barbiturate anesthetics:* decreased effects of both drugs
Buprenorphine, dezocine, nalbuphine: decreased analgesic effect
CNS depressants (antidepressants, other opioid analgesics, sedating antihistamines, sedative-hypnotics, skeletal muscle relaxants): profound sedation, hypoventilation, and hypotension
Erythromycin, ketoconazole, some protease inhibitors: decreased metabolism and increased effects of fentanyl, possibly leading to profound sedation, hypoventilation, and hypotension
MAO inhibitors: severe, unpredictable reactions
Opioid antagonists, partial-antagonist opioid analgesics: withdrawal in physically dependent patients
Drug-diagnostic tests. *Amylase, lipase:* increased levels
Granulocytes, hemoglobin, neutrophils, platelets, white blood cells: decreased levels
Drug-food. *Grapefruit juice:* decreased drug metabolism, increased risk of toxicity
Drug-herbs. *Chamomile, hops, kava, skullcap, valerian:* increased CNS depression
Drug-behaviors. *Alcohol use:* profound sedation, hypoventilation, and hypotension

Patient monitoring

🔊 Assess for muscle rigidity in patients receiving high doses; discuss need for neuromuscular blockers with prescriber. Patient will need ventilator if blocker is given.

- Monitor respiratory and cardiovascular function and urinary output.
- In patient using transdermal system, monitor pain level often to determine whether patch is effective for 72 hours or needs to be replaced after 48 hours. Know that drug level rises gradually for first 24 hours after patch is applied; supplemental analgesics may be needed during this period.
- If patient develops fever, assess for signs and symptoms of opioid toxicity, because more drug is absorbed at higher body temperatures.
- If patient has adverse reactions to transdermal system, monitor him for at least 12 hours after patch removal.
- Carefully monitor hematologic studies and hepatic enzyme levels.

Patient teaching

🔊 Caution patient to keep transmucosal (lozenge) form out of children's reach even though it's supplied in individually sealed, child-resistant pouch. One lozenge can be fatal to a child.

- Instruct patient to place lozenge between cheek and gum and suck on it for 15 minutes without chewing or swallowing.
- Tell patient that transdermal form is absorbed more rapidly if skin becomes warm by fever or hot environment. Instruct him to avoid electric blankets, heating pads, heat lamps, hot tubs, and heated water beds, and to promptly report fever or a move to a hot climate.
- Caution patient to avoid driving and other hazardous activities until he knows how drug affects concentration and alertness.
- As appropriate, review all significant and life-threatening adverse reactions and interactions, especially those related to the drugs, tests, foods, herbs, and behaviors mentioned above.

fexofenadine hydrochloride

Allegra

Pharmacologic class: Peripherally selective piperidine, selective histamine$_1$-receptor antagonist
Therapeutic class: Antihistamine (nonsedating type), second-generation
Pregnancy risk category C

Action

Blocks effects of histamine at peripheral histamine$_1$-receptor sites, decreasing allergy signs and symptoms

Availability

Capsules: 60 mg
Tablets: 30 mg, 60 mg, 180 mg

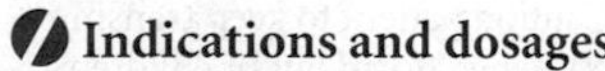

Indications and dosages

➢ Seasonal allergic rhinitis; chronic idiopathic urticaria
Adults and children older than age 12: 60 mg P.O. b.i.d. or 180 mg once daily
Children ages 6 to 12: 30 mg P.O. b.i.d.

Dosage adjustment

- Renal impairment

Contraindications

- Hypersensitivity to drug, terfenadine, or their components

Precautions

Use cautiously in:
- renal impairment
- concurrent ketoconazole or erythromycin therapy
- elderly patients
- pregnant or breastfeeding patients
- children younger than age 12 (safety not established).

Administration

- Don't give with apple, orange, or grapefruit juice.
- Don't give antacids within 2 hours of fexofenadine.

Route	Onset	Peak	Duration
P.O.	Within 1 hr	2-3 hr	12-24 hr

Adverse reactions

CNS: drowsiness, fatigue, headache
EENT: otitis media
GI: nausea, dyspepsia
Metabolic: dysmenorrhea
Respiratory: upper respiratory tract infection
Other: viral infection

Interactions

Drug-drug. *Antacids containing aluminum and magnesium:* decreased absorption and efficacy of fexofenadine
Drug-diagnostic tests. *Skin allergy tests:* false-negative results
Drug-food. *Apple, orange, and grapefruit juice:* decreased absorption and efficacy of fexofenadine

Patient monitoring

- Monitor renal function.
- Watch for signs and symptoms of viral infection.

Patient teaching

- Tell patient to stop taking drug 4 days before diagnostic skin tests, to avoid interference with test results.
- Advise patient to report signs or symptoms of viral infection, especially upper respiratory tract infection.
- Caution patient to avoid driving and other hazardous activities until he knows how drug affects concentration and alertness.
- Advise female patient to inform prescriber if she is pregnant or breastfeeding.
- As appropriate, review all other significant adverse reactions and interac-

tions, especially those related to the drugs, tests, and foods mentioned above.

filgrastim

Neupogen

Pharmacologic class: Granulocyte colony–stimulating factor

Therapeutic class: Hematopoietic stimulator, antineutropenic

Pregnancy risk category C

Action

Induces formation of neutrophil progenitor cells by binding directly to receptor on surface granulocyte, stimulating cell proliferation and differentiation. Also potentiates effects of mature neutrophils and reduces fever and risk of infection associated with severe neutropenia.

Availability

SingleJect prefilled syringes: 300 mcg, 480 mcg

Vial for injection: 300 mcg/ml, 480 mcg/1.6 ml

Indications and dosages

➢ To prevent infection after myelosuppressive chemotherapy

Adults: 5 mcg/kg/day by subcutaneous injection or I.V. infusion over 15 to 30 minutes, or continuous subcutaneous or continuous I.V. infusion, increased by 5 mcg/kg with each chemotherapy cycle if needed

➢ Neutropenia after bone marrow transplantation

Adults: 10 mcg/kg/day I.V. over 4 or 24 hours or as a continuous subcutaneous infusion over 24 hours

➢ To enhance peripheral blood progenitor cell collection in autologous hematopoietic stem cell transplantation

Adults: 10 mcg/kg/day by subcutaneous injection or as continuous subcutaneous infusion, starting 4 days before first leukapheresis procedure and continuing until last day of leukapheresis

➢ Neutropenia in congenital neutropenia

Adults: 6 mcg/kg subcutaneously b.i.d.

➢ Neutropenia in idiopathic or cyclic neutropenia

Adults: 5 mcg/kg/day subcutaneously

Off-label uses

- AIDS
- Aplastic anemia
- Hairy cell leukemia
- Myelodysplasia

Contraindications

- Hypersensitivity to drug, its components, or *Escherichia coli*–derived proteins

Precautions

Use cautiously in:

- patients receiving lithium or other drugs that can potentiate neutrophil release
- breastfeeding patients.

Administration

- Know that drug may be injected into venous return line of dialysis tubing after dialysis is completed.

🔊 To dilute for I.V. administration, use dextrose 5% in water. Never use saline solution, because it may cause drug to precipitate.

- Administer single dose intermittently over 15 to 30 minutes or by continuous infusion over 4 to 24 hours.
- Don't mix with other drugs, and don't shake.
- Don't give within 24 hours of chemotherapy, bone marrow transplantation, or radiation therapy.

Route	Onset	Peak	Duration
I.V.	5-60 min	24 hr	1-7 days
Subcut.	5-60 min	2-8 hr	1-7 days

Adverse reactions

CNS: headache, weakness
CV: chest pain, hypotension, transient supraventricular tachycardia, **myocardial infarction, arrhythmias**
EENT: sore throat
GI: nausea, vomiting, diarrhea, constipation, abdominal pain, splenomegaly, stomatitis
GU: bleeding
Hematologic: leukocytosis, sickle cell crisis, thrombocytopenia, splenic rupture
Metabolic: hyperuricemia
Musculoskeletal: bone, joint, muscle, arm, or leg pain
Respiratory: dyspnea, cough
Skin: pruritus, rash, erythema, alopecia, **cutaneous necrotic vasculitis**
Other: fever, mucositis, pain at injection site, edema, hypersensitivity reactions

Interactions

Drug-drug. *Lithium:* increased neutrophil production
Topotecan: prolonged neutropenia
Vincristine: increased risk of severe atypical peripheral neuropathy
Drug-diagnostic tests. *Alkaline phosphatase, creatinine, lactate dehydrogenase, uric acid:* increased levels
Platelets: decreased count

Patient monitoring

- Obtain CBC with platelet count before starting therapy; monitor these counts often thereafter.
- Monitor cardiovascular status carefully.
- Assess for signs and symptoms of sickle cell crisis and splenic rupture.

Patient teaching

- Teach patient how to recognize and promptly report signs and symptoms of allergic response.
- Caution patient to avoid driving and other hazardous activities until he knows how drug affects concentration and alertness.
- Advise patient to discuss possible need for iron supplements, vitamin B_{12}, and folic acid with prescriber.
- Teach patient how to monitor blood pressure at home.
- Advise patient to minimize GI upset by eating small, frequent servings of foods and drinking adequate fluids.
- Tell female patient to inform prescriber if she is breastfeeding.
- Inform patient that he'll undergo regular blood testing during therapy.
- As appropriate, review all other significant and life-threatening adverse reactions and interactions, especially those related to the drugs and tests mentioned above.

finasteride

Propecia, Proscar

Pharmacologic class: Androgen inhibitor
Therapeutic class: Sex hormone, hair regrowth stimulant
Pregnancy risk category X

Action

Suppresses dihydrotestosterone levels by inhibiting the hepatic enzyme 5-alpha reductase, which converts testosterone to dihydrotestosterone in prostate, liver, and skin

Availability

Tablets: 1 mg (Propecia), 5 mg (Proscar)

Indications and dosages

➢ Symptomatic benign prostatic hypertrophy (BPH)
Adults: 5 mg P.O. daily
➢ To reduce risk of progression of BPH symptoms
Adults: 5 mg P.O. daily (Proscar) given with doxazosin
➢ Male-pattern baldness
Adults: 1 mg P.O. daily

Off-label uses

- Acne in women
- Hirsutism

Contraindications

- Hypersensitivity to drug
- Females
- Children

Precautions

Use cautiously in:
- hepatic impairment, obstructive uropathy.

Administration

- Give with or without food.
- Know that female patients who are or may be pregnant shouldn't handle crushed or broken tablets. (Tablets are coated, so handling of intact tablets doesn't pose a problem).

Route	Onset	Peak	Duration
P.O. (BPH)	Unknown	8 hr	24 hr
P.O. (baldness)	3 mo	Unknown	Unknown

Adverse reactions

CNS: dizziness, headache, asthenia
EENT: lip swelling
GU: erectile dysfunction, decreased ejaculate volume, decreased libido, testicular pain, gynecomastia
Musculoskeletal: back pain
Skin: rash

Interactions

Drug-drug. *Theophylline:* increased theophylline clearance
Drug-diagnostic tests. *Prostate-specific antigen (PSA):* 50% decrease

Patient monitoring

- Carefully evaluate sustained PSA increases during therapy.
- Monitor fluid intake and output closely.

Patient teaching

- Tell patient he may take drug with or without food.
- Caution patient to avoid driving and other hazardous activities until he knows how drug affects concentration and alertness.
- Inform patient that he may experience erectile dysfunction and decreased ejaculate. Advise him to discuss these issues with prescriber.
- Caution female caregiver or companion who is or may be pregnant not to handle crushed or broken tablets.
- Tell patient he may need at least 6 months of therapy for BPH treatment and at least 3 months to see improvement in male-pattern baldness.
- Inform patient with BPH that he'll undergo periodic digital rectal exams.
- Instruct patient not to donate blood for at least 1 month after last dose.
- As appropriate, review all other significant adverse reactions and interactions, especially those related to the drugs and tests mentioned above.

flecainide acetate

Tambocor

Pharmacologic class: Cardiac benzamide local anesthetic

Therapeutic class: Antiarrhythmic (class IC)

Pregnancy risk category C

Action
Inhibits fast sodium channels of myocardial cell membrane. Also slows conduction, shortens action potential, stops paroxysmal reentrant supraventricular tachycardia, and decreases conduction in accessory pathways in Wolff-Parkinson-White syndrome.

Availability
Tablets: 50 mg, 100 mg, 150 mg

Indications and dosages
➢ Supraventricular tachyarrhythmias (including paroxysmal supraventricular tachycardia and paroxysmal atrial fibrillation or flutter)
Adults: Initially, 50 mg P.O. q 12 hours, increased by 50 mg b.i.d. q 4 days until desired response occurs or maximum daily dosage of 300 mg is reached.
➢ Sustained, life-threatening ventricular tachycardia
Adults: Initially, 100 mg P.O. q 12 hours, increased by 50 mg b.i.d. q 4 days until desired response occurs or maximum daily dosage of 400 mg is reached.

Dosage adjustment
- Heart failure
- Renal impairment

Off-label uses
- Ventricular arrhythmias
- Wolff-Parkinson-White syndrome

Contraindications
- Hypersensitivity to drug
- Preexisting atrioventricular block or right bundle-branch block
- Recent myocardial infarction
- Cardiogenic shock

Precautions
Use cautiously in:
- heart failure, renal impairment
- patients taking concurrent amiodarone, beta-adrenergic blockers, disopyramide, or verapamil
- pregnant or breastfeeding patients
- children (safety not established).

Administration
- Initiate therapy only in hospital setting with trained personnel and continuous ECG monitoring.
- Before giving, correct hypokalemia or hyperkalemia.
- Be aware that dosage may be reduced once arrhythmias have been adequately controlled.

Route	Onset	Peak	Duration
P.O.	Unknown	2-3 hr	12 hr

Adverse reactions
CNS: dizziness, anxiety, fatigue, headache, depression, malaise, tremor, weakness, hypoesthesia, paresthesia
CV: chest pain, palpitations, **second- or third-degree heart block, heart failure, new or worsening arrhythmias**
EENT: blurred vision, visual disturbances, corneal deposits
GI: nausea, vomiting, constipation, abdominal pain, dyspepsia, anorexia
Hepatic: hepatitis
Respiratory: dyspnea
Skin: rash, diaphoresis
Other: edema, fever

Interactions
Drug-drug. *Acidifying drugs:* increased renal elimination, decreased efficacy of flecainide (with urine pH below 5)
Alkalizing drugs: increased flecainide blood level, possible toxicity
Amiodarone: doubling of flecainide blood level
Beta-adrenergic blockers: increased blood levels of both drugs
Beta-adrenergic blockers, disopyramide, verapamil: additive myocardial depressant effect
Digoxin: 15% to 25% increase in digoxin blood level
Other antiarrhythmics (including calci-

um channel blockers): increased risk of arrhythmias
Drug-diagnostic tests. *Alkaline phosphatase:* increased level (with prolonged therapy)
Drug-food. *Foods that decrease urine pH below 5 (such as acidic juices):* increased renal elimination and possibly decreased efficacy of drug
Foods that increase urine pH above 7 (as in strict vegetarian diets): increased drug blood level
Drug-behaviors. *Smoking:* increased plasma clearance and decreased efficacy of drug

Patient monitoring

Monitor ECG for worsening arrhythmias.
- Measure pacing threshold 1 week before therapy starts and again after 1 week of therapy.
- Monitor potassium and flecainide blood levels.
- Assess respiratory status regularly.
- Monitor hepatic function tests.

Patient teaching

Instruct patient to immediately report cardiac or respiratory symptoms, unusual tiredness, or yellowing of skin or eyes.
- Tell patient drug may cause numbness. Advise him to avoid injury to areas with sensory impairment.
- Caution patient to avoid driving and other hazardous activities until he knows how drug affects concentration, alertness, and vision.
- Advise patient to minimize GI upset by eating small, frequent servings of food and drinking adequate fluids.
- Tell female patient to inform prescriber if she is pregnant or breastfeeding.
- Inform patient that he'll undergo regular blood testing during therapy.
- As appropriate, review all other significant and life-threatening adverse reactions and interactions, especially those related to the drugs, tests, foods, and behaviors mentioned above.

fluconazole
Diflucan

Pharmacologic class: Synthetic azole
Therapeutic class: Systemic antifungal
Pregnancy risk category C

f

Action

Alters cellular membrane, increasing permeability and leakage of essential elements needed for fungal growth. At higher concentrations, may be fungicidal.

Availability

Injection: 2 mg/ml in 100- or 200-ml bottles or containers
Powder for oral suspension: 50 mg/5 ml in 35-ml bottle, 200 mg/5 ml in 35-ml bottle
Tablets: 50 mg, 100 mg, 150 mg, 200 mg

Indications and dosages

➢ Oropharyngeal candidiasis
Adults: 200 mg P.O. or I.V. on first day, followed by 100 mg/day for at least 2 weeks
Children: 6 mg/kg P.O. or I.V. on first day, followed by 3 mg/kg/day for at least 2 weeks
➢ Esophageal candidiasis
Adults: 200 mg P.O. or I.V. on first day, followed by 100 mg/day for 3 weeks and then for 2 weeks after symptom resolution. Up to 400 mg/day may be used in severe cases.
Children: 6 mg/kg P.O. or I.V. on first day, followed by 3 mg/kg/day for 3 weeks and for at least 2 weeks after symptom resolution
➢ Systemic candidiasis
Adults: 400 mg P.O. or I.V. on first day, followed by 200 mg/day for 4 weeks

and for at least 2 weeks after symptom resolution
Children: 6 to 12 mg/kg/day P.O. or I.V.
➢ Vaginal candidiasis
Adults: 150 mg P.O. as a single dose
➢ Cryptococcal meningitis
Adults: 400 mg P.O. or I.V. on first day, followed by 200 or 400 mg/day for 10 to 12 weeks after cerebrospinal fluid (CSF) is negative
Children: 12 mg/kg P.O. or I.V. on first day, followed by 6 mg/kg/day for 10 to 12 weeks after CSF is negative
➢ Suppression of cryptococcal meningitis in patients with AIDS
Adults: 200 mg/day P.O. or I.V.
➢ To prevent candidiasis after bone marrow transplantation
Adults: 400 mg/day P.O. or I.V. for several days before and 7 days after neutrophil count rises above 1,000 cells/mm^3

Dosage adjustment
- Renal impairment
- Elderly patients

Contraindications
- Hypersensitivity to drug or its components

Precautions
Use cautiously in:
- hypersensitivity to other azole antifungals
- renal impairment or hepatic disease
- pregnant or breastfeeding patients
- children younger than 6 months.

Administration
🔈 Limit single I.V. infusion to 200 mg/hour or less, using infusion pump.
- Don't piggyback with other I.V. infusions.
- Keep overwrap on I.V. bag until just before use.
- Know that plastic container may be opaque (from moisture absorbed during sterilization). This doesn't affect drug and will decrease over time.

Route	Onset	Peak	Duration
P.O.	Slow	1-2 hr	2-4 days
I.V.	Rapid	1 hr	2-4 days

Adverse reactions
CNS: headache, dizziness
GI: nausea, vomiting, diarrhea, dyspepsia, abdominal discomfort
Hematologic: leukopenia, thrombocytopenia
Hepatic: hepatotoxicity
Skin: rash, pruritus, exfoliative skin disorders (including **Stevens-Johnson syndrome**)
Other: altered taste, **anaphylaxis**

Interactions
Drug-drug. *Alfentanil, cyclosporine, phenytoin, rifabutin, tacrolimus, theophylline, zidovudine:* increased blood levels of these drugs, greater risk of toxicity
Benzodiazepines, buspirone, losartan, nisoldipine, tricyclic antidepressants, zolpidem: increased blood levels and effects of these drugs
CYP3A4 inducers: inhibited CYP3A4 enzyme system, altered actions of CYP3A4 inducers (with fluconazole dosages above 200 mg/day)
Glipizide, glyburide, tolbutamide: increased hypoglycemic effect of these drugs
Rifampin: increased rifampin blood level, decreased fluconazole blood level
Thiazide diuretics: increased fluconazole blood level
Warfarin: increased warfarin activity
Drug-diagnostic tests. *Alanine aminotransferase, alkaline phosphatase, bilirubin, gamma-glutamyltransferase, hepatic enzymes:* increased levels
Platelets, white blood cells: decreased counts

Patient monitoring
🔈 Stay alert for signs and symptoms of anaphylaxis. Stop drug immediately if these occur.

• Monitor liver function test results and hematologic studies.
🔊 Assess for rash; if lesions develop, monitor patient. Stop drug and notify prescriber if lesions progress (may signal Stevens-Johnson syndrome).
• Be aware that patients with human immunodeficiency virus have greater risk of adverse reactions.

Patient teaching

🔊 Teach patient how to recognize and immediately report signs and symptoms of allergic response.
• Urge patient to contact prescriber if rash occurs, to determine whether Stevens-Johnson syndrome is developing.
• Caution patient to avoid driving and other hazardous activities until he knows how drug affects concentration and alertness.
• Advise patient to minimize GI upset by eating frequent, small servings of food and drinking adequate fluids.
• Tell female patient to inform prescriber if she is pregnant or breastfeeding.
• As appropriate, review all other significant and life-threatening adverse reactions and interactions, especially those related to the drugs and tests mentioned above.

flucytosine

Ancobon

Pharmacologic class: Fluorinated pyrimidine analog
Therapeutic class: Antifungal
Pregnancy risk category C

Action

Unclear. Thought to interfere with protein synthesis in cells of susceptible fungi after conversion to fluorouracil.

Availability

Capsules: 250 mg, 500 mg

Indications and dosages

➤ Severe fungal infections caused by susceptible strains of *Candida* species (including septicemia, endocarditis, urinary tract infections [UTIs]), and pulmonary infections) and *Cryptococcus* species (including meningitis, pulmonary infections, and UTIs)
Adults: 50 to 150 mg/kg P.O. daily in four equally divided doses q 6 hours

Dosage adjustment

• Renal impairment (glomerular filtration rate below 50 ml/minute)

Off-label uses

• Chromomycosis

Contraindications

• Hypersensitivity to drug or other antifungals

Precautions

Use cautiously in:
• renal impairment, underlying hepatic disease, bone marrow depression
• pregnant or breastfeeding patients
• children (safety not established).

Administration

• Give capsules a few at a time over 15 minutes to minimize nausea and vomiting.
• Know that drug is rarely used alone. Expect to give another antifungal or amphotericin B concurrently.

Route	Onset	Peak	Duration
P.O.	Variable	2 hr	10-12 hr

Adverse reactions

CNS: headache, dizziness, confusion, hallucinations, vertigo, psychosis, ataxia, paresthesia, parkinsonism, peripheral neuropathy
CV: chest pain, **cardiac arrest**
EENT: hearing loss

GI: nausea, vomiting, diarrhea, dyspepsia, ulcerative colitis, abdominal discomfort, anorexia, duodenal ulcer, **hemorrhage**
GU: azotemia, crystalluria, **renal failure**
Hematologic: eosinophilia, anemia, **leukopenia, aplastic anemia, thrombocytopenia, bone marrow depression, agranulocytosis**
Hepatic: jaundice
Metabolic: hypokalemia, **hypoglycemia**
Respiratory: dyspnea, **respiratory arrest**
Skin: rash, pruritus, urticaria, photosensitivity

Interactions

Drug-drug. *Amphotericin B:* synergistic effects, increased risk of toxicity
Drug-diagnostic tests. *Alanine aminotransferase, alkaline phosphatase, aspartate aminotransferase, bilirubin, gamma-glutamyltransferase:* increased levels
Glucose, granulocytes, hemoglobin, platelets, potassium, white blood cells: decreased levels

Patient monitoring

- Monitor kidney and liver function test results.
- Carefully monitor blood glucose level and hematologic test results.

◀ Assess for serious cardiovascular, renal, respiratory, and hematologic adverse reactions.

- Evaluate electrolyte levels, particularly potassium.
- Assess for signs and symptoms of bleeding.

Patient teaching

- Advise patient to take capsules over 15-minute period to reduce GI upset.

◀ Instruct patient to immediately report unusual bleeding or bruising.

- Caution patient to avoid driving and other hazardous activities until he knows how drug affects concentration and alertness.
- Instruct patient to minimize GI upset by eating frequent, small servings of food and drinking adequate fluids.
- Advise female patient to inform prescriber if she is pregnant or breastfeeding.
- Tell patient he'll undergo regular blood testing during therapy.
- As appropriate, review all other significant and life-threatening adverse reactions and interactions, especially those related to the drugs and tests mentioned above.

fludrocortisone acetate

Florinef Acetate

Pharmacologic class: Adrenocorticoid
Therapeutic class: Synthetic mineralocorticoid and glucocorticoid
Pregnancy risk category C

Action

Acts on renal distal tubule, increasing sodium reabsorption and potassium excretion

Availability

Tablets: 0.1 mg

Indications and dosages

➢ Addison's disease (adrenocortical insufficiency)
Adults: 0.1 mg P.O. daily
➢ Salt-losing adrenogenital syndrome
Adults: 0.1 to 0.2 mg P.O. daily

Off-label uses

- Hyponatremia
- Severe orthostatic hypotension

Contraindications

- Hypersensitivity to drug, tartrazine (some products), or sulfites (some products)
- Systemic fungal infection

Precautions

Use cautiously in:
- cardiovascular disease, cirrhosis, diverticulitis, ulcerative colitis, peptic ulcer, renal insufficiency, hypertension, myasthenia gravis, adrenal insufficiency
- pregnant or breastfeeding patients.

Administration

- Know that typical dosage may range from 0.1 mg three times weekly to 0.2 mg daily.
- Give with food to reduce GI upset.

◀ Reduce dosage, as ordered, if transient hypertension develops.

◀ Avoid abrupt discontinuation. Taper dosage gradually when withdrawing.

Route	Onset	Peak	Duration
P.O.	Variable	2 hr	1-2 days

Adverse reactions

CNS: headache, vertigo, **seizures**
CV: hypertension, cardiac hypertrophy, increased blood volume, **heart failure**
GU: glycosuria
Metabolic: hypernatremia, hypokalemia, hyperglycemia
Musculoskeletal: joint pain, tendon contractures, arm and leg weakness
Skin: urticaria, allergic rash, bruising, diaphoresis
Other: edema, infection, impaired wound healing, hypersensitivity reactions including **anaphylaxis**

Interactions

Drug-drug. *Amphotericin B, potassium-depleting diuretics:* enhanced hypokalemia
Anabolic steroids: increased risk of edema
Aspirin: increased ulcerogenic effect; decreased pharmacologic effect of aspirin; rarely, salicylate toxicity (in patients who discontinue fludrocortisone after concurrent high-dose aspirin therapy)
Barbiturates, phenytoin, rifampin: decreased fludrocortisone effects
Cardiac glycosides: increased risk of arrhythmias or digitalis toxicity associated with hypokalemia
Estrogen: increased risk of toxicity
Insulin, oral hypoglycemics: decreased hypoglycemic effect
Oral anticoagulants: decreased prothrombin time
Drug-diagnostic tests. *Cholesterol, urine glucose:* increased levels
Nitroblue tetrazolium test (for bacterial infection): false-negative result
Potassium, thyroxine, thyroid hormones: decreased levels
Drug-food. *Sodium-containing foods:* increased blood pressure
Drug-herbs. *Echinacea:* antagonism of fludrocortisone's immunosuppressive effect

Patient monitoring

◀ Monitor blood pressure. Report hypertension immediately.

- Assess for serious adverse reactions, particularly hypersensitivity and cardiovascular problems.
- Monitor sodium, potassium, and glucose levels carefully.
- Assess for signs and symptoms of infection.
- Weigh patient daily; report sudden gain.

Patient teaching

- Tell patient to take with meals or snack to minimize GI upset.

◀ Caution patient on long-term therapy not to stop taking drug abruptly.

- Advise patient on long-term therapy to wear or carry identification stating that he is receiving this drug.

◀ Teach patient to recognize and immediately report signs and symptoms of adrenal insufficiency (fatigue, appetite loss, nausea, vomiting, diarrhea, weight loss, weakness, dizziness, and low blood glucose level).

• Advise patient to consume a diet low in sodium and high in potassium and protein.
• Tell female patient to inform prescriber if she is pregnant or breastfeeding.
• As appropriate, review all other significant and life-threatening adverse reactions and interactions, especially those related to the drugs, tests, foods, and herbs mentioned above.

flunisolide

APO-Flunisolide✱, Nasarel, Novo-Flunisolide✱, PMS-Flunisolide✱, Ratio-Flunisolide✱, Rhinalar Nasal Mist✱

Pharmacologic class: Intranasal steroid
Therapeutic class: Respiratory inhalant
Pregnancy risk category C

Action

Unknown. Thought to diminish capillary permeability and suppress migration of polymorphonuclear leukocytes, decreasing inflammation.

Availability

Spray solution: 25 ml (each actuation delivers approximately 25 mcg)

Indications and dosages

➤ Relief of seasonal or perennial rhinitis
Adults: Two sprays in each nostril b.i.d.; may increase to two sprays in each nostril t.i.d. Maximum daily dose is eight sprays in each nostril. For maintenance, after desired clinical effect occurs, reduce dosage to smallest amount needed to control symptoms.
Children ages 6 to 14: One spray in each nostril t.i.d. or two sprays in each nostril b.i.d.; maximum daily dose is four sprays in each nostril. For maintenance, after desired clinical effect occurs, reduce dosage to smallest amount needed to control symptoms.

Contraindications

• Hypersensitivity to drug or its components
• Untreated local infections of nasal mucosa

Precautions

Use cautiously in:
• localized *Candida albicans* infection; tuberculosis; untreated fungal, bacterial, or systemic viral infections; ocular herpes simplex
• patients receiving immunosuppressive therapy.

Administration

• Don't increase dosage or discontinue drug abruptly.

Route	Onset	Peak	Duration
Inhalation (nasal)	Unknown	10-30 min	Unknown

Adverse reactions

CNS: headache, light-headedness, nervousness, dizziness
EENT: cataracts; glaucoma; blurred vision; conjunctivitis; increased intraocular pressure; lacrimation; dry, irritated eyes; tinnitus; otitis; otitis media; rhinorrhea; rhinitis; nasal irritation, burning, and dryness; nasal stuffiness and pain; sneezing; nasal ulcer; epistaxis; localized *Candida albicans* nasal infections; nasal mucosa ulcerations; nasal septum perforation; throat discomfort, soreness, and dryness; mild nasopharyngeal irritation; pharyngitis; dry mucous membranes; nasal and sinus congestion; sinusitis; hoarseness, voice changes
GI: nausea, vomiting, diarrhea, abdominal pain, dyspepsia, dry mouth
Metabolic: hyperadrenocorticism

Musculoskeletal: myalgia, arthralgia, aseptic necrosis of femoral head
Respiratory: wheezing, dyspnea, increased cough, bronchitis, **bronchospasm, asthma symptoms**
Skin: rash, pruritus, urticaria, contact dermatitis, alopecia, herpes simplex infection
Other: altered taste and smell, facial edema, fever, flulike symptoms, aches and pains, infections, **angioedema, anaphylaxis**

Interactions

Drug-diagnostic tests. *Aspartate aminotransferase:* increased level

Patient monitoring

Monitor patient closely for serious adverse reactions, including anaphylaxis, angioedema, hyperadrenocorticism, and serious infections.

Patient teaching

Teach patient to recognize and immediately report serious adverse reactions.

- Teach patient proper use of drug. Caution him not to use more than prescribed amount; doing so may cause serious side effects.
- Tell patient maximum drug effects may not occur for several weeks.
- Tell patient to avoid people with measles, chickenpox, and other transmissible infections.
- Caution patient to withhold dose and contact prescriber if infection occurs.
- Instruct female patient to tell prescriber if she becomes pregnant.
- Tell female patient not to breastfeed without consulting prescriber.
- As appropriate, review all other significant and life-threatening adverse reactions and interactions, especially those related to the tests mentioned above.

fluorouracil (5-fluorouracil, 5-FU)

Adrucil, Efudex, Fluoroplex

Pharmacologic class: Antimetabolite
Therapeutic class: Antineoplastic
Pregnancy risk category D

f

Action

Inhibits DNA and RNA synthesis, leading to death of rapid-growing neoplastic cells. Cell-cycle–S-phase specific.

Availability

Cream: 1%, 5%
Injection: 50 mg/ml in 10-ml ampules and 10-, 20-, and 100-ml vials
Solution: 1%, 2%, 5%

Indications and dosages

➤ Advanced colorectal cancer
Adults: 370 mg/m^2 I.V. for 5 days, preceded by leucovorin 200 mg/m^2 daily for 5 days; may be repeated q 4 to 5 weeks. No single daily dose should exceed 800 mg.
➤ Other cancers
Adults: Initially, 12 mg/kg/day I.V. for 4 days, followed by 1 day of rest; then 6 mg/kg I.V. every other day for four to five doses. Or 7 to 12 mg/kg/day I.V. for 4 days, followed by 3-day rest, then 7 to 10 mg/kg I.V. q 3 to 4 days for three doses. For maintenance, 7 to 12 mg/kg I.V. q 7 to 10 days, or 300 to 500 mg/m^2/day I.V. for 4 to 5 days, repeated monthly. No single daily dosage should exceed 800 mg.
Poor-risk patients: 3 to 6 mg/kg/day I.V. for 3 days, then 3 mg/kg/day I.V. on days 5, 7, and 9 (not to exceed 400 mg/dose)
➤ Actinic (solar) keratoses
Adults: 1% solution or cream applied once or twice daily to lesions on head,

neck, or chest; 2% to 5% solution or cream may be needed for other areas.
➢ Superficial basal cell carcinoma
Adults: 5% solution or cream applied b.i.d. for 3 to 6 weeks (up to 12 weeks)

Contraindications

- Hypersensitivity to drug or its components
- Bone marrow depression
- Dihydropyrimidine dehydrogenase enzyme deficiency (with topical route)
- Poor nutritional status
- Serious infection
- Pregnancy or breastfeeding

Precautions

Use cautiously in:
- renal or hepatic impairment, infections, edema, ascites
- obese patients.

Administration

🔊 Consult facility's cancer protocols to ensure correct dosage, administration technique, and cycle length.
- Give antiemetic before fluorouracil, as ordered, to reduce GI upset.
- Know that drug may be given without dilution by direct I.V. injection over 1 to 3 minutes.
- For I.V. infusion, dilute with dextrose 5% in water, sterile water, or normal saline solution in plastic bag (not glass bottle). Infusion may be given over a period of 24 hours or more.

🔊 Be aware of the importance of leucovorin rescue with fluorouracil therapy, if prescribed.
- Check infusion site frequently to detect extravasation.
- Use nonmetal applicator or appropriate gloves to apply topical form.
- Avoid applying topical form to mucous membranes or irritated skin.
- Don't use occlusive dressings over topical form.
- Know that pyridoxine may be given with fluorouracil to reduce risk of palmar-plantar erythrodysesthesia (hand-foot syndrome).

Route	Onset	Peak	Duration
I.V.	1-9 days	9-21 days	30 days
Topical	Unknown	Unknown	Unknown

Adverse reactions

CNS: confusion, disorientation, euphoria, ataxia, headache, weakness, malaise, **acute cerebellar syndrome or dysfunction**
CV: angina, **myocardial ischemia, thrombophlebitis**
EENT: vision changes, photophobia, lacrimation, lacrimal duct stenosis, nystagmus, epistaxis
GI: nausea, vomiting, diarrhea, stomatitis, anorexia, GI ulcer, **GI bleeding**
Hematologic: anemia, **leukopenia, thrombocytopenia**
Skin: alopecia, maculopapular rash, melanosis of nails, nail loss, palmar-plantar erythrodysesthesia, photosensitivity, local inflammation reaction (with cream), dermatitis
Other: fever, **anaphylaxis**

Interactions

Drug-drug. *Bone marrow depressants (including other antineoplastics):* additive bone marrow depression
Irinotecan: dehydration, neutropenia, sepsis
Leucovorin calcium: increased risk of fluorouracil toxicity
Live-virus vaccines: decreased antibody response to vaccine, increased risk of adverse reactions
Drug-diagnostic tests. *Alanine aminotransferase, alkaline phosphatase, aspartate aminotransferase, bilirubin, lactate dehydrogenase, urinary 5-hydroxyindoleacetic acid:* increased levels
Albumin, granulocytes, platelets, red blood cells, white blood cells (WBCs): decreased levels
Drug-behaviors. *Sun exposure:* increased risk of phototoxicity

Patient monitoring

🔊 Watch for signs and symptoms of toxicity, especially stomatitis and diarrhea. If these occur, stop drug and notify prescriber. Note that toxicity may take 1 to 3 weeks to develop.
- Monitor CBC, WBC and platelet counts, and kidney and liver function test results.
- Assess fluid intake and output.
- With long-term use, watch for serious rash on hands and feet. If it occurs, consult prescriber regarding need for pyridoxine.
- Assess for bleeding tendency.
- Monitor blood glucose level in patients at risk for hyperglycemia.

Patient teaching

🔊 Emphasize importance of taking leucovorin as prescribed with high-dose therapy.

🔊 Instruct patient to report signs and symptoms of toxicity, particularly stomatitis and diarrhea. Tell him that these may not occur for 1 to 3 weeks.
- Caution patient to avoid driving and other hazardous activities until he knows how drug affects concentration and alertness.
- Tell patient to avoid activities that can cause injury. Instruct him to use soft toothbrush and electric razor to avoid gum and skin injury.
- Advise patient to minimize GI upset by eating frequent, small servings of food and drinking adequate fluids.
- Tell patient that drug may cause reversible hair loss.
- Inform patient that he'll undergo regular blood testing during therapy.

🔊 Advise female to inform prescriber immediately if she is pregnant. Caution her not to breastfeed.
- As appropriate, review all other significant and life-threatening adverse reactions and interactions, especially those related to the drugs, tests, and behaviors mentioned above.

fluoxetine hydrochloride

Prozac, Prozac Weekly, Sarafem

Pharmacologic class: Selective serotonin reuptake inhibitor

Therapeutic class: Antidepressant

Pregnancy risk category B

f

Action

Selectively inhibits serotonin reuptake in CNS; has little to no effect on norepinephrine and dopamine reuptake

Availability

Capsules: 10 mg, 20 mg, 40 mg
Capsules (delayed-release): 90 mg
Oral solution: 20 mg/5 ml
Tablets: 10 mg

Indications and dosages

➢ Depression; obsessive-compulsive disorder

Adults: 20 mg/day P.O. in morning. After several weeks, may increase by 20 mg/day at weekly intervals. Give dosages above 20 mg/day in two divided doses (morning and noon); don't exceed 80 mg/day. In depression, patients stabilized on 20 mg/day may be switched to 90-mg/week delayed-release capsules (Prozac Weekly) 7 days after last 20-mg dose.

➢ Bulimia nervosa

Adults: 60 mg/day P.O.; may be titrated upward over several days

➢ Premenstrual dysphoric disorder

Adults: 20 mg/day P.O., not to exceed 80 mg/day

➢ Panic disorder

Adults: 10 mg/day P.O. for 1 week; then, if needed, increase to 20 mg/day. Dosage increases of up to 60 mg/day may be considered after several weeks if patient doesn't respond to lower dosage.

Dosage adjustment
- Hepatic impairment
- Elderly patients

Off-label uses
- Diabetic peripheral neuropathy
- Alcoholism
- Bipolar II disorder
- Borderline personality disorder
- Narcolepsy
- Posttraumatic stress disorder
- Schizophrenia
- Social phobia

Contraindications
- Hypersensitivity to drug
- MAO inhibitor use within past 14 days

Precautions
Use cautiously in:
- hepatic or renal impairment, diabetes mellitus, cardiovascular disease
- history of seizures
- pregnant or breastfeeding patients.

Administration
🔊 Be aware that drug should be discontinued 5 weeks before MAO inhibitor therapy begins.
- Give before 2 P.M. to prevent nighttime insomnia.

Route	Onset	Peak	Duration
P.O.	Unknown	6-8 hr	Unknown

Adverse reactions
CNS: anxiety, drowsiness, headache, insomnia, abnormal dreams, dizziness, fatigue, nervousness, hypomania, mania, weakness, tremor, **seizures, suicidal ideation**
CV: chest pain, palpitations, **prolonged QTc interval**
EENT: visual disturbances, stuffy nose, sinusitis, pharyngitis
GI: nausea, vomiting, diarrhea, constipation, abdominal pain, dyspepsia, dry mouth, anorexia
GU: urinary frequency, sexual dysfunction, dysmenorrhea
Metabolic: hypouricemia, hypocalcemia, hyponatremia, hyperglycemia, **hypoglycemia**
Musculoskeletal: joint, back, or muscle pain
Respiratory: cough, upper respiratory tract infection, dyspnea, **respiratory distress**
Skin: diaphoresis, pruritus, erythema nodosum, flushing, rash
Other: abnormal taste, weight loss, fever, flulike symptoms, hot flashes, allergic reactions, hypersensitivity reactions

Interactions
Drug-drug. *Adrenergics:* increased sensitivity to adrenergics, increased risk of serotonin syndrome
Alprazolam: decreased metabolism and increased effects of alprazolam
Antihistamines, opioids, other antidepressants, sedative-hypnotics: additive CNS depression
Buspirone: potentiation of fluoxetine effects, increased risk of seizures
Carbamazepine, clozapine, digoxin, haloperidol, lithium, phenytoin, warfarin: increased blood levels of these drugs, greater risk of adverse reactions
CYP450-2D6 inducers: increased effects of these drugs
Cyproheptadine: decrease in or reversal of fluoxetine effects
Digoxin, warfarin, other highly protein-bound drugs: increased risk of adverse reactions to either drug
Efavirenz, ritonavir, saquinavir, other CYP450 inhibitors: increased risk of serotonin syndrome
MAO inhibitors: confusion, agitation, seizures, hypertension, and hyperpyrexia (serotonin syndrome)
Other antidepressants, phenothiazines, risperidone, tryptophan: increased risk of adverse reactions
Ritonavir: increased ritonavir blood level

Drug-diagnostic tests. *Alanine aminotransferase, alkaline phosphatase, blood urea nitrogen, creatine kinase, electrolytes, glucose:* increased levels
Drug-herbs. *S-adenosylmethionine (SAM-e), St. John's wort:* increased risk of serotonin syndrome
Drug-behaviors. *Alcohol use:* additive CNS depression

Patient monitoring

- Monitor patient for signs and symptoms of depression. Assess for suicidal ideation.
- Evaluate neurologic status, watching especially for seizures.
- Monitor cardiovascular status, particularly for prolonged QTc interval.
- Assess weight regularly. Watch for signs of eating disorders.

Patient teaching

- Encourage patient to establish effective bedtime routine to minimize sleep disorders.
- Tell patient drug may take 4 weeks or longer to be fully effective.
- Instruct patient to contact prescriber if he develops worsening depression or has suicidal thoughts.
- Caution patient to avoid driving and other hazardous activities until he knows how drug affects concentration and alertness.
- Instruct patient to minimize adverse GI effects by eating frequent, small servings of healthy food and drinking adequate fluids.
- Advise patient to discuss anti-itching medicines with prescriber if rash develops.
- Tell female patient to inform prescriber if she is pregnant or breastfeeding.
- As appropriate, review all other significant and life-threatening adverse reactions and interactions, especially those related to the drugs, tests, herbs, and behaviors mentioned above.

fluoxymesterone

Halotestin

Pharmacologic class: Androgen, anabolic steroid
Therapeutic class: Sex hormone
Controlled substance schedule III
Pregnancy risk category X

f

Action

Responsible for normal growth and development of male sex organs; accelerates growth rate in children. Also has antiestrogen effect, helpful in treating estrogen-dependent tumors.

Availability

Tablets: 2 mg, 5 mg, 10 mg

Indications and dosages

➢ Hypogonadism caused by testicular deficiency
Adults: 5 to 20 mg/day P.O.
➢ Delayed puberty in boys
Adolescents: 2.5 to 10 mg/day P.O. in divided doses for 4 to 6 months. Individualize dosage and reduce to minimum when desired effects occur.
➢ Inoperable metastatic breast cancer
Adults: 10 to 40 mg/day P.O. in divided doses

Contraindications

- Hypersensitivity to drug, its components, or tartrazine
- Prostate cancer or breast cancer (other than inoperable breast cancer in women)
- Cardiac, renal, or hepatic disease
- Pregnancy or breastfeeding

Precautions

Use cautiously in:
- benign prostatic hypertrophy
- prepubertal boys.

Administration
- Give with food if GI upset occurs.
- Drug may contain tartrazine. Check patient history for allergies.

Route	Onset	Peak	Duration
P.O.	Unknown	2 hr	9 hr

Adverse reactions
CNS: headache, anxiety, depression, paresthesia
GI: nausea
GU: decreased urine output, increased libido, menstrual irregularities, gynecomastia
Hematologic: polycythemia, **leukopenia**
Hepatic: hepatic dysfunction, peliosis hepatitis, hepatocellular carcinoma
Metabolic: androgenic effects, hypoestrogenic effects, hypercalcemia, sodium and chloride retention
Skin: acne, hirsutism, male-pattern baldness, seborrhea
Other: fluid retention, edema, chills, premature epiphyseal closure, virilization (in females), hypersensitivity reaction

Interactions
Drug-drug. *Cyclosporine:* increased cyclosporine blood level
Hepatotoxic drugs: increased risk of hepatotoxicity
Insulin, oral antidiabetics: decreased blood glucose level
Oral anticoagulants: increased sensitivity to coagulants
Drug-diagnostic tests. *Calcium, creatinine, creatinine clearance, lipids, hepatic enzymes, red blood cells:* increased levels
Cholesterol: altered level
Drug-herbs. *Chaparral, comfrey, eucalyptus, germander, pennyroyal, skullcap, valerian:* increased risk of hepatotoxicity

Patient monitoring
- Watch for jaundice, and monitor liver function test results.
- Monitor hemoglobin, hematocrit, and cholesterol level.
- Evaluate for weight gain and edema.
- Monitor serum calcium level. Watch for signs and symptoms of hypercalcemia.
- Monitor skeletal maturation by X-ray in prepubertal male.
- Assess prepubertal male for excess hormonal effects (acne, priapism, increased body and facial hair, and phallic enlargement).
- Monitor postpubertal male for excess hormonal effects (testicular atrophy, erectile dysfunction, enlarged breasts, and epididymitis).

Patient teaching
- Advise patient to take with food to minimize GI upset.
- Instruct patient to consume high-calorie, high-protein diet and to eat frequent, small meals.
- Tell patient to weigh himself regularly and report sudden increases.

Caution female patient to stop taking drug and contact prescriber if menstrual irregularities develop.
- Instruct female patient to avoid pregnancy during therapy by using nonhormonal contraception.
- As appropriate, review all other significant and life-threatening adverse reactions and interactions, especially those related to the drugs, tests, and herbs mentioned above.

fluphenazine decanoate

Modecate, Prolixin Decanoate, Rho-Fluphenazine Decanoate✤

fluphenazine hydrochloride

Anatensol✤, Apo-Fluphenazine✤, Modecate Concentrate, Permitil Concentrate, PMS-Fluphenazine✤, Prolixin, Prolixin Concentrate

Pharmacologic class: Phenothiazine, dopaminergic blocker
Therapeutic class: Anxiolytic, antipsychotic
Pregnancy risk category C

Action

Unclear. May alter postsynaptic mesolimbic dopamine receptors in brain and reduce release of hypothalamic and hypophyseal hormones thought to depress reticular activating system, thereby preventing psychotic symptoms.

Availability

fluphenazine decanoate
Depot injection: 25 mg/ml
fluphenazine hydrochloride
Elixir: 2.5 mg/5 ml
Injection: 2.5 mg/ml
Oral concentrate: 5 mg/ml
Tablets: 1 mg, 2.5 mg, 5 mg, 10 mg

Indications and dosages

➢ Psychotic disorders

Adults: 2.5 to 10 mg/day (hydrochloride) P.O. in divided doses q 6 to 8 hours or as a single dose at bedtime; typical daily dosage is 1 to 5 mg; give oral doses above 20 mg/day with caution. Or initially, 1.25 mg I.M., divided and given q 6 to 8 hours. Parenteral hydrochloride dosage is one-third to one-half of oral dosage. Or 12.5 to 25 mg I.M. or subcutaneously (decanoate); base subsequent dosage and dosing intervals of 1 to 4 weeks on patient response; don't exceed 100 mg.

Dosage adjustment

- Elderly patients

Contraindications

- Hypersensitivity to drug, sulfites (with injectable form), or benzyl alcohol
- Angle-closure glaucoma
- Bone marrow depression
- Severe hepatic or cardiovascular disease

Precautions

Use cautiously in:

- diabetes, respiratory disease, prostatic hypertrophy, CNS tumors
- elderly patients
- pregnant or breastfeeding patients (safety not established)
- children with acute illnesses, infections, gastroenteritis, or dehydration.

Administration

- Don't give parenteral form to comatose or severely depressed patient.
- Use gloves when handling. To prevent contact dermatitis, keep drug away from clothing and skin.
- Dilute concentrated oral forms in juice, milk, or semisolid food just before administering.
- Give long-acting, oil-based preparations with dry needle of at least 21G.
- Be aware that antacids and adsorbent antidiarrheals may decrease adsorption of fluphenazine. Give 1 hour before or 2 hours after fluphenazine.

Route	Onset	Peak	Duration
P.O.	<1 hr	0.5 hr	6-8 hr
I.M. (HCl)	1 hr	1-5-2 hr	6-8 hr
I.M.	24-72 hr	Unknown	1-6 wk
Subcut.	Unknown	Unknown	Unknown

Adverse reactions

CNS: drowsiness, sedation, extrapyramidal reactions, tardive dyskinesia, pseudoparkinsonism, **neuroleptic malignant syndrome, seizures**
CV: hypotension, tachycardia
EENT: blurred vision, dry eyes, lens opacities, nasal congestion
GI: constipation, dry mouth, anorexia, **paralytic ileus**
GU: urinary retention, menstrual irregularities, inhibited ejaculation, priapism, gynecomastia, lactation
Hematologic: eosinophilia, **hemolytic anemia, aplastic anemia, agranulocytosis, leukopenia, thrombocytopenia**
Hepatic: jaundice, **hepatitis**
Metabolic: galactorrhea, hyperthermia
Skin: photosensitivity, rash
Other: allergic reactions, pain at injection site, sterile abscess

Interactions

Drug-drug. *Activated charcoal, adsorbent antidiarrheals, antacids:* decreased fluphenazine adsorption
Anticholinergics: decreased fluphenazine effects
Antidepressants, antihistamines, general anesthetics, MAO inhibitors, opioid analgesics, sedative-hypnotics: additive CNS depression
Antihistamines, disopyramide, quinidine, tricyclic antidepressants (TCAs): increased risk of anticholinergic effects
Antihypertensives: additive hypotension
Barbiturates: increased fluphenazine metabolism and decreased efficacy
Bromocriptine: decreased bromocriptine efficacy
Guanethidine: inhibition of antihypertensive effects
Lithium: disorientation, unconsciousness, extrapyramidal symptoms
Meperidine: excessive sedation and hypotension
Ofloxacin: increased QTc interval
Phenytoin: increased or decreased phenytoin blood level
Pimozide: increased risk of potentially serious cardiovascular reactions
Propranolol: increased blood levels of both drugs
TCAs: increased blood levels and effects of TCAs
Drug-diagnostic tests. *Alanine aminotransferase, alkaline phosphatase, aspartate aminotransferase, bilirubin:* increased levels
Granulocytes, hematocrit, hemoglobin, leukocytes, platelets: decreased values
Pregnancy tests: false-positive or false-negative result
Urine bilirubin: false-positive result
Drug-herbs. *Angel's trumpet, jimsonweed, scopolia:* increased anticholinergic effects
Chamomile, hops, kava, skullcap: increased CNS depression
St. John's wort: photosensitivity
Yohimbe: fluphenazine toxicity
Drug-behaviors. *Alcohol use:* increased CNS depression
Sun exposure: increased risk of photosensitivity

Patient monitoring

🔊 Monitor patient for signs and symptoms of neuroleptic malignant syndrome (extrapyramidal symptoms, hyperthermia, autonomic symptoms).
🔊 Stop giving drug and notify prescriber immediately if patient shows signs or symptoms of blood dyscrasias (fever, infection, sore throat, cellulitis, or weakness).
- Observe for tardive dyskinesia.
- Watch for bleeding tendency.
- Monitor CBC, bilirubin level, and liver function test results.
- Assess kidney function and ophthalmic test results in patients on long-term therapy.

Patient teaching

🔊 Tell patient not to stop taking drug suddenly, because serious adverse effects may occur.

• Advise patient to report urinary retention or constipation.
Instruct patient to immediately report unusual bleeding or bruising.
• Caution patient to avoid driving and other hazardous activities until he knows how drug affects concentration, alertness, and vision.
• Tell patient to avoid activities that can cause injury. Advise him to use soft toothbrush and electric razor to avoid gum and skin injury.
• Inform patient that he'll undergo regular blood testing during therapy.
• Tell female patient to inform prescriber if she is pregnant or breastfeeding.
• As appropriate, review all other significant and life-threatening adverse reactions and interactions, especially those related to the drugs, tests, herbs, and behaviors mentioned above.

flurazepam hydrochloride

Apo-Flurazepam✤, Dalmane, Novo-Flupam✤, Somnol✤

Pharmacologic class: Benzodiazepine
Therapeutic class: Sedative-hypnotic
Controlled substance IV
Pregnancy risk category X

Action

Depresses CNS at limbic, thalamic, and hypothalamic levels by enhancing inhibitory neurotransmitter effect of gamma-aminobutyric acid on neuronal excitability

Availability

Capsules: 15 mg, 30 mg

Indications and dosages

➢ Short-term management of insomnia (less than 4 weeks)
Adults: 15 to 30 mg P.O. at bedtime

Dosage adjustment

• Elderly or debilitated patients

Contraindications

• Hypersensitivity to drug or other benzodiazepines
• Preexisting CNS depression
• Angle-closure glaucoma
• Pregnancy or breastfeeding

Precautions

Use cautiously in:
• hepatic dysfunction
• history of suicide attempt or drug dependence
• elderly patients
• children younger than age 15 (safety not established).

Administration

• Before starting therapy, evaluate patient's mental status and check kidney and liver function tests and CBC.

Route	Onset	Peak	Duration
P.O.	15-45 min	0.5-1 hr	7-8 hr

Adverse reactions

CNS: dizziness, daytime drowsiness, headache, lethargy, confusion, poor concentration, depression, paradoxical excitation, ataxia
EENT: blurred vision
GI: nausea, vomiting, diarrhea, constipation, dyspepsia, abdominal pain
Respiratory: sleep apnea
Skin: rash
Other: abnormal taste, hangover, physical or psychological drug dependence, drug tolerance

Interactions

Drug-drug. *Antidepressants, antihistamines, opioids:* additive CNS depression
Barbiturates, rifampin: increased flurazepam metabolism, decreased efficacy
Cimetidine, disulfiram, fluoxetine, hormonal contraceptives, isoniazid, keto-

conazole, metoprolol, propoxyphene, propranolol, valproic acid: decreased flurazepam metabolism, enhanced efficacy
Levodopa: decreased levodopa efficacy
Theophylline: decreased sedative effects of flurazepam
Drug-diagnostic tests. *Alanine aminotransferase, alkaline phosphatase, aspartate aminotransferase, total and direct bilirubin:* increased levels
Drug-herbs. *Chamomile, hops, kava, skullcap, valerian:* additive CNS depression
Drug-behaviors. *Alcohol use:* additive CNS depression
Smoking: increased drug metabolism and clearance

Patient monitoring

- With long-term use, watch for signs and symptoms of physical or psychological dependence.
- Monitor patient's mental status, especially for depression and suicidal ideation.
- Watch for signs of drug hoarding or overuse.
- Monitor CBC and liver and kidney function tests.

Patient teaching

🔊 Urge patient (and significant other as appropriate) to report signs and symptoms of depression or suicidal thoughts or actions.
🔊 Advise female patient to immediately tell prescriber if she is pregnant. Caution her not to breastfeed.
- Inform patient that drug may cause physical or psychological dependence.
- Advise patient to minimize GI upset by eating frequent, small servings of food and drinking adequate fluids.
- As appropriate, review all other significant and life-threatening adverse reactions and interactions, especially those related to the drugs, tests, herbs, and behaviors mentioned above.

flutamide

Euflex✦, Eulexin, Novo-Flutamide✦

Pharmacologic class: Antiandrogen
Therapeutic class: Antineoplastic
Pregnancy risk category D

Action

Exerts potent antiandrogenic activity at cellular level by inhibiting androgen uptake or nuclear binding of androgen

Availability

Capsules: 125 mg

Indications and dosages

➢ Metastatic prostate cancer
Adults: 250 mg P.O. t.i.d. q 8 hours, given with luteinizing hormone-releasing hormone (LHRH) analog. Total daily dosage is 750 mg.

Off-label uses

- Benign prostatic hypertrophy

Contraindications

- Hypersensitivity to drug
- Severe hepatic impairment
- Sleep apnea
- Women

Precautions

None

Administration

- Be aware that leuprolide acetate is the most common LHRH analog given with flutamide.

Route	Onset	Peak	Duration
P.O.	Variable	2 hr	72 hr

Adverse reactions

CNS: drowsiness, confusion, depression, anxiety, nervousness, paresthesia
CV: peripheral edema, hypertension

GI: nausea, vomiting, diarrhea, constipation, abdominal pain, dyspepsia, anorexia, dry mouth
GU: erectile dysfunction, loss of libido, gynecomastia, hot flashes
Hematologic: anemia, **leukopenia, thrombocytopenia**
Hepatic: hepatitis
Skin: rash, photosensitivity

Interactions

Drug-drug. *Warfarin:* increased prothrombin time
Drug-diagnostic tests. *Alkaline phosphatase, alanine aminotransferase, aspartate aminotransferase, blood urea nitrogen, creatine kinase:* increased levels
Hemoglobin, platelets, white blood cells: decreased levels
Drug-herbs. *Chaparral, comfrey, eucalyptus, germander, pennyroyal, skullcap, valerian:* increased risk of hepatotoxicity
Drug-behaviors. *Sun exposure:* increased risk of photosensitivity

Patient monitoring

- Monitor CBC and liver function tests.

🔈 Watch for bleeding tendency and signs and symptoms of hepatic damage (jaundice, vomiting, dark yellow or brown urine).

- Monitor blood pressure.

Patient teaching

🔈 Instruct patient to immediately report unusual bleeding or bruising.

- Tell patient to avoid activities that can cause injury. Advise him to use soft toothbrush and electric razor to avoid gum and skin injury.
- Caution patient to avoid driving and other hazardous activities until he knows how drug affects concentration and alertness.
- Instruct patient to minimize GI upset by eating frequent, small servings of healthy food.
- Tell patient he'll undergo regular blood testing during therapy.
- As appropriate, review all other significant and life-threatening adverse reactions and interactions, especially those related to the drugs, tests, herbs, and behaviors mentioned above.

fluticasone propionate

Cutivate, Flonase, Flovent

f

Pharmacologic class: Corticosteroid
Therapeutic class: Respiratory inhalant (Flovent, Flonase), anti-inflammatory drug (Cutivate)
Pregnancy risk category C

Action

Unknown. Has potent vasoconstrictive and anti-inflammatory properties.

Availability

Inhalation aerosol (Flovent): 44 mcg, 110 mcg, 220 mcg
Nasal spray (Flonase): 50 mcg
Topical cream (Cutivate): 0.005%
Topical ointment (Cutivate): 0.005%

Indications and dosages

➢ Prophylaxis of asthma (Flovent)
Adults and children ages 12 and older: Initial dosage is based on previous therapy (see chart below). Once stability is achieved, titrate to lowest effective dosage.

Recommended Flovent dosages

Previous therapy	Starting dosage	Maximum dosage
Bronchodilator alone	88 mcg inhaled orally b.i.d.	440 mcg inhaled orally b.i.d.
Inhaled corticosteroid	88-220 mcg inhaled orally b.i.d.	440 mcg inhaled orally b.i.d.
Oral corticosteroid	880 mcg inhaled orally b.i.d.	880 mcg inhaled orally b.i.d.

➢ Seasonal and perennial allergic and nonallergic rhinitis (Flonase)
Adults: Two sprays in each nostril daily or one spray in each nostril b.i.d. After first few days, may reduce dosage to one spray in each nostril daily; some patients may find p.r.n. use of two sprays in each nostril daily effective for symptom control. Maximum dosage is 200 mcg daily (two sprays in each nostril).
Adolescents and children ages 4 and older: Initially, one spray in each nostril daily. If patient doesn't respond, may increase to two sprays in each nostril. Once adequate control is achieved, reduce dosage to one spray in each nostril daily.
➢ Inflammatory and pruritic manifestations of corticosteroid-responsive atopic dermatoses
Adults and children ages 3 months and older: Apply thin film of Cutivate cream to affected skin area once or twice daily.
➢ Other corticosteroid-responsive dermatoses
Adults and children ages 3 months and older: Apply thin film of Cutivate cream to affected skin area b.i.d.

Contraindications

• Hypersensitivity to drug or its components
• Primary treatment of status asthmaticus or other acute asthma episodes necessitating intensive measures (Flovent)
• Severe allergy to milk proteins

Precautions

Use cautiously in:
• recurrent epistaxis, recent nasal septal ulcer, nasal surgery, or nasal trauma
• elderly patients (Flonase)
• pregnant or breastfeeding patients (Flovent, Flonase)
• children (Flovent)
• children younger age than 4 (Flonase).

Administration

• Know that Flonase may cause immediate hypersensitivity reaction (contact dermatitis).
• Be aware that topical ointment should be used in adults only.

Route	Onset	Peak	Duration
Oral or nasal inhalation, topical	Unknown	Unknown	Unknown

Adverse reactions

CNS: *Cutivate ointment*—light-headedness; *Flonase*—headache, dizziness; *Flovent*—headache, dizziness, giddiness
EENT: *Flonase*—cataract, glaucoma, increased intraocular pressure (IOP), epistaxis, nasal burning or irritation, bloody nasal mucus, runny nose, pharyngitis; *Flovent*—nasal congestion, nasal septum perforation, nasal discharge, nasal sinus pain, sinusitis, rhinitis, allergic rhinitis, pharyngitis, dysphonia
GI: *Flonase*—nausea, vomiting, diarrhea, abdominal pain; *Flovent*—nausea, vomiting, diarrhea, dyspepsia, stomach disorder, oral candidiasis
GU: *Flovent*—dysmenorrhea
Musculoskeletal: *Flonase*—aches and pains; *Flovent*—joint pain, limb pain, sprain, strain, aches and pains
Respiratory: *Flonase*—cough, bronchitis, wheezing (rare), **asthma symptoms;** *Flovent*—upper respiratory tract infection, influenza, bronchitis, chest congestion, **bronchospasm**
Skin: *Cutivate cream*—pruritus, skin dryness, skin burning, erythematous rash, dusky erythema, eczema exacerbation, skin irritation, urticaria; *Cutivate ointment*—skin burning or irritation, hypertrichosis, increased erythema, hives; *Flovent*—urticaria, rash, skin eruption
Other: *Cutivate cream or ointment*—numbness of fingers, facial or nonfacial telangiectasia; *Flonase*—fever, flulike

symptoms, hypersensitivity reaction; *Flovent*—dental problems, fever, immediate or delayed hypersensitivity reactions, **angioedema**

Interactions

Drug-drug. *Ketoconazole:* increased fluticasone exposure (with Flonase, Flovent)
Ritonavir: increased systemic corticosteroid effects (with Flonase, Flovent)
Drug-diagnostic tests. *Adrenocorticotropic hormone stimulation test, plasma cortisol test, urinary free cortisol test:* interference with test results

Patient monitoring

Clinical alert: Monitor patient for withdrawal symptoms after Flovent is discontinued.
- Stay alert for systemic corticosteroid effects when administering Flovent or Flonase.
- Observe for reduced growth rate in child or adolescent using Flovent or Flonase.
- When giving Flovent, stay alert for eosinophilic conditions, such as Churg-Strauss syndrome.

Clinical alert: When giving Flonase, assess for wheezing, nasal septum perforation, cataracts, glaucoma, and increased IOP (rare).

Patient teaching

- Teach patient proper use of prescribed form.

Clinical alert: Advise patient to immediately report signs of allergic reaction.
- Caution patient to avoid exposure to people with chickenpox or measles.
- Advise female patient taking Flonase or Flovent to inform prescriber if she is pregnant or breastfeeding.
- As appropriate, review all other significant and life-threatening adverse reactions and interactions, especially those related to the drugs and tests mentioned above.

fluvastatin sodium

Lescol, Lescol XL

Pharmacologic class: HMG-CoA reductase inhibitor
Therapeutic class: Antihyperlipidemic
Pregnancy risk category X

Action

Competitively inhibits HMG-CoA reductase, an enzyme needed to synthesize cholesterol. This inhibition reduces cholesterol concentration in hepatic cells, which in turn increases synthesis of low-density lipoprotein (LDL) receptors, enhances LDL uptake, and ultimately reduces plasma cholesterol concentration.

Availability

Capsules: 20 mg, 40 mg
Tablets (extended-release): 80 mg

Indications and dosages

➢ Adjunctive therapy to reduce LDL cholesterol (LDL-C), total cholesterol, triglyceride, and apolipoprotein B levels
Adults: For LDL-C reduction of less than 25%, initial dosage is 20 mg daily at bedtime. For reduction of at least 25%, initial dosage is 40 mg P.O. (capsules) daily at bedtime; may increase if necessary to 40 mg (capsules) P.O. b.i.d. or 80 mg (extended-release tablet) P.O. daily in evening. Maximum dosage is 80 mg/day.
➢ Secondary prevention of cardiovascular events in patients with coronary heart disease who have undergone percutaneous intervention procedures
Adults: 40 mg (capsule) P.O. b.i.d.

Contraindications

- Hypersensitivity to drug
- Active hepatic disease

- Severe renal impairment
- Pregnancy or breastfeeding

Precautions

Use cautiously in:
- hypotension, mild to moderate renal impairment, severe metabolic disorders, visual disturbances, alcoholism
- patients receiving concurrent azole antifungals
- females of childbearing age
- children younger than age 18 (safety not established).

Administration

- Know that before starting drug, patient should be on standard cholesterol-lowering diet and weight-control and physical exercise programs, if appropriate.
- Give with or without food.
- Be aware that drug works better when taken in evening.
- If patient's also receiving bile-acid resin, give fluvastatin at bedtime at least 4 hours after resin.

Route	Onset	Peak	Duration
P.O.	1-2 wk	4-6 wk	Unknown
P.O. (extended)	2 wk	4 wk	Unknown

Adverse reactions

CNS: amnesia, malaise, drowsiness, weakness, emotional lability, facial paralysis, syncope, headache, poor coordination, hyperkinesia, paresthesia, peripheral neuropathy
CV: orthostatic hypotension, palpitations, phlebitis, **arrhythmias**
EENT: amblyopia, altered refraction, eye hemorrhage, glaucoma, dry eyes, hearing loss, tinnitus, epistaxis, sinusitis, pharyngitis
GI: nausea, vomiting, diarrhea, constipation, dyspepsia, flatulence, abdominal pain or cramps, gastroenteritis, colitis, stomach ulceration, dysphagia, esophagitis, stomatitis, melena, tenesmus, **rectal hemorrhage, pancreatitis**
GU: urinary frequency, urinary retention, nocturia, dysuria, hematuria, cystitis, decreased libido, epididymitis, erectile dysfunction, renal calculi, nephritis
Hematologic: anemia, **thrombocytopenia**
Hepatic: jaundice, **hepatitis**
Metabolic: hyperglycemia, **hypoglycemia**
Musculoskeletal: joint pain, back pain, leg cramps, gout, bursitis, myasthenia gravis, myositis, torticollis
Respiratory: dyspnea, pneumonia, bronchitis
Skin: acne, alopecia, contact dermatitis, eczema, diaphoresis, rash, urticaria, skin ulcers, seborrhea, photosensitivity
Other: gingival hemorrhage, appetite changes, weight gain, fever, facial or generalized edema, flulike symptoms, infection, allergic reaction

Interactions

Drug-drug. *Antacids, cholestyramine, colestipol:* decreased fluvastatin blood level
Antifungals, cyclosporine, erythromycin, niacin, other HMG-CoA inhibitors: increased risk of myopathy
Cimetidine, omeprazole, ranitidine: increased fluvastatin blood level
Digoxin: increased digoxin blood level
Phenytoin: increased blood levels of both drugs
Rifampin: increased fluvastatin metabolism, decreased blood level
Drug-diagnostic tests. *Alanine aminotransferase, aspartate aminotransferase, creatine kinase (CK):* increased levels
Drug-herbs. *Comfrey, germander, jin bu huan, pennyroyal, skullcap, valerian:* increased risk of hepatotoxicity
Red yeast rice: increased risk of adverse reactions
Drug-behaviors. *Alcohol use:* increased risk of hepatotoxicity

Patient monitoring

- Watch for allergic reaction to drug.
- Assess for myositis. If patient has muscle pain, monitor CK level.
- Monitor lipid levels and liver function test results.
- Watch for bleeding tendencies.
- In patients receiving phenytoin, monitor closely when fluvastatin therapy begins or fluvastatin dosage is changed.

Patient teaching

- Instruct patient to take in evening for best effect.
- Advise patient to maintain standard cholesterol-lowering diet and weight-control and physical exercise programs, as appropriate.

Clinical alert: Instruct patient to immediately report unusual bleeding or bruising, irregular heart beat, muscle aches or pains, yellowing of eyes or skin, or unusual tiredness.

- Teach patient how to recognize and report signs and symptoms of allergic response.
- Caution patient to avoid driving and other hazardous activities until he knows how drug affects concentration, alertness, and vision.
- Inform male patient that drug may cause erectile dysfunction and abnormal ejaculation.
- Tell patient that full effect of drug may take up to 4 weeks.
- Tell patient to move slowly when rising, to avoid dizziness from sudden blood pressure decrease.
- Tell patient that he'll undergo regular blood testing during therapy.
- As appropriate, review all other significant and life threatening adverse reactions and interactions, especially those related to the drugs, tests, herbs, and behaviors mentioned above.

fluvoxamine maleate

Apo-Fluvoxamine✤, Luvox

Pharmacologic class: Selective serotonin reuptake inhibitor (SSRI)

Therapeutic class: Antidepressant, antiobsessive agent

Pregnancy risk category C

Action

Selectively inhibits serotonin reuptake in neurons. This inhibition is thought to relieve depression and reduce behaviors related to obsessive-compulsive disorder (OCD).

Availability

Tablets: 25 mg, 50 mg, 100 mg

Indications and dosages

➤ OCD; depression

Adults: Initially, 50 mg P.O. daily at bedtime; may increase by 50 mg q 4 to 7 days until desired effect occurs (not to exceed 300 mg/day). If daily dosage exceeds 100 mg, give in two equally divided doses; if doses aren't equal, give larger dose at bedtime. As needed, adjust dosage periodically to maintain lowest effective dosage.

Children ages 8 to 17: Initially, 25 mg at bedtime; may increase by 25 mg/day q 4 to 7 days until desired effect occurs (up to 200 mg/day). If daily dosage exceeds 50 mg, give in divided doses, with larger dose at bedtime.

Dosage adjustment

- Hepatic impairment
- Elderly patients

Off-label uses

- Autism
- Anxiety disorders

Contraindications

- Hypersensitivity to drug or other SSRIs
- MAO inhibitor use within past 14 days

Precautions

Use cautiously in:

- cardiovascular disease, hepatic or renal impairment, mania, seizures, suicidal tendency
- elderly patients
- labor and delivery
- pregnant or breastfeeding patients.

Administration

- Give with or without food.
- Discontinue 5 weeks before MAO inhibitor therapy is set to begin.

Route	Onset	Peak	Duration
P.O.	Rapid	2-8 hr	Unknown

Adverse reactions

CNS: dizziness, drowsiness, headache, insomnia, nervousness, anxiety, apathy, manic or psychotic reactions, depression, hypokinesia or hyperkinesia, tremor, **suicide or suicidal ideation** (especially in child or adolescent)
CV: hypertension, orthostatic hypotension, palpitations, tachycardia
EENT: sinusitis
GI: nausea, vomiting, diarrhea, constipation, dyspepsia, flatulence, dry mouth, dysphagia, anorexia
GU: decreased libido, sexual dysfunction, anorgasmia
Musculoskeletal: hypertonia, myoclonus, twitching
Respiratory: cough, dyspnea
Skin: diaphoresis
Other: abnormal taste, tooth disorder, dental caries, edema, weight gain or loss, chills, fever, flulike symptoms, yawning, hot flashes, allergic reactions, hypersensitivity reaction

Interactions

Drug-drug. *Beta-adrenergic blockers (such as propranolol), carbamazepine, lithium, L-tryptophan, methadone, some benzodiazepines, theophylline, tolbutamide, warfarin:* decreased fluvoxamine metabolism, increased effects
Clozapine: increased clozapine blood level and risk of toxicity
MAO inhibitors: serotonin syndrome
Tricyclic antidepressants: increased fluvoxamine blood level
Drug-tests. *Hepatic enzyme levels:* increased
Drug-behaviors. *Smoking:* decreased fluvoxamine efficacy

Patient monitoring

Watch closely for signs and symptoms of depression and suicidal ideation (especially in child or adolescent).

- Assess patient's appetite. Report weight gain or loss.
- Monitor liver function test results.
- Monitor cardiovascular status, particularly blood pressure.

Patient teaching

Instruct patient or caregiver (especially with child or adolescent patient) to recognize and immediately report signs of suicidal intent or expressions of suicidal ideation.

- Inform patient that drug may take several weeks to be fully effective.
- Recommend establishing effective bedtime routine to minimize insomnia.
- Instruct female patient to notify prescriber if she becomes or intends to become pregnant. Caution her not to breastfeed.
- Caution patient to avoid driving and other hazardous activities until he knows how drug affects concentration and alertness.
- As appropriate, review all other significant and life-threatening adverse reactions and interactions, especially those related to the drugs, tests, and behaviors mentioned above.

fondaparinux sodium

Arixtra

Pharmacologic class: Selective factor Xa inhibitor

Therapeutic class: Anticoagulant, antithrombotic

Pregnancy risk category B

Action

Selectively inhibits factor Xa, disrupting blood coagulation and inhibiting thrombin formation and thrombus development

Availability

Injection: 2.5 mg/0.5 ml in single-dose syringe

Indications and dosages

➢ Prevention of deep-vein thrombosis after hip fracture surgery or hip or knee replacement surgery

Adults: 2.5 mg subcutaneously 6 to 8 hours after surgery, once hemostasis occurs; usual duration is 5 to 9 days (up to 11 days) given daily. After hip fracture surgery, extended prophylactic course of up to 24 additional days is recommended; some patients have tolerated a total course of 32 days.

➢ Deep-vein thrombosis and pulmonary emboli

Adults: 5 mg subcutaneously once daily for patients weighing less than 50 kg (110 lb), 7.5 mg subcutaneously for patients weighing 50 to 100 kg (110 to 220 lb) or 10 mg subcutaneously for patients weighing more than 100 kg (220 lb) for 5 days and until therapeutic oral anticoagulant effect occurs (as shown by International Normalized Ratio of 2 to 3). Usual duration of therapy is 5 to 9 days, but may continue for up to 26 days.

Dosage adjustment

- Renal impairment

Contraindications

- Hypersensitivity to drug
- Bacterial endocarditis
- Severe renal disease
- Active major bleeding
- Patients weighing less than 50 kg (110 lbs) who have undergone hip fracture, hip replacement, or knee replacement surgery

Precautions

Use cautiously in:

- diabetic retinopathy, hepatic disease, blood dyscrasias, heparin-induced thrombocytopenia, severe hypertension, alcoholism
- patients older than age 75
- pregnant or breastfeeding patients
- children (safety and efficacy not established).

Administration

🔊 Withhold for at least 6 to 8 hours after surgery, to minimize risk of major bleeding.

🔊 Give by subcutaneous injection only. Don't give I.M.

- Rotate injection sites among fatty tissue areas on left and right anterolateral and posterolateral abdominal walls.
- Don't expel air bubble from syringe; doing so may reduce amount of drug delivered.
- Listen for slight click when plunger is fully released. After drug has been injected, needle retracts and white safety indicator is visible.
- Don't mix with other injections or infusions.
- Know that when drug is used to treat deep-vein thrombosis and pulmonary emboli, concomitant warfarin treatment should begin as soon as possible (usually within 72 hours).

Route	Onset	Peak	Duration
Subcut.	Rapid	3 hr	72 hr

Adverse reactions

CNS: depression, dizziness, asthenia, headache, abnormal thinking, confusion, insomnia, neuropathy
CV: hypotension
GI: nausea, vomiting, diarrhea, constipation, abdominal pain, dyspepsia, dry mouth, anorexia
GU: urinary retention, urinary tract infection
Hematologic: anemia, hematoma, purpura, minor bleeding, **major bleeding, thrombocytopenia, retroperitoneal hemorrhage, postoperative hemorrhage**
Metabolic: hypokalemia
Skin: bullous eruption
Other: increased wound drainage, injection site bleeding, pain, edema, fever

Interactions

Drug-drug. *Anticoagulants:* increased risk of bleeding
Drug-herbs. *Anise, astragalus, bilberry, black currant, bladder wrack, bogbean, boldo, borage, buchu, capsaicin, cat's claw, celery, chaparral, cinchona, clove oil, dandelion, dong quai, fenugreek, feverfew, garlic, ginger, ginkgo, papaya, red clover, rhubarb, safflower oil, skullcap, tan-shen:* additive anticoagulant effect
St. John's wort: reduced anticoagulant effect

Patient monitoring

• Monitor CBC, platelet count, creatinine level, and renal function tests. Assess stools for occult blood.
• Monitor vital signs, temperature, and fluid intake and output.
[Clinical alert] Stay alert for bleeding tendency, especially postoperative hemorrhage.
• Check for increased wound drainage after surgery.
[Clinical alert] In patient undergoing concomitant neuraxial anesthesia or spinal puncture, watch for neurologic impairment (indicating possible spinal or epidural hematoma).
[Clinical alert] Discontinue drug if severe renal impairment occurs.

Patient teaching

[Clinical alert] Instruct patient to immediately report bleeding.
• Caution patient to avoid activities that can cause injury. Tell him to use soft toothbrush and electric razor to avoid gum and skin injury.
• Tell patient that he'll undergo regular blood testing during therapy.
• As appropriate, review all other significant and life-threatening adverse reactions and interactions, especially those related to the drugs and herbs mentioned above.

formoterol fumarate

Foradil Aerolizer

Pharmacologic class: Sympathomimetic; long-acting, selective beta$_2$-adrenergic receptor agonist
Therapeutic class: Bronchodilator
Pregnancy risk category C

Action

Stimulates intracellular adenylate cyclase, relaxing bronchial smooth muscle and inhibiting release of mediators of immediate hypersensitivity

Availability

Capsules for oral inhalation (used with Aerolizer inhaler): 12 mcg

Indications and dosages

➤ Long-term maintenance of asthma; prevention or long-term maintenance of bronchospasm in patients with chronic obstructive pulmonary disease
Adults and children ages 5 and older: Contents of 1 capsule inhaled orally via Aerolizer q 12 hours

➢ Acute prevention of exercise-induced bronchospasm (on occasional, as-needed basis)
Adults and children ages 5 and older: Contents of 1 capsule inhaled orally via Aerolizer at least 15 minutes before start of exercise. Wait 12 hours after initial dose before giving repeat dose.

Contraindications

- Hypersensitivity to drug or its components
- Tachyarrhythmias

Precautions

Use cautiously in:
- acute asthma symptoms, deteriorating asthma, cardiovascular disorders, seizure disorders, thyrotoxicosis, diabetes, possible hypokalemia
- patients older than age 75
- labor
- pregnant or breastfeeding patients
- children younger than age 5.

Administration

- Be aware that drug is not intended for acute asthma attacks.
- Use capsules only with Aerolizer inhaler supplied.
- Keep capsules in blister until immediately before use.

Make sure patient doesn't swallow capsules.

Route	Onset	Peak	Duration
Inhalation	Rapid	5 min	12 hr

Adverse reactions

CNS: tremor, dizziness, insomnia, anxiety
CV: chest pain
EENT: sinusitis, pharyngitis, tonsillitis
GI: dry mouth
Metabolic: hypokalemia, hyperglycemia
Musculoskeletal: muscle cramps, back pain, leg cramps
Respiratory: bronchitis, chest infection, dyspnea, upper respiratory tract infection, increased sputum
Skin: pruritus, rash
Other: dysphonia, viral infection, fever

Interactions

Drug-drug. *Adrenergics:* potentiation of formoterol's sympathomimetic effects
Beta-adrenergic blockers: partial or total inhibition of formoterol's effects
Cardiac glycosides, methylxanthines, potassium-wasting diuretics, steroids: potentiation of formoterol's hypokalemic effects, increased risk of arrhythmias
Disopyramide, MAO inhibitors, quinidine, phenothiazines, procainamide, tricyclic antidepressants: prolonged QTc interval, increased risk of ventricular arrhythmias
Halogenated hydrocarbon anesthetics: increased risk of arrhythmias
Levodopa, levothyroxine, oxytocin: impaired cardiac tolerance of formoterol
Drug-diagnostic tests. *Blood glucose:* increased level
Potassium: decreased level
Drug-behaviors. *Alcohol use:* impaired cardiac tolerance of formoterol

Patient monitoring

- Monitor pulmonary function test results.
- Monitor potassium and glucose levels.

Patient teaching

- Teach patient how to use capsules and Aerolizer inhaler provided.
- Instruct patient to keep capsules in blisters until immediately before use.
- Caution patient not to swallow capsules.
- Tell patient not to use drug for acute asthma attacks.

Instruct patient to contact prescriber immediately if difficulty breathing persists after using drug or if condition worsens.

• Caution patient to take drug exactly as prescribed and not to stop therapy even if he feels better.
• Tell patient to consult prescriber if he has been taking inhaled, short-acting drugs on a regular basis.
• Advise female patient to tell prescriber if she is pregnant or breastfeeding or if she plans to become pregnant.
• Caution patient to avoid alcohol during therapy.
• As appropriate, review all other significant adverse reactions and interactions, especially those related to the drugs, tests, and behaviors mentioned above.

foscarnet sodium

Foscavir

Pharmacologic class: Organic analog of inorganic pyrophosphate
Therapeutic class: Antiviral
Pregnancy risk category C

Action

Inhibits replication of pyrophosphate binding sites on virus-specific DNA polymerases and reverse transcriptases

Availability

Injection: 24 mg/ml in 250-ml and 500-ml bottles

Indications and dosages

➢ Acyclovir-resistant herpes simplex virus infection
Adults: 40 mg/kg I.V. given over 1 hour q 8 to 12 hours for 2 to 3 weeks or until infection heals
➢ Cytomegalovirus retinitis in patients with AIDS
Adults: 90 mg/kg I.V. given over 1 to 2 hours q 12 hours for 2 to 3 weeks, or 60 mg/kg I.V. given over at least 1 hour q 8 hours for 2 to 3 weeks, depending on response. Then a maintenance infusion of 90 to 120 mg/kg/day over 2 hours.

Dosage adjustment

• Renal impairment

Contraindications

• Hypersensitivity to drug

Precautions

Use cautiously in:
• hepatic or renal impairment, severe anemia
• history of seizures
• elderly patients
• breastfeeding or pregnant patients
• children.

Administration

• Administer by controlled I.V. infusion through central or peripheral line with good blood flow.
• Don't give by rapid I.V. infusion or bolus injection.
• For peripheral administration, dilute with dextrose 5% in water or normal saline solution to a concentration of 12 mg/ml.
• Administer induction treatment over at least 1 hour (or 1½ to 2 hours with 90-mg induction dose); give maintenance infusion over at least 2 hours.

Route	Onset	Peak	Duration
I.V.	Unknown	Unknown	Unknown

Adverse reactions

CNS: vertigo, abnormal gait, hypertonia, hemiparesis, hyporeflexia, hyperreflexia, speech disorders, headache, fatigue, tremor, ataxia, dementia, EEG abnormalities, neuralgia, neuritis, paresthesia, depression, confusion, anxiety, insomnia, amnesia, hallucinations, agitation, **coma, seizures, paralysis, tetany, cerebral edema**
CV: hypertension, hypotension, palpitations, ECG abnormalities, nonspecific ST-T segment changes

EENT: visual field defects, eye pain, conjunctivitis, tinnitus, otitis, sinusitis, pharyngitis, vocal cord paralysis
GI: nausea, vomiting, diarrhea, constipation, duodenal ulcer, dyspepsia, dysphagia, flatulence, esophageal ulcers, ulcerative stomatitis, glossitis, melena, enterocolitis, gastroenteritis, cholecystitis, tenesmus, proctitis, **rectal hemorrhage, pseudomembranous colitis, paralytic ileus, ulcerative colitis, pancreatitis**
GU: dysuria, polyuria, hematuria, albuminuria, pyelonephritis, **toxic nephropathy, renal tubular disorders, uremia, nephrosis, glomerulonephritis, acute renal failure**
Hepatic: jaundice, **hepatomegaly, hepatitis**
Metabolic: hypokalemia, hypocalcemia, hypercalcemia, hypomagnesemia, hypochloremia, hypophosphatemia, hyponatremia, dehydration, glycosuria, hypervolemia, **acidosis**
Musculoskeletal: joint, back, or muscle pain
Respiratory: hemoptysis, cough, dyspnea, pneumonia, bronchitis, **pneumothorax, respiratory depression, pleural effusion, pulmonary hemorrhage, pulmonary infiltration, bronchospasm**
Skin: alopecia, rash, diaphoresis, pruritus, urticaria, skin ulceration, seborrhea, skin discoloration, acne, dermatitis, dry skin
Other: facial edema, fever, infection, ascites, pain and inflammation at injection site

Interactions

Drug-drug. *Aminoglycosides, amphotericin, other nephrotoxic drugs:* increased risk of nephrotoxicity
Pentamidine: severe hypocalcemia
Zidovudine: increased risk of severe anemia
Drug-diagnostic tests. *Alanine aminotransferase, alkaline phosphatase, amylase, aspartate aminotransferase, bilirubin, creatinine, platelets:* increased values
Calcium, creatinine clearance, granulocytes, hemoglobin, magnesium, phosphate, potassium, red blood cells, sodium, white blood cells: decreased values

Patient monitoring

- Carefully monitor fluid intake and output and renal function tests (especially 24-hour creatinine clearance).
- Assess hematocrit, hemoglobin, and electrolyte levels.
- Monitor cardiovascular and respiratory status regularly.
- Evaluate neurologic status closely.
- Assess frequently for evidence of infection, including sepsis.

Patient teaching

- Tell patient to report numbness or tingling (especially around mouth or in arms or legs) and signs or symptoms of infection.

[Clinical alert] Instruct patient to immediately report difficulty breathing, yellowing of eyes or skin, unusual tiredness, change in urination pattern, bleeding, severe diarrhea, or abdominal pain.

- Advise patient to report unusual pain, redness, swelling, or other changes at infusion site.
- Inform patient that he'll undergo regular blood testing during therapy.
- As appropriate, review all other significant and life-threatening adverse reactions and interactions, especially those related to the drugs and tests mentioned above.

fosfomycin tromethamine
Monurol Sachet

Pharmacologic class: Phosphoric acid derivative
Therapeutic class: Antibacterial, urinary tract anti-infective
Pregnancy risk category B

Action
Interferes with bacterial cell-wall synthesis, blocking binding of bacteria to cells in urinary epithelium

Availability
Granule packet: 3 g

Indications and dosages
➢ Uncomplicated urinary tract infections (UTIs) caused by susceptible organisms in women
Women over age 18: One packet dissolved in water P.O. as a single dose

Contraindications
• Hypersensitivity to drug

Precautions
Use cautiously in:
• acute cystitis
• pregnant or breastfeeding patients
• children (safety and efficacy not established).

Administration
• Obtain specimens, as prescribed, for urine culture and sensitivity testing before starting therapy.
• Mix with 90 to 120 ml of cool water and stir to dissolve; administer immediately after dissolving.
• Give with or without food.
• Don't give more than one dose per UTI episode.

Route	Onset	Peak	Duration
P.O.	Rapid	2-4 hr	Unknown

Adverse reactions
CNS: dizziness, headache, paresthesia, weakness
EENT: rhinitis, pharyngitis
GI: nausea, vomiting, diarrhea, constipation, abdominal pain, dysphagia, dyspepsia, anorexia
GU: vaginitis, dysmenorrhea
Musculoskeletal: back pain
Skin: rash
Other: fever

Interactions
Drug-drug. *Metoclopramide, other drugs that increase GI motility:* decreased fosfomycin blood level and urinary excretion, increased GI motility

Patient monitoring
• Monitor patient for resolution of UTI symptoms within 2 to 3 days.

Patient teaching
• Teach patient proper technique for dissolving and taking drug.
• Instruct patient to take only one dose per UTI episode, with or without food.
• Tell patient to contact prescriber if symptoms don't resolve in 2 to 3 days.
• Caution patient to avoid driving and other hazardous activities until she knows how drug affects concentration and alertness.
• As appropriate, review all other significant adverse reactions and interactions, especially those related to the drugs mentioned above.

fosinopril sodium
Monopril

Pharmacologic class: Angiotensin-converting enzyme (ACE) inhibitor
Therapeutic class: Antihypertensive
Pregnancy risk category C (first trimester), *D* (second and third trimesters)

Action
Prevents conversion of angiotensin I to the vasoconstrictor angiotensin II, thereby reducing sodium and water retention and enhancing blood flow in circulatory system

Availability
Tablets: 10 mg, 20 mg, 40 mg

Indications and dosages
➢ Hypertension
Adults: 10 mg P.O. daily. May increase as required up to 80 mg/day; typical range is 20 to 40 mg P.O. daily.
➢ Heart failure
Adults: 10 mg P.O. daily. May increase over several weeks up to 40 mg/day; typical range is 20 to 40 mg/day.

Dosage adjustment
- Renal impairment

Off-label uses
- Adjunct in myocardial infarction
- Nephropathy

Contraindications
- Hypersensitivity to drug or other ACE inhibitors
- Angioedema (hereditary or idiopathic)
- Pregnancy

Precautions
Use cautiously in:
- aortic stenosis, cardiomyopathy, cerebrovascular or cardiac insufficiency, renal or hepatic impairment, hyponatremia, hypovolemia
- black patients with hypertension
- patients receiving diuretics concurrently
- elderly patients
- breastfeeding patients (safety not established)
- children (safety not established).

Administration
- Don't administer within 2 hours of antacids.
- Give with or without food, but avoid giving with high-potassium foods or potassium supplements.

Route	Onset	Peak	Duration
P.O.	Within 1 hr	2-6 hr	24 hr

Adverse reactions
CNS: dizziness, drowsiness, fatigue, headache, insomnia, weakness, vertigo
CV: hypotension, angina pectoris, tachycardia
EENT: sinusitis
GI: nausea, vomiting, diarrhea, anorexia
GU: proteinuria, erectile dysfunction, decreased libido, **renal failure**
Hematologic: agranulocytosis, bone marrow depression
Metabolic: hyperkalemia
Respiratory: cough, bronchitis, dyspnea, **asthma, eosinophilic pneumonitis**
Skin: rash, **angioedema**
Other: altered taste, fever, hypersensitivity reactions including **anaphylaxis**

Interactions
Drug-drug. *Allopurinol:* increased risk of hypersensitivity reaction
Antacids: decreased fosinopril absorption
Antihypertensives, diuretics, general anesthetics, nitrates, phenothiazines: additive hypotension
Cyclosporine, indomethacin, potassium-sparing diuretics, potassium supplements: hyperkalemia
Digoxin, lithium: increased blood levels of these drugs, greater risk of toxicity
Indomethacin: decreased hypotensive effects
Drug-diagnostic tests. *Alanine aminotransferase, alkaline phosphatase, aspartate aminotransferase, bilirubin, blood urea nitrogen, creatinine, potassium:* increased levels

Antinuclear antibody titer: false-positive result
Sodium: decreased level
Drug-food. *Salt substitutes containing potassium:* hyperkalemia
Drug-herbs. *Capsaicin:* increased incidence of cough
Drug-behaviors. *Acute alcohol ingestion:* additive hypotension

Patient monitoring

- Monitor cardiovascular, respiratory, and neurologic status.
- Monitor CBC and liver and kidney function tests.
- Measure blood pressure to assess drug efficacy and detect hypotension.
- Assess patient's potassium intake; monitor serum potassium level.

Monitor for signs and symptoms of angioedema and anaphylaxis. If these occur, withdraw drug and contact prescriber immediately.

Patient teaching

Instruct patient to immediately report rash or difficulty breathing.

- Tell patient to report dizziness, fainting, bleeding tendency, change in urination pattern, swelling, or persistent cough.
- Encourage patient to drink enough fluids to stay well hydrated.
- Caution patient to avoid driving and other hazardous activities until he knows how drug affects concentration and alertness.
- Instruct female patient to notify prescriber if she suspects she's pregnant.
- Tell patient that he'll undergo regular blood testing during therapy.
- As appropriate, review all other significant and life-threatening adverse reactions and interactions, especially those related to the drugs, tests, foods, herbs, and behaviors mentioned above.

fosphenytoin sodium

Cerebyx

Pharmacologic class: Hydantoin
Therapeutic class: Anticonvulsant
Pregnancy risk category D

Action

Thought to regulate neuronal membrane by promoting sodium excretion from neurons. This action prevents hyperexcitability and excessive stimulation, which inhibits spread of seizure activity. Lacks general CNS depressant effect.

Availability

Injection: 150 mg in 2-ml vials (100 mg phenytoin sodium), 750 mg in 10-ml vials (500 mg phenytoin sodium)

Indications and dosages

➢ Status epilepticus
Adults: 15 to 20 mg phenytoin sodium equivalent (PE)/kg I.V. at 100 to 150 mg PE/minute as a loading dose, then 4 to 6 mg (PE)/kg I.V. daily for maintenance

➢ To prevent seizures during neurosurgery
Adults: 10 to 20 mg PE/kg I.M. or I.V. as a loading dose, then 4 to 6 mg PE/kg I.M. or I.V. daily for maintenance

Dosage adjustment

- Hepatic disease
- Renal impairment
- Elderly patients

Contraindications

- Hypersensitivity to drug
- Adams-Stokes syndrome
- Arrhythmias

Precautions

Use cautiously in:

- hepatic or renal impairment, severe cardiac or respiratory disease
- elderly patients
- pregnant or breastfeeding patients (safety not established).

Administration

- Know that drug is a phenytoin prodrug and is given in PE units to avoid the need to perform molecular weight-based adjustments when converting between fosphenytoin and phenytoin sodium doses.
- For I.V. use, dilute in dextrose 5% in water or normal saline solution.
- Don't give faster than 150 mg PE/minute. Too-rapid infusion causes hypotension.

Check ECG, vital signs, and overall patient status continuously during infusion and for 10 to 20 minutes afterward.

- When giving I.M., rotate injection sites.

Route	Onset	Peak	Duration
I.V.	Rapid	Unknown	Up to 24 hr
I.M.	Unknown	30 min	Up to 24 hr

Adverse reactions

CNS: ataxia, agitation, dizziness, drowsiness, dysarthria, dyskinesia, speech disorder, extrapyramidal syndrome, headache, nervousness, weakness, confusion, hyperesthesia, paresthesia, **cerebral edema, coma, intracranial hypertension**
CV: hypotension, tachycardia
EENT: diplopia, nystagmus, tinnitus
GI: nausea, vomiting, constipation, dry mouth, anorexia
GU: pink, red, or reddish-brown urine
Hematologic: lymphadenopathy, **aplastic anemia, agranulocytosis, leukopenia, megaloblastic anemia, thrombocytopenia**
Hepatic: hepatitis
Metabolic: hypocalcemia, hypokalemia, hyperglycemia, increased glucose tolerance
Musculoskeletal: back or pelvic pain, osteomalacia
Skin: hypertrichosis, rash, pruritus, exfoliative dermatitis, **Stevens-Johnson syndrome**
Other: gingival hyperplasia, altered taste, fever, facial edema, weight loss, injection site pain, allergic reactions

Interactions

Drug-drug. *Amiodarone, benzodiazepines, chloramphenicol, cimetidine, disulfiram, estrogens, felbamate, fluconazole, fluoxetine, halothane, influenza vaccine, isoniazid, itraconazole, ketoconazole, methylphenidate, miconazole, omeprazole, phenothiazines, phenylbutazone, salicylates, sulfonamides, tolbutamide, trazodone:* increased fosphenytoin blood level
Antidepressants, antihistamines, opioids, sedative-hypnotics: additive CNS depression
Barbiturates, carbamazepine, reserpine: decreased fosphenytoin blood level
Corticosteroids, cyclosporine, doxycycline, estrogens, felbamate, methadone, quinidine, rifampin: altered effects of these drugs
Dopamine: additive hypotension
Lidocaine, propranolol: additive cardiac depression
Streptozocin, theophylline: decreased efficacy of these drugs
Warfarin: initial increase in warfarin effects in patients stabilized on warfarin therapy, followed by decreased response to warfarin
Drug-diagnostic tests. *Alkaline phosphatase, glucose, hepatic enzymes:* increased levels
Dexamethasone, metyrapone: test interference
Glucose tolerance test: decreased tolerance
Potassium, thyroxine: decreased levels
Thyroid function tests: decreased values

Drug-behaviors. *Acute alcohol ingestion:* increased drug blood level, additive CNS depression
Chronic alcohol ingestion: decreased drug blood level

Patient monitoring

• Be prepared to slow administration or stop therapy if significant cardiovascular reactions occur.
• Monitor neurologic status carefully, especially for evidence of increasing intracranial pressure.
🔊 Assess for rash. Withhold drug and notify prescriber if it occurs.
• Monitor phenytoin blood level after drug has metabolized to phenytoin (about 2 hours after I.V. dose or 4 hours after I.M. dose).
• Monitor electrolyte levels.
• Evaluate blood glucose level. Watch for hyperglycemia in patients with diabetes.

Patient teaching

• Inform patient that he may experience sensory disturbances during I.V. administration.
🔊 Advise patient to immediately report adverse effects, particularly rash.
• Tell patient that drug may turn his urine pink, red, or reddish brown.
• As appropriate, review all other significant and life-threatening adverse reactions and interactions, especially those related to the drugs, tests, and behaviors mentioned above.

frovatriptan succinate

Frova

Pharmacologic class: Serotonin 5-hydroxytryptamine $(5\text{-HT})_1$-receptor agonist
Therapeutic class: Antimigraine agent
Pregnancy risk category C

Action

Binds selectively to serotonin receptors on cranial arteries, causing vasoconstriction and decreased blood flow

Availability

Tablets: 2.5 mg

Indications and dosages

➢ Acute migraine
Adults: 2.5 mg P.O. as a single dose at first symptom of migraine. If migraine returns, may repeat after 2 hours. Maximum of three doses in 24 hours (7.5 mg/day).

Contraindications

• Hypersensitivity to drug or its components
• Cerebrovascular disorders
• Ischemic heart disease or history of myocardial infarction
• Uncontrolled hypertension
• Peripheral vascular disease
• Hemiplegic or basilar migraine
• Within 24 hours of another 5-HT_1-receptor agonist or ergotamine-containing or ergot-type drug

Precautions

Use cautiously in:
• patients receiving selective serotonin reuptake inhibitors (SSRIs)
• pregnant or breastfeeding patients
• children (safety and efficacy not established).

Administration

• Give one tablet with plenty of fluids at first symptom of migraine.
• If headache returns, administer another tablet after 2 hours.
• Don't exceed three tablets in 24-hour period.
• Give first dose under close supervision if patient has coronary artery disease or other risk factors.
• Don't give within 24 hours of another 5-HT_1-receptor agonist or ergotamine-containing or ergot-type drug.

Route	Onset	Peak	Duration
P.O.	Variable	2-4 hr	Unknown

Adverse reactions

CNS: dizziness, headache, anxiety, malaise, fatigue, weakness, drowsiness, paresthesia, sensation loss
CV: palpitations, tightness in chest, **myocardial infarction (MI)**
EENT: abnormal vision, tinnitus, rhinitis
GI: nausea, diarrhea, dyspepsia, abdominal pain
Musculoskeletal: skeletal or muscle pain
Skin: flushing, diaphoresis, photosensitivity
Other: altered taste, hot or cold sensations

Interactions

Drug-drug. *Ergot alkaloids, other serotonin 5-HT_1-receptor agonists:* prolonged vasoactive reactions
Hormonal contraceptives, propranolol: increased frovatriptan bioavailability
SSRIs: weakness, hyperreflexia, incoordination
Drug-behaviors. *Sun exposure:* increased risk of photosensitivity

Patient monitoring

- Assess for cardiovascular reactions, especially signs and symptoms of MI.
- Monitor neurologic status, particularly for indications of cerebrovascular accident.
- Check for rash and itching.

Patient teaching

- Instruct patient to take one tablet with plenty of fluids at first symptom of migraine.
- Tell patient he may take second tablet 2 hours after first if migraine returns.
- Advise patient to immediately report chest pain.
- Caution patient to avoid driving and other hazardous activities until he knows how drug affects concentration and alertness.
- As appropriate, review all other significant and life-threatening adverse reactions and interactions, especially those related to the drugs and behaviors mentioned above.

fulvestrant

Faslodex

Pharmacologic class: Estrogen receptor antagonist
Therapeutic class: Antineoplastic
Pregnancy risk category D

Action

Inhibits cell division by binding with and downgrading estrogen receptor protein in breast cancer cells

Availability

Prefilled syringes: 125 mg/2.5 ml, 250 mg/5 ml

Indications and dosages

➢ Hormone receptor–positive advanced metastatic breast cancer in postmenopausal women with disease progression who have received antiestrogen therapy
Adults: 250 mg I.M. q month as a single 5-ml injection or two concomitant 2.5-ml injections

Contraindications

- Hypersensitivity to drug
- Pregnancy

Precautions

Use cautiously in:
- bleeding disorders, hepatic dysfunction, thrombocytopenia
- breastfeeding patients.

Administration

- Expel air bubble from syringe before giving injection.
- Administer I.M. injection slowly.

Route	Onset	Peak	Duration
I.M.	Slow	2-3 days	Unknown

Adverse reactions

CNS: depression, light-headedness, dizziness, headache, hallucinations, vertigo, insomnia, paresthesia, anxiety, weakness
CV: chest pain, vasodilation, peripheral edema
EENT: pharyngitis
GI: nausea, vomiting, diarrhea, constipation, abdominal pain, anorexia
GU: urinary tract infection, pelvic pain
Hematologic: anemia
Musculoskeletal: back pain, bone pain, arthritis
Respiratory: dyspnea, increased cough
Skin: flushing, rash, diaphoresis
Other: food distaste, fever, hot flashes, injection site reactions, pain, flulike symptoms

Interactions

Drug-drug. *Anticoagulants:* increased bleeding risk

Patient monitoring

- Monitor CBC.
- Assess liver function test results.

Patient teaching

- Advise patient to report signs and symptoms of infection, especially urinary tract infection.
- Caution patient to avoid driving and other hazardous activities until she knows how drug affects concentration and alertness.

◀ Tell patient to notify prescriber immediately if she thinks she is pregnant.

- Teach patient comfort measures to minimize hot flashes and rash.
- Instruct patient to minimize GI upset and sore throat by eating frequent, small servings of healthy food and drinking adequate fluids.
- Tell patient that drug may cause headache, muscle aches, or bone pain. Encourage her to discuss activity recommendations and pain management with prescriber.
- Advise patient to establish effective bedtime routine to minimize sleep disorders.
- As appropriate, review all other significant adverse reactions and interactions, especially those related to the drugs mentioned above.

furosemide

Apo-Furosemide♣, Furoside♣, Lasix, Lasix Special♣, Novosemide♣

Pharmacologic class: Sulfonamide loop diuretic

Therapeutic class: Diuretic, antihypertensive

Pregnancy risk category C

Action

Unclear. Thought to inhibit sodium and chloride reabsorption from ascending loop of Henle and distal renal tubules. Increases potassium excretion and plasma volume, promoting renal excretion of water, sodium, chloride, magnesium, hydrogen, and calcium.

Availability

Injection: 10 mg/ml
Oral solution: 10 mg/ml, 40 mg/5 ml
Tablets: 20 mg, 40 mg, 80 mg

Indications and dosages

➢ Acute pulmonary edema

Adults: 40 mg I.V. given over 1 to 2 minutes. If adequate response doesn't occur within 1 hour, give 80 mg. I.V. over 1 to 2 minutes.

➢ Edema caused by heart failure, hepatic cirrhosis, or renal disease

Adults: Initially, 20 to 80 mg/day P.O. as a single dose; may increase in 20- to 40-mg increments P.O. q 6 to 8 hours until desired response occurs. Thereafter, may give once or twice daily. For maintenance, dosage may be reduced in some patients or carefully titrated upward to 600 mg P.O. daily in severe edema. Usual I.M. or I.V. dosage is 20 to 40 mg as a single injection; if response inadequate, second and each succeeding dose may be increased in 20-mg increments and given no more often than q 2 hours until desired response occurs. Single dose may then be given once or twice daily.

Infants and children: 2 mg/kg P.O. (oral solution) as a single dose. As necessary, increase in increments of 1 or 2 mg/kg q 6 to 8 hours to a maximum of 6 mg/kg/dose. For maintenance, give minimum effective dosage.

➢ Hypertension

Adults: 40 mg P.O. b.i.d. If satisfactory response doesn't occur, other antihypertensives may be added before furosemide dosage is increased. However, dosage may be titrated upward as needed and tolerated to a maximum of 240 mg P.O. daily in two or three divided doses.

Off-label uses

- Hypercalcemia associated with cancer

Contraindications

- Hypersensitivity to drug or other sulfonamides
- Anuria

Precautions

Use cautiously in:

- diabetes mellitus, severe hepatic disease
- elderly patients
- pregnant or breastfeeding patients
- neonates.

Administration

- Know that I.V. or I.M. injection is given when patient requires rapid onset of diuresis or can't receive oral doses.
- Be aware that I.V. dose may be given by direct injection over 1 to 2 minutes.
- For I.V. infusion, dilute in dextrose 5% in water, normal saline solution, or lactated Ringer's solution.

Clinical alert: Don't infuse more than 4 mg/minute.

- Give oral doses in morning with food. If second dose is prescribed, give in afternoon.

Route	Onset	Peak	Duration
P.O.	30-60 min	1-2 hr	6-8 hr
I.V.	5 min	20-60 min	2 hr
I.M.	10-30 min	30 min	4-8 hr

Adverse reactions

CNS: dizziness, headache, vertigo, weakness, lethargy, paresthesia, drowsiness, restlessness, light-headedness

CV: hypotension, orthostatic hypotension, tachycardia, volume depletion, **necrotizing angiitis, thrombophlebitis, arrhythmias**

EENT: blurred vision, xanthopsia, hearing loss, tinnitus

GI: nausea, vomiting, diarrhea, constipation, dyspepsia, oral and gastric irritation, cramping, anorexia, dry mouth, **acute pancreatitis**

GU: excessive and frequent urination, nocturia, glycosuria, bladder spasm, **oliguria, interstitial nephritis**

Hematologic: anemia, purpura, **leukopenia, thrombocytopenia, hemolytic anemia**

Hepatic: jaundice

Metabolic: hyperglycemia, hyperuricemia, dehydration, hypokalemia, hypomagnesemia, hypocalcemia, **hypochloremic alkalosis**

Musculoskeletal: muscle pain, muscle cramps
Skin: photosensitivity, rash, diaphoresis, urticaria, pruritus, exfoliative dermatitis, **erythema multiforme**
Other: fever, transient pain at I.M. injection site

Interactions

Drug-drug. *Aminoglycosides, ethacrynic acid, other ototoxic drugs:* increased risk of ototoxicity
Amphotericin B, corticosteroids, corticotropin, potassium-wasting diuretics, stimulant laxatives: additive hypokalemia
Antihypertensives, diuretics, nitrates: additive hypotension
Cardiac glycosides: increased risk of glycoside toxicity and fatal arrhythmias
Clofibrate: exaggerated diuretic response, muscle pain and stiffness
Hydantoins, nonsteroidal anti-inflammatory drugs, probenecid: diuresis inhibition
Insulin, oral hypoglycemics: decreased hypoglycemic effect
Lithium: decreased lithium excretion, possible toxicity
Norepinephrine: decreased arterial response to norepinephrine
Propranolol: increased propranolol blood level
Salicylates: increased risk of salicylate toxicity at lower dosages than usual
Succinylcholine: potentiation of succinylcholine effect
Sucralfate: decreased naturietic and antihypertensive effects of furosemide
Sulfonylureas: decreased glucose tolerance, resulting in hyperglycemia
Theophyllines: altered, enhanced, or inhibited theophylline effects
Tubocurarine: antagonism of tubocurarine effects
Drug-diagnostic tests. *Blood urea nitrogen (BUN):* transient increase
Calcium, magnesium, platelets, potassium, sodium: decreased levels
Cholesterol, creatinine, glucose, nitrogenous compounds: increased levels
Drug-herbs. *Dandelion:* interference with drug's diuretic effect
Ephedra (ma huang), ginseng: decreased furosemide efficacy
Licorice: rapid potassium loss
Drug-behaviors. *Acute alcohol ingestion:* additive hypotension
Sun exposure: increased risk of photosensitivity

Patient monitoring

- Watch for signs and symptoms of ototoxicity.

◀︎ Assess for other evidence of drug toxicity (arrhythmias, renal dysfunction, abdominal pain, sore throat, fever).

- Monitor CBC, BUN, and electrolyte, uric acid, and CO_2 levels.
- Monitor blood pressure, pulse, fluid intake and output, and weight.
- Assess blood glucose levels in patients with diabetes mellitus.
- Monitor dietary potassium intake. Watch for signs and symptoms of hypokalemia.

Patient teaching

- Instruct patient to take in morning with food (and second dose, if prescribed, in afternoon), to prevent nocturia.
- Tell patient that drug may cause serious interactions with many common drugs. Instruct him to tell all prescribers he's taking it.
- Instruct patient to report signs and symptoms of ototoxicity (hearing loss, ringing in ears, vertigo) and other drug toxicities.
- Caution patient to avoid driving and other hazardous activities until he knows how drug affects concentration and alertness.
- Instruct patient to move slowly when rising, to avoid dizziness from sudden blood pressure decrease.

• Encourage patient to discuss need for potassium and magnesium supplements with prescriber.
• Caution patient to avoid alcohol and herbs while taking this drug.
• Inform patient that he'll under regular blood testing during therapy.
• As appropriate, review all other significant and life-threatening adverse reactions and interactions, especially those related to the drugs, tests, herbs, and behaviors mentioned above.

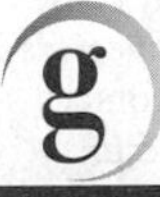

gabapentin

Neurontin

Pharmacologic class: 1-amino-methyl cyclohexoneacetic acid
Therapeutic class: Anticonvulsant
Pregnancy risk category C

Action

Unknown. Possesses properties resembling those of other anticonvulsants, which appear to stabilize cell membranes by altering cation (sodium, calcium, and potassium) transport, thereby decreasing excitability and suppressing seizure discharge or focus.

Availability

Capsules: 100 mg, 300 mg, 400 mg
Oral solution: 250 mg/5 ml
Tablets: 600 mg, 800 mg

Indications and dosages

➢ Adjunctive treatment of partial seizures
Adults and children older than age 12: Initially, 300 mg P.O. t.i.d. Usual range is 900 to 1,800 mg/day in three divided doses.
Children ages 5 to 12: Initially, 10 to 15 mg/kg/day P.O. in three divided doses, titrated upward over 3 days to 25 to 35 mg/kg/day in three divided doses
Children ages 3 to 4: Initially, 10 to 15 mg/kg/day P.O. in three divided doses, titrated upward over 3 days to 40 mg/kg/day in three divided doses
➢ Postherpetic neuralgia
Adults: Initially, 300 mg P.O. as a single dose on day 1; then 600 mg in two divided doses on day 2 and 900 mg in three divided doses on day 3. Then titrate upward as needed to 1,800 mg/day given in three divided doses.

g

Dosage adjustment

• Renal impairment

Off-label uses

• Bipolar disorder
• Migraine prophylaxis
• Tremor associated with multiple sclerosis

Contraindications

• Hypersensitivity to drug

Precautions

Use cautiously in:
• renal insufficiency
• elderly patients
• pregnant or breastfeeding patients
• children younger than age 3 (safety not established).

Administration

• Give with or without food.
• Administer first dose at bedtime to reduce adverse effects.
• Don't give within 2 hours of antacids.
• Give daily doses no more than 12 hours apart.

Route	Onset	Peak	Duration
P.O.	Rapid	2-4 hr	8 hr

Adverse reactions

CNS: drowsiness, anxiety, dizziness, malaise, vertigo, weakness, ataxia, altered reflexes, hyperkinesia, paresthesia, tremor, amnesia, abnormal thinking, difficulty concentrating, hostility, emotional lability
CV: hypertension, peripheral edema
EENT: abnormal vision, nystagmus, diplopia, amblyopia, rhinitis, pharyngitis, dry throat
GI: nausea, vomiting, constipation, flatulence, dyspepsia, anorexia, dry mouth
GU: erectile dysfunction
Hematologic: leukopenia
Musculoskeletal: joint, back, or muscle pain; fractures
Respiratory: cough
Skin: pruritus, abrasion
Other: dental abnormalities, gingivitis, facial edema, increased appetite, weight gain

Interactions

Drug-drug. *Antacids:* decreased gabapentin absorption
Antihistamines, CNS depressants, sedative-hypnotics: increased risk of CNS depression
Drug-diagnostic tests. *Urinary protein dipstick test:* false-positive result
White blood cells (WBCs): decreased count
Drug-herbs. *Chamomile, hops, kava, skullcap, valerian:* increased risk of CNS depression
Drug-behaviors. *Alcohol use:* increased risk of CNS depression

Patient monitoring

- Evaluate neurologic status and motor function.
- Assess WBC count.
- Monitor blood pressure.

Patient teaching

- Tell patient he may take with or without food.
- Advise patient to take first dose at bedtime to reduce adverse effects.

[Clinical alert] Caution patient not to stop taking drug suddenly. Dosage must be tapered to minimize seizure risk.

- Instruct patient to avoid driving and other hazardous activities until he knows how drug affects concentration, alertness, motor function, and vision.
- Tell patient that drug may cause joint pain, muscle aches, or bone pain. Encourage him to discuss activity recommendations and pain management with prescriber.
- Advise parents that drug may cause emotional lability and poor concentration in children. Tell them to contact prescriber if these problems occur.
- As appropriate, review all other significant and life-threatening adverse reactions and interactions, especially those related to the drugs, tests, herbs, and behaviors mentioned above.

galantamine hydrobromide

Reminyl

Pharmacologic class: Cholinesterase inhibitor

Therapeutic class: Anti-Alzheimer's agent

Pregnancy risk category B

Action

Unclear. May reversibly inhibit acetylcholinesterase, increasing concentration of acetylcholine (necessary for nerve impulse transmission) in brain synapses.

Availability

Oral solution: 4 mg/ml
Tablets: 4 mg, 8 mg, 12 mg

Indications and dosages

➣ Mild to moderate dementia of Alzheimer's disease

Adults: Initially, 4 mg P.O. b.i.d. If patient tolerates dosage well after at least 4 weeks of therapy, increase to 8 mg P.O. b.i.d. May increase to 12 mg P.O. b.i.d. after at least 4 weeks at previous dosage. Recommended range is 16 to 24 mg daily in two divided doses.

Dosage adjustment

- Moderate hepatic or renal impairment

Off-label uses

- Vascular dementia

Contraindications

- Hypersensitivity to drug
- Severe hepatic or renal impairment
- Pregnancy or breastfeeding
- Children

Precautions

Use cautiously in:

- asthma, chronic obstructive pulmonary disease, GI bleeding, moderate hepatic or renal impairment, Parkinson's disease, seizures.

Administration

- Before giving, make sure patient is well hydrated, to minimize GI upset.
- Give with morning and evening meals.
- Give with antiemetics as needed.
- Use pipette to add oral solution to beverage; have patient drink it right away.

Route	Onset	Peak	Duration
P.O.	Unknown	1 hr	Unknown

Adverse reactions

CNS: depression, dizziness, headache, tremor, insomnia, drowsiness, fatigue, syncope
CV: bradycardia
EENT: rhinitis
GI: nausea, vomiting, diarrhea, abdominal pain, dyspepsia, anorexia
GU: urinary tract infection, hematuria
Hematologic: anemia
Other: weight loss

Interactions

Drug-drug *Anticholinergics:* antagonism of anticholinergic activity
Cholinergics: synergistic effects
Cimetidine, erythromycin, ketoconazole, paroxetine: increased galantamine bioavailability

Patient monitoring

- Assess fluid intake and output to ensure adequate hydration, which helps reduce GI upset.
- Monitor cognitive status.
- Evaluate patient for cardiac conduction abnormalities. Assess pulse regularly for bradycardia.
- Observe for bleeding tendencies.
- (Clinical alert) Assess for depression and suicidal ideation.

Patient teaching

- Instruct caregiver in proper technique for using oral pipette.
- Teach caregiver how to measure patient's pulse. Tell him to report slow pulse right away.
- Recommend frequent, small servings of healthy food and adequate fluids to minimize GI upset.
- (Clinical alert) Tell patient or caregiver to watch for and report signs and symptoms of depression.
- Advise patient or caregiver to establish effective bedtime routine.
- Caution caregiver to prevent patient from performing hazardous activities until adverse reactions are known.
- As appropriate, review all other significant adverse reactions and interactions, especially those related to the drugs mentioned above.

ganciclovir (DHPG)

Cytovene, Vitrasert

Pharmacologic class: Acyclic purine nucleoside analog of 2′-deoxyguanosine
Therapeutic class: Antiviral
Pregnancy risk category C

Action

Inhibits binding of deoxyguanosine triphosphate to DNA polymerase by terminating DNA synthesis, thereby inhibiting viral replication

Availability

Capsules: 250 mg, 500 mg
Injection: 500 mg/vial
Intravitreal implant: 4.5 mg

Indications and dosages

➢ Prevention of cytomegalovirus (CMV) in advanced human immunodeficiency virus (HIV) infection
Adults: 1,000 mg P.O. t.i.d.
➢ Prevention of CMV in transplant recipients
Adults: 5 mg/kg I.V. q 12 hours for 7 to 14 days; then 5 mg/kg/day 7 days per week or 6 mg/kg/day 5 days per week
➢ CMV retinitis in immunocompromised patients
Adults and children ages 9 and older: Intravitreal implant (4.5 mg) placed during intraocular surgery
Adults and children older than 3 months: Initially, 5 mg/kg I.V. q 12 hours for 14 to 21 days, followed by a maintenance dosage of 5 mg/kg/day 7 days per week or 6 mg/kg 5 days per week. For P.O. maintenance, 1,000 mg P.O. t.i.d. or 500 mg P.O. q 3 hours while patient is awake.

Dosage adjustment

- Renal impairment
- Elderly patients

Off-label uses

- CMV gastroenteritis, CMV pneumonia

Contraindications

- Hypersensitivity to drug or acyclovir
- Neutropenia or thrombocytopenia
- Contraindications for intraocular surgery, such as external infections or thrombocytopenia (with intravitreal implant)
- Breastfeeding

Precautions

Use cautiously in:
- renal impairment
- history of cytopenic reactions
- pregnant patients
- children younger than age 9 (with intravitreal implant).

Administration

(Clinical alert) Follow facility policy for handling and disposing of antineoplastic drugs. (Drug shares some properties with antitumor agents.)
(Clinical alert) Don't let powder in capsules or I.V. solution contact skin, eyes, or mucous membranes. If contact occurs, wash skin thoroughly with soap and water, or flush eyes with water.
- Reconstitute 500-mg vial with 10 ml of sterile water; shake vial to dissolve drug. Then dilute drug again in 50 to 250 ml of compatible I.V. solution.
- If patient is on fluid restriction, dilute to a concentration of 10 mg/ml or less.

(Clinical alert) Administer a single dose by I.V. infusion slowly (over at least 1 hour), using infusion pump or microdrip (60 gtt/ml).
- Give I.V. solution within 24 hours of dilution to reduce risk of bacterial contamination.

(Clinical alert) Don't give by I.V. bolus or by I.M. or subcutaneous route.
- Administer oral doses with food.
- Be aware that intravitreal implant is designed to release drug over 5 to 8

months. Once drug is depleted (as shown by retinitis progression), implant may be removed and replaced.
🔊 Handle intravitreal implant carefully by suture tab only, to avoid damage to polymer coating. (Damage could increase rate of drug release.)

Route	Onset	Peak	Duration
P.O.	Slow	2-4 hr	Unknown
I.V., intravit.	Unknown	Unknown	Unknown

Adverse reactions

CNS: ataxia, confusion, dizziness, headache, drowsiness, tremor, abnormal thinking, agitation, amnesia, neuropathy, paresthesia, **seizures, coma**
CV: hypertension, hypotension, phlebitis, **arrhythmias**
EENT: vision loss for 2 to 4 weeks, vitreous loss, vitreous hemorrhage, cataract, retinal detachment, uveitis, endophthalmitis (all with intravitreal implant)
GI: nausea, vomiting, diarrhea, abdominal pain, dyspepsia, flatulence, anorexia, dry mouth
Hematologic: anemia, **agranulocytosis, thrombocytopenia, leukopenia**
Respiratory: pneumonia
Skin: rash, diaphoresis, pruritus
Other: fever; infection; chills; inflammation, pain, and phlebitis at injection site; **sepsis**

Interactions

Drug-drug. *Amphotericin B, cyclosporine, other nephrotoxic drugs:* increased risk of renal impairment and ganciclovir toxicity
Cilastatin, imipenem: increased seizure activity
Cytotoxic drugs: increased toxic effects
Immunosuppressants: increased immunologic and bone marrow depression
Probenecid: increased ganciclovir blood level
Zidovudine: increased risk of agranulocytosis

Drug-diagnostic tests. *Alanine aminotransferase, alkaline phosphatase, aspartate aminotransferase, creatinine, gamma-glutamyltransferase:* increased values
Granulocytes, hemoglobin, neutrophils, platelets, white blood cells: decreased values
Liver function tests: abnormal results

Patient monitoring

- Monitor liver function test results.
- Monitor neutrophil and platelet counts.
- Assess fluid intake and output to ensure adequate hydration.
- Make sure patent has regular ophthalmic examinations during both induction and maintenance therapy.

🔊 Monitor neurologic status closely; watch for seizures and coma.
🔊 Check for signs and symptoms of infection, particularly sepsis.

Patient teaching

🔊 Advise patient to immediately report signs and symptoms of infection, including those at infusion site.
🔊 Instruct patient to immediately report easy bruising or bleeding.
- Instruct patient to avoid driving and other hazardous activities until he knows how drug affects concentration and alertness.
- Caution female patient not to breastfeed.
- Inform patient that drug may cause birth defects. Tell females to use effective birth control during therapy; advise males to use barrier contraception during and for 90 days after therapy.

🔊 Caution patient not to open or crush capsule. If powder from capsule contacts skin or eyes, tell him to wash skin thoroughly with soap and water or flush eyes with water.
- Instruct patient to minimize GI upset by eating frequent, small servings of healthy food.

• Tell patient he'll undergo regular blood testing during therapy.
• Explain that drug doesn't cure CMV retinitis and that patient should have eye exams every 4 to 6 weeks during therapy.
• As appropriate, review all other significant and life-threatening adverse reactions and interactions, especially those related to the drugs and tests mentioned above.

ganirelix acetate

Pharmacologic class: Gonadotropin-releasing hormone (GnRH) antagonist
Therapeutic class: Sex hormone
Pregnancy risk category X

Action
Competitively blocks GnRH receptors on pituitary gonadotroph, suppressing secretion of gonadotropin and luteinizing hormone (LH) and thereby preventing ovulation

Availability
Prefilled syringe: 250 mcg/0.5 ml

Indications and dosages
➢ To inhibit premature LH surges during controlled ovarian hyperstimulation
Adult women: 250 mcg subcutaneously daily during early to mid-follicular phase

Contraindications
• Hypersensitivity to drug, its components, GnRH, or GnRH analogs
• Known or suspected pregnancy

Precautions
Use cautiously in:
• GnRH sensitivity
• latex sensitivity (packaging contains natural rubber latex)
• breastfeeding patients.

Administration
Know that pregnancy must be excluded before therapy begins.
• Inject into abdomen (around navel) or upper thigh.
• Be aware that drug is given with follicle-stimulating hormone (FSH). After starting FSH on day 2 or 3 of menstrual cycle, patient receives ganirelix on morning of day 7 or 8 and continues this drug until adequate follicular response occurs. Then human chorionic gonadotropin is given and FSH and ganirelix are discontinued.

Route	Onset	Peak	Duration
Subcut.	Unknown	Unknown	Unknown

Adverse reactions
CNS: headache
GI: nausea, abdominal pain of GI tract origin
GU: abdominal pain of gynecologic origin, vaginal bleeding, **ovarian hyperstimulation syndrome**
Other: injection site reaction, **fetal death**

Interactions
Drug-diagnostic tests. *Hematocrit, total bilirubin:* decreased values
Neutrophils: altered count (8.3/mm³ or greater)

Patient monitoring
Monitor patient for adverse effects, especially ovarian hyperstimulation.
• Monitor total bilirubin level and CBC with white cell differential.

Patient teaching
• Inform patient about possible adverse reactions.
• Teach patient about duration of treatment and required monitoring procedures.

Urge patient to tell prescriber if she is pregnant before starting drug.
- As appropriate, review all other significant and life-threatening adverse reactions and interactions, especially those related to the tests mentioned above.

gatifloxacin

Tequin, Zymar

Pharmacologic class: Fluoroquinolone
Therapeutic class: Anti-infective
Pregnancy risk category C

Action

Inhibits bacterial DNA gyrase (enzyme involved in replication, transcription, and repair of bacterial DNA) in susceptible gram-negative and gram-positive aerobic and anaerobic bacteria

Availability

Injection: 200 mg (2 mg/ml); 400 mg (2 mg/ml) in flexible containers
Injection, concentrate: 200-mg (10 mg/ml) vials, 400-mg (10 mg/ml) vials
Ophthalmic solution: 0.3% (5 ml in 8-ml bottle with dropper)
Tablets: 200 mg, 400 mg

Indications and dosages

➤ Acute bacterial exacerbation of chronic bronchitis caused by susceptible organisms
Adults: 400 mg P.O. or I.V. q 24 hours for 5 days
➤ Acute sinusitis
Adults: 400 mg P.O. or I.V. q 24 hours for 10 days
➤ Community-acquired pneumonia
Adults: 400 mg P.O. or I.V. q 24 hours for 7 to 14 days
➤ Uncomplicated urinary tract infections; cystitis
Adults: 400 mg P.O. or I.V. as a single dose, or 200 mg P.O. or I.V. q 24 hours for 3 days
➤ Uncomplicated urethral gonorrhea (in men); endocervical or rectal gonorrhea (in women)
Adults: 400 mg P.O. or I.V. as a single dose
➤ Bacterial conjunctivitis caused by susceptible organisms
Adults and children ages 1 and older: One drop of ophthalmic solution q 2 hours in affected eye(s) while awake, up to eight times daily on days 1 and 2. Then 1 drop up to q.i.d. while awake on days 3 to 7.

Dosage adjustment

- Renal impairment

Off-label uses

- Chronic prostatitis
- Atypical pneumonia
- Anthrax

Contraindications

- Hypersensitivity to drug
- Uncorrected hypokalemia
- Prolonged QTc interval
- Concurrent disopyramide or amiodarone therapy

Precautions

Use cautiously in:
- acute myocardial ischemia, arrhythmias, cirrhosis, renal impairment, CNS disease
- elderly patients
- pregnant or breastfeeding patients
- children younger than age 18 (except in postexposure inhalation or cutaneous anthrax)
- children younger than age 1 (ophthalmic use).

Administration

Administer single dose I.V. over 1 hour. Avoid rapid or bolus I.V. infusion.
- Dilute with compatible solution, such as dextrose 5% in water, normal

saline solution, or dextrose 5% and 0.9% sodium chloride injection. Don't dilute with sterile water for injection.
• Be aware that parenteral solution is for I.V. use only.
• Give P.O. doses at least 4 hours before ferrous sulfate, aluminum- or magnesium-containing antacids, or buffered tablets or solutions.

Route	Onset	Peak	Duration
P.O.	Rapid	1-2 hr	24 hr
I.V.	Rapid	End of infusion	24 hr
Ophthalmic	Unknown	Unknown	Unknown

Adverse reactions

CNS: dizziness, headache
EENT: with ophthalmic use—reduced visual acuity, conjunctival irritation or hemorrhage, increased lacrimation, keratitis, papillary conjunctivitis, chemosis, dry eye, eye discharge, eye irritation or redness, eye pain, eyelid edema; pharyngitis
GI: diarrhea, abdominal pain or discomfort, abdominal cramps
GU: vaginitis
Metabolic: hyperglycemia, **hypoglycemia**
Respiratory: dyspnea
Skin: photosensitivity, rash
Other: abnormal taste, pain or phlebitis at injection site, hypersensitivity reactions including **anaphylaxis**

Interactions

Drug-drug. *Amiodarone, bepridil, disopyramide, erythromycin, pentamidine, phenothiazines, pimozide, procainamide, quinidine, sotalol, tricyclic antidepressants:* increased risk of serious cardiovascular reactions
Antacids, bismuth subsalicylate, iron salts, sucralfate, zinc salts: decreased gatifloxacin absorption
Antineoplastics: decreased gatifloxacin blood level
Corticosteroids: increased risk of tendon rupture
Drug-diagnostic tests. *Bilirubin, hepatic enzymes, lactate dehydrogenase, platelets:* increased values
Hematocrit, hemoglobin: decreased values
Drug-food. *Milk, yogurt:* impaired drug absorption (but no interaction occurs with other dietary calcium sources)
Tube feedings: impaired drug absorption
Drug-herbs. *Dong quai, St. John's wort:* phototoxicity
Fennel: decreased drug absorption
Drug-behaviors. *Sun exposure:* phototoxicity

Patient monitoring

[Clinical alert] Stop drug and immediately report signs or symptoms of hypersensitivity reaction, including fever, rash, fatigue, nausea, vomiting, diarrhea, or abdominal pain.
• Monitor renal function test results in patients with renal insufficiency.
• Monitor blood glucose level in patient with diabetes mellitus.

Patient teaching

• Tell patient to take drug at least 4 hours before ferrous sulfate, antacids containing aluminum or magnesium, or buffered tablets and solutions.
[Clinical alert] Instruct patient to stop taking drug and contact prescriber immediately if fever, rash, nausea, vomiting, diarrhea, or abdominal pain occurs.
• Advise patient to avoid driving and other hazardous activities until he knows how drug affects concentration and alertness.
• Teach patient how to use eyedrops. Caution him not to let dropper tip touch eye, finger, or any other surface.
• Advise patient not to wear contact lenses if he has bacterial conjunctivitis.
• As appropriate, review all other significant and life-threatening adverse

reactions and interactions, especially those related to the drugs, tests, foods, herbs, and behaviors mentioned above.

gefitinib

Iressa

Pharmacologic class: Epidermal growth factor receptor inhibitor

Therapeutic class: Antineoplastic

Pregnancy risk category D

Action

Unclear. Inhibits tyrosine kinase action, which inhibits cell growth and reproduction. May also inhibit angiogenesis in tumor cells.

Availability

Tablets: 250 mg

Indications and dosages

➢ Locally advanced or metastatic non-small-cell lung cancer after failure of platinum-based and docetaxel chemotherapy

Adults: 250 mg P.O. daily

Dosage adjustment

- Patients with diarrhea or skin reactions, pulmonary symptoms, or ocular symptoms
- Patients taking CYP3A4 inducers concurrently

Contraindications

- Severe hypersensitivity to drug or its components

Precautions

Use cautiously in:

- hepatic impairment or hepatotoxicity
- pregnant or breastfeeding patients
- children.

Administration

- Give with or without food.

Route	Onset	Peak	Duration
P.O.	Unknown	3-7 hr	Unknown

Adverse reactions

CNS: asthenia

EENT: amblyopia, conjunctivitis, eye pain and corneal ulcer

GI: diarrhea, nausea, vomiting, mouth ulcers, anorexia

Respiratory: dyspnea, **interstitial lung disease**

Skin: acne, rash, dry skin, pruritus, vesiculobullous rash

Other: peripheral edema, weight loss

Interactions

Drug-drug. *Histamine$_2$-receptor antagonists (such as cimetidine, ranitidine), phenytoin, rifampin:* decreased gefitinib blood level

Itraconazole, ketoconazole: increased gefitinib blood level

Metoprolol: increased metoprolol exposure

Warfarin: increased International Normalized Ratio (INR), increased bleeding events

Drug-diagnostic tests. *Alkaline phosphatase, bilirubin, hepatic enzymes:* increased levels

Patient monitoring

- Monitor INR and watch for signs and symptoms of bleeding if patient is also receiving warfarin.
- Monitor liver function test results.

🔊 Watch for dehydration if patient has severe or persistent diarrhea, anorexia, nausea, or vomiting.

🔊 If patient experiences worsening pulmonary symptoms, severe diarrhea, skin reactions, or ocular symptoms, expect to stop therapy until cause is determined or problems resolve.

🔊 Discontinue therapy if interstitial lung disease is confirmed.

Patient teaching

- Tell patient to take with or without food.

Instruct patient to immediately report severe or persistent diarrhea, anorexia, nausea, vomiting, increased shortness of breath or cough, eye irritation, or new symptoms.

- Caution female of childbearing age not to become pregnant.
- As appropriate, review all other significant and life-threatening adverse reactions and interactions, especially those related to the drugs and tests mentioned above.

gemcitabine hydrochloride

Gemzar

Pharmacologic class: Antimetabolite (pyrimidine analog)
Therapeutic class: Antineoplastic
Pregnancy risk category D

Action

Kills malignant cells undergoing DNA synthesis; arrests progression of cells at G1/S border

Availability

Powder for injection: 200 mg in 10-ml vial, 1 g in 50-ml vial

Indications and dosages

➢ Pancreatic cancer

Adults: 1,000 mg/m² I.V. q week for 7 weeks, followed by 1 week of rest. May continue with cycles of once-weekly administration for 3 weeks, followed by 1 week of rest.

➢ Non-small-cell lung cancer (given with cisplatin)

Adults: 1,000 mg/m² I.V. on days 1, 8, and 15 of 28-day cycle; or 1,250 mg/m² on days 1 and 8 of 21-day cycle. Cisplatin also given on day 1.

➢ Breast cancer (combined with paclitaxel after failure of anthracycline-containing adjuvant chemotherapy, unless anthracyclines were contraindicated)

Adults: 1,250 mg/m² I.V. over 30 minutes on days 1 and 8 of 21-day cycle, with paclitaxel given on day 1 before gemcitabine

Dosage adjustment

- Bone marrow depression

Off-label uses

- Bladder cancer

Contraindications

- Hypersensitivity to drug

Precautions

Use cautiously in:

- hepatic or renal impairment
- females of childbearing age
- pregnant or breastfeeding patients.

Administration

- Follow facility policy for preparing, handling, and administering carcinogenic, mutagenic, and teratogenic drugs.
- Add 5 ml of preservative-free normal saline solution to 200-mg vial, or add 25 ml of this solution to 1-g vial. Shake vial to dissolve drug.
- Reconstitute drug to a concentration of 40 mg/ml. If necessary, dilute further to a concentration of 1 mg/ml.

Infuse each dose over 30 minutes. (Infusions lasting longer than 1 hour increase toxicity risk.)

Route	Onset	Peak	Duration
I.V.	Unknown	Unknown	Unknown

Adverse reactions

CNS: paresthesia
GI: nausea, vomiting, diarrhea, stomatitis

GU: hematuria, proteinuria, **hemolytic uremic syndrome, renal failure**
Hematologic: anemia, **leukopenia, thrombocytopenia**
Respiratory: dyspnea, **bronchospasm**
Skin: alopecia, rash, cellulitis
Other: flulike symptoms, fever, edema, injection site reactions, **anaphylactoid reactions**

Interactions

Drug-drug. *Live-virus vaccines:* decreased antibody response to vaccine, increased risk of adverse reactions
Other antineoplastics: additive bone marrow depression
Drug-diagnostic tests. *Alanine aminotransferase, alkaline phosphatase, aspartate aminotransferase, bilirubin:* transient increases
Blood urea nitrogen, serum creatinine: increased levels

Patient monitoring

Clinical alert: Stop infusion and notify prescriber immediately if patient has signs or symptoms of allergic reaction.
• Monitor liver and kidney function test results.
Clinical alert: Monitor CBC with white cell differential (particularly neutrophil and platelet counts) before each dose.
• Assess degree of bone marrow depression. Expect dosage changes based on blood counts.
Clinical alert: Watch for signs and symptoms of infection and bleeding tendencies, even after drug therapy ends.
• Evaluate respiratory status regularly.
• Monitor temperature, especially during first 12 hours of therapy.

Patient teaching

Clinical alert: Instruct patient to stop taking drug and immediately report signs or symptoms of allergic reaction.
Clinical alert: Advise patient to immediately report signs or symptoms of infection (especially flulike symptoms).
Clinical alert: Instruct patient to report unusual bleeding or bruising, change in urination pattern, or difficulty breathing.
• Caution patient to avoid driving and other hazardous activities until he knows how drug affects concentration and alertness.
• Advise patient to avoid activities that can cause injury. Tell him to use soft toothbrush and electric razor to avoid gum and skin injury.
• Tell patient to minimize GI upset by eating frequent, small servings of healthy food.
• Inform patient that he'll undergo blood testing periodically throughout therapy.
• As appropriate, review all other significant and life-threatening adverse reactions and interactions, especially those related to the drugs and tests mentioned above.

gemfibrozil

Apo-Gemfibrozil♣, Gen-Fibro♣, Lopid, Novo-Gemfibrozil♣, Nu-Gemfibrozil♣

Pharmacologic class: Fibric acid derivative
Therapeutic class: Antihyperlipidemic
Pregnancy risk category C

Action

Inhibits peripheral lipolysis, resulting in decreased triglyceride levels. Also inhibits synthesis and increases clearance of very-low-density lipoproteins.

Availability

Tablets: 600 mg

Indications and dosages

➢ Type IIb hyperlipidemia in patients without coronary artery disease who don't respond to other treatments; ad-

junctive therapy for types IV and V hyperlipidemia
Adults: 1,200 mg P.O. daily in two divided doses

Contraindications
- Hypersensitivity to drug
- Gallbladder disease
- Severe renal dysfunction
- Hepatic dysfunction

Precautions
Use cautiously in:
- renal impairment, cholelithiasis, diabetes, hypothyroidism
- pregnant or breastfeeding patients
- children (safety not established).

Administration
- Give 30 minutes before a meal.
- Know that before starting drug and throughout therapy, patient should use dietary measures and exercise, as appropriate, to control hyperlipidemia.

Route	Onset	Peak	Duration
P.O.	2-5 days	4 wk	Unknown

Adverse reactions
CNS: fatigue, hypoesthesia, paresthesia, drowsiness, syncope, vertigo, dizziness, headache, **seizures**
CV: vasculitis
EENT: cataracts, blurred vision, retinal edema, hoarseness
GI: nausea, vomiting, diarrhea, abdominal or epigastric pain, heartburn, flatulence, gallstones, dry mouth
GU: dysuria, erectile dysfunction, decreased male fertility
Hematologic: eosinophilia, anemia, **bone marrow hypoplasia, leukopenia, thrombocytopenia**
Hepatic: hepatotoxicity
Metabolic: hypoglycemia
Musculoskeletal: joint, back, or muscle pain; myasthenia; myopathy; synovitis; myositis; **rhabdomyolysis**
Respiratory: cough
Skin: alopecia, rash, urticaria, eczema, pruritus, angioedema
Other: abnormal taste, chills, weight loss, increased risk of bacterial and viral infection, lupuslike syndrome, **anaphylaxis**

Interactions
Drug-drug. *Chenodiol, ursodiol:* decreased gemfibrozil efficacy
Cyclosporine: decreased cyclosporine effects
HMG-CoA reductase inhibitors: increased risk of rhabdomyolysis
Sulfonylureas: increased hypoglycemic effects
Warfarin: increased bleeding risk
Drug-diagnostic tests. *Alanine aminotransferase, alkaline phosphatase, aspartate aminotransferase, bilirubin, creatine kinase (CK), glucose, lactate dehydrogenase:* increased values
Hematocrit, hemoglobin, potassium, white blood cells: decreased values

Patient monitoring
- Monitor kidney and liver function test results and serum lipid levels.
- [Clinical alert] Watch for signs and symptoms of adverse reactions, especially bleeding tendency and hypersensitivity reaction.
- Monitor periodic blood counts during first year of therapy.
- Check CK level if myopathy occurs.

Patient teaching
- Tell patient to take drug 30 minutes before breakfast and dinner.
- [Clinical alert] Advise patient to immediately report signs or symptoms of anaphylaxis (such as difficulty breathing or rash) or other allergic reactions.
- [Clinical alert] Instruct patient to immediately report unusual bleeding or bruising or muscle pain.
- Caution patient to avoid driving and other hazardous activities until he knows how drug affects concentration and alertness.

• Stress importance of diet and exercise in lowering lipid levels.
• Inform patient that he'll undergo regular blood testing during therapy.
• As appropriate, review all other significant and life-threatening adverse reactions and interactions, especially those related to the drugs and tests mentioned above.

gemifloxacin mesylate
Factive

Pharmacologic class: Quinolone
Therapeutic class: Broad-spectrum anti-infective
Pregnancy risk category C

Action
Inhibits DNA synthesis by inhibiting DNA gyrase and topoisomerase IV, enzymes needed for bacterial growth

Availability
Tablets: 320 mg

Indications and dosages
➢ Acute exacerbation of chronic bronchitis caused by susceptible organisms
Adults: 320 mg P.O. daily for 5 days
➢ Mild to moderate community-acquired pneumonia caused by susceptible organisms
Adults: 320 mg P.O. daily for 7 days

Dosage adjustment
• Renal impairment

Contraindications
• Hypersensitivity to drug
• History of prolonged QTc interval

Precautions
Use cautiously in:
• epilepsy or history of seizures
• pregnant or breastfeeding patients
• children younger than age 18 (safety not established).

Administration
• Give at same time every day with plenty of fluids, with or without food.
• Make sure patient swallows tablet whole without chewing.
• Don't give iron, multivitamins, didanosine, sucralfate, or antacids containing magnesium or aluminum within 3 hours of gemifloxacin.

Route	Onset	Peak	Duration
P.O.	Unknown	0.5-2 hr	Unknown

Adverse reactions
CNS: fatigue, headache, insomnia, drowsiness, nervousness, dizziness, tremor, vertigo, **seizures, loss of consciousness**
CV: hypotension, **prolonged QTc interval, cardiovascular collapse, shock**
EENT: vision abnormality, pharyngitis
GI: nausea, vomiting, diarrhea, constipation, abdominal pain, dyspepsia, gastritis, gastroenteritis, flatulence, anorexia, dry mouth, **pseudomembranous colitis**
GU: genital candidiasis, vaginitis, **acute renal insufficiency or failure, interstitial nephritis**
Hematologic: eosinophilia, anemia, **leukopenia, granulocytopenia, thrombocytopenia**
Hepatic: jaundice, **hepatitis, acute hepatic necrosis, hepatic failure**
Metabolic: hyperglycemia
Musculoskeletal: joint, back, or muscle pain; leg cramps; tendinitis; rupture of shoulder, hand, or Achilles tendon
Respiratory: dyspnea, pneumonia
Skin: rash, urticaria, pruritus, eczema, flushing, photosensitivity, angioedema
Other: altered taste, hot flashes, fungal infection, hypersensitivity reaction

Interactions
Drug-drug. *Antacids containing aluminum or magnesium, didanosine, iron,*

multivitamins, sucralfate: reduced gemifloxacin absorption
Antiarrhythmics (class IA, such as quinidine and procainamide, and class III, such as amiodarone and sotalol), antipsychotics, erythromycin, tricyclic antidepressants: increased risk of prolonged QTc interval
Sucralfate: decreased gemifloxacin bioavailability
Drug-diagnostic tests. *Alanine aminotransferase, aspartate aminotransferase, bilirubin:* increased levels
Drug-behaviors. *Sun exposure:* increased risk of photosensitivity

Patient monitoring

- Stay alert for signs and symptoms of hypersensitivity reaction and other serious adverse reactions.
- Monitor ECG in patients at risk for prolonged QTc interval.
- Watch for signs and symptoms of tendon rupture.

Patient teaching

- Instruct patient to take drug at same time each day, with or without food.
- Teach patient how to recognize and report signs and symptoms of allergic response.
- Advise patient to take iron, vitamins, antacids, didanosine, or sucralfate 3 hours before or 2 hours after gemifloxacin.

Instruct patient to stop taking drug and immediately report signs or symptoms of hypersensitivity reaction, severe diarrhea, change in urination pattern, easy bruising or bleeding, unusual tiredness, or yellowing of eyes or skin.

Tell patient that drug may cause tendon rupture. Advise him to immediately report sudden severe pain in shoulder, hand, or Achilles tendon.

- Caution patient to avoid driving and other hazardous activities until he knows how drug affects concentration and alertness.
- As appropriate, review all other significant and life-threatening adverse reactions and interactions, especially those related to the drugs, tests, and behaviors mentioned above.

gentamicin sulfate

Cidomycin✦, Garamycin, Genoptic, Gentacidin, Gentak

Pharmacologic class: Aminoglycoside
Therapeutic class: Anti-infective
Pregnancy risk category D (parenteral), ***C*** (topical)

Action

Destroys gram-negative bacteria by irreversibly binding to 30S subunit of bacterial ribosomes and blocking protein synthesis, resulting in misreading of genetic code and separation of ribosomes from messenger RNA

Availability

Cream: 0.1%
Injection: 10 mg/ml (pediatric), 40 mg/ml (adult)
I.V. infusion (premixed in normal saline solution): 40 mg, 60 mg, 70 mg, 80 mg, 90 mg, 100 mg, 120 mg
Ointment: 0.1%
Ointment (ophthalmic): 0.3% (base)
Solution (ophthalmic): 0.3% (base)

Indications and dosages

➤ Serious infections caused by *Pseudomonas aeruginosa, Escherichia coli,* and *Proteus, Klebsiella, Serratia, Enterobacter, Citrobacter,* or *Staphylococcus* species
Adults: 3 mg/kg/day in three divided doses I.M. or I.V. infusion q 8 hours. For life-threatening infections, up to 5 mg/kg/day in three to four divided doses; reduce to 3 mg/kg/day as indicated.

Children: 2 to 2.5 mg/kg q 8 hours I.M. or I.V. infusion
Infants older than 1 week: 2.5 mg/kg q 8 hours I.M. or I.V. infusion
Neonates younger than 1 week, preterm infants: 2.5 mg/kg q 12 hours I.M. or I.V. infusion. In preterm infants of less than 32 weeks' gestational age, 2.5 mg/kg q 18 hours or 3 mg/kg q 24 hours also may produce satisfactory peak and trough blood levels.

➢ Endocarditis prophylaxis before surgery
Adults: 1.5 mg/kg I.M. or I.V. 30 minutes before surgery, to a maximum of 80 mg. As prescribed, give with ampicillin or vancomycin.
Children: 2 mg/kg I.M. or I.V. 30 minutes before surgery, to a maximum of 80 mg

➢ External ocular infections caused by susceptible organisms
Adults and children: One to two drops of ophthalmic solution in eye q 4 hours. For serious infections, up to two drops q hour, or ophthalmic ointment applied to lower conjunctival sac two to three times daily.

➢ Treatment and prevention of superficial burns caused by susceptible bacteria
Adults and children older than age 1: Gently rub small a amount of drug topically on affected area three or four times daily.

Dosage adjustment

- Renal impairment
- Cystic fibrosis

Contraindications

- Hypersensitivity to drug or other aminoglycosides

Precautions

Use cautiously in:

- neuromuscular disease, renal impairment, hearing impairment
- sulfite sensitivity (with parenteral use)
- obese patients
- elderly patients
- pregnant or breastfeeding patients
- infants, neonates, and premature infants.

Administration

- Before starting therapy, obtain specimens as needed for culture and sensitivity testing.
- For I.V. infusion, dilute with 50 to 200 ml of dextrose 5% in water (D_5W) or normal saline solution, and administer over 30 minutes to 2 hours.
- After infusion, flush line with normal saline solution or D_5W.
- Obtain peak drug blood level 30 minutes after 30-minute infusion; obtain trough level within 30 minutes of next scheduled dose.
- Give cephalosporin or parenteral penicillin 1 hour before or after gentamicin, as prescribed.
- Know that for topical treatment of burns, gauze dressings may be applied.

Route	Onset	Peak	Duration
I.V.	Immediate	30-90 min	Unknown
I.M.	Unknown	30-90 min	Unknown
Topical, ophthalmic	Unknown	Unknown	Unknown

Adverse reactions

CNS: dizziness, vertigo, tremors, numbness, depression, confusion, lethargy, headache, paresthesia, **neuromuscular blockade, seizures, neurotoxicity**
CV: hypotension, hypertension, palpitations
EENT: visual disturbances, dry eyes, nystagmus, photophobia, ototoxicity, hearing loss, tinnitus
GI: nausea, vomiting, stomatitis, increased salivation, splenomegaly, anorexia
GU: increased urinary casts, polyuria, dysuria, erectile dysfunction, azotemia, **nephrotoxicity**

Hematologic: eosinophilia, **leukemoid reaction, hemolytic anemia, aplastic anemia, neutropenia, agranulocytosis, leukopenia, thrombocytopenia, pancytopenia**
Hepatic: hepatomegaly, hepatotoxicity, hepatic necrosis
Musculoskeletal: joint pain, muscle twitching
Respiratory: apnea
Skin: exfoliative dermatitis, rash, pruritus, urticaria, purpura, alopecia
Other: weight loss, superinfection, pain and irritation at I.M. injection site

Interactions

Drug-drug. *Acyclovir, amphotericin B, carboplatin, cephalosporins, cisplatin, loop diuretics, vancomycin, other ototoxic or nephrotoxic drugs:* increased risk of ototoxicity and nephrotoxicity
Dimenhydrinate, other antiemetics: masking of ototoxicity symptoms
General anesthetics, neuromuscular blockers: increased activity of these drugs
Indomethacin: increased gentamicin peak and trough levels
Penicillins (such as ampicillin, ticarcillin): synergistic effect
Tacrolimus: nephrotoxicity
Drug-diagnostic tests. *Alanine aminotransferase, aspartate aminotransferase, bilirubin, blood urea nitrogen (BUN), creatinine, lactate dehydrogenase:* increased values
Granulocytes, hemoglobin, platelets, white blood cells: decreased values
Reticulocytes: increased or decreased count

Patient monitoring

- Watch for signs and symptoms of hypersensitivity reactions.

◀ Know that drug blood level monitoring is especially important in therapy lasting more than 5 days, acute or chronic renal impairment, extracellular fluid volume changes, obesity, infants younger than 3 months, concomitant use of nephrotoxic drugs, patients requiring higher doses or dosage interval adjustments (such as those with cystic fibrosis, endocarditis, or critical illness), and patients with signs or symptoms of nephrotoxicity or ototoxicity.

- Assess fluid intake and output, urine specific gravity, and urinalysis for signs of nephrotoxicity.
- Monitor CBC, BUN, creatinine level, and creatinine clearance.
- Weigh patient regularly.
- Assess for signs and symptoms of ototoxicity (hearing loss, tinnitus, ataxia, and vertigo).

Patient teaching

◀ Teach patient to recognize and immediately report signs and symptoms of hypersensitivity reaction, infection, unusual tiredness, yellowing of skin or eyes, and muscle twitching.

- Advise patient to report signs and symptoms of ototoxicity (hearing loss, ringing in ears, vertigo).
- Instruct patient to drink plenty of fluids to ensure adequate urine output.
- Tell patient to monitor urine output and report significant changes.
- Caution patient to avoid driving and other hazardous activities until he knows how drug affects concentration and alertness.
- As appropriate, review all other significant and life-threatening adverse reactions and interactions, especially those related to the drugs and tests mentioned above.

glatiramer acetate

Copaxone

Pharmacologic class: Immunomodulator

Therapeutic class: Multiple sclerosis agent

Pregnancy risk category B

Action
Unknown. Thought to alter immune processes believed to be responsible for pathogenesis of multiple sclerosis.

Availability
Injection: 20 mg lyophilized glatiramer acetate and 40 mg mannitol in single-use 2-ml vial (1-ml vial of sterile water for injection included for reconstitution)

Indications and dosages
➢ To reduce frequency of relapses in relapsing-remitting multiple sclerosis
Adults: 20 mg/day subcutaneously

Contraindications
- Hypersensitivity to drug

Precautions
Use cautiously in:
- pregnant or breastfeeding patients
- children (safety and efficacy not established).

Administration
- Give only by subcutaneous injection into arms, abdomen, hips, or thighs.
- Administer immediately after preparing. Discard unused portion.

Route	Onset	Peak	Duration
Subcut.	Slow	Unknown	Unknown

Adverse reactions
CNS: abnormal dreams, agitation, anxiety, confusion, emotional lability, migraine, nervousness, speech disorder, stupor, tremor, weakness, vertigo
CV: chest pain, hypertension, palpitations, tachycardia, peripheral edema
EENT: eye disorder, nystagmus, ear pain, rhinitis
GI: nausea, vomiting, diarrhea, anorexia, gastroenteritis, other GI disorder, oral candidiasis, salivary gland enlargement, ulcerative stomatitis
GU: urinary urgency, hematuria, erectile dysfunction, amenorrhea, dysmenorrhea, menorrhagia, abnormal Papanicolaou smear, vaginal candidiasis, **vaginal hemorrhage**
Hematologic: ecchymosis, lymphadenopathy
Musculoskeletal: joint, back, or neck pain; foot drop; hypertonia
Respiratory: bronchitis, dyspnea, hyperventilation
Skin: eczema, erythema, diaphoresis, pruritus, rash, skin atrophy, skin nodules, urticaria, warts
Other: dental caries, facial edema, weight gain, herpes simplex, herpes zoster, cysts, chills, flulike symptoms, pain at injection site

Interactions
None reported

Patient monitoring
- [Clinical alert] Assess for immediate postinjection reaction, including flushing, chest pain, anxiety, breathing problems, and hives.
- Watch for transient chest pain, but be aware that this problem doesn't seem to be clinically significant.
- Check for vaginal bleeding.
- Watch for signs and symptoms of infection.

Patient teaching
- Teach patient how to prepare and self-administer drug. Supervise him the first time he does so.
- [Clinical alert] Teach patient to recognize and immediately report signs and symptoms of postinjection reaction. Tell him this reaction may occur right away or up to several months after first dose.
- Caution patient to avoid driving and other hazardous activities until he knows how drug affects concentration and alertness.
- [Clinical alert] Instruct patient to report signs or symptoms of infection or vaginal hemorrhage.

• Provide dietary counseling. Refer patient to dietitian if adverse GI effects significantly affect food intake.
• As appropriate, review all other significant and life-threatening adverse reactions.

glimepiride
Amaryl

Pharmacologic class: Sulfonylurea
Therapeutic class: Hypoglycemic
Pregnancy risk category C

Action
Lowers blood glucose level by stimulating insulin release from pancreas, increasing insulin sensitivity at receptor sites, and decreasing hepatic glucose production. Also increases peripheral tissue sensitivity to insulin and causes mild diuresis.

Availability
Tablets: 1 mg, 2 mg, 4 mg

Indications and dosages
➢ Adjunct to diet and exercise to lower blood glucose level in type 2 (non-insulin-dependent) diabetes mellitus
Adults: Initially, 1 to 2 mg P.O. daily given with first main meal; usual maintenance dosage is 1 to 4 mg P.O. daily. When patient reaches 2 mg/day, increase no more than 2 mg q 1 to 2 weeks, depending on glycemic control. Maximum dosage is 8 mg/day.
➢ Adjunct to insulin therapy in type 2 diabetes mellitus when diet, exercise, or glimepiride alone prove ineffective
Adults: 8 mg P.O. daily with low-dose insulin, given with first main meal. Based on glycemic control, raise insulin dosage weekly as prescribed.
➢ Adjunct to metformin therapy in type 2 diabetes mellitus when diet, exercise, and glimepiride or metformin alone prove ineffective
Adults: 1 to 4 mg/day P.O. with first main meal, increased gradually to a maximum of 8 mg/day P.O. Give with metformin if response to glimepiride monotherapy isn't adequate; adjust dosage based on glycemic response to determine minimum effective dosage.

Dosage adjustment
• Renal or hepatic impairment
• Adrenal or pituitary insufficiency

Contraindications
• Hypersensitivity to drug
• Diabetic coma or ketoacidosis
• Severe renal, hepatic, or endocrine disease
• Pregnancy or breastfeeding

Precautions
Use cautiously in:
• mild to moderate hepatic or renal disease; cardiovascular disease; impaired thyroid, pituitary, or adrenal function
• elderly patients.

Administration
• Check baseline creatinine level for normal renal function before giving first dose.
• Give with first meal of day.

Route	Onset	Peak	Duration
P.O.	1 hr	2-3 hr	>24 hr

Adverse reactions
CNS: dizziness, drowsiness, headache, weakness
CV: increased CV mortality risk
EENT: blurred vision
GI: nausea, vomiting, diarrhea, constipation, cramps, heartburn, epigastric distress, anorexia
Hematologic: aplastic anemia, leukopenia, pancytopenia, thrombocytopenia, agranulocytosis

Hepatic: cholestatic jaundice, **hepatitis**
Metabolic: hyponatremia, **hypoglycemia**
Skin: rash, erythema, maculopapular eruptions, urticaria, eczema, angioedema, photosensitivity
Other: increased appetite

Interactions

Drug-drug. *Androgens (such as testosterone), chloramphenicol, clofibrate, guanethidine, MAO inhibitors, nonsteroidal anti-inflammatory drugs (except diclofenac), salicylates, sulfonamides, tricyclic antidepressants:* increased risk of hypoglycemia
Beta-adrenergic blockers: altered response to glimepiride, necessitating dosage change; prolonged hypoglycemia (with nonselective agents)
Calcium channel blockers, corticosteroids, estrogens, hydantoins, hormonal contraceptives, isoniazid, nicotinic acid, phenothiazines, phenytoin, rifampin, sympathomimetics, thiazide diuretics, thyroid preparations: decreased hypoglycemic effect of glimepiride
Warfarin: initially increased, then decreased, effects of both drugs
Drug-diagnostic tests. *Alanine aminotransferase, alkaline phosphatase, aspartate aminotransferase, bilirubin, blood urea nitrogen, cholesterol, liver function tests:* increased values
Glucose, granulocytes, hemoglobin, platelets, white blood cells: decreased values
Drug-herbs. *Agoral marshmallow, aloe (oral), bitter melon, burdock, chromium, coenzyme Q10, dandelion, eucalyptus, fenugreek:* additive hypoglycemic effects
Glucosamine: impaired glycemic control
Drug-behaviors. *Alcohol use:* disulfiram-like reaction
Sun exposure: increased risk of photosensitivity

Patient monitoring

- Monitor CBC with white cell differential, electrolyte levels, and blood chemistry results.
- Monitor blood glucose level regularly. Assess glycosylated hemoglobin level every 3 to 6 months.
- Evaluate kidney and liver function test results frequently, especially in patients with impairments.
- Assess neurologic status. Report cognitive or sensory impairment.

Patient teaching

- Instruct patient to self-monitor his blood glucose level as prescribed.
- Teach patient how to recognize signs and symptoms of hypoglycemia and hyperglycemia.
- Stress importance of diet and exercise to help control diabetes.
- Instruct patient to wear or carry medical identification describing his condition.
- Advise patient to keep sugar source readily available at all times in case of hypoglycemia.
- Caution patient to avoid driving and other hazardous activities until he knows how drug affects concentration and alertness.
- Tell patient he'll undergo regular blood testing during therapy.
- As appropriate, review all other significant and life-threatening adverse reactions and interactions, especially those related to the drugs, tests, herbs, and behaviors mentioned above.

glipizide

Glucotrol, Glucotrol XL

Pharmacologic class: Sulfonylurea
Therapeutic class: Hypoglycemic
Pregnancy risk category C

Action

Lowers blood glucose level by stimulating insulin release from pancreas, increasing insulin sensitivity at receptor sites, and decreasing hepatic glucose production. Also increases peripheral tissue sensitivity to insulin and causes mild diuresis.

Availability

Tablets: 5 mg, 10 mg
Tablets (extended-release): 5 mg, 10 mg

Indications and dosages

➢ To control blood glucose in type 2 (non-insulin-dependent) diabetes mellitus in patients who have some pancreatic function and don't respond to diet therapy
Adults: 5 mg/day P.O. initially, increased as needed after several days (range is 2.5 to 40 mg/day). Give extended-release tablet once daily; maximum dosage is 20 mg/day. Give daily dosage above 15 mg in two divided doses.
➢ Conversion from insulin therapy
Adults: With insulin dosage above 20 units/day, start with usual glipizide dosage and reduce insulin dosage by 50%. With insulin dosage of 20 units/day or less, insulin may be discontinued when glipizide therapy starts.

Dosage adjustment

- Hepatic or renal impairment
- Elderly patients

Contraindications

- Hypersensitivity to drug
- Severe renal, hepatic, thyroid, or other endocrine disease
- Uncontrolled infection, serious burns, or trauma
- Diabetic ketoacidosis
- Pregnancy or breastfeeding

Precautions

Use cautiously in:
- mild to moderate hepatic, renal, or cardiovascular disease; impaired thyroid, pituitary, or adrenal function
- elderly patients.

Administration

- Check baseline creatinine level for normal renal function before giving first dose.
- Give daily dose (extended-release) at breakfast.
- Administer immediate-release tablets 30 minutes before a meal (preferably breakfast). If patient takes two daily doses, give second dose before dinner.

Route	Onset	Peak	Duration
P.O.	15-30 min	1-2 hr	Up to 24 hr

Adverse reactions

CNS: dizziness, drowsiness, headache, weakness
CV: increased CV mortality risk
EENT: blurred vision
GI: nausea, vomiting, diarrhea, constipation, cramps, heartburn, epigastric distress, anorexia
Hematologic: aplastic anemia, agranulocytosis, leukopenia, pancytopenia, thrombocytopenia
Hepatic: cholestatic jaundice, **hepatitis**
Metabolic: hyponatremia, **hypoglycemia**
Skin: rash, pruritus, erythema, urticaria, eczema, angioedema, photosensitivity
Other: increased appetite

Interactions

Drug-drug. *Androgens (such as testosterone), chloramphenicol, clofibrate, guanethidine, MAO inhibitors, nonsteroidal anti-inflammatory drugs (except diclofenac), salicylates, sulfonamides, tricyclic antidepressants:* increased risk of hypoglycemia
Beta-adrenergic blockers: altered response to glipizide, requiring dosage change; prolonged hypoglycemia (with nonselective beta blockers)

Calcium channel blockers, corticosteroids, estrogens, hydantoins, hormonal contraceptives, isoniazid, nicotinic acid, phenothiazines, phenytoin, rifampin, sympathomimetics, thiazide diuretics, thyroid preparations: decreased hypoglycemic effect
Warfarin: initially increased, then decreased, effects of both drugs
Drug-diagnostic tests. *Alanine aminotransferase, alkaline phosphatase, aspartate aminotransferase, bilirubin, blood urea nitrogen, cholesterol:* increased values
Glucose, granulocytes, hemoglobin, platelets, white blood cells: decreased values
Drug-herbs. *Aloe (oral), bitter melon, burdock, chromium, coenzyme Q10, dandelion, eucalyptus, fenugreek:* additive hypoglycemic effects
Glucosamine: impaired glycemic control
Drug-behaviors. *Alcohol use:* disulfiram-like reaction

Patient monitoring

- Monitor blood glucose level, especially during periods of increased stress.
- Evaluate CBC and renal function tests.
- If patient is ill or has abnormal laboratory values, monitor electrolyte, ketone, glucose, pH, lactate dehydrogenase, and pyruvate levels.
- Monitor cardiovascular status.

Patient teaching

- Advise patient to take daily dose of extended-release tablets with breakfast or immediate-release tablet 30 minutes before breakfast (and second dose, if prescribed, before dinner).
- Advise patient to monitor blood glucose level as instructed by prescriber.
- Tell patient he may need supplemental insulin during times of stress or when he can't maintain adequate oral intake.
- Teach patient how to recognize signs and symptoms of hypoglycemia and hyperglycemia.
- Stress importance of diet and exercise to help control diabetes.
- Instruct patient to wear or carry medical identification describing his condition.
- Advise patient to keep sugar source at hand at all times in case of hypoglycemia.
- Caution patient to avoid driving and other hazardous activities until he knows how drug affects concentration and alertness.
- Tell patient he'll undergo regular blood testing during therapy.
- As appropriate, review all other significant and life-threatening adverse reactions and interactions, especially those related to the drugs, tests, herbs, and behaviors mentioned above.

glucagon

GlucaGen Diagnostic Kit

Pharmacologic class: Antihypoglycemic
Therapeutic class: Insulin antagonist
Pregnancy risk category B

Action

Increases blood glucose concentration by converting glycogen in liver to glucose. Also relaxes GI smooth muscle.

Availability

Powder for injection: 1-mg vials

Indications and dosages

➢ Severe hypoglycemia
Adults and children weighing more than 20 kg (44 lb): 1 mg subcutaneously, I.M., or I.V.
Children weighing 20 kg (44 lb) or less: 20 to 30 mcg/kg or 0.5 mg dose subcutaneously, I.M., or I.V.

➢ Diagnostic aid for radiologic examination

Adults: 0.25 to 2 mg I.V. or 1 to 2 mg I.M. before radiologic procedure

Contraindications

- Hypersensitivity to drug
- Pheochromocytoma

Precautions

Use cautiously in:

- cardiac disease, adrenal insufficiency, chronic hypoglycemia
- history suggesting insulinoma or pheochromocytoma
- elderly patients
- pregnant or breastfeeding patients.

Administration

Clinical alert: Use only in hypoglycemic emergencies for patients with diabetes mellitus.

- Mix drug in 1-mg vial with 1 ml of diluent supplied by manufacturer.
- For I.V. injection, give 1 mg over 1 minute.
- Use drug immediately after preparing; discard unused portion.

Clinical alert: Patient should respond within 15 minutes. Because of potential serious adverse reactions linked to prolonged cerebral hypoglycemia, give I.V. glucose if patient fails to respond to glucagon.

- Give patient carbohydrate-rich foods as soon as he's alert.
- Dilute diagnostic aid doses above 2 mg with sterile water for injection.

Route	Onset	Peak	Duration
I.V.	Immediate	30 min	60-90 min
I.M., subcut.	4-10 min	Unknown	12-32 min

Adverse reactions

CV: hypotension

GI: nausea, vomiting

Metabolic: hypokalemia (with overdose)

Respiratory: bronchospasm, respiratory distress

Skin: urticaria, rash

Interactions

Drug-drug. *Anticoagulants:* enhanced anticoagulant effect

Drug-diagnostic tests. *Potassium:* decreased level

Patient monitoring

- Monitor blood glucose level.
- Monitor patient for aspiration.
- Assess blood pressure, electrolyte levels, and respiratory status.

Patient teaching

- Teach patient and family members the proper technique and timing for using this emergency drug.

Clinical alert: Emphasize importance of contacting prescriber right away if hypoglycemic emergency occurs.

Clinical alert: Tell caregiver or family member to arouse patient immediately and give additional carbohydrate by mouth as soon as patient can tolerate it.

- As appropriate, review all other significant and life-threatening adverse reactions and interactions, especially those related to the drugs and tests mentioned above.

glyburide

Albert Glyburide♣, Apo-Glyburide♣, DiaBeta, Euglucon♣, Gen-Glybe♣, Glynase PresTab, Micronase, Novo-Glyburide♣, Nu-Glyburide♣

Pharmacologic class: Sulfonylurea

Therapeutic class: Hypoglycemic

Pregnancy risk category B

Action

Increases insulin binding and sensitivity at receptor sites, stimulating insulin release from beta cells in pancreas and reducing blood glucose level. Also decreases production of basal glucose in liver, enhances sensitivity of peripheral tissue to insulin, inhibits platelet aggregation, and causes mild diuresis.

Availability

Tablets: 1.25 mg, 2.5 mg, 5 mg
Tablets (micronized): 1.5 mg, 3 mg, 6 mg

Indications and dosages

➢ To control blood glucose in type 2 (non-insulin-dependent) diabetes mellitus in patients who have some pancreatic function and don't respond to diet therapy
Adults: Initially, 2.5 to 5 mg (regular tablets) P.O. daily; range is 1.25 to 20 mg/day as a single dose or in divided doses. Or initially, 1.5 to 3 mg (micronized tablets) P.O. daily, with range of 0.75 to 12 mg/day; give dosages above 6 mg in two divided doses.
➢ Conversion from insulin therapy
Adults: If patient takes less than 20 units of insulin daily, give 2.5 to 5 mg glyburide daily; with insulin dosage of 20 to 40 units/day, give 5 mg glyburide; with insulin dosage above 40 units/day, give 5 mg glyburide daily or 3 mg (micronized tablets) P.O. daily and reduce insulin dosage by 50%.

Dosage adjustment

- Hepatic or renal failure
- Elderly patients

Contraindications

- Hypersensitivity to drug
- Type 1 (insulin-dependent) diabetes
- Severe renal, hepatic, thyroid or other endocrine disease
- Pregnancy or breastfeeding

Precautions

Use cautiously in:
- mild to moderate hepatic, renal, or cardiovascular disease; impaired thyroid, pituitary, or adrenal function
- infection, stress, or dietary changes
- elderly patients.

Administration

Know that micronized glyburide is not bioequivalent to regular glyburide.
- Check baseline creatinine level for normal renal function before giving first dose.
- Give daily dose at breakfast; for patient receiving drug b.i.d., give second dose at dinner.
- Adjust dosage slowly if patient is taking metformin.

Route	Onset	Peak	Duration
P.O.	45-60 min	1.5-3 hr	24 hr

Adverse reactions

CNS: dizziness, drowsiness, headache, weakness
CV: increased CV mortality risk
EENT: visual accommodation changes, blurred vision
GI: nausea, vomiting, diarrhea, constipation, cramps, heartburn, epigastric distress, anorexia
Hematologic: aplastic anemia, leukopenia, thrombocytopenia, agranulocytosis, pancytopenia
Hepatic: cholestatic jaundice, **hepatitis**
Metabolic: hyponatremia, **hypoglycemia**
Skin: rash, pruritus, urticaria, eczema, erythema, photosensitivity, angioedema
Other: increased appetite

Interactions

Drug-drug. *Androgens (such as testosterone), chloramphenicol, clofibrate, guanethidine, MAO inhibitors, nonsteroidal anti-inflammatory drugs (except diclofenac), salicylates, sulfonamides, tricyclic antidepressants:* increased risk of hypoglycemia
Beta-adrenergic blockers: altered response to glyburide, requiring increased

or decreased dosage; prolonged hypoglycemia (with nonselective agents)
Calcium channel blockers, corticosteroids, estrogens, hydantoins, hormonal contraceptives, isoniazid, nicotinic acid, phenothiazines, phenytoin, rifampin, sympathomimetics, thiazide diuretics, thyroid preparations: decreased hypoglycemic effect of glyburide
Warfarin: initially increased, then decreased, effects of both drugs
Drug-diagnostic tests. *Alanine aminotransferase, alkaline phosphatase, aspartate aminotransferase, bilirubin, blood urea nitrogen, cholesterol:* increased values
Glucose, granulocytes, hemoglobin, platelets, white blood cells: decreased values
Drug-herbs. *Agoral marshmallow, aloe (oral), bitter melon, burdock, chromium, coenzyme Q10, dandelion, eucalyptus, fenugreek:* increased hypoglycemic effect
Glucosamine: impaired glycemic control
Drug-behaviors. *Alcohol use:* disulfiram-like reaction

Patient monitoring

- Monitor blood glucose level, especially during periods of increased stress.
- Monitor CBC and renal function test results.
- If patient is ill or has abnormal laboratory findings, monitor electrolyte, ketone, glucose, pH, lactate dehydrogenase, and pyruvate levels.
- Evaluate cardiovascular status.

Patient teaching

- Advise patient to take daily dose with breakfast (and second dose, if prescribed, with dinner).
- Teach patient how to self-monitor his glucose level as prescribed; tell him to report significant changes.
- Inform patient that he may need supplemental insulin during times of stress or when he can't maintain adequate oral intake.
- Teach patient how to recognize signs and symptoms of hypoglycemia and hyperglycemia.
- Instruct patient to keep sugar source available at all times.
- Encourage patient to drink plenty of fluids.
- Stress importance of diet and exercise in helping to control diabetes.
- Advise patient to wear or carry medical identification stating he has diabetes.
- Caution patient to avoid driving and other hazardous activities until he knows how drug affects concentration and alertness.
- Tell patient he'll undergo regular blood testing during therapy.
- As appropriate, review all other significant and life-threatening adverse reactions and interactions, especially those related to the drugs, tests, herbs, and behaviors mentioned above.

glycopyrrolate

Robinul, Robinul Forte

Pharmacologic class: Anticholinergic
Therapeutic class: Antispasmodic, antimuscarinic, parasympatholytic
Pregnancy risk category B

Action

Inhibits action of acetylcholine on muscarinic receptors that mediate effects of parasympathetic postganglionic impulses. This inhibition relaxes cardiac smooth muscle, inhibits vagal reflexes, and decreases tracheal and bronchial secretions.

Availability

Injection: 0.2 mg/ml
Tablets: 1 mg, 2 mg

Indications and dosages

➢ Adjunct in peptic ulcer disorders
Adults: 1 mg P.O. t.i.d. or 2 mg (Forte) two to three times daily, to a maximum of 8 mg/day; or 0.1 to 0.2 mg I.M. or I.V. three or four times daily
➢ To diminish secretions and block cardiac vagal reflexes before surgery
Adults and children ages 2 and older: 0.0044 mg/kg I.M. 30 to 60 minutes before anesthesia
Children ages 1 month to 2 years: 0.0088 mg/kg I.M. 30 to 60 minutes before anesthesia
➢ To diminish secretions and block cardiac vagal reflexes during surgery
Adults: 0.1 mg I.V. May repeat as needed at 2- to 3-minute intervals.
Children: 0.004 mg/kg I.V., not to exceed 0.1 mg as a single dose. May repeat at 2- to 3-minute intervals.
➢ To diminish or block cholinergic effects caused by anticholinesterase
Adults and children: 0.2 mg I.V. for each 1 mg neostigmine or 5 mg pyridostigmine. May give I.V. undiluted or with dextrose injection by infusion.

Off-label uses

- Sweating

Contraindications

- Hypersensitivity to drug
- Arrhythmias
- Chronic obstructive pulmonary disease
- GI disease, infection, atony or ileus
- Myasthenia gravis
- Glaucoma
- Obstructive uropathy
- Severe prostatic hypertrophy

Precautions

Use cautiously in:
- cardiovascular disease, heart failure, hypertension, renal or hepatic disease, Down syndrome, hyperthyroidism, hiatal hernia, ulcerative colitis, mild to moderate prostatic hypertrophy, autonomic neuropathy, spasticity, suspected brain damage
- pregnant or breastfeeding patients.

Administration

- Give oral dose 30 to 60 minutes before meals.
- For I.V. injection, give either undiluted or diluted with dextrose 5% or 10% in water or saline solution. Give each 0.2 mg over 1 to 2 minutes.

Clinical alert: Keep resuscitation equipment on hand to treat curare-like effects of overdose.

Route	Onset	Peak	Duration
P.O.	Unknown	Unknown	8-12 hr
I.V.	1 min	Unknown	3-7 hr
I.M., subcut.	15-30 min	30-45 min	3-7 hr

Adverse reactions

CNS: weakness, nervousness, insomnia, drowsiness, dizziness, headache, confusion, excitement
CV: palpitations, tachycardia
EENT: blurred vision, photophobia, mydriasis, increased intraocular pressure, cycloplegia
GI: nausea, vomiting, constipation, abdominal distention, epigastric distress, heartburn, gastroesophageal reflux, dry mouth, **paralytic ileus**
GU: urinary hesitancy or retention, lactation suppression, erectile dysfunction
Skin: urticaria, decreased sweating or anhidrosis
Other: loss of taste, fever, allergic reaction, irritation at I.M. injection site, **anaphylaxis, malignant hyperthermia**

Interactions

Drug-drug. *Amantadine, antihistamines, antiparkinsonian drugs, disopyramide, glutethimide, meperidine, phenothiazines, procainamide, quinidine, tricyclic antidepressants:* additive anticholinergic effects

Patient monitoring

◀ Check for signs and symptoms of anaphylaxis and malignant hyperthermia.

- Monitor neurologic and cardiovascular status.

◀ Assess for curare-like effects (neuromuscular blockade leading to muscle weakness and possible paralysis), which indicate overdose.

- Assess fluid intake and output. Have patient void before each dose to avoid urinary retention.

Patient teaching

- Advise patient to take oral dose 30 to 60 minutes before meals.

◀ Tell patient to immediately report signs and symptoms of serious adverse effects, especially anaphylaxis.

- Caution patient to avoid driving and other hazardous activities until he knows how drug affects concentration, vision, and alertness.
- Tell patient to minimize GI upset by eating frequent, small servings of food and drinking adequate fluids.
- Advise patient to report urinary hesitancy or retention.
- As appropriate, review all other significant and life-threatening adverse reactions and interactions, especially those related to the drugs mentioned above.

goserelin acetate

Zoladex, Zoladex LA✱, Zoladex 3-Month

Pharmacologic class: Gonadotropin-releasing hormone analog

Therapeutic class: Antineoplastic, hormone

Pregnancy risk category D (breast cancer), ***X*** (endometriosis)

Action

Synthetic form of luteinizing hormone-releasing hormone (LHRH); inhibits gonadotropin production by acting directly on pituitary gland. Enhances release of luteinizing hormone (LH), follicle-stimulating hormone (FSH), and testosterone, lowering testosterone and estradiol levels.

Availability

Implant: 3.6 mg, 10.8 mg (in preloaded syringes)

Indications and dosages

➢ Palliative treatment of advanced prostate cancer

Adults: 3.6 mg subcutaneously q 4 weeks or 10.8 mg subcutaneously q 12 weeks into upper abdominal wall

➢ Adjunct to radiation therapy and flutamide in stage B2-C prostate cancer

Adults: 3.6 mg subcutaneously q 4 weeks starting on day 1 of radiation or during last week of radiation. Alternatively, 3.6 mg subcutaneously 8 weeks before radiation, then 10.8 mg on day 28 or 3.6 mg at 4-week intervals starting 8 weeks before radiation, for a total of four doses (two depots before and two during radiation therapy).

➢ Palliative treatment of advanced breast cancer in pre- and perimenopausal women

Adults: 3.6 mg subcutaneously q 4 weeks. If serum estradiol doesn't fall to postmenopausal levels, may increase to 7.2 mg q 4 weeks.

➢ Endometriosis

Adults ages 18 and older: 3.6 mg subcutaneously q 4 weeks, continued for 6 months

➢ Endometrial thinning before ablation for dysfunctional uterine bleeding

Adults: 3.6 mg subcutaneously 4 weeks before surgery. Alternatively, initial 3.6-mg dose may be followed 4 weeks later by a second 3.6-mg dose, with surgery 2 to 4 weeks after second dose.

Contraindications

- Hypersensitivity to drug or its components or to LHRH or LHRH-agonist analogs
- Undiagnosed vaginal bleeding
- Pregnancy or breastfeeding

Precautions

Use cautiously in:
- risk factors for osteoporosis
- chronic alcohol or tobacco use
- patients receiving drugs that affect bone density
- children younger than age 18 (safety not established).

Administration

- Administer pretreatment pregnancy test to female of childbearing age.
- Know that drug should be given only by a clinician experienced in its use.
- Implant is placed subcutaneously into upper abdominal wall using aseptic technique. Give local anesthetic and stretch skin with one hand. Insert needle into subcutaneous fat, then change needle angle until it parallels abdominal wall. Push needle in until hub touches patient's skin, and withdraw about 1 ml before depressing plunger all the way.
- Don't aspirate after inserting needle. Blood will be visible in syringe if needle enters blood vessel.

🔊 Don't give by I.V. route.

- Be aware that 10.8-mg implant should not be used in women.
- Be aware that if implant must be removed, it can be located by ultrasound.

Route	Onset	Peak	Duration
Subcut.	Unknown	2-4 wk	End of therapy

Adverse reactions

CNS: headache, anxiety, depression, dizziness, fatigue, insomnia, lethargy, pain, emotional lability, weakness, **cerebrovascular accident**
CV: vasodilation, chest pain, hypertension, palpitations, peripheral edema, **myocardial infarction, arrhythmias**
EENT: blurred vision
GI: nausea, vomiting, diarrhea, constipation, ulcer, anorexia
GU: urinary obstruction, lower urinary tract symptoms, breast swelling or tenderness, vaginitis, amenorrhea, infertility, decreased libido, erectile dysfunction, other sexual dysfunction, decreased testicular size, **renal insufficiency**
Hematologic: anemia
Musculoskeletal: increased bone pain, joint pain, decreased bone density
Metabolic: gout, hyperglycemia, hypercalcemia
Respiratory: dyspnea, chronic obstructive pulmonary disease, upper respiratory tract infection
Skin: rash, acne, diaphoresis, seborrhea
Other: hirsutism, chills, fever, hot flashes, infection, weight gain

Interactions

Drug-diagnostic tests. *Calcium, glucose, high- and low-density lipoproteins, triglycerides:* increased levels
FSH, LH: initially increased, then decreased, levels

Patient monitoring

- Assess menstrual symptoms and watch for breakthrough bleeding.
- Monitor neurologic status. Watch closely for signs and symptoms of cerebrovascular accident.
- Monitor cardiovascular and respiratory status.

Patient teaching

- Advise female patient to avoid pregnancy and to use a nonhormonal contraceptive method.
- Instruct patient to call prescriber if menstrual bleeding persists or breakthrough bleeding occurs.
- Inform patient that menstruation may be delayed after therapy ends.

• As appropriate, review all other significant and life-threatening adverse reactions and interactions, especially those related to the tests mentioned above.

granisetron hydrochloride

Kytril

Pharmacologic class: 5-hydroxytryptamine$_3$ antagonist
Therapeutic class: Antiemetic
Pregnancy risk category B

Action

Binds to serotonin receptors in chemoreceptor trigger zone and vagal nerve terminals, blocking serotonin release and controlling nausea and vomiting

Availability

Injection: 1 mg/ml
Oral solution: 2 mg/10 ml in 30-ml bottles
Tablets: 1 mg

Indications and dosages

➢ To prevent nausea and vomiting caused by chemotherapy

Adults and children ages 2 to 16: For I.V. use, 10 mcg/kg I.V. within 30 minutes before chemotherapy. For P.O. use (adults only), 1 mg P.O. b.i.d., with first dose given at least 1 hour before chemotherapy and second dose given 12 hours later on days when chemotherapy is administered; or 2 mg P.O. daily at least 1 hour before chemotherapy.

➢ To prevent nausea and vomiting caused by radiation therapy

Adults: 2 mg P.O. daily within 1 hour of radiation therapy

➢ Acute postoperative nausea and vomiting

Adults: 1 mg I.V. undiluted, administered over 30 seconds

Contraindications

• Hypersensitivity to drug

Precautions

Use cautiously in:
• pregnant or breastfeeding patients
• children younger than age 18 (safety of P.O. use not established)
• children younger than age 2 (safety of I.V. use not established).

Administration

• For I.V. infusion, dilute with 20 to 50 ml of normal saline solution or dextrose 5% in water.
• Infuse I.V. over 5 minutes, starting 30 minutes before chemotherapy.
• For direct I.V. injection, give undiluted over 30 seconds.
• Don't mix I.V. form with other drugs.
• For P.O. use, give first dose 1 hour before chemotherapy and second dose 12 hours after first.

Route	Onset	Peak	Duration
P.O.	Rapid	1 hr	24 hr
I.V.	Rapid	30 min	Up to 24 hr

Adverse reactions

CNS: headache, anxiety, stimulation, weakness, drowsiness, dizziness
CV: hypertension
GI: nausea, vomiting, diarrhea, constipation, abdominal pain
Hematologic: anemia, **leukopenia, thrombocytopenia**
Skin: alopecia
Other: altered taste, decreased appetite, fever, chills, shivering

Interactions

Drug-diagnostic tests. *Alanine aminotransferase, aspartate aminotransferase:* increased levels
Electrolytes: altered levels
Hemoglobin, platelets, white blood cells: decreased levels
Drug-herbs. *Horehound:* enhanced serotonergic effects

Patient monitoring
- Monitor hepatic enzyme levels and CBC with white cell differential.
- Monitor temperature and blood pressure. Have patient use caution when ambulating, to avoid orthostatic hypotension.

Patient teaching
- Caution patient to avoid driving and other hazardous activities until he knows how drug affects concentration and alertness.
- Advise patient to minimize GI upset by eating frequent, small servings of healthy food.
- Tell patient he'll undergo regular blood testing during therapy.
- As appropriate, review all other significant and life-threatening adverse reactions and interactions, especially those related to the tests and herbs mentioned above.

guaifenesin (glyceryl guaiacolate)
Anti-Tuss, Benylin-E✦, Breonesin, Calmylin Expectorant✦, Diabetic Tussin EX, Genatuss, GG-Cen, Glyate, Glycotuss, Glytuss, Guiatuss, Hytuss, Hytuss-2X, Monafed, Mucinex, Mytussin, Naldecon Senior EX, Organidin NR, Pneumomist, Resyl✦, Robitussin, Scot-tussin Expectorant, Siltussin SA, Tusibron, Uni-tussin

Pharmacologic class: Propanediol derivative

Therapeutic class: Expectorant

Pregnancy risk category C

Action
Exerts vasoconstrictive action that leads to decreased edema and congestion. Also increases respiratory secretions and reduces mucus viscosity.

Availability
Capsules: 200 mg
Oral solution: 100 mg/5 ml, 200 mg/5 ml
Syrup: 100 mg/5 ml
Tablets: 100 mg, 200 mg, 400 mg
Tablets (extended-release): 600 mg

Indications and dosages
➢ Cough due to upper respiratory tract infection

Adults: 200 to 400 mg P.O. q 4 hours (not to exceed 2,400 mg/day), or 600 to 1,200 mg P.O. (extended-release tablets) q 12 hours (not to exceed 2,400 mg/day)

Children ages 6 to 12: 100 to 200 mg P.O. q 4 hours (not to exceed 1,200 mg/day), or 600 mg P.O. (extended-release) q 12 hours (not to exceed 1,200 mg/day)

Children ages 2 to 6: 50 to 100 mg P.O. q 4 hours (not to exceed 600 mg/day)

Contraindications
- Hypersensitivity to drug
- Alcohol intolerance (with some products)

Precautions
Use cautiously in:
- diabetes mellitus, cough lasting more than 1 week or accompanied by fever, rash, or headache
- patients receiving disulfiram concurrently
- pregnant patients.

Administration
- Give with full glass of water.

Route	Onset	Peak	Duration
P.O.	30 min	Unknown	4-6 hr
P.O. (extended)	Unknown	Unknown	12 hr

Adverse reactions

CNS: headache, dizziness
GI: nausea, vomiting, diarrhea, stomach pain
Skin: rash, urticaria

Interactions

Drug-diagnostic tests. *Urinary 5-hydroxyindoleacetic acid, vanillylmandelic acid:* inaccurate results

Patient monitoring

- Assess cough quality and productivity. Reevaluate treatment if cough persists and is accompanied by fever or headache.

Patient teaching

- Tell patient to take with 8 oz of water and to drink plenty of fluids.
- Instruct patient to contact prescriber if cough lasts more than 1 week.
- Caution patient to avoid driving and other hazardous activities until he knows how drug affects concentration and alertness.
- As appropriate, review all other significant adverse reactions and interactions, especially those related to the tests mentioned above.

guanfacine

Tenex

Pharmacologic class: Centrally acting antiadrenergic

Therapeutic class: Antiadrenergic-sympatholytic, antihypertensive

Pregnancy risk category B

Action

Stimulates central alpha$_2$-adrenergic receptors, reducing sympathetic nerve impulses from vasomotor center to heart and blood vessels

Availability

Tablets: 1 mg, 2 mg

Indications and dosages

➢ Hypertension

Adults: 1 mg P.O. at bedtime. If response unsatisfactory after 3 to 4 weeks, increase to 2 mg P.O. at bedtime.

Off-label uses

- Attention deficit hyperactivity disorder
- Treatment of heroin withdrawal
- Hypertension in pregnancy

Contraindications

- Hypersensitivity to drug

Precautions

Use cautiously in:

- sedated patients (especially when given with centrally acting depressants)
- pregnant or breastfeeding patients
- children younger than age 12.

Administration

- Give at bedtime to reduce daytime sleepiness.
- Know that therapy shouldn't be stopped abruptly, because this may cause rebound plasma and urinary catecholamines, anxiety, and hypertension.
- Be aware that drug may be used alone or with other agents, especially thiazide diuretics.

Route	Onset	Peak	Duration
P.O.	Unknown	2.6 hr	Unknown

Adverse reactions

CNS: somnolence, insomnia, dizziness, headache, fatigue, amnesia, confusion, depression, hypokinesia, asthenia, malaise, paresthesia, paresis
CV: bradycardia, palpitations, substernal pain

EENT: conjunctivitis, iritis, vision disturbance, tinnitus, rhinitis
GI: nausea, diarrhea, constipation, abdominal pain, dyspepsia, dysphagia, dry mouth
GU: erectile dysfunction, decreased libido
Musculoskeletal: leg cramps
Respiratory: dyspnea
Skin: dermatitis, pruritus, purpura, sweating
Other: taste perversion

Interactions

Drug-drug. *CNS depressants:* additive sedation
Phenobarbital, phenytoin: decreased elimination half-life and blood level of guanfacine
Drug-behaviors. *Alcohol use:* additive sedation

Patient monitoring

- Monitor patient for evidence of drug efficacy.
- Monitor patient closely during drug withdrawal.

Patient teaching

- Tell patient to take drug at bedtime to reduce daytime sleepiness.
- Caution patient not to stop taking drug abruptly.
- Advise patient to avoid driving and other hazardous activities until he knows how drug affects concentration and alertness.
- Tell patient to avoid alcohol during therapy.
- As appropriate, review all other significant adverse reactions and interactions, especially those related to the drugs and behaviors mentioned above.

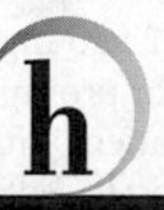

haloperidol

Apo-Haloperidol✤, Haldol, Novo-Peridol✤, Peridol✤, PMS Haloperidol✤

haloperidol decanoate

Haldol Decanoate 50, Haldol Decanoate 100, Haldol LA✤

haloperidol lactate

Haldol, Haldol Concentrate, Haloperidol Intensol

Pharmacologic class: Butyrophenone
Therapeutic class: Antipsychotic
Pregnancy risk category C

Action

Unknown. Thought to block postsynaptic dopamine receptors in brain and increase dopamine turnover rate, inhibiting signs and symptoms of psychosis.

Availability

Injection (decanoate): 50 mg/ml, 100 mg/ml
Injection (lactate): 5 mg/ml
Oral concentrate (lactate): 2 mg/ml
Tablets: 0.5 mg, 1 mg, 2 mg, 5 mg, 10 mg, 20 mg

Indications and dosages

➢ Symptomatic treatment of psychotic disorders or Tourette syndrome
Adults: For moderate symptoms, 0.5 to 2 mg P.O. two to three times daily. For severe symptoms or chronic or resistant disorder, 3 to 5 mg P.O. two to three times daily, to a maximum of 100 mg daily if needed. Adjust subsequent dosages carefully based on response

and tolerance. Alternatively, 2 to 5 mg I.M. (lactate) may be given for prompt control of acutely agitated patient with moderate to severe symptoms; based on response, subsequent doses may be given q hour.

➢ Schizophrenia in patients who need prolonged parenteral antipsychotic therapy

Adults: For patient previously stabilized on oral haloperidol, initial I.M. dose (decanoate) is 10 to 20 times the previous daily P.O. haloperidol equivalent, depending on patient's stability on low or high P.O. dosage. Initially, I.M. dosage shouldn't exceed 100 mg. If conversion requires dosage above 100 mg, give balance in 3 to 7 days. Maintenance dosage is 10 to 15 times the previous daily P.O. dosage, depending on response.

➢ Psychotic disorders

Children ages 3 to 12 or weighing 15 to 40 kg (33 to 88 lb): 0.05 to 0.15 mg/kg/day P.O. in two or three divided doses. May be increased by 0.5 mg daily given in two or three divided doses at 5- to 7-day intervals, depending on response and tolerance.

➢ Nonpsychotic behavior disorder; Tourette syndrome

Children ages 3 to 12 or weighing 15 to 40 kg (33 to 88 lb): 0.05 to 0.075 mg/kg/day P.O. in two or three divided doses

Dosage adjustment
- Elderly or debilitated patients

Off-label uses
- Nausea and vomiting
- Infantile autism
- Intractable hiccups

Contraindications
- Hypersensitivity to drug, tartrazine, sesame oil, or benzyl alcohol (with some products)
- Severe CNS depression

Precautions
Use cautiously in:
- hepatic disease, bone marrow depression, cardiac disease, respiratory insufficiency, CNS tumors, seizures, diabetes mellitus, angle-closure glaucoma, prostatic hypertrophy
- elderly patients
- pregnant or breastfeeding patients.
- children (parenteral form not recommended).

Administration
🔊 Don't give decanoate form I.V.
- Administer decanoate form by deep I.M. injection using 21G needle. Two injections may be necessary; maximum volume shouldn't exceed 3 ml.
- Know that recommended interval between I.M. injections is 4 weeks.
- Dilute oral concentrate in water, soda, or juice (orange, apple, tomato) immediately before administering.
- Be aware that patient should be switched from parenteral form to oral form as soon as possible.
- Know that parenteral form is not recommended in children.

Route	Onset	Peak	Duration
P.O.	Unknown	3-6 hr	Unknown
I.V. (lactate)	Unknown	Unknown	Unknown
I.M. (decanoate)	20-30 min	30-45 min	4-8 hr

Adverse reactions
CNS: confusion, drowsiness, restlessness, extrapyramidal reactions, sedation, lethargy, insomnia, vertigo, tardive dyskinesia, **seizures, neuroleptic malignant syndrome**

CV: hypotension, hypertension, tachycardia, ECG changes, **torsades de pointes** (with I.V. use)

EENT: blurred vision, dry eyes

GI: constipation, ileus, dry mouth, anorexia

GU: urinary retention, menstrual irregularities, gynecomastia, priapism
Hematologic: anemia, **leukocytosis, leukopenia**
Hepatic: jaundice, **drug-induced hepatitis**
Metabolic: galactorrhea
Respiratory: dyspnea, **respiratory depression, bronchospasm, laryngospasm**
Skin: diaphoresis, photosensitivity, rash
Other: hyperpyrexia, hypersensitivity reactions

Interactions

Drug-drug. *Antidepressants, antihistamines, atropine, disopyramide, phenothiazines, quinidine, other anticholinergics:* additive anticholinergic effects
Antihypertensives, nitrates: additive hypotension
CNS depressants (including antihistamines, opioid analgesics, sedative-hypnotics): additive CNS depression
Epinephrine: severe hypotension and tachycardia
Levodopa, pergolide: decreased therapeutic effects of haloperidol
Lithium: acute encephalopathic syndrome
Methyldopa: dementia
Drug-diagnostic tests. *Alanine aminotransferase, aspartate aminotransferase, thyroid function tests:* increased values
Arterial blood gases, bicarbonate: altered values
White blood cells: increased or decreased count
Drug-herbs. *Angel's trumpet, jimsonweed, scopolia:* antagonism of cholinergic effects
Chamomile, hops, kava, skullcap, valerian: increased CNS depression
Nutmeg: reduced haloperidol efficacy
Drug-behaviors. *Acute alcohol ingestion:* additive hypotension

Patient monitoring

🔊 Monitor CNS status closely, especially for seizures and neuroleptic malignant syndrome (shown by extrapyramidal symptoms, hyperthermia, and autonomic disturbances).
🔊 Monitor cardiovascular status, particularly for ECG changes, blood pressure changes, torsades de pointes, and atypical rapid ventricular tachycardia, which may progress to ventricular fibrillation (with I.V. use).
- Assess respiratory status.
- Monitor liver function test results and CBC with white cell differential.
- With prolonged use, assess for tardive dyskinesia (which may occur months or even years after starting drug).

Patient teaching

- Tell patient to dilute oral concentrate with water, cola, or juice immediately before taking.

🔊 Instruct patient to immediately report signs or symptoms of serious adverse reactions, such as unusual weakness, yellowing of skin or eyes, difficulty breathing, or symptoms of neuroleptic malignant syndrome (such as fever, muscle pain or rigidity, rapid or irregular pulse, increased sweating, change in urination pattern, or decreased mental acuity).
- Advise patient to minimize GI upset by eating frequent, small servings of food and drinking adequate fluids.
- As appropriate, review all other significant and life-threatening adverse reactions and interactions, especially those related to the drugs, tests, herbs, and behaviors mentioned above.

h

heparin sodium

Hepalean✤, Heparin Leo✤, Hep-Lock✤, Hep-Lock U/P, Hep-Pak, Uniparin

Pharmacologic class: Antithrombotic
Therapeutic class: Anticoagulant
Pregnancy risk category C

Action

Inhibits thrombus by preventing conversion of prothrombin to thrombin and fibrinogen to fibrin, preventing clot formation. Doesn't lyse existing clot, but prevents clot enlargement and extension.

Availability

Solution for injection: 10 units/ml, 100 units/ml, 1,000 units/ml, 5,000 units/ml, 7,500 units/ml, 10,000 units/ml, 20,000 units/ml, 40,000 units/ml

Indications and dosages

➢ Therapeutic anticoagulation

Adults: 10,000 units I.V. intermittent bolus, then 5,000 to 10,000 units I.V. q 4 to 6 hours. Or 5,000 units I.V. by continuous infusion, then 20,000 to 40,000 units I.V. over 24 hours (about 1,000 units/hour or 15 to 18 units/kg/hour). Or 5,000 units I.V., then initial subcutaneous dose of 10,000 to 20,000 units, then 8,000 to 10,000 units q 8 hours or 15,000 to 20,000 units q 12 hours.

Children: 50 units/kg I.V. intermittent bolus, then 50 to 100 units/kg I.V. q 4 hours. Or 50 units/kg I.V. by continuous infusion, then 100 units/kg/4 hours or 20,000 units/m^2/24 hours.

➢ To prevent thromboembolism

Adults: 5,000 units subcutaneously q 8 to 12 hours (may begin 2 hours before surgery) given for 7 days or until patient is fully ambulatory

➢ To prevent blood clotting during cardiovascular surgery

Adults: At least 150 units/kg I.V. (300 units/kg if procedure less than 60 minutes; 400 units/kg if more than 60 minutes)

➢ I.V. flush

Adults and children: 10 to 100 units/ml I.V. heparin sodium solution to fill heparin lock set

Off-label uses

- Prophylaxis of left ventricular thrombi
- Prophylaxis of cerebrovascular accident after myocardial infarction

Contraindications

- Hypersensitivity to drug
- Bleeding disorders
- Severe thrombocytopenia
- Patients who can't undergo regular blood coagulation tests

Precautions

Use cautiously in:

- severe hepatic or renal disease, bacterial endocarditis, hypertension, brain injury, retinopathy, ulcer disease
- recent CNS or ophthalmic surgery
- immediate postpartum period
- women older than age 60
- pregnant patients.

Administration

🔊 Know that heparin sodium is a high-alert drug.

- Draw baseline blood sample for clotting studies before starting drug.

🔊 Use infusion pump to administer I.V. dose. Check regularly to ensure that infusion rate is correct.

- For I.V. use, give each 1,000-unit dose or single-dose injection over at least 1 minute. Give continuous infusion over 4 to 24 hours, depending on dose and volume of infusion solution.
- Draw blood for partial thromboplastin time (PTT) from opposite arm 4 hours after continuous I.V. infusion begins.

• Put note at patient's bedside to remind personnel to apply pressure dressings after withdrawing blood.
• With intermittent I.V. drug infusion, withdraw blood 30 minutes before dose, using arm without I.V. infusion.
🔊 Don't mix heparin with other drugs or piggyback other drugs into heparin infusion line.
• For subcutaneous dose, inject slowly between iliac crests in lower abdomen, deep into subcutaneous fat layer. Leave needle in place for 10 seconds before withdrawing. Don't massage area after injection. Alternate subcutaneous sites every 12 hours.
• Have protamine available as heparin agonist.
🔊 Don't give I.M.
🔊 Don't give heparin products containing benzyl alcohol to premature infants.

Route	Onset	Peak	Duration
I.V.	Immediate	5-10 min	2-6 hr
Subcut.	20-60 min	2-4 hr	8-12 hr

Adverse reactions

EENT: rhinitis
Hematologic: anemia, **thrombocytopenia, bleeding, severely prolonged clotting time**
Hepatic: hepatitis
Metabolic: hyperkalemia
Musculoskeletal: osteoporosis (with long-term use)
Skin: irritation, rash, urticaria, hematoma, ulceration, cutaneous or subcutaneous necrosis, pruritus, alopecia (with long-term use)
Other: fever, pain at injection site, hypersensitivity reactions, **white clot syndrome, anaphylactoid reactions**

Interactions

Drug-drug. *Antihistamines, digoxin, nicotine, tetracyclines:* decreased anticoagulant effect of heparin
Cefamandole, cefmetazole, cefoperazone, cefotetan, plicamycin, quinidine, valproic acid, other drugs that cause hypoprothrombinemia; drugs that affect platelet function (including abciximab, aspirin, clopidogrel, dextran, dipyridamole, eptifibitide, nonsteroidal anti-inflammatory drugs, some penicillins, thrombolytics, ticlopidine, tirofiban): increased bleeding risk
Drug-diagnostic tests. *Alanine aminotransferase, aspartate aminotransferase, free fatty acids, thyroxine, triiodothyronine resin:* increased levels
Cholesterol, triglycerides: decreased levels
^{125}I fibrinogen uptake: false-negative result
Prothrombin time: prolonged
Drug-herbs. *Anise, arnica, chamomile, clove, dong quai, feverfew, garlic, ginger, ginseng:* increased bleeding risk
Drug-behaviors. *Smoking:* increased bleeding risk

Patient monitoring

• Monitor infusion rate closely, even when using infusion pump.
• Evaluate patient's vital signs.
🔊 Watch for signs and symptoms of anaphylactoid reaction.
🔊 Assess for white clot syndrome (new thrombus formation in association with thrombocytopenia caused by irreversible platelet aggregation).
🔊 Stay alert for signs and symptoms of bleeding tendency.
• Check PTT and platelet count frequently.
• Monitor liver function test results.
• In long-term therapy, periodically assess stool for occult blood.
• Monitor potassium level in patients with diabetes or renal disease. (Drug may cause hyperkalemia.)

Patient teaching

• If patient will self-administer drug, teach proper technique and emphasize need to rotate injection sites.

Advise patient that nosebleed, blood in urine, or black stools may be first sign of overdose and should be reported immediately.

Tell patient to immediately report other unusual bleeding or bruising.

- Urge patient to avoid activities that can cause injury. Advise him to use soft toothbrush and electric razor to avoid gum and skin injury.
- Tell patient he'll undergo regular blood testing during therapy.
- As appropriate, review all other significant and life-threatening adverse reactions and interactions, especially those related to the drugs, tests, herbs, and behaviors mentioned above.

hetastarch

Hespan

Pharmacologic class: Nonprotein colloid

Therapeutic class: Plasma volume expander

Pregnancy risk category C

Action

Expands plasma volume due to its osmotic effect. Increases erythrocyte sedimentation rate when added to whole blood.

Availability

Injection: 500 ml (6 g/100 ml in normal saline solution)

Indications and dosages

➢ Adjunctive therapy for plasma volume expansion in shock caused by burns, hemorrhage, surgery, sepsis, or other trauma

Adults: 500 to 1,000 ml I.V., depending on blood loss and hemoconcentration. Don't exceed total daily dosage of 1,500 ml.

➢ Continuous-flow centrifugation leukapheresis

Adults: 250 to 700 ml I.V. infused at a constant fixed ratio to venous whole blood (usually 1:8 to 1:13) up to twice weekly for a total of seven to ten treatments

Contraindications

- Hypersensitivity to drug
- Severe bleeding disorders
- Severe heart failure
- Renal failure

Precautions

Use cautiously in:

- hepatic disorders
- pregnant patients.

Administration

- Give by I.V. infusion only.
- Know that infusion rate depends on indication and patient response. For acute hemorrhagic shock, drug can be given at a rate of up to 20 ml/kg/hour.

Route	Onset	Peak	Duration
I.V.	Immediate	Immediate	24-36 hr

Adverse reactions

CNS: headache
CV: peripheral edema of legs
EENT: periorbital edema
GI: nausea, vomiting, submaxillary and parotid glandular enlargement
Hematologic: dilution of clotting factors, **increased bleeding and clotting times**
Musculoskeletal: muscle pain
Metabolic: fluid overload
Respiratory: wheezing
Skin: rash, urticaria
Other: chills, fever, flulike symptoms, hypersensitivity reaction

Interactions

Drug-diagnostic tests. *Partial thromboplastin time (PTT), prothrombin time (PT):* prolonged

Patient monitoring

- Stay alert for signs and symptoms of hypersensitivity reaction.
- Monitor vital signs and temperature.
- Assess for signs and symptoms of fluid overload, including peripheral edema of legs and periorbital edema.
- Check for adverse reactions, especially bleeding tendency.
- Monitor CBC, white blood cell count, platelet count, hematocrit, PT, and PTT.

Patient teaching

- Teach patient to recognize and report signs and symptoms of allergic response and other adverse reactions.
- Instruct patient to immediately report unusual bleeding or bruising.
- Tell patient to avoid activities that can cause injury. Advise him to use soft toothbrush and electric razor to avoid gum and skin injury.
- Tell patient he'll undergo regular blood testing during therapy.
- As appropriate, review all other significant and life-threatening adverse reactions and interactions, especially those related to the tests mentioned above.

hydralazine hydrochloride

Apo-Hydralazine✱, Apresoline, Novo-Hylazin✱, Nu-Hydral✱

Pharmacologic class: Peripheral vasodilator

Therapeutic class: Antihypertensive

Pregnancy risk category C

Action

Relaxes vascular smooth muscles of arteries and arterioles, causing peripheral vasodilation and decreasing peripheral vascular resistance. These actions decrease blood pressure and increase heart rate, stroke volume, and cardiac output.

Availability

Injection: 20 mg/ml
Tablets: 10 mg, 25 mg, 50 mg, 100 mg

Indications and dosages

➤ Hypertension

Adults: Initially, 10 mg P.O. q.i.d. After 2 to 4 days, may increase to 25 mg P.O. q.i.d. for remainder of first week; may then increase further to 50 mg P.O. q.i.d., up to 300 mg/day. Once maintenance dosage is established, may give in two daily doses.
Children: Initially, 0.75 mg/kg/day P.O. in four divided doses; may increase gradually over 3 to 4 weeks to 7.5 mg/kg or 200 mg/day
Neonates: 0.5 mg/kg P.O., I.M., or I.V. q 4 to 6 hours

➤ Heart failure

Adults: Initially, 50 to 75 mg P.O. q.i.d.; may increase up to 600 mg/day given in three to four divided doses

➤ Eclampsia

Adults: 5 mg I.V., followed by another 5 mg I.V. q 15 to 20 minutes until blood pressure decreases adequately. If no response occurs after a total dose of 20 mg, prescriber may consider alternative drug.

Contraindications

- Hypersensitivity to drug or tartrazine
- Coronary artery disease
- Mitral valvular rheumatic heart disease

Precautions

Use cautiously in:
- suspected CV or cerebrovascular disease, severe renal or hepatic disease
- pregnant or breastfeeding patients
- children.

h

Administration

• Administer oral form with food.

◀ Inject I.V. form slowly over 1 minute. Monitor blood pressure response continuously.

• Draw up and use parenteral drug immediately; solution changes color after contact with metal needle.

Route	Onset	Peak	Duration
P.O.	45 min	2 hr	3-8 hr
I.V.	10-20 min	15-30 min	3-8 hr
I.M.	10-30 min	1 hr	3-8 hr

Adverse reactions

CNS: dizziness, drowsiness, headache, peripheral neuritis
CV: tachycardia, angina, orthostatic hypotension, **arrhythmias**
EENT: lacrimation, nasal congestion
GI: nausea, vomiting, diarrhea, constipation, anorexia
Metabolic: sodium retention
Musculoskeletal: joint pain, arthritis
Skin: rash, blisters, flushing, pruritus, urticaria
Other: chills, fever, lymphadenopathy, edema, lupuslike syndrome

Interactions

Drug-drug. *Antihypertensives, nitrates:* additive hypotension
Beta-adrenergic blockers: decreased risk of hydralazine-induced tachycardia
Epinephrine: reduced pressor response to epinephrine
Metoprolol, propranolol: increased blood levels of both drugs
MAO inhibitors: increased hypotension
Nonsteroidal anti-inflammatory drugs: decreased antihypertensive response
Drug-diagnostic tests. *Coombs' test:* positive result
Granulocytes, hemoglobin, neutrophils, platelets, red blood cells, white blood cells: decreased levels
Drug-behaviors. *Alcohol use:* additive hypotensive response

Patient monitoring

• Monitor CBC, lupus erythematosus cell studies, and antinuclear antibody titers before and periodically during therapy.

• Monitor blood pressure, pulse rate and regularity, and daily weight.

• To avoid rapid blood pressure drop, taper dosage gradually before discontinuing.

◀ Assess for lupuslike signs and symptoms, including joint pain, fever, myalgia, pharyngitis, and splenomegaly.

• Watch for peripheral neuritis. If it occurs, expect to give pyridoxine.

Patient teaching

• Tell patient to take tablets with food.

• Instruct patient to move slowly when rising (especially in morning on awakening), to avoid dizziness from sudden blood pressure decrease.

◀ Instruct patient to immediately report fever, muscle and joint aches, or sore throat.

• Tell patient to report chest pain or numbness or tingling of hands or feet.

• To minimize GI upset, advise patient to eat small, frequent meals.

• Caution patient not to discontinue drug abruptly, because severe hypertension may result.

• As appropriate, review other significant and life-threatening adverse reactions and interactions, especially those related to the drugs, tests, and behaviors mentioned above.

hydrochlorothiazide

Apo-Hydro✤, Diuchlor H✤, Esidrix, Ezide, HydroDIURIL, Hydro-Par, Microzide, Neo-Codema✤, Novo-Hydrazide✤, Oretic, Urozide✤

Pharmacologic class: Thiazide diuretic
Therapeutic class: Diuretic, antihypertensive
Pregnancy risk category B

Action

Increases sodium and water excretion by inhibiting sodium reabsorption in distal tubules; promotes excretion of chloride, potassium, magnesium, and bicarbonate. Also may produce arteriolar dilation, reducing blood pressure.

Availability

Capsules: 12.5 mg
Oral solution: 10 mg/ml, 100 mg/ml
Tablets: 25 mg, 50 mg, 100 mg

Indications and dosages

➢ Edema caused by heart failure, renal dysfunction, cirrhosis, corticosteroid therapy, or estrogen therapy
Adults: 25 to 100 mg P.O. daily as a single dose or in divided doses. Maximum dosage is 200 mg/day.
➢ Mild to moderate hypertension
Adults: Initially, 12.5 mg daily P.O.; then, based on blood pressure response, may give 12.5 to 50 mg/day P.O. Higher dosages may be given in refractory cases.
Children ages 6 months to 12 years: 2.2 mg/kg P.O. daily in two divided doses
Children younger than 6 months: Up to 3.3 mg/kg P.O. daily in two divided doses

Off-label uses

- Hypercalcemia
- Ménière's disease

Contraindications

- Hypersensitivity to drug, other thiazides, sulfonamides, or tartrazine
- Renal decompensation or anuria

Precautions

Use cautiously in:
- renal or severe hepatic impairment, fluid or electrolyte imbalances, gout, systemic lupus erythematosus, hyperparathyroidism, glucose tolerance abnormalities, bipolar disorder
- pregnant or breastfeeding patients.

Administration

- Give with food or milk if GI upset occurs.
- Administer early in day so diuretic effect doesn't disturb sleep.

Route	Onset	Peak	Duration
P.O.	2 hr	3-6 hr	6-12 hr

Adverse reactions

CNS: dizziness, drowsiness, lethargy, headache, insomnia, nervousness, vertigo, asthenia, asterixis, paresthesias, confusion, fatigue, **encephalopathy**
CV: chest pain, orthostatic hypotension, ECG changes, **thrombophlebitis, arrhythmias**
EENT: nystagmus
GI: nausea, vomiting, epigastric distress, anorexia, **pancreatitis**
GU: polyuria, nocturia, erectile dysfunction, loss of libido, **renal failure**
Hematologic: anemia, **hemolytic anemia, agranulocytosis, leukopenia, thrombocytopenia**
Hepatic: jaundice, **hepatitis**
Metabolic: dehydration, gout, hyperglycemia, hypokalemia, hypocalcemia, hypovolemia, hypomagnesemia, hyponatremia, hypophosphatemia, hyperuricemia, **hypochloremic alkalosis**

Musculoskeletal: muscle cramps
Skin: photosensitivity, urticaria, rash, dermatitis, purpura, alopecia, flushing
Other: fever, weight loss, **anaphylaxis**

Interactions

Drug-drug. *Allopurinol:* increased risk of hypersensitivity reaction
Amphotericin B, corticosteroids, digoxin, mezlocillin, piperacillin, ticarcillin: increased risk of hypokalemia
Antihypertensives, barbiturates, nitrates, opioids: increased hypotension
Cholestyramine, colestipol: decreased hydrochlorothiazide absorption
Digoxin: increased risk of hypokalemia
Lithium: decreased excretion and increased blood level of lithium
Nonsteroidal anti-inflammatory drugs: decreased hydrochlorothiazide efficacy
Drug-diagnostic tests. *Bilirubin, blood and urine glucose (in diabetic patients), calcium, creatinine, uric acid:* increased levels
Cholesterol, low-density lipoproteins, magnesium, potassium, protein-bound iodine, sodium, triglycerides, urinary calcium: decreased levels
Drug-herbs. *Dandelion:* interference with diuretic activity
Ginkgo: decreased antihypertensive effect
Licorice, stimulant laxative herbs (aloe, cascara sagrada, senna): increased risk of hypokalemia
Drug-behaviors. *Alcohol use:* increased hypotension
Sun exposure: increased risk of photosensitivity

Patient monitoring

- Monitor blood pressure, fluid intake and output, and daily weight.
- Assess electrolyte levels, especially potassium. Monitor for signs and symptoms of hypokalemia.
- Monitor blood urea nitrogen and creatinine levels.
- Check blood glucose level in diabetic patients.
- Assess for signs and symptoms of gout attacks in patients with gouty arthritis.

Patient teaching

- Advise patient to take with food or milk if GI upset occurs.
- Tell patient to take early in day to avoid nighttime urination.
- Instruct patient to track intermittent doses on calendar.
- Tell patient to weigh himself daily, at same time on same scale and wearing same clothes.
- Instruct patient to report decreased urination, swelling, unusual bleeding or bruising, dizziness, fatigue, numbness, and muscle weakness or cramping.
- Instruct patient to move slowly when sitting up or standing, to avoid dizziness from sudden blood pressure decrease.
- Caution patient to avoid driving and other hazardous activities until he knows how drug affects concentration and alertness.
- As appropriate, review all other significant and life-threatening adverse reactions and interactions, especially those related to the drugs, tests, herbs, and behaviors mentioned above.

hydrocodone bitartrate

Hycodan✱, Robidone✱

hydrocodone bitartrate and acetaminophen

Anexsia, Ceta-Plus, Co-Gesic, Dolacet, Duocet, Hydrocet, Lorcet-HD, Lortab, Vicodin

hydrocodone bitartrate and aspirin

Azdone

hydrocodone bitartrate and ibuprofen

Vicoprofen

Pharmacologic class: Opioid agonist/ nonopioid analgesic combination

Therapeutic class: Opioid analgesic; allergy, cold, and cough remedy (antitussive)

Controlled substance schedule III

Pregnancy risk category C

Action

Blocks release of inhibitory neurotransmitters, altering perception of and emotional response to pain. Hydrocodone/ibuprofen combination raises pain threshold by nonselectively inhibiting cyclooxygenase; prostaglandin synthesis then decreases and anti-inflammatory and analgesic effects occur.

Availability

hydrocodone bitartrate

Suspension: 5 mg/5 ml, 10 mg/5 ml

Syrup: 5 mg/ml

Tablets: 5 mg

hydrocodone and acetaminophen

Capsules: 5 mg hydrocodone (hyd.)/ 500 mg acetaminophen (acet.)

Elixir/oral solution: 2.5 mg hyd./167 mg acet./5 ml

Tablets: 2.5 mg hyd./500 mg acet.; 5 mg hyd./325 mg acet.; 5 mg hyd./400 mg acet.; 5 mg hyd./500 mg acet.; 7.5 mg hyd./325 mg acet.; 7.5 mg hyd./400 mg acet.; 7.5 mg hyd./500 mg acet.; 7.5 mg hyd./650 mg acet.; 7.5 mg hyd./750 mg acet.; 10 mg hyd./325 mg acet.; 10 mg hyd./400 mg acet.; 10 mg hyd./500 mg acet.; 10 mg hyd./650 mg acet.; 10 mg hyd./660 mg acet.; 10 mg hyd./750 mg acet.

hydrocodone and aspirin

Tablets: 5 mg hyd./500 mg aspirin

hydrocodone and ibuprofen

Tablets: 7.5 mg hyd./200 mg ibuprofen

Indications and dosages

➢ Moderate to severe pain

Adults: 2.5 to 10 mg P.O. q 4 to 6 hours p.r.n. When giving hydrocodone/acetaminophen, don't exceed 60 mg/day; when giving hydrocodone/ ibuprofen, don't exceed 37.5 mg/day.

Children: 0.15 to 0.2 mg/kg P.O. q 6 hours

➢ Cough

Adults: 5 to 10 mg P.O. q 4 to 6 hours p.r.n. as a single dose, not to exceed 15 mg (usually given with decongestants)

Children: 0.6 mg/kg/day or 20 mg/m² P.O. in three to four divided doses. As a single dose, don't exceed 10 mg in children ages 12 and older, 5 mg in children ages 2 to 12, or 1.25 mg in children ages 2 and younger.

Contraindications

- Hypersensitivity to hydrocodone, acetaminophen, aspirin, or ibuprofen (for corresponding combination products) or to alcohol, aspartame, saccharine, sugar, or tartrazine (with some products)

Precautions

Use cautiously in:

- severe renal, hepatic, or pulmonary disease; increased intracranial pressure;

hypothyroidism; adrenal insufficiency; prostatic hypertrophy; thrombocytopenia; alcoholism
- elderly patients
- pregnant or breastfeeding patients.

Administration

Clinical alert: In patients receiving concurrent MAO inhibitors, know that hydrocodone may produce severe, unpredictable reactions. Initial dosage may need to be 25% lower than usual dosage.

Route	Onset	Peak	Duration
P.O.	10-30 min	30-60 min	4-6 hr

Adverse reactions

CNS: confusion, drowsiness, sedation, dysphoria, euphoria, floating feeling, hallucinations, headache, anxiety, depression, fatigue, insomnia, lethargy, nervousness, slurred speech, tremor, asthenia, unusual dreams
CV: orthostatic hypotension, bradycardia, peripheral edema, palpitations, **arrhythmias**
EENT: blurred vision, vision changes, diplopia, miosis, tinnitus, pharyngitis, rhinitis, sinusitis
GI: nausea, vomiting, constipation, dysphagia, esophagitis, dyspepsia, flatulence, gastritis, gastroenteritis, mouth ulcers, dry mouth, anorexia
GU: urinary retention or frequency, erectile dysfunction
Respiratory: respiratory depression, bronchitis, dyspnea
Skin: pruritus, urticaria, diaphoresis, flushing
Other: physical or psychological drug dependence, drug tolerance

Interactions

Drug-drug. *Angiotensin-converting enzyme inhibitors:* decreased therapeutic effects of these drugs
Antihistamines, sedative-hypnotics: additive CNS depression
Buprenorphine, butorphanol, nalbuphine, pentazocine: precipitation of opioid withdrawal in physically dependent patients
Buprenorphine, pentazocine: decreased analgesia
Lithium: increased lithium blood level (with hydrocodone/ibuprofen only)
MAO inhibitors: severe, unpredictable reactions
Methotrexate: increased methotrexate blood level
Naloxone: withdrawal symptoms
Oral anticoagulants: increased risk of GI bleeding (with hydrocodone/ibuprofen only)
Drug-diagnostic tests. *Amylase, lipase:* increased levels
Drug-herbs. *Chamomile, hops, kava, skullcaps, valerian:* increased CNS depression
Drug-behaviors. *Alcohol use:* increased CNS depression

Patient monitoring

- In prolonged use, monitor for psychological and physical dependence.
- Watch closely for withdrawal symptoms when drug is discontinued.
- Assess elderly patients carefully for adverse reactions.

Clinical alert: Monitor for signs and symptoms of drug overdose, including nausea, vomiting, blurred vision, cool and clammy skin, dizziness, confusion, dyspnea, respiratory depression, bradycardia, hearing loss, tinnitus, headache, and mood or behavior changes.

Patient teaching

- Tell patient drug may cause drowsiness. Caution him to avoid driving and other hazardous activities until CNS effects are known.
- Inform patient that prolonged use may lead to physical or psychological dependence.
- Caution patient to avoid alcohol during therapy.
- Instruct patient to move slowly when sitting up or standing, to avoid dizzi-

ness from sudden blood pressure decrease.
• As appropriate, review all other significant and life-threatening adverse reactions and interactions, especially those related to the drugs, tests, herbs, and behaviors mentioned above.

hydrocortisone
Cortef, Cortenema, Hycort♣, Hydrocortone

hydrocortisone acetate
Cortifoam

hydrocortisone butyrate
Locoid

hydrocortisone cypionate
Aquacort♣, Cortate♣, Cortef, Texacort♣

hydrocortisone sodium phosphate
Hydrocortone Phosphate

hydrocortisone sodium succinate
A-hydroCort, Solu-Cortef

hydrocortisone valerate
Westcort

Pharmacologic class: Short-acting corticosteroid
Therapeutic class: Anti-inflammatory (steroidal)
Pregnancy risk category C

Action
Suppresses inflammatory and immune responses, mainly by inhibiting migration of leukocytes and phagocytes and decreasing inflammatory mediators

Availability
Cream, gel, lotion, ointment, solution: various strengths
Injection: 25 mg/ml, 50 mg/ml; 100 mg/vial, 250 mg/vial, 500 mg/vial, 1,000 mg/vial
Intrarectal aerosol foam: 90 mg
Oral suspension: 10 mg/5 ml
Retention enema: 100 mg/60 ml
Spray (topical): 1%
Tablets: 5 mg, 10 mg, 20 mg

Indications and dosages
➤ Replacement therapy in adrenocortical insufficiency; hypercalcemia due to cancer; arthritis; collagen diseases; dermatologic diseases; autoimmune and hematologic disorders; trichinosis; ulcerative colitis; multiple sclerosis; proctitis; nephrotic syndrome; aspiration pneumonia
hydrocortisone, hydrocortisone cypionate—
Adults and children: 20 to 240 mg/day P.O.
hydrocortisone acetate (suspension)—
Adults and children: 5 to 75 mg by intra-articular injection (depending on joint size) q 2 to 3 weeks
hydrocortisone acetate (intrarectal foam)—
Adults and children: One applicatorful of intrarectal foam daily or b.i.d. for 2 to 3 weeks; then one applicatorful every other day
hydrocortisone sodium phosphate—
Adults and children: 15 to 240 mg/day subcutaneously, I.M., or I.V., adjusted according to response
hydrocortisone sodium succinate—
Adults and children: 100 to 500 mg I.M. or I.V.; may repeat at 2-, 4-, or 6-hour intervals, depending on response and condition
hydrocortisone retention enema—
Adults and children: 100 mg P.R. at bedtime for 21 nights or until desired response; patient should retain enema for at least 1 hour.

➢ Itching and inflammation caused by skin conditions
Adults and children: Thin film of topical preparation applied to affected area one to four times daily, depending on drug form and severity of condition

Off-label uses
- Phlebitis
- Stomatitis

Contraindications
- Hypersensitivity to drug, alcohol, bisulfites, or tartrazine (with some products)
- Systemic fungal infections
- Concurrent use of other immunosuppressant corticosteroids
- Concurrent administration of live-virus vaccines

Precautions
Use cautiously in:
- hypertension, osteoporosis, glaucoma, renal or GI disease, hypothyroidism, cirrhosis, thromboembolic disorders, myasthenia gravis, heart failure
- pregnant or breastfeeding patients
- children ages 6 and younger (safety not established).

Administration
- Give oral form with food or milk to avoid GI upset.
- Give I.V. injection of sodium succinate form over 30 seconds to a few minutes.
- Know that drug may be given as intermittent or continuous I.V. infusion. Dilute in normal saline solution, dextrose 5% in water, or dextrose 5% in normal saline solution.
- Inject I.M. deep into gluteal muscle. Rotate injection sites to prevent muscle atrophy.
- Be aware that subcutaneous administration may cause muscle atrophy or sterile abscess.

Never abruptly discontinue high-dose or long-term systemic therapy.
- Know that systemic forms typically are used for adrenal replacement rather than inflammation.
- Be aware that occlusive dressings, heat, hydration, inflammation, denuding, and thinning of skin increase topical drug absorption.

Route	Onset	Peak	Duration
P.O.	1-2 hr	1-2 hr	1-1.5 days
I.V.	Immediate	Unknown	1-1.5 days
I.M.	Rapid	4-8 hr	1-1.5 days
P.R.	Slow	3-5 days	4-6 days
Spray (topical), subcut.	Unknown	Unknown	Unknown

Adverse reactions
CNS: headache, nervousness, depression, euphoria, personality changes, psychoses, vertigo, paresthesia, insomnia, restlessness, conus medullaris syndrome, **meningitis, increased intracranial pressure, seizures**
CV: hypotension, hypertension, **thrombophlebitis, heart failure, shock, fat embolism, thromboembolism, arrhythmias**
EENT: cataracts, glaucoma, increased intraocular pressure, epistaxis, nasal congestion, perforated nasal septum, dysphonia, hoarseness, nasopharyngeal or oropharyngeal fungal infections
GI: nausea, vomiting, esophageal candidiasis or ulcer, abdominal distention, dry mouth, **rectal bleeding, peptic ulceration, pancreatitis**
Hematologic: purpura
Metabolic: sodium and fluid retention, hypokalemia, hypocalcemia, hyperglycemia, hypercholesterolemia, amenorrhea, growth retardation, diabetes mellitus, cushingoid appearance, **hypothalamic-pituitary-adrenal suppression with secondary adrenal insufficiency** (with abrupt withdrawal or high-dose, prolonged use)
Musculoskeletal: osteoporosis, aseptic joint necrosis, muscle pain or weak-

ness, steroid myopathy, loss of muscle mass, tendon rupture, spontaneous fractures
Respiratory: cough, wheezing, rebound congestion, **bronchospasm**
Skin: rash, pruritus, urticaria, contact dermatitis, acne, bruising, hirsutism, petechiae, striae, acneiform lesions, skin fragility and thinness, angioedema
Other: altered taste; anosmia; appetite changes; weight gain; facial edema; increased susceptibility to infection; masking or aggravation of infection; adhesive arachnoiditis; injection site pain, burning, or atrophy; immunosuppression; hypersensitivity reactions including **anaphylaxis**

Interactions

Drug-drug. *Amphotericin B, loop and thiazide diuretics, mezlocillin, piperacillin, ticarcillin:* additive hypokalemia
Fluoroquinolones: increased risk of tendon rupture
Hormonal contraceptives: prolonged half-life and increased effects of hydrocortisone
Insulin, oral hypoglycemics: increased requirements for these drugs
Live-virus vaccines: decreased antibody response to vaccine, increased risk of adverse reactions
Nonsteroidal anti-inflammatory drugs: increased risk of adverse GI reactions
Phenobarbital, phenytoin, rifampin: decreased hydrocortisone efficacy
Somatrem: inhibition of growth-promoting effect
Drug-diagnostic tests. *Calcium, potassium, thyroxine, triiodothyronine:* decreased levels
Cholesterol, glucose: increased levels
Digoxin assays: false elevation (with some test methods)
Nitroblue tetrazolium test: false-negative result
Drug-herbs. *Echinacea:* increased immunostimulation
Ginseng: potentiation of immunomodulation
Drug-behaviors. *Alcohol use:* increased risk of gastric irritation and GI ulcers

Patient monitoring

- [Clinical alert] In high-dose therapy (which should not exceed 48 hours), watch closely for signs and symptoms of depression or psychotic episodes.
- Monitor blood pressure, weight, and electrolyte levels regularly.
- Assess blood glucose levels in diabetic patients. Expect to increase insulin or oral hypoglycemic dosage.
- [Clinical alert] Monitor patient's response during weaning from drug. Watch for adrenal crisis, which may occur if drug is discontinued too quickly.

Patient teaching

- Instruct patient to take daily P.O. dose with food by 8 A.M.
- [Clinical alert] Urge patient to immediately report unusual weight gain, face or leg swelling, epigastric burning, vomiting of blood, black tarry stools, irregular menstrual cycles, fever, prolonged sore throat, cold or other infection, or worsening of symptoms.
- Tell patient using topical form not to apply occlusive dressing unless instructed by prescriber.
- Advise patient to discontinue topical drug and notify prescriber if local irritation occurs.
- Instruct patient to eat small, frequent meals and to take antacids as needed to minimize GI upset.
- Tell patient that response to drug will be monitored regularly.
- [Clinical alert] Caution patient not to stop taking drug abruptly.
- In long-term use, instruct patient to have regular eye exams.
- Instruct patient to wear medical identification stating that he's taking this drug.
- As appropriate, review all other significant and life-threatening adverse reactions and interactions, especially

h

those related to the drugs, tests, herbs, and behaviors mentioned above.

hydromorphone hydrochloride

Dilaudid, Dilaudid-5, Dilaudid-HP, Hydrostat IR, PMS-Hydromorphone✱

Pharmacologic class: Opioid agonist
Therapeutic class: Opioid analgesic, antitussive
Controlled substance schedule II
Pregnancy risk category C (with long-term use or at term with high doses: ***D***)

Action

Binds to opiate receptors in spinal cord and CNS, altering perception of and response to painful stimuli while producing generalized CNS depression. Also subdues cough reflex and decreases GI motility.

Availability

Injection: 1 mg/ml, 2 mg/ml, 4 mg/ml, 10 mg/ml
Oral solution: 5 mg/5 ml
Rectal suppositories: 3 mg
Tablets: 1 mg, 2 mg, 3 mg, 4 mg, 8 mg

Indications and dosages

➢ Moderate to severe pain

Adults weighing more than 50 kg (110 lb): 2 to 10 mg P.O. (tablets) q 4 to 6 hours p.r.n. or 2.5 to 10 mg P.O. (oral solution) q 4 to 6 hours p.r.n.; or 1 to 2 mg subcutaneously, I.M., or I.V. q 4 to 6 hours p.r.n., increased to 3 to 4 mg q 4 to 6 hours p.r.n. for severe pain; or 3 mg P.R. q 6 to 8 hours p.r.n.

Contraindications

- Hypersensitivity to narcotics or bisulfites
- Acute or severe bronchial asthma or upper respiratory tract obstruction
- Premature neonates

Precautions

Use cautiously in:

- increased intracranial pressure; severe renal, hepatic, or pulmonary disease; hypothyroidism; adrenal insufficiency; prostatic hypertrophy; alcoholism
- concurrent use of MAO inhibitors
- elderly patients
- pregnant or breastfeeding patients.

Administration

- For maximal analgesic effect, give before pain becomes severe.
- For I.V. infusion, mix with dextrose 5% in water, normal saline solution, or lactated Ringer's solution.
- Give single-dose I.V. injection slowly, over 2 to 5 minutes for each 2-mg dose.
- Rotate I.M. and subcutaneous sites to prevent muscle atrophy.
- Give oral form with food to avoid GI upset.

Route	Onset	Peak	Duration
P.O.	30 min	90-120 min	4 hr
I.V.	10-15 min	15-30 min	2-3 hr
I.M., subcut.	15 min	30-60 min	4-5 hr
P.R.	15-30 min	30-90 min	4-5 hr

Adverse reactions

CNS: confusion, sedation, dysphoria, euphoria, floating feeling, hallucinations, headache, unusual dreams, anxiety, dizziness, drowsiness
CV: hypotension, hypertension, palpitations, bradycardia, tachycardia
EENT: blurred vision, diplopia, miosis, nystagmus, tinnitus, laryngeal edema, **laryngospasm**
GI: nausea, vomiting, constipation, abdominal cramps, biliary tract spasm, anorexia
GU: urinary retention, dysuria
Hepatic: hepatotoxicity

Respiratory: dyspnea, wheezing, **bronchospasm, respiratory depression**
Skin: flushing, diaphoresis
Other: physical or psychological drug dependence; drug tolerance; injection site pain, redness, or swelling

Interactions

Drug-drug. *Antidepressants, antihistamines, MAO inhibitors, sedative-hypnotics:* additive CNS depression
Antihypertensives, diuretics, guanadrel, guanethidine, mecamylamine: increased risk of hypotension
Atropine, belladonna alkaloids, difenoxin, diphenoxylate, kaolin and pectin, loperamide, paregoric: increased risk of CNS depression, severe constipation
Barbiturates: increased sedation
Buprenorphine, butorphanol, nalbuphine, pentazocine: precipitation of opioid withdrawal in physically dependent patients
Nalbuphine, pentazocine: decreased analgesia
Drug-diagnostic tests. *Amylase, lipase:* increased levels
Drug-herbs. *Chamomile, hops, kava, skullcap, valerian:* increased CNS depression
Drug-behaviors. *Alcohol use:* increased CNS depression

Patient monitoring

With I.V. use, monitor for respiratory depression. Keep resuscitation equipment and naloxone nearby.
- Assess for signs and symptoms of physical or psychological drug dependence.
- Monitor for constipation.

Patient teaching

Instruct patient to take drug exactly as prescribed before pain becomes severe, but caution him that drug may be habit-forming.
- Tell patient to take oral form with food to avoid GI upset.
- Advise patient to report difficulty breathing, nausea, vomiting, or dizziness.
- Caution patient to avoid driving and other hazardous activities until he knows how drug affects concentration and alertness.
- Tell patient to avoid alcohol while taking drug.
- As appropriate, review all other significant and life-threatening adverse reactions and interactions, especially those related to the drugs, tests, herbs, and behaviors mentioned above.

h

hydroxychloroquine sulfate

Plaquenil

Pharmacologic class: 4-aminoquinolone
Therapeutic class: Antimalarial, antirheumatic, anti-inflammatory (disease-modifying)
Pregnancy risk category C

Action

Unknown. Thought to interfere with inhibition of protein synthesis and DNA replication, leading to parasitic death.

Availability

Tablets: 200 mg (155 mg base); 200 mg hydroxychloroquine sulfate is equivalent to 155 mg of hydroxychloroquine base

Indications and dosages

➤ Malaria prophylaxis (dosages expressed as mg of base)
Adults: 310 mg P.O. q week, starting 1 to 2 weeks before entering endemic area and continuing for 4 weeks after leaving area
Children: 5 mg/kg P.O. q week, starting 1 to 2 weeks before entering en

demic area and continuing for 4 weeks after leaving area

➢ Acute malarial attack (dosages expressed as mg of base)

Adults: Initially, 620 mg P.O., then 310 mg 6 hours, 24 hours, and 48 hours later

Children: Initially, 10 mg/kg P.O., then 5 mg/kg 6 hours, 24 hours, and 48 hours later

➢ Rheumatoid arthritis

Adults: 400 to 600 mg/day P.O. for 4 to 12 weeks, then reduced by 50%

➢ Systemic lupus erythematosus

Adults: 400 mg P.O. once or twice daily for several months, then reduced to 200 to 400 mg daily, depending on response

Contraindications

- Hypersensitivity to drug or chloroquine
- Retinal or visual field changes
- Long-term therapy in children

Precautions

Use cautiously in:

- hepatic or renal impairment, G6PD deficiency, psoriasis, bone marrow depression, alcoholism
- obese patients
- pregnant or breastfeeding patients
- children.

Administration

- Give with food or milk.
- For malaria prophylaxis, schedule doses on same day each week.

Route	Onset	Peak	Duration
P.O.	Unknown	2-4.5 hr	Unknown

Adverse reactions

CNS: anxiety, apathy, confusion, fatigue, headache, psychoses, mood swings, irritability, neuromyopathy, peripheral neuritis, **seizures**

CV: ECG changes, hypotension

EENT: visual disturbances, retinopathy, keratopathy, ototoxicity, tinnitus

GI: nausea, vomiting, diarrhea, abdominal cramps, anorexia

Hematologic: leukopenia, agranulocytosis, aplastic anemia, thrombocytopenia

Hepatic: jaundice, **hepatotoxicity**

Musculoskeletal: muscle weakness

Skin: dermatoses, rash, pruritus, pigmentation changes, pleomorphic skin eruption, worsened psoriasis, alopecia, bleaching of hair

Other: weight loss

Interactions

Drug-drug. *Aluminum salts, kaolin, magnesium salts:* decreased hydroxychloroquinine absorption

Cimetidine: decreased hepatic metabolism of hydroxychloroquinine

Hepatotoxic drugs: increased risk of hepatotoxicity

Drug-diagnostic tests. *Granulocytes, hemoglobin, platelets:* decreased values

Drug-behaviors. *Sun exposure:* exacerbation of drug-induced dermatoses

Patient monitoring

🔊 Monitor for signs and symptoms of overdose, such as nausea, vomiting, drowsiness, visual disturbances, cardiovascular collapse, and seizures.

- Watch for adverse reactions.

Patient teaching

- Advise patient to take with food or milk.

🔊 Instruct patient to immediately report such adverse reactions as vision changes, nausea, vomiting, drowsiness, mental changes, mood swings, headache, ringing in ears, muscle weakness, rash, bleeding, bruising, and yellowing of skin and eyes.

- In long-term therapy, advise patient to have regular eye exams.
- As appropriate, review all other significant and life-threatening adverse reactions and interactions, especially those related to the drugs, tests, and behaviors mentioned above.

hydroxyurea

Droxia, Hydrea

Pharmacologic class: Antimetabolite
Therapeutic class: Antineoplastic
Pregnancy risk category D

Action

Unknown. May inhibit enzyme necessary for DNA synthesis without disrupting RNA or protein synthesis.

Availability

Capsules: 200 mg, 250 mg, 300 mg, 400 mg, 500 mg

Indications and dosages

➢ Head and neck cancer; ovarian cancer; malignant melanoma
Adults: 60 to 80 mg/kg (2 to 3 g/m^2) P.O. as a single daily dose q 3 days, or 20 to 30 mg/kg/day P.O. as a single dose. Begin therapy begin 7 days before radiation.
➢ Resistant chronic myelogenous leukemia
Adults: 20 to 30 mg/kg/day P.O. in one or two divided doses
➢ Sickle cell anemia
Adults and children: 15 mg/kg/day P.O. as a single dose. May increase by 5 mg/kg/day P.O. q 12 weeks, up to 35 mg/kg/day.

Off-label uses

- Thrombocythemia
- Human immunodeficiency virus

Contraindications

- Hypersensitivity to drug or tartrazine
- Bone marrow depression
- Severe anemia or thrombocytopenia

Precautions

Use cautiously in:
- renal or hepatic impairment
- obese patients
- females of childbearing age
- elderly patients.

Administration

- Provide frequent mouth care.

Route	Onset	Peak	Duration
P.O.	Unknown	2 hr	24 hr

Adverse reactions

CNS: drowsiness, malaise, confusion, dizziness, headache
GI: nausea, vomiting, diarrhea, constipation, stomatitis, anorexia
GU: dysuria, hyperuricemia, infertility, **renal tubular dysfunction**
Hematologic: anemia, **megaloblastosis, leukopenia, thrombocytopenia, bone marrow depression**
Hepatic: hepatitis
Metabolic: hyperuricemia
Skin: alopecia, erythema, pruritus, rash, urticaria, exacerbation of postradiation erythema
Other: chills, fever

Interactions

Drug-drug. *Live-virus vaccines:* decreased antibody response to vaccine, increased risk of adverse reactions
Myelosuppressants: additive bone marrow depression
Drug-diagnostic tests. *Blood urea nitrogen, creatinine, uric acid:* increased values
Hemoglobin, platelets, red blood cells, white blood cells: decreased values
Mean corpuscular volume: transient increase

Patient monitoring

- Assess CBC weekly.
- Closely monitor patient with renal or hepatic impairment. Check kidney and liver function tests often.
- Assess fluid status. Make sure patient drinks 10 to 12 glasses of water daily.

Patient teaching

- Advise patient to mark dates for drug doses, diagnostic tests, and treatments on calendar.

🔊 Instruct patient to immediately report easy bruising, bleeding, unusual tiredness, or yellowing of skin or eyes.
- Tell patent to report such adverse effects as appetite loss, nausea, vomiting, oral lesions, constipation, diarrhea, confusion, dizziness, headache, and rash.
- Instruct female patient to use barrier contraception.
- Tell patient he'll undergo regular blood testing to monitor drug effects.
- As appropriate, review all other significant and life-threatening adverse reactions and interactions, especially those related to the drugs and tests mentioned above.

hydroxyzine hydrochloride

Apo-Hydroxyzine♣, Atarax, Novo-Hydroxyzin♣

hydroxyzine pamoate

Vistaril

Pharmacologic class: Piperazine derivative

Therapeutic class: Anxiolytic, antihistamine, sedative-hypnotic

Pregnancy risk category NR

Action

Unknown. Anxiolytic and sedative effects may stem from suppression of activity in subcortical levels of CNS. Antihistamine effects may result from histamine suppression at cellular receptor sites.

Availability

Capsules: 25 mg, 50 mg, 100 mg (pamoate)
Injection: 25 mg/ml, 50 mg/ml
Oral suspension: 25 mg/5 ml (pamoate)
Syrup: 10 mg/5 ml
Tablets: 10 mg, 25 mg, 50 mg, 100 mg

Indications and dosages

➤ Psychiatric emergencies; acute or chronic alcoholism
Adults: 50 to 100 mg I.M. immediately, then q 4 to 6 hours p.r.n.
➤ Nausea and vomiting; adjunct in pre- and postoperative sedation
Adults: 25 to 100 mg I.M. q 4 to 6 hours
Children: 1.1 mg/kg I.M. q 4 to 6 hours
➤ Anxiety
Adults and children ages 6 and older: 50 to 100 mg P.O. q.i.d.
Children younger than age 6: 50 mg P.O. daily in divided doses
➤ Pruritus
Adults: 25 mg P.O. three or four times daily
Children ages 6 and older: 50 to 100 mg P.O. daily in divided doses
Children younger than age 6: 50 mg P.O. daily in divided doses

Off-label uses

- Seasonal allergic rhinitis

Contraindications

- Hypersensitivity to drug or cetirizine

Precautions

Use cautiously in:
- severe hepatic dysfunction
- elderly patients.

Administration

🔊 Don't administer I.V. or subcutaneously (may cause tissue necrosis).
- Use Z-track method for I.M. injection. Inject deep into large muscle (preferably, upper outer quadrant of buttock).

Route	Onset	Peak	Duration
P.O., I.M.	15-30 min	2-4 hr	4-6 hr

Adverse reactions

CNS: drowsiness, agitation, dizziness, headache, asthenia, ataxia
GI: nausea, constipation, dry mouth
GU: urinary retention
Respiratory: wheezing
Skin: flushing
Other: bitter taste, hypersensitivity reaction, pain or abscess at I.M. injection site

Interactions

Drug-drug. *Anticholinergics, antidepressants, antihistamines, phenothiazines, quinidine:* additive effects of these drugs
Antidepressants, antihistamines, opioids, sedative-hypnotics, other CNS depressants: additive CNS depression
Drug-diagnostic tests. *Skin tests using allergen extracts:* false-negative results
Drug-herbs. *Angel's trumpet, jimsonweed, scopolia:* increased anticholinergic effects
Chamomile, hops, kava, skullcap, valerian: increased CNS depression
Drug-behaviors. *Alcohol use:* increased CNS depression

Patient monitoring

- Monitor closely for CNS depression and oversedation, especially if patient is receiving other CNS depressants.
- Assess for adverse effects, especially in elderly patients.
- Monitor liver function test results in patients with hepatic impairment.

Patient teaching

- Tell patient to contact prescriber if he experiences wheezing, muscle spasms, or incoordination.
- Caution patient to avoid driving and other hazardous activities until he knows how drug affects concentration and alertness.
- Instruct patient to avoid alcohol while taking drug.
- As appropriate, review all other significant adverse reactions and interactions, especially those related to the drugs, tests, herbs, and behaviors mentioned above.

hyoscyamine
Cystospaz

hyoscyamine sulfate
Anaspaz, A-Spas S/L, Cystospaz-M, Donnamar, ED-SPAZ, Gastrosed, Levbid, Levsin, Levsin Drops, Levsin/SL, Levsinex, Levsinex Timecaps, Neoquess, NuLev

Pharmacologic class: Anticholinergic
Therapeutic class: Antispasmodic
Pregnancy risk category C

Action

Competitively inhibits acetylcholine action at autonomic nerve sites, relaxing smooth muscle and decreasing glandular secretions

Availability

hyoscyamine
Tablets: 0.15 mg
hyoscyamine sulfate
Capsules (timed-release): 0.375 mg
Elixir: 0.125 mg/5 ml
Injection: 0.5 mg/ml
Oral solution: 0.125 mg/ml
Tablets: 0.125 mg
Tablets (extended-release): 0.375 mg
Tablets (orally disintegrating): 0.125 mg
Tablets (sublingual): 0.125 mg

Indications and dosages

➤ Adjunct in GI tract disorders; pain and hypersecretion in pancreatitis; cystitis; renal colic; infant colic; acute rhinitis; rigidity, tremors, and hyperhidrosis in Parkinson's disease; partial heart block due to vagal activity
Adults: 0.15 to 0.3 mg P.O. up to q.i.d.

Adults and children ages 12 and older: 0.125 to 0.25 mg (sulfate) P.O. or S.L. two to four times daily, or 0.375 to 0.75 mg (extended-release sulfate) P.O. q 12 hours, or 0.25 to 0.5 mg (sulfate) subcutaneously, I.M., or I.V. two to four times daily p.r.n.
Children ages 2 to 12: In children weighing approximately 50 kg (110 lb), 0.125 mg (sulfate) P.O. q 4 hours p.r.n.; in children weighing approximately 20 kg (40 lb), 0.0625 mg P.O. (sulfate); in children weighing approximately 10 kg (22 lb), 0.031 to 0.033 mg (sulfate) P.O. Don't exceed 0.75 mg/day.
Children ages 2 and younger: In children weighing approximately 7 kg (15 lb), 0.025 (sulfate) P.O. q 4 hours p.r.n.; in children weighing approximately 5 kg (11 lb), 0.0208 mg (sulfate) P.O. q 4 hours p.r.n.; in children weighing approximately 3.4 kg (7.5 lb), 0.0167 mg (sulfate) P.O. q 4 hours p.r.n.; in children weighing approximately 2.3 kg (5 lb), 0.0125 mg (sulfate) P.O. q 4 hours p.r.n.

➢ Before endoscopy or hypotonic duodenography
Adults: 0.25 to 0.5 mg (sulfate) subcutaneously, I.M., or I.V. 5 to 10 minutes before procedure

➢ Preoperatively to inhibit salivation and excessive respiratory secretions
Adults and children older than age 2: 5 mcg/kg (sulfate) I.M., I.V., or subcutaneously 30 to 60 minutes before anesthesia induction

➢ Muscarinic toxicity
Adults: 1 to 2 mg (sulfate) I.V. Additional 1-mg doses may be given I.M. or I.V. q 3 to 10 minutes until muscarinic signs and symptoms subside; doses may be repeated if needed. Patient may need up to 25 mg during first 24 hours. For maintenance, 0.5 to 1 mg P.O. at intervals of several hours until signs and symptoms disappear.

Contraindications

- Hypersensitivity to anticholinergics, alcohol, sulfites, or tartrazine
- Angle-closure glaucoma, synechia
- GU or GI obstructive disease, severe ulcerative colitis
- Renal or hepatic disease
- Neonates or premature infants

Precautions

Use cautiously in:

- cardiovascular disease, prostatic hypertrophy, reflux esophagitis, brain damage, autonomic neuropathy, hyperthyroidism, glaucoma, Down syndrome, spastic paralysis
- elderly patients
- pregnant (safety not established) or breastfeeding patients
- infants and small children.

Administration

- Administer 30 to 60 minutes before meals and at bedtime.
- Give bedtime dose at least 2 hours after last evening meal or snack.
- Be aware that hyoscyamine is given P.O. only, whereas hyoscyamine sulfate may be given P.O., I.M., I.V., sublingually, or subcutaneously.
- Know that a cholinerase reactivator (pralidoxime) is given concomitantly to treat muscarinic toxicity.

Route	Onset	Peak	Duration
P.O.	20-30 min	0.5-1 hr	4-12 hr
P.O. (extended)	20-30 min	40-90 min	12 hr
I.V.	2 min	15-30 min	4 hr
I.M., subcut.	Unknown	15-30 min	4-12 hr
S.L.	5-20 min	0.5-1 hr	4 hr

Adverse reactions

CNS: confusion, excitement, nervousness, dizziness, light-headedness, headache, insomnia
CV: palpitations, tachycardia

EENT: blurred vision, cycloplegia, increased intraocular pressure, mydriasis, photophobia
GI: nausea, vomiting, constipation, bloating, dry mouth, **paralytic ileus**
GU: urinary hesitancy or retention, erectile dysfunction, lactation suppression
Skin: flushing, decreased sweating, urticaria, local irritation (with I.M., I.V., or subcutaneous use)
Other: altered taste, allergic reactions (including fever), heat intolerance, **anaphylaxis**

Interactions

Drug-drug. *Amantadine, antihistamines, antiparkinsonian drugs, disopyramide, glutethimide, meperidine, procainamide, quinidine, tricyclic antidepressants:* increased anticholinergic effects
Antacids: decreased hyoscyamine absorption
Atenolol: increased atenolol effects
Ketoconazole: interference with absorption of both drugs
Methotrimeprazine: increased risk of extrapyramidal effects
Phenothiazines: decreased phenothiazine effects, increased anticholinergic effects
Drug-herbs. *Jimsonweed:* adverse cardiovascular effects

Patient monitoring

- Watch for adverse reactions.
- Check for mental status changes, such as confusion.
- Evaluate fluid intake and output.
- Assess patient's response to temperature changes (especially hot weather). Drug may cause heat intolerance, predisposing patient to heat stroke.

Patient teaching

- Tell patient to take on empty stomach 30 to 60 minutes before meals and at least 2 hours after last evening meal or snack.
- Instruct patient with urinary hesitancy to empty bladder before taking.
- Caution patient to avoid driving and other hazardous activities until he knows how drug affects concentration and alertness.
- As appropriate, review all other significant and life-threatening adverse reactions and interactions, especially those related to the drugs and herbs mentioned above.

ibritumomab tiuxetan

Zevalin

Pharmacologic class: Monoclonal antibody
Therapeutic class: Antineoplastic
Pregnancy risk category D

Action

Binds indium-111 (In-111) or yttrium-90 (Y-90) with free amino groups of lysines and arginines within antibody; binds specifically to CD20 antigen, found on surface of normal and malignant B lymphocytes. Radioactive component of Y-90 causes cellular damage via free radicals in target cells.

Availability

Injection: 3.2 mg/2 ml (two Zevalin kits containing four vials each)

Indications and dosages

➤ Non-Hodgkin's lymphoma
Adults: Two-step regimen that includes pre-dose of rituximab
Step 1: Single I.V. infusion of 250 mg/m² rituximab at 50 mg/hour; increase rate by 50 mg/hour q 30 minutes, to a

maximum of 400 mg/hour. If hypersensitivity or infusion-related reaction occurs, slow or interrupt infusion; if symptoms improve, may resume at 50% of previous rate. Within 4 hours of rituximab dose, 5 mCi of In-111 Zevalin I.V. should be given over 10 minutes.

Step 2: 7 to 9 days after step 1, I.V. infusion of 250 mg/m^2 rituximab at 100 mg/hour (50 mg/hour if infusion-related reaction occurred during first rituximab dose); increase by 100 mg/hour q 30 minutes, to a maximum of 400 mg/hour, as tolerated. Within 4 hours of rituximab dose, give 0.3 to 0.4 mCi/kg of Y-90 Zevalin I.V. over 10 minutes, not to exceed absolute maximum allowable dose of 32 mCi.

Contraindications

- Hypersensitivity to any drug in therapeutic regimen or its components or to murine products
- Pregnancy or breastfeeding

Precautions

Use cautiously in:

- cardiac conditions
- elderly patients.

Administration

🔈 Assess for human antimurine antibody before treatment. If result is positive, patient may experience hypersensitivity reaction.

- Premedicate patient with acetaminophen and diphenhydramine, as ordered, before each rituximab infusion.
- Know that ibritumomab should be used only as part of a regimen that combines ibritumomab and rituximab.

🔈 Give ibritumomab by slow I.V. infusion over 10 minutes; monitor closely.

🔈 Don't give by I.V. push.

🔈 Take steps to prevent extravasation of Y-90 Zevalin. If extravasation occurs, immediately stop infusion and restart in another vein.

- Don't give Y-90 Zevalin if platelet count is less than 100,000/mm^3.
- Follow facility policy on radiation precautions to protect patients, visitors, and medical personnel from radiation exposure.

Route	Onset	Peak	Duration
I.V.	Unknown	Unknown	Unknown

Adverse reactions

CNS: dizziness, anxiety, headache, insomnia, asthenia

CV: hypotension, peripheral edema

EENT: rhinitis, epistaxis, throat irritation

GI: nausea, vomiting, diarrhea, constipation, anorexia, dyspepsia, abdominal pain or enlargement, melena

Hematologic: anemia, **thrombocytopenia, neutropenia, pancytopenia, hemorrhage**

Musculoskeletal: joint pain, myalgia, back pain

Respiratory: increased cough, dyspnea, **apnea, bronchospasm**

Skin: flushing, bruising, diaphoresis, petechiae, pruritus, rash, urticaria, angioedema

Other: bacterial infection, I.V. site irritation, fever, chills, generalized pain, tumor pain, hypersensitivity reactions including **anaphylaxis, myeloid malignancies, dysplasias**

Interactions

None significant

Patient monitoring

🔈 Institute infection control protocols. Protect patient from potential sources of infection.

🔈 Assess CBC and platelet count before starting therapy. Monitor regularly during and after therapy.

🔈 Monitor patient for hypersensitivity reactions, which can be fatal and usually occur within 30 minutes to 2 hours of administration.

• Be alert for for unusual bleeding or bruising.

Patient teaching

🔊 Instruct patient to promptly report difficulty breathing, rash, fever, chills, severe GI distress, black tarry stools, illness or injury, or unusual bleeding or bruising.
• Tell patient that drug increases his risk of infection. Instruct him to avoid crowds and potential or known sources of infection.
• Advise patient to eat small, frequent meals and take antiemetic drugs to control nausea and vomiting, as needed and prescribed.
• Advise patient that he'll undergo blood testing during therapy to monitor drug effects.
• As appropriate, review all other significant and life-threatening adverse reactions mentioned above.

ibuprofen

Actiprofen Caplets✱, Advil, Advil Migraine, Apo-Ibuprofen✱, Children's Advil, Children's Motrin, Excedrin IB, Genpril, Haltran, Junior Strength Advil, Junior Strength Motrin, Medipren, Menadol, Midol IB, Motrin IB, Novo-Profen✱, Nu-Ibuprofen✱, Nuprin

Pharmacologic class: Nonsteroidal anti-inflammatory drug (NSAID)
Therapeutic class: Analgesic, antipyretic, anti-inflammatory
Pregnancy risk category B (third trimester: ***D***)

Action

Unknown. Thought to inhibit cyclooxygenase, an enzyme needed for prostaglandin synthesis.

Availability

Capsules (liquigels): 200 mg
Oral suspension: 100 mg/2.5 ml, 100 mg/5 ml
Pediatric drops: 50 mg/1.25 ml
Tablets: 100 mg, 200 mg, 400 mg, 600 mg, 800 mg
Tablets (chewable): 50 mg, 100 mg

Indications and dosages

➤ Rheumatoid arthritis; osteoarthritis
Adults: 1.2 to 3.2 g/day P.O. in three to four divided doses
➤ Mild to moderate pain
Adults: 400 mg P.O. q 4 to 6 hours p.r.n.
➤ Primary dysmenorrhea
Adults: 400 mg P.O. q 4 hours p.r.n.
➤ Juvenile arthritis
Children: 30 to 40 mg/kg/day P.O. in three or four divided doses. Daily dosages above 50 mg/kg aren't recommended.
➤ Fever reduction; pain relief
Children ages 6 to 12: 5 mg/kg P.O. if temperature is below 102.5° F (39.2° C) or 10 mg/kg if temperature is above 102.5° F. Maximum daily dosage is 40 mg/kg.

Off-label uses

• Migraine and tension headaches

Contraindications

• Hypersensitivity to drug or other NSAIDs
• Pregnancy

Precautions

Use cautiously in:
• severe cardiovascular, renal, or hepatic disease; GI disease; asthma; chronic alcohol use
• elderly patients
• breastfeeding patients.

Administration

• Ideally, give 1 hour before or 2 hours after meal. If GI upset occurs, give with meals.

Route	Onset	Peak	Duration
P.O. (analgesic)	30 min	1-2 hr	4-6 hr
P.O. (anti-inflam.)	7 days	1-2 wk	Unknown

Adverse reactions

CNS: headache, dizziness, drowsiness, nervousness, **aseptic meningitis**
CV: arrhythmias
EENT: amblyopia, blurred vision, tinnitus
GI: nausea, vomiting, constipation, dyspepsia, abdominal discomfort, **GI bleeding**
GU: cystitis, hematuria, azotemia, **renal failure**
Hematologic: anemia, **prolonged bleeding time, aplastic anemia, neutropenia, pancytopenia, thrombocytopenia, leukopenia, agranulocytosis**
Hepatic: hepatitis
Metabolic: hyperglycemia, **hypoglycemia**
Respiratory: bronchospasm
Skin: rash, pruritus, urticaria, **Stevens-Johnson syndrome**
Other: edema, allergic reactions including **anaphylaxis**

Interactions

Drug-drug. *Acetaminophen:* increased risk of adverse renal reactions
Antihypertensives, diuretics: decreased efficacy of these drugs
Antineoplastics: increased risk of adverse hematologic reactions
Aspirin and other NSAIDs, corticosteroids: additive adverse GI effects
Cefamandole, cefoperazone, cefotetan, drugs affecting platelet function (including abciximab, clopidogrel, eptifibatide, ticlopidine, tirofiban), plicamycin, thrombolytics, valproic acid, warfarin: increased risk of bleeding
Cyclosporine: increased risk of nephrotoxicity
Digoxin: slightly increased digoxin blood level
Lithium: increased lithium blood level, greater risk of lithium toxicity
Methotrexate: increased risk of methotrexate toxicity
Probenecid: increased risk of ibuprofen toxicity
Drug-diagnostic tests. *Alanine aminotransferase, alkaline phosphatase, aspartate aminotransferase, blood urea nitrogen, creatinine, lactate dehydrogenase, potassium:* increased values
Bleeding time: prolonged
Creatinine clearance, glucose, hematocrit, hemoglobin, platelets, white blood cells: decreased values
Drug-herbs. *Anise, arnica, chamomile, clove, dong quai, fenugreek, feverfew, garlic, ginger, ginkgo, ginseng, licorice:* increased risk of bleeding
White willow: additive adverse GI effects
Drug-behaviors. *Alcohol use:* additive adverse GI effects
Sun exposure: phototoxicity

Patient monitoring

- Monitor for desired effect.
- Watch for GI upset, adverse CNS effects (such as headache and drowsiness), and hypersensitivity reaction.
- Stay alert for GI bleeding and ulcers, especially in long-term therapy.
- In long-term therapy, assess renal and hepatic function regularly.

Patient teaching

- Tell patient to take with full glass of water, with food, or after meals to minimize GI upset.
- To help prevent esophageal irritation, instruct patient to avoid lying down for 30 to 60 minutes after taking dose.
- Instruct patient to immediately report irregular heartbeats, black tarry stools, vision changes, unusual tiredness, yellowing of skin or eyes, change in urination pattern, difficulty breathing, finger or ankle swelling, weight gain, itching, rash, fever, or sore throat.

• Caution patient to avoid driving and other hazardous activities until he knows how drug affects concentration, alertness, and balance.
• As appropriate, review all other significant and life-threatening adverse reactions and interactions, especially those related to the drugs, tests, herbs, and behaviors mentioned above.

ibutilide fumarate
Corvert

Pharmacologic class: Ibutilide derivative
Therapeutic class: Antiarrhythmic (class III)
Pregnancy risk category C

Action
Prolongs myocardial action potential by slowing repolarization and atrioventricular (AV) conduction

Availability
Solution: 0.1 mg/ml in 10-ml vials

Indications and dosages
➢ To convert atrial fibrillation or flutter to sinus rhythm
Adults weighing more than 60 kg (132 lb): 1 vial (1 mg) by I.V. infusion over 10 minutes. May repeat after 10 minutes if arrhythmia persists.
Adults weighing less than 60 kg (132 lb): 0.1 ml/kg (0.01 mg/kg) by I.V. infusion over 10 minutes. May repeat after 10 minutes if arrhythmia persists.

Contraindications
• Hypersensitivity to drug or its components

Precautions
Use cautiously in:
• ventricular and AV arrhythmias
• pregnant or breastfeeding patients.

Administration
Clinical alert: Monitor ECG continuously during and after infusion. Stop infusion immediately if ventricular tachycardia occurs.
• As appropriate, administer diluted or undiluted. To dilute, add 10-ml vial to 50 ml of normal saline solution or dextrose 5% in water, to yield a concentration of 0.017 mg/ml.
• Infuse over 10 minutes.
Clinical alert: Don't give with amiodarone, disopyramide, quinidine, procainamide, or sotalol, because of increased risk of dangerous arrhythmias.

Route	Onset	Peak	Duration
I.V.	Immediate	10 min	Unknown

Adverse reactions
CNS: headache, light-headedness, dizziness, numbness or tingling in arms
CV: hypotension, hypertension, bradycardia, **bundle-branch block, ventricular extrasystoles, ventricular arrhythmias, ventricular tachycardia, AV heart block, heart failure**
GI: nausea
GU: renal failure

Interactions
Drug-drug. *Amiodarone, disopyramide, quinidine, procainamide, sotalol:* increased risk of dangerous arrhythmias
Antihistamines, phenothiazines, tricyclic antidepressants: increased proarrhythmic effect (prolonged QT interval)

Patient monitoring
• Before giving, assess electrolyte levels and correct abnormalities (especially involving potassium and magnesium), because hypokalemia and hypomagnesemia can lead to arrhythmias.
Clinical alert: Watch for premature ventricular contractions, sinus tachycardia, sinus bradycardia, and heart block.
• Monitor ECG during and for at least 4 hours after infusion.

🔊 Keep emergency equipment (defibrillator, emergency cart and drug box, oxygen, suction, and intubation equipment) at hand during and for at least 4 hours after infusion.
• Monitor prothrombin time, International Normalized Ratio, and activated partial thromboplastin time if patient is receiving anticoagulant therapy.

Patient teaching

🔊 Instruct patient to immediately report chest pain, dizziness, numbness, palpitations, headache, or difficulty breathing.
• Tell patient he'll be monitored closely for at least 4 hours after drug administration.

idarubicin hydrochloride

Idamycin, Idamycin PFS

Pharmacologic class: Anthracycline antibiotic
Therapeutic class: Antineoplastic
Pregnancy risk category D

Action

Inhibits nucleic acid synthesis by disrupting DNA and RNA polymerase, causing cell death

Availability

Injection: 1 mg/ml

Indications and dosages

➢ Acute myeloid leukemia
Adults: 12 mg/m^2/day by slow I.V. injection over 10 to 15 minutes for 3 days. As prescribed, give with cytarabine by continuous I.V. infusion for 7 days, or give cytarabine as I.V. bolus followed by 5 days of cytarabine by continuous I.V. infusion. Second course may be given, depending on response.

Dosage adjustment

• Renal or hepatic impairment
• Severe mucositis

Off-label uses

• Acute nonlymphocytic and chronic myelogenous leukemias
• Non-Hodgkin's lymphoma
• Breast cancer

Contraindications

• Hypersensitivity to drug
• Cardiac disease
• Pregnancy or breastfeeding

Precautions

Use cautiously in:
• renal or hepatic impairment
• bone marrow depression
• previous treatment with anthracyclines or cardiotoxic drugs.

Administration

🔊 When preparing, wear goggles and gloves, because exposure may cause severe skin reaction. If exposure occurs, wash affected area immediately with soap and water. For eye exposure, follow standard eye irrigation procedure.
• Reconstitute 5-, 10-, or 20-mg vial with 5, 10, or 20 ml of normal saline solution, respectively, to yield a concentration of 1 mg/ml.
• Give slowly over 10 to 15 minutes into I.V. tubing that is infusing normal saline solution or dextrose 5% in water.
🔊 Don't administer subcutaneously or I.M. (may cause tissue necrosis).
• If severe mucositis occurs, delay second course (if prescribed) until full recovery; then reduce dosage by 25%.

Route	Onset	Peak	Duration
I.V.	Immediate	Several min	Unknown

Adverse reactions

CNS: headache, mental status changes, peripheral neuropathy, **seizures**
CV: chest pain, **heart failure, atrial**

fibrillation, myocardial infarction, arrhythmias
GI: nausea, vomiting, diarrhea, cramps, mucositis, **GI hemorrhage**
GU: red urine, **renal failure**
Hematologic: bone marrow depression
Hepatic: hepatic function changes
Metabolic: hyperuricemia
Skin: alopecia, urticaria, bullous erythematous rash on palms and soles, erythema at previously irradiated site, tissue necrosis or urticaria at injection site
Other: fever, infection, hypersensitivity reaction

Interactions

Drug-drug. *Alkaline solutions, heparin:* incompatibility

Patient monitoring

◀ Evaluate injection site for burning, stinging, and extravasation. If extravasation occurs, stop infusion and restart in another vein. Then rinse area with normal saline solution and apply cold compress. (Local infiltration with corticosteroids may be indicated.)
- Monitor patient's response to therapy regularly.
- Assess serum uric acid level and CBC.
- Monitor hemodynamic status and cardiac output. Assess for S_3 heart sound (which signals heart failure).
- Assess fluid intake and output. Make sure patient is adequately hydrated, to prevent hyperuricemia.

Patient teaching

◀ Instruct patient to immediately report unusual bleeding or bruising, difficulty breathing, or sudden weight gain.
- Tell patient to eat small, frequent meals.
- Advise patient to keep follow-up appointments for assessment, regular blood testing, and monitoring of drug effects.
- As appropriate, review all other significant and life-threatening adverse reactions and interactions, especially those related to the drugs mentioned above.

ifosfamide

Iflex

Pharmacologic class: Alkylating agent, nitrogen mustard
Therapeutic class: Antineoplastic
Pregnancy risk category D

Action

Alkylates DNA, interfering with replication and synthesis of susceptible cells and ultimately causing cell death

Availability

Injection: 1 g or 3 g in single-dose vials

Indications and dosages

➢ Germ-cell testicular cancer
Adults: 1.2 g/m²/day by I.V. infusion over 30 minutes for 5 days. May repeat q 3 weeks or after recovery from hematologic toxicity.

Off-label uses

- Acute leukemia
- Breast, lung, ovarian, and pancreatic cancer
- Malignant lymphomas
- Sarcomas

Contraindications

- Hypersensitivity to drug
- Severe bone marrow depression
- Pregnancy or breastfeeding

Precautions

Use cautiously in:
- impaired renal or hepatic function, mild to moderate bone marrow depression.

Administration

- Follow facility policy for handling antineoplastic agents.
- Know that drug is usually given with other antineoplastics and hemorrhagic cystitis agent.
- To reconstitute, add sterile water or bacteriostatic water to vial, and shake gently.
- Mix 20 ml of diluent with 1-g vial or 60 ml of diluent with 3-g vial, to yield a concentration of 50 mg/ml. For smaller concentrations, dilute solution further with normal saline solution, dextrose 5% in water, lactated Ringer's solution, or sterile water.
- Administer I.V. slowly over at least 30 minutes.

Route	Onset	Peak	Duration
I.V.	Immediate	Unknown	Unknown

Adverse reactions

CNS: drowsiness, confusion, ataxia, hallucinations, depressive psychosis, dizziness, disorientation, cranial nerve dysfunction, **coma, seizures**
CV: phlebitis
GI: nausea, vomiting, diarrhea, anorexia, stomatitis
GU: hematuria, bladder fibrosis, gonadal suppression, **nephrotoxicity, hemorrhagic cystitis**
Hematologic: anemia, **leukopenia, thrombocytopenia, bone marrow depression**
Metabolic: metabolic acidosis
Skin: alopecia
Other: infection, **secondary neoplasms**

Interactions

Drug-drug. *Anticoagulants, aspirin, nonsteroidal anti-inflammatory drugs:* increased risk of bleeding
Barbiturates, chloral hydrate, fosphenytoin, phenytoin: increased risk of toxicity
Corticosteroids: decreased ifosfamide effects
Cyclophosphamide: increased risk of cardiac tamponade
Myelosuppressants: increased hematologic toxicity
Drug-diagnostic tests. *Hepatic enzymes, uric acid:* increased levels
Platelets, white blood cells: decreased counts

Patient monitoring

- Monitor hematopoietic function tests (such as CBC with white cell differential) before therapy and weekly during therapy.
- Assess fluid intake and output. Ensure fluid intake of at least 2 L daily to prevent bladder toxicity.

🔊 Monitor urine output for hematuria and hemorrhagic cystitis. Administer mesna (protective drug), as indicated and prescribed.

Patient teaching

🔊 Tell patient to immediately report jaundice, unusual bleeding or bruising, bloody urine, pain on urination, fever, chills, sore throat, cough, difficulty breathing, unusual lumps or masses, mouth sores, or pain in flank, stomach, or joints.

- Instruct patient to maintain adequate hydration and nutrition. Advise him to drink 10 to 12 glasses of fluid each day.
- Inform patient that drug may cause hair loss.
- Advise both male and female patients to use reliable contraception during and immediately after therapy, because drug may cause severe birth defects.
- Urge patient to keep regular follow-up appointments for blood tests and monitoring of drug effects.
- As appropriate, review other significant and life-threatening adverse reactions and interactions, especially those related to the drugs and tests mentioned above.

imatinib mesylate

Gleevec

Pharmacologic class: Protein-tyrosine kinase inhibitor
Therapeutic class: Antineoplastic
Pregnancy risk category D

Action

Inhibits proliferation of Bcr-Abl tyrosine kinase, an abnormal chromosome protein found in most patients with chronic myeloid leukemia (CML). This inhibition suppresses tumor growth.

Availability

Tablets: 100 mg

Indications and dosages

➢ CML in chronic, accelerated, or blast-crisis phase (after interferon alpha therapy fails)
Adults: During chronic phase, 400 mg P.O. daily as a single dose; during accelerated phase or blast crisis, 600 mg P.O. daily as a single dose. May increase to 600 mg P.O. daily during chronic phase or to 800 mg P.O. daily (400 mg b.i.d.) during accelerated phase or blast crisis.
➢ Kit (CD117)-positive unresectable or metastatic malignant GI stromal tumors
Adults: 400 to 600 mg P.O. daily

Dosage adjustment

- Renal, hepatic, or hematologic impairment

Contraindications

- Hypersensitivity to drug or its components

Precautions

Use cautiously in:
- renal or hepatic impairment
- pregnant or breastfeeding patients
- children (safety and efficacy not established).

Administration

- Give with meal and large glass of water.

Route	Onset	Peak	Duration
P.O.	Unknown	2-4 hr	Unknown

Adverse reactions

CNS: headache, fatigue, asthenia, malaise, insomnia, headache, **cerebral hemorrhage**
GI: nausea, vomiting, diarrhea, constipation, anorexia, abdominal pain or cramps, dyspepsia, **GI hemorrhage**
Hematologic: anemia, **hemorrhage, neutropenia, thrombocytopenia**
Metabolic: hypokalemia, fluid retention
Musculoskeletal: myalgia, muscle cramps, musculoskeletal or joint pain
Respiratory: cough, dyspnea, pneumonia
Skin: rash, pruritus, night sweats, petechiae
Other: weight gain, edema, fever

Interactions

Drug-drug. *Cyclosporine, dihydropyridine calcium channel blockers, pimozide, some HMG-CoA reductase inhibitors, triazolobenzodiazepines:* increased blood levels of these drugs
CYP450-3A4 inducers (such as carbamazepine, dexamethasone, phenobarbital, phenytoin): increased metabolism and decreased blood level of imatinib
CYP450-3A4 inhibitors (such as clarithromycin, erythromycin, itraconazole, ketoconazole): decreased metabolism and increased blood level of imatinib
Warfarin: altered warfarin metabolism
Drug-diagnostic tests. *Alanine aminotransferase, alkaline phosphatase, aspartate aminotransferase, bilirubin, creatinine, hepatic enzymes:* increased values

Hemoglobin, neutrophils, platelets, potassium: decreased values
Drug-herbs. *St. John's wort:* decreased imatinib effects

Patient monitoring

- Monitor for GI distress. Provide small, frequent meals; consult dietitian if nausea and vomiting persist.

◀ Monitor CBC before therapy starts and regularly during therapy. Expect to adjust dosage if bone marrow depression occurs.

◀ Evaluate for signs and symptoms of bleeding, edema, and fluid retention.

- Measure daily weight and fluid intake and output.

Patient teaching

- Advise patient to take with a meal and a large glass of water.
- Instruct patient to avoid potential sources of infection, such as crowds and people with known infections.
- Tell patient drug may cause sudden weight gain and fluid retention. Instruct him to weigh himself daily.

◀ Advise patient to immediately report sudden weight gain, swelling, difficulty breathing, signs or symptoms of infection, unusual bleeding or bruising, or jaundice.

- Tell patient he'll undergo frequent blood testing to monitor drug effects.
- As appropriate, review all other significant and life-threatening adverse reactions and interactions, especially those related to the drugs, tests, and herbs mentioned above.

imipenem and cilastatin sodium

Primaxin

Pharmacologic class: Carbapenem
Therapeutic class: Anti-infective
Pregnancy risk category C

Action

Acts against many gram-positive and gram-negative organisms by binding to bacterial cell wall, causing cell death. Addition of cilastatin prevents renal inactivation of imipenem, resulting in increased urinary concentration. Imipenem resists actions of many enzymes that degrade most other penicillins and penicillin-like drugs.

Availability

Powder for I.M. injection: 500 mg imipenem/500 mg cilastatin, 750 mg imipenem/750 mg cilastatin
Powder for I.V. injection: 250 mg imipenem/250 mg cilastatin, 500 mg imipenem/500 mg cilastatin

Indications and dosages

➢ Lower respiratory tract infections, urinary tract infections, abdominal infections, gynecologic infections, skin infections, bone and joint infections, endocarditis, and polymicrobial infections

Adults: For mild infections, 250 to 500 mg I.V. q 6 hours; for moderate infections, 500 mg I.V. q 6 to 8 hours or 1 g I.V. q 8 hours; for serious infections, 500 mg I.V. q 6 hours to 1 g q 6 to 8 hours or 500 to 750 mg I.M. q 12 hours
Children: 15 to 25 mg/kg I.V. q 6 hours or 10 to 15 mg/kg I.M. q 6 hours
Infants ages 4 weeks to 3 months: 25 mg/kg I.V. q 6 hours

Infants ages 1 to 4 weeks: 25 mg/kg I.V. q 8 hours
Infants age 1 week and younger: 25 mg/kg I.V. q 12 hours

Dosage adjustment
• Renal impairment

Contraindications
• Hypersensitivity to drug, penicillins, or cephalosporins

Precautions
Use cautiously in:
• seizure disorders, renal impairment
• history of multiple hypersensitivity reactions
• elderly patients
• pregnant or breastfeeding patients.

Administration
• For I.V. use, reconstitute each 250- or 500-mg vial with 10 ml of diluent; shake well.
• For piggyback infusion, add 250- or 500-mg I.V. dose to 100 ml of diluent; shake solution until clear and drug has dissolved completely.
• Infuse doses of 500 mg or less over 20 to 30 minutes; infuse doses of 750 to 1,000 mg over 40 to 60 minutes.
• Slow infusion rate if patient experiences nausea, vomiting, dizziness or sweating.
• For I.M. use, inject into large muscle.

Route	Onset	Peak	Duration
I.V.	Rapid	End of infusion	6-8 hr
I.M.	Rapid	1-2 hr	12 hr

Adverse reactions
CNS: dizziness, drowsiness, **seizures**
CV: hypotension
GI: nausea, vomiting, diarrhea, **pseudomembranous colitis**
Hematologic: eosinophilia
Skin: rash, pruritus, diaphoresis, urticaria
Other: phlebitis at I.V. site, fever, superinfection, allergic reactions including **anaphylaxis**

Interactions
Drug-drug. *Aminoglycosides:* interference with imipenem effects
Cyclosporine, ganciclovir: increased risk of seizures
Probenecid: decreased renal excretion of imipenem
Drug-diagnostic tests. *Alanine aminotransferase, alkaline phosphatase, aspartate aminotransferase, bilirubin, blood urea nitrogen, creatinine, lactate dehydrogenase:* increased values
Direct Coombs' test: positive result
Hematocrit, hemoglobin: decreased

Patient monitoring
🔊 Stay alert for seizures in patients with brain lesions, head trauma, or other CNS disorders and in those receiving more than 2 g daily.
🔊 Monitor closely for severe diarrhea and hypersensitivity reaction.
• Assess tissue or fluid culture results obtained before and during therapy.
• Monitor for signs and symptoms of infection, such as fever and elevated white blood cell count. Also evaluate for bacterial and fungal superinfection.
• Monitor electrolyte levels, especially sodium.

Patient teaching
• Caution patient to report discomfort at I.V. site.
🔊 Instruct patient to report rash, hives, difficulty breathing, and signs or symptoms of superinfection (such as diarrhea, mouth sores, and vaginal itching or discharge).
• As appropriate, review all other significant and life-threatening adverse reactions and interactions, especially those related to the drugs and tests mentioned above.

imipramine hydrochloride
Apo-Imipramine✦, Impril✦, Novopramine✦, Tipramine, Tofranil

imipramine pamoate
Tofranil-PM

Pharmacologic class: Dibenzazepine derivative
Therapeutic class: Tricyclic antidepressant
Pregnancy risk category C

Action
Unknown. May block reuptake of norepinephrine and serotonin at neuronal membrane, potentiating their effects.

Availability
Capsules: 75 mg, 100 mg, 125 mg, 150 mg (pamoate)
Tablets: 10 mg, 25 mg, 50 mg (hydrochloride)

Indications and dosages
➢ Endogenous depression
Adults: 75 to 100 mg P.O. daily in divided doses. Don't exceed 200 mg/day for outpatients or 300 mg/day for inpatients.
Elderly patients, adolescents: 30 to 40 mg P.O. daily in divided doses, up to 100 mg/day
➢ Functional enuresis
Children: 25 mg P.O. daily 1 hour before bedtime. If necessary, increase by 25 mg/day at weekly intervals, up to 75 mg P.O. daily in children ages 12 and older or up to 50 mg P.O. daily in children younger than age 12.
➢ Attention deficit hyperactivity disorder
Children ages 6 and older: 2 to 5 mg/kg P.O. daily in two or three divided doses

Off-label uses
- Diabetic neuropathy

Contraindications
- Hypersensitivity to drug or bisulfites
- Untreated angle-closure glaucoma
- MAO inhibitor use within past 14 days

Precautions
Use cautiously in:
- cardiovascular disease, prostatic enlargement, seizures, urinary retention
- elderly patients
- pregnant or breastfeeding patients.

Administration
- Don't give concurrently with MAO inhibitors. Interaction may lead to hypotension, tachycardia, and potentially fatal reactions.
- Give with food or milk if GI upset occurs.

Route	Onset	Peak	Duration
P.O.	Unknown	30 min-2 hr	2-6 wk

Adverse reactions
CNS: fatigue, sedation, agitation, confusion, hallucinations, drowsiness, dizziness, syncope, extrapyramidal effects, poor concentration, **cerebrovascular accident, seizures, suicidal behavior or ideation** (especially in child or adolescent)
CV: hypotension, ECG changes, hypertension, vasculitis, palpitations, tachycardia, **arrhythmias, myocardial infarction, heart block**
EENT: blurred vision, increased intraocular pressure (IOP), lacrimation, tinnitus, nasal congestion
GI: nausea, constipation, dry mouth, **paralytic ileus**
GU: urinary retention, urinary tract dilation, gynecomastia, menstrual irregularities, galactorrhea, testicular swelling, libido changes, erectile dysfunction

Hematologic: eosinophilia, purpura, **bone marrow suppression, agranulocytosis, thrombocytopenia, leukopenia**
Hepatic: hepatitis
Metabolic: hyperthermia, hyperglycemia, **hypoglycemia**
Skin: flushing, diaphoresis, photosensitivity, rash, urticaria, pruritus, petechiae, alopecia
Other: increased appetite, weight gain or loss, edema, drug fever, chills, hypersensitivity reactions

Interactions

Drug-drug. *Adrenergics:* increased hypertensive effect
Carbamazepine, class IC antiarrhythmics, other antidepressants, phenothiazines: additive effects of imipramine
CNS depressants: additive CNS depression
Clonidine: decreased clonidine effects
CYP450-2D6 inhibitors (such as amiodarone, cimetidine, quinidine, ritonavir): increased imipramine effects
Guanethidine: prevention of therapeutic response to imipramine
Levodopa: delayed or decreased levodopa absorption, hypertension
MAO inhibitors: hypotension, tachycardia, potentially fatal reactions
Selective serotonin reuptake inhibitors: increased imipramine blood level
Sparfloxacin: increased risk of cardiovascular reactions
Drug-diagnostic tests. *Alkaline phosphatase, bilirubin:* elevated levels
Glucose: increased or decreased level
Liver function tests: altered values
Drug-herbs. *Angel's trumpet, jimsonweed, scopolia:* increased anticholinergic effects
Chamomile, hops, kava, skullcap, valerian: increased CNS depression
Evening primrose oil: additive or synergistic effects
S-adenosylmethionine (SAM-e), St. John's wort: serotonin syndrome
Drug-behaviors. *Alcohol use:* increased CNS depression
Smoking: increased metabolism and altered effects of imipramine
Sun exposure: increased risk of photosensitivity

Patient monitoring

🔈 Closely monitor patient's mood and assess his risk for self-harm. Limit drug access if he may be suicidal.
• Assess for urinary retention and increased IOP in patients with history of urinary retention or angle-closure glaucoma.
🔈 Monitor blood pressure before and during therapy and before dosage increases.
• Watch for arrhythmias in patients with history of cardiac disease.
• During withdrawal, monitor for adverse effects, such as headache, malaise, nausea, vomiting, and sleep disturbances.
• Assess for signs and symptoms of infection. Monitor CBC with white cell differential.

Patient teaching

🔈 Teach patient or caregiver to recognize and immediately report signs of suicidal intent or expressions of suicidal ideation (especially in child or adolescent).
• Instruct patient to eat small, frequent meals to minimize GI upset.
• Inform patient that drug may cause changes in sexual function, such as erectile dysfunction and decreased libido.
🔈 Tell patient to immediately report seizure, chest pain, abdominal pain or bloating, easy bruising or bleeding, unusual tiredness, or yellowing of skin or eyes.
• Advise patient to report fever, chills, sore throat, dry mouth, excessive sedation, difficulty urinating, or palpitations.

• Caution patient to avoid driving and other hazardous activities until he knows how drug affects concentration and alertness.
• As appropriate, review all other significant and life-threatening adverse reactions and interactions, especially those related to the drugs, tests, herbs, and behaviors mentioned above.

immune globulin for I.M. use (IGIM)

BayGam

immune globulin for I.V. use, human (IGIV)

Carimune, Carimune NF, Gamimune N 5% S/D, Gamimune N 10% S/D, Gammagard S/D, Gammagard S/D 0.5 g, Gammar-P IV, Iveegam EN, Panglobulin, Panglobulin NF, Polygam S/D, Sandoglobulin, Venoglobulin-I, Venoglobulin-S

Pharmacologic class: Immune serum
Therapeutic class: Antibody-production stimulator
Pregnancy risk category C

Action

Improves immunity by binding to and neutralizing pathogens, thereby increasing antibodies against bacterial, viral, parasitic, and mycoplasmic antigens. Acts through antimicrobial and antitoxin neutralization.

Availability

Injection: 2- and 10-ml vials (IGIM)
Powder for injection: 1-, 2.5-, 3-, 5-, 6-, 10-, and 12-g vials (IGIV)
Solution (5%): 10-, 50-, 100-, 200-, and 250-ml vials (IGIV)
Solution (10%): 10-, 25-, 50-, 100-, and 200-ml vials (IGIV)

Indications and dosages

➢ To prevent hepatitis A
Adults traveling to areas where hepatitis A is common: 0.02 ml/kg I.M. if staying less than 3 months; 0.06 ml/kg repeated q 4 to 6 months if staying 3 months or longer
Adults with household or institutional contacts: 0.02 ml/kg I.M.
➢ To prevent or reduce severity of measles in susceptible persons
Adults and children: 0.2 ml/kg to 0.25 ml/kg I.M. within 6 days of exposure to measles
➢ Exposure to measles in immunocompromised children
Children: 0.5 ml/kg I.M. as soon as possible after exposure
➢ Varicella in immunocompromised patients
Adults: 0.6 to 1.2 ml/kg I.M. as soon as possible if varicella-zoster immune globulin is unavailable
➢ To reduce risk of infection and fetal damage in females exposed to rubella during early pregnancy
Adults: 0.55 ml/kg I.M.
➢ Immunoglobulin deficiency
Adults: Initially, 1.3 ml/kg I.M., followed in 3 to 4 weeks by 0.66 ml/kg, up to 100 mg/kg q 3 to 4 weeks
➢ Immunodeficiency
Gamimune N—
Adults and children: 100 to 200 mg/kg I.V. or 2 to 4 ml/kg (10%) I.V. monthly
Gammagard S/D—
Adults and children: 200 to 400 mg/kg I.V., then monthly in doses based on response
Gammar-P IV—
Adults: 200 to 400 mg/kg I.V. q 3 to 4 weeks
Children and adolescents: 200 mg/kg I.V. q 3 to 4 weeks
Iveegam EN—
Adults and children: 200 mg/kg I.V. monthly; may increase up to 800 mg/kg/month based on response

Panglobulin—
Adults and children: 200 mg/kg I.V. monthly, increased to 300 mg/kg/month. In some patients, infusion frequency may be increased.
Panglobulin NF/Carimune NF—
Adults and children: 0.2 g/kg I.V. monthly. If response inadequate, dosage may be increased to 0.3 g/kg or infusion frequency may be increased.
Polygam S/D—
Adults and children: 100 to 400 mg/kg I.V. monthly
Sandoglobulin—
Adults and children: 100 to 400 mg/kg I.V. monthly. In patients with previously untreated agammaglobulinemia or hypogammaglobulinemia, first infusion may be increased to 300 mg/kg or infusion frequency may be increased.
Venoglobulin—
Adults and children: 200 mg/kg I.V. monthly, increased up to 400 mg/kg/month. In some patients, infusion frequency may be increased.

➤ Idiopathic thrombocytopenic purpura
Gamimune N—
Adults and children: 400 mg/kg I.V. for 5 consecutive days, or 1,000 mg/kg/day for 1 day or for 2 consecutive days
Gammagard S/D—
Adults and children: 1,000 mg/kg I.V. Up to three doses may be given on alternating days, dependent on platelet count.
Panglobulin—
Adults and children: Initially, 0.4 g/kg I.V. for 2 to 5 consecutive days
Polygam S/D—
Adults and children: 1 g/kg I.V. Depending on response, additional doses may be given.
Venoglobulin-S—
Adults and children: 2,000 mg/kg I.V. over 5 days or less for induction therapy; then 1,000 mg/kg p.r.n. to maintain platelet count of 30,000/mm³ in children or 20,000/mm³ in adults or to prevent bleeding episodes between infusions

➤ Kawasaki disease
Gammagard S/D—
Adults and adolescents: 1 g/kg I.V. as a single dose; alternatively, 400 mg/kg/day for 4 consecutive days with aspirin
Iveegam EN—
Adults and children: 400 mg/kg/day I.V. with aspirin
Polygam S/D—
Adults and children: 1 g/kg I.V. as a single dose, or 400 mg/kg I.V. for 4 consecutive days starting within 7 days of fever onset. Give with aspirin, as prescribed.
Sandoglobulin—
Adults and children: 400 mg/kg I.V. for 2 to 5 consecutive days. If platelet count falls below 30,000/mm³ or significant bleeding occurs, may give 0.4 g/kg as a single infusion, increased to 0.8 or 1 g/kg as a single infusion, depending on response.
Venoglobulin S—
Adults and children: 2 g/kg I.V. infused over 10 to 12 hours with aspirin

➤ To prevent bacterial infection in patients with hypogammaglobulinemia or recurrent bacterial infection associated with B-cell chronic lymphocytic leukemia
Adults and adolescents: 400 mg/kg I.V. (Gammagard S/D or Polygam S/D) q 3 to 4 weeks

➤ To reduce risk of graft-versus-host disease, interstitial pneumonia, septicemia, and other infections during first 100 days after bone marrow transplantation
Adults ages 20 and older: 500 mg/kg I.V. (Gamimune N) 7 days before and 2 days before transplantation, then weekly through 90th day after transplantation

➤ To prevent bacterial infection in children with human immunodeficiency virus
Children: 400 mg/kg I.V. (Gamimune N) q 28 days

Off-label uses

• Chronic inflammatory demyelinating polyneuropathy
• Guillain-Barré syndrome

Contraindications

• Hypersensitivity to drug or its components
• Selective immunoglobulin A deficiency

Precautions

Use cautiously in:
• bleeding disorders, renal impairment
• pregnant patients.

Administration

Before giving, determine if patient has risk factors for acute renal failure (such as use of nephrotoxic drugs; history of diabetes mellitus, renal insufficiency, sepsis, volume depletion, or paraproteinemia; age 65 or older).
• For I.V. use, decrease infusion rate by 50% to 25% for patients at risk for renal dysfunction.
Give IGIM by I.M. route only; give IGIV by I.V. route only.
• If sterile laminar airflow conditions aren't available for drug reconstitution, administer immediately; discard unused portion.
• Don't shake vigorously, because foaming may occur. Know that cold drug or diluent may take up to 20 minutes to dissolve.

Route	Onset	Peak	Duration
I.V.	Unknown	Unknown	21-28 days
I.M.	Unknown	2 days	Unknown

Adverse reactions

CNS: headache, malaise
CV: chest pain, tachycardia, **thromboembolism**
GI: nausea, vomiting, abdominal pain
Musculoskeletal: joint pain, back pain, myalgia
Respiratory: dyspnea
Skin: pruritus
Other: chills, lymphadenopathy, pain at injection site, **anaphylaxis**

Interactions

Drug-drug. *Live-virus vaccines:* decreased antibody response to vaccine

Patient monitoring

Watch for acute inflammatory reaction in patients receiving drug for first time (usually appears within 30 to 60 minutes after infusion begins), in those whose last treatment was more than 8 weeks earlier, and when initial infusion rate exceeds 1 ml/minute.
• Monitor vital signs continuously during I.V. infusion. Stay alert for hypotension.
• Assess fluid volume status and blood urea nitrogen and creatinine levels.
• After infusion ends, monitor patient closely for nausea, vomiting, drowsiness, and severe headache.

Patient teaching

• Instruct patient to report symptoms occurring during or after therapy.
• Advise patient to avoid live-virus vaccines for 3 months after therapy; drug may delay or inhibit body's response to vaccine.
• As appropriate, review all significant and life-threatening adverse reactions and interactions, especially those related to the drugs mentioned above.

inamrinone lactate

Amrinone

Pharmacologic class: Bipyridine derivative
Therapeutic class: Inotropic, vasodilator
Pregnancy risk category C

Action

Inhibits cyclic adenosine monophosphate (cAMP) phosphodiesterase activity in myocardium, increasing cellular levels of cAMP (which regulates intracellular and extracellular calcium levels). These actions increase myocardial contraction force. Also relaxes and dilates vascular smooth muscle, decreasing preload and afterload.

Availability

Injection: 5 mg/ml in 20-ml ampules

Indications and dosages

➢ Short-term management of heart failure

Adults: Initially, 0.75 mg/kg I.V. bolus over 2 to 3 minutes; may give additional bolus of 0.75 mg/kg over 30 minutes. Then begin maintenance infusion of 5 to 10 mcg/kg/minute. Maximum daily dosage is 10 mg/kg.

Off-label uses

- Open-heart surgery

Contraindications

- Hypersensitivity to drug or bisulfites

Precautions

Use cautiously in:

- renal or hepatic disease, atrial fibrillation or flutter, severe aortic or pulmonic valvular disease, acute phase of myocardial infarction
- elderly patients
- pregnant or breastfeeding patients
- children.

Administration

- Administer either undiluted or diluted in normal or half-normal saline solution to yield a concentration of 1 to 3 mg/ml, as prescribed. Don't mix with solutions containing dextrose.
- Give I.V. bolus over 2 to 3 minutes, followed by maintenance infusion using infusion pump or microdrip (60 gtt/ml) at recommended dosage.
- Protect drug from light.

Route	Onset	Peak	Duration
I.V.	2-5 min	10 min	30-120 min

Adverse reactions

CV: hypotension, **arrhythmias**
GI: nausea, vomiting
Hematologic: thrombocytopenia
Hepatic: hepatotoxicity
Other: hypersensitivity reaction

Interactions

Drug-drug. *Cardiac glycosides:* increased inotropic effects
Disopyramide: excessive hypotension
Drug-herbs. *Aloe, buckthorn bark, cascara sagrada, ephedra (ma huang), senna leaf:* increased drug action

Patient monitoring

◀ Monitor vital signs frequently. Expect to slow or stop infusion if significant hypotension occurs.
- Monitor hemodynamic indicators (including cardiac output, cardiac index, central venous pressure, and pulmonary artery wedge pressure) to assess drug efficacy.
- Assess daily weight and fluid intake and output.

◀ Watch closely for ventricular arrhythmias, especially if patient has atrial flutter or atrial fibrillation.
- Assess for signs and symptoms of thrombocytopenia, such as bleeding or bruising.
- Monitor platelet count and electrolyte levels before and during therapy.

Patient teaching

- Instruct patient to report dizziness or light-headedness.
- As appropriate, review all other significant and life-threatening adverse reactions and interactions, especially those related to the drugs and herbs mentioned above.

indapamide

Lozide✱, Lozol

Pharmacologic class: Thiazide-like diuretic

Therapeutic class: Diuretic, antihypertensive

Pregnancy risk category B

Action

Increases sodium and water excretion by inhibiting sodium reabsorption in distal tubule; enhances excretion of sodium, chloride, potassium, and water. May cause arteriolar vasodilation.

Availability

Tablets: 1.25 mg, 2.5 mg

Indications and dosages

➢ Edema caused by heart failure

Adults: 2.5 mg P.O. daily in morning. After 1 week, may increase to 5 mg/day.

➢ Mild to moderate hypertension

Adults: 1.25 mg P.O. daily in morning. May increase q 4 weeks, up to 5 mg/day.

Contraindications

- Hypersensitivity to drug, other thiazide-like drugs, or tartrazine
- Anuria

Precautions

Use cautiously in:

- renal or severe hepatic impairment, ascites, fluid or electrolyte imbalances, gout, systemic lupus erythematosus, impaired glucose tolerance, hyperparathyroidism, bipolar disorder
- pregnant or breastfeeding patients.

Administration

- Administer with food or milk to reduce GI upset.
- Give early in day to avoid nocturia.

Route	Onset	Peak	Duration
P.O. (single dose)	1-2 hr	2 hr	36 hr

Adverse reactions

CNS: dizziness, light-headedness, headache, restlessness, insomnia, lethargy, fatigue, drowsiness, asthenia, depression, anxiety, nervousness, paresthesia, irritability, agitation

CV: orthostatic hypotension, palpitations, premature ventricular contractions, **arrhythmias**

EENT: blurred vision, rhinorrhea

GI: nausea, vomiting, diarrhea, constipation, bloating, epigastric distress, gastric irritation, abdominal pain or cramps, dry mouth, anorexia

GU: nocturia, polyuria, glycosuria, erectile dysfunction

Metabolic: dehydration, gout, hyperglycemia, hypokalemia, hypocalcemia, hypomagnesemia, hyponatremia, hypovolemia, hypophosphatemia, hyperuricemia, **hypochloremic alkalosis**

Musculoskeletal: muscle cramps and spasms

Skin: flushing, rash, urticaria, pruritus, photosensitivity, cutaneous vasculitis, **necrotizing vasculitis**

Other: weight loss

Interactions

Drug-drug. *Amphotericin B, corticosteroids:* additive hypokalemia

Antihypertensives, nitrates: additive hypotension

Cholestyramine, colestipol: decreased indapamide absorption

Lithium: decreased lithium excretion, increased risk of lithium toxicity

Sulfonylureas: decreased hypoglycemic efficacy

Drug-diagnostic tests. *Bilirubin, blood and urine glucose (in diabetic patients), blood urea nitrogen (BUN), calcium, creatinine, uric acid:* increased values

Cholesterol, low-density lipoproteins, magnesium, potassium, protein-bound

iodine, sodium, triglycerides, urinary calcium: decreased values
Drug-herbs. *Ginkgo:* decreased antihypertensive effect
Licorice, stimulant laxative herbs (aloe, cascara sagrada, senna): increased risk of hypokalemia
Drug-behaviors. *Acute alcohol ingestion:* additive hypotension
Sun exposure: increased risk of photosensitivity

Patient monitoring

- Assess for signs and symptoms of hypokalemia, including ventricular arrhythmias, muscle weakness, and cramping.
- Monitor BUN, creatinine, and electrolyte levels.
- Assess daily weight and fluid intake and output.
- Monitor blood pressure response to drug.
- Watch for signs and symptoms of orthostatic hypotension.

Patient teaching

- Advise patient to consume potassium-rich foods, such as oranges, bananas, potatoes, and spinach.
- Instruct patient to move slowly when sitting up or standing, to avoid dizziness from sudden blood pressure decrease.
- Tell patient to weigh himself daily on same scale at same time of day while wearing similar clothing. Instruct him to report gain of more than 2 lb (0.9 kg) in 1 day or 5 lb (2.2 kg) in 1 week.
- Caution patient to avoid driving and other hazardous activities until he knows how drug affects concentration and alertness.
- As appropriate, review all other significant and life-threatening adverse reactions and interactions, especially those related to the drugs, tests, herbs, and behaviors mentioned above.

indinavir sulfate

Crixivan

Pharmacologic class: Protease inhibitor
Therapeutic class: Antiretroviral
Pregnancy risk category C

Action

Inhibits replication, function, and maturation of human immunodeficiency virus (HIV) protease, an enzyme essential to formation of infectious virus. As a result, further spread of virus is prevented.

Availability

Capsules: 100 mg, 200 mg, 333 mg, 400 mg

Indications and dosages

➢ HIV infection
Adults: 800 mg P.O. q 8 hours

Dosage adjustment

- Mild to moderate hepatic insufficiency secondary to cirrhosis

Contraindications

- Hypersensitivity to drug or its components
- Concurrent use of cisapride, ergot derivatives, midazolam, pimozide, or triazolam

Precautions

Use cautiously in:
- renal or severe hepatic impairment, history of renal calculi
- pregnant or breastfeeding patients
- children.

Administration

- Know that drug is usually given with other antiretrovirals.

• Give with full glass of water on empty stomach 1 hour before or 2 hours after meals.
• If GI upset occurs, give with a light meal.
Clinical alert: Don't give concurrently with cisapride (not available in U.S.), ergot derivatives, midazolam, pimozide, or triazolam.

Route	Onset	Peak	Duration
P.O.	Rapid	0.8 hr	8 hr

Adverse reactions

CNS: depression, dizziness, headache, drowsiness, malaise, asthenia
CV: angina, **myocardial infarction**
EENT: oral paresthesia
GI: nausea, vomiting, diarrhea, abdominal pain or distention, dyspepsia, acid regurgitation, **pancreatitis**
GU: dysuria, crystalluria, nephrolithiasis or urolithiasis leading to **renal insufficiency or failure, interstitial nephritis**
Hematologic: anemia, **acute hemolytic anemia, increased spontaneous bleeding** (in hemophiliacs)
Hepatic: jaundice, **hepatic dysfunction, hepatic failure**
Metabolic: new onset or exacerbation of diabetes mellitus, hyperglycemia
Musculoskeletal: joint or back pain
Respiratory: cough, dyspnea
Skin: urticaria, rash, pruritus
Other: abnormal taste, increased or decreased appetite, body fat redistribution or accumulation, fever, **anaphylactoid reactions**

Interactions

Drug-drug. *Azole antifungals, delavirdine, interleukins:* elevated indinavir blood level, greater risk of toxicity
Cisapride, ergot derivatives, midazolam, pimozide, triazolam: CYP3A4 inhibition by indinavir, leading to increased blood levels of these drugs and dangerous reactions
Didanosine, efavirenz, rifamycins: decreased indinavir effects
Drug-diagnostic tests. *Alanine aminotransferase, amylase, aspartate aminotransferase, bilirubin, cholesterol, glucose, triglycerides:* increased values
Hemoglobin, neutrophils, platelets: decreased values
Drug-food. *Any food:* decreased indinavir absorption
Drug-herbs. *St. John's wort:* decreased indinavir blood level

Patient monitoring

• Assess fluid intake and output to ensure adequate hydration and help prevent nephrolithiasis or urolithiasis.
• Monitor for adverse GI and CNS effects.
• Evaluate liver function test results. Assess for hyperbilirubinemia.
• Monitor cholesterol, glucose, and CBC with white cell differential.

Patient teaching

• Tell patient to take 1 hour before or 2 hours after meals with a full glass of water.
• If GI upset occurs, advise patient to take with a light meal.
Clinical alert: Instruct patient to report severe nausea or diarrhea, fever, chills, flank pain, urine or stool color changes, yellowing of skin or eyes, or personality changes.
• Tell patient that drug doesn't cure HIV infection and that its long-term effects are largely unknown.
• As appropriate, review all other significant and life-threatening adverse reactions and interactions, especially those related to the drugs, tests, foods, and herbs mentioned above.

indomethacin

Apo-Indomethacin✤, Indameth✤, Indocid✤, Indocin, Indocin SR, Indotec✤, Novo-Methacin✤, Nu-Indo✤, Rhodacine✤

Pharmacologic class: Nonsteroidal anti-inflammatory drug (NSAID)
Therapeutic class: Anti-inflammatory, analgesic, antipyretic
Pregnancy risk category B (third trimester: ***D***)

Action

Unknown. Thought to inhibit cyclooxygenase, an enzyme needed for prostaglandin synthesis.

Availability

Capsules: 25 mg, 50 mg
Capsules (sustained-release): 75 mg
Oral suspension: 25 mg/5 ml

Indications and dosages

➢ Rheumatoid arthritis; osteoarthritis; ankylosing spondylitis
Adults: 25 to 50 mg P.O. two or three times daily, not to exceed 200 mg daily; or one 75-mg sustained-release capsule P.O. once or twice daily
➢ Acute gouty arthritis
Adults: 50 mg P.O. t.i.d. until pain is tolerable; then reduce dosage rapidly and, finally, discontinue drug. Don't give sustained-release form.
➢ Acute bursitis or tendinitis of shoulder
Adults: 75 to 150 mg P.O. daily in three or four divided doses. Discontinue once inflammation is controlled.

Off-label uses

- Bartter's syndrome
- Pericarditis

Contraindications

- Hypersensitivity to drug, its components, or other NSAIDs
- Active GI bleeding
- Concurrent diflunisal use

Precautions

Use cautiously in:
- severe cardiovascular, renal, or hepatic disease
- history of ulcer disease
- elderly patients
- pregnant or breastfeeding patients
- children ages 14 and younger (efficacy not established).

Administration

- Give with food, full glass of water, or antacids to reduce GI upset.
- Don't open or crush capsules.
- For arthritis, give up to 100 mg of daily dose at bedtime as needed to reduce nighttime pain and morning stiffness.
- Don't give sustained-release form to patients with gouty arthritis.

Route	Onset	Peak	Duration
P.O. (analgesic)	30 min	0.5-2 hr	4-6 hr
P.O. (sustained, analgesic)	30 min	Unknown	4-6 hr
P.O. (regular or sustained, anti-inflam.)	Up to 7 days	1-2 wk	Unknown

Adverse reactions

CNS: headache, dizziness, drowsiness, fatigue, vertigo, depression, parkinsonism, **seizures**
EENT: tinnitus
GI: nausea, vomiting, diarrhea, constipation, abdominal pain or cramps, dyspepsia, ulcers, **GI bleeding**
Other: allergic reactions including **anaphylaxis**

Interactions

Drug-drug. *Antihypertensives, diuretics:* decreased efficacy of these drugs
Corticosteroids, other NSAIDs: additive adverse GI reactions
Cyclosporine: increased risk of nephrotoxicity
Diflunisal: potentially fatal GI hemorrhage
Lithium, methotrexate, zidovudine: increased risk of toxicity from these drugs
Probenecid: increased risk of indomethacin toxicity
Drug-diagnostic tests. *Dexamethasone suppression test:* false-negative result
Drug-herbs. *Anise, arnica, chamomile, clove, dong quai, feverfew, garlic, ginger, ginkgo, ginseng:* increased bleeding risk

Patient monitoring

- Assess for dizziness, drowsiness, headache, fatigue, and exacerbation of depression, epilepsy, or parkinsonism.
- Monitor for drug efficacy, indicated by improved joint mobility, pain relief, and decreased inflammation.
- Monitor urine output for marked reduction.
- Watch for signs and symptoms of GI bleeding and ulcers.

Patient teaching

- Tell patient to take with food, full glass of water, or antacid to reduce GI upset.
- Advise patient not to open or crush capsules.
- Inform breastfeeding patient that indomethacin enters breast milk and may cause seizures in infant. Advise her to use a different infant feeding method during therapy.
- Caution patient to avoid driving and other hazardous activities until he knows how drug affects concentration, balance, and alertness.
- As appropriate, review all other significant and life-threatening adverse reactions and interactions, especially those related to the drugs, tests, and herbs mentioned above.

infliximab

Remicade

Pharmacologic class: Monoclonal antibody
Therapeutic class: Antirheumatic, GI anti-inflammatory
Pregnancy risk category C

Action

Neutralizes and prevents activity of tumor necrosis factor-alpha (TNF-alpha) by binding to soluble and transmembrane forms of TNF and inhibiting its receptors, resulting in anti-inflammatory and antiproliferative activity. Reduces rate of joint destruction in rheumatoid arthritis and eases symptoms of Crohn's disease.

Availability

Powder for injection: 100 mg/vial

Indications and dosages

➢ Rheumatoid arthritis (given with methotrexate)
Adults: Initially, 3 mg/kg I.V., followed by 3 mg/kg 2 and 6 weeks after initial dose, then q 8 weeks. In partial responders, dosage may be adjusted up to 10 mg/kg or treatment may be repeated as often as q 4 weeks.
➢ Crohn's disease
Adults: 5 mg/kg I.V. as a single infusion, starting as induction regimen at 0, 2, and 6 weeks, then a maintenance regimen of 5 mg/kg q 8 weeks. For patients who respond initially but then stop responding, dosage of 10 mg/kg may be warranted.

Off-label uses

- Complicated ankylosing spondylitis
- Sarcoidosis

Contraindications

- Hypersensitivity to drug, murine proteins, or other drug components
- Heart failure (NYHA class III or IV)

Precautions

Use cautiously in:

- history of tuberculosis (TB), active infection, or exposure to TB
- elderly patients
- pregnant or breastfeeding patients
- children (safety not established).

Administration

- Know that latent TB should be treated before infliximab therapy begins.
- To reconstitute, use 21G or smaller needle to add 10 ml of sterile water to each vial. To mix, swirl (don't shake). Solution may foam and appear clear or light yellow.
- Withdraw volume equal to amount of reconstituted drug from 250-ml polypropylene or polyolefin infusion bag or glass bottle of normal saline solution. Slowly add reconstituted drug to infusion bag or bottle, and gently mix. Use within 3 hours.
- Know that concentration of infusion should be 0.4 mg/ml to 4 mg/ml.
- Give I.V. infusion over at least 2 hours. Use polyethylene-lined infusion set equipped with in-line filter, with pore size of 1.2 microns or less.
- Discard unused portions of infusion solution.
- Don't give to patient with active infection.
- Be aware that patient who doesn't respond by week 14 isn't likely to respond, and therapy should cease.

Route	Onset	Peak	Duration
I.V.	1-2 wk	Unknown	12-48 wk

Adverse reactions

CNS: fatigue, headache, anxiety, depression, dizziness, insomnia
CV: chest pain, hypertension, hypotension, tachycardia, peripheral edema, **worsening of heart failure**
EENT: conjunctivitis, rhinitis, sinusitis, laryngitis, pharyngitis
GI: nausea, vomiting, diarrhea, constipation, abdominal pain, dyspepsia, flatulence, ulcerative stomatitis, **intestinal obstruction**
GU: dysuria, urinary frequency, urinary tract infection
Hematologic: hematoma, **pancytopenia**
Musculoskeletal: arthritis, joint pain, back pain, myalgia, involuntary muscle contractions
Respiratory: upper respiratory tract infection, bronchitis, cough, dyspnea
Skin: acne, diaphoresis, dry skin, bruising, eczema, erythema, flushing, pruritus, urticaria, rash, alopecia
Other: oral pain, tooth pain, moniliasis, chills, hot flashes, flulike symptoms, herpes simplex, herpes zoster, lupuslike syndrome, infections, hypersensitivity reaction, **anaphylaxis**

Interactions

Drug-drug. *Vaccines:* decreased antibody response to vaccine
Drug-diagnostic tests. *Antinuclear antibodies:* positive titer
Hepatic enzymes: increased values
Hemoglobin: decreased value

Patient monitoring

🔊 Stay alert for signs and symptoms of hypersensitivity reaction, including fever, chills, itching, rash, chest pain, dyspnea, facial flushing, and headache.
🔊 Watch for evidence of infection, especially in patients who have chronic infections or are receiving immunosuppressants. Drug increases risk of life-threatening opportunistic infections and TB.
- Monitor platelets and CBC with white cell differential.

🔊 Assess for heart failure in patients with history of cardiac disease.

Patient teaching

Clinical alert: Instruct patient to report signs or symptoms of hypersensitivity reaction, such as fever, chills, itching, rash, chest pain, dyspnea, and facial flushing (may occur up to 12 days after therapy).
Clinical alert: Tell patient to report infection symptoms, such as fever, burning on urination, cough, or sore throat.
- Advise patient to avoid potential infection sources, such as crowds and people with known infections.
- As appropriate, review all other significant and life-threatening adverse reactions and interactions, especially those related to the drugs and tests mentioned above.

insulin, regular (insulin injection)

Humulin R, Humulin-R Regular U-500 (concentrate), Iletin II Regular, Insulin-Toronto ♣, Novolin ge Toronto ♣, Novolin R, Novolin R PenFill, Velosulin BR

insulin (lispro)

Humalog, Humalog Pen

insulin glulisine, recombinant

Apidra

insulin lispro protamine, human

Humalog Mix 50/50, Humalog Mix 75/25 Z

insulin zinc suspension (lente insulin)

Humulin L, Lente Iletin II, Novolin ge Lente ♣

insulin zinc suspension, extended (ultralente insulin)

Humulin U, Novolin ge Ultralente, Novolin U, Ultralente U

isophane insulin suspension (NPH insulin)

Humulin N, Novolin N, NPH-N, NPH Iletin II

isophane insulin suspension (NPH) and insulin injection (regular)

Humulin 50/50 (50% isophane insulin and 50% insulin injection), Humulin 70/30 (70% isophane insulin and 30% insulin injection), Humulin 70/30 PenFill, Novolin 70/30, Novolin 70/30 PenFill

Pharmacologic class: Pancreatic hormone
Therapeutic class: Hypoglycemic
Pregnancy risk category B

Action

Promotes glucose transport, which stimulates carbohydrate metabolism in skeletal and cardiac muscle and adipose tissue. Also promotes phosphorylation of glucose in liver, where it's converted to glycogen. Directly affects fat and protein metabolism, stimulates protein synthesis, inhibits release of free fatty acids, and indirectly decreases phosphate and potassium.

Availability

Glulisine, recombinant: 100 units/ml in 10-ml vials
Isophane suspension, injection (regular): 70 units NPH and 30 units regular insulin/ml (100 units/ml total), 50 units NPH and 50 units regular insulin/ml (100 units/ml total)

Isophane suspension (NPH insulin): 100 units/ml
Lispro: 100 units/ml in 10-ml vials and 1.5-ml cartridges
Regular insulin injection: 100 units/ml
Regular U-500 (concentrated), insulin human injection: 500 units/ml
Zinc suspension, extended (ultralente): 100 units/ml
Zinc suspension (lente insulin): 100 units/ml

Indications and dosages

➢ Type 1 (insulin-dependent) diabetes mellitus; type 2 (non-insulin-dependent) diabetes mellitus unresponsive to diet and oral hypoglycemics
Adults and children: In newly diagnosed diabetes, total of 0.5 to 1 unit/kg/day subcutaneously as part of multidose regimen of short- and long-acting insulin. Dosage individualized based on patient's glucose level, adjusted to premeal and bedtime glucose levels. Reserve concentrated insulin (500 units/ml) for patients requiring more than 200 units/day.
➢ Diabetic ketoacidosis
Adults and children: Loading dose of 0.15 units/kg (nonconcentrated regular insulin) I.V. bolus, followed by continuous infusion of 0.1 unit/kg/hour until glucose level drops. Then administer subcutaneously, adjusting dosage according to glucose level.

Contraindications

- Hypersensitivity to drug or its components
- Hypoglycemia

Precautions

Use cautiously in:
- hepatic or renal impairment, hypothyroidism, hyperthyroidism
- elderly patients
- pregnant or breastfeeding patients
- children.

Administration

Be aware that insulin is a high-alert drug whether given subcutaneously or I.V.
Don't give insulin I.V. (except nonconcentrated regular insulin), because anaphylactic reaction may occur.
- When mixing two types of insulin, draw up regular insulin into syringe first.
- For I.V. infusion, mix regular insulin only with normal or half-normal saline solution, as prescribed, to yield a concentration of 1 unit/ml. Give every 50 units I.V. over at least 1 minute.
- Rotate subcutaneous injection sites to prevent lipodystrophy.
- Administer mixtures of regular and NPH or regular and lente insulins within 5 to 15 minutes of mixing.

Route	Onset	Peak	Duration
I.V. (regular)	10-30 min	15-30 min	Unknown
Subcut. (glulisine)	Rapid	Unknown	Short
Subcut. (lente)	1-2.5 hr	7-15 hr	24 hr
Subcut. (lispro)	15 min	30-90 min	6-8 hr
Subcut. (lispro/ protamine mix; regular U-500 conc.)	Unknown	Unknown	Unknown
Subcut. (NPH)	1-1.5 hr	4-12 hr	24 hr
Subcut. (regular)	30-60 min	2-4 hr	Unknown
Subcut. (ultralente)	8 hr	10-30 hr	>36 hr

Adverse reactions

Metabolic: hypokalemia, sodium retention, **hypoglycemia, rebound hyperglycemia (Somogyi effect)**
Skin: urticaria, rash, pruritus
Other: edema; lipodystrophy; lipohypertrophy; erythema, stinging, or

warmth at injection site; allergic reactions including **anaphylaxis**

Interactions

Drug-drug. *Acetazolamide, albuterol, antiretrovirals, asparaginase, calcitonin, corticosteroids, cyclophosphamide, danazol, dextrothyroxine, diazoxide, diltiazem, diuretics, dobutamine, epinephrine, estrogens, hormonal contraceptives, isoniazid, morphine, niacin, phenothiazines, phenytoin, somatropin, terbutaline, thyroid hormones:* decreased hypoglycemic effect
Anabolic steroids, angiotensin-converting enzyme inhibitors, calcium, chloroquine, clofibrate, clonidine, disopyramide, fluoxetine, guanethidine, mebendazole, MAO inhibitors, octreotide, oral hypoglycemics, phenylbutazone, propoxyphene, pyridoxine, salicylates, sulfinpyrazone, sulfonamides, tetracyclines: increased hypoglycemic effect
Beta-adrenergic blockers (nonselective): masking of some hypoglycemia symptoms, delayed recovery from hypoglycemia
Lithium carbonate: decreased or increased hypoglycemic effect
Pentamidine: increased hypoglycemic effect, possibly followed by hyperglycemia
Drug-diagnostic tests. *Glucose, inorganic phosphate, magnesium, potassium:* decreased levels
Liver and thyroid function tests: interference with test results
Urine vanillylmandelic acid: increased level
Drug-herbs. *Basil, burdock, glucosamine, sage:* altered glycemic control
Chromium, coenzyme Q10, dandelion, eucalyptus, fenugreek, marshmallow: increased hypoglycemic effect
Garlic, ginseng: decreased blood glucose level
Drug-behaviors. *Alcohol use:* increased hypoglycemic effect
Marijuana use: increased blood glucose level
Smoking: increased blood glucose level, decreased response to insulin

Patient monitoring

- Monitor glucose level frequently to assess drug efficacy and appropriateness of dosage.
- Watch blood glucose level closely if patient is converting from one insulin type to another or is under unusual stress (as from surgery or trauma).

[Clinical alert] Monitor for signs and symptoms of hypoglycemia. Keep glucose source at hand in case hypoglycemia occurs.

[Clinical alert] Assess for signs and symptoms of hyperglycemia, such as polydipsia, polyphagia, polyuria, and diabetic ketoacidosis (as shown by blood and urinary ketones, metabolic acidosis, extremely elevated blood glucose level).

- Monitor for glycosuria.
- Closely evaluate kidney and liver function test results in patients with renal or hepatic impairment.

Patient teaching

- Teach patient how to administer insulin subcutaneously as appropriate.
- Advise patient to draw up regular insulin into syringe first when mixing two types of insulin. Caution him not to change order of mixing insulins.
- Instruct patient to rotate subcutaneous injection sites and keep a record of sites used, to prevent fatty tissue breakdown.

[Clinical alert] Teach patient how to recognize and report signs and symptoms of hypoglycemia and hyperglycemia. Advise him to carry a glucose source at all times.

- Instruct patient to store insulin in refrigerator (not freezer).
- Teach patient how to monitor and record blood glucose level and, if indicated, urine glucose and ketone levels.
- Tell patient that dietary changes, activity, and stress can alter blood glucose level and insulin requirements.

• Instruct patient to wear medical identification stating that he is diabetic and takes insulin.
• Advise patient to have regular medical, vision, and dental exams.
• As appropriate, review all other significant and life-threatening adverse reactions and interactions, especially those related to the drugs, tests, herbs, and behaviors mentioned above.

insulin aspart (rDNA origin)

NovoLog

insulin aspart and insulin aspart protamine

NovoLog Mix 70/30

Pharmacologic class: Pancreatic hormone
Therapeutic class: Hypoglycemic
Pregnancy risk category C

Action

Short-acting insulin form. Promotes glucose transport, which stimulates carbohydrate metabolism in skeletal and cardiac muscle and adipose tissue. Also promotes phosphorylation of glucose in liver, where it's converted to glycogen. Directly affects fat and protein metabolism, stimulates protein synthesis, inhibits release of free fatty acids, and indirectly decreases phosphate and potassium.

Availability

Injection (NovoLog): 100 units/ml in 10-ml vials and 3-ml PenFill cartridges
Injection (NovoLog Mix 70/30): 100 units/ml in 10-ml vials, 3-ml PenFill cartridges, and 3-ml FlexPen prefilled syringes

Indications and dosages

➢ Type 1 (insulin-dependent) diabetes mellitus; type 2 (non-insulin-dependent) diabetes mellitus
Adults and children ages 6 and older: *Insulin aspart*—Dosage tailored to patient's needs, given subcutaneously in divided doses 5 to 10 minutes before meals. Insulin aspart provides 50% to 70% of dose; intermediate or long-acting insulin provides remainder. Dosage range is 0.5 to 1 unit/kg/day in divided doses based on meals. *Insulin aspart and insulin aspart protamine*—Give subcutaneously b.i.d., 15 minutes before morning and evening meals. For monotherapy, initial dosage is 0.4 to 0.6 unit/kg/day in two divided doses. Titrate in increments of 2 to 4 units q 3 to 4 days to achieve target fasting plasma glucose level. When given with oral hypoglycemics, initial dosage is 0.2 to 0.3 unit/kg/day.

Contraindications

• Hypersensitivity to drug or its components
• Hypoglycemia

Precautions

Use cautiously in:
• hepatic or renal impairment, hypothyroidism, hyperthyroidism
• elderly patients
• pregnant or breastfeeding patients
• children.

Administration

Be aware that insulin is a high-alert drug.
• Know that drug is bioavailable as regular human insulin but has a faster onset and shorter duration.
• Give by subcutaneous route only, 5 to 10 minutes (15 minutes for Novolog Mix 70/30) before a meal.
• When mixing insulin aspart with intermediate or long-acting insulin, draw up insulin aspart into syringe first.

i

🔊 Don't mix insulin aspart protamine with any other insulin.
• When giving insulin aspart by pump, don't mix with other insulins.
• Rotate injection sites to prevent lipodystrophy.

Route	Onset	Peak	Duration
Subcut.	15 min	1-3 hr	3-5 hr

Adverse reactions

Metabolic: hypokalemia, sodium retention, **hypoglycemia, rebound hyperglycemia (Somogyi effect)**
Musculoskeletal: myalgia
Skin: urticaria, rash, pruritus
Other: edema; lipodystrophy; lipohypertrophy; redness, warmth, or stinging at injection site; allergic reactions including **anaphylaxis**

Interactions

Drug-drug. *Acetazolamide, albuterol, antiretrovirals, asparaginase, calcitonin, corticosteroids, cyclophosphamide, danazol, dextrothyroxine, diazoxide, diltiazem, diuretics, dobutamine, epinephrine, estrogens, hormonal contraceptives, isoniazid, morphine, niacin, phenothiazines, phenytoin, somatropin, terbutaline, thyroid hormones:* decreased hypoglycemic effect
Anabolic steroids, angiotensin-converting enzyme inhibitors, calcium, chloroquine, clofibrate, clonidine, disopyramide, fluoxetine, guanethidine, mebendazole, MAO inhibitors, octreotide, oral hypoglycemics, phenylbutazone, propoxyphene, pyridoxine, salicylates, sulfinpyrazone, sulfonamides, tetracyclines: increased hypoglycemic effect
Beta-adrenergic blockers (nonselective): masking of some hypoglycemia signs and symptoms, delayed recovery from hypoglycemia
Lithium carbonate: decreased or increased hypoglycemic effect
Pentamidine: increased hypoglycemic effect, possibly followed by hyperglycemia
Drug-diagnostic tests. *Glucose, inorganic phosphate, magnesium, potassium:* decreased levels
Liver and thyroid function studies: test interference
Urine vanillylmandelic acid: increased level
Drug-herbs. *Basil, bee pollen, burdock, glucosamine, sage:* altered glycemic control
Chromium, coenzyme Q10, dandelion, eucalyptus, fenugreek, marshmallow: increased hypoglycemic effect
Garlic, ginseng: decreased blood glucose level
Drug-behaviors. *Alcohol use:* increased hypoglycemic effect
Marijuana use: increased blood glucose level
Smoking: increased blood glucose level, decreased response to insulin

Patient monitoring

• Monitor blood glucose level frequently to gauge drug efficacy and appropriateness of dosage.
• Watch blood glucose level closely if patient is converting from one insulin type to another or is under unusual stress (as from surgery or trauma).
🔊 Stay alert for signs and symptoms of hypoglycemia. Keep glucose source at hand.
🔊 Assess for evidence of hyperglycemia, such as polydipsia, polyphagia, polyuria, and diabetic ketoacidosis (as shown by urine and blood ketones, metabolic acidosis, extremely elevated blood glucose level, and hypovolemia).
• Monitor for glycosuria.
• Closely monitor kidney and liver function test results in patients with renal or hepatic impairment.

Patient teaching

• Teach patient how to administer insulin subcutaneously or by injection pen.

• If patient must mix insulin aspart with intermediate or long-acting insulin, instruct him to draw up insulin aspart into syringe first.

Clinical alert: Tell patient not to mix any other insulin with mixture of insulin aspart and insulin aspart protamine.

• Advise patient to rotate subcutaneous injection sites and keep a record of sites used, to help prevent fatty tissue breakdown.

Clinical alert: Teach patient how to recognize and report signs and symptoms of hypoglycemia and hyperglycemia. Advise him to always carry a glucose source.

• Inform patient that changes in diet, activity, and stress level affect blood glucose levels and insulin requirements.

• Teach patient how to monitor and record blood glucose level and, if indicated, urine glucose and ketone levels.

• Tell patient to wear medical identification stating that he is diabetic and takes insulin.

• Instruct patient to have regular medical, vision, and dental exams.

• Tell female patient to contact prescriber if she is pregnant or plans to become pregnant.

• Advise patient to store insulin in refrigerator, not freezer.

• As appropriate, review all other significant and life-threatening adverse reactions and interactions, especially those related to the drugs, tests, herbs, and behaviors mentioned above.

insulin glargine (rDNA origin)

Lantus

Pharmacologic class: Pancreatic hormone
Therapeutic class: Hypoglycemic
Pregnancy risk category C

Action

Long-acting insulin form. Promotes glucose transport, which stimulates carbohydrate metabolism in skeletal and cardiac muscle and adipose tissue. Also promotes phosphorylation of glucose in liver, where it's converted to glycogen. Directly affects fat and protein metabolism, stimulates protein synthesis, inhibits release of free fatty acids, and indirectly decreases phosphate and potassium.

Availability

Injection: 100 units/ml in 10-ml vials and 3-ml cartridges

Indications and dosages

➢ Type 1 (insulin-dependent) diabetes mellitus and type 2 (non-insulin-dependent) diabetes mellitus in patients who need long-acting insulin
Adults and children ages 6 and older: Subcutaneous injection daily at same time each day, with dosage based on blood glucose level

➢ Conversion from another insulin type in patients with type 1 diabetes mellitus who need long-acting insulin
Adults and children ages 6 and older: For patients switching from once-daily NPH or ultralente human insulin, start glargine at same dosage as current insulin dosage. For patients taking twice-daily NPH or ultralente human insulin, reduce initial glargine dosage by approximately 20% of current insulin dosage during week 1; then adjust based on blood glucose level.

➢ Type 2 diabetes mellitus in patients receiving oral hypoglycemics
Adults: Dosage highly individualized based on glucose levels and response

Contraindications

• Hypersensitivity to drug or its components
• Hypoglycemia

Precautions

Use cautiously in:
- pregnant or breastfeeding patients
- children.

Administration

🔈 Be aware that insulin is a high-alert drug.
- Give by subcutaneous route only, at same time each day.

🔈 Don't mix in solution with other drugs, including other insulins.
- Before drawing up insulin into syringe, roll vial between hands to ensure uniform dispersion; don't shake.
- Rotate injection sites to prevent lipodystrophy.

Route	Onset	Peak	Duration
Subcut.	1.1 hr	5 hr	24 hr

Adverse reactions

Metabolic: rebound hyperglycemia (Somogyi effect), hypoglycemia
Skin: urticaria, rash, pruritus, redness, stinging, or warmth at injection site
Other: edema, lipodystrophy, lipohypertrophy, allergic reactions including **anaphylaxis**

Interactions

Drug-drug. *Acetazolamide, albuterol, antiretrovirals, asparaginase, calcitonin, corticosteroids, cyclophosphamide, danazol, dextrothyroxine, diazoxide, diltiazem, diuretics, dobutamine, epinephrine, estrogens, hormonal contraceptives, isoniazid, morphine, niacin, phenothiazines, phenytoin, somatropin, terbutaline, thyroid hormones:* decreased hypoglycemic effect
Anabolic steroids, angiotensin-converting enzyme inhibitors, calcium, chloroquine, clofibrate, clonidine, disopyramide, fluoxetine, guanethidine, mebendazole, MAO inhibitors, octreotide, oral hypoglycemics, phenylbutazone, propoxyphene, pyridoxine, salicylates, sulfinpyrazone, sulfonamides, tetracyclines: increased hypoglycemic effect
Beta-adrenergic blockers (nonselective): masking of some hypoglycemia signs and symptoms, delayed recovery from hypoglycemia
Lithium carbonate: altered hypoglycemic effect
Pentamidine: increased hypoglycemic effect, possibly followed by hyperglycemia
Drug-diagnostic tests. *Glucose, inorganic phosphate, magnesium, potassium:* decreased levels
Liver and thyroid function studies: test interference
Urine vanillylmandelic acid: increased level
Drug-herbs. *Basil, bee pollen, burdock, glucosamine, sage:* altered glycemic control
Chromium, coenzyme Q10, dandelion, eucalyptus, fenugreek, marshmallow: increased hypoglycemic effect
Garlic, ginseng: decreased blood glucose level
Drug-behaviors. *Alcohol use:* increased hypoglycemic effect
Marijuana use: increased blood glucose level
Smoking: increased blood glucose level, decreased response to insulin

Patient monitoring

- Monitor blood glucose level frequently to assess drug efficacy and appropriateness of dosage.
- Watch blood glucose level closely if patient is converting from one insulin type to another or is under unusual stress (as from surgery or trauma).

🔈 Check for signs and symptoms of hypoglycemia (such as CNS changes). Keep glucose source at hand.

🔈 Monitor for signs and symptoms of hyperglycemia, such as polydipsia, polyphagia, polyuria, and diabetic ketoacidosis (blood and urine ketones, metabolic acidosis, extremely elevated glucose level, hypovolemia).

• Monitor for glycosuria.
• Closely monitor kidney and liver function test results in patients with renal or hepatic impairment.

Patient teaching

• Instruct patient how to administer insulin subcutaneously.
Teach patient how to recognize and report signs and symptoms of hypoglycemia and hyperglycemia. Advise him to always carry glucose source.
• Advise patient to rotate subcutaneous injection sites and keep a record of sites used.
• Teach patient how to monitor and record blood glucose level and, if indicated, urine glucose and ketone levels.
• Inform patient that changes in diet, activity, and stress level can affect blood glucose level and insulin requirements.
• Advise patient to wear medical identification stating that he is diabetic and takes insulin.
• As appropriate, review all other significant and life-threatening adverse reactions and interactions, especially those related to the drugs, tests, herbs, and behaviors mentioned above.

interferon alfa-n3

Alferon N

Pharmacologic class: Immunomodulator
Therapeutic class: Immunologic agent, antiviral
Pregnancy risk category C

Action

Binds to membrane receptors on viral cells, inducing protein synthesis, inhibiting viral replication, and suppressing cell proliferation. Increases phagocytosis by macrophages, enhances expression of human leukocyte antigen, and augments lymphocyte cytotoxicity.

Availability

Injection: 5 million international units/ml

Indications and dosages

➤ Refractory or recurring external condylomata acuminata (genital warts)
Adults ages 18 and older: 0.05 ml (250,000 international units) injected intralesionally into base of each wart twice weekly for up to 8 weeks

Contraindications

• Hypersensitivity to human interferon alfa proteins or any product component
• Anaphylactic sensitivity to mouse immunoglobulin, egg protein, or neomycin

Precautions

Use cautiously in:
• fertile males and females
• debilitated patients
• pregnant or breastfeeding patients
• children younger than age 18.

Administration

• Use 30G needle to administer intralesional injection.

Route	Onset	Peak	Duration
Intrales.	Not measurable		

Adverse reactions

CNS: vasovagal reaction, fatigue, dizziness, insomnia, decreased concentration, depression, nervousness, malaise, headache
EENT: visual disturbances, nasal and sinus drainage, pharyngitis, epistaxis, throat tightness, tongue hyperesthesia
GI: increased salivation
GU: dysuria

Musculoskeletal: arthralgia, back pain, myalgia, muscle cramps
Skin: sweating, generalized pruritus, papular rash on neck, photosensitivity
Other: strange taste in mouth, fever, chills, swollen left inguinal lymph node, tingling sensation of legs and feet, hot sensation of soles, heat intolerance, hot flashes, flulike symptoms, itching and pain at injection site, hypersensitivity reactions including **anaphylaxis**

Interactions

Drug-diagnostic tests. *White blood cells (WBCs):* decreased

Patient monitoring

- Monitor WBC count.
- Watch closely for hypersensitivity reactions, including anaphylaxis.

Patient teaching

- Assure patient that flulike symptoms will subside with repeated doses.
- Tell patient to immediately report signs and symptoms of hypersensitivity reaction, such as hives, difficulty breathing, wheezing, and tightness in chest.
- Tell female patient to inform prescriber if she is or plans to become pregnant. Caution her not to breastfeed.
- As appropriate, review all other significant and life-threatening adverse reactions and interactions, especially those related to the tests mentioned above.

interferon alfa-2a, recombinant

Roferon-A

interferon alfa-2b, recombinant

Intron A

Pharmacologic class: Biological response modifier
Therapeutic class: Antineoplastic, antiviral
Pregnancy risk category C

Action

Unknown. Antitumor and antiviral activity may stem from direct antiproliferative action against tumor or viral cells, inhibition of viral replication, and modulation of host immune response.

Availability

alfa-2a
Injection (single-use vials): 3 million, 6 million, 9 million, and 36 million international units
Injection (multidose vials): 9 million and 18 million international units
Sterile powder for injection: 18 million international units with diluent
alfa-2b
Injection: 3 million international units/0.5-ml vial, 5 million international units/0.5-ml vial, 10 million international units/1-ml vial; 18 million international units/3.2-ml vial, 25 million international units/ 3.2 ml vial
Powder for injection (vial with diluent): 3 million, 5 million, 10 million, 18 million, 25 million, and 50 million international units

Indications and dosages

➢ Chronic hepatitis C
alfa-2a—
Adults: 3 million international units

subcutaneously or I.M. three times weekly for 48 to 52 weeks. Alternatively, induction dose of 6 million international units subcutaneously or I.M. three times weekly for first 12 weeks; then 3 million international units three times weekly for 36 weeks. Poor response after 3 months warrants withdrawal. Prescriber may order 6 to 12 months of retreatment with either 3 or 6 million international units three times weekly.
alfa-2b—
Adults: 3 million international units subcutaneously or I.M. three times weekly. If patient tolerates therapy and alanine aminotransferase (ALT) level is normal after 16 weeks, continue for 18 to 24 weeks. If ALT doesn't normalize, drug may be withdrawn.

➢ Chronic hepatitis B
alfa-2b—
Adults: 30 to 35 million international units subcutaneously or I.M. weekly for 16 weeks, given as 5 million international units daily or 10 million international units three times weekly

➢ Hairy cell leukemia
alfa-2a—
Adults: 3 million international units subcutaneously or I.M. daily for 16 to 24 weeks. Maintenance dosage is 3 million international units subcutaneously or I.M. three times weekly.
alfa-2b—
Adults: 2 million international units/m^2 I.M. or subcutaneously three times weekly for 6 months or longer

➢ AIDS-related Kaposi's sarcoma
alfa-2a—
Adults: 36 million international units subcutaneously or I.M. daily for 10 to 12 weeks. Maintenance dosage is 36 million international units subcutaneously or I.M. three times weekly. May start at 3 million international units and increase q 3 days, up to daily dosage of 36 million international units.
alfa-2b—
Adults: 30 million international units/m^2 subcutaneously or I.M. three times weekly. Continue dosage unless intolerance occurs or disease advances rapidly.

➢ Chronic myelogenous leukemia (Philadelphia chromosome–positive)
alfa-2a—
Adults: Initially, 3 million international units subcutaneously or I.M. daily for 3 days; then 6 million international units for 3 days; then 9 million international units daily for duration of treatment

➢ Malignant melanoma (as adjunct to surgery)
alfa-2b—
Adults: 20 million international units/m^2 I.V. for 5 consecutive days per week for 4 weeks; then a maintenance dosage of 10 million international units/m^2 subcutaneously three times weekly for 48 weeks. Withhold drug if adverse reactions occur; when reactions ease, resume at half of previous dosage. Withdraw if reactions persist.

➢ Condyloma acuminatum (genital or venereal warts)
alfa-2b—
Adults: 1 million international units/lesion given intralesionally three times weekly for 3 weeks

➢ Aggressive follicular non-Hodgkin's lymphoma
alfa-2b—
Adults: 5 million international units subcutaneously three times weekly for up to 18 months (given with chemotherapy regimen containing anthracycline)

Off-label uses

- Adjuvant treatment of malignant melanoma
- Hepatitis D

Contraindications

- Hypersensitivity to drug or its components

- Autoimmune disorders
- Female partners of males receiving drug

Precautions

Use cautiously in:
- cardiac or pulmonary disease; bone marrow, autoimmune, seizure, or psychiatric disorders
- diabetic patients prone to ketoacidosis
- pregnant or breastfeeding patients
- children.

Administration

- Give alfa-2a by subcutaneous or I.M. route. Reconstitute with 3 ml of diluent provided; swirl gently to dissolve.
- Administer alfa-2b by subcutaneous, I.M., or I.V. route. For I.V. use, reconstitute with diluent provided (bacteriostatic water for injection), according to chart provided. Mix gently, draw drug up into sterile syringe, and inject into 100 ml of normal saline solution. Infuse slowly over 20 minutes.
- Give antiemetics, as needed and prescribed, for nausea and vomiting.

Route	Onset	Peak	Duration
I.V. (alfa-2b)	Unknown	15-60 min	4 hr
I.M.	Unknown	2-12 hr	Unknown
Subcut.	Unknown	3-12 hr	Unknown
Intrales.	Unknown	Unknown	Unknown

Adverse reactions

CNS: dizziness, confusion, paresthesia, rigors, lethargy, depression, difficulty thinking or concentrating, insomnia, anxiety, fatigue, asthenia, amnesia, malaise, nervousness, drowsiness, **suicidal ideation**
CV: chest pain, hypertension, palpitations, **arrhythmias**
EENT: visual disturbances, stye, hearing disorders, nasal congestion, sinusitis, rhinitis, pharyngitis
GI: nausea, vomiting, diarrhea, constipation, abdominal pain, dyspepsia, flatulence, eructation, stomatitis, dry mouth, **intestinal obstruction**
GU: gynecomastia, impaired fertility in women, transient erectile dysfunction
Hematologic: anemia, **leukopenia, thrombocytopenia, neutropenia**
Metabolic: hyperglycemia, hypocalcemia
Musculoskeletal: joint pain, back pain, myalgia
Respiratory: cough, dyspnea
Skin: flushing, rash, dry skin, pruritus, alopecia, dermatitis, diaphoresis
Other: gingivitis, flulike symptoms, candidiasis, edema, weight loss

Interactions

Drug-drug. *Aminophylline, theophylline:* reduced clearance of these drugs
CNS depressants: additive CNS effects
Live-virus vaccines: decreased antibody response to vaccine, increased risk of adverse reactions
Zidovudine: synergistic effects
Drug-diagnostic tests. *Alkaline phosphatase, ALT, aspartate aminotransferase, bilirubin, blood urea nitrogen, calcium, creatinine, fasting glucose, lactate dehydrogenase, neutralizing antibodies, phosphate, uric acid:* increased levels
Hemoglobin, platelets, white blood cells: decreased values
International Normalized Ratio, partial thromboplastin time, prothrombin time: increased values

Patient monitoring

- Before therapy and monthly during therapy, assess CBC with white cell differential, bone marrow hairy cells, glucose and electrolyte levels, and liver and kidney function tests.
- Discontinue therapy if neutrophil count drops below 500 cells/mm^2.
- Monitor fluid intake and output. Keep patient well hydrated.
- Assess for GI upset. Provide small, frequent meals and antiemetics to ease severe nausea and vomiting.

Monitor for mental status changes, depression, and suicidal ideation.
- Assess for bleeding and bruising.
- Institute infection-control measures. Monitor for signs and symptoms of infection.

Patient teaching
- Teach patient or caregiver how to prepare and give drug subcutaneously or I.M., rotate injection sites, and track dosing schedule and injection sites on calendar.
- Caution patient to avoid driving and other hazardous activities until he knows how drug affects concentration, alertness, and vision.
- Inform female patient that drug is linked to fetal abnormalities. Advise her not to get pregnant during therapy, and to use barrier contraception.
- Tell female patient not to breastfeed.
- Advise patient to avoid potential infection sources, such as crowds and people with known infections.
- Tell patient to eat small, frequent meals to combat nausea, vomiting, and loss of appetite.
- Inform male patient that drug may cause transient erectile dysfunction.

Instruct patient to immediately report depression, suicidal thoughts, mental status changes, signs or symptoms of infection (such as fever, chills, sore throat), unusual bleeding or bruising, dizziness, palpitations, or chest pain.
- Tell patient he'll need regular follow-up examinations and blood tests to gauge drug effects.
- As appropriate, review all other significant and life-threatening adverse reactions and interactions, especially those related to the drugs and tests mentioned above.

interferon alfacon-1
Infergen

Pharmacologic class: Biological response modifier
Therapeutic class: Antiviral
Pregnancy risk category C

Action
Binds to membrane receptors on viral cells, inducing protein synthesis, inhibiting viral replication, and suppressing cell proliferation. Increases phagocytosis, enhances expression of human leukocyte antigen, and augments lymphocyte cytotoxicity.

Availability
Injection: 9-mcg/0.3-ml vials, 15-mcg/0.5-ml vials

Indications and dosages
➤ Chronic hepatitis C
Adults: 9 mcg subcutaneously as a single dose three times weekly for 24 weeks. Wait at least 48 hours between doses.

Off-label uses
- Hairy cell leukemia

Contraindications
- Hypersensitivity to drug or *Escherichia coli*–derived products

Precautions
Use cautiously in:
- thyroid disorders, bone marrow depression, hepatic or cardiac disease, seizure disorders, compromised CNS function, severe psychiatric disorders
- pregnant or breastfeeding patients
- children age 18 and younger.

Administration
- Give by subcutaneous route only.

• Give antiemetics for nausea and vomiting, as needed and prescribed.

Route	Onset	Peak	Duration
Subcut.	Unknown	24-36 hr	Unknown

Adverse reactions

CNS: dizziness, confusion, rigors, paresthesia, lethargy, depression, difficulty thinking or concentrating, insomnia, anxiety, fatigue, amnesia, nervousness, drowsiness, asthenia, malaise, **suicidal ideation**
CV: chest pain, hypertension, palpitations, **arrhythmias**
EENT: visual disturbances, stye, hearing disorders, nasal congestion, rhinitis, sinusitis, pharyngitis
GI: nausea, vomiting, diarrhea, constipation, abdominal pain, flatulence, eructation, stomatitis, dry mouth, anorexia, **intestinal obstruction**
GU: impaired fertility in women, gynecomastia, erectile dysfunction
Hematologic: anemia, **leukopenia, thrombocytopenia, neutropenia**
Metabolic: hyperglycemia, hypocalcemia
Musculoskeletal: joint pain, back pain, myalgia
Respiratory: cough, dyspnea
Skin: rash, dryness, pruritus, flushing, alopecia, candidiasis, dermatitis, diaphoresis
Other: gingivitis, flulike symptoms, edema, weight loss

Interactions

Drug-drug. *Drugs metabolized by CYP450:* altered blood levels of both drugs
Drug-diagnostic tests. *Granulocytes, hemoglobin, platelets, white blood cells:* decreased values
Alkaline phosphatase, aspartate aminotransferase, bilirubin, blood urea nitrogen, creatinine, International Normalized Ratio, lactate dehydrogenase, neutralizing antibodies, phosphorus, prothrombin time, triglycerides, uric acid: increased values

Patient monitoring

🔈 Before and regularly during therapy, assess CBC with white cell differential and hepatitis C virus antibodies.
• Assess fluid intake and output. Keep patient well hydrated.
• Monitor for GI upset. Provide small, frequent meals and give antiemetics, as prescribed, to ease severe nausea and vomiting.
🔈 Stay alert for depression, mental status changes, psychosis, and suicidal ideation (especially in patients with history of mental illness).
• Assess for bleeding and bruising.
• Institute infection-control measures. Monitor for signs and symptoms of infection.
• Watch for flulike symptoms.

Patient teaching

• Teach patient or caregiver how to administer drug subcutaneously, rotate injection sites, and track dosing schedule and injection sites on calendar.
• Advise patient to avoid sources of potential infection, such as crowds and people with known infections.
• Tell patient to eat small, frequent meals to combat nausea, vomiting, and appetite loss.
• Caution patient to avoid driving and other hazardous activities until he knows how drug affects concentration, alertness, and vision.
• Tell female patient that drug is linked to fetal abnormalities. Advise her not to get pregnant during therapy, and to use barrier contraception.
🔈 Instruct patient to immediately report symptoms of infection (fever, chills, sore throat), unusual bleeding or bruising, mental status changes, dizziness, palpitations, or chest pain.
• Tell patient he'll need regular follow-up examinations and blood tests to gauge drug effects.

• As appropriate, review all other significant and life-threatening adverse reactions and interactions, especially those related to the drugs and tests mentioned above.

interferon beta-1a
Avonex, Rebif

interferon beta-1b
Betaseron

Pharmacologic class: Biological response modifier
Therapeutic class: Antiviral, immunoregulator
Pregnancy risk category C

Action
Binds and competes with specific receptors on cell surface, inducing various interferon-induced gene products. Also inhibits proliferation of T cells.

Availability
Lyophilized powder for injection (beta-1a): 22 mcg (6 million international units; Rebif), 33 mcg (6.6 million international units; Avonex), 44 mcg (12 million international units; Rebif)
Powder for injection (beta-1b): 0.3 mg (9.6 million international units; Betaseron)
Prefilled syringes (beta-1a): 30 mcg/0.5 ml (Avonex)

Indications and dosages
➢ To reduce frequency of exacerbations in relapsing-remitting multiple sclerosis
Adults ages 18 and older: 8.8 mcg Rebif subcutaneously three times weekly, increased over a 4-week period to 44 mcg three times weekly. Or 30 mcg Avonex I.M. once a week. Or 8 million international units (0.25 mg) Betaseron subcutaneously every other day.

Contraindications
• Hypersensitivity to drug, its components, or albumin

Precautions
Use cautiously in:
• cardiac disease, seizure disorders, mental disorders, depression, suicidal tendencies
• women of childbearing age
• pregnant or breastfeeding patients
• children ages 18 and younger.

Administration
• Reconstitute Avonex (I.M. injection) and Rebif (subcutaneous injection) using diluent provided, according to instructions provided.
• Reconstitute Betaseron (subcutaneous injection) using 1.2 ml of diluent supplied by manufacturer, to yield a concentration of 0.25 mg/ml. Swirl gently to mix; don't shake. Use reconstituted drug within 3 hours; discard unused portion.

Route	Onset	Peak	Duration
I.M.	Unknown	Unknown	Unknown
Subcut.	Unknown	1-8 hr	Unknown

Adverse reactions
CNS: dizziness, confusion, rigors, paresthesia, lethargy, depression, difficulty thinking or concentrating, insomnia, anxiety, fatigue, amnesia, nervousness, drowsiness, asthenia, malaise, **suicidal ideation**
CV: chest pain, hypertension, palpitations, **arrhythmias**
EENT: visual disturbances, stye, hearing disorders, nasal congestion, sinusitis, rhinitis, pharyngitis
GI: nausea, vomiting, diarrhea, constipation, abdominal pain, dyspepsia, flatulence, eructation, stomatitis, dry mouth, **intestinal obstruction**

GU: gynecomastia, breast pain, early or delayed menses, menstrual bleeding or spotting, shortened duration of menstrual flow, menorrhagia
Hematologic: anemia, **neutropenia, leukopenia, thrombocytopenia**
Metabolic: hypocalcemia
Musculoskeletal: joint pain, back pain, myalgia, myasthenia
Respiratory: cough, dyspnea
Skin: rash, dry skin, pruritus, flushing, alopecia, dermatitis, diaphoresis
Other: gingivitis, flulike symptoms, weight loss, edema, candidiasis, lymphadenopathy, inflammation, pain

Interactions

Drug-diagnostic tests. *Alanine aminotransferase, alkaline phosphatase, aspartate aminotransferase, bilirubin, blood urea nitrogen, creatinine, glucose, lactate dehydrogenase, neutralizing antibodies, phosphorus, uric acid:* increased values
Hemoglobin, neutrophils, white blood cells: decreased values

Patient monitoring

Before therapy and monthly during therapy, assess CBC with white cell differential, glucose and electrolyte levels, and liver and kidney function tests.
• Assess fluid intake and output. Keep patient well hydrated.
• Watch for GI upset. Provide small, frequent meals to minimize nausea and vomiting.
Monitor for mental status changes, depression, and suicidal ideation.
• Evaluate for bleeding and bruising.
• Institute infection-control measures. Monitor for infection symptoms.

Patient teaching

• Teach patient or caregiver how to administer drug subcutaneously or I.M., rotate injection sites, and track dosing schedule and injection sites on calendar.
• Advise patient to avoid sources of potential infection, such as crowds and people with known infections.
• Tell patient to eat small, frequent meals to combat nausea, vomiting, and appetite loss.
• Caution patient to avoid driving and other hazardous activities until he knows how drug affects concentration, alertness, and vision.
Tell patient to contact prescriber immediately if depression or suicidal ideation occurs.
• Inform female patient that drug is linked to fetal abnormalities. Advise her not to get pregnant during therapy, and to use barrier contraception. Tell her to consult prescriber before breastfeeding.
Instruct patient to immediately report signs of symptoms of infection (such as fever, chills, sore throat, achiness), unusual bleeding or bruising, mental status changes, dizziness, palpitations, or chest pain.
• Tell patient he'll need regular follow-up examinations and blood tests to monitor drug effects.
• As appropriate, review all other significant and life-threatening adverse reactions and interactions, especially those related to the tests mentioned above.

interferon gamma-1b

Actimmune

Pharmacologic class: Biological response modifier
Therapeutic class: Antineoplastic
Pregnancy risk category C

Action

Enhances cellular toxicity and killer cell activity and promotes generation of oxygen metabolites in phagocytes, resulting in destruction of microorganisms.

Availability

Injection: 100 mcg (2 million international units)/0.5-ml vial

Indications and dosages

➤ Chronic granulomatous disease; severe malignant osteopetrosis

Adults with body surface area (BSA) above 0.5 m²: 50 mcg/m² (1 million international units/m²) subcutaneously three times weekly

Adults with BSA of 0.5 m² or less: 1.5 mcg/kg subcutaneously three times weekly in deltoid or anterior thigh

Contraindications

- Hypersensitivity to drug, its components, or *Escherichia coli*–derived products

Precautions

Use cautiously in:

- thyroid disorders, bone marrow depression, hepatic or cardiac disease, seizure disorders, compromised CNS function
- pregnant or breastfeeding patients
- children ages 18 and younger.

Administration

- Administer into deltoid muscle by subcutaneous route only.
- Give at bedtime if flulike symptoms occur.
- Provide antiemetics to ease nausea and vomiting, as prescribed.

Route	Onset	Peak	Duration
Subcut.	Unknown	7 hr	Unknown

Adverse reactions

CNS: dizziness, confusion, paresthesia, lethargy, depression, difficulty thinking or concentrating, insomnia, anxiety, fatigue, amnesia, nervousness, drowsiness, asthenia, malaise

CV: chest pain, hypertension, palpitations, **arrhythmias**

GI: nausea, vomiting, diarrhea, constipation, abdominal pain, **pancreatitis**

GU: proteinuria

Hematologic: anemia, **leukopenia, thrombocytopenia, neutropenia**

Musculoskeletal: joint pain, back pain, myalgia

Skin: flushing, rash, dry skin, erythema

Other: flulike symptoms, weight loss, edema, hypersensitivity reaction

Interactions

Drug-drug. *Bone marrow depressants:* increased bone marrow depression

Zidovudine: increased zidovudine blood level

Drug-diagnostic tests. *Hepatic enzymes:* increased levels

Neutrophils, platelets: decreased counts

Patient monitoring

🔊 Before and monthly during therapy, assess CBC with white cell differential, glucose and electrolyte levels, and liver and kidney function tests.

- Assess fluid intake and output. Keep patient well hydrated.
- Monitor for GI upset. Provide small, frequent meals or antiemetics to ease severe nausea and vomiting.

🔊 Monitor patient for mental status changes and depression.

- Assess for flulike symptoms. If these occur, give drug at bedtime and provide supportive care, such as rest and acetaminophen for headache and fever.

Patient teaching

- Teach patient or caregiver how to administer drug subcutaneously, rotate injection sites, and track dosing schedule and injection sites on calendar.

🔊 Tell patient to contact prescriber immediately if depression occurs.

- Advise patient to eat small, frequent meals to combat nausea, vomiting, and appetite loss.
- Caution patient to avoid driving and other hazardous activities until he knows how drug affects concentration and alertness.

• Inform female patient that drug is linked to fetal abnormalities. Advise her not to get pregnant during therapy, and to use barrier contraception.
• Tell female patient to consult prescriber before breastfeeding.
• Tell patient he'll need regular follow-up examinations and blood tests to monitor drug effects.
• As appropriate, review all other significant and life-threatening adverse reactions and interactions, especially those related to the drugs and tests mentioned above.

ipratropium bromide

Alti-Ipratropium✦, Apo-Ipravent✦, Atrovent, Novo-Ipramide✦

Pharmacologic class: Anticholinergic
Therapeutic class: Allergy, cold, and cough remedy; bronchodilator
Pregnancy risk category B

Action

Inhibits cholinergic receptors in bronchial smooth muscle, decreasing level of cyclic guanosine monophosphate and dilating bronchioles. When used locally, inhibits secretions from glands lining the nasal mucosa.

Availability

Aerosol inhaler: 18 mcg/spray in 14-g canister (200 inhalations)
Nasal spray: 0.03% solution (21 mcg/spray in 30-ml bottle, 345 sprays/bottle); 0.06% solution (42 mcg/spray in 15-ml bottle, 165 sprays/bottle)
Solution for inhalation: 0.02% in single-dose vials

Indications and dosages

➢ Chronic obstructive pulmonary disease; bronchospasm; asthma; perennial rhinitis; common cold

Aerosol—
Adults: Two inhalations (36 mcg) q.i.d. Don't exceed 12 inhalations in 24 hours.
Inhalation solution—
Adults: 500 mcg three to four times daily by oral nebulizer. Space doses 6 to 8 hours apart as needed.
Nasal spray (0.03% solution)—
Adults and children ages 6 and older: Two sprays (42 mcg) per nostril two to three times daily (total daily dosage of 168 to 252 mcg)
Nasal spray (0.06% solution)—
Adults and children ages 12 and older: Two sprays (84 mcg) per nostril three to four times daily (total daily dosage of 504 to 672 mcg)

Contraindications

• Hypersensitivity to drug, its components, atropine, belladonna alkaloids, bromide, fluorocarbons, or soy lecithin and related foods (such as soybeans, peanuts)

Precautions

Use cautiously in:
• acute bronchospasm, bladder neck obstruction, prostatic hypertrophy, glaucoma, urinary retention, undiagnosed abdominal pain
• elderly patients
• pregnant or breastfeeding patients
• children ages 5 and younger (safety not established).

Administration

• Give by inhalation or intranasal route as directed.
• When using nasal spray, prime with seven actuations to initiate pump. Give two actuations if spray hasn't been used within past 24 hours.
• With aerosol inhaler, prime new inhaler with three sprays. Also prime with three sprays if inhaler hasn't been used within past 24 hours.

Route	Onset	Peak	Duration
Inhalation	5-15 min	1-2 hr	3-4 hr (up to 8 hr)
Intranasal	15 min	Unknown	6-12 hr

Adverse reactions
CNS: dizziness, headache, nervousness
CV: hypotension, palpitations, chest pain
EENT: blurred vision, epistaxis, nasal dryness and irritation (with nasal spray), sore throat
GI: nausea, vomiting, GI irritation
Musculoskeletal: back pain
Respiratory: cough, upper respiratory tract infection, bronchitis, increased sputum, oropharyngeal edema, **bronchospasm**
Skin: rash
Other: flulike symptoms, hypersensitivity reactions including **anaphylaxis**

Interactions
Drug-drug. *Antihistamines, disopyramide, phenothiazines:* additive anticholinergic effects
Drug-herbs. *Jaborandi, pill-bearing spurge:* decreased drug effects

Patient monitoring
• Evaluate for urinary retention. Have patient void before giving drug.
• Ensure proper fit of mouthpiece or face mask.
• Monitor patient's response to therapy, vital signs, and neurologic, cardiovascular, and respiratory status.
• Monitor fluid intake and output. Keep patient well hydrated.
Monitor closely for hypersensitivity reactions, including anaphylaxis.

Patient teaching
• Teach patient how to use nasal spray or inhaler.
• Advise patient to rinse mouth after each dose to minimize throat irritation and dryness.
• Caution patient to keep drug out of eyes. If contact occurs, instruct him to rinse eyes with cool water and call prescriber right away.
• Caution patient to avoid driving and other dangerous activities if drug causes dizziness or blurred vision.
• Tell patient drug may cause GI upset, nausea, vomiting, or cough.
Instruct patient to promptly report vision changes, rash, or palpitations.
• As appropriate, review all other significant and life-threatening adverse reactions and interactions, especially those related to the drugs and herbs mentioned above.

irbesartan
Avapro

Pharmacologic class: Angiotensin II receptor antagonist
Therapeutic class: Antihypertensive
Pregnancy risk category C (first trimester), ***D*** (second and third trimesters)

Action
Blocks aldosterone-secreting and potent vasoconstrictive effects of angiotensin II at tissue receptor sites, which reduces vasoconstriction and lowers blood pressure

Availability
Tablets: 75 mg, 150 mg, 300 mg

Indications and dosages
➢ Hypertension
Adults: 150 mg/day P.O.; may increase to 300 mg/day
Children ages 13 to 16: 150 mg/day P.O.; may increase to 300 mg/day
Children ages 6 to 12: 75 mg/day P.O.; may increase to 150 mg/day

➢ Hypertension in volume-depleted or hemodialysis patients receiving diuretics
Adults: Initially, 75 mg/day P.O.

Off-label uses

• Nephropathy in patients with type 2 diabetes and hypertension

Contraindications

• Hypersensitivity to drug
• Bilateral renal artery stenosis
• Pregnancy (second and third trimesters)

Precautions

Use cautiously in:
• heart failure, volume or sodium depletion, renal disease, hepatic impairment
• black patients
• females of childbearing age
• breastfeeding patients
• children ages 18 and younger (safety not established).

Administration

• Administer with or without food.
• Know that drug may be given with other antihypertensive drugs.

Route	Onset	Peak	Duration
P.O.	Unknown	Within 2 hr	24 hr

Adverse reactions

CNS: dizziness, fatigue, headache, syncope
CV: orthostatic hypotension, chest pain, peripheral edema
EENT: sinus disorders
GI: nausea, diarrhea, constipation, abdominal pain, dry mouth
GU: albuminuria, **renal failure**
Metabolic: gout, **hyperkalemia**
Musculoskeletal: joint pain, back pain, muscle weakness
Respiratory: upper respiratory tract infection, cough, bronchitis
Other: dental pain

Interactions

Drug-drug. *Diuretics, other antihypertensives:* increased risk of hypotension
Lithium: increased lithium blood level
Nonsteroidal anti-inflammatory drugs: decreased antihypertensive effects
Potassium-sparing diuretics, potassium supplements: increased risk of hyperkalemia
Drug-diagnostic tests. *Albumin:* increased level
Drug-food. *Salt substitutes containing potassium:* increased risk of hyperkalemia

Patient monitoring

• Monitor vital signs, especially blood pressure.
• Watch for signs and symptoms of orthostatic hypotension.
• Watch blood pressure closely when volume depletion may cause hypotension (as in diaphoresis, nausea, vomiting, diarrhea, and postoperative period).
• Assess fluid intake and output. Keep patient well hydrated, especially if he's receiving diuretics concurrently.
• Monitor blood urea nitrogen and creatinine levels.

Patient teaching

• Tell patient he may take with or without food.
• Instruct patient to change position slowly and to stay well hydrated, to minimize blood pressure decrease when rising.
• Caution patient to avoid driving and other hazardous activities until he knows how drug affects concentration and alertness.
• Tell female patient that drug has been linked to fetal injury and deaths. Caution her not to get pregnant during therapy. Advise her to use barrier contraception.
• Instruct female patient to report pregnancy.

• Instruct patient to report fever, chills, dizziness, severe vomiting, diarrhea, and dehydration.
• As appropriate, review all other significant and life-threatening adverse reactions and interactions, especially those related to the drugs, tests, and foods mentioned above.

irinotecan hydrochloride

Camptosar

Pharmacologic class: Topoisomerase inhibitor

Therapeutic class: Hormonal antineoplastic

Pregnancy risk category D

Action

Inhibits topoisomerase 1 (an enzyme that allows DNA replication) by binding to it. This action prevents religation of DNA strand, which results in breakage of double-stranded DNA and cell death.

Availability

Injection: 20 mg/ml in 2-ml and 5-ml vials

Indications and dosages

➤ Metastatic colorectal cancer recurrence or progression after fluorouracil (5-FU) therapy

Adults: 125 mg/m² I.V. infused over 90 minutes on days 1, 8, 15, and 22, followed by a 2-week rest; given with leucovorin and 5-FU. Or, 180 mg/m² I.V. infused over 90 minutes on days 1, 15, and 29 with leucovorin, 5-FU bolus, and 5-FU infusion. Or as monotherapy, 125 mg/m² I.V. infused over 90 minutes weekly for 4 weeks, followed by a 2-week rest; or, 350 mg/m² I.V. infused over 90 minutes q 3 weeks as long as tolerable. Adjust dosage based on tolerance.

Off-label uses

• Most cancers

Contraindications

• Hypersensitivity to drug
• Concurrent atazanavir use
• Pregnancy or breastfeeding

Precautions

Use cautiously in:
• bone marrow depression, severe diarrhea
• patients undergoing radiation therapy
• elderly patients
• children.

Administration

Clinical alert: Follow facility policy for handling antineoplastics. If skin contact occurs, wash with soap and water immediately and thoroughly. If mucous membrane contact occurs, flush with water.
• Dilute in dextrose 5% in water or normal saline solution, to a concentration of 0.12 to 1.1 mg/ml.
• Infuse within 6 hours if drug is stored at room temperature or within 24 hours if refrigerated.
• Give single dose by I.V. infusion over 90 minutes.
• Administer antiemetic to ease nausea and vomiting, as needed and prescribed.

Route	Onset	Peak	Duration
I.V.	Immediate	1-2 hr	Unknown

Adverse reactions

CNS: insomnia, dizziness, asthenia, headache, akathisia
CV: vasodilation, orthostatic hypotension
EENT: rhinitis
GI: nausea, vomiting, constipation, diarrhea, flatulence, dyspepsia, abdominal pain or enlargement, stomatitis, anorexia
Hematologic: anemia, **neutropenia, leukopenia, thrombocytopenia**
Hepatic: hepatotoxicity

Metabolic: dehydration
Musculoskeletal: back pain
Respiratory: dyspnea, increased cough
Skin: alopecia, diaphoresis, rash
Other: weight loss, edema, fever, pain, chills, minor infections

Interactions

Drug-drug. *Dexamethasone:* increased risk of lymphocytopenia
Diuretics: increased risk of dehydration
Laxatives: increased risk of diarrhea
Other antineoplastics: additive adverse effects
Drug-diagnostic tests. *Alkaline phosphatase:* increased level
Hemoglobin, neutrophils, white blood cells: decreased values

Patient monitoring

- Assess CBC before each infusion. Withhold dose if neutrophil count is below 1,500 cells/mm^3.
- Monitor infusion site for extravasation; if it occurs, flush with sterile water and apply ice.
- Assess fluid intake and output. Keep patient well hydrated.
- Monitor oral intake. Evaluate for nausea and vomiting.
- Assess for diarrhea. In severe diarrhea, expect to decrease dosage or withhold dose.
- Institute infection-control protocols to help prevent infection.
- Monitor liver function test results.

Patient teaching

- Inform patient that blood tests will be done before each dose.
- Instruct patient to report pain at infusion site; severe nausea or vomiting; severe, increased, or bloody diarrhea; infection; or injury.
- Instruct patient to immediately report unusual tiredness or yellowing of skin or eyes.
- Tell patient that drug increases his risk of infection. Advise him to avoid crowds and other potential infection sources.
- Caution female patient not to breastfeed or become pregnant during therapy. Recommend barrier contraception.
- As appropriate, review all other significant and life-threatening adverse reactions and interactions, especially those related to the drugs and tests mentioned above.

iron dextran

DexFerrum, InFeD

Pharmacologic class: Trace element
Therapeutic class: Iron supplement
Pregnancy risk category C

Action

Replenishes depleted stores of iron (a component of hemoglobin) in bone marrow

Availability

Injection: 50 mg/ml

Indications and dosages

➢ Iron-deficiency anemia in patients who can't tolerate oral iron
Adults and children weighing more than 15 kg (33 lb): Dosage individualized based on patient's weight and hemoglobin (Hgb) value, using the following formula: Dosage (ml) = 0.0442 (desired Hgb minus patient's Hgb) times lean body weight (LBW) plus the product of 0.26 times LBW

Give test dose before starting I.V. or I.M. therapy: For I.V. use, administer test dose of 0.5 ml (25 mg) I.V. over 30 seconds to 5 minutes; if no reactions occur within 1 hour, give remainder of therapeutic dose I.V.; repeat this dose daily. For I.M. use, give test dose of 0.5 ml (25 mg) by Z-track method; if no reactions occur, give daily doses not exceeding 100 mg I.M. in adults,

50 mg I.M. in children weighing more than 10 kg (22 lb), or 25 mg in infants weighing less than 5 kg (11 lb).

➢ Iron replacement caused by blood loss

Adults: Dosage individualized based on the following formula: Replacement iron (in mg) = blood loss (in ml) times hematocrit

Contraindications

- Hypersensitivity to drug, alcohol, tartrazine, or sulfites
- Acute phase of infectious renal disease or hemolytic anemia

Precautions

Use cautiously in:

- autoimmune disorders, arthritis, severe hepatic impairment
- elderly patients
- breastfeeding patients
- children.

Administration

- For I.M. administration, inject by Z-track method into upper outer quadrant of gluteal muscle.
- For intermittent I.V. infusion, administer undiluted at a rate no faster than 1 ml/minute.
- Don't give with oral iron preparations.

Route	Onset	Peak	Duration
I.V., I.M.	4 days	1-2 wk	Wks-mos

Adverse reactions

CNS: dizziness, headache, syncope, **seizures**

CV: chest pain, tachycardia, hypotension

GI: nausea, vomiting

Hematologic: hemochromatosis, hemolysis, **hemosiderosis**

Musculoskeletal: joint pain, myalgia

Respiratory: dyspnea

Other: abnormal or metallic taste, tooth discoloration, fever, lymphadenopathy, hypersensitivity reactions including **anaphylaxis**

Interactions

None significant

Patient monitoring

- Monitor for hypersensitivity reaction. Keep epinephrine and other emergency supplies on hand in case reaction occurs.
- Assess serum ferritin levels regularly, because these levels correlate with iron stores.
- In patients with rheumatoid arthritis, monitor for acute exacerbation of joint pain and swelling. Provide appropriate comfort measures.
- Watch for signs and symptoms of iron overload, including decreased activity, sedation, and GI or respiratory tract bleeding.

Patient teaching

- Caution patient not to take oral iron preparations or vitamins containing iron during therapy.
- Instruct patient to report difficulty breathing, itching, or rash.
- Tell patient he'll undergo periodic blood testing to monitor his response to therapy.
- As appropriate, review all other significant and life-threatening adverse reactions mentioned above.

iron sucrose

Venofer

Pharmacologic class: Trace element

Therapeutic class: Iron supplement

Pregnancy risk category B

Action

Replenishes depleted stores of iron (a component of hemoglobin) in bone marrow

Availability

Aqueous complex for injection: 20 mg elemental iron/ml in 5-ml single-use vials (100 mg of elemental iron)

Indications and dosages

➢ Iron-deficiency anemia in hemodialysis patients concurrently receiving erythropoietin

Adults: 100 mg of elemental iron (5 ml) I.V. directly into dialysis line or by slow injection or infusion during dialysis session (up to three times weekly) for 10 doses (total of 1,000 mg)

Off-label uses

- Autologous blood donation
- Bloodless surgery

Contraindications

- Hypersensitivity to drug, alcohol, tartrazine, or sulfites
- Hemolytic anemias and other anemias not caused by iron deficiency
- Primary hemochromatosis

Precautions

Use cautiously in:

- autoimmune disorders, arthritis, severe hepatic impairment
- elderly patients
- breastfeeding patients
- children.

Administration

- Give test dose only if ordered: 50 mg (2.5 ml) I.V. over 3 to 10 minutes.
- Dilute 100 mg of elemental iron in no more than 100 ml of normal saline solution; infuse slowly I.V. over at least 15 minutes.
- Administer I.V. directly into dialysis line or by infusion at 20 mg/minute, not to exceed 100 mg/injection.
- Don't give with oral iron preparations.

Route	Onset	Peak	Duration
I.V.	4 days	1-2 wk	Wks-mos

Adverse reactions

CNS: dizziness, headache, syncope, **seizures**

CV: chest pain, tachycardia, hypotension

GI: nausea, vomiting

Hematologic: hemochromatosis, hemolysis, **hemosiderosis**

Musculoskeletal: muscle cramps, aches, or weakness; joint pain

Respiratory: dyspnea

Other: abnormal or metallic taste, tooth discoloration, fever, lymphadenopathy, allergic reactions including **anaphylaxis**

Interactions

None significant

Patient monitoring

- 🔈 Monitor for hypersensitivity reaction. Keep epinephrine and other emergency supplies available in case reaction occurs.
- Assess hemoglobin, hematocrit, serum ferritin, and transferrin saturation levels before, during, and after therapy.
- 🔈 Monitor blood pressure. Stay alert for hypotension.
- Watch for signs and symptoms of iron overload, such as decreased activity, sedation, and GI or respiratory tract bleeding.

Patient teaching

- Caution patient not to take oral iron preparations or vitamin supplements containing iron during therapy.
- Instruct patient to report dyspnea, itching, or rash.
- Tell patient he'll undergo periodic blood testing to monitor his response to therapy.
- As appropriate, review all other significant and life-threatening adverse reactions mentioned above.

isocarboxazid
Marplan

Pharmacologic class: MAO inhibitor
Therapeutic class: Antidepressant
Pregnancy risk category C

Action
Nonselectively inhibits hydrazine MAO, an enzyme system thought to raise biogenic amine levels in brain

Availability
Tablets: 10 mg

Indications and dosages
➢ Depression
Adults: Initially, 10 mg P.O. b.i.d. If tolerated, may increase in increments of 1 tablet q 2 to 4 days, to achieve dosage of 4 tablets/day by end of week. May then increase in increments of up to 20 mg/week, if needed and tolerated, to a maximum of 60 mg/day given in two to four divided doses. Once maximum clinical response occurs, dosage may be lowered slowly over several weeks if it doesn't jeopardize therapeutic response.

Contraindications
- Hypersensitivity to drug
- Concurrent use of other MAO inhibitors, dibenzazepine derivatives, selective serotonin reuptake inhibitors (SSRIs), tricyclic antidepressants (TCAs), sympathomimetics (including amphetamines), certain CNS depressants (including opioids), sedatives, antihypertensives, antihistamines, thiazide diuretics, anesthetics, bupropion, buspirone, or dextromethorphan
- Known or suspected cerebrovascular defect
- Hypertension, cardiovascular disease
- Severe or frequent headache
- Pheochromocytoma
- Hepatic disease, abnormal liver function tests
- Renal disease
- Consumption of tyramine-rich foods (such as aged cheeses) or excessive amounts of caffeine

Precautions
Use cautiously in:
- hyperthyroidism, seizure disorders, hypotension, diabetes mellitus, myocardial ischemia, hypomania
- patients switching MAO inhibitors
- suicidal or drug-dependent patients
- elderly patients
- pregnant or breastfeeding patients
- children younger than age 16 (safety and efficacy not established).

Administration
- If hypertensive crisis occurs, withdraw drug immediately and give phentolamine 5 mg I.V. slowly, as ordered.
- Ask patient about other drugs he's using. MAO inhibitors can cause dangerous interactions with many drugs.
- Know that psychotropics should be withheld for 14 days after isocarboxazid withdrawal.

Route	Onset	Peak	Duration
P.O.	Unknown	Unknown	Unknown

Adverse reactions
CNS: drowsiness, anxiety, forgetfulness, hyperactivity, lethargy, sedation, syncope, headache, insomnia, sleep disturbance, tremor, myoclonic jerks, paresthesia, dizziness, **suicidal behavior or ideation** (especially in child or adolescent)
CV: orthostatic hypotension, palpitations, **hypertensive crisis**
GI: nausea, diarrhea, constipation, dry mouth
GU: urinary frequency, urinary hesitancy, erectile dysfunction
Hepatic: jaundice, **hepatotoxicity**
Musculoskeletal: heavy feeling

Skin: sweating
Other: chills

Interactions

Drug-drug. *Amphetamines, CNS depressants, dextromethorphan, dibenzazepine derivatives and other TCAs, other MAO inhibitors, SSRIs (such as fluoxetine, paroxetine), sympathomimetics:* hypertensive crisis, seizures, fever, diaphoresis, excitation, delirium, tremor, coma, circulatory collapse
Anesthetics: severe hypotension
Antidepressants, bupropion, buspirone: hypertension
Antihypertensives, beta-adrenergic blockers, thiazide diuretics: increased hypotensive effects
Dextromethorphan, tryptophan: hypertension, excitation, hyperpyrexia
Disulfiram: severe toxicity
Epinephrine, guanadrel, guanethidine, norepinephrine, reserpine, vasoconstrictors: hypertensive crisis
Insulin, oral hypoglycemics: additive hypoglycemia
Meperidine: severe hypertension or hypotension, respiratory depression, seizures, malignant hyperpyrexia, excitation, peripheral vascular collapse, coma, death
Drug-diagnostic tests. *Liver function tests:* altered results
Drug-food. *Excessive caffeine consumption:* nervousness, shakiness, rapid heartbeat, anxiety
Foods high in tyramine, such as cheese (especially aged cheeses), sour cream, Chianti wine, sherry, beer (including nonalcoholic beer), liqueurs, pickled herring, anchovies, caviar, liver, canned figs, raisins, bananas, avocados, soy sauce, sauerkraut, pods of broad beans (such as fava beans), yeast extracts, yogurt, meat extracts, meat prepared with tenderizers, dry sausage: hypertensive crisis
Drug-behaviors. *Alcohol use:* potential for severe hypertension, excitation, seizures, delirium, hyperpyrexia, circulatory collapse, coma, death

Patient monitoring

🔊 Monitor blood pressure frequently. Drug may cause hypertensive crisis.
🔊 Watch for increased depression and suicidal ideation, especially in child or adolescent.
🔊 Monitor liver function tests. Assess for jaundice and signs and symptoms of hepatic dysfunction; discontinue drug and notify prescriber if these occur.

Patient teaching

- Explain importance of taking drug exactly as prescribed.

🔊 Caution patient not to stop therapy suddenly. Dosage must be tapered.
🔊 Instruct patient to immediately report occipital headache, palpitations, stiff neck, nausea, sweating, dilated pupils, and photophobia (indications of hypertensive crisis).
🔊 Tell patient to immediately report rash, hives, itching, shortness of breath, wheezing, cough, or swelling of face, lips, tongue, or throat.
🔊 Advise patient (or caregiver, as appropriate) to monitor his mental status carefully and immediately report increased depression or suicidal thoughts or behavior (especially in child or adolescent).
🔊 Stress importance of avoiding certain foods and beverages (especially those containing tyramine) and over-the-counter preparations during and for 14 days after therapy. Inform patient that pharmacist can provide complete list of foods to avoid.

- Instruct patient to tell all prescribers he's taking drug.

🔊 Caution patient not drink alcohol or consume excessive amounts of caffeine.

- Advise patient to rise slowly from a lying or sitting position, to avoid dizziness.
- Caution patient to avoid driving and other hazardous activities until he

knows how drug affects concentration, vision, and alertness.
• Tell patient to discontinue drug at least 10 days before elective surgery.
• As appropriate, review all other significant and life-threatening adverse reactions and interactions, especially those related to the drugs, tests, foods, and behaviors mentioned above.

isoniazid (INH)

Isotamine✦, Laniazid, Nydrazid, PMS Isoniazid✦

Pharmacologic class: Isonicotinic acid hydrazide
Therapeutic class: Antitubercular
Pregnancy risk category C

Action

Inhibits cell-wall biosynthesis by interfering with lipid and nucleic acid DNA synthesis in tubercle bacilli cells

Availability

Injection: 100 mg/ml
Syrup: 50 mg/5 ml
Tablets: 100 mg, 300 mg

Indications and dosages

➢ Active tuberculosis (TB)
Adults: 5 mg/kg P.O. or I.M. (maximum of 300 mg/day) daily as a single dose, or 15 mg/kg (maximum of 900 mg/day) two to three times weekly; given with other agents
Children: 10 to 15 mg/kg P.O. or I.M. (maximum of 300 mg/day) daily as a single dose, or 20 to 40 mg/kg (maximum of 900 mg/day) two to three times weekly
➢ To prevent TB in patients exposed to active disease
Adults: 300 mg P.O. daily as a single dose for 6 to 12 months
Children and infants: 10 mg/kg P.O. daily as a single dose for up to 12 months

Off-label uses

• *Mycobacterium kansasii* infection

Contraindications

• Hypersensitivity to drug
• Acute hepatic disease or previous hepatitis caused by isoniazid therapy

Precautions

Use cautiously in:
• severe renal impairment, diabetes, diabetic retinopathy, ocular defects, chronic alcoholism, hepatic damage
• Black or Hispanic women
• pregnant or breastfeeding patients
• children ages 13 and younger.

Administration

• Give on empty stomach 1 hour before or 2 hours after meals. If GI upset occurs, administer with food.
• Administer parenterally only if patient can't receive oral form.
• Use cautiously in diabetic or alcoholic patients and those at risk for neuropathy.

Route	Onset	Peak	Duration
P.O., I.M.	Rapid	1-2 hr	Up to 24 hr

Adverse reactions

CNS: peripheral neuropathy, dizziness, memory impairment, slurred speech, psychosis, **toxic encephalopathy, seizures**
EENT: visual disturbances
GI: nausea, vomiting
GU: gynecomastia
Hematologic: eosinophilia, **methemoglobinemia, hemolytic anemia, aplastic anemia, agranulocytosis, thrombocytopenia**
Hepatic: hepatitis
Metabolic: pyridoxine deficiency, hyperglycemia, **metabolic acidosis**
Respiratory: dyspnea

Other: fever, pellagra, lupuslike syndrome, injection site irritation, hypersensitivity reaction

Interactions

Drug-drug. *Aluminum-containing antacids:* decreased isoniazid absorption
Bacille Calmette-Guérin vaccine: ineffective vaccination
Carbamazepine: increased carbamazepine blood level
Disulfiram: psychotic reactions, incoordination
Hepatotoxic drugs: increased risk of hepatotoxicity
Ketoconazole: decreased ketoconazole blood level and efficacy
Other antituberculars: additive CNS toxicity
Phenytoin: inhibition of phenytoin metabolism
Drug-diagnostic tests. *Albumin:* increased level
Drug-food. *Foods containing tyramine:* hypertensive crisis, other severe reactions
Drug-behaviors. *Alcohol use:* increased risk of hepatitis

Patient monitoring

- Assess hepatic enzyme levels.
- Watch for adverse reactions, such as peripheral neuropathy.

Patient teaching

- Advise patient to take once daily on empty stomach, 1 hour before or 2 hours after meals. If GI upset occurs, tell him to take with small amount of food.
- Caution patient to avoid foods containing tyramine (such as cheese, fish, salami, red wine, and yeast extracts), because drug-food interaction may cause chills, diaphoresis, and palpitations.
- Teach patient with peripheral neuropathy to take care to prevent burns and other injuries.
- Instruct patient to report anorexia, nausea, vomiting, jaundice, dark urine, and numbness or tingling of hands or feet.
- Tell patient he'll need periodic medical and eye examinations and blood tests to gauge drug effects.
- As appropriate, review all other significant and life-threatening adverse reactions and interactions, especially those related to the drugs, tests, foods, and behaviors mentioned above.

isoproterenol hydrochloride

Isuprel

Pharmacologic class: Sympathomimetic, $beta_1$-adrenergic and $beta_2$-adrenergic agonist

Therapeutic class: Vasopressor, bronchodilator, antiasthmatic

Pregnancy risk category C

Action

Acts on $beta_2$-adrenergic receptors, causing relaxation of bronchial smooth muscle; acts on $beta_1$-adrenergic receptors in heart, causing positive inotropic and chronotropic effects and increasing cardiac output. Also lowers peripheral vascular resistance in skeletal muscle and inhibits antigen-induced histamine release.

Availability

Injection: 20 mcg/ml, 200 mcg/ml

Indications and dosages

➢ Shock

Adults and children: 0.5 to 5 mcg/minute by continuous I.V. infusion

➢ Heart block; ventricular arrhythmias

Adults: Initially, 0.02 to 0.06 mg I.V., then 0.01 to 0.2 mg I.V. or 5 mcg/

minute I.V. Or initially, 0.2 mg I.M., then 0.02 to 1 mg I.M., depending on response. Or initially, 0.2 mg subcutaneously, then 0.15 to 0.2 mg subcutaneously, depending on response.

➢ Bronchospasm during anesthesia
Adults: 0.01 to 0.02 mg I.V., repeated when necessary

➢ Status asthmaticus
Children: 0.08 to 1.7 mcg/kg/minute by I.V. infusion

Contraindications

- Angina pectoris
- Angle-closure glaucoma
- Tachyarrhythmias
- Tachycardia or heart block caused by digitalis intoxication
- Ventricular arrhythmias that warrant inotropic therapy
- Labor, delivery, breastfeeding

Precautions

Use cautiously in:

- renal impairment, unstable vasomotor disorders, hypertension, coronary insufficiency, chronic obstructive pulmonary disease, diabetes mellitus, hyperthyroidism
- history of cerebrovascular accident or seizures
- elderly patients.

Administration

- Give each 0.02-mg I.V. dose by direct injection over 1 minute, or by I.V. infusion, as ordered. Always use continuous infusion pump to deliver infusion.

Route	Onset	Peak	Duration
I.V.	Immediate	Unknown	<1 hr
I.M.	Unknown	Unknown	Unknown
Subcut.	Immediate	Unknown	2hr

Adverse reactions

CNS: tremors, anxiety, insomnia, headache, dizziness, asthenia
CV: palpitations, tachycardia, angina, rapid blood pressure changes, **arrhythmias, cardiac arrest, Stokes-Adams attacks**
EENT: pharyngitis
GI: nausea, vomiting, heartburn
Metabolic: hyperglycemia
Respiratory: bronchitis, increased sputum, **pulmonary edema, bronchospasm**
Skin: diaphoresis
Other: parotid gland swelling (with prolonged use)

Interactions

Drug-drug. *Cyclopropane, epinephrine, halogenated general anesthetics:* increased risk of arrhythmias
Propranolol, other beta-adrenergic blockers: antagonism of bronchodilating effects
Drug-diagnostic tests. *Glucose:* increased level

Patient monitoring

- During I.V. administration, monitor ECG and vital signs carefully.
- Assess patient's response to drug and adjust I.V. infusion rate accordingly.
- Closely monitor arterial blood gas values, urine output, and central venous pressure.

🔊 Stay alert for rebound bronchospasm.

Patient teaching

- Assure patient that he'll be monitored closely.

isosorbide dinitrate

Apo-ISDN✱, Cedocard-SR✱, Dilatrate-SR, Isordil, Isordil Tembids, Isordil Titradose

isosorbide mononitrate

Imdur, ISMO, Monoket

Pharmacologic class: Nitrate
Therapeutic class: Antianginal
Pregnancy risk category C

Action

Promotes peripheral vasodilation and reduces preload and afterload, decreasing myocardial oxygen consumption and increasing cardiac output. Also dilates coronary arteries, increasing blood flow and improving collateral circulation.

Availability

isosorbide dinitrate
Capsules: 40 mg
Capsules (extended-release): 40 mg
Tablets: 2.5 mg, 5 mg, 10 mg, 20 mg, 30 mg, 40 mg
Tablets (chewable): 5 mg, 10 mg
Tablets (extended-release): 20 mg, 40 mg
Tablets (sublingual): 2.5 mg, 5 mg, 10 mg
isosorbide mononitrate
Tablets: 10 mg, 20 mg
Tablets (extended-release): 30 mg, 60 mg, 120 mg

Indications and dosages

➢ Treatment and prophylaxis in situations likely to provoke acute angina pectoris
Adults: 2.5 to 5 mg S.L. May repeat dose q 5 to 10 minutes for a total of three doses in 15 to 30 minutes.
➢ Prophylaxis of angina pectoris
Adults: 5 to 40 mg P.O. (dinitrate conventional tablets) two to three times daily. Or 5 to 20 mg (mononitrate conventional tablets) b.i.d. Or 30 to 60 mg (mononitrate extended-release tablets) once daily. Maximum dosage is 120 mg/day.

Off-label uses

- Heart failure

Contraindications

- Hypersensitivity to drug
- Severe anemia
- Acute myocardial infarction
- Angle-closure glaucoma
- Concurrent sildenafil therapy

Precautions

Use cautiously in:
- head trauma, volume depletion
- elderly patients
- pregnant or breastfeeding patients
- children.

Administration

- Give oral form 30 minutes before or 1 to 2 hours after a meal. Make sure patient swallows tablets or capsules whole.
- Have patient wet S.L. tablet with saliva before placing it under tongue. To avoid tingling sensation, have him place tablet in buccal pouch.

Route	Onset	Peak	Duration
P.O. (dinitrate)	15-40 min	Unknown	4 hr
P.O. (dinitrate, extended)	30 min	Unknown	≤12 hr
P.O. (mononitrate)	30-60 min	Unknown	7 hr
P.O. (mononitrate, extended)	Unknown	Unknown	12 hr
S.L. (dinitrate)	2-5 min	Unknown	1-2 hr

Adverse reactions

CNS: dizziness, headache, apprehension, asthenia, syncope
CV: orthostatic hypotension, tachycardia, paradoxical bradycardia
EENT: sublingual burning (with S.L. route)
GI: nausea, vomiting, abdominal pain
Skin: flushing

Interactions

Drug-drug. *Aspirin:* increased isosorbide blood level and effects
Beta-adrenergic blockers, calcium channel blockers, phenothiazines: additive hypotension
Dihydroergotamine: antagonism of dihydroergotamine effects
Sildenafil: severe and potentially fatal hypotension
Drug-diagnostic tests. *Cholesterol:* decreased level
Methemoglobin, urine vanillylmandelic acid: increased levels

Patient monitoring

- Monitor ECG and vital signs closely, especially blood pressure.

Clinical alert: In suspected overdose, assess for signs and symptoms of increased intracranial pressure.

- Monitor arterial blood gas values and methemoglobin levels.

Patient teaching

- Teach patient to take oral drug 30 minutes before or 1 to 2 hours after a meal.
- Inform patient that drug may cause headache. Advise him to treat headache as usual and not to alter drug schedule. If headache persists, tell him to contact prescriber.
- Instruct patient to move slowly when sitting up or standing, to avoid dizziness or light-headedness from sudden blood pressure decrease.
- As appropriate, review all other significant adverse reactions and interactions, especially those related to the drugs and tests mentioned above.

isradipine

DynaCirc, DynaCirc CR

Pharmacologic class: Calcium channel blocker
Therapeutic class: Antihypertensive
Pregnancy risk category C

Action

Inhibits calcium ion movement across cell membranes of cardiac and arterial muscles, relaxing coronary and peripheral vascular smooth muscle. This action reduces diastolic blood pressure, enhances left ventricular function, and improves ejection rates; it also reduces mean vascular and systemic vascular resistance, increasing cardiac output and improving stroke volume.

Availability

Capsules: 2.5 mg, 5 mg
Tablets (controlled-release): 5 mg, 10 mg

Indications and dosages

➢ Hypertension

Adults: Initially, 2.5 mg P.O. b.i.d. as monotherapy or combined with a thiazide diuretic (regular-release capsules); may increase in increments of 5 mg/day at 2- to 4-week intervals, to a maximum of 20 mg/day. Or, 5 to 10 mg P.O. (controlled-release) daily as monotherapy or combined with a thiazide diuretic.

Contraindications

- Hypersensitivity to drug or other calcium channel blockers

Precautions

Use cautiously in:

- heart disease, hypotension, hepatic

or renal disease, GI hypermotility or obstruction (controlled-release form)
• concurrent use of beta-adrenergic blockers
• elderly patients
• pregnant or breastfeeding patients
• children.

Administration
• Give with or without food.
• Don't give with grapefruit juice.
• Don't crush or break controlled-release tablets. Make sure patient swallows them whole.

Route	Onset	Peak	Duration
P.O.	2 hr	Unknown	Unknown
P.O. (controlled)	Unknown	Unknown	Unknown

Adverse reactions
CNS: dizziness, headache, fatigue, syncope, sleep disturbances
CV: peripheral edema, tachycardia, hypotension, chest pain, **arrhythmias**
GI: nausea, vomiting, constipation, abdominal pain or distention, dry mouth
GU: nocturia, urinary frequency
Hematologic: leukopenia
Hepatic: hepatitis
Skin: rash, pruritus, urticaria
Other: flushing

Interactions
Drug-drug. *Atracurium, gallamine, pancuronium, tubocurarine, vecuronium:* increased respiratory depression
Beta-adrenergic blockers: increased cardiac depression
Carbamazepine, digoxin, prazosin, quinidine: increased blood levels of these drugs
Drug-food. *Grapefruit juice:* increased drug absorption

Patient monitoring
• Monitor vital signs closely, especially blood pressure.
• Assess liver function test results.
• Monitor for arrhythmias and peripheral edema.

Patient teaching
• Tell patient he may take with or without food, but not with grapefruit juice.
• Instruct patient to move slowly when sitting up or standing, to avoid dizziness or light-headedness from sudden blood pressure decrease.
• Caution patient to avoid driving and other hazardous activities until he knows how drug affects concentration and alertness.
• Teach patient with heart, kidney, or liver disease to watch for and promptly report adverse reactions.
• As appropriate, review all other significant and life-threatening adverse reactions and interactions, especially those related to the drugs and foods mentioned above.

itraconazole
Sporanox

Pharmacologic class: Synthetic triazole
Therapeutic class: Antifungal
Pregnancy risk category C

Action
Prevents ergosterol synthesis in fungal cell membranes, altering membrane permeability

Availability
Capsules: 100 mg
Injection: 10 mg/ml, 250-mg ampules
Oral solution: 10 mg/ml

Indications and dosages
➤ Aspergillosis; blastomycosis; histoplasmosis
Adults: 200 to 400 mg P.O. daily for at least 3 months until patient is cured. In

life-threatening infections, loading dose of 200 mg P.O. t.i.d. for 3 days, then 200 to 400 mg P.O. daily until cured. Or 200 mg I.V. b.i.d. for four doses, then 200 mg P.O. daily; continue combination of I.V. and P.O. regimen for at least 3 months.

➢ Esophageal candidiasis

Adults: 100 to 200 mg of oral solution daily, swished in mouth for several seconds and swallowed, for at least 3 weeks; continue for 2 weeks after symptoms resolve.

➢ Oropharyngeal candidiasis

Adults: 200 mg of oral solution daily, swished in mouth for several seconds and swallowed, for 1 to 2 weeks

➢ Febrile neutropenic patients with suspected fungal infections

Adults: 200 mg I.V. b.i.d. for four doses, then 200 mg daily for up to 14 days. Continue with 200 mg of oral solution b.i.d. until neutropenia resolves.

➢ Onychomycosis; tinea unguium

Adults: For toenails, 200 mg P.O. daily for 12 weeks. For fingernails, 200 mg b.i.d. for 1 week; wait 3 weeks, then repeat dosage for 1 week.

Contraindications

- Hypersensitivity to drug or its components
- Fungal meningitis
- Ventricular dysfunction, heart failure (in onychomycosis use)
- Concomitant use of astemizole, cisapride, dofetilide, lovastatin, midazolam, pimozide, quinidine, simvastatin, or triazolam
- Pregnancy or anticipated pregnancy (in onychomycosis use)

Precautions

Use cautiously in:

- hypersensitivity to other azole derivatives
- renal impairment (with I.V. use), hepatic disorders, achlorhydria, hypochlorhydria
- breastfeeding patients
- children (safety and efficacy not established).

Administration

- Obtain specimens for fungal cultures, as needed, before starting therapy.
- Administer capsule with a full meal.
- Give oral solution without food when possible.
- For I.V. use, dilute contents of 250-mg ampule in 50-ml bag of normal saline solution, to yield a final concentration of 75 ml of 3.33 mg/ml. Infuse over 1 hour. Don't mix with or give in same I.V. line with other drugs. After infusion, flush through two-way stopcock with 15 to 20 ml of normal saline solution for 30 seconds to 15 minutes.
- Be aware that liquid and tablets aren't interchangeable.

Route	Onset	Peak	Duration
P.O.	Slow	4-6 hr	4-6 days
I.V.	Rapid	Unknown	End of infusion

Adverse reactions

CNS: dizziness, headache, fatigue, malaise

CV: peripheral edema, tachycardia, **heart failure**

EENT: rhinitis

GI: nausea, vomiting, constipation, abdominal pain, flatulence, anorexia, dyspepsia

GU: albuminuria, erectile dysfunction

Hepatic: jaundice, **hepatotoxicity** (including **hepatic failure and death**)

Metabolic: hypokalemia

Musculoskeletal: myalgia, bursitis, **rhabdomyolysis**

Respiratory: pulmonary edema

Skin: flushing, rash, pruritus, urticaria, increased sweating, herpes zoster infection

Other: fever, pain

Interactions

Drug-drug. *Alfentanil, antihistamines (minimally sedating agents, such as fexofenadine, loratadine), antineoplastics (busulfan, docetaxel, vinca alkaloids), anxiolytics, benzodiazepines, cyclosporine, delavirdine, digoxin, immunosuppressants, methylprednisolone, protease inhibitors, tacrolimus, tolterodine, tretinoin:* increased blood levels of these drugs
Amiodarone, anabolic steroids, androgens, antithyroid drugs, carmustine, chloroquine, dantrolene, daunorubicin, disulfiram, estrogens, gold salts, hormonal contraceptives, hydroxychloroquine, mercaptopurine, methotrexate, methyldopa, naltrexone (with long-term use), valproic acid: increased risk of hepatic damage
Amphotericin B: reduced or inhibited amphotericin B effects
Antacids, anticonvulsants, antimycobacterials, cyclobenzaprine, histamine$_2$-receptor blockers, isoniazid, proton pump inhibitors (such as lansoprazole, omeprazole), reverse transcriptase inhibitors, sucralfate: reduced itraconazole blood level
Antipsychotics, antiarrhythmics (such as quinidine, dofetilide), anxiolytics, astemizole, cisapride: increased risk of serious cardiovascular effects
Calcium channel blockers: increased risk of edema, possible increase in itraconazole's effect
Carbamazepine, carbidopa, levodopa: altered blood levels of these drugs
Didanosine, vinblastine, vincristine, xanthine bronchodilators: decreased efficacy of these drugs
Digoxin: increased digoxin blood level, possible digoxin toxicity
HMG-CoA reductase inhibitors, miconazole: inhibited metabolism of these drugs, increased risk of skeletal muscle toxicity (including rhabdomyolysis)
Macrolide antibiotics: increased itraconazole blood level
Oral hypoglycemics: severe blood glucose decrease
Quetiapine, sildenafil: increased efficacy of these drugs
Warfarin: enhanced anticoagulant effect
Drug-diagnostic tests. *Alanine aminotransferase, alkaline phosphatase, aspartate aminotransferase, blood urea nitrogen, gamma-glutamyltransferase, serum creatinine:* increased levels
Lactate dehydrogenase: increased level (with I.V. use)
Potassium, magnesium: decreased levels
Drug-food. *Any food, cola:* increased itraconazole blood level
Grapefruit juice: decreased blood level and reduced therapeutic effects of itraconazole
Drug-herbs. *Chaparral, comfrey, germander, jin bu huan, kava:* increased risk of hepatic damage
Drug-behaviors. *Alcohol consumption:* toxic reaction, hepatic damage

Patient monitoring

- In patient with hepatic dysfunction, monitor hepatic enzyme levels.

◀ Monitor for signs and symptoms of hepatic dysfunction (jaundice, fatigue, nausea, vomiting, dark urine, pale stools), heart failure, muscle disorder, and pulmonary or peripheral edema.

- Monitor potassium level. Stay alert for hypokalemia.

Patient teaching

- Tell patient he may take capsule with a full meal. If he's using oral solution, advise him to take it without food.
- Inform patient that drug interacts with many other drugs. Advise him to tell all prescribers he's taking it.

◀ Teach patient to recognize and immediately report signs and symptoms of hepatic dysfunction, persistent muscle pain, and heart failure.

- Caution patient to avoid driving and other hazardous activities until he

knows how drug affects concentration and alertness.

- Advise female patient of childbearing potential to use effective contraception during and for 1 month after therapy. Caution her not to breastfeed.
- As appropriate, review all other significant and life-threatening adverse reactions and interactions, especially those related to the drugs, tests, foods, herbs, and behaviors mentioned above.

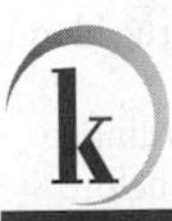

kanamycin sulfate

Kantrex

Pharmacologic class: Aminoglycoside
Therapeutic class: Anti-infective
Pregnancy risk category D

Action

Interferes with protein synthesis in bacterial cells by binding to 30S ribosomal subunit, causing misreading of genetic code. Inaccurate peptide sequence in protein chain leads to bacterial death.

Availability

Capsules: 500 mg
Injection: 75 mg/2 ml, 500 mg/2 ml, 1,000 mg/3 ml

Indications and dosages

➢ Serious infections caused by susceptible organisms
Adults and children: 7.5 mg/kg I.V. or I.M. q 12 hours. If a continuously high drug blood level is desired, may give 15 mg/kg/day in equally divided doses q 6 or 8 hours, not to exceed 1.5 g/day.

➢ Hepatic coma
Adults: 8 to 12 g/day P.O. in divided doses q 6 hours

➢ Bowel sterilization
Adults: 1 g P.O. q hour for 4 hours, then 1 g q 6 hours for 36 to 72 hours

Dosage adjustment

- Renal impairment
- Elderly patients

Contraindications

- Hypersensitivity or toxic reaction to drug or other aminoglycosides
- Intestinal obstruction

Precautions

Use cautiously in:

- renal impairment, neuromuscular diseases (such as myasthenia gravis), hearing impairment, obesity
- elderly patients
- pregnant or breastfeeding patients
- infants and neonates (safety not established).

Administration

- Collect specimens for culture and sensitivity testing, as appropriate, before therapy starts.
- Keep patient well hydrated; drug may cause nephrotoxicity.
- Administer I.M. injection deep into a large muscle.
- Reconstitute I.V. dose by mixing 500 mg in 100 to 200 ml of normal saline solution or dextrose 5% in water, or by adding 1g to 200 to 400 ml of either solution.
- Infuse total single dose I.V. over 30 to 60 minutes at a rate no faster than 3 to 4 ml/minute.

Route	Onset	Peak	Duration
P.O.	Slow	Unknown	Unknown
I.V.	Immediate	15-30 min	Unknown
I.M.	Rapid	30-90 min	Unknown

Adverse reactions

CNS: dizziness, vertigo, tremors, numbness, depression, confusion, lethargy, headache, paresthesia, **neuro-**

muscular blockade, seizures, neurotoxicity
CV: hypotension, hypertension, palpitations
EENT: visual disturbances, dry eyes, nystagmus, photophobia, hearing loss, tinnitus, ototoxicity
GI: nausea, vomiting, anorexia, splenomegaly, stomatitis, increased salivation
GU: polyuria, dysuria, azotemia, increased urinary cast excretion, erectile dysfunction, **nephrotoxicity**
Hematologic: purpura, eosinophilia, **leukemoid reaction, hemolytic anemia, aplastic anemia, neutropenia, agranulocytosis, leukopenia, thrombocytopenia, pancytopenia**
Hepatic: hepatomegaly, hepatic necrosis, hepatotoxicity
Musculoskeletal: joint pain, muscle twitching
Respiratory: apnea
Skin: rash, urticaria, pruritus, exfoliative dermatitis, alopecia
Other: weight loss, superinfection, pain and irritation at I.M. site

Interactions

Drug-drug. *Acyclovir, amphotericin B, cisplatin, potent diuretics, vancomycin:* increased risk of ototoxicity and nephrotoxicity
Dimenhydrinate: masking of ototoxicity symptoms
General anesthetics, neuromuscular junction blockers: increased neuromuscular blockade
Indomethacin: increased kanamycin peak and trough blood levels
Parenteral penicillins (such as ampicillin, ticarcillin), cephalosporins: kanamycin inactivation
Drug-diagnostic tests. *Alanine aminotransferase, aspartate aminotransferase, bilirubin, blood urea nitrogen (BUN), creatinine, low-density lipoproteins, nonprotein nitrogen:* increased levels
Granulocytes, hemoglobin, platelets, white blood cells: decreased levels
Reticulocytes: increased or decreased count

Patient monitoring

- Monitor urine output, urinalysis, BUN, and creatinine level.
- Evaluate cardiovascular status carefully.
- Assess neurologic status. Institute safety measures as needed to prevent injury.
- Monitor peak and trough drug blood levels.
- Check for hearing loss according to baseline audiogram recorded before first dose.
- Assess for bleeding tendency.

Patient teaching

- 🔊 Instruct patient to immediately report unusual bleeding or bruising, unusual tiredness, or yellowing of skin or eyes.
- Tell patient to promptly report tinnitus or difficulty hearing.
- Instruct patient to maintain adequate hydration and report change in urination pattern.
- Tell patient to avoid activities that can cause injury. Advise him to use soft toothbrush and electric razor to avoid gum and skin injury.
- Caution patient to avoid driving and other hazardous activities until he knows how drug affects concentration and alertness.
- Tell patient he'll undergo regular blood testing during therapy.
- As appropriate, review all other significant and life-threatening adverse reactions and interactions, especially those related to the drugs and tests mentioned above.

kaolin and pectin

Donnagel MB✱, Kao-Spen, Kapectolin, K-P

Pharmacologic class: Adsorbent
Therapeutic class: Antidiarrheal
Pregnancy risk category NR

Action

Kaolin is thought to adsorb bacteria and toxins and reduce water loss. Pectin action is unknown.

Availability

Oral suspension: 5.2 g kaolin/260 mg pectin per 30 ml, 5.85 g kaolin/130 mg pectin per 30 ml

Indications and dosages

➤ Mild to moderately acute diarrhea
Adults: 60 to 120 ml P.O. after each loose bowel movement
Children ages 12 and older: 45 to 60 ml P.O. after each loose bowel movement
Children ages 6 to 12: 30 to 60 ml P.O. after each loose bowel movement
Children ages 3 to 6: 15 to 30 ml P.O. after each loose bowel movement

Contraindications

None

Precautions

Use cautiously in:

- dehydration, acute dysentery, suspected parasite-associated diarrhea
- elderly patients
- infants and children younger than age 3 with diarrhea.

Administration

- Give 2 to 3 hours before or after other oral drugs.
- Know that in children, drug should be accompanied by rehydration therapy.
- Be aware that in acute dysentery, sole treatment with kaolin/pectin (or other adsorbent diarrheals) may be inadequate and patient may need antibiotics.
- Know that in suspected parasite-associated diarrhea, use of kaolin/pectin may complicate recognition of parasitic cause. If parasite is suspected, stools should be analyzed before adsorbent therapy begins.

Route	Onset	Peak	Duration
P.O.	NA	NA	NA

Adverse reactions

GI: constipation, fecal impaction

Interactions

Drug-drug. *Anticholinergics, antidyskinetics, cardiac glycosides, lincomycins, loxapine, phenothiazines, thioxanthenes:* decreased efficacy of these drugs
Other oral drugs: reduced absorption of these drugs

Patient monitoring

- Assess frequency and consistency of bowel movements.
- Watch for signs and symptoms of dehydration, especially in children. Be aware that children should receive rehydration therapy.
- Know that kaolin/pectin may make feces more solid and decrease frequency of evacuation.

Patient teaching

- Advise patient to consume plenty of clear liquids (such as gelatin, broth, and ginger ale) for first 24 hours.
- Tell patient to consume bland foods (such as bread, cooked cereals, and applesauce) and avoid spicy or sweet foods, bran, fruits, vegetables, caffeine, and alcohol during second 24 hours.
- Instruct patient to contact physician if he experiences fever, bloody stools, or signs and symptoms of dehydration (such as decreased urination, dry skin,

increased thirst, dizziness, or lightheadedness), or if diarrhea is not controlled within 48 hours.

• As appropriate, review all other significant adverse reactions and interactions, especially those related to the drugs mentioned above.

ketoconazole

Ketozole, Nizoral, Nizoral A-D

Pharmacologic class: Imidazole
Therapeutic class: Antifungal
Pregnancy risk category C

Action

Alters fungal cell membranes, resulting in increased permeability, growth inhibition, and ultimately, cell death

Availability

Cream: 2%
Shampoo: 1%, 2%
Tablets: 200 mg

Indications and dosages

➢ Blastomycosis; chronic mucocutaneous candidiasis; oral thrush; candiduria; coccidioidomycosis; histoplasmosis; chromomycosis; paracoccidioidomycosis; mucocutaneous or vaginal candidiasis
Adults: 200 to 400 mg P.O. daily
Children ages 2 and older: 3.3 to 6.6 mg/kg P.O. as a single daily dose. Duration depends on infection: for candidiasis, 1 to 2 weeks; other systemic mycoses, 6 months; recalcitrant dermatophyte infections involving glabrous skin, 4 weeks. Chronic mucocutaneous candidiasis requires maintenance therapy.

➢ Scaling caused by dandruff or seborrheic dermatitis
Adults: 2% shampoo applied topically twice weekly for 4 weeks, then as needed to control symptoms; or 1% shampoo applied topically q 3 to 4 days for up to 8 weeks, then as needed to control dandruff

➢ Tinea corporis; tinea cruris; tinea versicolor; tinea pedis
Adults: 2% cream applied topically to affected areas daily for 2 weeks (except for tinea pedis, which may require 6 weeks of therapy)

Contraindications

• Hypersensitivity to drug or its components
• Concurrent oral astemizole, cisapride, triazolam, or terfenadine therapy

Precautions

Use cautiously in:
• renal or hepatic disease, achlorhydria
• pregnant or breastfeeding patients
• children younger than age 2.

Administration

• Apply cream to damp skin of affected area and wide surrounding area.
• To use shampoo, wet hair, then apply shampoo and massage into scalp for 1 minute. Leave on for 5 minutes before rinsing. Rinse and repeat, this time leaving shampoo on scalp for 3 minutes before rinsing.
• Don't apply shampoo to broken or inflamed skin.
• In achlorhydria, dissolve 200-mg tablet in 4 ml of 0.2N hydrochloric acid solution.
• Withhold antacids for at least 2 hours after giving oral ketoconazole.
Clinical alert: Don't give concurrently with cisapride, available in U.S. for compassionate use only. (Astemizole and terfenadine are not available in U.S.)

Route	Onset	Peak	Duration
P.O.	Unknown	1-2 hr	Unknown
Topical	Unknown	Unknown	Unknown

Adverse reactions

CNS: headache, nervousness, dizziness, drowsiness, severe depression, **suicidal ideation**
EENT: photophobia
GI: nausea, vomiting, diarrhea, abdominal pain, anorexia
GU: erectile dysfunction, gynecomastia
Hematologic: purpura, **hemolytic anemia, thrombocytopenia, leukopenia**
Hepatic: hepatotoxicity
Metabolic: hyperlipidemia
Skin: pruritus, rash, dermatitis, urticaria, severe irritation, stinging, alopecia, abnormal hair texture, scalp pustules, oily skin, dry hair and scalp
Other: fever, chills, allergic reaction

Interactions

Drug-drug. *Antacids, anticholinergics, histamine$_2$-receptor antagonists:* decreased ketoconazole absorption
Cyclosporine: increased cyclosporine blood level
Isoniazid, rifampin: increased ketoconazole metabolism
Theophylline: decreased theophylline blood level
Topical corticosteroids: increased corticosteroid absorption
Triazolam (oral): increased triazolam effects
Drug-diagnostic tests. *Alanine aminotransferase, alkaline phosphatase, aspartate aminotransferase:* increased levels
Hemoglobin, platelets, white blood cells: decreased levels
Drug-herbs. *Yew:* inhibited ketoconazole metabolism

Patient monitoring

🔊 Assess for suicidal ideation and signs and symptoms of depression.
🔊 Monitor for evidence of hepatotoxicity, such as nausea, fatigue, jaundice, dark urine, and pale stools.
- With long-term therapy, stay alert for adrenal crisis.

Patient teaching

🔊 Advise patient to watch for signs and symptoms of depression and to immediately report suicidal thoughts.
🔊 Teach patient to recognize and immediately report signs and symptoms of hepatotoxicity, such as unusual tiredness or yellowing of skin or eyes.
- Advise patient not to take antacids for at least 2 hours after oral ketoconazole.
- Instruct patient to apply cream to damp skin of affected area and wide surrounding area.
- Tell patient to wet hair before applying shampoo and to massage into scalp for 1 minute; then leave on for 5 minutes before rinsing off. Tell him to shampoo again, leaving it on for 3 minutes this time before rinsing.
- Caution patient not to apply shampoo to broken or inflamed skin.
- As appropriate, review all other significant and life-threatening adverse reactions and interactions, especially those related to the drugs, tests, and herbs mentioned above.

k

ketoprofen

Actron, Apo-Keto✱, Apo-Keto-E✱, Orudis KT, Orudis-SR✱, Oruvail, Rhodis✱

Pharmacologic class: Nonsteroidal anti-inflammatory drug (NSAID)
Therapeutic class: Analgesic, antipyretic, anti-inflammatory
Pregnancy risk category B (first and second trimesters), ***D*** (third trimester)

Action

Unknown. Thought to inhibit prostaglandin and leukotriene synthesis and possibly help stabilize lysosomal membranes. Also inhibits platelet aggregation and synthesis.

Availability

Capsules: 25 mg, 50 mg, 75 mg
Capsules (extended-release): 100 mg, 150 mg, 200 mg
Tablets: 12.5 mg

Indications and dosages

➤ Rheumatoid arthritis; osteoarthritis
Adults: 75 mg P.O. t.i.d. or 50 mg q.i.d. Maximum dosage is 200 mg/day (Oruvail) or 300 mg/day (Orudis).
➤ Primary dysmenorrhea
Adults: 25 to 50 mg P.O. q 6 to 8 hours p.r.n. If optimal response doesn't occur, may give up to 75 mg as a single dose. Maximum is 300 mg/day.
➤ Fever
Adults: One 12.5-mg tablet P.O. q 4 to 6 hours; give second dose if fever persists after 1 hour. Or initially, two 12.5-mg tablets P.O. Maximum dosage is two 12.5-mg tablets in 4 hours or six 12.5-mg tablets in 24 hours, continued no more than 3 days.
➤ Pain
Adults: 25 to 50 mg P.O. q 6 to 8 hours p.r.n.

Dosage adjustment

- Renal impairment
- Cirrhosis
- Elderly patients

Contraindications

- Hypersensitivity to drug, its components, or other NSAIDs
- Severe renal or hepatic disease
- Bleeding disorders

Precautions

Use cautiously in:

- tartrazine intolerance
- hepatic or renal disease (extended-release form), ulcer disease, GI bleeding or perforation, asthma, rhinitis, urticaria, chronic alcohol use or abuse
- elderly patients (extended-release form)
- pregnant patients in second or third trimester
- breastfeeding patients
- children.

Administration

- Give tablets either 30 minutes before or 2 hours after meals.
- Give capsules with food, milk, or antacids to minimize GI upset.

Route	Onset	Peak	Duration
P.O.	Within 1 hr	1-2 hr	4-6 hr
P.O. (extended)	Unknown	6-7 hr	≤24 hr

Adverse reactions

CNS: headache, dizziness, irritability
EENT: visual disturbances, tinnitus
GI: nausea, vomiting, diarrhea, constipation, abdominal pain or cramps, dyspepsia, flatulence, stomatitis, anorexia, **GI bleeding**
GU: urinary tract infection, renal impairment, **nephrotoxicity**
Hematologic: agranulocytosis
Skin: rash
Other: edema

Interactions

Drug-drug. *Angiotensin-converting enzyme inhibitors, beta-adrenergic blockers:* decreased antihypertensive effect
Anticoagulants: prolonged prothrombin time
Aspirin: altered ketoprofen distribution, metabolism, and excretion; increased risk of serious adverse reactions
Cholestyramine: decreased ketoprofen absorption
Corticosteroids, other NSAIDs: additive GI adverse reactions
Diuretics: decreased diuretic effect
Hydantoins, lithium: increased blood levels of these drugs, greater risk of toxicity
Methotrexate: increased risk of methotrexate toxicity

Probenecid: increased risk of ketoprofen toxicity
Drug-diagnostic tests. *Bleeding time:* prolonged
Blood urea nitrogen: increased
Drug-herbs. *Anise, arnica, chamomile, clove, dong quai, feverfew, garlic, ginger, ginkgo, ginseng:* increased bleeding risk

Patient monitoring

- Watch for adverse renal effects.
- Monitor closely for fluid retention in elderly patients and those with heart failure.

Patient teaching

Instruct patient to immediately report bleeding or change in urination pattern.

- Caution patient to avoid driving and other hazardous activities until he knows how drug affects concentration and alertness.
- Tell patient to consult prescriber before taking over-the-counter preparations (especially aspirin-containing products) or herbs.
- As appropriate, review all other significant and life-threatening adverse reactions and interactions, especially those related to the drugs, tests, and herbs mentioned above.

ketorolac tromethamine

Acular, Acular LS, Toradol

Pharmacologic class: Nonsteroidal anti-inflammatory drug (NSAID)

Therapeutic class: Analgesic, antipyretic, anti-inflammatory

Pregnancy risk category C (first and second trimesters), ***D*** (third trimester)

Action

Interferes with prostaglandin biosynthesis by inhibiting cyclooxygenase pathway of arachidonic acid metabolism; also acts as potent inhibitor of platelet aggregation

Availability

Injection: 15 mg/ml in 1-ml preloaded syringes, 30 mg/ml in 1- and 2-ml preloaded syringes
Ophthalmic solution: 0.4%, 0.5%
Tablets: 10 mg

Indications and dosages

➢ Moderately severe pain

Adults younger than age 65: Initially, 30 mg I.V. or 60 mg I.M. as a single dose, or 30 mg I.M. or I.V. q 6 hours, not to exceed 120 mg/day. To switch to P.O. therapy, 20 mg P.O. initially for patients who received single 30-mg I.V. or 60-mg I.M. dose, followed by 10 mg P.O. q 4 to 6 hours as needed (not to exceed 40 mg/day).
Children ages 2 to 16: 1 mg/kg I.M. as a single dose, to a maximum of 30 mg; or one dose of 0.5 mg/kg, to a maximum of 15 mg

➢ Ocular itching caused by seasonal allergic conjunctivitis

Adults and children ages 3 and older: One drop of 0.5% ophthalmic solution (Acular) instilled into affected eye q.i.d.

➢ Postoperative ocular inflammation related to cataract extraction

Adults and children ages 3 and older: One drop of 0.5% ophthalmic solution (Acular) instilled into operative eye q.i.d., starting 24 hours after surgery and continuing for 2 weeks

➢ To reduce ocular pain, burning, or stinging after corneal refractive surgery

Adults and children ages 3 and older: One drop of 0.4% ophthalmic solution (Acular LS) instilled into operative eye q.i.d. for up to 4 days

Dosage adjustment

- Mild to moderate renal impairment
- Elderly patients
- Patients weighing less than 50 kg (110 lb)

k

Contraindications

- Hypersensitivity to drug, its components, aspirin, or other NSAIDs
- Concurrent use of aspirin, other NSAIDs, or probenecid
- Peptic ulcer disease
- GI bleeding or perforation
- Advanced renal impairment, risk of renal failure
- Increased risk of bleeding, suspected or confirmed cerebrovascular bleeding, hemorrhagic diathesis, incomplete hemostasis
- Prophylactic use before major surgery, intraoperative use when hemostasis is critical
- Labor and delivery
- Breastfeeding

Precautions

Use cautiously in:

- mild to moderate renal impairment, cardiovascular disease
- elderly patients
- pregnant patients
- children.

Administration

- Be aware that oral therapy is indicated only as continuation of parenteral therapy.

Clinical alert: Know that parenteral therapy shouldn't exceed 20 doses in 5 days.

- For I.V. use, dilute with normal saline solution, dextrose 5% in water, dextrose 5% and normal saline solution, Ringer's solution, or lactated Ringer's solution.
- Administer single I.V. bolus over 1 to 2 minutes.
- Inject I.M. dose slowly and deeply.
- Don't give by epidural or intrathecal injection.

Route	Onset	Peak	Duration
P.O.	Unknown	2-3 hr	≥4-6 hr
I.V., I.M.	10 min	1-2 hr	≥6 hr
Ophthalmic	Unknown	Unknown	Unknown

Adverse reactions

CNS: drowsiness, headache, dizziness
CV: hypertension
EENT: tinnitus
GI: nausea, vomiting, diarrhea, constipation, flatulence, dyspepsia, epigastric pain, stomatitis
Hematologic: thrombocytopenia
Skin: rash, pruritus, diaphoresis
Other: excessive thirst, edema, injection site pain

Interactions

Drug-drug. *Angiotensin-converting enzyme inhibitors, beta-adrenergic blockers:* decreased antihypertensive effect
Anticoagulants: prolonged prothrombin time
Aspirin: altered ketorolac distribution, metabolism, and excretion; increased risk of serious adverse reactions
Cholestyramine: decreased ketorolac absorption
Corticosteroids, other NSAIDs: additive adverse GI effects
Diuretics: decreased diuretic effect
Hydantoins, lithium: increased blood levels and greater risk of toxicity of these drugs
Methotrexate: increased risk of methotrexate toxicity
Probenecid: increased risk of ketorolac toxicity
Drug-diagnostic tests. *Bleeding time:* prolonged for 24 to 48 hours after therapy ends
Drug-herbs. *Anise, arnica, chamomile, clove, dong quai, feverfew, garlic, ginger, ginkgo, ginseng:* increased risk of bleeding

Patient monitoring

- Monitor for adverse reactions, especially prolonged bleeding time and CNS reactions.
- Check I.M. injection site for hematoma and bleeding.
- Monitor fluid intake and output.

Patient teaching

- Inform patient that drug is meant only for short-term pain management.

Tell patient to immediately report bleeding and adverse CNS reactions.
- Advise patient to minimize GI upset by eating small, frequent servings of healthy foods.
- Instruct patient to avoid aspirin products and herbs during therapy.
- Teach patient how to use eye drops, if prescribed.
- Caution female patient not to take drug if she's breastfeeding.
- Advise patient to avoid driving and other hazardous activities until he knows how drug affects concentration and alertness.
- As appropriate, review all other significant and life-threatening adverse reactions and interactions, especially those related to the drugs, tests, and herbs mentioned above.

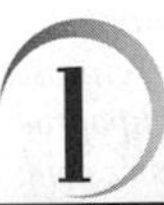

labetalol hydrochloride

Normodyne, Trandate

Pharmacologic class: Beta-adrenergic blocker (nonselective), alpha-adrenergic blocker (selective)
Therapeutic class: Antihypertensive
Pregnancy risk category C

Action

Blocks stimulation of $beta_1$- and $beta_2$-adrenergic receptor sites and $alpha_1$-adrenergic receptors, decreasing myocardial contractile force and enhancing coronary artery blood flow and myocardial perfusion. Net effect is decreased heart rate and blood pressure.

Availability

Injection: 5 mg/ml
Tablets: 100 mg, 200 mg, 300 mg

Indications and dosages

➤ Hypertension

Adults: Initially, 100 mg P.O. b.i.d., alone or combined with a diuretic; may increase by 100 mg b.i.d. q 2 to 3 days as needed. Usual range is 400 to 800 mg/day in two divided doses; up to 2.4 g/day have been given.

➤ Hypertensive crisis

Adults: Initially, 20 mg I.V. bolus over 2 minutes, then I.V. injection of 40 to 80 mg q 10 minutes until blood pressure falls to desired level; maximum dosage is 300 mg. Alternatively, 50 to 200 mg by continuous I.V. infusion at 2 mg/minute; continue infusion until desired blood pressure is reached. Follow I.V. dosing with P.O. dosing.

➤ Conversion from I.V. to P.O. dosing

Hospitalized adults: Discontinue I.V. therapy when desired blood pressure is reached; start P.O. dosing when supine diastolic pressure begins to rise. Initial P.O. dosage is 200 mg, followed 6 to 12 hours later with additional dose of 200 to 400 mg P.O., depending on blood pressure response. Then titrate at 1-day intervals to dosage ranging from 400 to 2,400 mg/day P.O. in two or three divided doses.

Dosage adjustment

- Chronic hepatic disease
- Elderly patients

Off-label uses

- Hypertension secondary to pheochromocytoma or clonidine withdrawal

Contraindications

- Hypersensitivity to drug
- Bronchospastic disease
- Overt heart failure, cardiogenic shock
- Second or third-degree atrioventricular block

• Severe bradycardia
• Conditions associated with severe and prolonged hypotension

Precautions

Use cautiously in:
• hepatic impairment, pulmonary disease, diabetes mellitus, hyperthyroidism, thyrotoxicosis
• elderly patients
• pregnant or breastfeeding patients
• children.

Administration

• Know that drug may be given as I.V. bolus or continuous infusion.
• Be aware that drug may be given undiluted for I.V. bolus injection. For continuous infusion, dilute in dextrose 5% in water or normal saline solution, and deliver with infusion control pump.
• Don't mix with 5% sodium bicarbonate injection.
• Give direct I.V. injection over 2 minutes at 10-minute intervals.

Route	Onset	Peak	Duration
P.O.	20 min-2 hr	1-4 hr	8-12 hr
I.V.	2-5 min	5 min	16-18 hr

Adverse reactions

CNS: fatigue, asthenia, anxiety, depression, dizziness, paresthesia, drowsiness, insomnia, memory loss, nightmares, mental status changes
CV: orthostatic hypotension, peripheral vasoconstriction, bradycardia, **arrhythmias, heart failure**
EENT: blurred vision, dry eyes, nasal congestion
GI: nausea, diarrhea, constipation
GU: erectile dysfunction, decreased libido
Hematologic: purpura, **agranulocytosis, thrombocytopenia**
Metabolic: hyperglycemia, **hypoglycemia**
Musculoskeletal: joint pain, back pain, muscle cramps
Respiratory: wheezing, **bronchospasm, pulmonary edema**
Skin: rash, pruritus

Interactions

Drug-drug. *Adrenergic bronchodilators, theophylline:* decreased efficacy of these drugs
Antihypertensives, nitrates: additive hypotension
Cimetidine, propranolol: increased labetalol effects
Digoxin: additive bradycardia
Dobutamine, dopamine: reduced beneficial cardiovascular effects of these drugs
General anesthetics, verapamil: additive myocardial depression
Insulin, oral hypoglycemics: altered hypoglycemic efficacy
MAO inhibitors: hypertension
Nonsteroidal anti-inflammatory drugs: decreased antihypertensive action
Drug-diagnostic tests. *Alanine aminotransferase, alkaline phosphatase, antinuclear antibodies, aspartate aminotransferase, blood urea nitrogen, glucose, liver function tests, low-density lipoproteins, potassium, triglycerides, uric acid:* increased values

Patient monitoring

• Monitor ECG and vital signs, especially blood pressure.
• Assess cardiovascular, respiratory, and neurologic status closely to detect adverse reactions.
• Monitor CBC, blood glucose level, and liver function tests.

Patient teaching

🔊 Instruct patient to immediately report adverse reactions, such as easy bruising or bleeding or respiratory problems.
• Tell patient he may feel dizzy when starting therapy, especially if he's also taking a diuretic.
• Advise patient to move slowly when sitting up or standing, to avoid dizzi-

ness or light-headedness from sudden blood pressure decrease.
• Caution patient to avoid driving and other hazardous activities until he knows how drug affects concentration, vision, and alertness.
• Emphasize need for follow-up care and regular blood pressure monitoring.
Caution patient not to stop taking drug abruptly, because this may cause myocardial infarction or worsen angina.
• As appropriate, review all other significant and life-threatening adverse reactions and interactions, especially those related to the drugs and tests mentioned above.

lactulose

Acilac, Apo-Lactulose✤, Cephulac, Cholac, Constilac, Constulose, Enulose, Evalose, Euro-Lac✤, Generlac, Gen-Lac✤, Heptalac, Lactulax✤, Laxilose, PMS-Lactulose✤, Ratio-Lactulose✤

Pharmacologic class: Osmotic
Therapeutic class: Laxative
Pregnancy risk category B

Action

Produces osmotic effect, which increases water content in colon and enhances peristalsis. Breakdown products in colon lead to acidification of colonic contents, softening of feces, and decreased ammonia absorption from colon to systemic circulation. These effects reduce blood ammonia level in portal-system encephalopathy.

Availability

Powder (single-use packets): 10 g, 20 g
Syrup: 10 g/15 ml

Indications and dosages

➢ Constipation
Adults: 10 to 20 g (15 to 30 ml) P.O. daily; may increase to 60 ml daily p.r.n.
➢ Portal-system encephalopathy
Adults: 20 to 30 g (30 to 45 ml) P.O. three or four times daily until two or three soft stools are produced daily. Therapy may continue long term.

Contraindications

• Patients requiring low-galactose diet

Precautions

Use cautiously in:
• diabetes mellitus
• elderly patients
• pregnant or breastfeeding patients
• children.

Administration

• Don't give concurrently with other laxatives.
• Dissolve contents of single-use packet in 4 oz of water or juice.
• Dilute syrup with water or fruit juice to mask taste.

Route	Onset	Peak	Duration
P.O.	24-48 hr	Unknown	Unknown

Adverse reactions

GI: diarrhea, intestinal cramps, abdominal distention, flatulence
Metabolic: hyperglycemia (in diabetic patients)

Interactions

Drug-drug. *Anti-infectives:* decreased lactulose efficacy
Other laxatives: interference with response to lactulose (in patients with hepatic encephalopathy)
Drug-diagnostic tests. *Blood ammonia:* 25% to 50% decrease
Glucose: increased level (in diabetic patients)

Patient monitoring

• Watch for adverse GI reactions.
• Check stool consistency and frequency.
• Monitor electrolyte levels, especially in elderly patients.
• Check blood glucose level in diabetic patients.

Patient teaching

• Instruct patient to dissolve contents of single-use packet in 4 oz of water or juice.
• Suggest that patient dilute syrup with water or juice to mask taste.
• Tell patient drug may cause flatulence and intestinal cramps at first, but these symptoms usually subside.
• Inform patient that excessive use may cause diarrhea and excessive fluid loss.
• Encourage patient to drink adequate fluids and to report signs and symptoms of dehydration.
• As appropriate, review all other significant adverse reactions and interactions, especially those related to the drugs and tests mentioned above.

lamivudine

Epivir, Epivir-HBV, 3TC✤

Pharmacologic class: Nucleoside reverse transcriptase inhibitor
Therapeutic class: Antiretroviral
Pregnancy risk category C

Action

Inhibits human immunodeficiency virus (HIV) reverse transcription by viral DNA chain termination. Impedes RNA- and DNA-dependent DNA polymerase activities.

Availability

Oral solution: 5 mg/ml and 10 mg/ml in 240-ml bottles
Tablets: 100 mg, 150 mg, 300 mg

Indications and dosages

➢ HIV infection (given with other antiretrovirals)
Adults and children older than age 16: 150 mg P.O. b.i.d. or 300 mg P.O. daily
Children ages 3 months to 16 years: 4 mg/kg P.O. b.i.d. to a maximum of 150 mg P.O. b.i.d.
➢ Chronic hepatitis B virus (HBV)
Adults: 100 mg (Epivir-HBV) P.O. once daily
Children ages 2 to 17: 3 mg/kg (Epivir-HBV) P.O. once daily, to a maximum of 100 mg P.O. daily

Dosage adjustment

• Renal impairment

Contraindications

• Hypersensitivity to drug or its components

Precautions

Use cautiously in:
• impaired renal function, history of hepatic disease, obesity, granulocyte count below 1,000/mm^3
• long-term therapy
• elderly patients
• women (especially if pregnant)
• children.

Administration

• Give with or without food.
Be aware that Epivir contains 150 mg lamivudine and Epivir-HBV contains 100 mg lamivudine. Strengths are not interchangeable.
Know that when given to patients with unrecognized or untreated HIV, Epivir-HBV is likely to cause rapid emergence of HIV resistance.

Route	Onset	Peak	Duration
P.O.	Unknown	0.9 hr	12 hr

Adverse reactions

CNS: fatigue, headache, insomnia, malaise, asthenia, depression, dizziness,

paresthesia, peripheral neuropathy, **seizures**
GI: nausea, vomiting, diarrhea, anorexia, abdominal discomfort, dyspepsia, splenomegaly, **pancreatitis**
Hematologic: anemia, **neutropenia**
Hepatic: hepatomegaly with steatosis
Metabolic: hyperglycemia, **lactic acidosis**
Musculoskeletal: muscle, joint, or bone pain; muscle weakness; myalgia; **rhabdomyolysis**
Respiratory: cough, abnormal breath sounds, wheezing
Skin: alopecia, rash, urticaria, **erythema multiforme, Stevens-Johnson syndrome**
Other: lymphadenopathy, body fat redistribution, hypersensitivity reactions including **anaphylaxis**

Interactions

Drug-drug. *Co-trimoxazole:* increased lamivudine blood level
Zalcitabine: interference with effects of both drugs
Drug-diagnostic tests. *Alanine aminotransferase, alkaline phosphatase, aspartate aminotransferase, bilirubin, creatine kinase, liver function tests:* increased levels
Hemoglobin, hematocrit, neutrophils: decreased levels

Patient monitoring

- Check vital signs regularly.
- Monitor CBC and platelet count frequently. Watch for evidence of bone marrow toxicity.
- Monitor blood glucose level and kidney and liver function test results.
- Assess neurologic and mental status. Report signs or symptoms of depression.
- Closely monitor obese patients, women, and patients with a history of hepatic disease; they're at increased risk for lactic acidosis and severe hepatomegaly with steatosis.
- Monitor HIV patients for co-infection with HBV (which may recur when drug is withdrawn).

Patient teaching

- Tell patient he may take with or without food.
- Advise patient to minimize GI upset by eating small, frequent servings of healthy food and drinking plenty of fluids.
- Tell HIV patient that drug doesn't cure virus or prevent its transmission and that opportunistic infections may occur. Advise him to take appropriate precautions during sex.
- Caution patient to avoid driving and other hazardous activities until he knows how drug affects concentration and alertness.
- Caution HIV patient not to breastfeed, because of risk of passing infection to infant.
- As appropriate, review all other significant and life-threatening adverse reactions and interactions, especially those related to the drugs and tests mentioned above.

lamotrigine

Lamictal, Lamictal Chewable Dispersible

Pharmacologic class: Phenyltriazine
Therapeutic class: Anticonvulsant
Pregnancy risk category C

Action

Unknown. Thought to block sodium channel membranes, which in turn inhibits release of the neurotransmitters glutamate and aspartate in brain.

Availability

Tablets: 25 mg, 100 mg, 150 mg, 200 mg
Tablets (chewable): 2 mg, 5 mg, 25 mg

Indications and dosages

➢ Seizures of Lennox-Gastaut syndrome in patients receiving valproate

Adults and children ages 12 and older: 25 mg P.O. every other day during weeks 1 and 2, then 25 mg daily during weeks 3 and 4. To achieve maintenance dosage of 100 to 200 mg daily in divided doses, increase subsequent doses q 1 to 2 weeks, as ordered.

Children ages 2 to 12: 0.15 mg/kg/day P.O. (rounded down to nearest whole tablet) in one or two divided doses during weeks 1 and 2; then 0.3 mg/kg/day P.O. (rounded down to nearest whole tablet) in one or two divided doses during weeks 3 and 4. Alternatively, 2 mg P.O. every other day during weeks 1 and 2, then 2 mg daily during weeks 3 and 4 for children weighing 6.7 to 14 kg (14.7 to 30.8 lb); or 2 mg P.O. daily during weeks 1 and 2, then 4 mg daily during weeks 3 and 4 for children weighing 14.1 to 27 kg (31 to 59.5 lb); or 4 mg P.O. daily during weeks 1 and 2, then 8 mg daily during weeks 3 and 4 for children weighing 27.1 to 34 kg (59.7 to 74.9 lb); or 5 mg P.O. daily during weeks 1 and 2, then 10 mg daily during weeks 3 and 4 for children weighing 34.1 to 40 kg (75.1 to 88 lb). To achieve maintenance dosage of 1 to 3 mg/kg/day in divided doses, increase subsequent doses q 1 to 2 weeks, as ordered.

➢ Seizures of Lennox-Gastaut syndrome in patients receiving carbamazepine, phenytoin, phenobarbital, or primidone

Adults and children ages 12 and older: 50 mg/day P.O. during weeks 1 and 2, then 100 mg/day in two divided doses during weeks 3 and 4. To achieve maintenance dosage of 300 to 500 mg/day in divided doses, increase subsequent doses q 1 to 2 weeks, as ordered.

Children ages 2 to 12: 0.6 mg/kg/day P.O. in two divided doses (rounded down to nearest whole tablet) during weeks 1 and 2, then 1.2 mg/kg/day P.O. in two divided doses (rounded down to nearest whole tablet) during weeks 3 and 4. To achieve maintenance dosage of 5 to 15 mg/kg/day (maximum 400 mg daily) in divided doses, increase subsequent doses q 1 to 2 weeks, as ordered.

➢ Conversion to monotherapy for seizures in patients receiving valproate

Adults and children ages 16 and older: 25 mg P.O. every other day during weeks 1 and 2, then 25 mg daily during weeks 3 and 4. Then increase subsequent doses, as ordered, q 1 to 2 weeks to 200 mg/day. Keep lamotrigine dosage at 200 mg/day and gradually decrease valproate to 500 mg/day in weekly decrements no greater than 500 mg/day; maintain regimen for 1 week. Then increase lamotrigine dosage to 300 mg/day while simultaneously decreasing valproate to 250 mg/day; maintain regimen for 1 week. Then discontinue valproate completely and increase lamotrigine dosage by 100 mg/day q week to 500 mg/day.

➢ Conversion to monotherapy for seizures in patients receiving carbamazepine, phenytoin, phenobarbital, or primidone as a single agent

Adults and children ages 16 and older: 50 mg/day P.O. during weeks 1 and 2, then 100 mg/day in two divided doses during weeks 3 and 4. Then increase by 100 mg/day q 1 to 2 weeks until maintenance dosage of 500 mg/day is reached. Taper concomitant drug in 20% decrements weekly over 4 weeks.

➢ Bipolar I disorder

Adults: Target dosage is 200 mg P.O. daily (or 100 mg daily in patients taking valproate, or 400 mg daily in patients not taking valproate who are receiving carbamazepine, rifampin, phenytoin, phenobarbital, or primidone).

Dosage adjustment

- Hepatic dysfunction
- Renal impairment
- Heart disease

Off-label uses
• Absence, generalized tonic-clonic, and myoclonic seizures
• Drug-resistant seizures
• Mood stabilization in rapid-cycling bipolar II disorder

Contraindications
• Hypersensitivity to drug or its components

Precautions
Use cautiously in:
• renal or hepatic impairment
• concurrent use of other anticonvulsants
• pregnant or breastfeeding patients
• children.

Administration
• Give with or without food.
• Don't crush or break regular tablets; make sure patient swallows them whole.
• Crush chewable tablets or mix in diluted fruit juice if patient can't chew them.
Clinical alert: Be aware that abrupt withdrawal may induce seizures. If drug must be discontinued, decrease dosage 50% per week over at least 2 weeks.
Clinical alert: Don't confuse Lamictal with other drugs having sound-alike names (such as Lamisil, Lomotil, and Ludiomil).

Route	Onset	Peak	Duration
P.O.	Unknown	1.4-4.8 hr	Unknown

Adverse reactions
CNS: dizziness, vertigo, headache, drowsiness, ataxia, incoordination, insomnia, sleep disorders, tremor, depression, anxiety, irritability, impaired memory, poor concentration, emotional lability, racing thoughts, dysarthria, malaise, **seizures**
CV: palpitations
GI: nausea, vomiting, diarrhea, constipation, abdominal pain, dyspepsia, dry mouth, anorexia
GU: dysmenorrhea, amenorrhea, vaginitis
Hepatic: hepatotoxicity
Musculoskeletal: muscle spasm, neck pain
Respiratory: cough, dyspnea
Skin: alopecia, rash, urticaria, **erythema multiforme, Stevens-Johnson syndrome**
Other: hypersensitivity reactions (rare) including **anaphylaxis**

Interactions
Drug-drug. *Carbamazepine, phenobarbital, phenytoin, primidone:* decreased lamotrigine steady-state level
Folate inhibitors (such as methotrexate, co-trimoxazole): additive effects of lamotrigine
Valproic acid: decreased lamotrigine clearance, increased steady-state level
Drug-behaviors. *Sun exposure:* photosensitivity

l

Patient monitoring
Clinical alert: Watch for signs and symptoms of hypersensitivity reaction (Stevens-Johnson syndrome, anaphylaxis).
• Monitor vital signs regularly.
• Monitor CNS status carefully, noting adverse reactions and changes in seizure pattern.
• Check liver function tests frequently. Watch for signs and symptoms of hepatotoxicity.

Patient teaching
• Tell patient he may take with or without food.
• Instruct patient taking regular tablets to swallow them whole without crushing or breaking.
• Instruct patient taking chewable tablets to crush them or mix in diluted fruit juice if he can't chew them.
• Inform patient that dosage is adjusted slowly, as indicated.
Clinical alert: Advise patient to stop taking drug and notify prescriber immediately at first sign of rash.

• Caution patient to avoid driving and other hazardous activities until he knows how drug affects concentration and alertness.
• As appropriate, review all other significant and life-threatening adverse reactions and interactions, especially those related to the drugs and behaviors mentioned above.

lansoprazole

Prevacid, Prevacid I.V., Prevacid NapraPAC, Prevacid SoluTab, Prevpac

Pharmacologic class: Gastric acid pump inhibitor
Therapeutic class: Antiulcer drug
Pregnancy risk category B

Action

Inhibits activity of proton pump in gastric parietal cells, decreasing gastric acid production

Availability

Capsules (delayed-release): 15 mg, 30 mg
Granules for oral suspension (delayed-release, enteric-coated): 15 mg, 30 mg
Powder for injection: 30 mg/vial
Prevpac (combination product for Helicobacter pylori *infection):* daily pack containing two 30-mg lansoprazole capsules, four 500-mg amoxicillin capsules, and two 500-mg clarithromycin tablets
Prevacid NapraPAC 375 (combination product for reducing risk of ulcers from nonsteroidal anti-inflammatory drugs [NSAIDs]): weekly pack containing seven 15-mg Prevacid capsules and fourteen 375-mg Naprosyn tablets
Prevacid NapraPAC 500 (combination product for reducing risk of ulcers from NSAIDs): weekly pack containing seven 15-mg Prevacid capsules and fourteen 500-mg Naprosyn tablets
Prevacid SoluTab (delayed-release, orally disintegrating tablet): 15 mg, 30 mg

Indications and dosages

➢ Active duodenal ulcer
Adults: 15 mg P.O. daily for 4 weeks
➢ *H. pylori* eradication, to reduce risk of duodenal ulcer recurrence
Adults: In triple therapy, 30 mg lansoprazole P.O., 1 g amoxicillin P.O., and 500 mg clarithromycin P.O. q 12 hours for 10 or 14 days. In dual therapy, 30 mg lansoprazole P.O. and 1 g amoxicillin P.O. q 8 hours for 14 days.
➢ Benign gastric ulcer
Adults: 30 mg P.O. daily for up to 8 weeks
➢ Gastric ulcer associated with NSAIDs
Adults: 30 mg P.O. once daily for up to 8 weeks
➢ To reduce risk of NSAID-associated gastric ulcer
Adults: 15 mg P.O. daily for up to 12 weeks
➢ Gastroesophageal reflux disease
Adults and children ages 12 to 17: 15 mg P.O. daily for up to 8 weeks
Children ages 1 to 11 weighing more than 30 kg (66 lb): 30 mg P.O. daily for up to 12 weeks
Children ages 1 to 11 weighing 30 kg (66 lb) or less: 15 mg P.O. daily for up to 12 weeks
➢ Erosive esophagitis
Adults and children ages 12 to 17: 30 mg P.O. daily for up to 8 weeks. Some patients may require 8 additional weeks.
Children ages 12 to 17: 30 mg P.O. daily for up to 8 weeks
Children ages 1 to 11 weighing more than 30 kg (66 lb): 30 mg P.O. daily for up to 12 weeks
Children ages 1 to 11 weighing 30 kg (66 lb) or less: 15 mg P.O. daily for up to 12 weeks

➢ Erosive esophagitis in patients who can't take drugs orally
Adults: 30 mg/day I.V. infused over 30 minutes for up to 7 days
➢ To maintain healing of erosive esophagitis
Adults: 15 mg P.O. daily
➢ Pathologic hypersecretory conditions (including Zollinger-Ellison syndrome)
Adults: Initially, 60 mg P.O. daily, to a maximum of 90 mg P.O. b.i.d. Divide daily dosages over 120 mg.

Dosage adjustment

- Significant hepatic insufficiency

Contraindications

- Hypersensitivity to drug or its components

Precautions

Use cautiously in:

- phenylketonuria (orally disintegrating tablets), severe hepatic impairment
- elderly patients
- pregnant or breastfeeding patients
- children younger than age 18.

Administration

- To reconstitute for I.V. infusion, inject 5 ml of sterile water for injection into 30-mg vial; resulting solution contains 6 mg/ml. Mix gently until powder dissolves; then dilute reconstituted solution in 50 ml of 0.9% sodium chloride injection, lactated Ringer's injection, or 5% dextrose injection.
- Infuse I.V. dose over 30 minutes (using in-line filter provided) within 24 hours if reconstituted drug was diluted with 0.9% sodium chloride injection or lactated Ringer's injection, or over 12 hours if 5% dextrose injection was used.
- Don't give I.V. with other drugs or with diluents other than those listed above.
- Give oral form before meals.
- If patient has difficulty swallowing delayed-release capsule, open it and sprinkle contents onto small amount of soft food, such as applesauce or pudding. Don't crush or let patient chew drug.
- When giving orally disintegrating tablet, place tablet on patient's tongue and let it disintegrate until particles can be swallowed.
- Know that orally disintegrating tablet contains phenylalanine.
- When giving oral suspension, empty packet contents into container with 2 tbsp water. Stir contents well, and have patient drink immediately. Don't give oral suspension through nasogastric (NG) tube.
- When injecting contents of delayed-release capsule through NG tube, open capsule and mix granules with 40 ml apple juice. Then rinse tube with additional apple juice to clear.

Route	Onset	Peak	Duration
P.O.	Rapid	Unknown	>24 hr

Adverse reactions

CNS: headache, confusion, anxiety, malaise, paresthesia, abnormal thinking, depression, dizziness, syncope, **cerebrovascular accident**
CV: chest pain, hypertension, hypotension, **myocardial infarction, shock**
EENT: visual field deficits, otitis media, tinnitus, epistaxis
GI: nausea, diarrhea, abdominal pain, cholelithiasis, ulcerative colitis, esophageal ulcer, hematemesis, stomatitis, dysphagia, **GI hemorrhage**
GU: renal calculi, erectile dysfunction, abnormal menses, breast tenderness, gynecomastia
Hematologic: anemia
Respiratory: cough, bronchitis, **asthma**
Skin: urticaria, alopecia, acne, pruritus, photosensitivity

Interactions

Drug-drug. *Drugs requiring acidic pH (such as ampicillin esters, digoxin, iron salts, itraconazole, ketoconazole):* decreased absorption of these drugs
Sucralfate: decreased lansoprazole absorption
Theophylline: increased theophylline clearance
Drug-food. *Any food:* decreased rate and extent of GI drug absorption
Drug-herbs. *Male fern:* inactivation of herb
St. John's wort: increased risk of photosensitivity

Patient monitoring

- Monitor for GI adverse reactions.
- Assess nutritional status and fluid balance to identify significant problems.

Patient teaching

- Instruct patient to take before meals.
- If patient has difficulty swallowing, tell him to open delayed-release capsule and sprinkle contents onto small amount of soft food (such as applesauce or pudding). Emphasize that he must not crush or chew drug.
- Tell patient to take orally disintegrating tablet by placing it on tongue and letting it disintegrate.
- Instruct patient to take oral suspension by emptying packet contents into container with 2 tbsp water. Tell him to stir contents well and drink immediately.
- Advise patient to minimize GI upset by eating small, frequent servings of food and drinking plenty of fluids.
- As appropriate, review all other significant and life-threatening adverse reactions and interactions, especially those related to the drugs, foods, and herbs mentioned above.

leflunomide

Arava

Pharmacologic class: Immune modulator
Therapeutic class: Antirheumatic
Pregnancy risk category X

Action

Inhibits T-cell pyrimidine biosynthesis, tyrosine kinases, and dihydroorotate dehydrogenase, blocking structural damage caused by inflammatory response to autoimmune process. Also shows analgesic, antipyretic, and histamine-blocking activity.

Availability

Tablets: 10 mg, 20 mg, 100 mg

Indications and dosages

➢ Active rheumatoid arthritis
Adults: 100 mg P.O. daily for 3 days, then a maintenance dosage of 20 mg daily. If intolerance occurs, decrease to 10 mg daily.

Dosage adjustment

- Hepatic enzyme elevations

Contraindications

- Hypersensitivity to drug or its components
- Immunocompromised state, including bone marrow dysplasia and severe uncontrolled infection
- Hepatic impairment, evidence of hepatitis B or C
- Live-virus vaccinations
- Pregnancy or breastfeeding

Precautions

Use cautiously in:
- renal insufficiency
- men attempting to father a child
- children younger than age 18.

Administration
• Give with or without food.
• Be aware that drug has a long half-life. To eliminate from bloodstream, give 8 g cholestyramine P.O. t.i.d. for 11 days.

Route	Onset	Peak	Duration
P.O.	1 mo	3-6 mo	Unknown

Adverse reactions
CNS: headache, dizziness, asthenia
CV: chest pain, hypertension
EENT: rhinitis, sinusitis, pharyngitis
GI: nausea, vomiting, diarrhea, abdominal pain, dyspepsia, gastroenteritis, mouth ulcers, anorexia
GU: urinary tract infection
Hepatic: hepatotoxicity
Metabolic: hypokalemia
Musculoskeletal: joint pain or disorders, back pain, leg cramps, synovitis, tenosynovitis
Respiratory: bronchitis, increased cough, pneumonia, respiratory infection
Skin: alopecia, rash, dry skin, eczema, pruritus
Other: weight loss, pain, infection, allergic reactions, flulike symptoms

Interactions
Drug-drug. *Activated charcoal, cholestyramine:* rapid, steep drop in blood level of leflunomide's active metabolite
Methotrexate, other hepatotoxic drugs: increased risk of hepatotoxicity
Rifampin: increased blood level of leflunomide's active metabolite
Drug-diagnostic tests. *Alanine aminotransferase, aspartate aminotransferase:* increased levels

Patient monitoring
• Check vital signs closely.
🔊 Watch for signs and symptoms of hepatotoxicity.
• Assess cardiovascular and respiratory status carefully to detect adverse reactions.
• Monitor electrolyte levels and liver function tests.
• Stay alert for signs and symptoms of urinary tract infection.
• Observe patient closely after dosage reduction. Metabolite levels may take several weeks to fall.

Patient teaching
• Tell patient he may take with or without food.
🔊 Advise patient to immediately report unusual tiredness or yellowing of skin or eyes.
• Tell patient to minimize GI upset by eating small, frequent servings of food and drinking plenty of fluids.
• Caution patient to avoid driving and other hazardous activities until he knows how drug affects concentration and alertness.
🔊 Inform female of childbearing age that drug may harm fetus. Tell her to contact prescriber immediately if she suspects pregnancy.
• Caution female not to breastfeed without consulting prescriber.
• Advise male planning to father a child to consult prescriber, because drug can harm fetus.
• Tell patient he'll undergo regular blood testing to check liver function.
• As appropriate, review all other significant and life-threatening adverse reactions and interactions, especially those related to the drugs and tests mentioned above.

lepirudin
Refludan

Pharmacologic class: Thrombin inhibitor
Therapeutic class: Anticoagulant
Pregnancy risk category B

l

Action
Binds with thrombin, blocking its thrombogenic activity

Availability
Powder for injection: 50 mg

Indications and dosages
➤ Heparin-induced thrombocytopenia and associated thromboembolic disease

Adults: Initially, 0.4 mg/kg by I.V. bolus over 15 to 20 seconds (to a maximum of 44 mg), followed by 0.15 mg/kg as a continuous I.V. infusion for 2 to 10 days, or longer if needed

Dosage adjustment
- Renal impairment
- Elderly patients

Contraindications
- Hypersensitivity to drug, its components, or hirudin

Precautions
Use cautiously in:
- renal or hepatic disease, bleeding, bacterial endocarditis
- recent cerebrovascular accident or neurosurgery
- pregnant or breastfeeding patients
- children.

Administration
- Check activated partial thromboplastin time (APTT) before therapy starts.

Administer I.V. bolus slowly, over at least 15 to 20 seconds.
- Follow bolus with continuous I.V. infusion for 2 to 10 days.
- To reconstitute, mix with sterile water for injection or 0.9% sodium chloride injection.
- For further dilution, use 0.9% sodium chloride injection or 5% dextrose injection.

Base dosage adjustments on APTT measured 4 hours after drug initiation and then at least once daily.

Route	Onset	Peak	Duration
I.V.	Immediate	Unknown	Unknown

Adverse reactions
CNS: depression
CV: heart failure, pericardial effusion, ventricular fibrillation
GI: GI bleeding
GU: hematuria, **abnormal renal function**
Hematologic: hemorrhage, thrombocytopenia
Respiratory: pneumonia, hemoptysis
Skin: rash, pruritus, urticaria
Other: chills, fever, bleeding at injection site, excessive wound bleeding, **multisystem failure, sepsis, anaphylaxis**

Interactions
Drug-drug. *Cefamandole, cefoperazone, cefotetan, clopidogrel, eptifibatide, nonsteroidal anti-inflammatory drugs, oral anticoagulants, platelet aggregation inhibitors, plicamycin, thrombolytics, ticlopidine, tirofiban, valproic acid:* increased risk of bleeding

Drug-diagnostic tests. *Liver function tests:* increased values

Patient monitoring
- Check vital signs frequently.

Monitor APTT at least daily. Target range is 1.5 to 2.5.
- Assess fluid intake and output and monitor creatine clearance.

Watch closely for signs and symptoms of bleeding.
- Monitor CBC with white cell differential; assess liver function tests.

Check for adverse effects, particularly signs and symptoms of infection, multisystem failure, and cardiovascular or respiratory problems.

Patient teaching
- Explain bleeding precautions that patient should take.

◀ Teach patient to recognize and immediately report signs and symptoms of bleeding.
- Inform patient that he'll undergo frequent blood testing during therapy.
- As appropriate, review all other significant and life-threatening adverse reactions and interactions, especially those related to the drugs and tests mentioned above.

letrozole

Femara

Pharmacologic class: Aromatase inhibitor
Therapeutic class: Antineoplastic
Pregnancy risk category D

Action

Inhibits aromatase, an enzyme that promotes conversion of estrogen precursors to estrogen. This inhibition reduces circulating estrogen levels and stops progression of breast cancer.

Availability

Tablets: 2.5 mg

Indications and dosages

➤ Metastatic or advanced breast cancer in postmenopausal women; early breast cancer in postmenopausal women who have received 5 years of antiestrogen therapy
Adults: 2.5 mg P.O. daily

Contraindications

- Hypersensitivity to drug or its components

Precautions

Use cautiously in:
- severe hepatic impairment
- pregnant or breastfeeding patients
- children (safety not established).

Administration

- Give with or without meals.

Route	Onset	Peak	Duration
P.O.	Unknown	2-3 days	Unknown

Adverse reactions

CNS: anxiety, depression, dizziness, drowsiness, fatigue, headache, vertigo, asthenia
CV: chest pain, hypertension
GI: nausea, vomiting, diarrhea, constipation, abdominal pain, dyspepsia, anorexia
Metabolic: hypercalcemia
Musculoskeletal: musculoskeletal or joint pain, fractures
Respiratory: cough, dyspnea, **pleural effusion**
Skin: alopecia, pruritus, rash, diaphoresis
Other: hot flashes, edema, weight gain

Interactions

Drug-diagnostic tests. *Cholesterol, gamma-glutamyltransferase:* increased levels

Patient monitoring

- Check vital signs and assess cardiovascular and respiratory status.
- Monitor renal and hepatic function, electrolyte levels, and lipid panels.
- Assess for adverse CNS effects, including depression. Institute safety measures as needed to prevent injury.

Patient teaching

- Tell patient she can take with or without food.
- Instruct patient to weigh herself regularly and report significant changes.
- Advise patient and family to watch for signs and symptoms of depression.
- Tell patient to minimize GI upset by eating small, frequent servings of healthy food and drinking plenty of fluids.
- Caution patient to avoid driving and other hazardous activities until she

knows how drug affects concentration and alertness.

• Inform patient that treatment is long term. Urge her to keep follow-up appointments with prescriber.

• Tell patient to inform prescriber if she is pregnant or breastfeeding.

• As appropriate, review all other significant and life-threatening adverse reactions and interactions, especially those related to the tests mentioned above.

leucovorin calcium (citrovorum factor, folinic acid)

Pharmacologic class: Water-soluble vitamin

Therapeutic class: Vitamin, antidote to folic acid antagonist, antianemic, antineoplastic adjunct

Pregnancy risk category C

Action

Counteracts therapeutic and toxic effects of folic acid antagonists; may enhance therapeutic and toxic effects of fluoropyrimidines used in cancer therapy. Also supplements folic acid in folic acid deficiency.

Availability

Injection (expressed as base): 10 mg/vial, 50 mg/vial, 100 mg/vial, 200 mg/vial, 350 mg/vial, 500 mg/vial

Injection, preservative-free (expressed as base): 10 mg/vial, 50 mg/vial, 200 mg/vial, 350 mg/vial, 500 mg/vial

Tablets: 5 mg, 15 mg, 25 mg

Indications and dosages

➤ Leucovorin rescue after high-dose methotrexate therapy

Adults: 15 mg (approximately 10 mg/m²) P.O., I.M. , or I.V. q 6 hours, starting 24 hours after methotrexate infusion begins and continuing until serum methotrexate level drops below 10^{-8} M. If 24-hour serum creatinine level rises 50% over baseline or if 24-hour methotrexate level exceeds 5×10^{-6} M or 48-hour level exceeds 9×10^{-7} M, increase leucovorin dosage to 100 mg/m² I.V. q 3 hours and continue hydration and urinary alkalization until methotrexate level drops below 10^{-8} M.

➤ To reduce toxicity and counteract effects of impaired methotrexate elimination or inadvertent overdose of folic acid antagonist

Adults: 15 mg (roughly 10 mg/m²) I.M., I.V., or P.O. q 6 hours until serum methotrexate level drops below 10^{-8} M. If 24-hour serum creatinine level rises 50% over baseline or if 24-hour methotrexate level exceeds 5×10^{-6} M or 48-hour level exceeds 9×10^{-7} M, increase leucovorin dosage to 100 mg/m² I.V. q 3 hours and continue hydration and urinary alkalization until methotrexate level drops below 10^{-8} M.

➤ Advanced colorectal cancer

Adults: Usually given in one of the following regimens: 200 mg/m² slow I.V. injection over at least 3 minutes, followed by I.V. injection of 5-fluorouracil (5-FU); or 20 mg/m² I.V. injection, followed by I.V. injection of 5-FU. Treatment is repeated daily for 5 days, and may then be repeated at 28-day intervals for two courses and then at 4- to 5-week intervals, as prescribed.

➤ Megaloblastic anemia secondary to folic acid deficiency

Adults: Up to 1 mg I.M. daily

Dosage adjustment

• In leucovorin rescue after high-dose methotrexate therapy: delayed early or late methotrexate elimination (serum methotrexate level still above 0.2 µM at 72 hours and above 0.05 µM [5×10^{-8}] at 96 hours after administration)

• Evidence of acute renal injury

Contraindications

• Treatment of pernicious anemia and other megaloblastic anemias caused by vitamin B_{12} deficiency

Precautions

Use cautiously in:
• anemia (when vitamin B_{12} deficiency has been ruled out)
• patients receiving 5-FU concomitantly
• pregnant or breastfeeding patients
• children.

Administration

🔊 Recheck leucovorin dosage in current published protocols before giving as methotrexate rescue.
• Give parenterally in patients with GI toxicity, nausea, or vomiting.
• Reconstitute leucovorin injection with sterile or bacteriostatic water for injection containing benzyl alcohol. (When giving with 5-FU for colorectal cancer in dosages above 10 mg/m^2, reconstitute only with sterile water for injection.)
🔊 Don't mix leucovorin injection with 5-FU, because precipitation will occur.
🔊 Give I.V. leucovorin slowly (no faster than 160 mg/minute) because of calcium content. Large doses may be infused over 1 to 6 hours as directed.
🔊 Don't give intrathecally; drug may be harmful or fatal by this route.
• Be aware that P.O. dosages above 25 mg are not recommended.

Route	Onset	Peak	Duration
P.O.	20-30 min	60 to 90 min	3-6 hr
I.V.	<5 min	Unknown	3-6 hr
I.M.	10-20 min	35 to 60 min	3-6 hr

Adverse reactions

Skin: urticaria
Other: allergic sensitization reactions, **anaphylactoid reactions**

Interactions

Drug-drug. *5-FU:* enhanced fluorouracil toxicity
Methotrexate, other folic acid antagonists: negated therapeutic and toxic effects of these drugs
Phenobarbital, phenytoin, primidone: negated anticonvulsant effect, increased frequency of seizures in susceptible children

Patient monitoring

🔊 Monitor serum creatinine and methotrexate levels every 24 hours.
🔊 Monitor closely for adverse reactions. Continue leucovorin therapy, hydration, and urinary alkalization until serum methotrexate level drops below 10^{-8} M.
🔊 Monitor CBC with white cell differential and platelet count before leucovorin/5-FU therapy starts. Repeat weekly during first two courses and then once each cycle at anticipated white blood cell nadir.
• Check electrolyte levels and liver function tests before each treatment for first three cycles. Thereafter, check before every other cycle.
• Assess for adequate hydration when giving with 5-FU or high-dose methotrexate.
• Watch for hypersensitivity reactions, especially anaphylactoid reactions.

Patient teaching

• Teach patient about drug and protocol.
🔊 Stress importance of taking leucovorin as prescribed with high-dose methotrexate therapy. Emphasize that it's not just a vitamin.
• Tell patient to immediately report signs or symptoms of allergic reaction, such as hives.
• As appropriate, review all other significant and life-threatening adverse reactions and interactions, especially those related to the drugs mentioned above.

L

leuprolide acetate

Eligard, Lupron, Lupron Depot, Lupron Depot-Ped, Lupron Depot-3 Month, Lupron Depot-4 Month, Lupron-3 Month SR Depot, Viadur

Pharmacologic class: Gonadotropin-releasing hormone (GnRH) analog
Therapeutic class: Antineoplastic
Pregnancy risk category X

Action

Inhibits and desensitizes GnRH receptors, thus inhibiting gonadotropin secretion when given continuously. This inhibition causes initial increase and then profound decrease in luteinizing hormone and follicle-stimulating hormone levels and, ultimately, reduces testosterone and estrogen sex hormones.

Availability

Eligard Depot: 7.5 mg, 22.5 mg, 30 mg
Implant (12-month): 72 mg (65 mg free base)
Injection: 1 mg/0.2 ml
Lupron Depot injection: 3.75 mg/ml, 7.5 mg/ml
Lupron Depot-3 month injection: 11.25 mg, 22.5 mg
Lupron Depot-4 month injection: 30 mg
Lupron Depot-Ped injection: 7.5 mg, 11.25 mg, 15 mg

Indications and dosages

➢ Advanced prostate cancer
Adults: 1 mg subcutaneously daily or 7.5 mg I.M. monthly (depot injection). Or 22.5 mg I.M. q 3 months, 30 mg I.M. q 4 months, or one 72-mg implant q 12 months.
➢ Endometriosis
Adults: 3.75 mg I.M. (depot injection) as a single injection once monthly, or 11.25 mg I.M. q 3 months. Duration is up to 6 months.
➢ Adjunct to iron therapy in anemia caused by uterine leiomyomas
Adults: 3.75 mg I.M. monthly or 11.25 mg I.M. q 3 months as a single dose. Recommended duration is 6 months or less.
➢ Central precocious puberty
Children: 50 mcg/kg/day subcutaneously as a single injection, increased in increments of 10 mcg/kg/day as needed
Children weighing more than 37.5 kg (82.5 lb): Initially, 15 mg of Depot-Ped I.M. q 4 weeks, increased in increments of 3.75 mg q 4 weeks as needed
Children weighing 25 to 37.5 kg (55 to 82.5 lb): Initially, 11.25 mg of Depot-Ped I.M. q 4 weeks, increased in increments of 3.75 mg q 4 weeks as needed
Children weighing less than 25 kg (55 lb): Initially, 7.5 mg of Depot-Ped I.M. q 4 weeks, increased in increments of 3.75 mg q 4 weeks as needed

Contraindications

- Hypersensitivity to drug, its components, GnRH, or other GnRH analogs
- Undiagnosed abnormal vaginal bleeding
- Pregnancy or breastfeeding

Precautions

Use cautiously in:
- renal, hepatic, or cardiac impairment.

Administration

- Give Eligard within 30 minutes of mixing. After this time, discard.
- Administer Lupron injection immediately after mixing. Otherwise, discard.
- Administer Lupron Depot-Ped only under prescriber's supervision.

Route	Onset	Peak	Duration
I.M. depot	4 hr	Variable	1, 3, 4 mo
Implant	Unknown	Unknown	1 yr
Subcut. (prec. puberty)	1 wk	Unknown	4-12 wk after therapy
Subcut. (endometriosis, cancer)	2-4 wk	After 1-2 mo	2-3 mo after therapy

Adverse reactions

CNS: anxiety, depression, dizziness, drowsiness, asthenia, fatigue, headache, vertigo, syncope, mood changes
CV: palpitations, angina, **arrhythmias, myocardial infarction**
EENT: blurred vision
GI: nausea, vomiting, diarrhea, constipation, abdominal pain, dyspepsia, anorexia
GU: urinary frequency, hematuria, decreased testes size, erectile dysfunction, decreased libido, gynecomastia
Hematologic: anemia, **thrombocytopenia**
Respiratory: dyspnea, pleural rub, **worsening of pulmonary fibrosis, pulmonary embolism**
Skin: alopecia, pruritus, rash, diaphoresis
Other: sour taste, edema, hot flashes, **anaphylaxis**

Interactions

Drug-diagnostic tests. *Blood urea nitrogen, creatinine:* increased levels
Pituitary-gonadal system tests: misleading results during and for up to 3 months after therapy

Patient monitoring

- Observe injection site for local reactions.

Clinical alert: Monitor cardiovascular and respiratory status carefully to detect serious adverse reactions.

- Evaluate neurologic status. Institute safety measures as needed to prevent injury.
- Periodically monitor serum testosterone and prostate-specific antigen levels.

Patient teaching

- Inform patient that localized reaction may occur at injection site. Tell him to contact prescriber if symptoms don't resolve.
- Advise patient and family to watch for and report signs or symptoms of depression.
- Tell patient drug may cause libido changes or erectile dysfunction. Encourage him to discuss these problems with prescriber.
- Teach patient to minimize GI upset by eating small, frequent servings of food and drinking plenty of fluids.

Clinical alert: Instruct female of childbearing age to use reliable contraception during therapy. Tell her to stop drug immediately and contact prescriber if she suspects pregnancy.

Clinical alert: Tell female patient not to breastfeed.

- Caution patient to avoid driving and other hazardous activities until he knows how drug affects concentration and alertness.
- As appropriate, review all other significant and life-threatening adverse reactions and interactions, especially those related to the tests mentioned above.

levalbuterol hydrochloride

Xopenex

Pharmacologic class: Adrenergic $beta_2$ agonist
Therapeutic class: Bronchodilator
Pregnancy risk category C

Action

Binds to $beta_2$-adrenergic receptors on bronchial cell membrane, stimulating the intracellular enzyme adenylate cyclase to convert adenosine triphosphate to cyclic-3′,5′-adenosine monophosphate. This action relaxes smooth muscles, dilates bronchioles, and increases diuresis.

Availability

Solution for inhalation: 0.31 mg/3 ml, 0.63 mg/3 ml, 1.25 mg/3 ml

Indications and dosages

➢ Prevention and treatment of bronchospasm

Adults and children ages 12 and older: 0.63 to 1.25 mg by oral inhalation via nebulizer q 6 to 8 hours

Children ages 6 to 11: 0.31 to 0.63 mg by oral inhalation via nebulizer t.i.d.

Contraindications

- Hypersensitivity to drug or racemic albuterol

Precautions

Use cautiously in:

- renal, hepatic, or cardiac impairment; hyperthyroidism; diabetes mellitus; hypertension; prostatic hypertrophy; angle-closure glaucoma; seizures
- pregnant patients.

Administration

- Use only with nebulizer system designed for this drug.
- Keep unopened vials in foil pouch. Once pouch is opened, use within 2 weeks.
- If vial is removed from pouch, protect from light and use within 1 week.

Route	Onset	Peak	Duration
Inhalation	10-17 min	1.5 hr	5-6 hr

Adverse reactions

CNS: anxiety, dizziness, hypertonia, insomnia, migraine, headache, nervousness, paresthesia, syncope, tremor
CV: chest pain, hypertension, hypotension, tachycardia
EENT: rhinitis, sinusitis, dry throat
GI: nausea, vomiting, diarrhea, constipation, abdominal pain, dyspepsia, anorexia, dry mouth
Metabolic: hypokalemia
Musculoskeletal: muscle cramps, myalgia
Respiratory: cough, dyspnea, **asthma exacerbation, paradoxical bronchospasm**
Other: sour taste, flulike symptoms, lymphadenopathy, chills

Interactions

Drug-drug. *Aerosol bronchodilators:* increased action of both drugs
Antidepressants: increased risk of adverse cardiovascular effects
Beta-adrenergic blockers: inhibition of levalbuterol effect
Digoxin: decreased digoxin blood level
Loop and thiazide diuretics: increased risk of hypokalemia
Drug-food. *Caffeine-containing foods and beverages:* increased stimulation
Drug-herbs. *Cola nut, ephedra (ma huang), guarana, yerba maté:* increased stimulation

Patient monitoring

- Monitor vital signs and ECG closely.
- Assess cardiovascular and neurologic status. Institute safety measures as needed to prevent injury.

[Clinical alert] Monitor for paradoxical bronchospasm. If it occurs, stop drug therapy and notify prescriber immediately.

- Check electrolyte levels for hypokalemia.
- Assess patient's response to drug. Contact prescriber if patient needs more frequent doses for same effect.

Patient teaching

- Teach patient how to prepare drug, administer it with nebulizer, and maintain and clean nebulizer.
- Advise patient to continue treatment for about 5 to 15 minutes or until mist no longer forms in nebulizer reservoir.

⚠ Tell patient to immediately report increased difficulty breathing or tightness in chest.

- Caution patient to avoid driving and other hazardous activities until he knows how drug affects concentration and alertness.
- As appropriate, review all other significant and life-threatening adverse reactions and interactions, especially those related to the drugs, foods, and herbs mentioned above.

levetiracetam

Keppra

Pharmacologic class: Pyrrolidine derivative

Therapeutic class: Anticonvulsant

Pregnancy risk category C

Action

Unknown. Thought to prevent seizures by inhibiting nerve impulses in hippocampus of brain. Chemically unrelated to other anticonvulsants.

Availability

Oral solution: 100 mg/ml

Tablets: 250 mg, 500 mg, 750 mg

Indications and dosages

➤ Adjunctive treatment of partial seizures

Adults and children ages 16 and older: 500 mg P.O. b.i.d. May increase by 1,000 mg/day q 2 weeks to a maximum daily dosage of 3,000 mg, as needed.

Dosage adjustment

- Renal impairment (especially in dialysis patients)

Contraindications

- Hypersensitivity to drug or its components

Precautions

Use cautiously in:

- renal, hepatic, or cardiac impairment
- psychosis
- pregnant or breastfeeding patients
- children.

Administration

- Give with or without food.

⚠ Don't discontinue suddenly. Instead, taper dosage gradually.

Route	Onset	Peak	Duration
P.O.	Rapid	1 hr	Unknown

Adverse reactions

CNS: aggression, anger, irritability, mental or mood changes, asthenia, ataxia, dizziness, drowsiness, headache, paresthesia, vertigo

EENT: diplopia, pharyngitis, rhinitis, sinusitis

GI: nausea, vomiting, anorexia

Hematologic: neutropenia, leukopenia

Respiratory: cough, sinusitis

Other: infection

Interactions

Drug-drug. *Phenytoin:* increased phenytoin blood level

Drug-herbs. *Evening primrose oil:* lowered seizure threshold

Patient monitoring

- Measure temperature and watch for signs and symptoms of infection.

⚠ Monitor neurologic status. Report signs that patient is dangerous to himself or others.

- Evaluate nutritional status. Report signs of anorexia.

Patient teaching

• Tell patient to take with or without food.

Advise family to contact prescriber if patient poses a danger to himself or others.

Caution patient not to stop taking drug abruptly, because doing so may increase seizure activity.

• Teach patient and family about adverse CNS reactions, and tell them to report these promptly. Urge them to take safety measures to prevent injury.

• Instruct patient to avoid activities that require mental alertness until CNS reactions are known.

• Inform patient that he'll undergo periodic blood testing during therapy.

• As appropriate, review all other significant and life-threatening adverse reactions and interactions, especially those related to the drugs and herbs mentioned above.

levofloxacin

Iquix, Levaquin, Quixin

Pharmacologic class: Fluoroquinolone
Therapeutic class: Anti-infective
Pregnancy risk category C

Action

Inhibits the enzyme DNA gyrase in susceptible gram-negative and gram-positive aerobic and anaerobic bacteria, interfering with bacterial DNA synthesis

Availability

Ophthalmic solution: Quixin—0.5% (5 mg/ml), Iquix—1.5%
Premixed solution for injection: 250 mg/50 ml, 500 mg/100 ml, 750 mg/150 ml
Solution for injection (concentrated): 500 mg/20 ml
Tablets: 250 mg, 500 mg, 750 mg

Indications and dosages

➤ Acute bacterial exacerbation of chronic bronchitis
Adults: 500 mg I.V. or P.O. q 24 hours for 7 days

➤ Community-acquired pneumonia
Adults: 500 mg I.V. or P.O. q 24 hours for 7 to 14 days, or 750 mg I.V. or P.O. q 24 hours for 5 days

➤ Nosocomial pneumonia caused by methicillin-susceptible strains of *Staphylococcus aureus, Pseudomonas aeruginosa, Serratia marcescens, Escherichia coli, Klebsiella pneumoniae, Haemophilus influenzae,* or *Streptococcus pneumoniae;* complicated skin and skin-structure infections
Adults: 750 mg I.V. or P.O. q 24 hours for 7 to 14 days

➤ Acute maxillary sinusitis
Adults: 500 mg I.V. or P.O. q 24 hours for 10 to 14 days

➤ Uncomplicated skin and skin-structure infections
Adults: 500 mg I.V. or P.O. q 24 hours for 7 to 10 days

➤ Complicated urinary tract infections; acute pyelonephritis caused by *E. coli*
Adults: 250 mg I.V. or P.O. q 24 hours for 10 days

➤ Uncomplicated urinary tract infections
Adults: 250 mg I.V. or P.O. q 24 hours for 3 days

➤ Chronic bacterial prostatitis
Adults: 500 mg I.V. or P.O. q 24 hours for 28 days.

➤ Conjunctivitis
Adults and children ages 1 and older: One or two drops of 0.5% ophthalmic solution into affected eye q 2 hours while awake on days 1 and 2 (up to eight times daily); then one or two drops q 4 hours while awake on days 3 through 7 (up to four times daily)

➤ Corneal ulcers
Adults and children ages 6 and older: On days 1 to 3, one or two drops of

1.5% ophthalmic solution instilled into affected eye(s) q 30 minutes to 1 hour while awake and q 4 to 6 hours after retiring; thereafter, one or two drops q 1 to 4 hours while awake until treatment completion

Dosage adjustment
• Renal impairment

Contraindications
• Hypersensitivity to drug, its components, or other quinolones

Precautions
Use cautiously in:
• bradycardia, acute myocardial ischemia, prolonged QTc interval, cirrhosis, renal impairment, underlying CNS disease, uncorrected hypocalcemia
• elderly patients
• pregnant or breastfeeding patients
• children younger than age 18 (except in ophthalmic use).

Administration
• Be aware that oral and I.V. dosages are identical.
• Give parenteral form by I.V. route only. Drug isn't for I.M., subcutaneous, intrathecal, or intraperitoneal use.
• To prepare I.V. infusion, use compatible solution, such as 0.9% sodium chloride injection, dextrose 5% and 0.9% sodium chloride injection, dextrose 5% in water, or dextrose 5% in lactated Ringer's solution.
• Infuse over 60 to 90 minutes, depending on dosage. Don't infuse with other drugs.
Avoid rapid or bolus I.V. administration, because this may cause severe hypotension
• Flush I.V. line before and after infusion.
• Give oral doses 2 hours before or after sucralfate, iron, antacids containing magnesium or aluminum, or multivitamins with zinc.
• Give oral form without regard to food, but don't give with milk or yogurt alone.
• Be aware that the two ophthalmic preparations have different indications.

Route	Onset	Peak	Duration
P.O.	Rapid	1-2 hr	24 hr
I.V.	Rapid	End of infusion	24 hr
Ophth.	Unknown	Unknown	Unknown

Adverse reactions
CNS: dizziness, headache, insomnia, **seizures**
CV: chest pain, palpitations, hypotension
EENT: photophobia, sinusitis, pharyngitis
GI: nausea, vomiting, diarrhea, constipation, abdominal pain, dyspepsia, flatulence, **pseudomembranous colitis**
GU: vaginitis
Hematologic: lymphocytopenia
Metabolic: hyperglycemia, **hypoglycemia**
Musculoskeletal: back pain, tendon rupture, tendinitis
Skin: photosensitivity
Other: altered taste, reaction and pain at I.V. site, hypersensitivity reactions including **Stevens-Johnson syndrome**

Interactions
Drug-drug. *Antacids containing aluminum or magnesium, didanosine (tablets), iron salts, sucralfate, zinc salts:* decreased levofloxacin absorption
Cimetidine: interference with levofloxacin elimination
Nonsteroidal anti-inflammatory drugs: increased risk of CNS stimulation and seizures
Drug-diagnostic tests. *Glucose:* increased or decreased level
Lymphocytes: decreased count
EEG: abnormal findings

Drug-food. *Concurrent tube feedings, milk, yogurt:* impaired levofloxacin absorption
Drug-herbs. *Dong quai, St. John's wort:* phototoxicity
Fennel: decreased levofloxacin absorption
Drug-behaviors. *Sun exposure:* phototoxicity

Patient monitoring

- Check vital signs, especially blood pressure. Too-rapid infusion can cause hypotension.
- Closely monitor patients with renal insufficiency
- Monitor blood glucose level closely in diabetic patients.

🔊 Assess for severe diarrhea, which may indicate pseudomembranous colitis.
🔊 Watch for hypersensitivity reaction. Discontinue drug immediately if rash or other signs or symptoms occur.

Patient teaching

🔊 Tell patient to stop taking drug and contact prescriber if he experiences signs or symptoms of hypersensitivity reaction (rash, hives, or other skin reactions) or severe diarrhea (which may indicate pseudomembranous colitis).

- Instruct patient not to take with milk, yogurt, multivitamins containing zinc or iron, or antacids containing aluminum or magnesium.
- Teach patient proper use of eye drops. Tell him to avoid touching applicator tip to eye, finger, or any other object.
- Caution patient to avoid driving and other activities that require mental alertness until CNS effects of drug are known.
- As appropriate, review all other significant and life-threatening adverse reactions and interactions, especially those related to the drugs, tests, foods, herbs, and behaviors mentioned above.

levonorgestrel

Mirena, Plan B

Pharmacologic class: Contraceptive, intrauterine device (Mirena); oral contraceptive, progestin-only pill (Plan B)
Therapeutic class: Contraceptive
Pregnancy risk category X (Mirena), ***NR*** (Plan B)

Action

Unclear. Mirena may enhance local contraceptive efficacy by thickening the cervical mucus (which prevents passage of sperm into uterus), inhibiting sperm capacitation or survival, and altering the endometrium. Plan B is thought to prevent ovulation or fertilization.

Availability

Intrauterine system (Mirena): 52 mg levonorgestrel
Two-tablet, single course of treatment (Plan B): 0.75 mg levonorgestrel per tablet

Indications and dosages

➢ Intrauterine contraception for up to 5 years
Adults: One intrauterine system (Mirena) inserted into uterus for up to 5 years
➢ Emergency contraception to prevent pregnancy
Adults: One tablet (Plan B) P.O. within 72 hours after unprotected intercourse, with second tablet taken 12 hours after first tablet

Contraindications

Mirena—

- Hypersensitivity to drug or its components
- Known or suspected pregnancy

• Congenital or acquired uterine anomaly
• Acute pelvic inflammatory disease (PID) or history of PID (unless patient had subsequent intrauterine pregnancy)
• Postpartum endometritis or infected abortion within past 3 months
• Known or suspected uterine or cervical neoplasia or unresolved abnormal Papanicolaou (Pap) test
• Untreated acute cervicitis or vaginitis
• Acute hepatic disease or hepatic tumor (benign or malignant)
• Genital bleeding of unknown cause
• Conditions associated with increased risk of infection
• Genital actinomycosis
• Previously inserted intrauterine device that has not been removed
• Known or suspected breast cancer
• History of ectopic pregnancy or conditions that predispose to it

Plan B —
• Hypersensitivity to drug or its components
• Known or suspected pregnancy
• Undiagnosed abnormal genital bleeding

Precautions

Use Mirena cautiously in:
• diabetes mellitus
• breastfeeding patients.

Use Plan B cautiously in:
• coagulopathy
• diabetes mellitus
• patients receiving anticoagulants concurrently.

Administration

• Know that Mirena should be inserted under aseptic conditions by health care professional familiar with procedure.
• Verify that patient isn't pregnant before Mirena insertion.
• Know that Plan B should be given as soon as possible within 72 hours of unprotected sexual intercourse. Drug isn't suitable as long-term contraceptive.

Route	Onset	Peak	Duration
P.O.	Unknown	1.6 ± 0.7 hr	Unknown
Intrauterine	No peaks or troughs		

Adverse reactions

CNS: headache (Mirena, Plan B), fatigue, dizziness (Plan B), severe headache, migraine, nervousness, depression (Mirena)
CV: hypertension (Mirena)
EENT: sinusitis (Mirena)
GI: nausea, vomiting, abdominal pain (Mirena, Plan B), diarrhea (Plan B), **intestinal perforation or obstruction** (Mirena)
GU: breast tenderness (Mirena, Plan B); lighter or heavier menstrual bleeding (Plan B); breast pain; increased progesterone levels; ovarian cysts; dysmenorrhea; amenorrhea; spotting; erratic or prolonged menstrual bleeding; pelvic infection; vaginitis; cervicitis; dyspareunia; leukorrhea; decreased libido; abnormal Pap smear; expulsion, embedment in myometrium, adhesions, **cervical or ureteral perforation** (Mirena)
Hematologic: anemia (Mirena)
Hepatic: jaundice (Mirena)
Musculoskeletal: back pain (Mirena)
Respiratory: upper respiratory tract infection (Mirena)
Skin: skin disorder, acne, eczema, hair loss (Mirena)
Other: water retention, weight gain, **sepsis** (Mirena)

Interactions

Drug-drug. *Hepatic enzyme-inducing drugs (such as barbiturates, carbamazepine, phenytoin, rifampin):* decreased Plan B efficacy
Drug-diagnostic tests. *Glucose:* altered level (Mirena)

Patient monitoring

• Monitor blood pressure.

• Watch for adverse reactions, especially changes in menstrual bleeding.
• Monitor blood glucose level in diabetic patients.
• Check liver function tests frequently.

Patient teaching

• Tell patient taking either product that drug does not prevent HIV or other sexually transmitted diseases.
• Teach patient using Mirena how to check (after menstrual period) to make sure thread still protrudes from cervix. Caution her not to pull on thread, because this could cause displacement.
Instruct patient using Mirena to immediately report fever, chills, unusual vaginal discharge, or abdominal or pelvic pain or tenderness.
• Explain that for maximum efficacy, patient should take Plan B as soon as possible after unprotected sex.
• Inform patient that Plan B isn't intended for routine contraception and doesn't terminate existing pregnancy.
• Tell patient to report adverse reactions.
• As appropriate, review all other significant and life-threatening adverse reactions and interactions, especially those related to the drugs and tests mentioned above.

levorphanol tartrate

Levo-Dromoran

Pharmacologic class: Synthetic opioid agonist
Therapeutic class: Opioid analgesic
Controlled substance schedule II
Pregnancy risk category C

Action

Inhibits adenylate cyclase, which regulates release of pain neurotransmitters (acetylcholine, dopamine, substance P, and gamma-aminobutyric acid). Also stimulates mu and kappa opioid receptors, altering perception of and emotional response to pain.

Availability

Injection: 2 mg/ml
Tablets: 2 mg

Indications and dosages

➤ Pain
Adults: 2 mg P.O. q 3 to 6 hours p.r.n., provided patient is assessed for hypoventilation and excessive sedation. Range is 8 to 16 mg over 24 hours in nontolerant patients (daily dosages above 16 mg aren't recommended). Alternatively, 2 mg subcutaneously or I.V.; may increase to 3 mg p.r.n. For cancer patients and in other situations in which long-term opioid therapy is indicated, daily dosage is approximately one-twelfth of daily oral morphine dosage; however, therapy should be individualized.
➤ Preoperative analgesia
Adults: 1 to 2 mg subcutaneously 90 minutes before surgery

Dosage adjustment

• Hepatic or renal insufficiency
• Elderly patients

Contraindications

• Hypersensitivity to drug or other opioid agonists
• Bronchial asthma
• Increased intracranial pressure
• Respiratory depression
• Acute alcoholism

Precautions

Use cautiously in:
• renal or hepatic dysfunction, chronic obstructive pulmonary disease, acute abdominal conditions, cardiovascular disease, seizure disorders, cerebral arteriosclerosis, Addison's disease, prostatic hypertrophy, toxic psychosis
• pregnant or breastfeeding patients
• children.

Administration

Make sure resuscitation equipment is available before starting therapy.

- Give I.V. injection slowly, administering each 2 mg over at least 4 to 5 minutes. Monitor patient response.
- Know that I.V. route is preferred in emergencies only.
- After parenteral administration, place patient in supine position with legs elevated to minimize adverse reactions.
- Be aware that 2 mg of levorphanol tartrate is analgesically equivalent to 10 to 15 mg of morphine and 100 mg of meperidine.

Route	Onset	Peak	Duration
P.O.	10-60 min	90-120 min	4-5 hr
I.V.	Unknown	20 min	4-5 hr
I.M.	Unknown	60 min	4-5 hr
Subcut.	Unknown	60-90 min	4-5 hr

Adverse reactions

CNS: personality disorders, nervousness, insomnia, hypokinesia, dyskinesia, drowsiness, light-headedness, dizziness, depression, delusions, confusion, amnesia, sedation, euphoria, delirium, mood changes, **coma, seizures**
CV: palpitations, hypotension, tachycardia, bradycardia, **shock, peripheral circulatory collapse, cardiac arrest**
EENT: diplopia, abnormal vision
GI: nausea, vomiting, constipation, abdominal pain, dyspepsia, increased colonic motility (in patients with chronic ulcerative colitis), dry mouth
GU: dysuria, urinary retention or hesitancy, ureteral or vesicle sphincter spasms, decreased libido, **oliguria**
Hepatic: biliary tract spasms, **hepatic failure**
Respiratory: suppressed cough reflex, hyperventilation, **periodic apnea**
Skin: urticaria, rash, pruritus, cyanosis, facial flushing
Other: injection site pain, redness, or swelling; physical or psychological drug dependence

Interactions

Drug-drug. *Alfentanil, fentanyl, sufentanil, other CNS depressants:* increased CNS and respiratory depression, increased risk of hypotension
Anticholinergics: increased risk of severe constipation
Antidiarrheals (such as atropine, difenoxin, kaolin, loperamide), antihypertensives: increased risk of hypotension
Buprenorphine, naloxone, naltrexone: decreased levorphanol efficacy
Metoclopramide: antagonism of metoclopramide effects
Neuromuscular blockers: increased risk of prolonged CNS and respiratory depression
Drug-diagnostic tests. *Amylase, lipase:* increased levels
Drug-behaviors. *Alcohol use:* increased CNS depression

Patient monitoring

- Check vital signs and respiratory status, and monitor ECG carefully.
- Evaluate fluid intake and output.
- Assess neurologic status. Institute safety precautions as needed to prevent injury.
- Watch for signs and symptoms of depression.
- Monitor liver and kidney function tests.

Patient teaching

- With parenteral use, explain need for continuous vital sign and ECG monitoring.
- To minimize adverse effects, instruct patient to lie supine after parenteral administration, if possible.

Instruct patient or caregiver to report adverse reactions immediately.

- Tell patient or caregiver to use safety measures as needed to prevent injury and to report significant problems.

• Instruct patient to minimize GI upset by eating small, frequent servings of food and drinking plenty of fluids.
• Caution patient to avoid driving and other hazardous activities until he knows how drug affects concentration and alertness.
• As appropriate, review all other significant and life-threatening adverse reactions and interactions, especially those related to the drugs, tests, and behaviors mentioned above.

levothyroxine sodium (L-thyroxine, T_4)

Eltroxin✦, Levolet, Levo-T, Levothroid, Levoxyl, PMS-Levothyroxine Sodium✦, Synthroid, Thyro-Tabs, Unithroid

Pharmacologic class: Synthetic thyroxine hormone
Therapeutic class: Thyroid hormone replacement
Pregnancy risk category A

Action

Synthetic form of thyroxine that replaces endogenous thyroxine, increasing thyroid hormone levels. Thyroid hormones help regulate cell growth and differentiation and increase metabolism of lipids, protein, and carbohydrates.

Availability

Powder for injection: 200 mcg/vial in 6- and 10-ml vials, 500 mcg/vial in 6- and 10-ml vials
Tablets: 25 mcg, 50 mcg, 75 mcg, 88 mcg, 100 mcg, 112 mcg, 125 mcg, 137 mcg, 150 mcg, 175 mcg, 200 mcg, 300 mcg

Indications and dosages

➢ Hypothyroidism; treatment or prevention of euthyroid goiter
Adults: For healthy adults younger than age 50 and those over age 50 who have recently been treated or undergone short-term therapy, start at full replacement dosage of 1.7 mcg/kg P.O. daily, given 30 minutes to 1 hour before breakfast. For patients older than age 50 or younger than age 50 with heart disease, 25 to 50 mcg P.O. daily, increased q 4 to 6 weeks. In severe hypothyroidism, initial dosage is 12.5 to 25 mcg P.O. daily, adjusted by 25 mcg daily q 2 to 4 weeks. For patients who can't tolerate oral doses, adjust I.M. or I.V. dosage to roughly half of oral dosage.

➢ Congenital hypothyroidism
Children older than age 12 who have completed puberty and growth: 1.7 mcg/kg P.O. daily
Children older than age 12 who have not completed puberty and growth: Up to 150 mcg or 2 to 3 mcg/kg P.O. daily
Children ages 6 to 12: 4 to 5 mcg/kg P.O. daily
Children ages 1 to 5: 5 to 6 mcg/kg P.O. daily
Infants ages 6 to 12 months: 6 to 8 mcg/kg P.O. daily
Infants ages 3 to 6 months: 8 to 10 mcg/kg P.O. daily
Infants up to 3 months old: 10 to 15 mcg/kg P.O. daily

➢ Myxedema coma or stupor
Adults: 200 to 500 mcg I.V. as a solution containing 100 mcg/ml. Additional 100 to 300 mcg may be given on day 2 if significant improvement has not occurred. Convert to P.O. therapy when patient is clinically stable.

➢ Thyroid-stimulating hormone suppression in well-differentiated thyroid cancers and thyroid nodules
Adults: Dosage individualized based on disease and patient

Dosage adjustment

- Cardiovascular disease
- Psychosis or agitation
- Elderly patients

Contraindications

- Hypersensitivity to drug, its components, or tartrazine
- Acute myocardial infarction
- Thyrotoxicosis
- Adrenal insufficiency

Precautions

Use cautiously in:

- cardiovascular disease, severe renal insufficiency, diabetes mellitus
- elderly patients
- pregnant or breastfeeding patients.

Administration

- Be aware that all dosages are highly individualized.
- Give tablets on an empty stomach 30 minutes to 1 hour before first meal of day.
- If patient can't swallow tablets, crush them and sprinkle onto small amount of food, such as applesauce. For infants and children, dissolve tablets in small amount of water, nonsoybean formula, or breast milk and administer immediately.
- Don't give oral form within 4 hours of bile acid sequestrants or antacids.
- Reconstitute Synthroid powder for injection with 5 ml of 0.9% sodium chloride injection. Shake until clear and use immediately.
- For I.V. administration, give each 100 mcg over at least 1 minute.
- Be aware that the various levothyroxine preparations aren't bioequivalent. Patient should consistently use same brand or generic product, with dosing based on weight, age, physical condition, and symptom duration.
- When drug is given for thyroid-stimulating hormone (TSH) suppression test, TSH suppression level is not well established and radioactive iodine (^{131}I) is given before and after treatment course.

Route	Onset	Peak	Duration
P.O.	Unknown	Unknown	Unknown
I.V.	6-8 hr	24 hr	Unknown
I.M.	Unknown	Unknown	Unknown

Adverse reactions

CNS: insomnia, irritability, nervousness, headache
CV: tachycardia, angina pectoris, hypotension, hypertension, increased cardiac output, **arrhythmias, cardiovascular collapse**
GI: vomiting, diarrhea, abdominal cramps
GU: menstrual irregularities
Metabolic: hyperthyroidism
Musculoskeletal: accelerated bone maturation (in children), decreased bone density (in women on long-term therapy)
Skin: alopecia (in children), diaphoresis
Other: heat intolerance, weight loss

Interactions

Drug-drug. *Aminoglutethimide, amiodarone, anabolic steroids, antithyroid drugs, asparaginase, barbiturates, carbamazepine, chloral hydrate, cholestyramine, clofibrate, colestipol, corticosteroids, danazol, diazepam, estrogens, ethionamide, fluorouracil, heparin (with I.V. use), insulin, lithium, methadone, mitotane, nitroprusside, oxyphenbutazone, perphenazine, phenylbutazone, phenytoin, propranolol, salicylates (large doses), sulfonylureas, thiazides:* altered thyroid function test results
Antacids, bile acid sequestrants: interference with levothyroxine absorption
Anticoagulants: increased anticoagulant action
Beta-adrenergic blockers (selected): decreased beta blocker action
Cardiac glycosides: decreased cardiac glycoside blood level

L

Cholestyramine, colestipol: levothyroxine inefficacy
Theophyllines: decreased theophylline clearance
Drug-diagnostic tests. *Thyroid function tests:* decreased values
Drug-food. *Foods high in iron or fiber, soybeans:* decreased drug absorption

Patient monitoring

- Check vital signs and ECG routinely.
- Monitor thyroid and liver function tests.

🔈 Evaluate for signs and symptoms of overdose, including those of hyperthyroidism (weight loss, cardiac symptoms, abdominal cramps).

- Monitor closely for drug efficacy.
- Check patients with Addison's disease or diabetes mellitus for worsening of these conditions.

🔈 Watch for signs and symptoms of bleeding tendency, especially in patients receiving anticoagulants concurrently.

Patient teaching

- Explain that patient may require lifelong therapy and must undergo regular blood testing.
- Tell patient or parent to report adverse effects, including signs or symptoms of hyperthyroidism or hypothyroidism.
- Caution patient to avoid driving and other hazardous activities until he knows how drug affects concentration and alertness.
- Advise patient to avoid getting overheated, as in hot environments or during vigorous exercise.
- Tell parents that child being treated may lose hair during first few months of therapy. Reassure them that this effect usually is transient.
- As appropriate, review all other significant and life-threatening adverse reactions and interactions, especially those related to the drugs, tests, and foods mentioned above.

lidocaine hydrochloride

Anestacon, Lidoderm, LidoPen Auto-Injector, Xylocaine, Xylocaine-MPF, Xylocaine Viscous, Xylocard✦

Pharmacologic class: Amide
Therapeutic class: Antiarrhythmic (class IB), local anesthetic
Pregnancy risk category B

Action

Suppresses automaticity of ventricular cells, decreasing diastolic depolarization and increasing ventricular fibrillation threshold. Produces local anesthesia by reducing sodium permeability of sensory nerves, which blocks impulse generation and conduction.

Availability

Injection for I.M. use: 300 mg/3 ml (automatic injection device)
Injection for direct I.V. use: 1% and 2% in syringes and vials
Injection for I.V. infusion: 2 mg/ml, 4 mg/ml, 8 mg/ml
Injection for I.V injection admixtures: 40 mg/ml, 100 mg/ml, 200 mg/ml
Patch: 5%
Topical cream: 0.5%, 4%
Topical gel: 0.5%, 2.5%
Topical jelly: 2%
Topical liquid, ointment: 2.5%, 5%
Topical solution: 4%
Topical solution (viscous): 2%
Topical spray: 0.5%

Indications and dosages

➢ Ventricular arrhythmias
Adults: Initially, 50 to 100 mg I.V. bolus given at rate of 25 to 50 mg/minute. If desired response doesn't occur after 5 minutes, give repeat dose at 25 to 50 mg/minute; maximum dosage is 300 mg given over 1 hour. Mainte-

nance dosage is 1 to 4 mg/minute by continuous I.V. infusion for no more than 24 hours.
Children: Initially, 1 mg/kg I.V. bolus, then repeated based on patient response; don't exceed 5 mg/kg. Maintenance dosage is 30 mcg/kg/minute by continuous I.V. infusion.
➢ Caudal anesthesia (without epinephrine)
Adults: For obstetric analgesia, 200 to 300 mg caudally as 1% solution. For surgical anesthesia, 225 to 300 mg as 1.5% solution. For continuous caudal anesthesia, don't repeat maximum dosage at intervals of less than 90 minutes.
➢ Epidural anesthesia (without epinephrine)
Adults: For lumbar analgesia, 250 to 300 mg epidurally as 1% solution, 225 to 300 mg as 1.5% solution, or 200 to 300 mg as 2% solution. For thoracic anesthesia, 200 to 300 mg as 1% solution. For continuous epidural anesthesia, don't repeat maximum dosage at intervals of less than 90 minutes.
➢ I.V. regional infiltration (without epinephrine)
Adults: 50 to 300 mg I.V. as 0.5% solution. For I.V. regional anesthesia, maximum dosage is 4 mg/kg.
➢ I.V. local infiltration (without epinephrine)
Children: Up to 4.5 mg/kg I.V. as 0.25% to 1% solution
➢ Spinal anesthesia (without epinephrine)
Adults: For obstetric low-spinal or saddle-block anesthesia (normal vaginal delivery), 50 mg of 5% Xylocaine-MPF with glucose 7.5%, or 9 to 15 mg of 1.5% Xylocaine-MPF with dextrose 7.5%. For cesarean section, 75 mg of 5% Xylocaine-MPF with glucose 7.5%. For surgical anesthesia, 75 to 100 mg of 5% Xylocaine-MPF with glucose 7.5%.
➢ Paracervical anesthesia (without epinephrine)
Adults: For obstetric analgesia, 100 mg paracervically as 1% solution (each side). For paracervical block, maximum dosage is 200 mg over each 90-minute period (half administered on each side).
➢ Peripheral nerve block
Adults: For brachial nerve block, 225 to 300 mg as 1.5% solution. For dental nerve block, 20 to 100 mg as 2% solution with epinephrine 1:100,000 or 1:50,000. For intercostal nerve block, 30 mg as 1% solution. For pudendal nerve block, 100 mg as 1% solution. For paravertebral nerve block, 30 mg to 50 mg as 1% solution.
➢ Sympathetic nerve block (without epinephrine)
Adults: For cervical nerve block, 50 mg as 1% solution. For lumbar nerve block, 50 to 100 mg as 1% solution.
➢ Dental anesthesia
Adults: 1 to 5 ml of lidocaine 2% with epinephrine 1:50,000 or 1:100,000. Maximum dosage is less than 500 mg (7 mg/kg).
Children: 20 to 30 mg as 2% solution with epinephrine 1:100,000
➢ Topical anesthesia for skin or mucous membranes
Adults: Apply thin layer of gel, jelly, or ointment to skin or mucous membranes as needed before procedure; or apply 5% patch to most painful areas and intact skin (up to three patches at a time for up to 12 hours within a 24-hour period). For new denture fittings, use 5-g ointment (250 mg) per single dose or 20 g/day. For oropharyngeal use, apply to desired area or to instrument before insertion.
Children: Apply thin layer of ointment to skin or mucous membranes p.r.n. before procedure. Maximum dosage is 2.5 g ointment per 6 hours or 4.5 mg/kg.
➢ Prevention or treatment of pain during procedures involving male or female urethra
Adults: For female urethral examination, apply 3 to 5 ml of 2% jelly topi-

L

cally several minutes before exam. For male sounding or cystoscopy, apply 5 to 10 ml of 2% jelly topically before procedure, or apply 30 ml to fill or dilate urethra in divided doses using penile clamp for several minutes between doses. For male catheterization, apply 5 to 10 ml of 2% jelly to anterior urethra before procedure. Don't use more than 600 mg/12 hours.

➢ Oral cavity disorders; pharyngeal disorders

Adults: For oral cavity disorders, 300 mg (15 ml) of viscous oral topical solution swished and then expelled, or applied with cotton swab q 3 hours p.r.n. For pharyngeal disorders, use same dosage, but solution may be swallowed.

Children older than age 3: Dosage individualized based on age, weight, and physical condition. Maximum dosage is 4.5 mg/kg q 3 hours.

Children up to age 3: 1.25 ml applied with swab q 3 hours

➢ Local anesthesia (oral or nasal mucosa)

Adults: 0.6 to 3 mg/kg or 40 to 200 mg of 4% topical solution, not to exceed 4.5 mg/kg or 300 mg (7.5 ml)

Children: Dosage individualized

Off-label uses

- Pediatric patients with cardiac arrest who develop frequent premature ventricular contractions
- Status epilepticus

Contraindications

- Hypersensitivity to drug, its components, or other amide local anesthetics
- Heart failure, cardiogenic shock, second- or third-degree heart block, intraventricular block in absence of a pacemaker
- Wolff-Parkinson-White or Adams-Stokes syndrome
- Severe hemorrhage, shock, or heart block (lidocaine with dextrose)
- Local infection at puncture site (lidocaine with dextrose)
- Septicemia (lidocaine with dextrose)

Precautions

Use cautiously in:

- renal or hepatic disorders, inflammation or sepsis in injection area
- labor or delivery
- breastfeeding patients.

Administration

🔊 Know that I.V. lidocaine is a high-alert drug.

🔊 Make sure resuscitation equipment and oxygen are available before giving I.V. lidocaine.

- Dilute injection in additive syringe and single-use vial according to manufacturer's instructions before administering as I.V. infusion.
- Add 1 g lidocaine to 1 L dextrose 5% in water to yield a solution of 1 mg/ml.
- For I.V. bolus injection, give doses of 25 to 50 mg over at least 1 minute. Deliver continuous infusion by infusion pump no faster than 4 mg/minute.

🔊 Know that too-rapid infusion may cause seizures.

- Be aware that drug can be given I.M. using 10% parenteral solution only.

Route	Onset	Peak	Duration
I.V.	45-90 sec	Immediate	10-20 min
I.M.	5-15 min	Unknown	60-90 min
Topical	2-5 min	Unknown	30-60 min

Adverse reactions

CNS: anxiety; confusion; difficulty speaking; dizziness; hallucinations; lethargy; paresthesia; light-headedness; fatigue; drowsiness; headache; persistent sensory, motor, or **autonomic deficit of lower spinal segment; septic meningitis; seizures**

CV: bradycardia, hypotension, new or worsening **arrhythmias, cardiac arrest**

EENT: diplopia, abnormal vision

GI: nausea, vomiting, dry mouth

GU: urinary retention
Metabolic: methemoglobinemia
Respiratory: suppressed cough reflex, **respiratory depression, respiratory arrest**
Skin: rash; urticaria; pruritus; erythema; contact dermatitis; cutaneous lesions; tissue irritation, sloughing, and necrosis
Other: fever; edema; infection, burning, stinging, tenderness, and swelling at injection site; **anaphylaxis**

Interactions

Drug-drug. *Beta-adrenergic blockers, cimetidine:* increased lidocaine blood level
MAO inhibitors, tricyclic antidepressants: prolonged hypertension
Mexiletine, tocainide: additive cardiac effects
Phenytoin, procainamide: increased cardiac depression
Drug-diagnostic tests. *Creatine kinase:* increased level (with I.M. use)

Patient monitoring

- Monitor vital signs and ECG continuously. Watch for cardiac depression.
- Evaluate level of consciousness closely.
- Watch for adverse reactions, particularly anaphylaxis.
- Stay alert for seizures.
- Monitor neurologic status for lower spinal segment deficits.
- Give supportive oxygen therapy, as indicated and prescribed.
- Monitor electrolyte, blood urea nitrogen, and creatinine levels.
- Assess topical site for adverse reactions.

Patient teaching

- Discuss reason for drug therapy with patient and family, when appropriate.
- Explain that patient will be monitored continuously during therapy.
- Instruct patient to promptly report discomfort at I.V. site as well as adverse effects, especially cardiovascular, respiratory, or neurologic problems or allergic reactions.
- As appropriate, review all other significant and life-threatening adverse reactions and interactions, especially those related to the drugs and tests mentioned above.

lindane

Hexit Lotion*, Hexit Shampoo 1*, Kwell, PMS-Lindane LOT 1*, PMS-Lindane SHP 1*

Pharmacologic class: Chlorinated hydrocarbon
Therapeutic class: Scabicide, pediculocide
Pregnancy risk category C

Action

Absorbed through parasitic ova and arthropods, which stimulates parasitic nervous system and results in seizures and death of parasite

Availability

Lotion: 1%
Shampoo: 1%

Indications and dosages

➢ Secondary treatment of scabies
Adults and children: Apply enough lotion on dry skin to cover entire surface from neck down. Rub in well, and leave in place 12 hours. Then wash skin thoroughly.
➢ Secondary treatment of *Pediculosis capitis* (head lice) or *Pediculosis pubis* (pubic lice)
Adults and children: Apply enough shampoo to dry hair (1 oz or less for short hair, 1½ oz for medium length

hair, up to 2 oz for long hair) to thoroughly wet hair and skin or scalp of affected and surrounding hairy areas. Leave in place 12 hours. Then wash hair thoroughly.

Contraindications

- Hypersensitivity to drug or its components
- Seizure disorder
- Crusted (Norwegian) scabies and other conditions that may increase systemic drug absorption
- Premature neonates

Precautions

Use cautiously in:
- conditions that increase seizure risk (such as history of seizures, head injury, AIDS)
- skin conditions
- concurrent use of skin creams, oils, or ointments
- patients weighing less than 50 kg (110 lb)
- elderly patients
- breastfeeding patients
- infants or children.

Administration

- To apply, wear gloves made of nitrile, latex with neoprene, or sheer vinyl.
- Before applying lindane shampoo, use regular shampoo without conditioner; rinse and dry hair completely. Wait 1 hour before using lindane shampoo.
- Don't use lindane lotion or shampoo with other lotions, creams, or oils.
- Thoroughly wash skin after lotion has been in place for 12 hours.

Route	Onset	Peak	Duration
Topical	Unknown	6 hr	Unknown

Adverse reactions

CNS: dizziness, **seizures**, headache, anxiety, paresthesia
EENT: irritation of eyes, nose, and throat (from vapor inhalation)
GI: nausea and vomiting (from vapor inhalation)
Hematologic: aplastic anemia (with prolonged use)
Skin: dermatitis, urticaria, pruritus, alopecia
Other: pain

Interactions

Drug-drug. *Drugs that lower seizure threshold, antidepressants:* increased seizure activity

Patient monitoring

- Monitor drug efficacy.

Patient teaching

- 🔊 Emphasize that drug is for external use only, and that ingesting even small amounts can be fatal.
- If drug will be applied by another person, tell patient that this person must wear gloves made of nitrile, latex with neoprene, or sheer vinyl.
- Instruct patient using lindane lotion to wash, rinse, and dry skin well before applying lindane if skin has cream, lotion, ointment, or oil on it. If he takes a warm bath or shower before applying lindane, instruct him to let skin dry and cool down. Then tell him to apply lindane to dry skin, rub in well, leave on skin for 8 to 12 hours, and then remove it by washing thoroughly.
- Instruct patient using lindane shampoo to apply enough shampoo to dry hair to thoroughly wet the hair and skin or scalp of affected and surrounding hairy areas, and then rub shampoo thoroughly into hair and skin or scalp and let it sit for 4 minutes. Then tell him to add just enough water to work up a good lather, then rinse thoroughly and dry hair with clean towel. When hair is completely dry, instruct him to comb it with a fine-toothed comb to remove any remaining nits or nit shells. Tell him not to use shampoo in combination with oils, lotions, or creams.

• To avoid reinfestation, instruct patient to launder all recently worn or used clothing, bed linens, and towels in hot water.
• Caution patient to avoid contact with eyes when applying lotion or shampoo.
• Tell patient with scabies that sexual contacts and other close personal contacts should be examined and, if necessary, treated.
• Advise female patient to inform prescriber if she plans to breastfeed.
• As appropriate, review all other significant and life-threatening adverse reactions and interactions, especially those related to the drugs mentioned above.

linezolid

Zyvox

Pharmacologic class: Oxazolidinone
Therapeutic class: Anti-infective
Pregnancy risk category C

Action

Selectively binds to bacterial 23S ribosomal RNA of 50S subunit, preventing formation of essential component of bacterial protein synthesis. Bacteriostatic or bactericidal against gram-positive and some gram-negative bacteria.

Availability

Injection: 2 mg/ml
Powder for oral suspension: 100 mg/5 ml
Tablets: 400 mg, 600 mg

Indications and dosages

➤Vancomycin-resistant *Enterococcus faecium* infections
Adults and children ages 12 and older: 600 mg P.O. or I.V. infusion q 12 hours for 14 to 28 days
Children from birth to age 11: 10 mg/kg I.V. q 8 hours for 14 to 28 days
➤Nosocomial pneumonia; community-acquired pneumonia; complicated skin and skin-structure infections
Adults and children ages 12 and older: 600 mg P.O. or I.V. infusion q 12 hours for 10 to 14 days
Children from birth to age 11: 10 mg/kg P.O. or I.V. q 8 hours for 10 to 14 days
➤Uncomplicated skin and soft-tissue infections
Adults: 400 mg P.O. q 12 hours for 10 to 14 days
Adolescents: 600 mg P.O. or I.V. q 12 hours for 10 to 14 days
Children ages 5 to 11: 10 mg/kg P.O. or I.V. q 12 hours for 10 to 14 days
Children younger than age 5: 10 mg/kg P.O. or I.V. q 8 hours for 10 to 14 days

Contraindications

• Hypersensitivity to drug or its components

Precautions

Use cautiously in:
• hepatic dysfunction, hypertension, hyperthyroidism, pheochromocytoma, bone marrow depression, pseudomembranous colitis
• phenylketonuria (oral suspension only)
• pregnant or breastfeeding patients.

Administration

• Give oral drug with or without food.
• For I.V. injection, use single-use, ready-to-use infusion bag. Check for particulate matter before giving. Infuse over 30 minutes to 2 hours.
• For I.V. infusion, mix with dextrose 5% in water, normal saline solution, or lactated Ringer's injection.
• Flush I.V. line before and after administering, to avoid incompatibilities.

Route	Onset	Peak	Duration
P.O.	Rapid	1-2 hr	Unknown
I.V.	Unknown	Unknown	Unknown

Adverse reactions

CNS: anxiety, confusion, difficulty speaking, dizziness, hallucinations, lethargy, paresthesia, light-headedness, fatigue, drowsiness, headache, **seizures**
GI: nausea, vomiting, diarrhea, gastritis, anorexia, dry mouth, **pseudomembranous colitis**
Hematologic: thrombocytopenia
Skin: rash, photosensitivity, diaphoresis
Other: fever, fungal infections

Interactions

Drug-drug. *Antiplatelet drugs (such as aspirin, dipyridamole, nonsteroidal anti-inflammatory drugs):* increased bleeding risk
MAO inhibitors, pseudoephedrine: increased risk of hypertension and associated adverse effects
Serotonergics: serotonin syndrome
Drug-diagnostic tests. *Prothrombin time:* altered
Drug-food. *Tyramine-containing foods and beverages (such as beer; Chianti and certain other red wines; aged cheese; bananas; aged, cured, or spoiled meats; salted herring and other dried fish; avocado; bananas; bean curd; red plums; soy sauce; spinach; tofu, tomatoes; yeast):* hypertension

Patient monitoring

- Monitor neurologic status. Institute safety measures as needed to prevent injury.
- Check I.V. site for infiltration.

◀ Watch for bleeding and signs and symptoms of other adverse reactions (especially pseudomembranous colitis).

- Monitor CBC, coagulation studies, and culture and sensitivity tests.

Patient teaching

- Tell patient he may take with or without food, but should avoid foods containing tyramine.

◀ Tell patient to promptly report bleeding or severe diarrhea.

- Instruct patient to minimize adverse GI effects by eating small, frequent servings of healthy foods.
- Caution patient to avoid driving and other hazardous activities until he knows how drug affects concentration and alertness.
- As appropriate, review all other significant and life-threatening adverse reactions and interactions, especially those related to the drugs, tests, and foods mentioned above.

liothyronine sodium (T_3)

Cytomel, Triostat

Pharmacologic class: Synthetic thyroxine hormone
Therapeutic class: Thyroid hormone replacement
Pregnancy risk category A

Action

Synthetic form of triiodothyronine (T_3). Regulates cell growth and differentiation; increases metabolism of lipids, proteins, and carbohydrates; and enhances aerobic mitochondrial function. Also reduces tissue lactic acidosis.

Availability

Injection: 10 mcg/ml in 1-ml vials
Tablets: 5 mcg, 25 mcg, 50 mcg

Indications and dosages

➤ Thyroid hormone replacement in mild hypothyroidism
Adults: All dosages individualized. Initially, 25 mcg P.O. daily; may increase in increments of 12.5 to 25 mcg/day q 1 to 2 weeks. Usual maintenance dosage is 25 to 75 mcg P.O. daily.
➤ Myxedema
Adults: All dosages individualized. Initially, 5 mcg P.O. daily; increase in increments of 5 to 10 mcg/day q 1 to 2 weeks, up to 25 mcg/day. If response

still isn't adequate, increase by 5 mcg to 25 mcg P.O. daily q 1 to 2 weeks until desired response occurs. Usual maintenance dosage is 50 to 100 mcg/day P.O.

➢ Myxedema coma

Adults: Initially, 25 to 50 mcg I.V.; after 4 hours, reassess patient's need for subsequent doses (up to 65 mcg in 24 hours). In cardiovascular disease, initial dosage is 10 to 20 mcg I.V.

➢ Simple goiter

Adults: All dosages individualized. Initially, 5 mcg P.O. daily. Increase by 5 to 10 mcg/day q 1 to 2 weeks, up to 25 mcg/day; then increase by 12.5 to 25 mcg P.O. daily q week until desired effect occurs. Usual maintenance dosage is 75 mcg P.O. daily.

Children or elderly adults: Initially, 5 mcg P.O once daily. Increase by 5 mcg q 1 to 2 weeks until desired effect occurs.

➢ T_3 suppression test to distinguish hyperthyroidism from thyroid gland autonomy

Adults: 75 to 100 mcg P.O. daily for 7 days in conjunction with radioactive iodine

Dosage adjustment

- Severe, long-standing hypothyroidism
- Cardiovascular disease
- Psychosis or agitation
- Elderly patients

Contraindications

- Hypersensitivity to drug or its components
- Acute myocardial infarction
- Untreated thyrotoxicosis
- Uncorrected adrenal insufficiency and coexisting hypothyroidism
- Artificial rewarming (I.V. form only)

Precautions

Use cautiously in:

- cardiovascular disease, severe renal insufficiency, uncorrected adrenocortical disorders, diabetes mellitus
- elderly patients
- pregnant or breastfeeding patients.

Administration

- Know that all dosages are highly individualized.
- Administer single oral dose in morning with or without food.
- Injectable form is for I.V. use only. Don't give I.M.
- Infuse each 10-mcg dose over 1 minute.
- Give repeat I.V. doses more than 4 hours but less than 12 hours apart.
- Be aware that in T_3 suppression test, radioactive iodine (^{131}I) is given before and after 7-day liothyronine course.

Route	Onset	Peak	Duration
P.O.	Unknown	24-72 hr	72 hr
I.V.	Unknown	Unknown	Unknown

Adverse reactions

CNS: insomnia, irritability, nervousness, headache

CV: tachycardia, angina pectoris, hypotension, hypertension, increased cardiac output, **arrhythmias, cardiovascular collapse**

GI: vomiting, diarrhea, cramps

GU: menstrual irregularities

Metabolic: hyperthyroidism, hyperglycemia

Musculoskeletal: accelerated bone maturation (in children), decreased bone density (with long-term use in women)

Skin: alopecia (in children), diaphoresis

Other: weight loss, heat intolerance

Interactions

Drug-drug. *Anabolic steroids, antithyroid drugs, asparaginase, barbiturates, carbamazepine, chloral hydrate, clofibrate, corticosteroids, danazol, estrogens, fluorouracil, heparin (with I.V. use), lithium, methadone, mitotane, oxyphenbutazone, perphenazine, phenylbutazone, phenytoin, propranolol, salicylates*

(large doses), sulfonylureas: altered thyroid function test results
Anticoagulants: increased anticoagulant action
Beta-adrenergic blockers (selected): impaired beta blocker action
Cardiac glycosides: decreased cardiac glycoside blood level
Cholestyramine, colestipol: liothyronine inefficacy
Theophyllines: decreased theophylline clearance
Drug-diagnostic tests. *Thyroid function tests:* altered values
Drug-food. *Foods high in iron or fiber, soybeans:* decreased drug absorption

Patient monitoring

- Monitor for evidence of overdose, including signs and symptoms of hyperthyroidism (weight loss, cardiac symptoms, and abdominal cramps).
- In patients with Addison's disease or diabetes mellitus, assess for evidence that these conditions are worsening. In diabetic patients, also monitor blood glucose level.
- Monitor vital signs and ECG routinely.
- Check thyroid and liver function tests.

Patient teaching

- Teach patient to take in morning with or without food.
- Explain that patient may require lifelong therapy and will need to undergo regular blood testing.
- Caution patient to avoid driving and other hazardous activities until he knows how drug affects concentration and alertness.
- Inform parents that hair loss may occur in children during first few months but that this effect is usually transient.
- As appropriate, review all other significant and life-threatening adverse reactions and interactions, especially those related to the drugs, tests, and foods mentioned above.

liotrix

Thyrolar

Pharmacologic class: Synthetic thyroid hormone
Therapeutic class: Thyroid hormone replacement
Pregnancy risk category A

Action

Increases basal metabolic rate, helps regulate cell growth and differentiation, and enhances metabolism of lipids, proteins, and carbohydrates

Availability

Tablets: 12.5 mcg levothyroxine sodium and 3.1 mcg liothyronine sodium (Thyrolar-¼); 25 mcg levothyroxine sodium and 6.25 mcg liothyronine sodium (Thyrolar-½); 50 mcg levothyroxine sodium and 12.5 mcg liothyronine sodium (Thyrolar-1); 100 mcg levothyroxine sodium and 25 mcg liothyronine sodium (Thyrolar-2); 150 mcg levothyroxine sodium and 37.5 mcg liothyronine sodium (Thyrolar-3)

Indications and dosages

➢ Hypothyroidism
Adults: All dosages individualized. Initially, one tablet Thyrolar-½ P.O., increased by one tablet Thyrolar-¼ P.O. daily until desired effect occurs. Usual maintenance dosage is one tablet Thyrolar-1 or Thyrolar-2 P.O. daily, adjusted within first 4 weeks based on laboratory results.
➢ Congenital hypothyroidism
Children older than age 12: 18.75/75 mcg P.O. daily
Children ages 6 to 11: 12.5/50 to 18.75/75 mcg P.O. daily
Children ages 1 to 5: 9.35/37.5 to 12.5/50 mcg P.O. daily

Children ages 6 to 12 months: 6.25/25 to 9.35/37.5 mcg P.O. daily
Children up to 6 months: 3.1/12.5 to 6.25/25 mcg (Thyrolar-¼) P.O. daily

Dosage adjustment

- Severe, long-standing hypothyroidism
- Cardiovascular disease
- Psychosis or agitation
- Elderly patients

Contraindications

- Hypersensitivity to drug or its components
- Acute myocardial infarction
- Uncorrected thyrotoxicosis
- Uncorrected adrenal insufficiency and coexisting hypothyroidism

Precautions

Use cautiously in:

- cardiovascular disease, severe renal insufficiency, diabetes mellitus, uncorrected adrenocortical disorders
- elderly patients
- pregnant or breastfeeding patients.

Administration

- Know that all dosages are highly individualized.
- Administer single daily dose in morning with or without food.

Route	Onset	Peak	Duration
P.O. (levothyroxine)	Unknown	Unknown	Unknown
P.O. (liothyronine)	Unknown	24-72 hr	72 hr

Adverse reactions

CNS: insomnia, irritability, nervousness, headache
CV: angina pectoris, hypotension, hypertension, increased cardiac output, tachycardia, **arrhythmias, cardiovascular collapse**
GI: vomiting, diarrhea, cramps
GU: menstrual irregularities
Metabolic: hyperthyroidism
Musculoskeletal: accelerated bone maturation (in children), decreased bone density (with long-term use in women)
Skin: alopecia (in children), diaphoresis
Other: weight loss, heat intolerance

Interactions

Drug-drug. *Aminoglutethimide, amiodarone, anabolic steroids, antithyroid drugs, asparaginase, barbiturates, carbamazepine, chloral hydrate, cholestyramine, clofibrate, colestipol, corticosteroids, danazol, diazepam, estrogens, ethionamide, fluorouracil, heparin (with I.V. use), insulin, lithium, methadone, mitotane, nitroprusside, oxyphenbutazone, P-aminosalicyclic acid, perphenazine, phenylbutazone, phenytoin, propranolol, salicylates (large doses), sulfonylureas, thiazides:* altered thyroid function test results
Anticoagulants: increased anticoagulant action
Beta-adrenergic blockers (selected): decreased beta blocker action
Cardiac glycosides: decreased cardiac glycoside blood level
Cholestyramine, colestipol: liotrix inefficacy
Theophyllines: decreased theophylline clearance
Drug-diagnostic tests. *Thyroid function tests:* decreased values
Drug-food. *Foods high in iron or fiber, soybeans:* decreased drug absorption

Patient monitoring

- Monitor for evidence of overdose, such as signs and symptoms of hyperthyroidism (weight loss, cardiac symptoms, abdominal cramps).
- Watch closely for signs and symptoms of undertreatment.
- In patients with Addison's disease or diabetes mellitus, assess for signs that these conditions are worsening. In dia-

L

betic patients, monitor blood glucose level.
• Check vital signs and ECG routinely.
• Monitor thyroid and liver function tests.
• Assess for signs and symptoms of bleeding tendency, especially if patient's taking anticoagulants.

Patient teaching

• Inform patient or parents that drug should be taken in morning with or without food.
• Explain that patient may require lifelong therapy and will need to undergo regular blood testing.
• Advise diabetic patient (or his parents) to monitor patient's blood glucose level closely.
• Caution patient to avoid driving and other hazardous activities until he knows how drug affects concentration and alertness.
• Inform parents that hair loss may occur in children during first few months of therapy but that this effect is usually transient.
• As appropriate, review all other significant and life-threatening adverse reactions and interactions, especially those related to the drugs, tests, and foods mentioned above.

lisinopril

Prinivil, Zestril

Pharmacologic class: Angiotensin-converting enzyme (ACE) inhibitor

Therapeutic class: Antihypertensive

Pregnancy risk category C (first trimester), ***D*** (second and third trimesters)

Action

Inhibits conversion of angiotensin I to angiotensin II (a potent vasoconstrictor), decreasing systemic vascular resistance, blood pressure, preload, and afterload. Also inactivates bradykinin and other vasodilatory prostaglandins, increases plasma renin levels, and reduces aldosterone levels.

Availability

Tablets: 2.5 mg, 5 mg, 10 mg, 20 mg, 30 mg, 40 mg

Indications and dosages

➢ Hypertension

Adults: Initially, 10 mg P.O. daily, increased to a maintenance dosage of 20 to 40 mg/day. Maximum daily dosage is 80 mg. In patients on diuretics, start with 5 mg/day P.O.

➢ Heart failure

Adults: 5 mg/day P.O. (Prinivil), increased in increments, as ordered, to a maximum of 20 mg/day as a single dose. Or 5 to 40 mg P.O. (Zestril) as a single daily dose given with digitalis and diuretics, increased in increments of no more than 10 mg at intervals of at least 2 weeks, to highest dosage tolerated; maximum dosage is 40 mg/day P.O.

➢ Adjunctive therapy after acute myocardial infarction

Adults: Initially, 5 mg P.O., followed by 5 mg after 24 hours, 10 mg after 48 hours, and then 10 mg daily for 6 weeks (given with standard thrombolytic, aspirin, or beta-adrenergic blocker therapy). If systolic pressure is 120 mm Hg or lower, initial dosage is 2.5 mg for 2 days, then 2.5 to 5 mg/day.

Dosage adjustment

• Impaired renal function
• Heart failure with hyponatremia

Contraindications

• Hypersensitivity to drug or other ACE inhibitors
• Angioedema (hereditary, idiopathic, or ACE-inhibitor induced)
• Pregnancy (second and third trimesters)

Precautions

Use cautiously in:
- renal impairment, hypertension, cerebrovascular or cardiac insufficiency
- family history of angioedema
- concurrent diuretic therapy
- black patients (in whom drug may be less effective in treating hypertension)
- elderly patients
- pregnant patients in first trimester
- breastfeeding patients
- children (safety not established).

Administration

- Give once a day in morning, with or without food.

🔊 Measure blood pressure before administering. Withhold drug, if appropriate, according to prescriber's blood pressure parameters. Adjust dosage according to blood pressure response.
- Expect prescriber to add low-dose diuretic if lisinopril alone doesn't control blood pressure.

Route	Onset	Peak	Duration
P.O.	1 hr	6 hr	24 hr

Adverse reactions

CNS: dizziness, fatigue, headache, asthenia
CV: hypotension, orthostatic hypotension, syncope, chest pain, angina pectoris
GI: nausea, diarrhea, abdominal pain, anorexia
GU: erectile dysfunction, decreased libido, **renal dysfunction**
Metabolic: hyponatremia, **hyperkalemia**
Musculoskeletal: myalgia
Respiratory: cough, upper respiratory tract infection, bronchitis, dyspnea, **asthma**
Skin: rash, pruritus, angioedema
Other: altered taste, fever, **anaphylaxis**

Interactions

Drug-drug. *Cyclosporine, potassium-sparing diuretics, potassium supplements:* hyperkalemia
Diuretics, other antihypertensives: excessive hypotension
Indomethacin: reduced antihypertensive effect
Lithium: increased lithium blood level, greater risk of lithium toxicity
Nonsteroidal anti-inflammatory drugs: further deterioration in patients with renal compromise, decreased antihypertensive effects
Thiazides: hypokalemia
Drug-diagnostic tests. *Blood urea nitrogen, creatinine, hematocrit, hemoglobin:* slightly increased levels
Liver function tests, potassium: increased levels
Sodium: decreased level
Drug-food. *Salt substitutes containing potassium:* hyperkalemia
Drug-herbs. *Capsaicin:* cough
Ephedra (ma huang), licorice, yohimbine: antagonistic effects
Drug-behaviors. *Acute alcohol ingestion:* excessive hypotension

Patient monitoring

- Before and periodically during therapy, monitor CBC with white cell differential and kidney and liver function tests.

🔊 Monitor for signs and symptoms of angioedema or anaphylaxis. If these occur, discontinue drug and contact prescriber immediately.
- Check blood pressure frequently to assess drug efficacy. Monitor closely for hypotension, especially in patients also taking diuretics.
- Check vital signs and ECG regularly. Assess cardiovascular status carefully.
- Monitor respiratory and neurologic status.
- Assess potassium intake and blood potassium level.

Patient teaching

- Advise patient to take once a day in morning, with or without food.

🔊 Tell patient to immediately report fainting, continuing cough, rash, itching, swelling (especially of face, lips, tongue, or throat), severe dizziness, difficulty breathing, extreme tiredness, or continuing nausea.

🔊 Instruct female patient to notify prescriber if she becomes pregnant.

- Tell patient that drug may cause temporary blood pressure decrease if he stands up suddenly. Advise him to rise slowly and carefully.
- Explain that drug may cause muscle aches or headache. Encourage patient to discuss activity recommendations and pain relief with prescriber.
- Caution patient to avoid driving and other hazardous activities until he knows how drug affects concentration and alertness.
- Instruct patient to avoid potassium-based salt substitutes or potassium supplements.
- Tell patient he'll undergo regular blood testing during therapy.
- As appropriate, review all other significant and life-threatening adverse reactions and interactions, especially those related to the drugs, tests, foods, herbs, and behaviors mentioned above.

lithium carbonate

Eskalith, Eskalith CR, Lithizine✱, Lithobid

lithium citrate

Pharmacologic class: Miscellaneous CNS drug
Therapeutic class: Antimanic drug
Pregnancy risk category D

Action

Unknown. Thought to disrupt sodium exchange and transport in nerves and muscles and control reuptake of neurotransmitters.

Availability

Capsules: 150 mg, 300 mg, 600 mg
Capsules (slow-release): 150 mg, 300 mg
Syrup (citrate): 300 mg (8 mEq lithium)/5 ml
Tablets: 300 mg
Tablets (controlled-release): 450 mg
Tablets (extended-release): 300 mg, 450 mg
Tablets (slow-release): 300 mg

Indications and dosages

➤ Manic episodes of bipolar disorder

Adults and children ages 12 and older: 900 to 1,800 mg P.O. daily in divided doses (for example, 300 to 600 mg t.i.d. or 450 to 900 mg b.i.d. of controlled- or slow-release form) to achieve blood level of 1 to 1.5 mEq/L; measure blood level twice weekly until patient stabilizes. Maintenance dosage is 900 to 1,200 mg/day in divided doses (for example, 300 to 400 mg t.i.d. or 450 to 600 mg b.i.d. of controlled- or slow-release form) to maintain blood level of 0.6 to 1.2 mEq/L. Monitor blood level at least q 2 months.

Dosage adjustment

- Impaired renal function
- Elderly patients

Off-label uses

- Acute manic episodes in children
- Corticosteroid-induced psychosis
- Neutropenia secondary to antineoplastic therapy
- Tardive dyskinesia
- Alcoholism
- Bulimia

Contraindications

None

Precautions

Use cautiously in:
- hepatic or thyroid disease, severe cardiovascular or renal disease, diabetes mellitus, seizure disorders, systemic infections, brain trauma, organic brain syndrome, urinary retention, severe sodium depletion
- elderly patients
- pregnant or breastfeeding patients
- children (safety not established).

Administration

(Clinical alert) Be aware that dosages are individualized according to lithium blood level and response.
- Give with food or milk to minimize GI upset.
- Make sure patient swallows slow-release tablet whole without chewing or crushing.
- When switching patient from immediate-release to controlled- or slow-release form, give same total daily dosage.
- Know that immediate-release tablets typically are given three or four times daily, whereas controlled-release forms usually are given twice daily, roughly 12 hours apart.

Route	Onset	Peak	Duration
P.O.	Unknown	0.5-3 hr	Unknown
P.O. (controlled, slow-release)	Unknown	3-12 hr	Unknown

Adverse reactions

CNS: dizziness, drowsiness, headache, tremor, tics, EEG changes, ataxia, choreoathetotic movements, abnormal tongue movements, extrapyramidal reactions, cogwheel rigidity, blackout spells, psychomotor retardation, slow mental functioning, slurred speech, startled response, restlessness, agitation, confusion, hallucinations, poor memory, worsening of organic brain syndrome, stupor, **coma, epileptiform seizures**
CV: bradycardia, ECG changes, hypotension, **sinus node dysfunction with severe bradycardia and syncope, arrhythmias, peripheral circulatory collapse**
EENT: blurred vision, nystagmus, tinnitus
GI: nausea, vomiting, diarrhea, abdominal pain, fecal incontinence, gastritis, flatulence, dyspepsia, anorexia, increased salivation, salivary gland swelling, dry mouth
GU: urinary incontinence, glycosuria, albuminuria, erectile or other sexual dysfunction, polyuria or other signs of nephrogenic diabetes insipidus, **oliguria**
Hematologic: leukocytosis
Metabolic: hypothyroidism or hyperthyroidism, goiter, hyperglycemia, hypercalcemia, hyponatremia, hyperparathyroidism
Musculoskeletal: swollen or painful joints, muscle weakness, muscle fasciculations and twitching, clonic arm or leg movements, hypertonicity, hyperactive deep tendon reflexes, polyarthralgia
Skin: dry thin hair, alopecia, diminished or absent skin sensations, chronic folliculitis, eczema with dry skin, new onset or exacerbation of psoriasis, pruritus (with or without rash), cutaneous ulcers, angioedema
Other: altered, metallic, or salty taste; dental caries; weight gain; excessive thirst; polydipsia; fever; edema of lips, ankles, and wrists

Interactions

Drug-drug. *Acetazolamide, alkalinizing agents (such as sodium bicarbonate), urea, verapamil, xanthines:* decreased lithium blood level
Calcium channel blockers, carbamazepine, haloperidol, methyldopa: increased risk of neurotoxicity
Diuretics: increased sodium loss, increased risk of lithium toxicity
Fluoxetine, loop diuretics, metronida-

zole, nonsteroidal anti-inflammatory drugs: increased risk of lithium toxicity
Iodide salts: synergistic effects, increased risk of hypothyroidism
Neuromuscular blockers: prolonged neuromuscular blockade, severe respiratory depression
Phenothiazines: decreased phenothiazine blood level or increased lithium blood level, greater risk of neurotoxicity
Selective serotonin reuptake inhibitors: increased risk of tremor, confusion, dizziness, agitation, and diarrhea
Sympathomimetics: decreased pressor sensitivity
Tricyclic antidepressants: increased antidepressant effects
Drug-diagnostic tests. *Albumin, creatinine, sodium, thyroxine, triiodothyronine:* decreased levels
Calcium, glucose, ^{131}I *uptake, white blood cells (WBCs):* increased levels
Drug-food. *Caffeine-containing foods and beverages:* decreased lithium blood level and efficacy
Drug-herbs. *Caffeine-containing herbs (cola nut, guarana, yerba maté):* decreased lithium blood level and efficacy

Patient monitoring

- Obtain baseline ECG and electrolyte levels before and periodically during therapy.
- Assess neurologic and psychiatric status. Institute safety measures as needed to prevent injury.
- Monitor lithium blood level, WBC count, and thyroid and kidney function tests.
- Assess cardiovascular status regularly.
- Monitor fluid intake and output. Watch for edema and weight gain.

Patient teaching

- Advise patient to take with food or milk to minimize GI upset.
- Instruct patient to swallow slow-release tablet whole without chewing or crushing.
- Tell patient that beneficial effects may take 1 to 3 weeks to appear.
- Advise patient to limit foods and beverages containing caffeine, because they may interfere with drug action.
- Tell patient to maintain adequate fluid intake.
- Explain that drug may cause adverse CNS effects. Advise patient to avoid activities requiring mental alertness until effects are known.

[Clinical alert] Emphasize importance of having regular blood tests, to help detect and prevent serious adverse reactions.

- Instruct patient to carry appropriate medical identification at all times.
- As appropriate, review all other significant and life-threatening adverse reactions and interactions, especially those related to the drugs, tests, foods, and herbs mentioned above.

lomefloxacin hydrochloride

Maxaquin

Pharmacologic class: Fluoroquinolone
Therapeutic class: Anti-infective
Pregnancy risk category C

Action

Inhibits the enzyme DNA gyrase in susceptible gram-negative and gram-positive aerobic and anaerobic bacteria, interfering with bacterial DNA synthesis

Availability

Tablets: 400 mg

Indications and dosages

➢ Acute bacterial exacerbation of chronic bronchitis
Adults: 400 mg P.O. daily for 10 days
➢ Complicated urinary tract infections
Adults: 400 mg P.O. daily for 14 days

➢ Uncomplicated cystitis
Adults: 400 mg P.O. daily for 3 days
➢ Perioperative prophylaxis (transurethral surgery)
Adults: 400 mg P.O. 2 to 6 hours before surgery
➢ Perioperative prophylaxis (transrectal prostate biopsy)
Adults: 400 mg P.O. 1 to 6 hours before surgery

Dosage adjustment
• Renal impairment

Contraindications
• Hypersensitivity to drug or other fluoroquinolones

Precautions
Use cautiously in:
• bradycardia, acute myocardial ischemia, cirrhosis, renal impairment, underlying CNS disease
• elderly patients
• pregnant or breastfeeding patients
• children under age 18.

Administration
• Give on empty stomach when possible.
• Know that drug shouldn't be used in *Streptococcus pneumoniae*–induced acute bacterial exacerbation of chronic bronchitis.

Route	Onset	Peak	Duration
P.O.	Rapid	Unknown	24 hr

Adverse reactions
CNS: dizziness, headache
CV: chest pain, **cardiopulmonary arrest, cerebral thrombosis**
Hematologic: agranulocytosis
Hepatic: hepatic disease
GI: nausea, diarrhea, constipation, abdominal pain, **pseudomembranous colitis**
Skin: photosensitivity
Other: hypersensitivity reactions including **anaphylaxis**

Interactions
Drug-drug. *Antacids, iron salts, sucralfate:* decreased lomefloxacin absorption
Nonsteroidal anti-inflammatory drugs: increased risk of CNS stimulation and seizures
Probenecid: decreased urinary excretion of lomefloxacin
Drug-food. *Any food:* delayed drug absorption
Drug-herbs. *Dong quai, St. John's wort:* increased risk of photosensitivity
Fennel: decreased drug absorption

Patient monitoring
🔊 Watch for signs and symptoms of anaphylaxis.
🔊 Monitor for signs and symptoms of serious adverse reactions (such as cardiopulmonary arrest, cerebral thrombosis, and agranulocytosis).
• Assess for drug efficacy.
• Monitor vital signs and ECG. Assess cardiovascular status carefully.
• Monitor liver and kidney function tests, CBC, blood glucose level, and urinalysis. Know that other quinolones have caused changes in blood glucose level and hematologic and kidney function tests.

Patient teaching
• Instruct patient to take on empty stomach, if possible.
🔊 Advise patient to report rash immediately so prescriber can determine if it reflects a hypersensitivity reaction.
🔊 Tell patient to report diarrhea, which may be first sign of pseudomembranous colitis.
• Caution patient to avoid driving and other hazardous activities until he knows how drug affects concentration and alertness.
• Instruct patient to minimize GI upset by eating small, frequent servings of healthy food.
• Tell patient he'll need to undergo regular blood testing during therapy.

• As appropriate, review all other significant and life-threatening adverse reactions and interactions, especially those related to the drugs, foods, and herbs mentioned above.

lomustine

CeeNU

Pharmacologic class: Alkylating drug (nitrosourea)

Therapeutic class: Antineoplastic

Pregnancy risk category D

Action

Inactivates neoplastic cells by alkylating DNA, causing DNA structural modification and fragmentation. Thought to act in late G1 or early S phase of cell cycle.

Availability

Capsules: 10 mg, 40 mg, 100 mg
Dose pack: two 10-mg capsules, two 40-mg capsules, and 100-mg capsules

Indications and dosages

➤ Adjunctive therapy in primary and metastatic brain tumors; secondary therapy in Hodgkin's disease

Adults and children: As monotherapy, 130 mg/m^2 P.O. as a single dose q 6 weeks in previously untreated patients. In bone marrow suppression, initial dosage is 100 mg/m^2 P.O. q 6 weeks; don't repeat dose until platelet count exceeds 100,000/mm^3 and white blood cell (WBC) count exceeds 4,000/mm^3. When given with other myelosuppressive drugs, adjust dosage accordingly.

Dosage adjustment

• Bone marrow depression (based on WBC and platelet counts)

Contraindications

• Hypersensitivity to drug

Precautions

Use cautiously in:
• renal or hepatic dysfunction, bone marrow depression
• pregnant or breastfeeding patients.

Administration

• Obtain CBC with white cell differential before starting therapy.
• Administer antiemetic before giving drug, as prescribed, to minimize nausea.
• Give 2 to 4 hours after meals to enhance absorption.
• If vomiting occurs shortly after administration, notify prescriber.

Route	Onset	Peak	Duration
P.O.	10 min	3 hr	48 hr

Adverse reactions

CNS: anxiety, confusion, dizziness, hallucinations, lethargy, headache, paresthesia, light-headedness, drowsiness, fatigue, **seizures**
GI: nausea; vomiting; anorexia; sore mouth, lips, and throat; **GI bleeding**
GU: amenorrhea, azoospermia, progressive azotemia, **nephrotoxicity, renal failure**
Hematologic: anemia, **leukopenia, thrombocytopenia, bone marrow depression**
Hepatic: hepatotoxicity
Skin: alopecia
Other: secondary cancers

Interactions

Drug-drug. *Anticoagulants, nonsteroidal anti-inflammatory drugs:* increased bleeding risk
Myelosuppressants: increased bone marrow depression
Drug-diagnostic tests. *Hemoglobin, platelets, red blood cells, WBCs:* decreased values
Liver function tests, nitrogenous compounds: increased values

Patient monitoring

🔊 Watch for evidence of overdose, including bone marrow depression, nausea, and vomiting.
🔊 Monitor CBC and platelet counts closely. Watch for signs and symptoms of bleeding and bruising.
- Avoid I.M. injections if platelet count is below 100,000/mm^3.
- Check kidney, liver, and pulmonary function tests frequently.
- Assess neurologic status carefully. Institute safety measures as needed to prevent injury.

🔊 Watch for signs and symptoms of secondary cancers.

Patient teaching

- Instruct patient to contact prescriber if he vomits shortly after taking drug.

🔊 Tell patient to immediately report easy bruising or bleeding, which may signal low platelet count.
- Advise patient to report changes in urination pattern.
- Instruct patient to avoid exposure to people with infections, because drug may make him more susceptible to infection.

🔊 Caution female of childbearing age to use reliable contraception and to immediately report suspected or confirmed pregnancy.
- Advise female patient to inform prescriber if she is breastfeeding.
- Caution patient to avoid driving and other hazardous activities until he knows how drug affects concentration and alertness.
- Advise patient to minimize GI side effects by eating small, frequent servings of healthy food.
- Inform patient that drug may cause hair loss.
- Tell patient he'll undergo frequent blood testing during therapy.
- As appropriate, review all other significant and life-threatening adverse reactions and interactions, especially those related to the drugs and tests mentioned above.

loperamide hydrochloride

Apo-Loperamide✦, Diarr-Eze✦, Imodium, Imodium A-D, Kaopectate II, Loperacap✦, Novo-Loperamide✦, Pepto Diarrhea Control, PMS-Loperamide✦, Rho-Loperamide✦, Riva-Loperamide✦

Pharmacologic class: Piperidine derivative

Therapeutic class: Antidiarrheal

Pregnancy risk category B

Action

Inhibits peristalsis of intestinal wall musculature and intestinal contents. Also reduces fecal volume, increases fecal bulk, and minimizes fluid and electrolyte loss.

Availability

Capsules: 2 mg
Solution: 1 mg/5 ml
Tablets: 2 mg
Tablets (chewable): 2 mg

Indications and dosages

➢ Acute diarrhea

Adults: Initially, 4 mg P.O., then 2 mg after each loose stool. Usual maintenance dosage is 4 to 8 mg P.O. daily in divided doses, not to exceed 16 mg daily.

Children ages 8 to 12 or weighing more than 30 kg (66 lb): Initially, 2 mg P.O. t.i.d., then 1 mg/10 kg after each loose stool, not to exceed 6 mg daily

Children ages 6 to 8 or weighing 20 to 30 kg (44 to 66 lb): Initially, 2 mg P.O. b.i.d., then 1 mg/10 kg after each loose stool, not to exceed 4 mg daily

Children ages 2 to 5 or weighing 13 to 20 kg (29 to 44 lb): Initially, 1 mg P.O. t.i.d., then 1 mg/10 kg after each loose stool, not to exceed 3 mg daily

➢ Acute diarrhea (treated with over-the-counter loperamide)

Adults and children ages 12 and older: Two caplets with 4 to 8 oz water after first loose stool, then one caplet (with 4 to 8 oz water) after each subsequent loose stool. Don't exceed four caplets in 24 hours. Or give equivalent dosage in liquid form.

Children ages 9 to 11 who weigh 27 to 43 kg (60 to 95 lbs): One caplet with 4 to 8 oz water after first loose stool, then ½ caplet (with 4 to 8 oz water) after each subsequent loose stool. Don't exceed three caplets in 24 hours. Or give equivalent dosage in liquid form.

Children ages 6 to 8 who weigh 22 to 27 kg (48 to 59 lbs): One caplet with 4 to 8 oz water after first loose stool, then ½ caplet with 4 to 8 oz water after each subsequent loose stool. Don't exceed two caplets in 24 hours. Or give equivalent dosage in liquid form.

Children younger than age 6: Consult physician.

➢ Chronic diarrhea

Adults: Initially, 4 mg P.O., then 2 mg after each loose stool; reduce dosage as tolerated. Don't exceed 16 mg daily for more than 10 days.

Contraindications

- Hypersensitivity to drug
- Abdominal pain of unknown cause (especially with fever)
- Acute diarrhea caused by enteroinvasive *Escherichia coli, Salmonella,* or *Shigella*
- Acute ulcerative colitis
- Bloody diarrhea with temperature above 38.3° C (101° F) (with OTC product)
- Pseudomembranous colitis associated with broad-spectrum anti-infectives
- Children younger than age 6

Precautions

Use cautiously in:

- hepatic disease
- elderly patients
- pregnant or breastfeeding patients
- children.

Administration

- Use patient's weight to determine appropriate dosage (especially in children).

Route	Onset	Peak	Duration
P.O.	1 hr	2.5-5 hr	10 hr

Adverse reactions

CNS: drowsiness, dizziness

GI: nausea; vomiting; constipation; abdominal pain, distention, or discomfort; dry mouth; **toxic megacolon** (in patients with acute ulcerative colitis)

Other: allergic reactions

Interactions

Drug-drug. *Antidepressants, antihistamines, other anticholinergics:* additive anticholinergic effects

CNS depressants (including antihistamines, opioid analgesics, sedative-hypnotics): additive CNS depression

Drug-herbs. *Chamomile, hops, kava, skullcap, valerian:* increased CNS depression

Drug-behaviors. *Alcohol use:* increased CNS depression

Patient monitoring

- 🔊 Watch for signs and symptoms of abdominal distention, which may signal toxic megacolon in patient with ulcerative colitis.
- Assess bowel movements to evaluate drug efficacy and determine need for repeat doses.
- Monitor stool cultures as indicated.
- Check stool for occult blood as indicated.
- Evaluate fluid intake and output.
- Stay alert for CNS effects, especially in children.

Patient teaching

- Stress importance of maintaining high fluid intake to prevent dehydration.

Clinical alert: Instruct patient or parents to report fever, mucus in stool, or history of hepatic disease before using drug.

Clinical alert: Caution patient or parents to discontinue drug if symptoms worsen or diarrhea lasts longer than 2 days.

- As appropriate, review all other significant and life-threatening adverse reactions and interactions, especially those related to the drugs, herbs, and behaviors mentioned above.

loracarbef

Lorabid

Pharmacologic class: Second-generation cephalosporin
Therapeutic class: Anti-infective
Pregnancy risk category B

Action

Binds to essential proteins of bacterial cell wall, interfering with cell-wall synthesis in susceptible strains of gram-positive and gram-negative bacteria

Availability

Capsules: 200 mg, 400 mg
Oral suspension: 100 mg/5 ml
Powder for oral solution: 100 mg/5 ml, 200 mg/5 ml

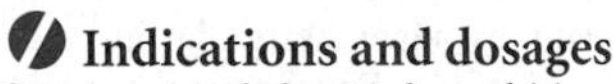

Indications and dosages

➢ Acute and chronic bronchitis
Adults and children ages 13 and older: 200 to 400 mg P.O. q 12 hours for 7 days

➢ Pneumonia; uncomplicated pyelonephritis
Adults and children ages 13 and older: 400 mg P.O. q 12 hours for 14 days

➢ Pharyngitis or tonsillitis
Adults and children ages 13 and older: 200 mg P.O. q 12 hours for 10 days
Infants and children ages 6 months to 12 years: 15 mg/kg/day P.O. (oral suspension) in divided doses q 12 hours for 10 days

➢ Sinusitis
Adults and children ages 13 and older: 400 mg P.O. q 12 hours for 10 days

➢ Uncomplicated skin and skin-structure infections
Adults and children ages 13 and older: 200 mg P.O. q 12 hours for 7 days

➢ Uncomplicated cystitis
Adults and children ages 13 and older: 200 mg P.O. q 24 hours for 7 days

➢ Acute otitis media or acute maxillary sinusitis
Children ages 6 months to 12 years: 30 mg/kg/day P.O. (oral suspension) in divided doses q 12 hours for 10 days

➢ Impetigo
Children ages 6 months to 12 years: 15 mg/kg/day P.O. (oral suspension) in divided doses q 12 hours for 7 days

Dosage adjustment

- Renal impairment
- Elderly patients

Contraindications

- Hypersensitivity to drug or other cephalosporins

Precautions

Use cautiously in:

- renal impairment, phenylketonuria (with products containing aspartame)
- history of GI disease (especially colitis)
- elderly patients
- pregnant or breastfeeding patients.

Administration

- Give 1 hour before or 2 hours after a meal.
- Reconstitute oral suspension as follows: For 50-ml bottle, add 15 ml of

water twice to dry mixture; shake well after each addition. For 100-ml bottle, add 30 ml of water twice; shake well after each addition.
• Use oral suspension for patients with otitis media, because it's more rapidly absorbed than capsules.

Route	Onset	Peak	Duration
P.O.	Rapid	0.5-1.2 hr	12 hr

Adverse reactions
CNS: headache, nervousness, drowsiness, dizziness, insomnia
CV: vasodilation
GI: nausea, vomiting, diarrhea, epigastric distress, **pseudomembranous colitis**
GU: vaginal candidiasis, vaginitis
Hematologic: eosinophilia, **transient thrombocytopenia, leukopenia**
Skin: rash, urticaria, pruritus, **erythema multiforme, Stevens-Johnson syndrome**
Other: allergic reaction, superinfection, **anaphylaxis**

Interactions
Drug-drug. *Potent diuretics:* increased risk of renal dysfunction
Probenecid: increased loracarbef blood level
Drug-diagnostic tests. *Alanine aminotransferase, alkaline phosphatase, aspartate aminotransferase, blood urea nitrogen, creatinine, eosinophils:* transient elevations
Coombs' test, urine glucose tests using Benedict's or Fehling's solution or Clinitest tablets: false-positive results
Platelets, white blood cells: transient decreases
Drug-food. *Moderate- or high-fat meal:* increased drug bioavailability
Drug-herbs. *Anise, arnica, asafetida, bogbean, boldo, celery, chamomile, clove, danshen, fenugreek, feverfew, garlic, ginger, ginkgo, ginseng, horse chestnut, horseradish, licorice, meadowsweet, onion, papain, passionflower, poplar, prickly ash, quassia, red clover, turmeric, wild carrot, wild lettuce, willow:* increased risk of bleeding

Patient monitoring
🔊 Watch for signs and symptoms of anaphylaxis, Stevens-Johnson syndrome, and hepatic dysfunction. Withhold drug and contact prescriber immediately if these occur.
• Monitor for signs and symptoms of toxicity, including rash, vomiting, diarrhea, and epigastric distress.
• Measure patient's temperature. Watch for signs and symptoms of superinfection.
🔊 Check bowel movements for early signs of pseudomembranous colitis.
• Monitor CBC with white cell differential and kidney function tests, as appropriate.
• Obtain and monitor cultures as indicated.

Patient teaching
🔊 Tell patient (or parents) to monitor bowel movements and report significant diarrhea.
• Instruct patient to increase fluid intake as tolerated.
🔊 Caution patient to stop taking drug and immediately report rash, yellowing of skin or eyes, or signs or symptoms of toxicity (such as vomiting, diarrhea, or epigastric distress).
• Advise patient to eat low-fat diet, because high-fat meals alter drug's action.
• Explain that many herbs may increase risk of bleeding when taken with this drug. Discourage their use.
• As appropriate, review all other significant and life-threatening adverse reactions and interactions, especially those related to the drugs, tests, foods, and herbs mentioned above.

loratadine

Alavert, Claritin, Claritin Hives Relief, Claritin RediTabs

Pharmacologic class: Histamine$_1$-receptor antagonist (second-generation)

Therapeutic class: Antihistamine (nonsedating)

Pregnancy risk category B

Action

Selective histamine$_1$-receptor antagonist. Blocks peripheral effects of histamine release during allergic reactions, decreasing or preventing allergy symptoms.

Availability

Syrup: 1 mg/ml
Tablets: 10 mg
Tablets (rapidly disintegrating): 10 mg

Indications and dosages

➢ Seasonal allergies; chronic idiopathic urticaria

Adults and children ages 6 and older: 10 mg P.O. daily

Children ages 2 to 5: 5 mg P.O. daily

Dosage adjustment

- Renal or hepatic impairment

Contraindications

- Hypersensitivity to drug

Precautions

Use cautiously in:
- renal or hepatic impairment
- elderly patients
- pregnant patients
- children younger than age 2 (safety not established).

Administration

- Give once a day on empty stomach.
- Place rapidly disintegrating tablet on tongue; give with or without water.
- Use rapidly disintegrating tablets within 6 months of opening foil pouch and immediately after opening individual tablet blister.

Route	Onset	Peak	Duration
P.O.	1-3 hr	8-12 hr	>24 hr

Adverse reactions

CNS: headache, nervousness, insomnia
EENT: conjunctivitis, earache, epistaxis, pharyngitis
GI: abdominal pain; dry mouth; diarrhea, stomatitis (in children)
Skin: rash, photosensitivity, angioedema
Other: tooth disorder (in children), fever, flulike symptoms, viral infections

Interactions

Drug-food. *Any food:* increased drug absorption

Patient monitoring

- Watch for adverse reactions, especially in children.
- Assess patient's response to drug.
- Watch for new symptoms or exacerbation of existing symptoms.

Patient teaching

- Advise patient to take exactly as prescribed, once a day on empty stomach.
- Tell patient to report persistent or worsening symptoms.
- Instruct patient to report adverse reactions, such as headache or nervousness.
- Caution patient to avoid driving and other hazardous activities until he knows how drug affects concentration and alertness.
- As appropriate, review all other significant adverse reactions and interactions, especially those related to the foods mentioned above.

lorazepam

Apo-Lorazepam✤, Ativan, Novo-Lorazem✤, Nu-Loraz✤

Pharmacologic class: Benzodiazepine
Therapeutic class: Anxiolytic
Controlled substance schedule IV
Pregnancy risk category D

Action

Unknown. Thought to depress CNS at limbic system and disrupt neurotransmission in reticular activating system.

Availability

Injection: 2 mg/ml, 4 mg/ml
Solution (concentrated): 2 mg/ml
Tablets: 0.5 mg, 1 mg, 2 mg

Indications and dosages

➢ Anxiety
Adults: 2 to 3 mg P.O. daily in two or three divided doses. Maximum dosage is 10 mg daily.
➢ Insomnia
Adults: 2 to 4 mg P.O. at bedtime
➢ Premedication before surgery (as antianxiety agent, sedative-hypnotic, or amnestic)
Adults: 0.05 mg/kg (not to exceed 4 mg) deep I.M. injection at least 2 hours before surgery, or 0.044 mg/kg (not to exceed 2 mg) I.V. 15 to 20 minutes before surgery. For greater amnestic effect, give up to 0.05 mg/kg (not to exceed 4 mg) I.V. 15 to 20 minutes before surgery.
➢ Status epilepticus
Adults: 4 mg I.V. given slowly (no faster than 2 mg/minute). If seizures continue or recur after 10 to 15 minutes, repeat dose. If seizure control isn't established after second dose, other measures should be used. Don't exceed 8 mg in 12 hours.

Dosage adjustment

- Elderly or debilitated patients

Off-label uses

- Acute alcohol withdrawal syndrome

Contraindications

- Hypersensitivity to drug, other benzodiazepines, polyethylene or propylene glycol, or benzyl alcohol
- Acute angle-closure glaucoma
- Coma or CNS depression
- Hepatic or renal failure

Precautions

Use cautiously in:
- hepatic or renal impairment
- history of suicide attempt, drug abuse, depressive disorder, or psychosis
- elderly patients
- pregnant or breastfeeding patients.

Administration

- For I.V. use, dilute with equal volume of compatible diluent, such as normal saline solution or dextrose 5% in water. Keep resuscitation equipment and oxygen at hand.

Clinical alert: Give each 2 mg of I.V. dose slowly, over 2 to 5 minutes. Don't exceed rate of 2 mg/minute.

- Don't give parenteral form to children younger than age 18.

Route	Onset	Peak	Duration
P.O.	15-45 min	1-6 hr	Up to 48 hr
I.V.	Rapid	15-20 min	Up to 48 hr
I.M.	15-30 min	1-2 hr	Up to 48 hr

Adverse reactions

CNS: amnesia, agitation, ataxia, depression, disorientation, dizziness, drowsiness, headache, incoordination, asthenia
CV (with too rapid I.V. administration): hypotension, bradycardia, tachycardia, apnea, **cardiac arrest, cardiovascular collapse**

EENT: blurred vision, diplopia, nystagmus
GI: nausea, abdominal discomfort
Other: increased or decreased appetite

Interactions

Drug-drug. *CNS depressants (including antidepressants, antihistamines, benzodiazepines, sedative-hypnotics):* additive CNS depression
Hormonal contraceptives: increased lorazepam clearance
Drug-herbs. *Chamomile, hops, kava, skullcap, valerian:* increased CNS depression
Drug-behaviors. *Alcohol use:* increased CNS depression
Smoking: increased metabolism and decreased efficacy of lorazepam

Patient monitoring

During I.V. administration, monitor ECG and cardiovascular and respiratory status.
- Monitor vital signs closely.
- Evaluate for amnesia.
- Watch closely for CNS depression. Institute safety precautions as needed to prevent injury.

Monitor for signs and symptoms of overdose (such as confusion, hypotension, coma, and labored breathing).
- Assess liver function tests and CBC.

Patient teaching

- Tell patient and family about drug's possible CNS effects. Recommend appropriate safety precautions.
- Explain that with long-term use, drug must be discontinued slowly (typically over 8 to 12 weeks).
- Instruct patient to avoid alcohol, because it increases drowsiness and other CNS effects.
- Caution patient to avoid smoking, because it speeds drug breakdown in body.
- Advise female patient to inform prescriber if she is pregnant or breastfeeding.
- As appropriate, review all other significant and life-threatening adverse reactions and interactions, especially those related to the drugs, herbs, and behaviors mentioned above.

losartan potassium

Cozaar

Pharmacologic class: Angiotensin II receptor antagonist
Therapeutic class: Antihypertensive
Pregnancy risk category C (first trimester), ***D*** (second and third trimesters)

Action

Blocks vasoconstricting and aldosterone-secreting effects of angiotensin II at various receptor sites, including vascular smooth muscle and adrenal glands. Also increases urinary flow and enhances excretion of chloride, magnesium, calcium, and phosphate.

l

Availability

Tablets: 25 mg, 50 mg, 100 mg

Indications and dosages

➢ Hypertension
Adults: Initially, 50 mg/day P.O.; range is 25 to 100 mg/day as a single dose or in two divided doses. May be used alone or with other drugs.
➢ To prevent cerebrovascular accident (stroke) in hypertensive patients with left ventricular hypertrophy (LVH)
Adults: Initially, 50 mg P.O. daily, increased to 100 mg P.O. daily. May be given concurrently with hydrochlorothiazide.

Dosage adjustment

- Hepatic impairment
- Concurrent diuretic therapy

Off-label uses
• Type 2 diabetes with nephropathy

Contraindications
• Hypersensitivity to drug or its components

Precautions
Use cautiously in:
• heart failure, renal or hepatic impairment, obstructive biliary disorders
• high-dose diuretic therapy
• black patients
• pregnant or breastfeeding patients
• children younger than age 18 (safety not established).

Administration
• Administer with or without food.
• Know that if drug efficacy (measured at trough) is inadequate with once-daily dosing, prescriber may switch to twice-daily regimen using same or higher daily dosage.
• Be aware that drug may take 3 to 6 weeks to reach maximal efficacy.

Route	Onset	Peak	Duration
P.O.	Unknown	1 hr	Unknown

Adverse reactions
CNS: dizziness, insomnia, headache, asthenia, fatigue
CV: hypotension
EENT: sinus disorders
GI: nausea, vomiting, diarrhea, dyspepsia, abdominal pain
Metabolic: hyperkalemia
Musculoskeletal: joint pain, back pain, muscle cramps
Respiratory: symptoms of upper respiratory infection, dry cough
Other: hypersensitivity reactions including **angioedema**

Interactions
Drug-drug. *Diuretics, other antihypertensives:* increased risk of hypotension
Fluconazole: inhibited losartan metabolism, increased antihypertensive effects
Indomethacin: decreased losartan effects
Phenobarbital, rifamycins: enhanced losartan metabolism, decreased antihypertensive effects
Potassium-sparing diuretics, potassium supplements: hyperkalemia
Drug-diagnostic tests. *Albumin:* increased level
Drug-food. *Salt substitutes containing potassium:* hyperkalemia

Patient monitoring
🔈 Watch for angioedema and other hypersensitivity reactions.
• Monitor blood pressure to evaluate drug efficacy.
• Assess liver and kidney function tests and electrolyte levels.
• Stay alert for oliguria, progressive azotemia, and renal failure in patients with severe heart failure whose renal function depends on the renin-angiotensin-aldosterone system.
• Know that in black patients, losartan and other ACE inhibitors may be ineffective when used alone. Drug isn't indicated for stroke prevention in black hypertensive patients with LVH.
• Be aware that drug may cause fetal injury or death when used during second or third trimester of pregnancy.

Patient teaching
• Instruct patient to avoid potassium supplements and salt substitutes containing potassium, unless directed by prescriber.
🔈 Caution female patient not to take drug during second or third trimester of pregnancy. Advise her to contact prescriber immediately if she suspects pregnancy.
• Tell female patient to discuss breastfeeding with prescriber before taking.
🔈 Instruct patient to immediately report hypersensitivity reactions, espe-

cially lip or eyelid swelling, throat tightness, and difficulty breathing.
• As appropriate, review all other significant and life-threatening adverse reactions and interactions, especially those related to the drugs, tests, and foods mentioned above.

lovastatin

Altocor, Apo-Lovastatin✦, Dom-Lovastatin✦, Gen-Lovastatin✦, Mevacor, Novo-Lovastatin✦, PMS-Lovastatin✦

Pharmacologic class: HMG-CoA reductase inhibitor
Therapeutic class: Antihyperlipidemic
Pregnancy risk category X

Action

Inhibits HMG-CoA reductase, an enzyme crucial to cholesterol synthesis. Decreases total cholesterol and low-density lipoprotein (LDL) levels and increases high-density lipoprotein level.

Availability

Tablets: 10 mg, 20 mg, 40 mg
Tablets (extended-release): 10 mg, 20 mg, 40 mg, 60 mg

Indications and dosages

➢ To reduce LDL, total cholesterol, triglyceride, and apolipoprotein B levels

Adults: Initially, 20 mg P.O. daily. May be increased, as needed, at 4-week intervals to a maximum of 80 mg/day as a single dose or in divided doses. Or 20 mg P.O. (extended-release) daily. May be increased, as needed, at 4-week intervals to a maximum daily dosage of 60 mg.

Dosage adjustment

• Severe renal insufficiency

Off-label uses

• High-risk patients with diabetic dyslipidemia, familial dysbetalipoproteinemia, familial combined hyperlipidemia, or nephrotic hyperlipidemia

Contraindications

• Hypersensitivity to drug, its components, or angiotensin-converting enzyme inhibitors
• Active hepatic disease or unexplained persistent hepatic enzyme elevation
• Concurrent gemfibrozil or azole antifungal therapy
• Females of childbearing age
• Pregnancy or breastfeeding

Precautions

Use cautiously in:
• cerebral arteriosclerosis, heart disease, renal impairment, severe acute infection, severe hypotension or hypertension, uncontrolled seizures, myopathy, visual disturbances, major surgery, trauma, alcoholism
• severe metabolic, endocrine, or electrolyte problems
• children.

Administration

• Give daily dose with evening meal.
• Increase dosage at intervals of 4 weeks or longer, as ordered.
• Don't give with grapefruit juice (may increase drug blood level).
[Clinical alert] Discontinue if alanine aminotransferase (ALT) or aspartate aminotransferase (AST) level exceeds three times the upper limit of normal.
• Be aware that drug may be used to treat heterozygous familial hypercholesterolemia in boys and postmenarchal girls ages 10 and older who have high LDL and cholesterol levels despite adequate trial of diet therapy.

Route	Onset	Peak	Duration
P.O.	Unknown	2 hr	Unknown
P.O. (extended)	Unknown	Unknown	Unknown

Adverse reactions

CNS: headache, dizziness, asthenia
EENT: blurred vision, eye irritation
GI: nausea, vomiting, constipation, diarrhea, abdominal pain or cramps, dyspepsia, flatulence
Hepatic: hepatotoxicity
Musculoskeletal: myalgia, cramps, **rhabdomyolysis**
Skin: pruritus, rash, photosensitivity
Other: hypersensitivity reaction

Interactions

Drug-drug. *Antifungals, cyclosporine, erythromycin, folic acid derivatives, gemfibrozil, niacin, other HMG-CoA inhibitors:* increased risk of myopathy and rhabdomyolysis
Bile acid sequestrants: decreased lovastatin blood level
Isradipine: increased lovastatin clearance
Warfarin: increased prothrombin time, bleeding
Drug-diagnostic tests. *ALT, AST:* increased levels
Drug-food. *Grapefruit juice:* increased lovastatin blood level
Drug-herbs. *Red yeast rice:* increased risk of adverse reactions
Chaparral, comfrey, germander, jin bu huan, kava, pennyroyal, St. John's wort: increased risk of hepatotoxicity

Patient monitoring

- Obtain liver function tests before starting therapy, 6 and 12 weeks after therapy begins or dosage is increased, and periodically thereafter.

Patient teaching

- Tell patient to take immediate-release tablets with evening meal or extended-release tablets at bedtime.
- Instruct patient not to break, crush, or chew extended-release tablets.
- Emphasize importance of cholesterol-lowering diet and other therapies, such as exercise and weight control.
- [Clinical alert] Instruct patient to report unexplained muscle pain, tenderness, or weakness, as well as signs or symptoms of hepatotoxicity (fever, malaise, abdominal pain, yellowing of skin or eyes, clay-colored stools, or tea-colored urine).
- [Clinical alert] Advise patient to contact prescriber immediately if she is breast-feeding or suspects pregnancy.
- Tell patient not to use herbs without consulting prescriber.
- Inform patient that drug may cause photosensitivity. Caution him to avoid excessive sun or heat lamp light.
- As appropriate, review all other significant and life-threatening adverse reactions and interactions, especially those related to the drugs, tests, foods, and herbs mentioned above.

loxapine succinate

Apo-Loxapine✱, Loxapac✱, Loxitane, Nu-Loxapine✱

Pharmacologic class: Tricyclic dibenzoxazepine derivative

Therapeutic class: Antipsychotic

Pregnancy risk category C

Action

Unknown. Thought to block neurotransmission of postsynaptic dopamine receptors in brain, alleviating psychotic symptoms.

Availability

Capsules: 5 mg, 10 mg, 25 mg, 50 mg

Indications and dosages

➤ Psychotic disorders
Adults: 10 mg P.O. b.i.d. Dosage may be increased over first 7 to 10 days, up to 100 mg/day P.O. in two to four divided doses. Maximum dosage is 250 mg/day.

Dosage adjustment
• Elderly patients

Contraindications
• Hypersensitivity to drug or other dibenzoxazepines
• Coma or severe CNS depression from any cause

Precautions
Use cautiously in:
• seizures, cardiovascular or respiratory disorders, circulatory collapse, cerebral arteriosclerosis, severe hypotension, hypertension, glaucoma, prostatic hypertrophy, breast cancer, thyrotoxicosis, peptic ulcer, renal impairment, hepatic disease, bone marrow depression, subcortical brain damage, Parkinson's disease, blood dyscrasias
• pregnant or breastfeeding patients
• children younger than age 16.

Administration
• Give with or without food.

Route	Onset	Peak	Duration
P.O.	30 min	1.5-3 hr	12 hr

Adverse reactions
CNS: drowsiness, insomnia, vertigo, headache, dizziness, weakness, akinesia, staggering or shuffling gait, slurred speech, agitation, extrapyramidal reactions, sedation, syncope, tardive dyskinesia, numbness, confusion, pseudoparkinsonism, EEG changes, **seizures, neuroleptic malignant syndrome**
CV: orthostatic hypotension, hypertension, ECG changes
EENT: blurred vision, ptosis, nasal congestion
GI: nausea, vomiting, constipation, dry mouth, **paralytic ileus**
GU: urinary retention
Hematologic: leukopenia, agranulocytosis, thrombocytopenia
Hepatic: hepatocellular injury with hepatic enzyme elevations
Metabolic: polydipsia
Musculoskeletal: muscle twitching
Skin: rash, pruritus, seborrhea, photosensitivity, alopecia
Other: weight gain or loss, hyperpyrexia, facial edema, hypersensitivity reactions

Interactions
Drug-drug. *Anticholinergics, CNS depressants:* additive effects
Epinephrine: severe hypotension, tachycardia, decreased epinephrine effects
Drug-diagnostic tests. *Granulocytes, platelets, white blood cells:* decreased counts
Liver function tests: increased values
Drug-behaviors. *Alcohol use:* increased CNS depression

Patient monitoring
• Measure blood pressure before and periodically during therapy.
• Monitor hematologic studies and liver function tests.
Stay alert for evidence of neuroleptic malignant syndrome (extrapyramidal symptoms, hyperpyrexia, muscle rigidity, altered mental status, irregular pulse or blood pressure, tachycardia, arrhythmias, diaphoresis).
• Assess for tardive dyskinesia (involuntary jerky movements of face, tongue, jaws, trunk, arms, and legs), especially in elderly women.

Patient teaching
• Tell patient to take with or without food.
• Inform patient that drug may cause tardive dyskinesia. Describe symptoms.
• Caution patient to avoid activities requiring mental concentration until drug's effects are known.
Teach patient to immediately report sore throat, fever, rash, impaired vision, tremors, involuntary muscle twitching, muscle stiffness, or yellowing of eyes or skin.

• Instruct patient to move slowly when sitting up or standing, to avoid dizziness from sudden blood pressure decrease.
• Caution patient to avoid alcohol use.
• As appropriate, review all other significant and life-threatening adverse reactions and interactions, especially those related to the drugs, tests, and behaviors mentioned above.

lymphocyte immune globulin (antithymocyte globulin equine, ATG, ATG equine, LIG)

Atgam

Pharmacologic class: Immunoglobulin
Therapeutic class: Immunosuppressant
Pregnancy risk category C

Action

Unknown. Thought to inhibit cell-mediated immune response by altering function of or eliminating T lymphocytes in circulation.

Availability

Injection: 50 mg /ml in 5-ml ampules

Indications and dosages

➢ To prevent acute renal allograft rejection
Adults: 15 mg/kg/day I.V. for 14 days, then switch to alternate-day dosing for 14 days (for a total of 21 doses in 28 days). Give first dose within 24 hours of transplantation.
➢ Acute renal allograft rejection
Adults and children: 10 to 15 mg/kg/day I.V. for 14 days, then may switch to alternate-day dosing for 14 days (for a total of 21 doses in 28 days). Start therapy at first sign of rejection.
➢ Aplastic anemia in patients ineligible for bone marrow transplantation
Adults: 10 to 20 mg/kg/day I.V. for 8 to 14 days; then may give additional alternate-day doses for a total of up to 21 doses in 28 days

Off-label uses

• Bone marrow, liver, and heart transplantation
• Multiple sclerosis
• Myasthenia gravis
• Scleroderma

Contraindications

• History of severe systemic reaction to lymphocyte immune globulin or other equine preparation

Precautions

Use cautiously in:
• severe renal or hepatic disease
• pregnant or breastfeeding patients
• children.

Administration

Know that drug should be given only by health care professionals experienced in immunosuppressive therapy for treating aplastic anemia or renal transplant patients, in facilities equipped and staffed with adequate laboratory and supportive resources.
Because of high risk of anaphylaxis, perform intradermal skin test before first dose. Inject 0.1-ml dose of 1:1,000 dilution of LIG intradermally; a control test using 0.9% sodium chloride injection is injected contralaterally. Observe site every 15 to 20 minutes during first hour after injection, and monitor patient for systemic manifestations. Local reaction of 10 mm or greater with wheal, erythema, or both (with or without pseudopod formation and itching or marked local swelling) indicates positive test (which warrants consideration of alternate therapy). Systemic reaction (such as tachycardia,

dyspnea, hypotension, or anaphylaxis) precludes LIG therapy.

- Premedicate with antipyretic, antihistamine, or corticosteroid, as prescribed, to minimize reactions.
- For I.V. infusion, dilute prescribed dose in 250 to 1,000 ml of 0.45% or 0.9% sodium chloride injection. (Don't dilute in dextrose solutions or highly acidic solutions.) Final concentration shouldn't exceed 4 mg/ml. Infuse total daily dose over at least 4 hours.
- When adding drug to infusion container, invert container so air doesn't enter. Gently swirl or rotate container to mix solution.
- Using in-line filter with pore size of 0.2 to 1 micron, infuse into central vein, shunt, or arteriovenous fistula over at least 4 hours.
- Be aware that drug is usually given concurrently with azathioprine and corticosteroids when used for allograft rejection.

Route	Onset	Peak	Duration
I.V.	Immediate	5 days	Unknown

Adverse reactions

CNS: malaise, agitation, headache, dizziness, weakness, syncope, **encephalitis, seizures**
CV: hypotension, hypertension, chest pain, bradycardia, tachycardia, cardiac irregularities, phlebitis, **myocarditis, thrombophlebitis, heart failure**
EENT: periorbital edema
GI: nausea, vomiting, diarrhea, stomatitis
Hematologic: leukopenia, agranulocytosis, thrombocytopenia, aplastic anemia
Hepatic: hepatosplenomegaly
Metabolic: hyperglycemia
Musculoskeletal: joint pain or stiffness, myalgia, back pain
Respiratory: dyspnea, **pleural effusion**
Skin: rash, pruritus, urticaria, diaphoresis, night sweats
Other: burning soles and palms, fever, chills, pain at infusion site, edema, lymphadenopathy, hypersensitivity reactions including **serum sickness** and **anaphylaxis**

Interactions

Drug-diagnostic tests. *Creatinine, glucose, hepatic enzymes:* increased values
Hemoglobin, platelets, white blood cells: decreased values
Kidney and liver function tests: abnormal results

Patient monitoring

- [Clinical alert] During infusion, watch for signs and symptoms of hypersensitivity reaction, such as rash, respiratory distress, or chest, flank, or back pain. Be aware that this reaction may occur even with a negative skin test.
- [Clinical alert] Discontinue drug if renal transplant patient develops signs or symptoms of anaphylaxis or severe thrombocytopenia or leukopenia.
- Be aware that product derives from equine and human blood components and may transmit infections.
- Monitor for signs and symptoms of infection, such as fever, malaise, and sore throat (caused by immunosuppression).

Patient teaching

- [Clinical alert] Tell patient to immediately report adverse reactions during infusion (such as pain at infusion site) as well as systemic complaints (such as easy bruising or bleeding or signs of hypersensitivity reaction).
- Instruct patient to avoid sources of infection, such as people with known infections. Tell him to promptly report signs or symptoms of infection.
- [Clinical alert] Advise patient to immediately report evidence of serum sickness, including fever, joint pain, nausea, vomiting, lymphadenopathy, and rash.
- [Clinical alert] Caution female patient not to take drug if she is pregnant.

• Tell female patient to inform prescriber if she is breastfeeding.
• As appropriate, review all other significant and life-threatening adverse reactions and interactions, especially those related to the tests mentioned above.

magaldrate (aluminum magnesium hydroxide sulfate)

Lowsium, Lowsium Plus, Riopan

Pharmacologic class: GI drug
Therapeutic class: Antacid
Pregnancy risk category NR

Action

Increases gastric pH and elasticity of esophageal sphincter, decreasing pepsin activity and acid production in GI tract.

Availability

Oral solution: 540 mg/5 ml, 1,080 mg/ 5 ml

Indications and dosages

➢ Antacid
Adults: 5 to 10 ml P.O.

Contraindications

• Hypersensitivity to drug or its components
• Severe renal disease

Precautions

Use cautiously in:
• renal disease, decreased GI motility, GI obstruction, fluid restriction, dehydration, sodium-restricted diet
• elderly patients
• pregnant patients.

Administration

• Give between meals with water, or at bedtime.

Route	Onset	Peak	Duration
P.O.	20 min	Unknown	20-180 min

Adverse reactions

GI: mild constipation, diarrhea
Metabolic: hypermagnesemia, hypophosphatemia, hypokalemia

Interactions

Drug-drug. *Diazepam, digoxin, indomethacin, iron salts, isoniazid, pseudoephedrine, tetracycline:* decreased effects of these drugs
Enteric-coated drugs: premature gastric release of these drugs
Drug-diagnostic tests. *Gastrin, urine pH:* increased levels
Potassium: decreased level

Patient monitoring

Stay alert for signs and symptoms of magnesium toxicity, including hypotension, nausea, vomiting, ECG changes, CNS or respiratory depression, and coma.
• With long-term or repeated use, monitor potassium, phosphorus, and magnesium levels.

Patient teaching

• Tell patient to shake oral solution well and to drink water after taking dose.
• Caution patient not to use drug for more than 2 weeks unless directed by prescriber.
• Advise patient to inform prescriber if he's taking other drugs; magaldrate may delay or enhance absorption of concurrent drugs.
• Tell patient to report change in bowel habits.

• As appropriate, review all other significant adverse reactions and interactions, especially those related to the drugs and tests mentioned above.

magnesium chloride

magnesium citrate
Citro-Mag✤, Citroma, Evac-Q-Mag

magnesium gluconate
Magonate

magnesium hydroxide
Phillips Chewable, Phillips Milk of Magnesia, Phillips Milk of Magnesia Concentrate

magnesium oxide
Mag-ox, Maox, Uro-Mag

magnesium sulfate
Epsom Salts

Pharmacologic class: Mineral

Therapeutic class: Electrolyte replacement, laxative, antacid, anticonvulsant

Pregnancy risk category A (magnesium sulfate), ***NR*** (magnesium citrate, hydroxide, oxide), ***unknown*** (magnesium chloride, gluconate)

Action
Increases osmotic gradient in small intestine, which draws water into intestines and causes distention. These effects stimulate peristalsis and bowel evacuation. In antacid action, reacts with hydrochloric acid in stomach to form water and increase gastric pH. In anticonvulsant action, depresses CNS and blocks transmission of peripheral neuromuscular impulses.

Availability
magnesium chloride
Injection: 20%
magnesium citrate
Oral solution: 240-ml, 296-ml, and 300-ml bottles
magnesium gluconate
Liquid: 1,000 mg/5 ml
Tablets: 500 mg
magnesium hydroxide
Liquid: 400 mg/5 ml
Liquid concentrate: 800 mg/5 ml
Tablets (chewable): 300 mg
magnesium oxide
Capsules: 140 mg
Tablets: 400 mg, 420 mg, 500 mg
magnesium sulfate
Granules (for oral use): 120 g, 4 lb
Injection: 10%, 12.5%, 25%, 50%

Indications and dosages
➢ Mild magnesium deficiency
Adults: 1 g (2 ml of 50% sulfate solution) I.M. q 6 hours for four doses
➢ Severe hypomagnesemia
Adults: 250 mg (2 mEq)/kg (sulfate) I.M. within 4-hour period, or 5 g (approximately 40 mEq) in 1 liter 5% dextrose injection or 0.9% sodium chloride solution by I.V. infusion over 3 hours
➢ Hypomagnesemia treatment
Adults and children: Dosage individualized based on severity of deficiency; may give citrate, gluconate, hydroxide, oxide, or sulfate.
➢ Hypomagnesemia prophylaxis
Adults and children: Dosage based on normal recommended daily magnesium intake; may give citrate, gluconate, hydroxide, oxide, or sulfate.
➢ Supplemental magnesium in total parenteral nutrition (TPN)
Adults: 8 to 24 mEq/day (sulfate) by I.V. infusion, added to TPN solution
➢ Constipation
Adults and children ages 12 and older: 15 g (sulfate granules) in 240 ml water; or 30 to 60 ml/day P.O. (hydroxide)

m

given with water; or a single dose of 10 to 30 ml P.O. (hydroxide concentrate); or one bottle of oral solution (citrate), as directed
Children ages 6 to 11: 5 to 10 g (sulfate granules) in 120 ml water; or a single dose of 2.5 to 5 ml P.O. (sulfate) in a half-glass of water; or 15 to 30 ml P.O. daily (hydroxide) given with water; or a single dose of 7.5 to 15 ml P.O. (hydroxide concentrate); or three to four tablets (hydroxide); or 50 to 100 ml, as directed, of oral solution (citrate)
Children ages 2 to 5: Single dose of 5 to 15 ml P.O. (hydroxide); or 2.5 to 7.5 ml P.O. daily (hydroxide concentrate); or one to two tablets (hydroxide); or 4 to 12 ml oral solution (citrate), as directed
➢ Indigestion
Adults and children ages 12 and older: 5 to 15 ml P.O. (hydroxide liquid) up to q.i.d. with water; or 2.5 to 7.5 ml P.O. (hydroxide liquid concentrate) up to q.i.d. with water; or 622 to 1,244 mg P.O. (hydroxide tablets) up to q.i.d.; or 400 to 800 mg P.O. (oxide tablets) daily
➢ To prevent and control seizures in preeclampsia or eclampsia
Adults: 4 to 5 g 50% sulfate solution I.M. q 4 hours, as necessary; or 4 g 10% to 20% sulfate solution I.V., not to exceed 1.5 ml/minute of 10% solution; or 4 to 5 g I.V. infusion in 250 ml of 5% dextrose or sodium chloride solution, not to exceed 3 ml/minute
➢ Acute nephritis to control hypertension, encephalopathy, and seizures in children
Children: 100 mg/kg 50% sulfate solution I.M. q 4 to 6 hours as needed; or 20 to 40 mg/kg 20% solution I.M., repeated as necessary

Off-label uses
• Bronchodilation in some asthmatic patients
• Post–myocardial infarction hypomagnesemia

Contraindications
• Hypermagnesemia
• Heart block
• Myocardial damage
• Active labor or within 2 hours of delivery

Precautions
Use cautiously in:
• renal insufficiency, abdominal pain, nausea and vomiting, rectal bleeding, anuria, hypocalcemia
• pregnant patients.

Administration
🔊 Be aware that magnesium sulfate injection is a high-alert drug.
• Know that I.V. use is reserved for life-threatening seizures.
• When giving magnesium sulfate I.V., don't exceed concentration of 20% or infusion rate of 150 mg/minute, except in seizures caused by severe eclampsia. Too-rapid I.V. infusion may cause hypotension and asystole.
• When giving magnesium sulfate I.M. to adults, use concentration of 25% to 50%; when giving to infants and children, don't exceed 20%.

Route	Onset	Peak	Duration
P.O.	3-6 hr	4 hr	Unknown
I.V.	Immediate	Unknown	30 min
I.M.	60 min	Unknown	3-4 hr

Adverse reactions
CNS (with I.V. use): confusion, decreased reflexes, dizziness, syncope, sedation, hypothermia, **paralysis**
CV (with I.V. use): hypotension, **arrhythmias, circulatory collapse**
GI: nausea, vomiting, cramps, flatulence, anorexia
Metabolic: hypermagnesemia, hypocalcemia
Musculoskeletal (with I.V. use): muscle weakness, flaccidity
Respiratory: respiratory paralysis
Skin: diaphoresis

Other: allergic reaction, injection site reaction, laxative dependence (with repeated or prolonged use)

Interactions

Drug-drug. *Aminoquinolones, nitrofurantoin, penicillamine, tetracyclines:* decreased absorption of these drugs (with oral magnesium)
CNS depressants: additive effects
Digoxin: heart block, conduction changes (with I.V. use)
Enteric-coated drugs: faster dissolution of these drugs
Neuromuscular blockers: increased effects of these drugs (with I.V. use)
Drug-diagnostic tests. *Calcium, magnesium:* increased levels (with I.V. use)

Patient monitoring

🔊 When giving prolonged or repeated I.V. infusions, assess patellar reflex and monitor for respiratory rate of 16 breaths/minute or more.
🔊 With I.V. use, monitor blood magnesium level (desired level is 3 to 6 mg/dl or 2.5 to 5 mEq/L). Check for signs and symptoms of magnesium toxicity (hypotension, nausea, vomiting, ECG changes, muscle weakness, mental or respiratory depression, coma). Keep injectable calcium on hand to counteract magnesium toxicity.
• Monitor urine output, which should measure 100 ml or more every 4 hours.
🔊 If I.V. magnesium was given before delivery, assess neonate for signs and symptoms of magnesium toxicity, such as neuromuscular or respiratory depression.
• Monitor electrolyte levels and liver function tests.

Patient teaching

🔊 Teach patient about adverse reactions. Instruct him to report symptoms that occur during I.V. administration.
• Advise patient to consult prescriber before using magnesium if he's taking other drugs. Magnesium may delay or enhance absorption of other drugs.
• Inform patient that repeated or prolonged use of magnesium citrate, hydroxide, or sulfate may cause laxative dependence. Inform him that healthy diet and exercise can reduce need for laxatives.
• Tell pregnant female to make sure prescriber knows she's pregnant before taking drug.
• As appropriate, review all other significant and life-threatening adverse reactions and interactions, especially those related to the drugs and tests mentioned above.

mannitol

Osmitrol, Resectisol

Pharmacologic class: Osmotic diuretic
Therapeutic class: Diuretic
Pregnancy risk category C

m

Action

Increases osmotic pressure of plasma in glomerular filtrate, inhibiting tubular reabsorption of water and electrolytes (including sodium and potassium). These actions enhance water flow from various tissues and ultimately decrease intracranial and intraocular pressures; serum sodium level rises while potassium and blood urea levels fall. Also protects kidneys by preventing toxins from forming and blocking tubules.

Availability

Injection: 5%, 10%, 15%, 20%, 25%
Solution: 5 g/100 ml

Indications and dosages

➢ Test dose for marked oliguria or suspected inadequate renal function
Adults: 0.2 g/kg I.V. infusion (approximately 50 ml of 25% solution, 75 ml of

20% solution, or 100 ml of 15% solution) over 3 to 5 minutes. If urine flow doesn't increase, second dose may be given; if response is inadequate after second dose, reevaluate patient.

➢ To prevent acute renal failure during cardiovascular and other surgeries
Adults: 50 to 100 g I.V. infusion as 5% to 25% solution, up to 6 g/kg/day

➢ Acute renal failure
Adults: 50 to 100 g I.V. infusion as 15% to 25% solution, up to 6 g/kg/day

➢ To reduce intracranial pressure and brain mass
Adults: 0.5 to 2 g/kg I.V. infusion as 15% to 25% solution given over 30 to 60 minutes

➢ To reduce intraocular pressure
Adults: 0.5 to 2 g/kg I.V. infusion as 15% to 25% solution given over 30 to 60 minutes. For preoperative use, give 60 to 90 minutes before surgery.

➢ To promote diuresis in drug toxicity
Adults: 25 g I.V. infusion as loading dose, followed by infusion of 5% to 25% solution given continuously to maintain high urine output

➢ Irrigation during transurethral resection of prostate
Adults: 2.5% to 5% solution instilled into bladder via indwelling urethral catheter, as needed

Contraindications

- Active intracranial bleeding (except during craniotomy)
- Anuria secondary to severe renal disease
- Progressive heart failure, pulmonary congestion, renal damage, or renal dysfunction after mannitol therapy begins
- Severe pulmonary congestion or pulmonary edema
- Severe dehydration

Precautions

Use cautiously in:

- severe renal disease, heart failure, mild to moderate dehydration
- pregnant or breastfeeding patients.

Administration

[Clinical alert] Withhold drug until adequate renal function and urinary output are established.

- Be aware that at low temperatures, solution may crystallize (especially concentrations above 15%). If crystals form, warm bottle in hot-water bath or dry-heat oven or autoclave, then cool to body temperature or lower before giving.
- Don't give electrolyte-free mannitol solutions with blood; when giving blood with mannitol, add 20 mEq or more of sodium chloride solution to each liter of mannitol solution to avoid pseudoagglutination.
- Know that drug may be given as continuous or intermittent I.V. infusion. Infuse at prescribed rate using infusion device and in-line filter. Give single I.V. dose over 30 to 90 minutes in adults.

[Clinical alert] Avoid extravasation, because it may cause local edema and tissue necrosis.

Route	Onset	Peak	Duration
I.V. (diuresis)	1-3 hr	Unknown	Up to 8 hr
I.V. (intraocular press.)	30-60 min	Unknown	4-8 hr
I.V. (intracranial press.)	15 min	Unknown	3-8 hr

Adverse reactions

CNS: dizziness, headache, **seizures**
CV: chest pain, hypotension, hypertension, tachycardia, **thrombophlebitis, heart failure, vascular overload**
EENT: blurred vision, rhinitis
GI: nausea, vomiting, diarrhea, dry mouth
GU: polyuria, urinary retention, **osmotic nephrosis**
Metabolic: dehydration, water intoxication, hypernatremia, hyponatremia, hypovolemia, hypokalemia, **hyperkalemia, metabolic acidosis**

Respiratory: pulmonary congestion
Skin: rash, urticaria
Other: chills, fever, thirst, edema, extravasation with edema and tissue necrosis

Interactions

Drug-drug. *Digoxin:* increased risk of digoxin toxicity
Diuretics: increased therapeutic effects of mannitol
Lithium: increased urinary excretion of lithium
Drug-diagnostic tests. *Electrolytes:* increased or decreased levels

Patient monitoring

- Monitor I.V. site carefully to avoid extravasation and tissue necrosis.
- In comatose patient, insert indwelling urinary catheter as ordered to monitor urine output.
- Monitor renal function tests, urinary output, fluid balance, central venous pressure, and electrolyte levels (especially sodium and potassium).
- Watch for excessive fluid loss and signs and symptoms of hypovolemia and dehydration.
- Assess for evidence of circulatory overload, including pulmonary edema, water intoxication, and heart failure.

Patient teaching

- Teach patient about importance of monitoring exact urinary output.
- Advise patient to report pain at infusion site as well as adverse reactions, such as increased shortness of breath or pain in back, legs, or chest.
- Tell patient drug may cause thirst or dry mouth. Emphasize that fluid restrictions are necessary, but that frequent mouth care should ease these symptoms.
- As appropriate, review all other significant and life-threatening adverse reactions and interactions, especially those related to the drugs and tests mentioned above.

mebendazole

Vermox

Pharmacologic class: Benzimidazole
Therapeutic class: Antihelmintic
Pregnancy risk category C

Action

Blocks glucose and other nutrient uptake in susceptible helminths, interfering with absorption

Availability

Tablets (chewable): 100 mg

Indications and dosages

➢ Pinworm (*Enterobius vermicularis*)
Adults and children older than age 2: 100 mg P.O. as a single dose. Repeat in 2 to 3 weeks, if necessary.
➢ Whipworm *(Trichuris trichiura),* roundworm *(Ascaris lumbricoides),* American hookworm *(Necator americanus),* common hookworm *(Ancylostoma duodenale),* and mixed infections
Adults and children older than age 2: 100 mg P.O. in morning and evening for 3 days. Repeat in 3 weeks, if necessary.

Contraindications

- Hypersensitivity to drug

Precautions

Use cautiously in:

- impaired hepatic function, Crohn's ileitis, ulcerative colitis
- pregnant patients (use in first trimester only if benefit justifies risk to fetus)
- breastfeeding patients
- children younger than age 2.

m

Administration

• Know that tablets may be chewed, swallowed, or crushed and mixed with food.

Route	Onset	Peak	Duration
P.O.	Unknown	2-5 hr	Unknown

Adverse reactions

GI: abdominal pain, diarrhea
Other: fever

Interactions

Drug-drug. *Carbamazepine, phenytoin:* increased mebendazole metabolism and decreased efficacy (with high doses)
Cimetidine: inhibited mebendazole metabolism and increased blood level

Patient monitoring

• In prolonged therapy, monitor hematologic and hepatic studies.
• Ask family members if they have signs or symptoms of pinworm; infection spreads easily.

Patient teaching

• Tell patient he may chew tablets, swallow them whole, or crush and mix with food.
• Inform patient that parasite removal from GI tract may take up to 3 days after treatment. If he's not cured after 3 weeks, he may need a second course.
• Advise patient not to prepare food for others.
• Teach patient to maintain strict hygiene to prevent reinfection. Instruct him to disinfect bathroom daily and change and launder clothing, bed linens, and towels daily.
• Advise patient that dietary restrictions, fasting, and laxatives aren't necessary.
• Tell female patient to inform prescriber if she is pregnant or breastfeeding.
• As appropriate, review all other significant adverse reactions and interactions, especially those related to the drugs mentioned above.

mechlorethamine hydrochloride (HN_2, mustine, nitrogen mustard)

Mustargen

Pharmacologic class: Alkylating agent, nitrogen mustard agent
Therapeutic class: Antineoplastic
Pregnancy risk category D

Action

Interferes with DNA and RNA synthesis by cross-linking strands of cellular DNA. Cell-cycle-phase nonspecific.

Availability

Powder for injection: 10 mg/vial

Indications and dosages

➢ Chronic myelocytic or chronic lymphocytic leukemia; lymphosarcoma; polycythemia vera; mycosis fungoides; bronchogenic carcinoma
Adults: 0.4 mg/kg I.V. given as a single dose or in divided doses of 0.1 to 0.2 mg/kg/day I.V., with subsequent doses given after hematologic recovery (usually 3 to 6 weeks)
➢ Advanced Hodgkin's disease (stages III and IV)
Adults: 6 mg/m^2 I.V. on days 1 and 8 of 28-day cycle as part of MOPP regimen (mechlorethamine, vincristine, procarbazine, prednisone). During subsequent cycles, blood counts determine dosage.
➢ Metastatic cancer with effusion
Adults: 0.4 mg/kg intrapleurally or intraperitoneally or 0.2 mg/kg intrapericardially

Contraindications
- Hypersensitivity to drug
- Active infection

Precautions
Use cautiously in:
- chronic lymphocytic leukemia, decreased bone marrow reserve, hematopoietic depression, amyloidosis, infections, severe edema, obesity
- previous radiation therapy or chemotherapy
- elderly or debilitated patients
- patients with childbearing potential
- pregnant or breastfeeding patients
- children (safety and efficacy not established).

Administration
🔊 Follow facility policy when handling and preparing. Drug is carcinogenic, mutagenic, and teratogenic.
- Know that severe nausea and vomiting may occur 1 to 3 hours after administration. Premedicate with antiemetics and sedatives, as prescribed.

🔊 Be aware that drug has narrow margin of safety. Use extreme caution with dosages.
- Reconstitute with 10 ml of sterile water or sodium chloride for injection, to yield a concentration of 1 mg/ml. Give immediately after reconstitution.
- Withdraw calculated dosage and inject either directly into vein or into port of free-flowing I.V. line (preferred) over 3 to 5 minutes.

🔊 Monitor I.V. site for infiltration. Drug is potent vesicant.
- If extravasation occurs, infiltrate area with sterile isotonic sodium thiosulfate; then apply ice compresses for 6 to 12 hours and notify prescriber.

🔊 Neutralize equipment or unused solution in equal volumes of 5% sodium thiosulfate and 5% sodium bicarbonate. Soak for 45 minutes, then discard unused solution according to facility policy.
- Consult current published protocols before intracavitary use.
- After intracavitary administration, change patient's position every 5 to 10 minutes to promote uniform drug distribution.

Route	Onset	Peak	Duration
I.V., intracavitary	Unknown	Unknown	Unknown

Adverse reactions
GI: nausea, vomiting, diarrhea
GU: infertility, delayed menses, oligomenorrhea, amenorrhea
Hematologic: anemia, **leukopenia, thrombocytopenia, lymphocytopenia, granulocytopenia, agranulocytosis, persistent pancytopenia**
Metabolic: hyperuricemia
Skin: rash, alopecia, **erythema multiforme**
Other: herpes zoster reactivation; chromosome abnormalities; tissue necrosis and phlebitis at I.V. site with extravasation; hypersensitivity reactions, including **anaphylaxis; amyloidosis; secondary cancers**

Interactions
Drug-drug. *Other antineoplastics:* additive bone marrow depression
Live-virus vaccines: decreased antibody response to vaccine, increased risk of adverse reactions
Drug-diagnostic tests. *Granulocytes, lymphocytes, platelets, red blood cells:* decreased counts
Uric acid: increased level

Patient monitoring
🔊 Check I.V. site carefully to avoid extravasation and tissue necrosis.
- Monitor hematologic, kidney, and liver function tests.
- Watch for hyperuricemia. Maintain adequate hydration to prevent uric acid elevation.
- Monitor patient for infection. Lymphocytopenia occurs within 24 hours;

m

significant granulocytopenia occurs in 6 to 8 days and lasts 10 to 21 days, with recovery within 2 weeks after nadir.

Patient teaching

- 🔊 Teach patient to immediately report pain or burning at injection site.
- 🔊 Advise patient to immediately report signs or symptoms of infection, including fever, malaise, or sore throat.
- 🔊 Teach patient to report bleeding gums, dark stools, or easy bruising or bleeding.
- Instruct patient to avoid crowds and practice good handwashing.
- Tell patient to avoid pregnancy or breastfeeding.
- Inform patient that drug may cause sterility.
- As appropriate, review all other significant and life-threatening adverse reactions and interactions, especially those related to the drugs and tests mentioned above.

meclizine hydrochloride

Antivert, Bonamine✤, Bonine, Dramamine Less Drowsy Formula

Pharmacologic class: Anticholinergic
Therapeutic class: Antiemetic, antivertigo drug
Pregnancy risk category B

Action

Decreases excitability of middle-ear labyrinth and depresses conduction in vestibular-cerebellar pathways

Availability

Tablets: 12.5 mg, 25 mg, 50 mg
Tablets (chewable): 25 mg

Indications and dosages

➢ Motion sickness
Adults: 25 to 50 mg P.O. 1 hour before travel. May repeat q 24 hours for duration of travel.

➢ Vertigo associated with diseases affecting the vestibular system
Adults: 25 to 100 mg P.O. daily in divided doses

Contraindications

- Hypersensitivity to drug
- Children younger than age 12

Precautions

Use cautiously in:
- prostatic hypertrophy, stenosing peptic ulcer, bladder neck obstruction, pyloroduodenal obstruction, arrhythmias, angle-closure glaucoma, bronchial asthma
- pregnant or breastfeeding patients
- children.

Administration

- Know that tablets may be chewed or swallowed whole.

Route	Onset	Peak	Duration
P.O.	1 hr	Unknown	8-24 hr

Adverse reactions

CNS: drowsiness, fatigue, confusion, excitement, euphoria, nervousness, restlessness, insomnia, vertigo, visual and auditory hallucinations, **seizures**
CV: hypotension, palpitations, tachycardia
EENT: blurred vision, diplopia, tinnitus, dry nose, dry throat
GI: nausea, vomiting, diarrhea, constipation, dry mouth, anorexia
GU: difficulty urinating, urinary retention, urinary frequency
Skin: rash, urticaria

Interactions

Drug-drug. *Anticholinergics (including some antihistamines, antidepressants, atropine, haloperidol, phenothiazines):* additive anticholinergic effects

Antihistamines, CNS depressants (such as opioids, sedative-hypnotics): additive CNS depression
Drug-diagnostic tests. *Skin tests using allergen extracts:* false-negative results
Drug-behaviors. *Alcohol use:* additive CNS depression

Patient monitoring

- Discontinue drug, as ordered, at least 4 days before skin testing.
- Know that drug has anticholinergic effects.

Patient teaching

- Tell patient to take as prescribed to minimize adverse effects.
- Caution patient to avoid driving and other hazardous activities until he knows how drug affects concentration and alertness.
- Advise patient to relieve dry mouth with hard candy or frequent sips of fluids.
- As appropriate, review all other significant and life-threatening adverse reactions and interactions, especially those related to the drugs, tests, and behaviors mentioned above.

medroxyprogesterone acetate

Alti-MPA♣, Amen, Depo-Provera, Gen-Medroxy♣, Novo-Medrone♣, Provera

Pharmacologic class: Hormone
Therapeutic class: Progestin
Pregnancy risk category X

Action

Inhibits pituitary gonadotropin secretion, preventing follicular maturation, ovulation, and pregnancy

Availability

Suspension for depot injection: 150 mg/ml, 400 mg/ml
Tablets: 2.5 mg, 5 mg, 10 mg

Indications and dosages

➢ Secondary amenorrhea
Adults: 5 to 10 mg/day P.O. for 5 to 10 days, starting at any time during menstrual cycle
➢ Dysfunctional uterine bleeding; menses induction
Adults: 5 to 10 mg/day P.O. for 5 to 10 days, starting on day 16 or 21 of menstrual cycle
➢ To prevent estrogen-related endometrial changes in postmenopausal women
Adults: 2.5 to 5 mg/day P.O. given with 0.625 mg conjugated estrogens P.O. (monophasic regimen); or 5 mg/day P.O. on days 15 to 28 of cycle, given with 0.625 mg conjugated estrogens P.O. daily throughout cycle (biphasic regimen)
➢ To prevent pregnancy
Adults: 150 mg (Depo-Provera) deep I.M. injection q 13 weeks. Give first injection during first 5 days of normal menstrual period or first 5 postpartal days if patient isn't breastfeeding, or during sixth postpartal week if patient is breastfeeding exclusively.
➢ Renal or endometrial cancer
Adults: 400 to 1,000 mg I.M.; may repeat weekly. If improvement occurs, decrease to 400 mg q month.

Off-label uses

- Advanced breast cancer

Contraindications

- Hypersensitivity to drug or its components
- Cerebrovascular or thromboembolic disease
- Hepatic dysfunction or disease
- Breast or genital cancer
- Undiagnosed vaginal bleeding
- Known or suspected pregnancy

m

Precautions

Use cautiously in:
- seizure disorder, renal or cardiovascular disease, asthma, diabetes mellitus, depression, migraine
- history of hepatic disease.

Administration

- Before starting therapy, obtain thorough history and physical examination, with emphasis on breast and pelvic organs. Also obtain Pap smear, and repeat annually during therapy.
- With contraceptive use, rule out pregnancy before first dose and when more than 14 weeks have passed since previous dose.
- For I.M. injection, inject deep into gluteal, deltoid, or anterior thigh muscle. Rotate injection sites.
- Be aware that when drug is used to prevent estrogen-related endometrial changes in postmenopausal women, lowest dosage should be used for shortest time, because treatment exceeding 1 year correlates with cancer. (Some combination products have 0.3 mg estrogen/1.5 mg progesterone or 0.45 mg estrogen/1.5 mg progesterone.)

Route	Onset	Peak	Duration
P.O.	Unknown	Unknown	Unknown
I.M.	Wks-1 mo	1 mo	Unknown

Adverse reactions

CNS: insomnia, migraine, nervousness, drowsiness, dizziness, fatigue, depression, mood changes
CV: thrombophlebitis, thromboembolism
EENT: diplopia, proptosis, retinal vascular lesions, **papilledema**
GI: abdominal pain, bloating
GU: amenorrhea, leukorrhea, spotting, cervical secretions, galactorrhea, breast tenderness and secretion, cervical erosions, pelvic pain, infertility
Hepatic: jaundice
Metabolic: fluid retention, hyperglycemia
Musculoskeletal: leg cramps, back pain
Respiratory: pulmonary embolism
Skin: pruritus, urticaria, rash, acne, alopecia, hirsutism, cholasma, melasma, sterile abscesses, induration at I.M. site
Other: weight and appetite changes, edema, angioedema, allergic reactions including **anaphylaxis**

Interactions

Drug-drug. *Bromocriptine:* decreased bromocriptine efficacy
Carbamazepine, phenobarbital, phenytoin, rifampin: decreased contraceptive efficacy
Drug-diagnostic tests. *Alkaline phosphatase, low-density lipoproteins:* increased levels
High-density lipoproteins, pregnanediol excretion: decreased levels
Thyroid hormone assays: altered results
Drug-behaviors. *Alcohol use:* additive CNS depression

Patient monitoring

- Monitor patient for fluid retention and for signs and symptoms of thrombophlebitis, including pain, swelling, and redness of lower legs.

[Clinical alert] Assess for visual disturbances and headache. If ocular exam shows papilledema or retinal vascular lesions, drug should be discontinued.
- Evaluate liver function tests.

[Clinical alert] Watch for abdominal pain, fever, malaise, jaundice, darkened urine, and clay-colored stools.

Patient teaching

- Advise patient that drug may cause nausea, vomiting, headache, abdominal pain, painful breast swelling, and abnormal bleeding pattern. Instruct her to report these effects if pronounced.

Tell patient to promptly report bloating, swelling, appetite loss, rash, yellowed skin, mood changes or depression, nervousness, dizziness, chest pain, shortness of breath, visual disturbances, or severe headache.
- Teach patient how to perform breast self-exams.
- Tell patient she must undergo yearly physical examinations with Pap smear.
- As appropriate, review all other significant and life-threatening adverse reactions and interactions, especially those related to the drugs, tests, and behaviors mentioned above.

mefloquine hydrochloride

Lariam

Pharmacologic class: 4-quinoline-methanol derivative, quinine analog
Therapeutic class: Antimalarial
Pregnancy risk category C

Action

Unknown. Thought to increase intravesicular pH in parasite acid vesicles and form complexes with hemin, inhibiting parasite development.

Availability

Tablets: 250 mg

Indications and dosages

➢ Acute malarial infection

Adults: 1,250 mg P.O. as a single dose
Children: 20 to 25 mg/kg P.O. in two divided doses given 6 to 8 hours apart

➢ Malaria prophylaxis

Adults and children weighing more than 45 kg (99 lb): 250 mg P.O. once weekly on same day each week, starting 1 week before entering endemic area and continuing for 4 weeks after leaving area
Children weighing 31 to 45 kg (67 to 99 lb): 187.5 mg P.O. q week
Children weighing 20 to 30 kg (44 to 66 lb): 125 mg P.O. q week
Children weighing 10 to 20 kg (22 to 44 lb): 62.5 mg P.O. q week
Children weighing 5 to 10 kg (11 to 22 lb): 31.25 mg P.O. q week

Contraindications

- Hypersensitivity to drug, related agents (quinine, quinidine), or excipients

Precautions

Use cautiously in:
- cardiac disorders, seizure disorders
- pregnant or breastfeeding patients
- children.

Administration

- Don't give on empty stomach. Administer with at least 240 ml of water.
- Know that after completing mefloquine therapy for acute malarial infection, patient should receive primaquine (or other 8-aminoquinolone) to prevent relapse.

Route	Onset	Peak	Duration
P.O.	Unknown	7-24 hr	Unknown

Adverse reactions

CNS: dizziness, syncope, headache, psychotic changes, depression, hallucinations, confusion, anxiety, fatigue, vertigo, **seizures**
EENT: blurred vision, tinnitus
GI: nausea, vomiting, diarrhea, loose stools, abdominal discomfort, anorexia
Hematologic: leukopenia, thrombocytopenia
Musculoskeletal: myalgia
Skin: rash
Other: fever, chills

Interactions

Drug-drug. *Beta-adrenergic blockers, quinidine, quinine:* ECG abnormalities, cardiac arrest

m

Chloroquine, quinine: increased risk of seizures
Valproic acid: decreased valproic acid blood level, loss of seizure control
Drug-diagnostic tests. *Hematocrit, platelets, white blood cells:* decreased values
Transaminases: transient increases

Patient monitoring

- Clinical alert: Monitor patient with acute *Plasmodium vivax* malaria who is at high risk for relapse. Because drug doesn't eliminate exoerythrocytic (hepatic-phase) parasites, patient should receive primaquine after mefloquine therapy.
- Clinical alert: Watch for psychiatric symptoms, such as acute anxiety, depression, restlessness, or confusion. These may precede more serious psychiatric events.
- Evaluate hepatic function during prolonged prophylactic therapy.
- Clinical alert: In patients receiving related drugs (such as quinine, quinidine, or chloroquine) concurrently, be alert for ECG abnormalities and seizures. Separate administration times by at least 12 hours.
- Clinical alert: Closely monitor patients with serious or life-threatening *Plasmodium falciparum* infection. Be aware that they should receive I.V. antimalarial drugs and that mefloquine may be used to complete course of therapy.

Patient teaching

- Tell patient to take with full glass of water and not on empty stomach.
- In prophylactic use, instruct patient to take first dose 1 week before departure and to continue therapy as prescribed upon return. Tell him to take drug on same day each week.
- Advise patient to report fever after returning from malarious area.
- Inform patient that malaria prophylaxis should include protective clothing, insect repellent, and bed netting.
- Clinical alert: Tell patient to immediately report psychiatric symptoms (such as acute anxiety, depression, restlessness, or confusion) and to stop taking drug.
- Caution patient to avoid driving and other hazardous activities because drug may cause dizziness.
- Instruct patient to have periodic ophthalmic exams, because drug may cause eye damage.
- Tell female patient to inform prescriber if she is pregnant.
- Advise female patient not to breastfeed while taking drug.
- As appropriate, review all other significant and life-threatening adverse reactions and interactions, especially those related to the drugs and tests mentioned above.

megestrol acetate

Apo-Megestrol (Canada), Megace, Megace-OS (Canada)

Pharmacologic class: Hormone
Therapeutic class: Progestin, antineoplastic, appetite stimulant
Pregnancy risk category D (tablets), *X* (suspension)

Action

Unknown. Thought to suppress growth of progestin-sensitive breast and endometrial tumors by inhibiting pituitary and adrenal function.

Availability

Oral suspension: 40 mg/ml
Tablets: 20 mg, 40 mg

Indications and dosages

➢ Breast cancer
Adults: 160 mg/day P.O. as a single dose, or 40 mg P.O. q.i.d.
➢ Endometrial cancer
Adults: 40 to 320 mg/day P.O. in divided doses

➢ Anorexia, cachexia, or unexplained significant weight loss in AIDS patients
Adults: 800 mg (suspension only) P.O. daily

Off-label uses

- Endometriosis, endometrial hyperplasia
- Prostatic hypertrophy
- Contraception

Contraindications

- Hypersensitivity to drug or its components
- Known or suspected pregnancy (suspension only)

Precautions

Use cautiously in:
- diabetes mellitus, severe hepatic disease, renal disease, cardiovascular disease, seizure disorders, cerebral hemorrhage, migraine, asthma, undiagnosed vaginal bleeding, depression
- history of thrombophlebitis
- breastfeeding.

Administration

- Give with meals if GI upset occurs.

Route	Onset	Peak	Duration
P.O.	Wks-1 mo	2 mo	Unknown

Adverse reactions

CNS: headache, insomnia, drowsiness, asthenia, confusion, neuropathy, hyperesthesia, abnormal thinking, paresthesias, depression, **seizures**
CV: hypertension, chest pain, **thrombophlebitis**
EENT: amblyopia, retinal thrombosis, pharyngitis
GI: nausea, vomiting, constipation, abdominal pain, flatulence, dyspepsia, dry mouth, increased salivation, oral candidiasis
GU: breast tenderness, breakthrough bleeding, decreased libido
Hematologic: anemia, **leukopenia**
Hepatic: hepatomegaly
Metabolic: hyperglycemia
Musculoskeletal: carpal tunnel syndrome, back pain
Respiratory: dyspnea, cough, pneumonia, **pulmonary embolism**
Skin: alopecia, rash, pruritus, sweating
Other: edema, fever, weight gain, herpes infection

Interactions

Drug-diagnostic tests. *Lactate dehydrogenase:* increased level

Patient monitoring

🔊 Watch for signs and symptoms of thromboembolic disorders.
🔊 Stay alert for visual disturbances, headache, abdominal pain, and hepatomegaly.
- Monitor glucose level in diabetic patients.

Patient teaching

- Inform patient that drug may cause back or abdominal pain, headache, nausea, vomiting, or breast tenderness.

🔊 Tell patient to immediately report pain, swelling or redness of lower legs, chest or back pain, or shortness of breath.
- Advise patient to contact prescriber if adverse effects become pronounced or if other troublesome signs or symptoms occur.
- Urge patient to use reliable contraception.

🔊 Instruct patient to immediately report suspected pregnancy.
- Caution female patient to avoid breastfeeding.
- Advise diabetic patient to monitor blood glucose level.
- As appropriate, review all other significant and life-threatening adverse reactions and interactions, especially those related to the tests mentioned above.

m

meloxicam

Mobic, Mobicox✱

Pharmacologic class: Nonopioid analgesic, nonsteroidal anti-inflammatory drug (NSAID)
Therapeutic class: Analgesic, anti-inflammatory drug
Pregnancy risk category C

Action

Unknown. Thought to reduce inflammation and pain by inhibiting prostaglandin synthesis of the enzyme cyclooxygenase.

Availability

Oral suspension: 7.5 mg/5 ml
Tablets: 7.5 mg, 15 mg

Indications and dosages

➢ Osteoarthritis; rheumatoid arthritis
Adults: 7.5 mg P.O. once daily; may increase to 15 mg/day

Contraindications

• Hypersensitivity to drug, its components, or other NSAIDs

Precautions

Use cautiously in:
• bleeding disorders, GI or cardiac disorders, severe renal impairment, severe hepatic disease, asthma, peptic ulcer disease
• concurrent aspirin, oral anticoagulant, or corticosteroid therapy
• elderly or debilitated patients
• pregnant or breastfeeding patients
• children younger than age 18 (safety and efficacy not established).

Administration

• Before starting therapy, ask patient about aspirin sensitivity and allergies to other NSAIDs. If patient is dehydrated, provide adequate fluids.

Route	Onset	Peak	Duration
P.O.	Unknown	5-6 hr	24 hr

Adverse reactions

CNS: headache, dizziness, syncope, malaise, fatigue, asthenia, depression, confusion, nervousness, drowsiness, insomnia, vertigo, tremor, paresthesia, anxiety, **seizures**
CV: hypertension, hypotension, palpitations, angina, vasculitis, **heart failure, arrhythmias, myocardial infarction**
EENT: abnormal vision, conjunctivitis, hearing loss, tinnitus, pharyngitis
GI: nausea, vomiting, diarrhea, constipation, colitis, GI ulcers with perforation, abdominal pain, dyspepsia, gastroesophageal reflux, esophagitis, flatulence, ulcerative stomatitis, dry mouth, **pancreatitis, GI hemorrhage**
GU: urinary frequency, urinary tract infection, albuminuria, hematuria, **renal failure**
Hematologic: anemia, purpura, **leukopenia, thrombocytopenia**
Hepatic: hepatitis
Musculoskeletal: joint pain, back pain
Metabolic: dehydration
Respiratory: upper respiratory infection, dyspnea, coughing, asthma, **bronchospasm**
Skin: rash, urticaria, pruritus, bullous eruption, sweating, alopecia, photosensitivity, angioedema
Other: altered taste, increased appetite, weight gain or loss, hot flashes, fluid retention and edema, masking of infection symptoms, hypersensitivity reactions including **anaphylaxis**

Interactions

Drug-drug. *Angiotensin-converting enzyme inhibitors:* decreased antihypertensive effect
Anticoagulants: increased risk of bleeding
Aspirin: increased meloxicam blood level, increased risk of toxicity

Cholestyramine: decreased meloxicam blood level
Furosemide, thiazides: decreased diuretic effect
Lithium: increased lithium blood level
Drug-diagnostic tests. *Alanine aminotransferase, aspartate aminotransferase, bilirubin, blood urea nitrogen, creatinine, gamma-glutamyl transferase:* increased levels
Hemoglobin, platelets, white blood cells: decreased values
Drug-behaviors. *Alcohol use, smoking:* increased risk of GI irritation and bleeding

Patient monitoring

Clinical alert: Closely monitor patient with aspirin-sensitivity asthma, because of risk of severe bronchospasm.

- In prolonged therapy, monitor CBC and kidney and liver function tests.

Clinical alert: Assess for cardiovascular disorders and hepatotoxicity.

- Monitor patient for fluid retention and weight gain.

Patient teaching

Clinical alert: Instruct patient to immediately report signs and symptoms of hepatotoxicity, including right upper quadrant pain, nausea, fatigue, lethargy, pruritus, and jaundice.

- Tell patient to report abdominal pain, blood in stool or emesis, or black tarry stools.
- Instruct patient to avoid alcohol and smoking.
- Caution pregnant patient to avoid drug, especially during third trimester.
- Tell patient to consult prescriber before taking over-the-counter preparations.
- As appropriate, review all other significant and life-threatening adverse reactions and interactions, especially those related to the drugs, tests, and behaviors mentioned above.

melphalan (L-PAM, L-phenylalanine mustard, L-sarcolysin)

Alkeran

melphalan hydrochloride

Alkeran

Pharmacologic class: Alkylator
Therapeutic class: Antineoplastic
Pregnancy risk category D

Action

Forms cross-links between strands of cellular DNA, disrupting DNA and RNA transcription and causing cell death

Availability

Powder for injection (melphalan hydrochloride): 50 mg
Tablets: 2 mg

Indications and dosages

➢ Multiple myeloma

Adults: Initially, 6 mg P.O. daily for 2 to 3 weeks, then discontinue drug for up to 4 weeks or until white blood cell (WBC) and platelet counts increase; then give maintenance dosage of 2 mg/day or 0.15 mg/kg/day P.O. for 7 days or 0.25 mg/kg for 4 days, repeated q 4 to 6 weeks. For those who can't tolerate oral therapy, 16 mg/m^2 by I.V. infusion over 15 to 20 minutes at 2-week intervals for four doses (usually with prednisone); I.V. dose can be repeated q 4 weeks after recovery from toxicity.

➢ Nonresectable advanced ovarian cancer

Adults: 0.2 mg/kg/day P.O. for 5 days q 4 to 5 weeks

Dosage adjustment

- Renal impairment

m

Contraindications

- Hypersensitivity to drug
- Patients whose disease has shown previous drug resistance

Precautions

Use cautiously in:

- bone marrow depression, infection, renal disease
- previous radiation therapy
- patients with childbearing potential
- pregnant or breastfeeding patients
- children (safety and efficacy not established).

Administration

- Before starting therapy, obtain CBC with white cell differential and platelet count. Repeat periodically before each course.
- For I.V. use, reconstitute by rapidly injecting 10 ml of supplied diluent into vial with lyophilized powder. Shake until solution is clear (yields a concentration of 5 mg/ml).
- Dilute desired dosage in 0.9% sodium chloride injection to a concentration no greater than 0.45 mg/ml. Administer over 15 minutes, being sure to give entire dose within 60 minutes of reconstitution.

🔊 Minimize time between reconstitution, dilution, and administration, because solution is unstable.

Route	Onset	Peak	Duration
P.O.	5 days	2-3 wk	5-6 wk
I.V.	Unknown	Unknown	Unknown

Adverse reactions

CV: hypotension, tachycardia, vasculitis
GI: nausea, vomiting, diarrhea, oral ulcers, stomatitis
GU: hyperuricemia, amenorrhea, gonadal suppression, infertility
Hematologic: anemia, purpura, **bone marrow depression, leukopenia, thrombocytopenia**
Hepatic: hepatotoxicity
Metabolic: hyperuricemia
Respiratory: dyspnea, **interstitial pneumonitis, bronchospasm, fibrosis**
Skin: rash, urticaria, pruritus, alopecia, sweating
Other: edema, extravasation at I.V. site, allergic reactions including **anaphylaxis**

Interactions

Drug-drug. *Carmustine:* increased pulmonary toxicity
Cimetidine: decreased GI absorption of melphalan
Cisplatin: increased risk of renal dysfunction, decreased melphalan clearance
Cyclosporine: increased risk of nephrotoxicity, severe renal failure
Interferon alfa: decreased melphalan blood level
Live-virus vaccines: decreased antibody response to vaccine
Myelosuppressants: additive toxicity
Nalidixic acid: increased risk of severe hemorrhagic necrotic enterocolitis (in children)
Drug-diagnostic tests. *Hemoglobin, platelets, red blood cells, WBCs:* decreased values
Nitrogenous compounds: increased levels
Drug-food. *Any food:* decreased absorption of oral melphalan

Patient monitoring

🔊 Monitor patient for thrombocytopenia and leukopenia. If platelet count exceeds 100,000/mm^3 or WBC count is below 3,000/mm^3, discontinue drug until peripheral blood counts recover.

🔊 Watch closely for indications of bone marrow depression, including infection, anemia, and bleeding.

🔊 After multiple courses, watch for acute hypersensitivity reaction. If it occurs, discontinue drug and administer volume expanders, corticosteroids, or antihistamines, as prescribed.

- Watch for signs and symptoms of GI or pulmonary toxicity.
- Evaluate renal and hepatic function.

Patient teaching

- Tell patient to take oral tablets without food, because food may decrease drug absorption.
- Instruct patient to take entire daily oral dose at one time on empty stomach.

Clinical alert: Advise patient to immediately report unusual bleeding or bruising, fever, chills, sore throat, shortness of breath, yellowing of skin or eyes, persistent cough, flank or stomach pain, joint pain, black tarry stools, rash, or unusual lumps or masses.

- Tell patient to consult prescriber before using over-the-counter medications.
- Advise patient to use reliable contraception.
- Caution patient to avoid breastfeeding.
- As appropriate, review all other significant and life-threatening adverse reactions and interactions, especially those related to the drugs, tests, and foods mentioned above.

memantine

Namenda

Pharmacologic class: N-methyl-D-aspartate receptor antagonist (NMDA)

Therapeutic class: Anti-Alzheimer's agent

Pregnancy risk category B

Action

Unclear. Thought to act as a low- to moderate-affinity NMDA receptor antagonist, binding to NMDA receptor-operated channels. (Activation of these channels is thought to contribute to Alzheimer's symptoms.)

Availability

Tablets: 5 mg, 10 mg
Tablets (titration pack): 28 tablets of 5 mg and 21 tablets of 10 mg

Indications and dosages

➢ Moderate to severe Alzheimer's-type dementia

Adults: Initially, 5 mg P.O. daily. Then titrate at intervals of at least 1 week in 5-mg increments, to a maximum of 10 mg P.O. b.i.d.

Dosage adjustment

- Moderate renal impairment

Contraindications

- Hypersensitivity to drug or its components

Precautions

Use cautiously in:

- neurologic conditions, moderate to severe renal impairment, genitourinary conditions that increase pH
- pregnant or breastfeeding patients.

Administration

- Give with or without food.

Route	Onset	Peak	Duration
P.O.	Unknown	3-7 hr	Unknown

Adverse reactions

CNS: dizziness, headache, syncope, aggressive reaction, confusion, somnolence, hallucinations, agitation, insomnia, vertigo, ataxia, abnormal gait, hypokinesia, anxiety, **transient ischemic attack, cerebrovascular accident** (CVA)
CV: hypertension, **cardiac failure**
EENT: cataract, conjunctivitis
GI: nausea, vomiting, diarrhea, constipation, anorexia
GU: frequent voiding, urinary incontinence, urinary tract infection
Hematologic: anemia
Musculoskeletal: back pain, arthralgia

Respiratory: cough, dyspnea, bronchitis, pneumonia
Skin: rash
Other: weight loss, fatigue, pain, falls, flulike symptoms, peripheral edema

Interactions

Drug-drug. *Cimetidine, hydrochlorothiazide, nicotine, quinidine, ranitidine, triamterene:* altered blood levels of both drugs
Urine-alkalizing drugs (carbonic anhydrase inhibitors, sodium bicarbonate): decreased memantine elimination
Drug-diagnostic tests. *Alkaline phosphatase:* increased level

Patient monitoring

Check for heart failure and signs and symptoms of CVA.
• Monitor kidney function tests.

Patient teaching

• Tell patient to take with or without food.
• Make sure patient or caregiver knows exactly how drug should be taken and understands dose escalation.
• As appropriate, review all other significant and life-threatening adverse reactions and interactions, especially those related to the drugs and tests mentioned above.

menotropins

Repronex

Pharmacologic class: Hormone
Therapeutic class: Exogenous gonadotropin
Pregnancy risk category X

Action

Simulates action of follicle-stimulating hormone (FSH) by promoting follicular growth and maturation

Availability

Injection (powder or pellet for reconstitution): 75 international units luteinizing hormone (LH); 150 international units LH and 150 international units FSH activity/vial

Indications and dosages

➢ Controlled ovarian stimulation in patients with oligoanovulation
Women: Dosage individualized. Recommended dosage is 150 international units I.M. or subcutaneously daily during first 5 days of treatment, with subsequent dosages adjusted based on response. Adjust dosage no more often than every 2 days, and don't exceed 75 to 150 international units per adjustment. Maximum daily dosage is 450 international units. Dosing beyond 12 days is not recommended. If response is appropriate, human chorionic gonadotropin (hCG) should be given I.M. 1 day after last menotropins dose.
➢ Assisted reproductive technologies
Women: In patients who've received gonadotropin-releasing hormone agonists or antagonist pituitary suppression, recommended initial dosage is 225 international units I.M. or subcutaneously, with subsequent dosage adjustments based on response. Adjust dosage no more often than every 2 days, and don't exceed 75 to 150 international units per adjustment. Maximum daily dosage is 450 international units. Dosing beyond 12 days isn't recommended. Once adequate follicular development appears, hCG is given to induce follicular maturation in preparation for oocyte retrieval.

Contraindications

• Hypersensitivity to drug
• High FSH levels (indicating primary ovarian failure)
• Abnormal bleeding of undetermined origin
• Uncontrolled thyroid or adrenal dysfunction

2006 Nursing Spectrum Drug Handbook Photogallery of common tablets and capsules

This special section helps you identify unlabeled drugs that patients bring from home. It can also serve as a visual aid for patients who can't recall the names of the drugs they're taking. (Note: For more help in identifying medications, see the drug imprint codes at www.nursesdrughandbook.com.) Drugs are shown alphabetically by generic name; corresponding trade names also appear. Dosage forms appear in increasing order of strength.

alendronate sodium	**Fosamax** 5 mg, 10 mg, 35 mg, 70 mg
alprazolam	**Xanax** 0.25 mg, 0.5 mg, 1 mg, 2 mg
amlodipine besylate	**Norvasc** 2.5 mg, 5 mg, 10 mg
amlodipine besylate and benazepril hydrochloride	**Lotrel** 2.5 mg/10 mg, 5 mg/10 mg, 5 mg/20 mg, 10 mg/20 mg
amoxicillin trihydrate	**Amoxil** 125 mg, 250 mg, 500 mg, 875 mg

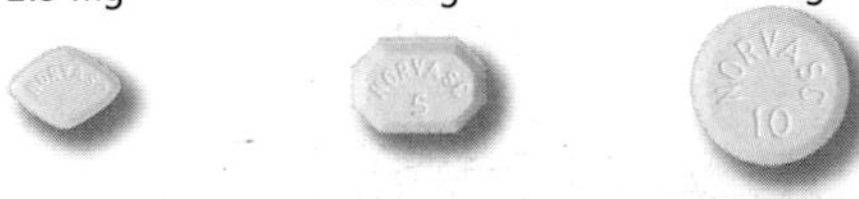

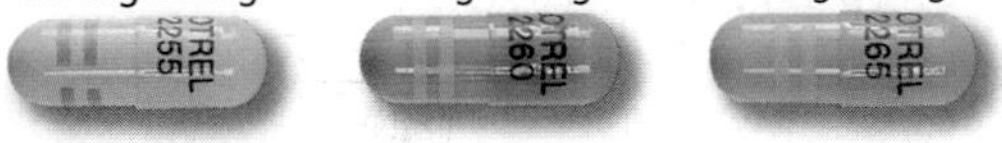

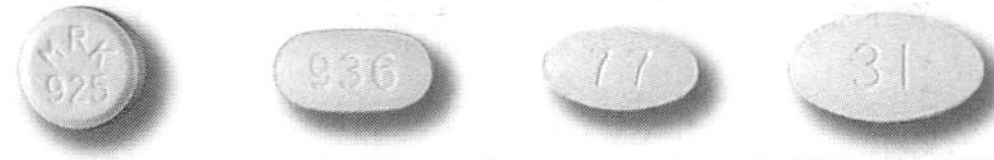

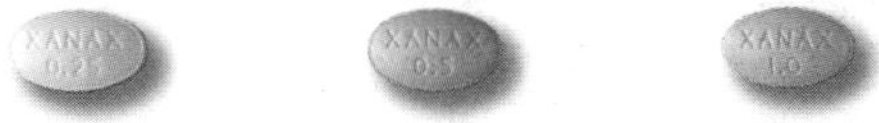

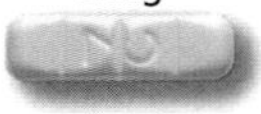

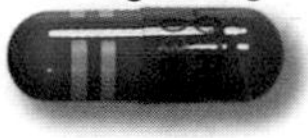

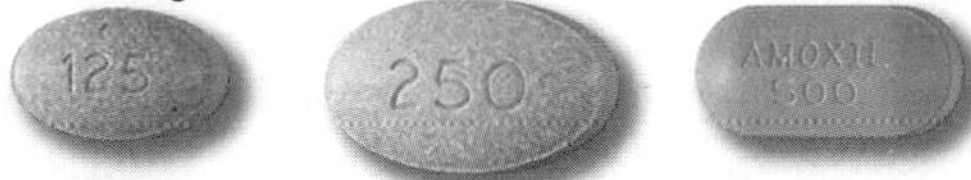

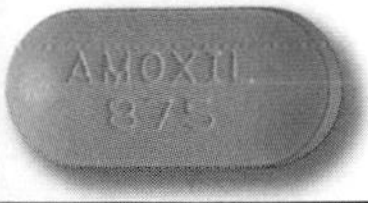

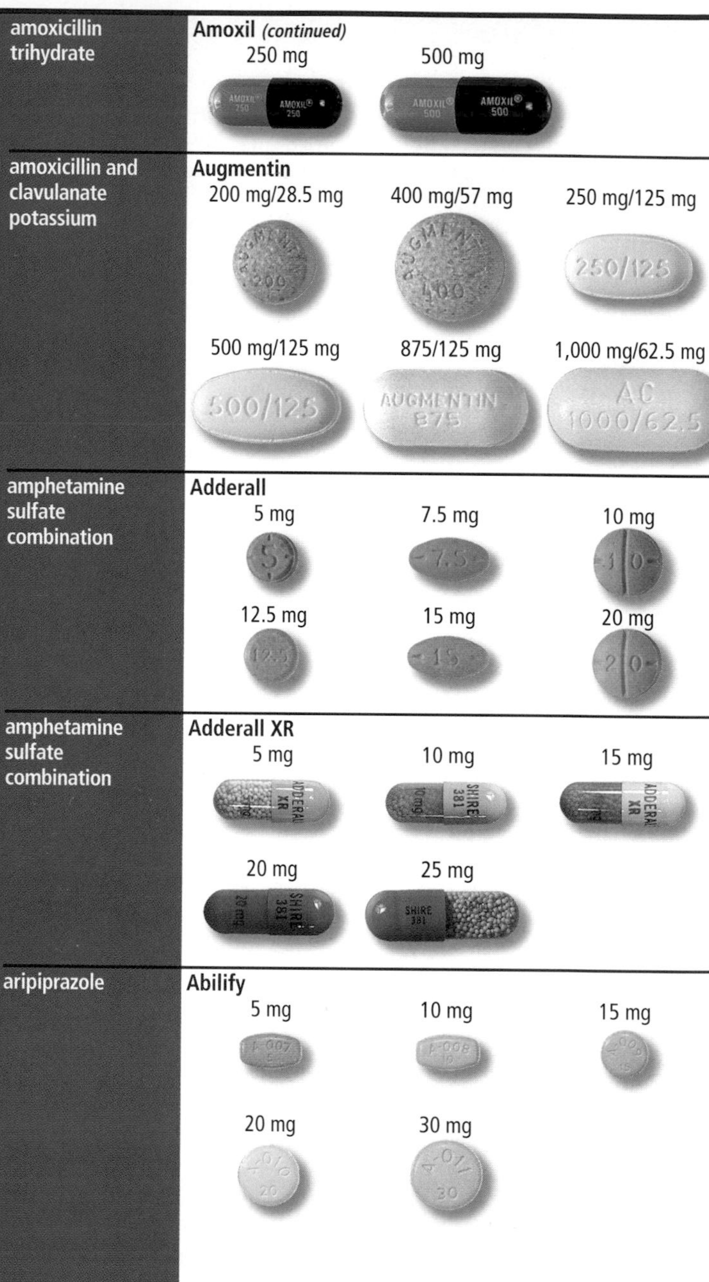
amoxicillin trihydrate
Amoxil (continued)
250 mg
500 mg
amoxicillin and clavulanate potassium
Augmentin
200 mg/28.5 mg
400 mg/57 mg
250 mg/125 mg
500 mg/125 mg
875/125 mg
1,000 mg/62.5 mg
amphetamine sulfate combination
Adderall
5 mg
7.5 mg
10 mg
12.5 mg
15 mg
20 mg
amphetamine sulfate combination
Adderall XR
5 mg
10 mg
15 mg
20 mg
25 mg
aripiprazole
Abilify
5 mg
10 mg
15 mg
20 mg
30 mg

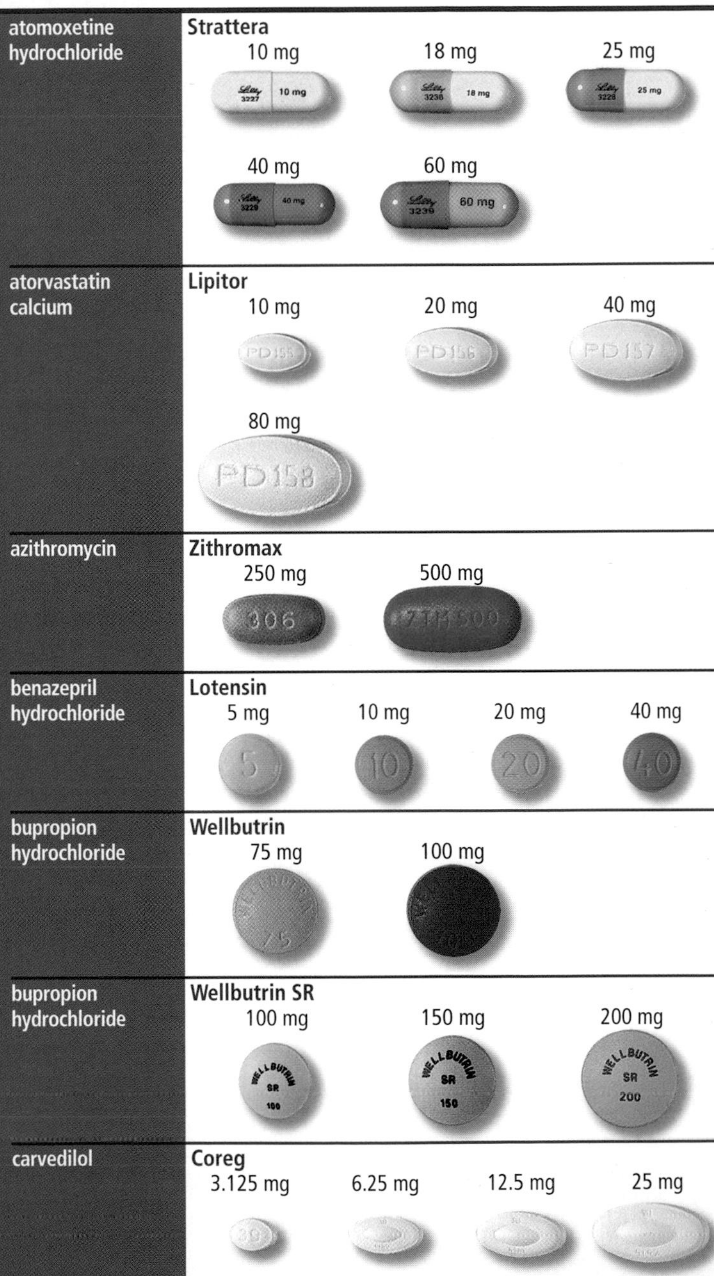
atomoxetine hydrochloride
Strattera
10 mg
18 mg
25 mg
40 mg
60 mg
atorvastatin calcium
Lipitor
10 mg
20 mg
40 mg
80 mg
azithromycin
Zithromax
250 mg
500 mg
benazepril hydrochloride
Lotensin
5 mg
10 mg
20 mg
40 mg
bupropion hydrochloride
Wellbutrin
75 mg
100 mg
bupropion hydrochloride
Wellbutrin SR
100 mg
150 mg
200 mg
carvedilol
Coreg
3.125 mg
6.25 mg
12.5 mg
25 mg

cefprozil	**Cefzil** 250 mg · 500 mg
celecoxib	**Celebrex** 100 mg · 200 mg · 400 mg
cephalexin monohydrate	**Keflex** 250 mg · 500 mg
cetirizine hydrochloride	**Zyrtec** 5 mg · 10 mg
ciprofloxacin hydrochloride	**Cipro** 100 mg · 250 mg · 500 mg 750 mg
citalopram hydrobromide	**Celexa** 10 mg · 20 mg · 40 mg
clarithromycin	**Biaxin** 250 mg · 500 mg
clarithromycin	**Biaxin XL** 500 mg
clopidogrel bisulfate	**Plavix** 75 mg

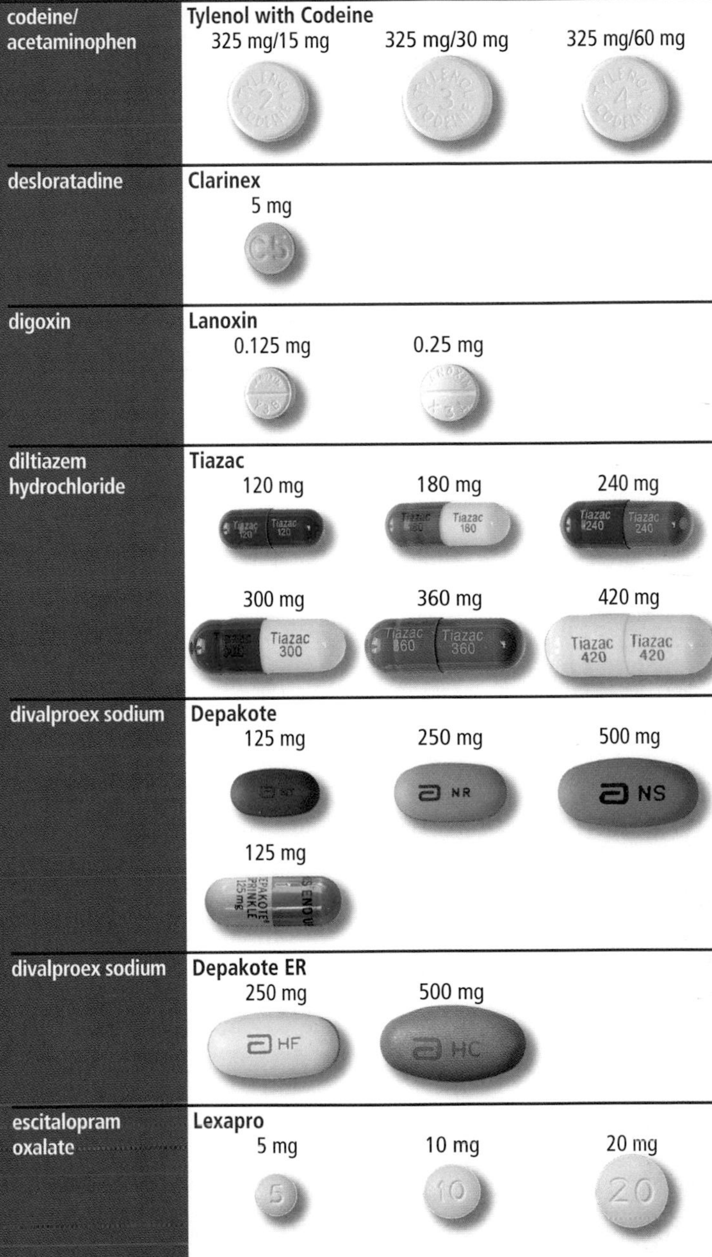
codeine/
acetaminophen
Tylenol with Codeine
325 mg/15 mg
325 mg/30 mg
325 mg/60 mg
desloratadine
Clarinex
5 mg
digoxin
Lanoxin
0.125 mg
0.25 mg
diltiazem
hydrochloride
Tiazac
120 mg
180 mg
240 mg
300 mg
360 mg
420 mg
divalproex sodium
Depakote
125 mg
250 mg
500 mg
125 mg
divalproex sodium
Depakote ER
250 mg
500 mg
escitalopram
oxalate
Lexapro
5 mg
10 mg
20 mg

esomeprazole magnesium	**Nexium** 20 mg, 40 mg
estrogens, conjugated	**Premarin** 0.3 mg, 0.625 mg, 0.9 mg, 1.25 mg, 2.5 mg
ezetimibe	**Zetia** 10 mg
fenofibrate	**Tricor** 54 mg, 160 mg
fexofenadine hydrochloride	**Allegra** 30 mg, 60 mg, 180 mg
fexofenadine hydrochloride and pseudoephedrine hydrochloride	**Allegra-D** 60 mg/120 mg
fluconazole	**Diflucan** 50 mg, 100 mg, 150 mg, 200 mg

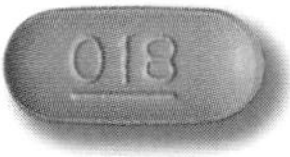

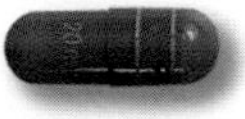

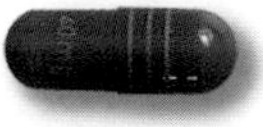

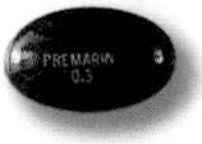

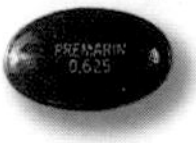

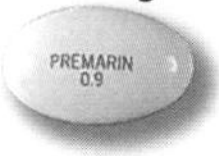

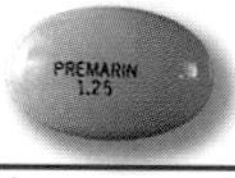

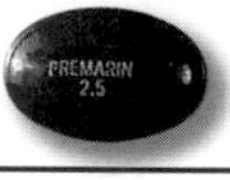

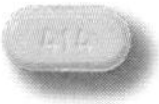

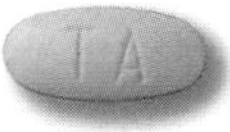

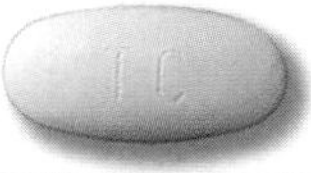

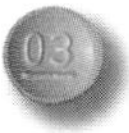

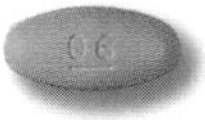

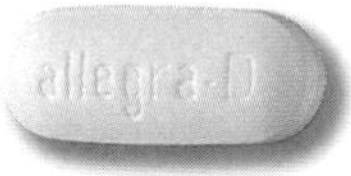

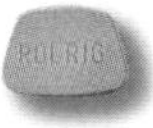

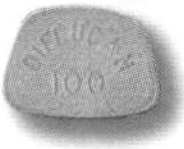

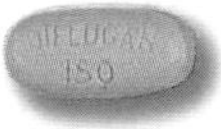

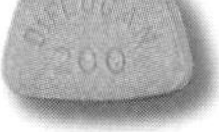

fluoxetine hydrochloride	Prozac	10 mg, 10 mg, 20 mg, 40 mg, 90 mg
fosinopril sodium	Monopril	10 mg, 20 mg, 40 mg
furosemide	Lasix	20 mg, 40 mg, 80 mg
gabapentin	Neurontin	100 mg, 300 mg, 400 mg, 600 mg, 800 mg
glimepiride	Amaryl	1 mg, 2 mg, 4 mg
glipizide	Glucotrol	5 mg, 10 mg
glipizide	Glucotrol XL	2.5 mg, 5 mg, 10 mg

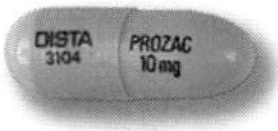

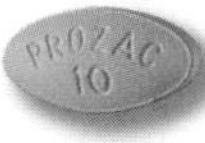

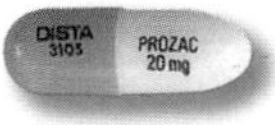

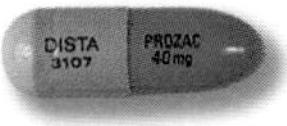

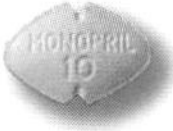

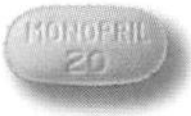

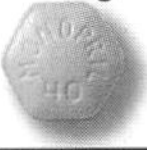

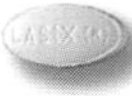

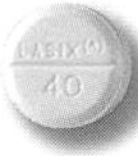

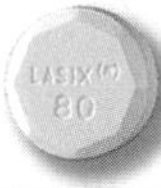

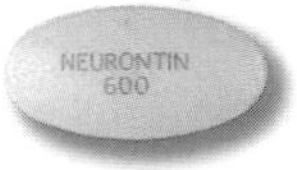

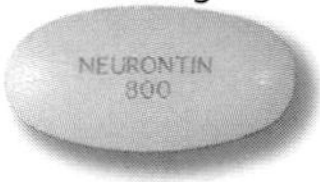

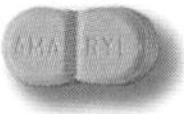

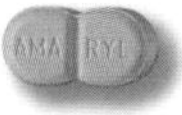

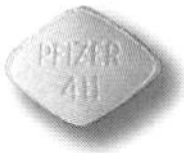

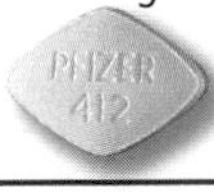

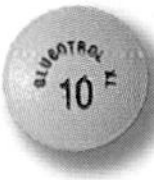

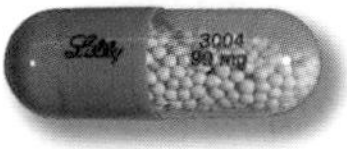

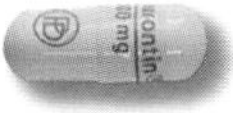

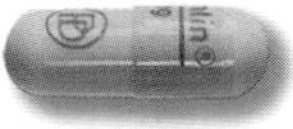

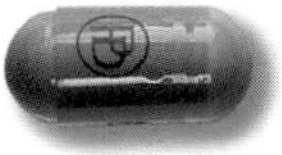

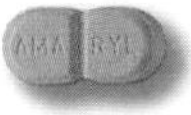

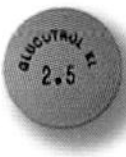

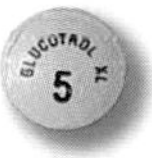

glyburide and metformin hydrochloride	**Glucovance**	1.25 mg/250 mg; 2.5 mg/500 mg; 5 mg/500 mg
hydrocodone bitartrate and acetaminophen	**Lortab**	2.5 mg/500 mg; 5 mg/500 mg; 7.5 mg/500 mg; 10 mg/500 mg
ibuprofen	**Motrin**	400 mg; 600 mg; 800 mg
irbesartan	**Avapro**	75 mg; 150 mg; 300 mg
lansoprazole	**Prevacid**	15 mg; 30 mg
levofloxacin	**Levaquin**	250 mg; 500 mg; 750 mg
levothyroxine sodium	**Levoxyl**	25 mcg; 50 mcg; 75 mcg; 88 mcg; 100 mcg; 112 mcg; 125 mcg; 137 mcg; 150 mcg; 175 mcg; 200 mcg; 300 mcg

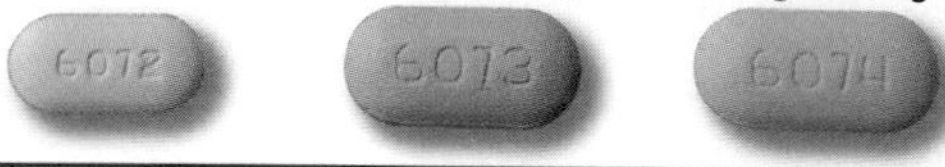

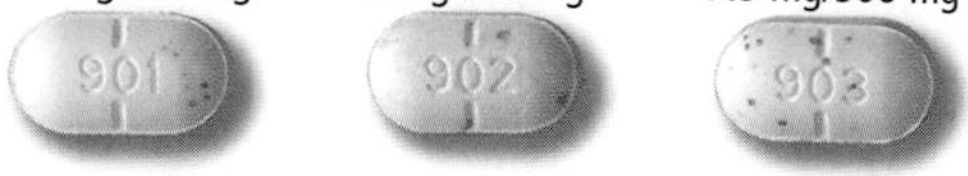

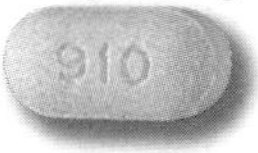

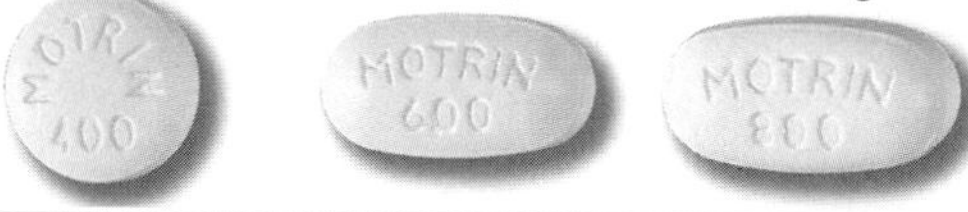

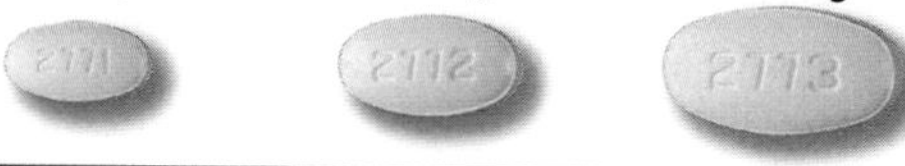

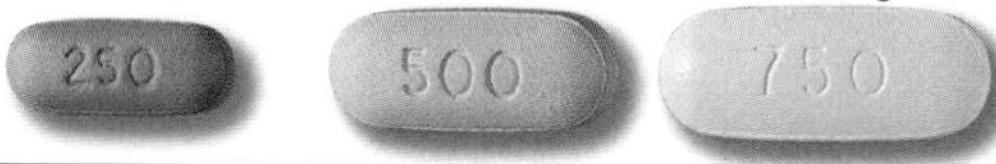

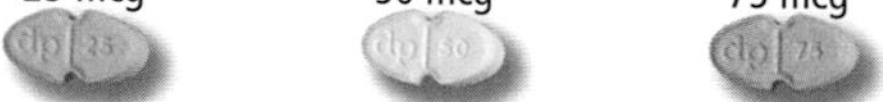

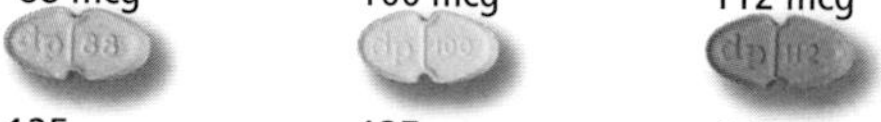

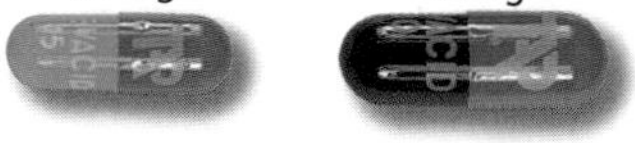

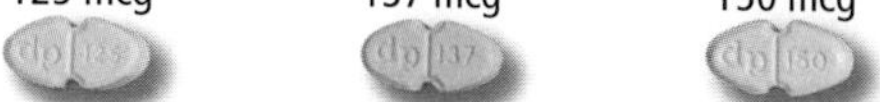

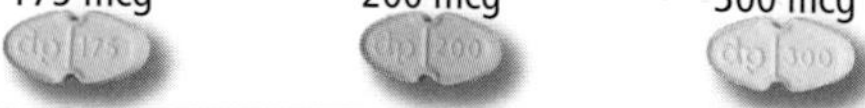

Generic	Brand		
levothyroxine sodium	**Synthroid**		
	25 mcg	50 mcg	75 mcg
	88 mcg	100 mcg	112 mcg
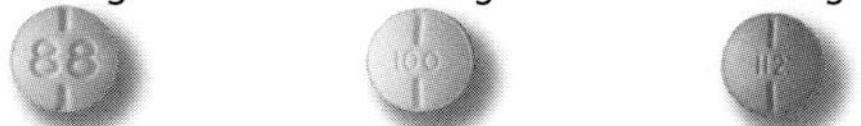	125 mcg	137 mcg	150 mcg
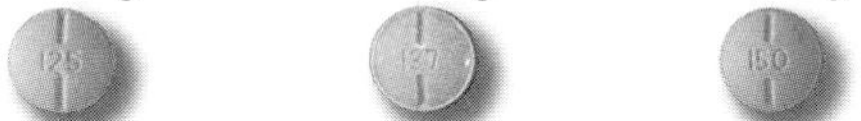	175 mcg	200 mcg	300 mcg
lisinopril	**Prinivil**		
	2.5 mg	5 mg	10 mg
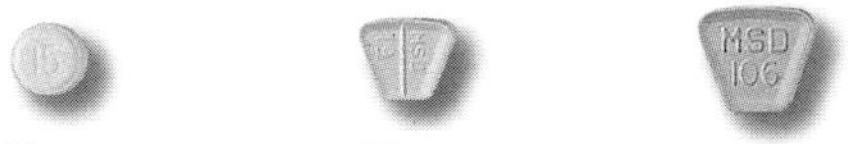	20 mg	40 mg	
lisinopril	**Zestril**		
	2.5 mg	5 mg	10 mg
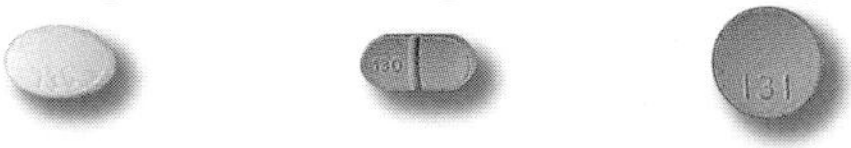	20 mg	30 mg	40 mg
lisinopril and hydrochlorothiazide	**Zestoretic**		
	10 mg/12.5 mg	20 mg/12.5 mg	20 mg/25 mg
lorazepam	**Ativan**		
	0.5 mg	1 mg	2 mg
losartan potassium	**Cozaar**		
	25 mg	50 mg	100 mg

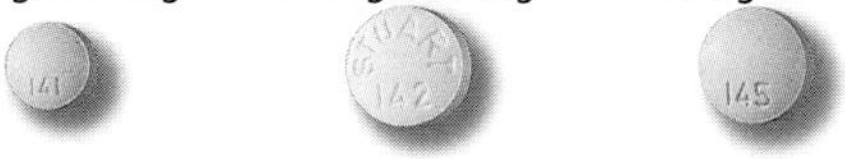

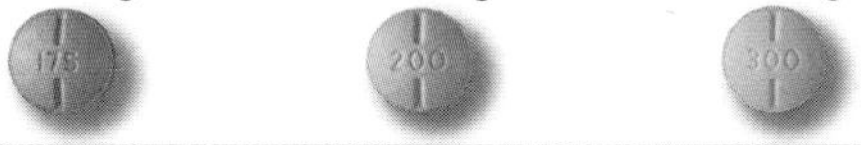

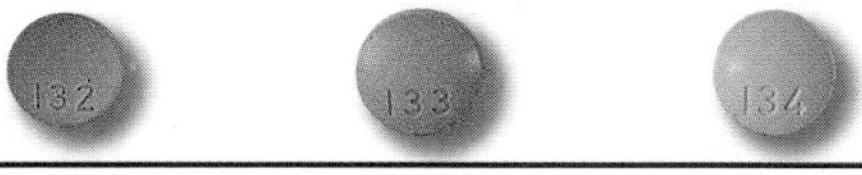

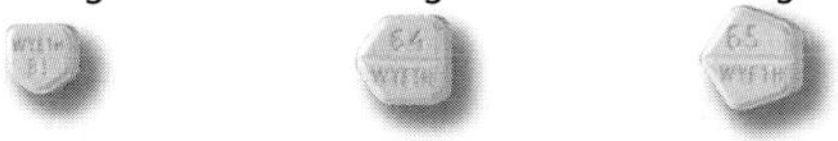

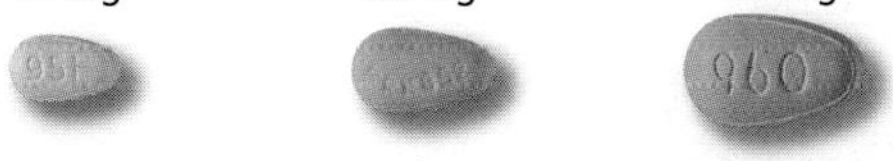

losartan potassium and hydrochlorothiazide	**Hyzaar**		
	50 mg/12.5 mg	100 mg/25 mg	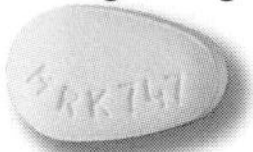
memantine hydrochloride	**Namenda**		
	5 mg	10 mg	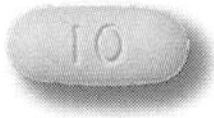
metformin hydrochloride	**Glucophage**		
	500 mg	850 mg	1,000 mg
metformin hydrochloride	**Glucophage XR**		
	500 mg	750 mg	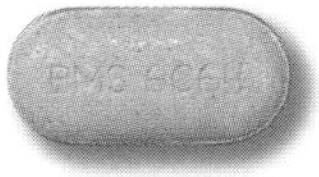
methylphenidate hydrochloride	**Concerta**		
	18 mg	27 mg	36 mg
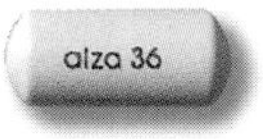	54 mg		
metoprolol succinate	**Toprol-XL**		
	25 mg	50 mg	100 mg
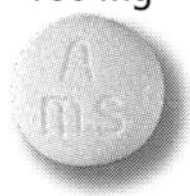	200 mg		
montelukast sodium	**Singulair**		
	4 mg	5 mg	10 mg

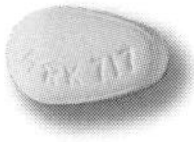

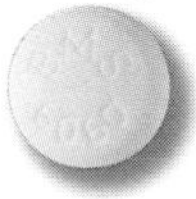

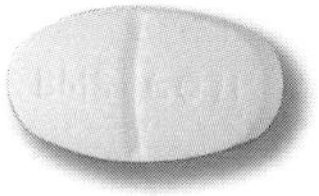

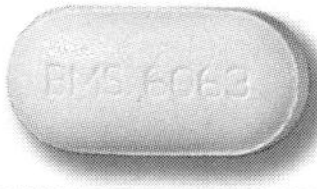

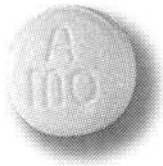

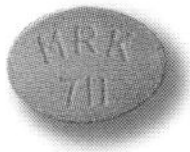

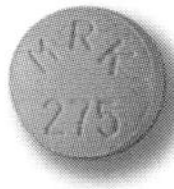

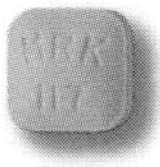

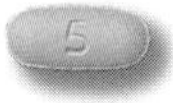

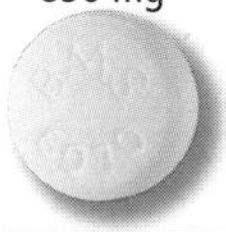

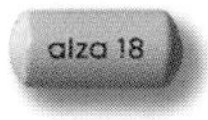

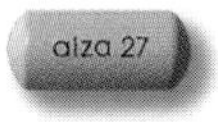

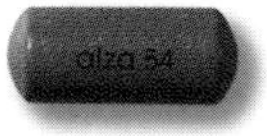

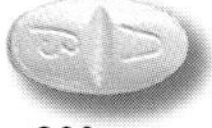

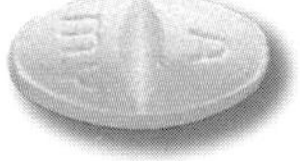

nitrofurantoin macrocrystals	**Macrodantin** 25 mg, 50 mg, 100 mg
nitrofurantoin monohydrate	**Macrobid** 100 mg
olanzapine	**Zyprexa** 2.5 mg, 5 mg, 7.5 mg, 10 mg, 15 mg, 20 mg
olmesartan medoxomil	**Benicar** 5 mg, 20 mg, 40 mg
omeprazole	**Prilosec** 10 mg, 20 mg, 40 mg
oxcarbazepine	**Trileptal** 150 mg, 300 mg, 600 mg
oxybutynin chloride	**Ditropan XL** 5 mg, 10 mg, 15 mg
oxycodone hydrochloride	**OxyContin** 10 mg, 20 mg, 40 mg, 80 mg
pantoprazole sodium	**Protonix** 40 mg

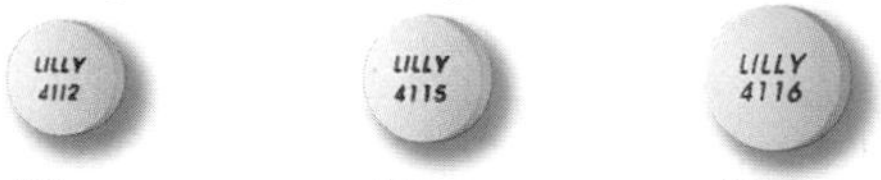

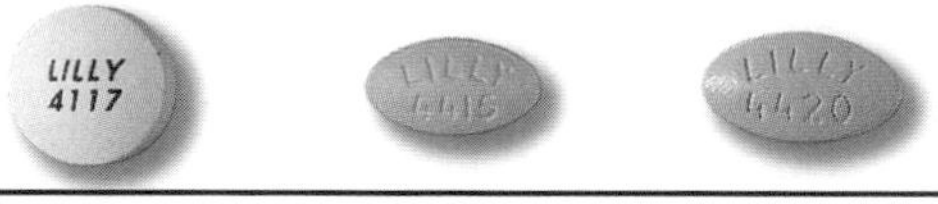

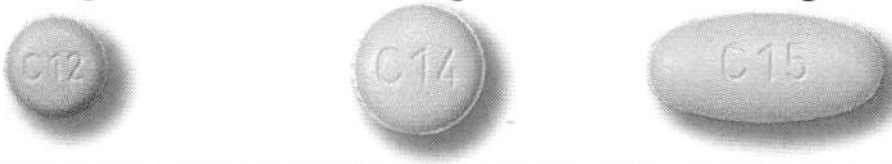

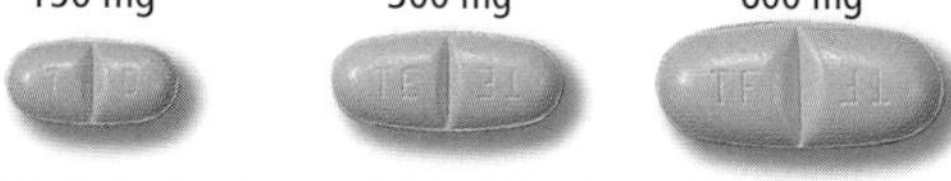

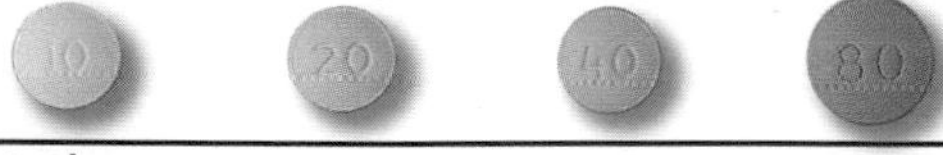

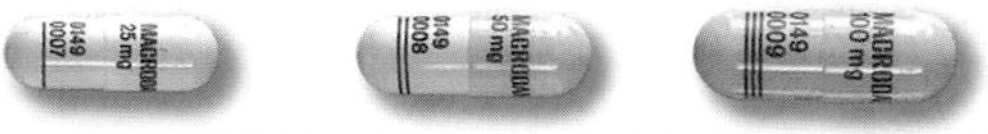

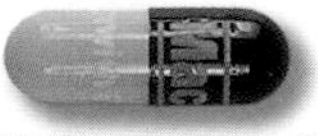

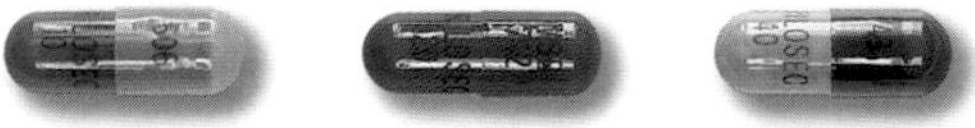

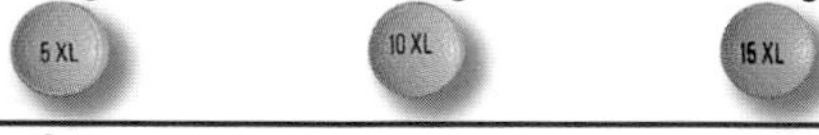

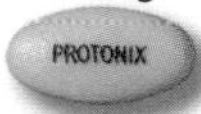

paroxetine hydrochloride	**Paxil** 10 mg, 20 mg, 30 mg, 40 mg
paroxetine hydrochloride	**Paxil CR** 12.5 mg, 25 mg, 37.5 mg
penicillin V potassium	**Veetids** 250 mg, 500 mg
phenytoin sodium (extended)	**Dilantin** 30 mg, 100 mg
pioglitazone hydrochloride	**Actos** 15 mg, 30 mg, 45 mg
pravastatin sodium	**Pravachol** 10 mg, 20 mg, 40 mg, 80 mg
propoxyphene napsylate and acetaminophen	**Darvocet-N 50** 50 mg; **Darvocet-N 100** 100 mg
quetiapine fumarate	**Seroquel** 25 mg, 100 mg, 200 mg, 300 mg

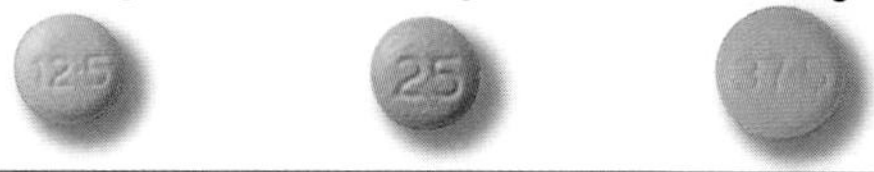

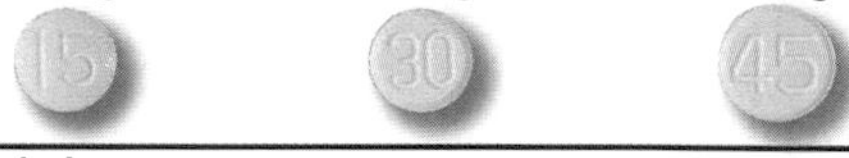

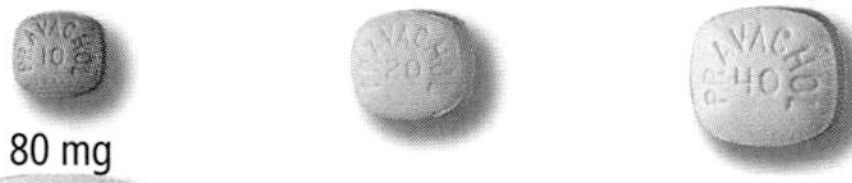

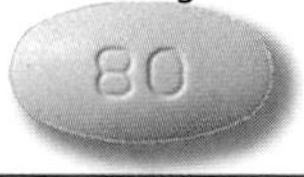

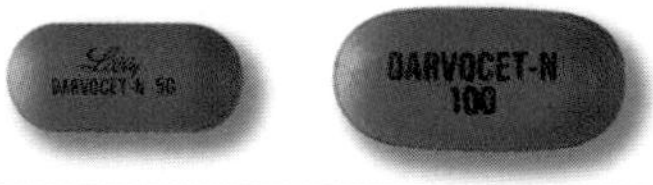

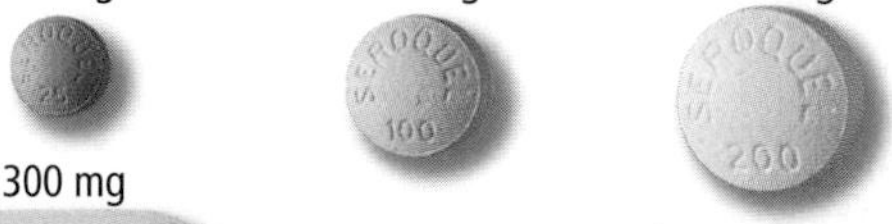

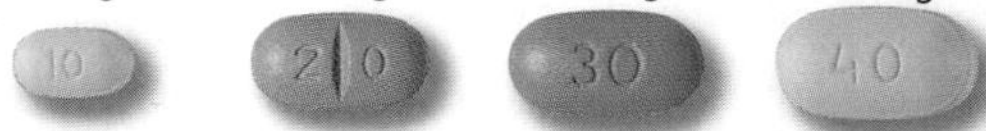

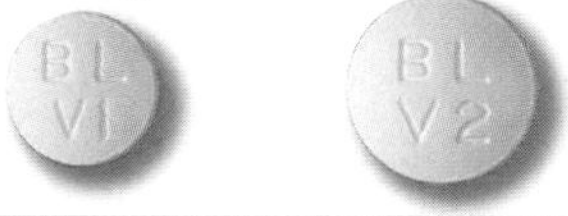

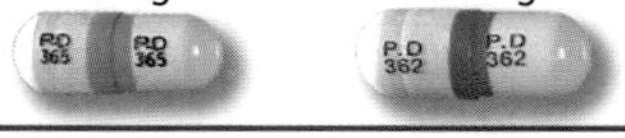

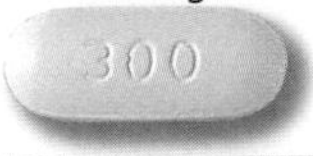

Generic name	Brand and strengths
quinapril hydrochloride	**Accupril** 5 mg, 10 mg, 20 mg 40 mg
rabeprazole sodium	**Aciphex** 20 mg
raloxifene hydrochloride	**Evista** 60 mg
ramipril	**Altace** 1.25 mg, 2.5 mg, 5 mg 10 mg
risedronate sodium	**Actonel** 5 mg, 30 mg, 35 mg
risperidone	**Risperdal** 0.25 mg, 0.5 mg, 1 mg 2 mg, 3 mg, 4 mg
rosiglitazone maleate	**Avandia** 2 mg, 4 mg, 8 mg

Generic name	Brand and strengths
rosuvastatin calcium	**Crestor** 5 mg, 10 mg, 20 mg, 40 mg
sertraline hydrochloride	**Zoloft** 25 mg, 50 mg, 100 mg
sildenafil citrate	**Viagra** 25 mg, 50 mg, 100 mg
simvastatin	**Zocor** 5 mg, 10 mg, 20 mg, 40 mg, 80 mg
sumatriptan succinate	**Imitrex** 25 mg, 50 mg, 100 mg
tadalafil	**Cialis** 5 mg, 10 mg, 20 mg
tamsulosin hydrochloride	**Flomax** 0.4 mg

tolterodine tartrate	**Detrol**		
	1 mg	2 mg	
tolterodine tartrate	**Detrol LA**		
	2 mg	4 mg	
topiramate	**Topamax**		
	25 mg	100 mg	200 mg
topiramate	**Topamax Sprinkle**		
	15 mg	25 mg	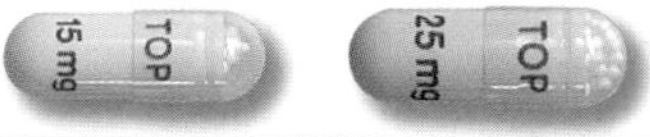
tramadol hydrochloride	**Ultram**		
	50 mg		
tramadol hydrochloride and acetaminophen	**Ultracet**		
	37.5 mg/325 mg		
triamterene and hydrochlorothiazide	**Maxzide**		
	37.5 mg/25 mg	75 mg/50 mg	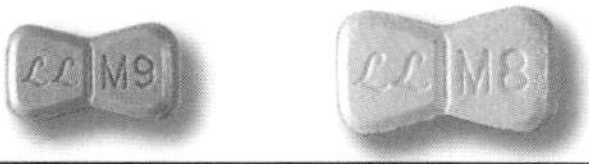
valacyclovir hydrochloride	**Valtrex**		
	500 mg	1,000 mg	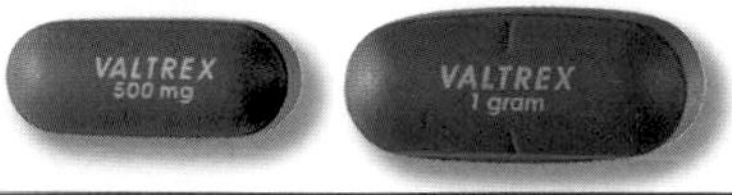
valdecoxib	**Bextra**		
	10 mg	20 mg	

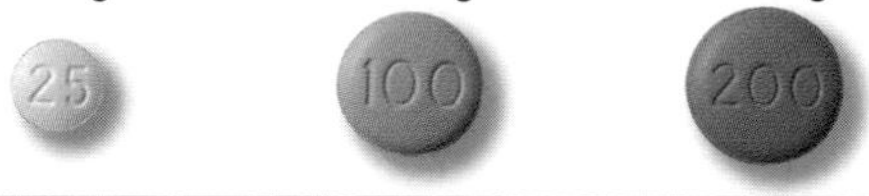

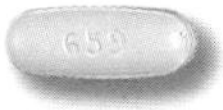

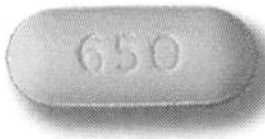

valsartan	**Diovan** 80 mg, 160 mg, 320 mg
valsartan and hydrochlorothiazide	**Diovan HCT** 80 mg/12.5 mg, 160 mg/12.5 mg, 160 mg/25 mg
vardenafil hydrochloride	**Levitra** 2.5 mg, 5 mg, 10 mg, 20 mg
venlafaxine hydrochloride	**Effexor** 25 mg, 37.5 mg, 50 mg, 75 mg, 100 mg
venlafaxine hydrochloride	**Effexor XR** 37.5 mg, 75 mg, 150 mg
warfarin sodium	**Coumadin** 1 mg, 2 mg, 2.5 mg, 3 mg, 4 mg, 5 mg, 6 mg, 7.5 mg, 10 mg
zolpidem tartrate	**Ambien** 5 mg, 10 mg

• Organic intracranial lesion (such as pituitary tumor)
• Causes of infertility other than anovulation (unless patient is candidate for in vitro fertilization)
• Ovarian cysts or enlargement not caused by polycystic ovarian syndrome
• Pregnancy

Precautions

Use cautiously in:
• renal or hepatic insufficiency (safety and efficacy not established)
• breastfeeding patients.

Administration

• Know that drug may be given either I.M. or subcutaneously.
• To reconstitute powder or pellet for injection, add accompanying 2 ml of 0.9% sodium chloride injection to vial.
• Inject immediately after reconstitution. Discard unused portion.
• Rotate injection sites.
• Use lower abdomen for subcutaneous injection.
• Withhold hCG if serum estradiol level exceeds 2,000 pg/ml or abdominal pain occurs.

Route	Onset	Peak	Duration
I.M.	Unknown	Unknown	Unknown
Subcut.	Unknown	Unknown	Unknown

Adverse reactions

CNS: headache, malaise, dizziness, **cerebrovascular accident**
CV: tachycardia, **venous thrombophlebitis, arterial occlusion, arterial thromboembolism**
GI: nausea, vomiting, diarrhea, abdominal cramps and distention, **hemoperitoneum**
GU: ovarian enlargement with pain, gynecomastia, ovarian cysts, multiple births, **ovarian hyperstimulation syndrome (OHSS), ectopic pregnancy**
Metabolic: electrolyte imbalances
Musculoskeletal: muscle aches, joint pain
Respiratory: dyspnea, tachypnea, **atelectasis, adult respiratory distress syndrome, pulmonary embolism, pulmonary infarction**
Skin: rash
Other: fever, hypersensitivity reaction, **anaphylaxis**

Interactions

None significant

Patient monitoring

• Know that before starting menotropins/hCG therapy to induce ovulation and pregnancy, patient should undergo gynecologic and endocrine evaluation with hysterosalpingogram to rule out pregnancy and neoplastic lesions.
• Assess patient to confirm anovulation. Obtain urinary gonadotropin levels as ordered to rule out primary ovarian failure. (Male partner's fertility should be evaluated, also).
• In older females (who have greater risk of anovulatory disorders and endometrial cancer), assess cervical dilation and curettage results.
• Evaluate patient for expected ovarian stimulation without hyperstimulation.
Monitor for early indications of OHSS—severe pelvic pain, nausea, vomiting, and weight gain. OHSS usually occurs 2 weeks after treatment ends, peaks 7 to 10 days after ovulation, and resolves with menses onset.
If OHSS occurs, drug is withdrawn and patient is hospitalized for bed rest, fluid and electrolyte management, and analgesics. Monitor daily fluid intake and output, weight, abdominal girth, hematocrit, serum and urinary electrolytes, urine specific gravity, blood urea nitrogen, and creatinine. Watch for hemoconcentration caused by fluid loss into peritoneal, pleural, and pericardial cavities.
Stay alert for pulmonary and thromboembolic complications.

m

• Assess male patient for pituitary insufficiency as possible cause of infertility.

Patient teaching

• Before therapy, teach patient about duration of treatment and necessary monitoring.
• Inform patient about risk of multiple births with menotropins and hCG use.
• For infertile females, encourage daily intercourse starting on day before hCG administration.
• As appropriate, review all other significant and life-threatening adverse reactions.

meperidine hydrochloride (pethidine hydrochloride)

Demerol

Pharmacologic class: Opioid agonist
Therapeutic class: Analgesic, adjunct to anesthesia
Controlled substance schedule II
Pregnancy risk category C

Action

Binds to and depresses opiate receptors in spinal cord and CNS, altering perception of and response to pain

Availability

Injection: 10 mg/ml, 25 mg/ml, 50 mg/ml, 75 mg/ml, 100 mg/ml
Syrup: 50 mg/5 ml
Tablets: 50 mg, 100 mg

Indications and dosages

➢ Moderate to severe pain
Adults: 50 to 150 mg P.O., I.M., or subcutaneously q 3 to 4 hours as needed
Children: 1.1 to 1.8 mg/kg P.O., I.M., or subcutaneously q 3 to 4 hours, not to exceed 100 mg/dose

➢ Preoperative sedation
Adults: 50 to 100 mg I.M. or subcutaneously 30 to 90 minutes before anesthesia, or 15 to 35 mg/hour I.V. as a continuous infusion
Children: 1 to 2.2 mg/kg I.M. or subcutaneously 30 to 90 minutes before anesthesia. Don't exceed adult dosage.

➢ Analgesia during labor
Adults: 50 to 100 mg I.M. or subcutaneously when contractions are regular. May repeat q 1 to 3 hours.

Contraindications

• Hypersensitivity to drug or bisulfites (with some injectable products)
• MAO inhibitor use within past 14 days

Precautions

Use cautiously in:
• head trauma; increased intracranial pressure (ICP); severe renal, hepatic, or pulmonary disease; hypothyroidism; adrenal insufficiency; extensive burns; alcoholism
• undiagnosed abdominal pain or prostatic hyperplasia
• elderly or debilitated patients
• pregnant patients (not recommended before labor)
• labor (drug may cause respiratory depression in neonate)
• breastfeeding patients
• children.

Administration

• Give I.M. injection slowly into large muscle. Preferably, use diluted solution.
• Be aware that drug is compatible with 5% dextrose and lactated Ringer's solution, dextrose-saline solution combinations, and 2.5%, 5%, or 10% dextrose in water.
Know that drug is not compatible with soluble barbiturates, aminophylline, heparin, morphine sulfate, methicillin, phenytoin, sodium bicarbonate, iodide, sulfadiazine, or sulfisoxazole.

• Don't give for chronic pain control, because of potential toxicity and dependence.

Route	Onset	Peak	Duration
P.O.	15 min	60 min	2-4 hr
I.V.	Immediate	5-7 min	2-4 hr
I.M.	10-15 min	30-50 min	2-4 hr
Subcut.	10-15 min	40-60 min	2-4 hr

Adverse reactions

CNS: confusion, sedation, dysphoria, euphoria, floating feeling, hallucinations, headache, unusual dreams, **seizures**
CV: hypotension, **bradycardia, cardiac arrest, shock**
EENT: blurred vision, diplopia, miosis
GI: nausea, vomiting, constipation, ileus, biliary tract spasms
GU: urinary retention
Respiratory: respiratory depression, respiratory arrest
Skin: flushing, sweating, induration
Other: pain at injection site, local irritation, physical or psychological drug dependence, drug tolerance

Interactions

Drug-drug. *Antihistamines, sedative-hypnotics:* additive CNS depression
Barbiturates, cimetidine, protease inhibitor antiretrovirals: increased respiratory and CNS depression
Chlorpromazine, thioridazine: increased risk of meperidine toxicity
MAO inhibitors, procarbazine: potentially fatal reaction
Opioid agonist-antagonists: precipitation of opioid withdrawal in physically dependent patients
Phenytoin: increased meperidine metabolism and decreased effects
Drug-diagnostic tests. *Amylase, lipase:* increased levels
Drug-herbs. *Chamomile, hops, kava, skullcap, valerian:* increased CNS depression
Drug-behaviors. *Alcohol use:* increased CNS depression

Patient monitoring

[Clinical alert] Monitor vital signs. Don't give drug if patient has significant respiratory or CNS depression.
• Reassess patient's pain level after administration.
[Clinical alert] Watch for seizures, agitation, irritability, nervousness, tremors, twitches, and myoclonus in patients at risk for normeperidine accumulation (such as those with renal or hepatic impairment).
[Clinical alert] Use with extreme caution in patients with head injury. Drug may increase ICP and cause adverse reactions that obscure clinical course.
• Closely monitor patients with acute abdominal pain. Drug may obscure diagnosis and clinical course of GI condition.
• Evaluate bowel and bladder function.
• With long-term or repeated use, watch for psychological and physical drug dependence and tolerance.
[Clinical alert] With pediatric patients, stay alert for increased risk of seizures.

Patient teaching

• Tell patient using oral syrup to take drug with a half-glass of water to minimize local anesthetic effect.
• Caution patient to avoid driving and other hazardous activities, because drug may cause dizziness or drowsiness.
• Advise patient to avoid alcohol.
• Instruct ambulatory patient to change position slowly to avoid orthostatic hypotension.
• Tell female patient to inform prescriber if she is pregnant or breastfeeding.
• As appropriate, review all other significant and life-threatening adverse reactions and interactions, especially those related to the drugs, tests, herbs, and behaviors mentioned above.

m

mercaptopurine (6-mercaptopurine, 6-MP)

Purinethol

Pharmacologic class: Antimetabolite
Therapeutic class: Antineoplastic
Pregnancy risk category D

Action

Inhibits DNA and RNA synthesis, suppressing growth of certain cancer cells

Availability

Tablets: 50 mg

Indications and dosages

➤ Acute lymphatic, myelogenous, or myelomonocytic leukemia
Adults and children: 2.5 mg/kg/day P.O. as a single dose, increased to 5 mg/kg/day after 4 weeks if response inadequate or if no toxicity occurs. On complete hematologic remission, give maintenance dosage of 1.5 to 2.5 mg/kg/day P.O. as a single dose (combined with other agents as prescribed).

Contraindications

- Hypersensitivity to drug or its components
- Prior resistance to drug or thioguanine
- Breastfeeding

Precautions

Use cautiously in:

- renal or hepatic impairment
- decreased platelet or neutrophil counts after chemotherapy or radiation
- pregnant patients.

Administration

- Follow facility protocols regarding proper handling and disposal of drug.

◀ Don't handle drug if you're pregnant.

- Be aware that total daily dosage is calculated to nearest multiple of 25 mg and given once daily.

◀ Withdraw drug immediately if white blood cell (WBC) or platelet count falls rapidly or steeply.

Route	Onset	Peak	Duration
P.O.	Unknown	2 hr	Unknown

Adverse reactions

GI: nausea, vomiting, anorexia, diarrhea, GI ulcers, painful oral ulcers, **pancreatitis**
Hematologic: anemia, **leukopenia**, **thrombocytopenia**
Hepatic: jaundice, **hepatotoxicity**
Metabolic: hyperuricemia
Skin: rash, hyperpigmentation

Interactions

Drug-drug. *Allopurinol (more than 300 mg), aminosalicylate derivatives (mesalazine, olsalazine, sulfasalazine):* increased bone marrow depression
Warfarin: decreased anticoagulant effect
Drug-diagnostic tests. *Hemoglobin, platelets, red blood cells, uric acid, WBCs:* increased values

Patient monitoring

◀ Watch for signs and symptoms of hepatotoxicity.

- Monitor weekly CBC with white cell differential and platelet count.
- Assess bone marrow aspiration and biopsy results, as necessary, to aid assessment of disease progression, resistance to therapy, and drug-induced marrow hypoplasia.
- Monitor serum uric acid level.
- Evaluate fluid intake and output.
- Monitor liver function tests and bilirubin level weekly at start of therapy, then monthly.

Patient teaching

◀ Instruct patient to immediately report fever, sore throat, increased

bleeding or bruising, or signs or symptoms of liver problems (right-sided abdominal pain, yellowing of skin or eyes, nausea, vomiting, clay-colored stools, or dark urine).
• Advise both male and female patients to use reliable contraception.
• Encourage patient to maintain adequate fluid intake.
• Caution patient not to get vaccinations without consulting prescriber.
• As appropriate, review all other significant and life-threatening adverse reactions and interactions, especially those related to the drugs and tests mentioned above.

meropenem

Merrem I.V.

Pharmacologic class: Carbapenem
Therapeutic class: Anti-infective
Pregnancy risk category B

Action

Inhibits bacterial cell-wall synthesis and penetrates gram-negative and gram-positive bacteria

Availability

Powder for injection: 500-mg and 1-g vials

Indications and dosages

➢ Intra-abdominal infections
Adults: 1 g I.V. q 8 hours over 15 to 30 minutes by infusion or over 3 to 5 minutes as a bolus injection
Children weighing 50 kg (110 lb) or more: 1 g I.V. q 8 hours over 15 to 30 minutes by infusion or over 3 to 5 minutes as a bolus injection
Children ages 3 months and older weighing less than 50 kg (110 lb): 20 mg/kg q 8 hours over 15 to 30 minutes by infusion or over 3 to 5 minutes as a bolus injection
➢ Bacterial meningitis
Children weighing 50 kg (110 lb) or more: 2 g I.V. q 8 hours over 15 to 30 minutes by infusion or over 3 to 5 minutes as a bolus injection
Children ages 3 month and older weighing less than 50 kg (110 lb): 40 mg/kg q 8 hours over 15 to 30 minutes by infusion or over 3 to 5 minutes as a bolus injection, to a maximum of 2 g q 8 hours

Dosage adjustment

• Renal impairment

Off-label uses

• Acute pulmonary exacerbation caused by respiratory tract infection with susceptible organisms in cystic fibrosis patients

Contraindications

• Hypersensitivity to drug, its components, or other beta-lactams

Precautions

Use cautiously in:
• sulfite sensitivity, renal disease, seizure disorder
• pregnant or breastfeeding patients
• children.

Administration

• For I.V. bolus, add 10 or 20 ml of sterile water to 500-mg or 1-g vial, respectively, to yield a concentration of 50 mg/ml. Shake until clear. Administer single dose over 3 to 5 minutes.
• For intermittent I.V. infusion, piggyback vials can be reconstituted with compatible I.V. solution (0.9% sodium chloride or 5% dextrose) to yield a concentration of 2.5 to 50 mg/ml. Or vials can be reconstituted as for direct I.V. injection and added to compatible I.V. solution for further dilution. To reconstitute and administer ADD-Vantage systems, follow manufacturer's instructions. Infuse drug over 15 to 30 minutes.

• Use diluted solution immediately, if possible.

Route	Onset	Peak	Duration
I.V.	Unknown	1 hr	Unknown

Adverse reactions

CNS: headache, insomnia, dizziness, drowsiness, weakness, **seizures**
CV: hypotension, phlebitis, palpitations, **heart failure, cardiac arrest, myocardial infarction**
GI: nausea, vomiting, diarrhea, constipation, tongue discoloration, oral candidiasis, glossitis, **pseudomembranous colitis**
GU: vaginal candidiasis
Hematologic: anemia, eosinophilia, **leukopenia, bone marrow depression, thrombocytopenia, neutropenia**
Musculoskeletal: myoclonus
Respiratory: chest discomfort, dyspnea, hyperventilation
Skin: rash, urticaria, pruritus, erythema at injection site
Other: altered taste, fever, pain, fungal infection, **anaphylaxis**

Interactions

Drug-drug. *Probenecid:* increased meropenem blood level
Drug-diagnostic tests. *Alanine aminotransferase, alkaline phosphatase, amylase, aspartate aminotransferase, bilirubin, blood urea nitrogen, eosinophils, gamma-glutamyl transpeptidase, lactate dehydrogenase, lipase:* increased values
Hematocrit, hemoglobin, platelets, neutrophils, white blood cells: decreased values
International Normalized Ratio, partial thromboplastin time, prothrombin time: increased or decreased values

Patient monitoring

• Collect specimens for culture and sensitivity testing as needed. However, be aware that drug therapy may start pending results.
◀ Monitor patient for hypersensitivity reaction or anaphylaxis. If either occurs, stop infusion immediately and initiate emergency treatment.
• Monitor for CNS irritability and seizures.
• In prolonged therapy, evaluate hematopoietic, renal, and hepatic function and watch for overgrowth of nonsusceptible organisms.
• If diarrhea occurs, check for pseudomembranous colitis and obtain stool cultures.
• Obtain hearing tests in child being treated for bacterial meningitis.

Patient teaching

• Advise patient to report such adverse reactions as CNS irritability, diarrhea, rash, shortness of breath, or pain at infusion site.
• As appropriate, review all other significant and life-threatening adverse reactions and interactions, especially those related to the drugs and tests mentioned above.

mesalamine (5-aminosalicylic acid, 5-ASA, mesalazine)

Asacol, Canasa, Mesasal✦, Pentasa, Rowasa, Salofalk✦

Pharmacologic class: 5-amino-2-hydroxybenzoic acid
Therapeutic class: GI anti-inflammatory drug
Pregnancy risk category B

Action

Unknown. Thought to act in colon, where it blocks cyclooxygenase and inhibits prostaglandin synthesis.

Availability

Capsules (extended-release): 250 mg, 500 mg
Rectal suspension: 4 g/60 ml
Suppositories: 500 mg, 1,000 mg
Tablets (delayed-release): 400 mg

Indications and dosages

➢ Active ulcerative colitis
Adults: 800 mg P.O. (Asacol delayed-release tablets) t.i.d. for 6 weeks
➢ To induce remission in active ulcerative colitis
Adults: 1 g P.O. (Pentasa extended-release capsules) q.i.d. for a total dosage of 4 g daily for up to 8 weeks
➢ Active distal ulcerative colitis, proctosigmoiditis, or proctitis
Adults: 4-g enema (Rowasa 60 ml) P.R. daily at bedtime, retained for 8 hours. Continue for 3 to 6 weeks.
➢ Active ulcerative proctitis
Adults: 500 mg (Canasa suppository) P.R. b.i.d., increased to t.i.d. if response inadequate after 2 weeks. Or 1,000 mg (suppository) P.R. at bedtime, continued for 3 to 6 weeks.
➢ To maintain remission of ulcerative colitis
Adults: 1.6 g (Asacol) P.O. daily in divided doses

Contraindications

• Hypersensitivity to drug, its components, or salicylates

Precautions

Use cautiously in:
• severe hepatic or renal impairment
• pregnant or breastfeeding patients.

Administration

• Make sure patient swallows tablets whole without crushing or chewing.
• For best effect, have patient retain suppository for 1 to 3 hours.

Route	Onset	Peak	Duration
P.O.	Unknown	Unknown	6-8 hr
P.R.	Unknown	Unknown	24 hr

Adverse reactions

CNS: headache, dizziness, malaise, weakness
CV: chest pain
EENT: rhinitis, pharyngitis
GI: nausea, vomiting, diarrhea, eructation, flatulence, anal irritation (with rectal use), **pancreatitis**
GU: interstitial nephritis, renal failure
Musculoskeletal: back pain
Skin: alopecia, rash
Other: fever, acute intolerance syndrome, **anaphylaxis**

Interactions

None significant

Patient monitoring

Closely monitor patients with history of allergic reactions to sulfasalazine or sulfite sensitivity (if using enema).
• Assess kidney and liver function before and periodically during therapy.
• Monitor for suppository efficacy, which should appear in 3 to 21 days. However, know that treatment usually continues for 3 to 6 weeks.
Watch for signs and symptoms of intolerance syndrome, such as cramping, acute abdominal pain, bloody diarrhea, fever, headache, and rash. If these occur, discontinue drug and notify prescriber.

Patient teaching

• Instruct patient to swallow tablets or capsules whole.
• Tell patient to contact prescriber if partially intact tablets repeatedly appear in stools.
• Advise patient using suppository to avoid excessive handling and to retain suppository for 1 to 3 hours or longer for maximum benefit.
• Teach patient about proper enema administration. Tell him to stay in position for at least 30 minutes and, if possible, retain medication overnight.

m

Advise patient to promptly report cramping, acute abdominal pain, bloody diarrhea, fever, headache, or rash.
- As appropriate, review all other significant and life-threatening adverse reactions.

mesna

Mesnex, Uromitexan✤

Pharmacologic class: Detoxifying agent

Therapeutic class: Hemorrhagic cystitis inhibitor

Pregnancy risk category B

Action

Reacts in kidney with urotoxic ifosfamide metabolites (acrolein and 4-hydroxy-ifosfamide), resulting in their detoxification. Also binds to double bonds of acrolein and to other urotoxic metabolites.

Availability

Injection: 100 mg/ml in 2-ml and 10-ml vials

Tablets (coated): 400 mg

Indications and dosages

➢ To prevent hemorrhagic cystitis in patients receiving ifosfamide

Adults: *Combination I.V. and P.O. regimen*—Single I.V. bolus dose of mesna at 20% of ifosfamide dosage, given at same time as ifosfamide, followed by two doses of mesna tablets P.O. at 40% of ifosfamide dosage given 2 and 6 hours after ifosfamide dose. *I.V. regimen*—I.V. bolus of mesna at 20% of ifosfamide dosage given at same time as ifosfamide, repeated 4 and 8 hours after each ifosfamide dose.

Dosage adjustment

- Children

Contraindications

- Hypersensitivity to drug or other thiol compounds

Precautions

Use cautiously in:
- autoimmune disorders
- pregnant or breastfeeding patients.

Administration

- Dilute with dextrose 5% in water, dextrose 5% in normal saline solution, or lactated Ringer's solution for injection.
- Give I.V. bolus over at least 1 minute with ifosfamide dose and at prescribed intervals after ifosfamide doses.

Don't use multidose vial (contains benzyl alcohol) in neonates or infants. In older children, use with caution.
- If patient vomits within 2 hours of oral mesna dose, repeat oral dose or switch to I.V. route.

Route	Onset	Peak	Duration
P.O.	Unknown	4-8 hr	24 hr
I.V.	Unknown	1 hr	24 hr

Adverse reactions

CNS: fatigue, malaise, irritability, headache, dizziness, drowsiness, hyperesthesia, rigors

CV: hypertension, hypotension, ST-segment elevation, tachycardia

EENT: conjunctivitis, pharyngitis, rhinitis

GI: nausea, vomiting, diarrhea, constipation, anorexia, flatulence

Hematologic: hematuria

Musculoskeletal: back pain, joint pain, myalgia

Respiratory: coughing, tachypnea, **bronchospasm**

Skin: flushing, rash

Other: arm or leg pain, injection site reactions, fever, flulike symptoms, allergic reactions

Interactions

Drug-diagnostic tests. *Hepatic enzymes:* increased levels
Urinary erythrocytes: false-positive or false-negative results
Urine tests using Ames Multistix: false-positive for ketonuria

Patient monitoring

- Monitor nutritional and hydration status.
- Monitor vital signs and ECG. Watch closely for blood pressure changes and tachycardia.
- Assess body temperature. Stay alert for fever, flulike symptoms, and EENT infections.
- Monitor respiratory status carefully. Watch closely for cough, bronchospasm, and tachypnea.

Patient teaching

- Inform patient that drug may cause significant adverse effects. Reassure him that he'll be monitored closely.
- Encourage patient to request analgesics or other pain-relief measures for headache, back or joint pain, hyperesthesia, or muscle ache.

Advise patient to immediately report breathing difficulties and allergic symptoms.

- Inform patient about drug's adverse CNS effects. Explain safety measures used to prevent injury.
- As appropriate, review all other significant and life-threatening adverse reactions and interactions, especially those related to the tests mentioned above.

metaproterenol sulfate

Alupent

Pharmacologic class: Sympathomimetic, selective $beta_2$-adrenergic agonist
Therapeutic class: Bronchodilator
Pregnancy risk category C

Action

Relaxes $beta_2$ (pulmonary) receptors, causing bronchodilation and inhibiting histamine release. Acts on $beta_1$ (cardiac) receptors with weaker effect.

Availability

Aerosol solution for inhalation: 0.65 mg/metered spray
Nebulizer inhaler: 0.4%, 0.6%
Syrup: 10 mg/5 ml
Tablets: 10 mg, 20 mg

m

Indications and dosages

➢ Bronchial asthma and reversible bronchospasm

Adults and children ages 9 and older or weighing more than 27 kg (59.5 lb): 20 mg P.O. three or four times daily
Children ages 6 to 9 or weighing less than 27 kg (59.5 lb): 10 mg P.O. three or four times daily
Aerosol solution for inhalation—
Adults and children ages 12 and older: Two or three inhalations by metered aerosol (1.3 or 1.9 mg) q 3 to 4 hours, to a maximum of 12 inhalations (7.8 mg) in 24 hours. Alternatively, one plastic ampule of 0.4% or 0.6% solution for nebulization by intermittent positive-pressure breathing device (usually not given more than q 4 hours).

Contraindications

- Hypersensitivity to drug or its components
- Tachyarrhythmias

Precautions

Use cautiously in:

- unstable vasomotor system disorders, hypertension, coronary artery disease, peripheral or mesenteric vascular thrombosis, hyperthyroidism, chronic obstructive pulmonary disease complicated by degenerative heart disease, hypoxia, hypercapnia
- history of cerebrovascular accident or seizure disorders
- patients who've received general anesthesia
- labor and delivery
- pregnant or breastfeeding patients.

Administration

- If patient's using aerosol metered-dose inhaler, place mouthpiece well into his mouth and have him close lips tightly around it. Tell him to exhale completely through nose and then inhale slowly and deeply through mouth while activating inhaler. Have him hold his breath for a few seconds and then remove mouthpiece and exhale slowly. Wait about 2 minutes between inhalations. Rinse mouthpiece with water after use.
- Know that use of Aero-Chamber may aid proper drug delivery.

Route	Onset	Peak	Duration
P.O.	15 min	1 hr	4 hr or more
Inhalation (aerosol)	1 min	1 hr	4 hr or more
Inhalation (nebulizer)	5-30 min	Unknown	4 hr or more

Adverse reactions

CNS: drowsiness, tremor, vertigo, headache, nervousness, restlessness, apprehension, anxiety, fear, CNS stimulation, hyperkinesia, insomnia, irritability, weakness
CV: tachycardia, hypertension, palpitations, anginal pain, **cardiac arrest** (with excessive use)
GI: nausea, vomiting, diarrhea, heartburn, dry mouth
Respiratory: cough, respiratory difficulty, **bronchospasm, pulmonary edema, paradoxical bronchiolar constriction** (with excessive use)
Skin: rash, sweating, pallor, flushing
Other: abnormal or bad taste, hypersensitivity reaction

Interactions

Drug-drug. *Epinephrine, other sympathomimetics:* increased risk of arrhythmias
MAO inhibitors, tricyclic antidepressants: potentiation of metaproterenol effects
Propranolol and other beta-adrenergic blockers: inhibition of bronchodilating effect

Patient monitoring

🔊 Monitor patient for hypersensitivity reaction or paradoxical bronchospasm. If either occurs, discontinue drug immediately and implement alternative therapy and airway control measures.

- Monitor patient for effective use of aerosol inhaler or hand-held nebulizer.
- Assess for drug efficacy. Be aware that efficacy may decrease with prolonged use.
- Check for adverse effects.

Patient teaching

- Tell patient to take tablets with food if GI distress occurs.
- Teach patient proper use of metered-dose aerosol inhaler.
- Advise patient to remove canister and wash mouthpiece frequently.

🔊 Caution patient not to increase number or frequency of inhalations without prescriber's consent; cardiac arrest may occur with excessive use.

- If patient uses multiple drugs to control asthma, assess level of understanding regarding administration. Tell him

to continue taking each drug as prescribed even if he feels better.
• As appropriate, review all other significant and life-threatening adverse reactions and interactions, especially those related to the drugs mentioned above.

metaxalone

Skelaxin

Pharmacologic class: Skeletal muscle relaxant
Therapeutic class: Autonomic agent
Pregnancy risk category C

Action
Unclear. Thought to depress CNS.

Availability
Tablets: 400 mg, 800 mg

Indications and dosages
➢ Acute, painful musculoskeletal conditions
Adults and children older than age 12: 800 mg P.O. t.i.d. to q.i.d.

Contraindications
• Hypersensitivity to drug or its components
• Significant renal or hepatic impairment
• History of drug-induced, hemolytic, or other anemias

Precautions
Use cautiously in:
• preexisting hepatic damage
• pregnant or breastfeeding patients
• children ages 12 and younger (safety not established).

Administration
• Give with full glass of water, with or without food.
• Know that drug should be used in conjunction with rest and physical therapy.

Route	Onset	Peak	Duration
P.O.	Unknown	2-4.5 hr	Unknown

Adverse reactions
CNS: drowsiness, dizziness, headache, nervousness, irritability
GI: nausea, vomiting, GI upset
Hematologic: leukopenia, hemolytic anemia
Hepatic: jaundice
Skin: rash (with or without pruritus)
Other: hypersensitivity reaction, **anaphylactoid reaction**

Interactions
Drug-drug. *Barbiturates, CNS depressants:* enhanced sedative effect
Drug-diagnostic tests. *Benedict's tests:* false-positive results
Cephalin flocculation tests: elevated results
Drug-behaviors. *Alcohol use:* increased sedation

Patient monitoring
• Monitor liver function tests and CBC with white cell differential.
Watch for severe adverse reactions, such as leukopenia, hemolytic anemia, and anaphylactoid reactions.

Patient teaching
• Tell patient to take with full glass of water, with or without food.
Advise patient to immediately report severe rash, difficulty breathing, unusual bruising or bleeding, yellowing of skin or eyes, or unusual tiredness or weakness.
• Instruct patient to take missed dose as soon as he remembers. However, if it's almost time for next dose, tell him to skip missed dose and continue with regular dosing schedule.

- Emphasize that drug should be used along with rest, physical therapy, and other measures to relieve discomfort.
- Advise patient to use caution while driving or operating heavy machinery.
- Caution female patient not to breastfeed while taking drug.
- Tell patient to avoid alcohol during therapy because it increases drowsiness.
- As appropriate, review all other significant and life-threatening adverse reactions and interactions, especially those related to the drugs, tests, and behaviors mentioned above.

metformin hydrochloride

Apo-Metformin✦, Glucophage, Glucophage XR, Glycon✦, Novo-Metformin✦, Riomet

Pharmacologic class: Biguanide
Therapeutic class: Hypoglycemic
Pregnancy risk category B

Action

Increases insulin sensitivity by decreasing glucose production and absorption in liver and intestines and enhancing glucose uptake and utilization

Availability

Oral solution: 100 mg/ml, 500 mg/5 ml
Tablets: 500 mg, 850 mg, 1,000 mg
Tablets (extended-release): 500 mg, 750 mg

Indications and dosages

➢ Adjunct to diet and exercise to improve glycemic control in type 2 (non-insulin-dependent) diabetes mellitus
Adults and children ages 17 and older: Initially, 500 mg P.O. b.i.d.; may increase by 500 mg/week, up to 2,000 mg/day. If patient needs more than 2,000 mg/day, give in three divided doses (not to exceed 2,500 mg/day). Alternatively, 850 mg P.O. daily, increased by 850 mg q 2 weeks, up to 2,550 mg/day in divided doses (850 mg t.i.d.). *Extended-release tablets*—500 mg/day P.O. with evening meal; may increase by 500 mg weekly, up to 2,000 mg/day. If 2,000 mg once daily is inadequate, 1,000 mg may be given b.i.d.
Children ages 10 to 16: 500 mg P.O. b.i.d. Increase in increments of 500 mg weekly to a maximum of 2,000 mg daily in divided doses.
➢ Concurrent use with sulfonylurea or insulin in type 2 diabetes mellitus
Adults and children ages 17 and older: If patient hasn't responded to maximum metformin dosage of 2,000 mg/day in 4 weeks, sulfonylurea may be added while metformin therapy continues at highest dosage (even if patient experienced primary or secondary failure on sulfonylurea). Adjust dosages of both drugs until glycemic control adequate. If response inadequate within 1 to 3 months of concurrent therapy, consider alternatives.
➢ Concurrent use with insulin in type 2 diabetes mellitus
Adults ages 17 and older: Continue current insulin dosage while starting metformin at 500 mg P.O. once daily. If response inadequate, increase metformin dosage by 500 mg after approximately 1 week and then by 500 mg weekly until glycemic control is achieved. Maximum metformin dosage is 2,500 mg. Optimally, decrease insulin dosage 10% to 25% when fasting plasma glucose level is below 120 mg/dl. Individualize dosage adjustments based on glycemic response.

Dosage adjustment

- Elderly or debilitated patients

Contraindications

- Hypersensitivity to drug
- Acute or chronic metabolic acidosis (including diabetic ketoacidosis) with or without coma

- Underlying renal dysfunction
- Heart failure requiring drug therapy

Precautions

Use cautiously in:

- renal impairment, myocardial infarction, cerebrovascular accident, hypoxia, sepsis, pituitary deficiency or hyperthyroidism, dehydration, hypoxemia, chronic alcohol use
- elderly or debilitated patients
- pregnant or breastfeeding patients
- children (safety not established).

Administration

- Administer with a meal.
- Make sure patient swallows extended-release tablets whole without crushing or chewing.
- Don't administer extended-release tablets to children.
- Know that drug is given with diet therapy, sulfonylureas, or both.

Route	Onset	Peak	Duration
P.O.	Unknown	2-4 hr	12 hr
P.O. (extended)	Unknown	4-8 hr	24 hr

Adverse reactions

GI: diarrhea, nausea, vomiting, abdominal bloating
Metabolic: lactic acidosis
Other: unpleasant metallic taste, decreased vitamin B_{12} level

Interactions

Drug-drug. *Amiloride, calcium channel blockers, digoxin, morphine, procainamide, quinidine, ranitidine, triamterene, trimethoprim, vancomycin:* altered response to metformin
Cimetidine, furosemide, nifedipine: increased metformin effects
Iodinated contrast media: increased risk of lactic acidosis
Drug-diagnostic tests. *Urine ketones:* false-positive results
Drug-herbs. *Glucosamine:* decreased glycemic control
Chromium, coenzyme Q10, fenugreek: additive hypoglycemic effects
Drug-behaviors. *Alcohol use:* increased metformin effects

Patient monitoring

- When switching from chlorpropamide, stay alert for hypoglycemia during first 2 weeks of metformin therapy; chlorpropamide may stay in body for prolonged time. Conversion from other standard oral hypoglycemics requires no transition period.
- Monitor blood glucose level closely. If it isn't controlled after 4 weeks at maximum dosage, oral sulfonylurea may be added.
- Monitor kidney and liver function tests, particularly in elderly patients.
- Assess hematologic parameters and vitamin B_{12} levels at start of therapy and periodically thereafter.

🔊 Watch for signs and symptoms of lactic acidosis. Stop drug if acidosis occurs. To aid differential diagnosis, check electrolyte, ketone, glucose, blood pH, lactate, and metformin blood levels.

- Periodically monitor glucose and glycosylated hemoglobin levels to evaluate drug efficacy.

Patient teaching

- Teach patient about diabetes and importance of proper diet, exercise, weight control, and blood glucose monitoring.
- Inform patient that drug may cause diarrhea, nausea, and upset stomach. Advise him to take it with meals to reduce these effects, and tell him that adverse effects often subside over time.

🔊 Teach patient to recognize and immediately report signs and symptoms of acidosis, such as weakness, fatigue, muscle pain, dyspnea, abdominal pain, dizziness, light-headedness, and slow or irregular heartbeat.

- Advise patient to report changes in health status (such as infection, persistent vomiting and diarrhea, or need for

m

surgery). These may warrant dosage decrease or drug withdrawal.
- As appropriate, review all other significant and life-threatening adverse reactions and interactions, especially those related to the drugs, tests, herbs, and behaviors mentioned above.

methadone hydrochloride

Dolophine, Methadone HCl Diskets, Methadone HCl Intensol, Methadose

Pharmacologic class: Opioid agonist
Therapeutic class: Analgesic, opioid detoxification adjunct
Controlled substance schedule II
Pregnancy risk category C

Action

Binds to and depresses opiate receptors in spinal cord and CNS, altering perception of and response to pain

Availability

Injection: 10 mg/ml
Oral solution: 5 mg/5 ml, 10 mg/5 ml, 10 mg/ml (concentrate)
Tablets: 5 mg, 10 mg
Tablets (dispersible diskettes): 40 mg

Indications and dosages

➢ Opioid detoxification
Adults: Initially, 15 to 20 mg/day P.O. to suppress withdrawal. Additional doses may be necessary if symptoms aren't suppressed or if they reappear. Most patients are adequately stabilized on total daily dosage of 40 mg given in single or divided doses; however, some may need higher dosages. When patient is stable for 2 to 3 days, decrease dosage gradually at 2-day intervals. If patient can't tolerate oral doses, give I.M. or subcutaneously (usually at about 25% of total daily P.O. dosage) in two injections.

➢ To maintain opioid abstinence
Adults: Oral dosage highly individualized based on control of abstinence symptoms without respiratory depression or marked sedation. If patient can't tolerate oral doses, give I.M. or subcutaneously (usually at about 25% of total daily P.O. dosage) in two injections.

➢ Chronic and severe pain
Adults: For chronic pain, 2.5 to 10 mg P.O., I.M., or subcutaneously q 3 to 4 hours as needed; adjust dosage and dosing interval as needed. For severe chronic pain (as in terminal illness), 5 to 20 mg P.O. q 6 to 8 hours.
Children: Dosage individualized.

Contraindications

- Hypersensitivity to drug or other opioid agonists

Precautions

Use cautiously in:
- head trauma; severe renal, hepatic, or pulmonary disease; hypothyroidism; adrenal insufficiency; undiagnosed abdominal pain; prostatic hypertrophy; urethral stricture; toxic psychosis; Addison's disease; cor pulmonale; increased intracranial pressure; severe inflammatory bowel disease; severe CNS depression; hypercapnia; seizures; fever; alcoholism
- recent renal or hepatic surgery
- elderly or debilitated patients
- pregnant patients, patients in labor, or breastfeeding patients.

Administration

- Mix dispersible tablets with 120 ml of water or orange juice, citrus Tang, or other acidic fruit beverage.
- Dilute 10 mg/ml of oral solution with water or other liquid to at least 30 ml. In detoxification and maintenance of opioid withdrawal, dilute solution in at least 90 ml of fluid.
- When used parenterally, I.M. route is preferred. Rotate injection sites.

• For detoxification and maintenance, give oral solution only, to reduce potential for parenteral abuse, hoarding, and accidental ingestion.
• Know that patients who can't take oral drugs because of nausea or vomiting during detoxification or maintenance should be hospitalized and given methadone parenterally.

Route	Onset	Peak	Duration
P.O.	30-60 min	1.5-2 hr	4-6 hr
I.M., subcut.	10-20 min	1-2 hr	4-5 hr

Adverse reactions

CNS: amnesia, anxiety, confusion, poor concentration, delirium, delusions, depression, dizziness, drowsiness, euphoria, fever, hallucinations, headache, insomnia, lethargy, lightheadedness, malaise, psychosis, restlessness, sedation, clouded sensorium, syncope, tremor, **seizures, coma**
CV: hypotension, palpitations, edema, bradycardia, **shock, cardiac arrest**
EENT: visual disturbances
GI: nausea, vomiting, constipation, ileus, biliary tract spasm, gastroesophageal reflux, indigestion, dysphagia, dry mouth, anorexia
GU: urinary hesitancy, urinary retention, prolonged labor, difficult ejaculation, erectile dysfunction
Hematologic: anemia, **leukopenia, thrombocytopenia**
Musculoskeletal: joint pain
Respiratory: depressed cough reflex, hypoventilation, wheezing, **asthma exacerbation, atelectasis, pulmonary edema, bronchospasm, respiratory depression or arrest, apnea**
Skin: urticaria, pruritus, flushing, pallor, diaphoresis
Other: allergic reaction, hiccups, facial or injection site edema, pain, physical or psychological drug dependence, withdrawal symptoms

Interactions

Drug-drug. *Amitriptyline, antihistamines, chloral hydrate, clomipramine, glutethimide, methocarbamol, MAO inhibitors, nortriptyline:* increased CNS and respiratory depression
Anticholinergics: increased risk of severe constipation leading to ileus
Antiemetics, general anesthetics, phenothiazines, sedative-hypnotics, tranquilizers: coma, hypotension, respiratory depression, severe sedation
Ascorbic acid, phenytoin, phosphate, potassium, rifampin: decreased methadone blood level
Cimetidine, fluvoxamine, protease inhibitors: increased analgesia, CNS and respiratory depression
Diuretics: increased diuresis
Hydroxyzine: increased analgesia, CNS depression, and hypotension
Paregoric, loperamide: increased CNS depression, severe constipation
Naloxone: antagonism of methadone's analgesic, CNS, and respiratory effects
Naltrexone: induction or worsening of withdrawal symptoms (when given within 7 days of methadone)
Neuromuscular blockers: increased or prolonged respiratory depression
Drug-diagnostic tests. *Amylase, liver function tests:* increased levels
Drug-behaviors. *Alcohol use:* increased CNS and respiratory depression

Patient monitoring

• Assess patient for relief of severe, chronic pain requiring around-the-clock dosing. Tailor dosage to patient's pain level and drug tolerance.
• Monitor CNS, respiratory, and cardiovascular status.
• Watch for deepening sedation, which may increase with successive doses.
• Evaluate bowel and bladder function. Give laxatives if appropriate.
• Monitor detoxification treatment closely. Short-term detoxification shouldn't exceed 30 days; long-term detoxification, 180 days.

m

• Assess patient on maintenance therapy for successful rehabilitation. Know that maintenance therapy should be part of comprehensive treatment plan that includes medical, vocational rehabilitative, employment, educational, and counseling services.

Patient teaching

🔈 Instruct patient to promptly report severe adverse reactions.
• Tell patient he may take drug with food if GI upset occurs.
• Tell ambulatory patient to change positions slowly to avoid orthostatic hypotension.
🔈 Caution patient not to discontinue drug abruptly.
• Advise patient to avoid driving and other hazardous activities, because drug may cause drowsiness or dizziness.
• Tell female patient to inform prescriber if she's pregnant or breastfeeding.
• As appropriate, review all other significant and life-threatening adverse reactions and interactions, especially those related to the drugs, tests, and behaviors mentioned above.

methimazole

Tapazole

Pharmacologic class: Thiomidazole derivative

Therapeutic class: Antithyroid drug

Pregnancy risk category D

Action

Directly interferes with thyroid synthesis by preventing iodine from combining with thyroglobulin, leading to decreased thyroid hormone levels

Availability

Tablets: 5 mg, 10 mg

Indications and dosages

➢ Mild hyperthyroidism

Adults and adolescents: Initially, 15 mg P.O. daily in three equally divided doses at approximately 8-hour intervals. For maintenance, 5 to 15 mg/day in equally divided doses at approximately 8-hour intervals.

Children: Initially, 0.4 mg/kg/day in three divided doses at 8-hour intervals. For maintenance, approximately 0.2 mg/kg/day in three divided doses at 8-hour intervals.

➢ Moderate hyperthyroidism

Adults and adolescents: Initially, 30 to 40 mg P.O. daily in three equally divided doses at approximately 8-hour intervals. For maintenance, 5 to 15 mg/day in three equally divided doses at approximately 8-hour intervals.

Children: 0.4 mg/kg/day P.O. as a single dose or in divided doses at 8-hour intervals. For maintenance, approximately 0.2 mg/kg/day as a single dose or in three divided doses at 8-hour intervals.

➢ Severe hyperthyroidism

Adults and adolescents: Initially, 60 mg/day P.O. in three equally divided doses at approximately 8-hour intervals. For maintenance, 5 to 15 mg/day in three equally divided doses at approximately 8-hour intervals.

Children: Initially, 0.4 mg/kg/day P.O. as a single dose or in three divided doses at 8-hour intervals. For maintenance, approximately 0.2 mg/kg/day as a single dose or in three divided doses at 8-hour intervals.

Contraindications

• Hypersensitivity to drug
• Breastfeeding

Precautions

Use cautiously in:
• bone marrow depression
• patients older than age 40
• pregnant patients.

Administration

- Give with meals as needed to reduce GI upset.

Route	Onset	Peak	Duration
P.O.	30-40 min	60 min	2-4 hr

Adverse reactions

CNS: headache, vertigo, paresthesia, neuritis, depression, neuropathy, CNS stimulation
GI: nausea, vomiting, constipation, epigastric distress, ileus, salivary gland enlargement, dry mouth, anorexia
GU: nephritis
Hematologic: thrombocytopenia, agranulocytosis, leukopenia, aplastic anemia
Hepatic: jaundice, **hepatic dysfunction, hepatitis**
Metabolic: hypothyroidism
Musculoskeletal: joint pain, myalgia
Skin: rash, urticaria, skin discoloration, pruritus, erythema nodosum, exfoliative dermatitis, abnormal hair loss
Other: fever, lymphadenopathy, lupus-like syndrome

Interactions

Drug-drug. *Aminophylline, oxtriphylline, theophylline:* decreased clearance of both drugs
Amiodarone, iodine, potassium iodide: decreased response to methimazole
Anticoagulants: altered requirements for both drugs
Beta-adrenergic blockers: altered beta blocker clearance
Digoxin: increased digoxin blood level
Drug-diagnostic tests. *Granulocytes, hemoglobin, platelets, white blood cells:* decreased values

Patient monitoring

- Check for agranulocytosis in patients older than age 40 and in those receiving more than 40 mg/day.
- Assess hematologic studies. Agranulocytosis usually occurs within first 2 months of therapy and is rare after 4 months.
- Monitor thyroid function tests periodically. Once hyperthyroidism is controlled, elevated thyroid-stimulating factor indicates need for dosage decrease.
- Assess liver function tests and check for signs and symptoms of hepatic dysfunction.
- Monitor patient for fever, sore throat, and other evidence of infection as well as for unusual bleeding or bruising.
- Assess patient for signs and symptoms of hypothyroidism, such as hard edema of subcutaneous tissue, drowsiness, slow mentation, dryness or loss of hair, decreased temperature, hoarseness, and muscle weakness.

Patient teaching

- Tell patient to take with meals if GI upset occurs.
- Advise patient to take exactly as prescribed to maintain constant blood level.
- Tell patient to report rash, fever, sore throat, unusual bleeding or bruising, headache, rash, yellowing of skin or eyes, abdominal pain, vomiting, or flu-like symptoms.
- Caution female patient not to breastfeed while taking drug.
- As appropriate, review all other significant and life-threatening adverse reactions and interactions, especially those related to the drugs and tests mentioned above.

m

methocarbamol

Methocarbamol✱, Robaxin

Pharmacologic class: Autonomic nervous system agent
Therapeutic class: Skeletal muscle relaxant (centrally acting)
Pregnancy risk category C

Action

Unknown. Thought to depress central perception of pain without directly relaxing skeletal muscles or directly affecting motor endplate or motor nerves.

Availability

Injection: 100 mg/ml in 10-ml ampules, 100 mg/ml in 10-ml vials
Tablets: 500 mg, 750 mg

Indications and dosages

➢ Adjunct in muscle spasms caused by acute, painful musculoskeletal conditions

Adults: Initially, 1.5 g P.O. q.i.d. (up to 8 g/day) for 2 to 3 days, then 4 to 4.5 g/day P.O. in three to six divided doses; or 750 mg P.O. q 4 hours or 1 g P.O. q.i.d. or 1.5 g P.O. t.i.d. If oral dosing isn't feasible or if condition is severe, give 1 to 3 g/day I.M. or I.V. for maximum of 3 days.

Off-label uses

- Tetanus

Contraindications

- Hypersensitivity to drug, its components, or polyethylene glycol (with parenteral form)
- Renal impairment (with parenteral form)

Precautions

Use cautiously in:
- seizure disorders (with parenteral use)
- pregnant or breastfeeding patients
- children (safety not established).

Administration

- For direct I.V. injection, administer slowly. Keep patient supine for 10 to 15 minutes afterward.
- For I.V. infusion, dilute 1 g with up to 250 ml 5% dextrose or 0.9% sodium chloride injection.
- Avoid extravasation; drug is hypertonic.
- Don't give subcutaneously.
- For I.M. use, inject no more than 500 mg (5 ml of 10% injection) into each gluteal area.
- Don't use parenteral form in patients with renal impairment. Polyethylene glycol vehicle may irritate kidneys.
- When giving for tetanus, crush and suspend tablets in water or saline solution, and give via nasogastric tube, if necessary.
- Be aware that drug is usually given as part of regimen that includes rest and physical therapy.

Route	Onset	Peak	Duration
P.O.	30 min	2 hr	Unknown
I.V.	Immediate	End of infusion	Unknown
I.M.	Unknown	Unknown	Unknown

Adverse reactions

CNS: dizziness, light-headedness, drowsiness, syncope, **seizures** (with I.V. use)
CV: bradycardia or hypotension (with I.V. use)
EENT: blurred vision, conjunctivitis, nasal congestion
GI: nausea, GI upset, anorexia
GU: brown, black, or green urine
Musculoskeletal: mild muscle incoordination (with I.V. or I.M. use)
Skin: flushing (with I.V. use), pruritus, rash, urticaria
Other: fever, pain at I.M. injection site, phlebitis at I.V. site, allergic reactions including **anaphylaxis** (with I.M. or I.V. use)

Interactions

Drug-drug. *Antihistamines, CNS depressants (such as opioids, sedative-hypnotics):* additive CNS depression
Drug-diagnostic tests. *Urinary 5-hydroxyindoleacetic acid, urine vanillylmandelic acid:* false elevations

Drug-herbs. *Chamomile, hops, kava, skullcap, valerian:* increased CNS depression
Drug-behaviors. *Alcohol use:* increased CNS depression

Patient monitoring

• Assess for orthostatic hypotension, especially with parenteral use. Keep patient supine for 10 to 15 minutes after I.V. administration.
◀ Watch for anaphylaxis after I.M. or I.V. administration.
◀ Stay alert for bradycardia and syncope after I.V. or I.M. dose. As needed and prescribed, give epinephrine, corticosteroids, or antihistamines.
• Monitor I.V. site frequently to prevent sloughing and thrombophlebitis.

Patient teaching

• Tell patient that drug may turn urine brown, black, or green.
• Caution patient to avoid driving and other hazardous activities, because drug may cause drowsiness or dizziness.
• Instruct patient to move slowly when changing position, to avoid dizziness from sudden blood pressure decrease.
• As appropriate, review all other significant and life-threatening adverse reactions and interactions, especially those related to the drugs, tests, herbs, and behaviors mentioned above.

methotrexate (amethopterin, MTX)

methotrexate sodium

Pharmacologic class: Antimetabolite, folic acid antagonist
Therapeutic class: Antineoplastic
Pregnancy risk category X

Action

Binds to dihydrofolate reductase, interfering with folic acid metabolism and inhibiting DNA synthesis and cellular replication

Availability

Injection: 20-mg, 25-mg, 50-mg, 100-mg, 250-mg, and 1,000-mg vials *(lyophilized powder, preservative-free)*
Tablets: 2.5 mg, 5 mg, 7.5 mg, 10 mg, 15 mg

Indications and dosages

➢ Acute lymphoblastic leukemia
Adults and children: 3.3 mg/m² P.O. or I.M. daily for 4 to 6 weeks, then 20 to 30 mg/m² P.O. or I.M. weekly in two divided doses; given with corticosteroid. Alternatively, 2.5 mg/kg I.V. q 14 days.
➢ Meningeal leukemia
Adult and children: 12 mg/m² (maximum of 15 mg) intrathecally at intervals of 2 to 5 days, repeated until cerebrospinal fluid cell count is normal
➢ Burkitt's lymphoma
Adults: In stages I and II, 10 to 25 mg P.O. daily for 4 to 8 days; in stage III, combined with other neoplastic drugs. Patients in all stages usually require several courses of therapy, with 7- to 10-day rest periods between courses.
➢ Mycosis fungoides
Adults: 2.5 to 10 mg/day P.O. or 50 mg I.M. q week or 25 mg I.M. twice weekly
➢ Osteosarcoma
Adults: As part of adjunctive regimen with other antineoplastics, initially 12 g/m² I.V. as 4-hour infusion, then 12 to 15 g/m² I.V. in subsequent 4-hour infusions given at weeks 4, 5, 6, 7, 11, 12, 15, 16, 29, 30, 44, and 45 until peak blood level reaches 1,000 micromoles. Leucovorin rescue must start 24 hours after methotrexate infusion begins; if patient can't tolerate oral leucovorin, dose must be given I.M. or I.V. on same schedule.

m

➢ Trophoblastic tumors (choriocarcinoma, hydatidiform mole)
Adults: 15 to 30 mg P.O. or I.M. daily for 5 days. Repeat course three to five times as required, with rest periods of at least 1 week between courses, until toxic symptoms subside.
➢ Lymphosarcoma (stage III)
Adults: 0.625 to 2.5 mg/kg/day P.O., I.M., or I.V.
➢ Psoriasis
Adults: After test dose, 2.5 mg P.O. at 12-hour intervals for three doses weekly, to a maximum of 30 mg weekly. Alternatively, 10 to 25 mg P.O., I.M., or I.V. as a single weekly dose, to a maximum of 30 mg weekly; decrease dosage when adequate response occurs.
➢ Rheumatoid arthritis
Adults: 7.5 mg P.O. weekly as a single dose or divided as 2.5 mg q 12 hours for three doses weekly. May gradually increase, if needed, up to 20 mg/week; decrease when adequate response occurs.

Dosage adjustment
• Renal or hepatic impairment
• Elderly patients

Off-label uses
• Relapsing-remitting multiple sclerosis
• Refractory Crohn's disease

Contraindications
• Hypersensitivity to drug
• Psoriasis or rheumatoid arthritis in pregnant patients
• Breastfeeding

Precautions
Use cautiously in:
• severe myocardial, hepatic, or renal disease; decreased bone marrow reserve; active infection; hypotension; coma
• elderly patients
• patients with childbearing potential
• young children.

Administration
🔊 Be aware that methotrexate is a high-alert drug.
🔊 Know that patient must be adequately hydrated before therapy and urine must be alkalized using sodium bicarbonate.
• Follow facility policy for handling, preparing, and administering carcinogenic, mutagenic, and teratogenic drugs.
• Be aware that oral administration is preferred. Give oral dose 1 hour before or 2 hours after meals. (Food decreases absorption of tablets and reduces peak blood level.)
• Reconstitute powder for injection with preservative-free solution, such as 5% dextrose solution or 0.9% sodium chloride injection. Reconstitute 20-mg and 50-mg vials to yield a concentration no greater than 25 mg/ml. Reconstitute 1-g vial with 19.4 ml to yield a concentration of 50 mg/ml.
• For high-dose I.V. infusion, dilute in 5% dextrose solution. Administer each 10 mg over 1 minute or by infusion over 30 minutes to 4 hours as directed.
• For intrathecal use, reconstitute immediately before administration, using preservative-free solution (such as 0.9% sodium chloride for injection), to a concentration of 1 mg/ml.
🔊 For intrathecal or high-dose therapy, use preservative-free injection form.
• Avoid I.M. injections if platelet count is below 50,000/mm³.
🔊 For osteosarcoma, make sure leucovorin rescue is used appropriately in patients receiving high methotrexate doses. Rescue usually starts 24 hours after methotrexate infusion begins.

Route	Onset	Peak	Duration
P.O.	Unknown	1-2 hr	Unknown
I.V.	Immediate	Immediate	Unknown
I.M.	Unknown	0.5-1 hr	Unknown
Intrathecal	Unknown	Unknown	Unknown

Adverse reactions

CNS: malaise, fatigue, drowsiness, dizziness, headache, aphasia, hemiparesis, demyelination, **seizures, leukoencephalopathy, chemical arachnoiditis** (with intrathecal use)
EENT: blurred vision, pharyngitis
GI: nausea, vomiting, stomatitis, hematemesis, melena, GI ulcers, enteritis, gingivitis, pharyngitis, anorexia, **GI bleeding**
GU: hematuria, cystitis, infertility, menstrual dysfunction, defective spermatogenesis, abortion, **tubular necrosis, severe nephropathy, renal failure**
Hematologic: anemia, **leukopenia, thrombocytopenia, severe bone marrow depression**
Hepatic: hepatotoxicity
Metabolic: hyperuricemia, diabetes mellitus
Musculoskeletal: joint pain, myalgia, osteonecrosis, osteoporosis (with long-term use in children)
Respiratory: dry nonproductive cough, **pneumonitis, pulmonary fibrosis, pulmonary interstitial infiltrates**
Skin: pruritus, rash, urticaria, alopecia, painful plaque erosions, photosensitivity
Other: chills, fever, increased susceptibility to infection, **septicemia, anaphylaxis, sudden death**

Interactions

Drug-drug. *Activated charcoal:* decreased blood level of oral or I.V. methotrexate
Folic acid derivatives: antagonism of methotrexate effects
Fosphenytoin, phenytoin: decreased blood levels of these drugs
Hepatotoxic drugs: increased risk of hepatotoxicity
Nonsteroidal anti-inflammatory drugs, phenylbutazone, probenecid, salicylates, sulfonamides: increased methotrexate toxicity
Oral antibiotics: decreased methotrexate absorption
Penicillin, sulfonamide: increased methotrexate blood level
Procarbazine: increased nephrotoxicity
Theophylline: increased theophylline level
Vaccines: vaccine inefficacy
Drug-diagnostic tests. *Hemoglobin, platelets, red blood cells, white blood cells:* decreased values
Pregnancy tests: false-positive result
Protein-bound iodine, transaminases, uric acid: increased levels
Drug-food. *Any food:* delayed methotrexate absorption and decreased peak blood level
Drug-herbs. *Astragalus, echinacea, melatonin:* interference with methotrexate-induced immunosuppression
Drug-behaviors. *Alcohol use:* increased hepatotoxicity
Sun exposure: photosensitivity

Patient monitoring

- Watch for vomiting, diarrhea, or stomatitis, which may cause dehydration.
- Know that high-dose therapy may cause nephrotoxicity. Monitor renal function, hydration status, urine alkalization (for pH above 6.5), and methotrexate blood level.
- Assess for fever, sore throat, bleeding, increased bruising, and other signs and symptoms of hematologic compromise or infection.
- With high-dose or intrathecal therapy, watch for CNS toxicity.
- Monitor creatinine and methotrexate blood levels 24 hours after therapy starts and then daily. Adjust leucovorin dosage as prescribed.
- Check hematologic studies at least monthly; blood or platelet transfusions may be necessary.
- Monitor liver and kidney function studies every 1 to 3 months. Evaluate uric acid levels.

m

🔊 Watch for signs and symptoms of pulmonary toxicity, such as fever, dry nonproductive cough, dyspnea, hypoxemia, and infiltrates on chest X-ray.
• Know that methotrexate exits slowly from third-space compartments (ascites, pleural effusions). Before therapy starts, fluid should be evacuated; during therapy, monitor drug blood level.

Patient teaching
🔊 Review dosing instructions carefully with patient to avoid toxicity. Tell patient with rheumatoid arthritis or psoriasis to take doses weekly.
• Advise patient to take oral doses 1 hour before or 2 hours after meals.
• Instruct patient to report diarrhea, abdominal pain, clay-colored or black tarry stools, fever, chills, sore throat, unusual bleeding or bruising, sores in or around mouth, cough or shortness of breath, yellowing of skin or eyes, dark or bloody urine, swelling of feet or legs, or joint pain.
• Tell patient to take temperature daily and to report fever or other signs or symptoms of infection.
• Instruct patient to drink 2 to 3 L of fluid each day.
• Advise male patients to use reliable contraception during and for at least 3 months after therapy. Advise female patients to use reliable contraception during and for one ovulatory cycle after therapy; also caution them not to breastfeed.
• Advise patient to avoid sun exposure and to use sunscreen and protective clothing (especially if he has psoriasis).
• Instruct patient to avoid alcohol.
• Tell patient he'll need to undergo blood tests during therapy.
• As appropriate, review all other significant and life-threatening adverse reactions and interactions, especially those related to the drugs, tests, foods, herbs, and behaviors mentioned above.

methylcellulose
Citrucel, Entrocel🍁, Prodiem🍁

Pharmacologic class: Semisynthetic cellulose derivative
Therapeutic class: Bulk laxative
Pregnancy risk category NR

Action
Stimulates peristalsis by promoting water absorption into fecal matter and increasing bulk, resulting in bowel evacuation

Availability
Powder: 105 mg/g, 196 mg/g

Indications and dosages
➢ Chronic constipation
Adults and children ages 12 and older: Up to 6 g P.O. daily in divided doses of 0.45 to 3 g
Children ages 6 to 11: Up to 3 g P.O. daily in divided doses of 0.45 to 1.5 g

Contraindications
• Signs or symptoms of appendicitis or undiagnosed abdominal pain
• Partial bowel obstruction
• Dysphagia

Precautions
Use cautiously in:
• hepatitis
• intestinal ulcers
• laxative-dependent patients.

Administration
• Give with 8 oz of fluid.
• If patient's receiving maximum daily dosage, give in divided doses to reduce risk of esophageal obstruction.

Route	Onset	Peak	Duration
P.O.	12-24 hr	<3 days	Unknown

Adverse reactions

GI: nausea; vomiting; diarrhea; severe constipation; abdominal distention; cramps; esophageal, gastric, small-intestine, or colonic strictures (with dry form); **GI obstruction**
Other: laxative dependence (with long-term use)

Interactions

Drug-drug. *Antibiotics, digitalis, nitrofurantoin, oral anticoagulants, salicylates, tetracyclines:* decreased absorption and action of these drugs

Patient monitoring

- Assess patient's dietary habits. Consider factors that promote constipation, such as certain diseases and medications.
- Monitor patient for signs and symptoms of esophageal obstruction.
- Evaluate fluid and electrolyte balance in patients using laxatives excessively.

Patient teaching

- Instruct patient to take with a full glass (8 oz) of water.
- Advise patient to prevent or minimize constipation through adequate fluid intake (four to six glasses of water daily), proper diet, increased fiber intake, daily exercise, and prompt response to urge to defecate.

Instruct patient to report chest pain or pressure, vomiting, and difficulty breathing (possible symptoms of GI obstruction).

- Caution patient not to use drug for more than 1 week without prescriber's approval.
- Inform patient that chronic laxative use may lead to dependence.
- Tell patient to contact prescriber if constipation persists or if rectal bleeding or symptoms of electrolyte imbalance (muscle cramps, weakness, dizziness) occur.
- As appropriate, review all other significant and life-threatening adverse reactions and interactions, especially those related to the drugs mentioned above.

methyldopa

Apo-Methyldopa♣, Dopamet♣, Novomedopa♣, Nu-Medopa♣

methyldopate hydrochloride

Pharmacologic class: Centrally acting antiadrenergic
Therapeutic class: Antihypertensive
Pregnancy risk category B

Action

Stimulates CNS alpha-adrenergic receptors, decreasing sympathetic stimulation to heart and blood vessels. Also reduces arterial pressure and plasma renin.

Availability

Injection: 50 mg/ml in 5- and 10-ml vials
Oral suspension (contains bisulfites): 250 mg/5 ml
Tablets: 125 mg, 250 mg, 500 mg

Indications and dosages

➢ Hypertension

Adults: 250 mg P.O. two to three times daily for 2 days (not to exceed 500 mg/day in divided doses if used with other agents); may increase q 2 days as needed. Usual maintenance dosage is 500 mg to 2 g/day (not to exceed 3 g/day) P.O. in two to four divided doses or 250 to 500 mg I.V. q 6 hours (up to 1 g q 6 hours).
Children: 10 mg/kg/day (300 mg/m²/day) P.O. in two to four divided doses. May increase q 2 days up to 65 mg/kg/

day (2 g/m²/day), or 3 g/day in divided doses (whichever is lower) or 5 to 10 mg/kg I.V. q 6 hours; up to 65 mg/kg/day (2 g/m²/day), or 3 g/day in divided doses (whichever is lower).

Contraindications

- Hypersensitivity to drug or its components
- Pheochromocytoma
- Active hepatic disease or history of methyldopa-associated hepatic disorders
- MAO inhibitor use within past 14 days

Precautions

Use cautiously in:

- heart failure, edema, hemolytic anemia, hypotension, severe bilateral cerebrovascular disease
- dialysis patients
- elderly patients
- pregnant or breastfeeding patients.

Administration

🔊 Don't give within 14 days of MAO inhibitors.

- To prepare I.V. infusion, add prescribed dosage to 100 ml 5% dextrose injection. Or administer in 5% dextrose injection in a concentration of 100 mg/10 ml. Give each dose over 30 to 60 minutes.
- Dilute and administer ADD-Vantage vials containing 50 mg/ml according to manufacturer's instructions.

🔊 Don't stop drug therapy abruptly.

Route	Onset	Peak	Duration
P.O.	Unknown	4-6 hr	24-48 hr
I.V.	Unknown	4-6 hr	10-16 hr

Adverse reactions

CNS: headache, asthenia, weakness, dizziness, sedation, decreased mental acuity, depression, paresthesia, parkinsonism, Bell's palsy, involuntary choreoathetotic movements
CV: bradycardia, edema, orthostatic hypotension, **myocarditis**
EENT: nasal congestion
GI: nausea, vomiting, diarrhea, constipation, abdominal distention, colitis, dry mouth, sialadenitis, sore or black tongue, **pancreatitis**
GU: breast enlargement, gynecomastia, failure to ejaculate, erectile dysfunction
Hematologic: eosinophilia, **hemolytic anemia**
Hepatic: hepatitis
Other: fever

Interactions

Drug-drug. *Adrenergics, MAO inhibitors:* excessive sympathetic stimulation
Amphetamines, barbiturates, nonsteroidal anti-inflammatory drugs, phenothiazines, tricyclic antidepressants: decreased antihypertensive effect
Anesthetics, antihypertensives, nitrates: additive hypotension
Ferrous gluconate, ferrous sulfate: decreased methyldopa blood level
Haloperidol: increased haloperidol effects, increased risk of psychoses
Levodopa: additive hypotension and CNS toxicity
Lithium: increased risk of lithium toxicity
Nonselective beta-adrenergic blockers: paradoxical hypertension
Tolbutamide: increased tolbutamide effects
Drug-diagnostic tests. *Alanine aminotransferase, alkaline phosphatase, aspartate aminotransferase, bilirubin, blood urea nitrogen, creatinine, potassium, prolactin, sodium, uric acid:* increased levels
Direct Coombs' test: positive result
Liver function tests: abnormal results
Prothrombin time: prolonged
Drug-herbs. *Capsicum:* reduced antihypertensive effects
Drug-behaviors. *Alcohol use:* increased hypotension

Patient monitoring

- Obtain direct Coombs' test before therapy starts and 6 and 12 months later.
- Monitor periodic blood counts to detect adverse hematologic reactions.
- Monitor liver function tests and check for signs and symptoms of hepatic dysfunction (particularly during first 6 to 12 weeks of therapy).
- Check for edema or weight gain to help determine if diuretic should be added to regimen.
- Monitor blood pressure. Drug tolerance may occur during second and third months of therapy.

Patient teaching

- Tell patient that sedation usually occurs when therapy starts and during dosage titration. To lessen this effect, advise him to begin dosage titration in evening.

Tell patient not to stop taking drug abruptly.

Instruct patient to report fever, yellowing of skin or eyes, fatigue, abdominal pain, flulike symptoms, swelling, or significant weight gain.

- Inform patient that urine may darken after exposure to air.
- Advise patient to move slowly when changing position, to avoid dizziness from sudden blood pressure decrease.
- Caution patient to avoid driving and other hazardous activities until effects of drug are known or dosage titration is completed.
- As appropriate, review all other significant and life-threatening adverse reactions and interactions, especially those related to the drugs, tests, herbs, and behaviors mentioned above.

methylergonovine maleate

Methergine

Pharmacologic class: Ergot alkaloid
Therapeutic class: Oxytocic
Pregnancy risk category C

Action

Directly stimulates vascular smooth-muscle contractions in uterus and cervix and decreases bleeding after delivery

Availability

Injection: 0.2 mg/ml
Tablets: 0.2 mg

Indications and dosages

➢ Prevention and treatment of postpartum hemorrhage

Adults: 0.2 mg I.M.; repeat q 2 to 4 hours as needed to a total of five doses. In emergencies, 0.2 mg I.V. over 1 minute. After initial I.M. or I.V. dose, 0.2 mg P.O. q 6 to 8 hours for 2 to 7 days; decrease dosage if cramping occurs.

Contraindications

- Hypersensitivity to drug
- Hypertension
- Toxemia
- Pregnancy (except during third stage of labor)

Precautions

Use cautiously in:

- severe hepatic or renal disease, vascular disease, jaundice, sepsis
- patients in second stage of labor.

Administration

- Be aware that drug isn't routinely given I.V. because of risk of severe hypertension and cerebrovascular accident (CVA). Monitor blood pressure and uterine contractions during administration.

m

• If I.V. use is necessary, give dose over 1 minute. Dose may be diluted in 5 ml of 0.9% sodium chloride injection.
• Be aware that prolonged therapy should be avoided because of ergotism risk.

Route	Onset	Peak	Duration
P.O.	5-10 min	30 min	3 hr
I.V.	Immediate	Unknown	45 min
I.M.	2-5 min	Unknown	3 hr

Adverse reactions

CNS: dizziness, headache, hallucination, **seizures, CVA** (with I.V. use)
CV: hypertension, hypotension, transient chest pain, palpitations, **thrombophlebitis**
EENT: tinnitus, nasal congestion
GI: nausea, vomiting, diarrhea
GU: hematuria
Musculoskeletal: leg cramps
Respiratory: dyspnea
Skin: diaphoresis, rash, allergic reactions
Other: foul taste

Interactions

Drug-drug. *Dopamine, ergot alkaloids, oxytocin, regional anesthetics, vasoconstrictors:* excessive vasoconstriction
Drug-diagnostic tests. *Prolactin:* increased level

Patient monitoring

Know that if used during third stage of labor, drug increases risk of hemorrhage and infection.
• When giving I.V., closely monitor blood pressure, pulse, uterine contractions, and bleeding.
• Monitor patient for adverse effects.

Patient teaching

• Inform patient and family of reason for using drug, and provide reassurance.
• Tell patient drug may cause nausea, vomiting, dizziness, increased blood pressure, headache, ringing in ears, chest pain, or shortness of breath. Advise her to report severe or troublesome symptoms.
• As appropriate, review all other significant and life-threatening adverse reactions and interactions, especially those related to the drugs and tests mentioned above.

methylphenidate hydrochloride

Concerta, Metadate CD, Metadate ER, Methylin, Methylin ER, PHL-Methylphenidate✱, PMS-Methylphenidate✱, Riphenidate✱, Ritalin, Ritalin LA, Ritalin-SR

Pharmacologic class: Piperidine derivative
Therapeutic class: CNS stimulant
Controlled substance schedule II
Pregnancy risk category C

Action

Increases release of norepinephrine, which stimulates impulse transmission in respiratory system and CNS. Net effect is increased mental alertness.

Availability

Capsules (extended-release): 10 mg, 20 mg, 30 mg, 40 mg
Tablets (chewable): 2.5 mg, 5 mg, 10 mg
Tablets (extended-release): 10 mg, 18 mg, 20 mg, 27 mg, 36 mg, 54 mg
Tablets (prompt-release): 5 mg, 10 mg, 20 mg
Tablets (sustained-release): 20 mg

Indications and dosages

➢ Adjunctive treatment of attention deficit hyperactivity disorder (ADHD)
Adults: 5 to 20 mg P.O. (prompt-release tablets) two to three times daily.

Once maintenance dosage is determined, may switch to extended-release.
Children older than age 6: Initially, 5 mg P.O. (prompt-release tablets) before breakfast and lunch; increase by 5 to 10 mg at weekly intervals, not to exceed 60 mg/day. Once maintenance dosage is determined, may switch to extended-release.

If previous methylphenidate dosage was 10 mg b.i.d. or 20 mg sustained-release, give Ritalin LA 20 mg P.O. once daily. If previous dosage was 15 mg b.i.d., give Ritalin LA 30 mg P.O. once daily. If previous dosage was 20 mg b.i.d. or 40 mg sustained-release, give Ritalin LA 40 mg P.O. once daily. If previous dosage was 30 mg b.i.d. or 60 mg sustained-release, give Ritalin LA 60 mg P.O. once daily.

In all patients, Ritalin-SR or Metadate ER may be prescribed instead of prompt-release tablets when 8-hour dosage of those forms corresponds to titrated 8-hour dosage of prompt-release tablets.

Concerta—
Children ages 6 and older who haven't used methylphenidate previously: Initially, 18 mg P.O. once daily in morning; may be titrated weekly up to 54 mg/day
Children ages 6 and older using other methylphenidate forms: 18 mg P.O. once daily in morning if previous dosage was 5 mg two to three times daily, or 20 mg P.O. daily (sustained-release); 36 mg once daily in morning if previous dosage was 10 mg two to three times daily or 40 mg daily (sustained-release); or 54 mg once daily in morning if previous dosage was 15 mg two to three times daily or 60 mg once daily (sustained-release)
Metadate CD—
Children ages 6 and older: Initially, 20 mg once daily; may adjust in weekly increments of 10 to 20 mg, to a maximum of 60 mg/day taken in morning

➢ Narcolepsy
Adults: 10 mg P.O. (Ritalin, Ritalin SR, or Metadate ER) two to three times daily, 30 to 45 minutes before a meal. Some patients may require up to 60 mg daily.

Off-label uses

- Depression in ill, elderly patients (such as those with cerebrovascular accident)
- To enhance analgesia and sedation in patients receiving opioids

Contraindications

- Hypersensitivity to drug or its components
- Glaucoma
- Motor tics, Tourette syndrome (or family history of syndrome)
- Psychosis
- Suicidal or homicidal tendencies
- MAO inhibitor use within past 14 days

m

Precautions

Use cautiously in:
- hypertension, cardiovascular disease, diabetes mellitus, seizure disorders
- elderly or debilitated patients
- pregnant or breastfeeding patients.

Administration

- Don't crush extended-release tablets or extended-release trilayer core tablets (Concerta).
- Have patient swallow extended-release capsules (Metadate CD, Ritalin LA) intact; or, if desired, sprinkle entire contents onto small amount (1 tbsp) of applesauce immediately before administration. (However, don't sprinkle Ritalin LA onto warm applesauce because its release properties may be affected.) Give water after patient swallows dose.
- Don't give extended-release tablets to initiate therapy or for daily use until dosage has been titrated using conventional tablets.

Don't give within 14 days of MAO inhibitor use.
- To help prevent insomnia, give last daily dose of conventional tablets several hours before bedtime.
- Discontinue drug periodically in children who have responded to therapy, to assess patient's condition. After withdrawal, improvement may be temporary or permanent.
- Be aware that therapy shouldn't continue indefinitely.

Route	Onset	Peak	Duration
P.O.	Unknown	1-3 hr	4-6 hr
P.O. (extended)	Unknown	Unknown	Up to 8 hr

Adverse reactions

CNS: restlessness, tremor, dizziness, headache, irritability, hyperactivity, insomnia, akathisia, dyskinesia, **toxic psychosis**
CV: hypertension, hypotension, palpitations, tachycardia
EENT: blurred vision
GI: nausea, vomiting, diarrhea, constipation, cramps, dry mouth, anorexia
Skin: rash
Other: metallic taste, fever, suppression of weight gain (in children), hypersensitivity reactions, physical or psychological drug dependence, drug tolerance

Interactions

Drug-drug. *Anticonvulsants, selective serotonin reuptake inhibitors, tricyclic antidepressants, warfarin:* inhibited metabolism and increased effects of these drugs
Guanethidine: antagonism of hypotensive effect
MAO inhibitors, vasopressors: hypertensive crisis
Drug-food. *Caffeine-containing foods and beverages (such as coffee, cola, chocolate):* increased CNS stimulation
Drug-herbs. *Ephedra (ma huang), caffeine-containing herbs (such as cola nut, guarana, maté):* increased CNS stimulation
Drug-behaviors. *Alcohol use:* additive hypotension

Patient monitoring

- Monitor patient periodically for drug tolerance and psychological dependence.
- Watch for adverse effects. Know that these usually can be controlled by adjusting schedule or dosage.
- Stay alert for tachycardia, abdominal pain, insomnia, anorexia, and weight loss (more common in children).
- Consider periodic hematologic and liver function tests, especially during prolonged therapy.
- Monitor blood pressure, especially in patients with history of hypertension.
- Evaluate child's weight and growth patterns.
- Assess child for tics, which may develop in 15% to 30% of children using drug.

Patient teaching

- Inform patient or parent that last daily dose should be taken several hours before bedtime to avoid insomnia.
- Make sure patient or parent understands how drug should be taken.
- Tell patient taking Concerta not to be concerned if tablet-like substance appears in stool.
- Advise patient or parent to report insomnia, palpitations, vomiting, fever, or rash.
- Caution patient or parent that continual use may lead to psychological or physical dependence.
- Instruct patient to avoid driving and other hazardous tasks until drug effects are known.
- As appropriate, review all other significant and life-threatening adverse reactions and interactions, especially those related to the drugs, foods, herbs, and behaviors mentioned above.

methylprednisolone
Medrol

methylprednisolone acetate
Depo-Medrol, Methysone✱, Unimed✱

methylprednisolone sodium succinate
A-Methapred, Solu-Medrol

Pharmacologic class: Glucocorticoid
Therapeutic class: Antiasthmatic, anti-inflammatory (steroidal), immunosuppressant
Pregnancy risk category C

Action
Unclear. Reduces inflammation and prevents edema by stabilizing membranes and reducing permeability of leukocytic cells. Suppresses immune system by interfering with antigen-antibody interactions of macrophages and T cells.

Availability
Solution for injection: 40 mg, 125 mg, 500 mg, 1 g, 2 g
Suspension for injection: 20 mg/ml, 40 mg/ml, 80 mg/ml
Tablets: 2 mg, 4 mg, 8 mg, 16 mg, 24 mg, 32 mg

Indications and dosages
➢ Diseases and disorders of endocrine system, collagen, skin, eye, GI tract, respiratory system, or hematologic system; neoplastic diseases; allergies; edema; multiple sclerosis; tuberculous meningitis; trichinosis; rheumatic disorders; osteoarthritis; bursitis; localized inflammatory lesions
Adults: *Methylprednisolone*—4 to 160 mg P.O. daily in four divided doses, depending on disease or disorder. *Acetate*—40 to 120 mg I.M., or 4 to 80 mg by intra-articular or soft-tissue injection, or 20 to 60 mg by intralesional injection (depending on type, size, and location of inflammation); may be repeated at 1 to 5 weeks. *Sodium succinate high-dose therapy*—30 mg/kg I.V. over at least 30 minutes. May be repeated q 4 to 6 hours for 48 hours.

Off-label uses
- Lupus nephritis
- *Pneumocystis jiroveci* pneumonia in AIDS patients

Contraindications
- Hypersensitivity to drug or its component
- Systemic fungal infections
- Use in premature infants (with sodium succinate form, which contains benzyl alcohol)

Precautions
Use cautiously in:
- cardiovascular, hepatic, renal, or GI disease; active untreated infections; thromboembolitic tendency; idiopathic thrombocytopenic purpura; osteoporosis; myasthenia gravis; hypothyroidism; glaucoma; ocular herpes simplex; vaccinia or varicella; seizure disorders; metastatic cancer
- pregnant or breastfeeding patients
- children.

Administration
- As needed and prescribed, give prophylactic antacids to prevent peptic ulcers in patients receiving high doses.
- When methylprednisolone acetate is substituted for oral form, know that I.M. dosage should equal oral dosage and should be given once daily.
- Know that methylprednisolone acetate is not for I.V. use. It may be giv-

m

en I.M. or by intra-articular, intralesional, or soft-tissue injection.
• Be aware that methylprednisolone sodium succinate may be given I.M. or I.V. Reconstitute with bacteriostatic water for injection containing 0.9% benzyl alcohol, per manufacturer's instructions.
• In long-term methylprednisolone therapy, alternate-day therapy should be considered.
• For direct I.V. injection, inject each 500-mg dose over 2 to 3 minutes or more. For I.V. infusion, further dilute in compatible I.V. solution (such as 5% dextrose, 0.9% sodium chloride, or 5% dextrose in 0.9% sodium chloride injection) and give over 10 to 20 minutes.
• Maintain patient on lowest effective dosage, to minimize adverse effects.

Route	Onset	Peak	Duration
P.O.	Rapid	2-3 hr	30-36 hr
I.M., I.V. (succinate)	Rapid	Unknown	Unknown
I.M. (acetate)	6-48 hr	4-8 days	1-4 wk

Adverse reactions

CNS: headache, restlessness, nervousness, depression, euphoria, personality changes, psychoses, vertigo, paresthesias, insomnia, adhesive arachnoiditis, conus medullaris syndrome, **increased intracranial pressure, seizures, meningitis**
CV: hypotension, hypertension, **arrhythmias, heart failure, shock, fat embolism, thrombophlebitis, thromboembolism**
EENT: cataracts, glaucoma, increased intraocular pressure, nasal irritation, nasal septum perforation, sneezing, epistaxis, nasopharyngeal or oropharyngeal fungal infection, dysphonia, hoarseness, throat irritation
GI: nausea, vomiting, abdominal distention, rectal bleeding, dry mouth, anorexia, esophageal candidiasis, **esophageal ulcer, peptic ulcer, pancreatitis**
GU: amenorrhea, irregular menses
Respiratory: cough, wheezing, **bronchospasm**
Metabolic: decreased growth (in children), reduced carbohydrate tolerance, diabetes mellitus, hyperglycemia, sodium and fluid retention, hypokalemia, hypocalcemia, cushingoid state (with long-term use), **hypothalamic-pituitary-adrenal suppression** (with systemic use beyond 5 days), **adrenal suppression** (with long-term, high-dose use), **acute adrenal insufficiency** (with abrupt withdrawal)
Musculoskeletal: muscle wasting, osteoporosis, osteonecrosis, tendon rupture, aseptic joint necrosis, muscle pain and weakness, steroid myopathy, spontaneous fractures (with long-term use)
Skin: facial edema, rash, pruritus, urticaria, contact dermatitis, acne, decreased wound healing, bruising, hirsutism, thin and fragile skin, petechiae, purpura, striae, subcutaneous fat atrophy, skin atrophy, acneiform lesions, angioedema
Other: anosmia, bad taste, increased appetite, weight gain (with long-term use), Churg-Strauss syndrome, increased susceptibility to infection, aggravation or masking of infections, impaired wound healing, atrophy at injection site, local pain and burning, irritation, hypersensitivity reaction

Interactions

Drug-drug. *Amphotericin B, mezlocillin, piperacillin, thiazide and loop diuretics, ticarcillin:* additive hypokalemia
Fluoroquinolones: increased risk of tendon rupture
Isoniazid, phenobarbital, phenytoin, rifampin: decreased methylprednisolone efficacy
Ketoconazole: decreased methylprednisolone clearance

Live-virus vaccines: decreased antibody response to vaccine, increased risk of adverse reactions
Nonsteroidal anti-inflammatory drugs: increased risk of adverse GI effects
Oral anticoagulants: altered anticoagulant requirement
Drug-diagnostic tests. *Calcium, potassium, thyroxine, triiodothyronine:* decreased levels
Cholesterol, glucose: increased levels
Nitroblue tetrazolium test for bacterial infection: false-negative result
Drug-herbs. *Echinacea:* increased immune stimulation
Ginseng: immunomodulation
Drug-behaviors. *Alcohol use:* increased risk of gastric irritation and ulcers

Patient monitoring

- Monitor fluid and electrolyte balance, weight, and blood pressure.
- With long-term or high-dose use, assess for cushingoid effects, such as moon face, central obesity, acne, abdominal striae, hypertension, osteoporosis, myopathy, hyperglycemia, fluid and electrolyte imbalances, and increased susceptibility to infection.

◀ Check for signs and symptoms of steroid-induced psychosis (delirium, euphoria, insomnia, mood swings, personality changes, and depression).

- Monitor growth and development in children on prolonged therapy.
- Know that therapy beyond 6 months increases risk of osteoporosis. Obtain baseline bone density mass, and provide teaching about lifestyle factors (such as weight-bearing exercise, proper diet, moderation of alcohol intake, and smoking cessation) and possible need for calcium, vitamin D, or bisphosphonate therapy.
- With long-term use, withdraw drug gradually.

◀ After dosage reduction or drug withdrawal, monitor patient for signs and symptoms of adrenal insufficiency.

Patient teaching

- Tell patient to take with food to minimize GI upset.
- Advise patient on chronic therapy to have periodic eye exams and to carry medical identification that states he's taking drug.
- Inform patient that drug increases risk for infection. Urge him to avoid exposure to people with infections such as measles and chickenpox. Tell him to contact prescriber if exposure occurs.
- Advise patient to report unusual weight gain, swelling, muscle weakness, black tarry stools, vomiting of blood, menstrual irregularities, sore throat, fever, or infection.

◀ Tell patient to immediately report signs or symptoms of adrenal insufficiency (including fatigue, appetite loss, nausea, vomiting, diarrhea, weight loss, weakness, and dizziness) after dosage reduction or drug withdrawal.

- Advise diabetic patient to monitor blood glucose level carefully.
- As appropriate, review all other significant and life-threatening adverse reactions and interactions, especially those related to the drugs, tests, herbs, and behaviors mentioned above.

metoclopramide hydrochloride

Apo-Metoclop✤, Maxeran✤, Nu-Metoclopramide✤, Octamide, Octamide-PFS, Reglan

Pharmacologic class: Dopamine antagonist

Therapeutic class: Antiemetic, GI stimulant

Pregnancy risk category B

m

Action

Blocks dopamine receptors by disrupting CNS chemoreceptor trigger zone, increasing peristalsis and promoting gastric emptying

Availability

Injection: 5 mg/ml
Solution: 5 mg/5 ml
Solution (concentrated): 10 mg/ml
Tablets: 5 mg, 10 mg

Indications and dosages

➢ To prevent chemotherapy-induced vomiting
Adults: 1 to 2 mg/kg I.V. 30 minutes before chemotherapy, then q 2 hours for two doses, then q 3 hours for three additional doses
➢ To facilitate small-bowel intubation; radiologic examination when delayed gastric emptying interferes
Adults and children older than age 14: 10 mg I.V. as a single dose
Children ages 6 to 14: 2.5 to 5 mg I.V. as a single dose
Children younger than age 6: 0.1 mg/kg I.V. as a single dose
➢ Diabetic gastroparesis
Adults: 10 mg P.O. 30 minutes before meals and at bedtime for 2 to 8 weeks. If patient can't tolerate P.O. doses, give same dosage I.V. or I.M.
➢ Gastroesophageal reflux
Adults: 10 to 15 mg P.O. 30 minutes before meals and at bedtime for up to 12 weeks. For prevention, single dose of 20 mg (some patients may respond to doses as small as 5 mg).
➢ Prevention of postoperative nausea and vomiting
Adults: 10 to 20 mg I.M. near end of surgical procedure. Repeat dose q 4 to 6 hours, as needed.

Dosage adjustment

- Renal impairment

Off-label uses

- Hiccups

Contraindications

- Hypersensitivity to drug
- Pheochromocytoma
- Parkinson's disease
- Suspected GI obstruction, perforation, or hemorrhage
- History of seizure disorders

Precautions

Use cautiously in:
- diabetes mellitus
- history of depression
- elderly patients
- pregnant or breastfeeding patients
- children.

Administration

- Mix oral solution with water, juice, carbonated beverage, or semisolid food (such as applesauce or pudding) just before administration.
- Give I.M. or direct I.V. without further dilution.
- Administer low doses (10 mg or less) by direct I.V. injection slowly over 2 minutes. (Rapid injection may cause intense anxiety and restlessness followed by drowsiness.)
- For I.V. infusion, dilute with 50 ml of 5% dextrose in 0.9% sodium chloride solution, 5% dextrose in 0.45% sodium chloride solution, or lactated Ringer's solution. Infuse over at least 15 minutes.

Route	Onset	Peak	Duration
P.O.	30-60 min	Unknown	1-2 hr
I.V.	1-3 min	Immediate	1-2 hr
I.M.	10-15 min	Unknown	1-2 hr

Adverse reactions

CNS: drowsiness, restlessness, anxiety, depression, irritability, fatigue, lassitude, insomnia, tardive dyskinesia, parkinsonian-like reactions, extrapyramidal reactions, akathisia, dystonia
CV: hypertension, hypotension, **arrhythmias**

GI: nausea, constipation, diarrhea, dry mouth
GU: gynecomastia

Interactions

Drug-drug. *Anticholinergics, opioids:* antagonism of metoclopramide's GI motility effect
Antidepressants, antihistamines, other CNS depressants (such as opioids, sedative-hypnotics): additive CNS depression
Cimetidine, digoxin: decreased blood levels of these drugs
General anesthetics: exaggerated hypotension
Haloperidol, phenothiazines: increased risk of extrapyramidal reactions
Levodopa: decreased metoclopramide efficacy
MAO inhibitors: increased catecholamine release
Drug-diagnostic tests. *Aldosterone, prolactin:* increased levels
Drug-behaviors. *Alcohol use:* increased blood alcohol level, increased CNS depression

Patient monitoring

- Monitor blood pressure during I.V. administration.
- Stay alert for depression and other adverse CNS effects.

Watch for extrapyramidal reactions, which usually occur within first 24 to 48 hours of therapy. To reverse these symptoms, give diphenhydramine 50 mg I.M. or benztropine 1 to 2 mg I.M., as prescribed.

- Check for development of parkinsonian-like symptoms, which may occur within first 6 months of therapy and usually subside within 2 to 3 months after withdrawal.
- With long-term use, assess patient for tardive dyskinesia.
- In diabetic patient, stay alert for gastric stasis. Insulin dosage may need to be adjusted.

Patient teaching

- Tell patient to take 30 minutes before meals.
- Instruct patient to report involuntary movements of face, eyes, or limbs.
- Caution patient to avoid driving and other hazardous activities until drug's effects are known.
- As appropriate, review all other significant and life-threatening adverse reactions and interactions, especially those related to the drugs, tests, and behaviors mentioned above.

metolazone

Zaroxolyn

Pharmacologic class: Thiazide-like diuretic
Therapeutic class: Diuretic, antihypertensive
Pregnancy risk category B

Action

Inhibits electrolyte reabsorption from ascending loop of Henle and decreases reabsorption of sodium and potassium in distal renal tubules, increasing plasma osmotic pressure and promoting diuresis

Availability

Tablets: 2.5 mg, 5 mg, 10 mg

Indications and dosages

➢ Hypertension
Adult: 2.5 to 5 mg P.O. daily.
➢ Edema caused by heart failure or renal disease
Adults: 5 to 20 mg P.O. daily

Contraindications

- Hypersensitivity to drug
- Hepatic coma or precoma
- Anuria

m

Precautions

Use cautiously in:
- severe hepatic or renal impairment, gout, hyperparathyroidism, glucose tolerance abnormalities, fluid or electrolyte imbalances, bipolar disorders
- elderly patients
- pregnant or breastfeeding patients
- children (safety not established).

Administration

- Give in morning to avoid frequent nighttime urination.
- Discontinue drug before parathyroid function tests are performed.
- Be aware that metolazone is the only thiazide-like diuretic that may cause diuresis in patients with glomerular filtration rates below 20 ml/minute.

Route	Onset	Peak	Duration
P.O.	1 hr	2 hr	12-24 hr

Adverse reactions

CNS: drowsiness, lethargy, vertigo, paresthesia, weakness, headache, fatigue
CV: chest pain, hypotension, palpitations, **venous thrombosis, arrhythmias**
GI: nausea, vomiting, bloating, cramping, anorexia, **pancreatitis**
GU: polyuria, nocturia, erectile dysfunction, decreased libido
Hematologic: aplastic anemia, leukopenia, agranulocytosis
Hepatic: hepatitis
Metabolic: dehydration, hypercalcemia, hypomagnesemia, hyponatremia, hypophosphatemia, hypovolemia, hyperglycemia, hyperuricemia, **hypokalemia, hypochloremic alkalosis**
Musculoskeletal: muscle cramps
Skin: photosensitivity, rashes
Other: chills

Interactions

Drug-drug. *Amphotericin B, corticosteroids, mezlocillin, piperacillin, ticarcillin:* additive hypokalemia
Antigout drugs: increased uric acid level
Antihypertensives, nitrates: additive hypotension
Digoxin: increased risk of digoxin toxicity
Lithium: decreased lithium excretion, increased risk of lithium toxicity
Drug-diagnostic tests. *Bilirubin, calcium, cholesterol, creatinine, low-density lipoproteins, triglycerides, uric acid:* increased levels
Blood glucose, urine glucose: increased levels in diabetic patients
Magnesium, potassium, protein-bound iodine, sodium, urinary calcium: decreased levels
Drug-food. *Any food:* increased metolazone absorption
Drug-herbs. *Aloe, cascara sagrada, senna:* increased risk of hypokalemia
Drug-behaviors. *Sun exposure:* increased risk of photosensitivity

Patient monitoring

- Monitor baseline and periodic electrolyte, blood urea nitrogen, glucose, and uric acid levels.
- Evaluate blood pressure regularly.

🔊 Watch for signs and symptoms of hypokalemia, which may necessitate potassium supplements, potassium-rich diet, or potassium-sparing diuretic. Hypokalemia is particularly dangerous to patients who are on digitalis or have had ventricular arrhythmias.
- Assess patient for fluid and electrolyte imbalances.

Patient teaching

- Advise patient to take in morning to avoid frequent nighttime urination.
- Tell patient he may take with food or milk to prevent GI upset.

🔊 Instruct patient to report muscle pain, weakness, or cramps; nausea; vomiting; diarrhea; dizziness; restlessness; excessive thirst; fatigue; drowsiness; increased pulse; or irregular heart beats.

• Inform patient that drug may cause gout attacks. Advise him to report sudden joint pain.
• Instruct patient to use sunscreen and protective clothing to avoid photosensitivity.
• As appropriate, review all other significant and life-threatening adverse reactions and interactions, especially those related to the drugs, tests, foods, herbs, and behaviors mentioned above.

metoprolol succinate
Toprol-XL

metoprolol tartrate
Apo-Metoprolol✤, Betaloc✤, Betaloc Durules✤, Lopresor SR✤, Lopressor, Novo-Metoprol✤, Nu-Metop✤, PMS-Metoprolol-L✤

Pharmacologic class: Beta-adrenergic blocker (selective)

Therapeutic class: Antihypertensive, antianginal

Pregnancy risk category C

Action
Blocks stimulation of $beta_1$ (myocardial) adrenergic receptors, usually without affecting $beta_2$ (pulmonary, vascular, uterine) adrenergic receptor sites

Availability
Injection (tartrate): 1 mg/ml
Tablets: 50 mg, 100 mg
Tablets (extended-release, succinate): 25 mg, 50 mg, 100 mg, 200 mg

Indications and dosages
➢ Hypertension
Adults: 50 to 100 mg P.O. daily as a single dose or in two divided doses (conventional tablets) or once daily (extended-release tablets). May be increased q 7 days as needed, up to 450 mg/day (tartrate) or 400 mg (succinate extended-release).
➢ Angina pectoris
Adults: 100 mg P.O. daily as a single dose or in two divided doses (conventional tablets) or once daily (extended-release tablets). May be increased q 7 days as needed, up to 400 mg.
➢ Acute myocardial infarction (MI)
Adults: Three bolus injections of 5 mg I.V. given at 2-minute intervals. If patient tolerates I.V. dose, give 50 mg P.O. 15 minutes after last I.V. dose, and continue P.O. doses q 6 hours for 48 hours. For maintenance, 100 mg P.O. b.i.d. If patient doesn't tolerate full I.V. dose, give 25 to 50 mg P.O. (depending on degree of intolerance), starting 15 minutes after last I.V. dose or when clinical condition allows; discontinue drug if patient shows severe intolerance. As late treatment, 100 mg P.O. b.i.d. when clinical condition allows, continued for at least 3 months.
➢ Symptomatic heart failure
Adults: 25 mg P.O. daily (extended-release tablets) in patients with NYHA Class II heart failure. Dosage may be doubled q 2 weeks, up to 200 mg/day or until highest tolerated dosage is reached. For more severe heart failure, start with 12.5 mg P.O. daily.

Off-label uses
• Ventricular arrhythmias, tachycardia
• Tremors
• Anxiety

Contraindications
• Sinus bradycardia, heart block greater than first degree, cardiogenic shock, overt cardiac failure (with Lopressor used for hypertension or angina)
• Heart rate below 45 beats/minute, second- or third-degree heart block, significant first-degree heart block; systolic pressure below 100 mm Hg; or moderate-to-severe cardiac failure (when Lopressor is used for MI)

• Hypersensitivity to drug or its components, severe bradycardia, heart block greater than first degree, cardiogenic shock, decompensated cardiac failure, sick sinus syndrome (unless permanent pacemaker is in place) (with Toprol-XL)

Precautions

Use cautiously in:
• renal or hepatic impairment, pulmonary disease, diabetes mellitus, thyrotoxicosis
• MAO inhibitor use within past 14 days
• pregnant or breastfeeding patients
• children (safety not established).

Administration

• Give metoprolol tartrate with or immediately after meals, because food enhances its absorption.
• Know that succinate extended-release tablets are scored and can be divided. However, tablet or half-tablet should be swallowed whole and not crushed or chewed.
• For I.V. administration, give each dose undiluted by direct injection over at least 1 minute.

Route	Onset	Peak	Duration
P.O.	15 min	1 hr	6-12 hr
P.O. (extended)	15 min	6-12 hr	24 hr
I.V.	Immediate	20 min	5-8 hr

Adverse reactions

CNS: fatigue, weakness, anxiety, depression, dizziness, drowsiness, insomnia, memory loss, mental status changes, nervousness, nightmares
CV: orthostatic hypotension, peripheral vasoconstriction, bradycardia, **heart failure, pulmonary edema**
EENT: blurred vision, stuffy nose
GI: nausea, vomiting, constipation, diarrhea, flatulence, gastric pain, heartburn, dry mouth
GU: urinary frequency, erectile dysfunction, decreased libido
Hepatic: hepatitis
Metabolic: hyperglycemia, **hypoglycemia**
Respiratory: wheezing, **bronchospasm**
Musculoskeletal: back pain, joint pain
Skin: rash
Other: drug-induced lupus syndrome

Interactions

Drug-drug. *Amphetamines, ephedrine, epinephrine, norepinephrine, phenylephrine, pseudoephedrine:* unopposed alpha-adrenergic stimulation (excessive hypertension, bradycardia)
Antihypertensives, nitrates: additive hypotension
Digoxin: additive bradycardia
Dobutamine, dopamine: reduced cardiovascular benefits of these drugs
General anesthestics, phenytoin (I.V.), verapamil: additive myocardial depression
Insulin, oral hypoglycemics: altered efficacy of these drugs
MAO inhibitors: hypertension
Drug-diagnostic tests. *Alanine aminotransferase, alkaline phosphatase, aspartate aminotransferase, blood urea nitrogen, glucose, lactate dehydrogenase, lipoproteins, potassium, triglycerides, uric acid:* increased levels
Drug-food. *Any food:* enhanced drug absorption
Drug-behaviors. *Acute alcohol ingestion:* additive hypotension
Cocaine use: unopposed alpha-adrenergic stimulation (excessive hypertension, bradycardia)

Patient monitoring

• Measure blood pressure closely when starting therapy and titrating dosage. Once patient stabilizes, measure blood pressure every 3 to 6 months.
• Monitor blood pressure and pulse before I.V. administration. If patient is

hypotensive or has bradycardia, consult prescriber before giving dose.
• Watch for orthostatic hypotension in at-risk patients, particularly the elderly.
• Assess glucose levels in diabetic patient. Be aware that drug may mask signs and symptoms of hypoglycemia.
• Monitor for signs and symptoms of hyperthyroidism. Know that drug may mask these. Reduce dosage gradually in hyperthyroid patients.
Clinical alert: When discontinuing drug, reduce dosage gradually over 1 to 2 weeks.

Patient teaching

• Advise patient to take with or immediately after meals.
• Tell patient that extended-release tablets are scored and can be divided, but that he should swallow tablets or half-tablets whole and not crush or chew them.
Clinical alert: Advise patient with heart failure to report signs or symptoms of worsening condition, including weight gain and increasing shortness of breath.
• Caution patient to avoid driving and other hazardous activities until drug effects are known.
• Instruct patient to notify health care providers (including dentists) that he is taking drug before having surgery.
• As appropriate, review all other significant and life-threatening adverse reactions and interactions, especially those related to the drugs, tests, foods, and behaviors mentioned above.

metronidazole

Apo-Metronidazole♣, Flagyl, Flagyl ER, Flagyl IV RTU, Metric 21, Metro IV, MetroCream, MetroGel, MetroGel-Vaginal, MetroLotion, Metromidol, Metryl, Nidagel♣, Noritate, PMS-Metronidazole♣, Protostat

metronidazole hydrochloride

Flagyl IV

Pharmacologic class: Nitroimidazole derivative
Therapeutic class: Anti-infective, antiprotozoal
Pregnancy risk category B

Action

Disturbs DNA synthesis in susceptible bacterial organisms

Availability

Capsules: 375 mg
Powder for injection: 5 mg/ml, 500-mg vials
Premixed injection: 500 mg/100 ml
Tablets: 250 mg, 500 mg
Tablets (extended-release): 750 mg
Topical cream, topical gel: 0.75% in 28.4-g tubes
Topical lotion: 0.75% in 59-ml bottle
Vaginal gel: 0.75% (37.5 mg/5-g applicator) in 70-g tubes

Indications and dosages

➢ Trichomoniasis
Adults: 2 g P.O. as a single dose or in two 1-g doses given on same day. Alternatively, 500 mg P.O. b.i.d. for 7 days.
➢ Bacterial infections
Adults: Initially, 15 mg/kg I.V., fol-

m

lowed by 7.5 mg/kg I.V. q 6 hours, not to exceed 4 g/day for 7 to 10 days
➢ Amebiasis
Adults: 750 mg P.O. q 8 hours for 5 to 10 days
➢ Amebic liver abscess
Adults: 500 to 750 mg P.O. t.i.d. for 5 to 10 days. If drug can't be given orally, administer 500 mg I.V. q 6 hours for 10 days.
Children: 35 to 50 mg/kg/day P.O. in three divided doses for 10 days, to a maximum of 750 mg/dose
➢ Bacterial vaginosis
Adults: In nonpregnant patients, 750 mg/day P.O. (extended-release) for 7 days or 5 g of 0.75% vaginal gel b.i.d. for 5 days. In pregnant patients, 250 mg P.O. t.i.d. for 7 days.
➢ Perioperative prophylaxis in colorectal surgery
Adults: Initially, 15 mg/kg I.V. infusion over 30 to 60 minutes, completed 1 hour before surgery; if necessary, 7.5 mg/kg I.V. infusion over 30 to 60 minutes at 6 and 12 hours after initial dose
➢ Rosacea
Adults: Rub a thin layer of topical lotion, gel, or cream onto entire affected area morning and evening. Improvement should occur within 3 weeks.

Contraindications
- Hypersensitivity to drug, other nitroimidazole derivatives, or parabens (topical form only)
- First-trimester pregnancy in patients with trichomoniasis

Precautions
Use cautiously in:
- severe hepatic impairment
- history of blood dyscrasias, seizures, or other neurologic problems
- breastfeeding patients
- children.

Administration
- Reconstitute powder for injection by adding 4.4 ml of sterile or bacteriostatic water for injection, 0.9% sodium chloride injection, or bacteriostatic sodium chloride injection to 500-mg vial. Further dilute resulting concentration (100 mg/ml) in 0.9% sodium chloride injection, 5% dextrose injection, or lactated Ringer's injection solution to a concentration of 8 mg/ml or less. Infuse each I.V. dose over 1 hour.
- Be aware that for I.V. injection, drug need not be diluted or neutralized.
- Don't use equipment containing aluminum to reconstitute or transfer reconstituted solution to diluent; solution may turn reddish-brown.
- Don't interchange vaginal gel with topical gel, cream, or lotion.

Route	Onset	Peak	Duration
P.O.	Rapid	1-3 hr	8 hr
P.O. (extended)	Rapid	Unknown	Up to 24 hr
I.V.	Rapid	End of infusion	6-8 hr
Topical	Unknown	6-12 hr	Unknown
Vaginal	Unknown	6-12 hr	12 hr

Adverse reactions
CNS: dizziness, headache, ataxia, vertigo, incoordination, insomnia, fatigue
EENT: rhinitis, sinusitis, pharyngitis
GI: nausea, vomiting, diarrhea, abdominal pain, furry tongue, glossitis, dry mouth, anorexia
GU: dysuria, dark urine, incontinence
Hematologic: leukopenia
Skin: rash, urticaria, burning, mild skin dryness, skin irritation, transient redness (with topical forms)
Other: unpleasant or metallic taste, superinfection, phlebitis at I.V. site

Interactions
Drug-drug. *Azathioprine, fluorouracil:* increased risk of leukopenia
Cimetidine: decreased metronidazole metabolism, increased risk of toxicity
Disulfiram: acute psychosis and confusion

Lithium: increased lithium blood level
Phenobarbital: increased metronidazole metabolism, decreased efficacy
Warfarin: increased warfarin effects
Drug-diagnostic tests. *Alanine aminotransferase, aspartate aminotransferase, lactate dehydrogenase:* altered levels
Drug-behaviors. *Alcohol use:* disulfiram-like reaction

Patient monitoring

- Monitor I.V. site. Avoid prolonged use of indwelling catheter.
- Evaluate hematologic studies, especially in patients with history of blood dyscrasias.

Patient teaching

- Advise patient to take drug with food if it causes GI upset. However, instruct him to take extended-release tablets 1 hour before or 2 hours after meals.
- Tell patient with trichomoniasis to refrain from sexual intercourse or to have male partner wear a condom to prevent reinfection. Explain that asymptomatic sex partners should be treated simultaneously.
- Advise patient to report fever, sore throat, bleeding, or bruising.
- Inform patient that drug may cause metallic taste and may discolor urine deep brownish-red.
- Tell patient using topical form to clean area thoroughly with mild cleanser before use and then wait 15 to 20 minutes before applying drug. Tell her she may apply cosmetics to skin after applying drug; with topical lotion, instruct her to let skin dry at least 5 minutes before applying cosmetics.
- Tell female patient to consult prescriber if she is pregnant or plans to become pregnant.
- As appropriate, review all other significant and life-threatening adverse reactions and interactions, especially those related to the drugs, tests, and behaviors mentioned above.

mexiletine hydrochloride

Mexitil, Novo-Mexiletine✤

Pharmacologic class: Lidocaine-like agent
Therapeutic class: Antiarrhythmic (class IB)
Pregnancy risk category C

Action

Decreases duration of action potential and effective refractory period in cardiac conduction tissue by altering sodium transport across myocardial cell membranes

Availability

Capsules: 150 mg, 200 mg, 250 mg

Indications and dosages

➢ Serious ventricular arrhythmias, including sustained ventricular tachycardia
Adults: Initially, 200 mg P.O. q 8 hours when rapid control isn't essential; may adjust dosage by 50 to 100 mg q 2 to 3 days. When rapid control is needed, give initial loading dose of 400 mg P.O., followed by 200 mg in 8 hours.

Off-label uses

- Pain, dysesthesias, paresthesias associated with diabetes mellitus

Contraindications

- Cardiogenic shock
- Second- or third-degree heart block (in patients without pacemakers)

Precautions

Use cautiously in:
- sinus node or intraventricular conduction abnormalities, heart failure, hypotension, seizure disorder, severe hepatic impairment
- pregnant or breastfeeding patients
- children (safety not established).

m

Administration

🔊 Be aware that therapy should be initiated in hospital setting. Also, drug is reserved for life-threatening ventricular arrhythmias and shouldn't be used to treat asymptomatic premature ventricular contractions.

- When switching patient to mexiletine from lidocaine, stop lidocaine infusion as soon as first oral mexiletine dose is given, but maintain I.V. line until heart rhythm is satisfactory.
- When switching patient to mexiletine from other class I oral antiarrhythmics, give mexiletine as prescribed and titrate to response.

Route	Onset	Peak	Duration
P.O.	30 min-2 hr	2-3 hr	8-12 hr

Adverse reactions

CNS: dizziness, nervousness, confusion, fatigue, headache, sleep disorder, tremor, poor coordination, paresthesia
CV: chest pain, edema, palpitations, **new or increased arrhythmias**
EENT: blurred vision, tinnitus
GI: nausea, vomiting, heartburn
Hematologic: leukopenia, neutropenia, agranulocytosis, thrombocytopenia
Hepatic: hepatic necrosis
Respiratory: dyspnea
Skin: rash

Interactions

Drug-drug. *Antacids, atropine, opioids:* slow mexiletine absorption
Cimetidine: increased or decreased mexiletine blood level
Metoclopramide: increased mexiletine absorption
Other antiarrhythmics: additive cardiac effects
Phenobarbital, phenytoin, rifampin: increased mexiletine metabolism, decreased efficacy
Theophylline: increased theophylline blood level, greater risk of toxicity
Urine acidifiers: increased mexiletine excretion, decreased blood level
Urine alkalizers: decreased mexiletine excretion, increased blood level
Drug-diagnostic tests. *Antinuclear antibodies:* positive titers
Aspartate aminotransferase: transient increase
Platelets: decreased count (usually returns to normal within 1 month after drug withdrawal)
Drug-food. *Foods that drastically alter urine pH:* altered mexiletine blood level
Caffeine: 50% decrease in caffeine clearance
Drug-behaviors. *Cigarette smoking:* increased mexiletine metabolism, decreased efficacy

Patient monitoring

- Monitor vital signs and ECG frequently when initiating therapy.
- Evaluate liver function tests and hematologic studies.

🔊 Watch for early evidence of toxicity (dizziness, tremor, poor coordination). With increasing toxicity, patient may develop hypotension, sinus bradycardia, ventricular arrhythmias, and seizures. Therapeutic mexiletine blood level is 0.5 to 2 mcg/ml.

Patient teaching

- Tell patient to take with food or antacids if adverse GI reactions occur.
- Advise patient to avoid dietary changes that would markedly alter urine pH.
- Inform patient that drug may cause nausea, vomiting, diarrhea, constipation, heartburn, dizziness, tremor, nervousness, poor coordination, changes in sleep pattern, headache, visual disturbances, tingling or numbness, ringing in ears, and palpitations or chest pain. Tell him to contact prescriber if these effects are bothersome or severe.

🔊 Tell patient to immediately report tiredness, yellowing of skin or eyes, flu-like symptoms, fever, or sore throat.

• As appropriate, review all other significant and life-threatening adverse reactions and interactions, especially those related to the drugs, tests, foods, and behaviors mentioned above.

midazolam hydrochloride

Apo-Midazolam✦, Versed, Versed Syrup

Pharmacologic class: Benzodiazepine
Therapeutic class: Anxiolytic, sedative-hypnotic, adjunct for general anesthesia induction
Controlled substance schedule IV
Pregnancy risk category D

Action

Unknown. Thought to suppress CNS stimulation at limbic and subcortical levels by enhancing the effects of gamma-aminobutyric acid, an inhibitory neurotransmitter.

Availability

Injection: 1 mg/ml, 5 mg/ml
Syrup: 2 mg/ml

Indications and dosages

➢ To induce general anesthesia
Adults younger than age 55: 0.3 to 0.35 mg/kg I.V. over 20 to 30 seconds if patient hasn't received premedication, or 0.15 to 0.35 mg/kg (usual dosage of 0.25 mg/kg) I.V. over 20 to 30 seconds if patient has received premedication. Wait 2 minutes to evaluate effect. Additional increments of 25% of initial dosage may be needed to complete induction.

➢ Continuous infusion to initiate sedation
Adults: When rapid sedation is required, give loading dose of 0.01 to 0.05 mg/kg I.V. slowly; repeat dose q 10 to 15 minutes until adequate sedation occurs. To maintain sedation, infuse at initial rate of 0.02 to 0.10 mg/kg/hour (1 to 7 mg/hour). Adjust infusion rate as needed.

➢ Preoperative sedation, anxiolysis, and amnesia
Adults: 0.07 to 0.08 mg/kg I.M. 30 minutes to 1 hour before surgery. For I.V. administration in healthy adults younger than age 60, give initial dose of 1 mg and titrate slowly to effect. Some patients may respond adequately to 1-mg dose. Don't give more than 2.5 mg over a 2-minute period. Total dosage above 5 mg is rarely necessary. Wait at least 2 minutes after additional doses to assess effect.

➢ Anxiolysis and amnesia before diagnostic, therapeutic, and endoscopic procedures or anesthesia induction
Children: 0.25 to 0.5 mg/kg P.O. as a single dose. Maximum dosage is 20 mg.

Dosage adjustment

• Elderly patients
• Children or neonates

Contraindications

• Hypersensitivity to drug, its components, or other benzodiazepines
• Acute closed-angle glaucoma
• Allergy to cherries (syrup preparation)

Precautions

Use cautiously in:
• pulmonary disease, heart failure, renal impairment, severe hepatic impairment
• obese pediatric patients
• elderly or debilitated patients
• pregnant or breastfeeding patients
• children and neonates.

Administration

Keep oxygen and resuscitation equipment at hand in case severe respiratory depression occurs.
• Inject I.M. deep into large muscle mass.

• Know that drug may be mixed in same syringe as meperidine, atropine, scopolamine, or morphine.
• Dilute concentrate for I.V. infusion to 0.5 mg/ml using dextrose 5% in water or normal saline solution. Infuse over at least 2 minutes; then wait at least 2 minutes before giving second dose. Be aware that excessive dosage or rapid I.V. delivery may cause severe respiratory depression.
• Give oral form with liquid, but never with grapefruit juice.

Route	Onset	Peak	Duration
P.O.	10-20 min	45-60 min	2-6 hr
I.V.	1.5-5 min	Rapid	2-6 hr
I.M.	15 min	15-60 min	2-6 hr

Adverse reactions

CNS: headache, oversedation, drowsiness, agitation and excitement (in children)
CV: hypotension, irregular pulse, bradycardia, **arrhythmias, cardiac arrest**
GI: nausea, vomiting
Respiratory: decreased respiratory rate, hiccups, **apnea, respiratory arrest**
Other: pain and tenderness at injection site

Interactions

Drug-drug. *CNS depressants (such as some antidepressants, antihistamines, barbiturates, opioids, tranquilizers), respiratory depressants:* potentiation of CNS effects of these drugs
Diltiazem, verapamil: increased midazolam blood level
Erythromycin: decreased midazolam clearance
Hormonal contraceptives: prolonged midazolam half-life
Rifampin: decreased midazolam blood level
Theophylline: increased sedative effect of midazolam
Drug-food. *Grapefruit juice:* increased bioavailability of oral midazolam
Drug-herbs. *Chamomile, kava, skullcap, valerian:* increased CNS depression
Drug-behaviors. *Alcohol use:* potentiation of midazolam effects

Patient monitoring

• Monitor vital signs, ECG, respiratory status, and oxygen saturation.
• Assess neurologic status closely, especially in pediatric patient.
• Watch for nausea and vomiting.

Patient teaching

• Advise patient that drug causes perioperative amnesia.
• If patient will use oral drug at home, instruct him to take it with liquid but never grapefruit juice.
• Caution patient to avoid driving and other hazardous activities until he knows how drug affects concentration and alertness.
• Tell female patient to inform prescriber is she is pregnant or breastfeeding.
• As appropriate, review all other significant and life-threatening adverse reactions and interactions, especially those related to the drugs, foods, herbs, and behaviors mentioned above.

midodrine hydrochloride

Amatine✤, ProAmatine

Pharmacologic class: Alpha$_1$-adrenergic agonist

Therapeutic class: Antihypotensive, vasopressor

Pregnancy risk category C

Action

Forms active metabolite, desglymidodrine, an alpha$_1$-adrenergic agonist that activates alpha-adrenergic receptors in arteriolar and venous vasculature. This effect increases vascular resistance and ultimately raises blood pressure.

Availability

Tablets: 2.5 mg, 5 mg

Indications and dosages

➢ Symptomatic orthostatic hypotension

Adults: 10 mg P.O. t.i.d. during daytime hours with patient in upright position. Give first dose when patient arises in morning, second dose at midday, and third dose in late afternoon.

Dosage adjustment

- Renal impairment

Contraindications

- Severe coronary artery disease or organic heart disease
- Acute renal disease, urinary retention
- Pheochromocytoma
- Thyrotoxicosis
- Persistent, excessive supine hypertension

Precautions

Use cautiously in:

- renal or hepatic impairment, diabetes mellitus, vision problems
- pregnant or breastfeeding patients.

Administration

- Don't give within 4 hours of bedtime.

Route	Onset	Peak	Duration
P.O.	Rapid	1-2 hr	Unknown

Adverse reactions

CNS: paresthesia
CV: vasodilation, bradycardia, **supine hypertension**
GI: abdominal pain, dry mouth
GU: urinary retention, frequency, or urgency
Skin: rash, pruritus, piloerection
Other: chills, increased pain

Interactions

Drug-drug. *Alpha- and beta-adrenergic blockers, cardiac glycosides, steroids:* increased risk of bradycardia, atrioventricular block
Alpha-adrenergic blockers, fludrocortisone: increased risk of supine hypertension

Patient monitoring

- Monitor supine and sitting blood pressures closely. Report marked rise in supine blood pressure.
- Stay alert for paresthesias.
- Monitor kidney function studies and fluid intake and output. Watch for urinary frequency, urgency, or retention.

Patient teaching

🔊 Instruct patient to take while in upright position.

- Tell patient to take first dose as soon as he arises for the day, second dose at midday, and third dose in late afternoon (before 6 P.M.). Stress that doses must be taken at least 3 hours apart. Advise patient not to take drug after dinner or within 4 hours of bedtime.

🔊 Instruct patient to promptly report symptoms of supine hypertension (pounding in ears, blurred vision, headache).

- Caution patient to avoid driving and other hazardous activities until he knows how drug affects concentration, vision, and alertness.
- As appropriate, review all other significant and life-threatening adverse reactions and interactions, especially those related to the drugs mentioned above.

m

mifepristone (RU-486)

Mifeprex

Pharmacologic class: Synthetic steroid
Therapeutic class: Antiprogestational agent, abortifacient
Pregnancy risk category NR

Action

Antagonizes progesterone receptor sites, inhibiting activity of endogenous and exogenous progesterone and stimulating uterine contractions, which causes fetus to separate from placental wall

Availability

Tablets: 200 mg

Indications and dosages

➢ Termination of intrauterine pregnancy through day 49 of pregnancy
Adults: On day 1, mifepristone 600 mg P.O. as a single dose. On day 3, misoprostol 400 mcg P.O. (unless abortion has been confirmed).

Contraindications

- Hypersensitivity to drug, misoprostol, or other prostaglandins
- Confirmed or suspected ectopic pregnancy or adnexal mass
- Chronic adrenal failure
- Bleeding disorders
- Concurrent anticoagulant therapy or long-term corticosteroid therapy
- Presence of intrauterine device (IUD)
- Inherited porphyrias

Precautions

Use cautiously in:
- cardiovascular, respiratory, renal, or hepatic disorders; hypertension; type 1 diabetes mellitus; anemia; jaundice; seizure disorder; cervicitis; infected endocervical lesions; acute vaginitis; uterine scarring.

Administration

- Before giving, make sure patient doesn't have an IUD in place.
- Give only in health care facility under supervision of health care provider qualified to assess pregnancy stage and rule out ectopic pregnancy.
- Administer with fluids, but not with grapefruit juice.
- Confirm pregnancy termination 14 days after initial dose.

Route	Onset	Peak	Duration
P.O.	Rapid	90 min	11 days

Adverse reactions

CNS: dizziness, fainting, headache, weakness, fatigue, insomnia, asthenia, anxiety, syncope, rigors
EENT: sinusitis
GI: nausea, vomiting, diarrhea, abdominal cramping, dyspepsia
GU: vaginitis, leukorrhea, uterine cramping, pelvic pain, **uterine hemorrhage**
Hematologic: anemia
Musculoskeletal: leg pain, back pain
Skin: fever
Other: viral infections

Interactions

Drug-drug. *Carbamazepine, dexamethasone, phenobarbital, phenytoin, rifampin:* decreased mifepristone blood level and effects
Drugs metabolized by CYP450-3A4: decreased mifepristone metabolism and increased effects
Erythromycin, itraconazole, ketoconazole: inhibited mifepristone metabolism and increased blood level
Drug-diagnostic tests. *Hematocrit, hemoglobin:* decreased values
Red blood cells: decreased count
Drug-food. *Grapefruit juice:* decreased mifepristone blood level and effects

Patient monitoring

- Assess vital signs, breath sounds, and bowel sounds.

- Monitor uterine contractions and type and amount of vaginal bleeding.
- Evaluate CBC.

Patient teaching

- After administration, tell patient she'll need to return in 48 hours for a prostaglandin drug or to verify pregnancy termination.
- Tell patient she'll have contractions for 3 or more hours after receiving drug and that vaginal bleeding may last 9 to 16 days.
- Instruct patient to contact prescriber if she has persistent or extremely heavy vaginal bleeding, extreme fatigue, or orthostatic hypotension.
- Caution patient that vaginal bleeding does not prove that complete abortion has occurred. Tell her she'll need follow-up appointment 2 weeks later to verify pregnancy termination.
- Inform patient that she's at risk for pregnancy right after abortion is complete. Encourage appropriate contraceptive decision.
- As appropriate, review all other significant and life-threatening adverse reactions and interactions, especially those related to the drugs, tests, and foods mentioned above.

miglitol

Glyset

Pharmacologic class: Alpha-glucosidase inhibitor
Therapeutic class: Hypoglycemic
Pregnancy risk category B

Action

Inhibits alpha-glucosidases, which convert oligosaccharides and disaccharides to glucose. This inhibition causes blood glucose reduction (especially in postprandial hyperglycemia).

Availability

Tablets: 25 mg, 50 mg, 100 mg

Indications and dosages

➢ Adjunct to diet in non-insulin-dependent (type 2) diabetes mellitus or combined with a sulfonylurea when diet plus either miglitol or a sulfonylurea alone doesn't control hyperglycemia

Adults: 25 mg P.O. t.i.d. with first bite of each main meal. After 4 to 8 weeks, may increase to 50 mg P.O. t.i.d. After 3 months, adjust dosage further based on glycosylated hemoglobin (HbA1c) level, to a maximum of 100 mg P.O. t.i.d.

Contraindications

- Hypersensitivity to drug or its components
- Insulin-dependent (type 1) diabetes mellitus, diabetic ketoacidosis
- Chronic intestinal disorder associated with marked digestive or absorptive disorders or conditions that may deteriorate due to increased gas formation
- Inflammatory bowel disease, colonic ulceration, partial intestinal obstruction, or predisposition to intestinal obstruction

Precautions

Use cautiously in:
- significant renal impairment (safety not established)
- fever, infection, trauma, stress
- pregnant or breastfeeding patients
- children (safety not established).

Administration

- Give with first bite of three main meals.

Route	Onset	Peak	Duration
P.O.	Unknown	2-3 hr	Unknown

Adverse reactions

GI: abdominal pain, diarrhea, flatulence
Skin: rash

Interactions

Drug-drug. *Digestive enzyme preparations (such as amylase), intestinal absorbents (such as charcoal):* reduced miglitol efficacy
Digoxin, propranolol, ranitidine: decreased bioavailability of these drugs
Drug-diagnostic tests. *Serum iron:* below-normal level
Drug-food. *Carbohydrates:* increased diarrhea

Patient monitoring

- Monitor CBC, blood glucose, and HBA1c levels.
- Watch for hyperglycemia or hypoglycemia, especially if patient also takes insulin or oral sulfonylureas.

Patient teaching

- Instruct patient to take drug three times daily with first bite of three main meals.
- Advise patient to take drug as prescribed. If appropriate, tell him he may need insulin during periods of increased stress, infection, or surgery.
- Teach patient about diabetes. Stress importance of proper diet, exercise, weight control, and blood glucose monitoring.
- Inform patient that sucrose (as in table sugar) and fruit juice don't effectively treat miglitol-induced hypoglycemia. Advise him to use dextrose or glucagon instead to raise blood glucose level quickly.
- Tell patient drug may cause abdominal pain, diarrhea, and gas. Reassure him that these effects usually subside after several weeks.
- As appropriate, review all other significant adverse reactions and interactions, especially those related to the drugs, tests, and foods mentioned above.

milrinone lactate

Primacor

Pharmacologic class: Bipyridine phosphodiesterase inhibitor
Therapeutic class: Inotropic
Pregnancy risk category C

Action

Increases cellular levels of cyclic adenosine monophosphate, causing inotropic action that relaxes vascular smooth muscle and increases myocardial contractility

Availability

Injection: 1 mg/ml in 10-, 20-, and 50-ml vials
Injection (premixed): 200 mcg/ml in dextrose 5% in water (D_5W)

Indications and dosages

➢ Heart failure

Adults: Initially, 50 mcg/kg I.V. bolus given slowly over 10 minutes, followed by continuous I.V. infusion of 0.375 to 0.75 mcg/kg/minute. Don't exceed total daily dosage of 1.13 mg/kg.

Dosage adjustment

- Renal impairment

Contraindications

- Hypersensitivity to drug

Precautions

Use cautiously in:

- atrial flutter or fibrillation, supraventricular and ventricular arrhythmias, renal impairment, electrolyte abnormalities, decreased blood pressure, severe aortic or pulmonic valvular disease, acute phase of myocardial infarction (not recommended), electrolyte abnormalities, abnormal blood digoxin level

- elderly patients
- pregnant or breastfeeding patients
- children (safety and efficacy not established).

Administration

- Dilute 1 mg/ml solution with half-normal saline solution, normal saline solution, or D_5W per manufacturer's instructions.

Clinical alert: Don't administer through same I.V. line as furosemide or torsemide (precipitate will form).

- Deliver I.V. slowly over 10 minutes.
- Expect to titrate infusion rate depending on response.

Route	Onset	Peak	Duration
I.V.	5-15 min	1-2 hr	3-6 hr

Adverse reactions

CNS: headache

CV: hypotension, chest pain, angina, **ventricular or supraventricular arrhythmias, ventricular tachycardia or fibrillation**

Interactions

None significant

Patient monitoring

- Monitor vital signs and ECG. Watch closely for ventricular arrhythmias, sustained tachycardia, and fibrillation.
- Assess cardiovascular status closely. Stay alert for complaints of chest pain.

Clinical alert: Stop drug and contact prescriber immediately if patient's systolic pressure drops 30 mm Hg or more.

Patient teaching

- Instruct patient to change position slowly, to avoid light-headedness or dizziness from hypotension.
- As appropriate, review all other significant and life-threatening adverse reactions.

minocycline hydrochloride

Alti-Minocycline (Canada), Arestin, Gen-Minocycline (Canada), Minocin, Novo-Minocycline (Canada), Vectrin

Pharmacologic class: Tetracycline
Therapeutic class: Anti-infective
Pregnancy risk category D

Action

Binds reversibly to 30S ribosome, inhibiting bacterial protein synthesis

Availability

Capsules: 50 mg, 75 mg, 100 mg
Capsules (pellet-filled): 50 mg, 100 mg
Microspheres (sustained-release): 1 mg
Powder for injection: 100 mg/vial
Suspension: 50 mg/5 ml
Tablets: 50 mg, 75 mg, 100 mg

m

Indications and dosages

➢ Infections caused by susceptible organisms

Adults: Initially, 200 mg P.O. or I.V., then 100 mg P.O. q 12 hours or 50 mg P.O. q 6 hours

Children ages 8 and older: 4 mg/kg P.O. or I.V., followed by 2 mg/kg q 12 hours

➢ Gonorrhea in penicillin-sensitive patients

Adults: Initially, 200 mg P.O., then 100 mg q 12 hours for at least 4 days

➢ Uncomplicated gonococcal urethritis in men

Adults: 100 mg P.O. q 12 hours for 5 days

➢ Syphilis

Adults: Initially, 200 mg P.O., then 100 mg q 12 hours for 10 to 15 days

➢ Acne

Adults: 50 mg P.O. one to three times daily

Dosage adjustment
• Renal impairment

Contraindications
• Hypersensitivity to drug, its components, or tetracyclines

Precautions
Use cautiously in:
• sulfite sensitivity, renal disease, hepatic impairment, nephrogenic diabetes insipidus
• cachectic or debilitated patients
• pregnant (last half of pregnancy) or breastfeeding patients
• children younger than age 8 (not recommended).

Administration
• Ask patient about sulfite sensitivity before giving.
• Give oral form with 8 oz. of water, with or without food.
• For I.V. use, add 5 ml of sterile water to 100 mg of powder for injection. Dilute further in 500 to 1,000 ml, to a final concentration of 100 to 200 mcg/ml. Infuse over 6 hours.
• Know that drug is used in penicillin-sensitive patients.

Route	Onset	Peak	Duration
P.O.	Unknown	1-4 hr	Unknown
I.V.	Immediate	End of infusion	Unknown

Adverse reactions
CNS: headache
CV: pericarditis
EENT: pharyngitis
GI: nausea, vomiting, diarrhea, oral candidiasis, stomatitis, mouth ulcers
GU: bladder or vaginal yeast infection
Metabolic: eosinophilia, **hemolytic anemia, thrombocytopenia**
Skin: photosensitivity, rash
Other: dental caries; dental infection; gingivitis; periodontitis; tooth disorder, pain, or discoloration; phlebitis at I.V. site; superinfection; hypersensitivity reactions including **anaphylaxis**

Interactions
Drug-drug. *Adsorbent antidiarrheals:* decreased minocycline absorption
Antacids containing aluminum, calcium, or magnesium; calcium, iron, and magnesium supplements; sodium bicarbonate: decreased minocycline absorption (with oral use)
Cholestyramine, colestipol: decreased oral absorption of minocycline
Hormonal contraceptives: decreased contraceptive efficacy
Methoxyflurane: nephrotoxicity
Penicillin: interference with bactericidal action of penicillin
Sucralfate: blocked absorption of minocycline
Warfarin: increased anticoagulant effect
Drug-diagnostic tests. *Alanine aminotransferase, alkaline phosphatase, amylase, aspartate aminotransferase, bilirubin, blood urea nitrogen:* increased levels
Hemoglobin, platelets, neutrophils, white blood cells: decreased levels
Urinary catecholamines: false elevation
Drug-food. *Dairy products:* decreased minocycline absorption
Drug-behaviors. *Alcohol use:* decreased antibiotic effect
Sun exposure: increased risk of photosensitivity reaction

Patient monitoring
• Assess patient's oral health closely for dental problems.
• Monitor patient for superinfection, especially oral, bladder, and vaginal yeast infections.
• Evaluate CBC and renal and liver function tests frequently.
Watch closely for hypersensitivity reactions, including anaphylaxis.

Patient teaching

- Tell patient he may take oral form with or without food, followed by a full glass of water. Instruct him to space doses evenly over 24 hours and to take one dose 1 hour before bedtime.
- Advise patient not to take oral form with antacids or iron, calcium, or magnesium products.

Instruct patient to immediately report fever, chills, skin rash, unusual bleeding or bruising, sore throat, or mouth pain or discomfort.

- Stress importance of good oral hygiene to minimize adverse oral and dental effects.
- Tell patient to complete entire course of therapy even after symptoms improve.

Caution patient not to use outdated minocycline because it may cause serious kidney disease.

- Inform female patient that drug may make hormonal contraceptives ineffective. Urge her to use barrier contraception.
- Tell pregnant patient that drug may stain fetus' teeth if taken during last half of pregnancy.
- Advise female patient to tell prescriber if she's breastfeeding.
- As appropriate, review all other significant and life-threatening adverse reactions and interactions, especially those related to the drugs, tests, foods, and behaviors mentioned above.

minoxidil

Apo-Gain✱, Gen-Minoxidil✱, Hairgro✱, Loniten, Minodyl, Minox✱, Minoxigaine✱, Rogaine, Rogaine Extra Strength

Pharmacologic class: Peripheral vasodilator (direct-acting)

Therapeutic class: Antihypertensive, hair growth stimulant

Pregnancy risk category C

Action

Reduces blood pressure by relaxing vascular smooth muscle, causing vasodilation. Action in hair growth stimulation unclear; vasodilatory action may enhance microcirculation around hair follicles.

m

Availability

Tablets: 2.5 mg, 10 mg
Topical solution: 2%, 5%

Indications and dosages

➤ Severe symptomatic hypertension; hypertension associated with end-organ damage

Adults and children ages 12 and older: 5 mg/day as a single dose, increased carefully q 3 days. Usual range is 10 to 40 mg/day in single or divided doses. For rapid blood pressure control with careful monitoring, dosage may be adjusted q 6 hr. Maximum dosage is 100 mg/day.

Children younger than age 12: 0.2 mg/kg/day P.O. as a single dose. May increase in increments of 50% to 100% until blood pressure control is optimal. Usual range is 0.25 to 1 mg/kg/day; maximum recommended dosage is 50 mg/day.

➤ Male-pattern baldness; diffuse hair loss or thinning in women; adjunct to hair transplantation

Adults: Apply 1 ml of 2% or 5% topical solution to affected area b.i.d. for 4 months or longer.

➢ Alopecia areata

Adults: Apply 1 ml of 2% or 5% topical solution to scalp b.i.d.

Contraindications

- Hypersensitivity to drug or its components
- Dissecting aortic aneurysm
- Pheochromocytoma

Precautions

Use cautiously in:

- recent MI, malignant hypertension, heart failure, angina pectoris, severe renal impairment
- concurrent guanethidine therapy
- pregnant or breastfeeding patients.

Administration

- Give oral form with meals to decrease GI upset.

🔊 If patient is also receiving guanethidine, discontinue that drug 1 to 3 days before starting minoxidil, to avoid severe orthostatic hypotension.

- Know that oral form usually is given with a beta-adrenergic blocker or diuretic to control hypertension.

Route	Onset	Peak	Duration
P.O.	30 min	2-3 hr	2-5 days
Topical	Unknown	Unknown	Unknown

Adverse reactions

CV: ECG changes (such as T-wave changes), tachycardia, angina, **pericardial effusion, cardiac tamponade, heart failure**

GI: nausea, vomiting

Respiratory: pulmonary edema

Skin: hypertrichosis

Other: weight gain, edema

Interactions

Drug-drug. *Antihypertensives, nitrates:* additive hypotension

Guanethidine: severe orthostatic hypotension

Nonsteroidal anti-inflammatory drugs: decreased minoxidil efficacy

Drug-diagnostic tests. *Alkaline phosphatase, blood urea nitrogen, creatinine, plasma renin activity, sodium:* increased levels

Hematocrit, hemoglobin, red blood cells: decreased levels

Patient monitoring

- Monitor vital signs and ECG.
- Assess daily weight and fluid intake and output.

🔊 Monitor cardiovascular status carefully. Stay alert for signs and symptoms of heart failure.

- Watch for hypertrichosis.
- Know that hematologic and renal values usually return to pretreatment levels with continued therapy.

Patient teaching

- Instruct patient to take oral form with meals to decrease GI upset.
- Advise patient to weigh himself daily and report sudden gains.
- Tell patient taking oral form that drug may darken, lengthen, and thicken body hair. Tell him to shave or use depilatory to reduce unwanted hair growth. Reassure him that unwanted growth will disappear 1 to 6 months after he stops taking drug.

🔊 Instruct patient to immediately report difficulty breathing (especially when lying down) or pain in chest, arm, or shoulder.

- Teach patient how to use topical form. Urge him to read package insert carefully.
- Caution patient not to use topical form on other body parts and not to let it contact mucous membranes.
- Tell patient using topical form that new scalp hair will be soft and barely visible. Caution him to use only 1 ml twice daily, regardless of amount of

balding. Remind him not to stop using drug suddenly, because new hair growth will be lost.
• As appropriate, review all other significant and life-threatening adverse reactions and interactions, especially those related to the drugs and tests mentioned above.

mirtazapine

Remeron, Remeron RD✤, Remeron Soltab

Pharmacologic class: Piperazino-azepine derivative
Therapeutic class: Tetracyclic antidepressant
Pregnancy risk category C

Action

Potentiates effects of norepinephrine and serotonin by blocking their synaptic reuptake. Also exerts anticholinergic activity by disrupting muscarinic receptors.

Availability

Tablets: 15 mg, 30 mg, 45 mg
Tablets (orally disintegrating): 15 mg, 30 mg, 45 mg

Indications and dosages

➢ Depression
Adults: Initially, 15 mg/day as a single dose at bedtime; may increase dosage q 1 to 2 weeks up to 45 mg/day. For maintenance, 15 to 45 mg/day.

Dosage adjustment

• Renal or hepatic impairment
• Elderly patients

Contraindications

• Hypersensitivity to drug
• MAO inhibitor use within past 14 days

Precautions

Use cautiously in:
• hepatic or renal impairment
• history of seizures, cardiovascular or cerebrovascular disease, or psychiatric illness
• elderly patients
• pregnant or breastfeeding patients
• children (safety not established).

Administration

• Administer orally disintegrating tablet without water. Have patient place it on tongue until it melts. Make sure tablet isn't broken.
• Be aware that drug is usually used in conjunction with psychotherapy.
Clinical alert: Don't give within 14 days of MAO inhibitors.

Route	Onset	Peak	Duration
P.O.	1-2 wk	≥6 wk	Unknown

Adverse reactions

CNS: drowsiness, dizziness, abnormal dreams, abnormal thinking, asthenia, tremor, confusion, **suicidal behavior or ideation (especially in child or adolescent)**
CV: orthostatic hypotension, chest pain
EENT: sinusitis
GI: constipation, dry mouth
GU: urinary frequency, urinary tract infection
Hematologic: agranulocytosis
Musculoskeletal: back pain, myalgia
Respiratory: increased cough, dyspnea
Skin: photosensitivity
Other: flulike symptoms, edema, increased appetite, weight gain, increased thirst

Interactions

Drug-drug. *Benzodiazepines, other CNS depressants:* additive CNS depression
Drugs metabolized by CYP450 enzyme: altered metabolism of these drugs
MAO inhibitors: hypertension, seizures, death

Drug-diagnostic tests. *Alanine aminotransferase, cholesterol, triglycerides:* increased levels
Drug-herbs. *Chamomile, hops, kava, skullcap, valerian:* increased CNS depression
S-adenosylmethionine (SAM-e), St. John's wort: increased risk of serotonergic adverse effects (including serotonin syndrome)
Drug-behaviors. *Alcohol use:* additive CNS effects

Patient monitoring

- Monitor vital signs, especially for orthostatic hypotension.
- Assess neurologic status.
- Watch for weight gain caused by edema or increased appetite.
- Stay alert for urinary tract infection, sinusitis, and flulike symptoms.

◀ Monitor CBC with white cell differential. Stay alert for agranulocytosis.
◀ Watch for suicidal behavior or ideation (especially in child or adolescent).

Patient teaching

- Advise patient to take with food or milk to reduce GI upset.
- Tell patient he may crush conventional tablets if he can't swallow them whole.
- Instruct patient to take orally disintegrating tablet without water. Tell him to place it on tongue until it melts and to make sure tablet isn't broken.
- Advise patient that therapeutic effects may take 2 to 3 weeks.

◀ Tell patient to immediately report sore throat, fever, mouth sores, or other signs or symptoms of infection.
◀ Instruct patient (or parent) to immediately report suicidal thoughts or actions (especially in child or adolescent).
◀ Caution patient not to discontinue drug abruptly. Dosage must be tapered.

- If drug causes oversedation, tell patient to consult prescriber about taking entire daily dose at bedtime.
- Caution patient to avoid driving and other hazardous activities until he knows how drug affects concentration and alertness.
- Tell patient to avoid alcohol and to discuss herbal use with prescriber.
- Instruct patient to avoid exposure to excessive sunlight or sun lamps.
- As appropriate, review all other significant and life-threatening adverse reactions and interactions, especially those related to the drugs, tests, herbs, and behaviors mentioned above.

misoprostol

Apo-Misoprostol✱, Cytotec

Pharmacologic class: Prostaglandin E_1 analog
Therapeutic class: Antiulcerative, cytoprotective agent
Pregnancy risk category X

Action

Reduces gastric acid secretion and increases gastric mucus and bicarbonate production, creating a protective coating on gastric mucosa

Availability

Tablets: 100 mcg, 200 mcg

Indications and dosages

➤ To prevent gastric ulcers caused by nonsteroidal anti-inflammatory drugs (NSAIDs)
Adults: 200 mcg q.i.d. with food, with last daily dose given at bedtime. If intolerance occurs, decrease to 100 mcg q.i.d.

Off-label uses

- Duodenal ulcer
- Pregnancy termination

Contraindications
- Prostaglandin hypersensitivity
- Pregnancy

Precautions
Use cautiously in:
- females of childbearing age
- breastfeeding patients
- children younger than age 18 (safety not established).

Administration
Before starting therapy, make sure female patient understands dangers of taking drug while pregnant or breastfeeding.
- Be aware that drug should not be used in females of childbearing age, except those who need NSAIDs and are at high risk for complications from NSAID-associated gastric ulcers.
- For antiulcer use in females, start therapy on day 2 or 3 of normal menses.

Route	Onset	Peak	Duration
P.O.	Rapid	14-20 min	3-6 hr

Adverse reactions
CNS: headache
GI: nausea, vomiting, diarrhea, constipation, abdominal pain, dyspepsia, flatulence
GU: miscarriage, menstrual disorders, postmenopausal bleeding

Interactions
Drug-drug. *Magnesium-containing antacids:* increased risk of diarrhea

Patient monitoring
- Assess GI status. Report significant adverse reactions.
- Monitor menstrual pattern or postmenopausal bleeding. Report significant problems.

Patient teaching
- Instruct patient to take with food.
- Advise patient to report diarrhea, abdominal pain, and menstrual irregularities.

Tell patient drug may cause spontaneous abortion. Stress importance of using reliable contraception.
- Instruct female patient using drug for ulcer treatment to start therapy on second or third day of normal menses.
- Caution patient not to take magnesium-containing antacids, which may worsen diarrhea.
- As appropriate, review all other significant adverse reactions and interactions, especially those related to the drugs mentioned above.

mitomycin
Mutamycin, Mytozytrex

Pharmacologic class: Antitumor antibiotic

Therapeutic class: Antineoplastic

Pregnancy risk category C

Action
Selectively inhibits DNA synthesis by causing cross-linking of DNA strands and suppressing RNA and protein synthesis, resulting in cell death

Availability
Injection: 5-mg, 20-mg, and 40-mg vials

Indications and dosages
➤ Disseminated adenocarcinoma of stomach or pancreas (given with other chemotherapeutic agents); palliative treatment when other therapies fail

Adults: 20 mg/m^2 I.V. as a single dose. Repeat cycle q 6 to 8 weeks, adjusting dosage if necessary.

Dosage adjustment
- Reduced white blood cell or platelet count

Contraindications

- Hypersensitivity to drug
- Thrombocytopenia, coagulation disorders, increased bleeding tendency

Precautions

Use cautiously in:
- active infections, decreased bone marrow reserve, impaired hepatic function
- history of pulmonary disorders
- elderly patients
- pregnant or breastfeeding patients.

Administration

🔊 Follow facility policy for handling, administering, and disposing of mutagenic, teratogenic, and carcinogenic drugs.
- Reconstitute 5-mg vial with 10 ml of sterile water. Shake, let mixture stand, and administer by direct I.V. injection through Y-tube or three-way stopcock. Infuse over 5 to 10 minutes through line with running infusion of normal saline solution or dextrose 5% in water.

🔊 Avoid extravasation and contact with skin, mucous membranes, and eyes.

Route	Onset	Peak	Duration
I.V.	Unknown	Unknown	Unknown

Adverse reactions

GI: nausea, vomiting, anorexia, mouth ulcers, stomatitis
GU: renal failure, hemolytic uremic syndrome
Hematologic: anemia, **leukopenia, thrombocytopenia**
Respiratory: pulmonary toxicity, interstitial pneumonitis
Skin: reversible alopecia; pruritus; desquamation; phlebitis, necrosis, and sloughing with I.V. site extravasation
Other: fever

Interactions

Drug-drug. *Live-virus vaccines:* decreased antibody response to vaccine, increased risk of adverse reactions
Other antineoplastics: additive bone marrow depression
Vinca alkaloids: respiratory toxicity

Patient monitoring

🔊 Closely monitor CBC with white cell differential and platelet count. Stay alert for evidence of blood dyscrasias.
- Assess kidney function tests. Measure fluid intake and output and evaluate fluid balance.

🔊 Watch for signs and symptoms of hemolytic uremic syndrome (irritability, fatigue, pallor, and decreased urinary output).
🔊 Closely monitor I.V. site and skin integrity to prevent extravasation.
🔊 Assess respiratory status carefully to detect severe pulmonary problems.

Patient teaching

🔊 Teach patient to recognize and immediately report signs and symptoms of hemolytic uremic syndrome, blood dyscrasias, and renal failure.
🔊 Instruct patient to report cough or shortness of breath, even if it occurs several months after therapy ends.
- Advise patient to limit exposure to infections and to avoid live vaccines.
- Tell patient drug may cause hair loss. Discuss options for dealing with this problem.
- As appropriate, review all other significant and life-threatening adverse reactions and interactions, especially those related to the drugs mentioned above.

mitoxantrone hydrochloride

Novantrone

Pharmacologic class: Antibiotic antineoplastic

Therapeutic class: Antineoplastic, immune modifier

Pregnancy risk category D

Action

Selectively inhibits DNA synthesis by causing cross-linking of DNA strands and suppressing RNA and protein synthesis, resulting in cell death

Availability

Injection: 2 mg/ml in 10-ml, 12.5-ml, and 15-ml vials

Indications and dosages

➢ Acute nonlymphocytic leukemia (given with other agents)

Adults: For induction—12 mg/m²/day I.V. on days 1 to 3, with 100 mg/m² of cytosine arabinoside given for 7 days as a continuous I.V. infusion (over 24 hours) on days 1 through 7. If remission doesn't occur, second course may follow, with mitoxantrone given for 2 days and cytosine arabinoside for 5 days at same daily dosages. For consolidation therapy—12 mg/m²/day mitoxantrone I.V. on days 1 and 2 and 100 mg/m² cytosine arabinoside I.V. as a continuous infusion over 24 hours on days 1 through 5, given 6 weeks after induction therapy.

➢ Pain in patients with advanced hormone-refractory prostatic cancer (given with corticosteroids)

Adults: 12 to 14 mg/m² I.V. given over 15 to 30 minutes q 21 days

➢ Multiple sclerosis

Adults: 12 mg/m² I.V. given over 5 to 15 minutes q 3 months. Maximum cumulative lifetime dosage is 140 mg/m².

Contraindications

- Hypersensitivity to drug

Precautions

Use cautiously in:

- bone marrow depression, heart failure, chronic debilitating illness, hepatobiliary dysfunction
- elderly patients
- pregnant or breastfeeding patients
- children.

Administration

◀ Follow facility policy for handling, administering, and disposing of mutagenic, teratogenic, and carcinogenic drugs.

- Dilute with 50 ml or more of normal saline solution or dextrose 5% in water (D_5W). Infuse I.V. over 3 to 5 minutes into running line of normal saline solution or D_5W.
- Alternatively, dilute drug further in normal saline solution or D_5W and infuse intermittently I.V. over 15 to 30 minutes.

◀ If extravasation occurs, stop infusion immediately.

◀ Avoid contact with skin, mucous membranes, and eyes.

- Be aware that drug isn't indicated for primary progressive multiple sclerosis.

Route	Onset	Peak	Duration
I.V.	Unknown	Unknown	Unknown

Adverse reactions

CNS: headache, **seizures**

CV: heart failure, arrhythmias, cardiotoxicity

EENT: conjunctivitis, mucositis

GI: nausea, vomiting, diarrhea, abdominal pain, stomatitis, **GI bleeding**

GU: urinary tract infection, blue-green urine, **renal failure**

Hematologic: anemia, **bone marrow**

depression, leukopenia, thrombocytopenia
Hepatic: jaundice, **hepatotoxicity**
Metabolic: hyperuricemia
Respiratory: cough, dyspnea
Skin: rash, petechiae, bruising, alopecia
Other: fever, infection, hypersensitivity reaction

Interactions

Drug-drug. *Anthracycline antineoplastics (daunorubicin, doxorubicin, idarubicin):* increased risk of cardiomyopathy
Live-virus vaccines: decreased antibody response to vaccine
Other antineoplastics: additive bone marrow depression
Drug-diagnostic tests. *Alanine aminotransferase, aspartate aminotransferase, bilirubin, uric acid:* increased levels

Patient monitoring

- Monitor CBC with white cell differential. Watch for evidence of blood dyscrasias.
- Assess vital signs, ECG, and respiratory and cardiovascular status.
- Monitor kidney and liver function tests. Measure fluid intake and output and evaluate fluid balance.
- Monitor temperature. Stay alert for fever and signs and symptoms of urinary tract and other infections.

Patient teaching

- Advise patient to immediately report chest pain, seizure, easy bruising or bleeding, change in urination pattern, yellowing of skin or eyes, or difficulty breathing.
- Instruct patient to limit exposure to infections and to avoid live vaccines.
- Tell patient drug may turn urine blue-green.
- Advise patient to minimize GI upset by eating small, frequent servings of food and drinking plenty of fluids.
- Tell female patient to inform prescriber if she's pregnant or breastfeeding.
- As appropriate, review all other significant and life-threatening adverse reactions and interactions, especially those related to the drugs and tests mentioned above.

modafinil

Alertec✱, Provigil

Pharmacologic class: Nonamphetamine CNS stimulant
Therapeutic class: Analeptic
Controlled substance schedule IV
Pregnancy risk category C

Action

Unknown. Thought to stimulate CNS by decreasing the release of gamma-aminobutyric acid (a CNS depressant), thereby increasing mental alertness.

Availability

Tablets: 100 mg, 200 mg

Indications and dosages

➢ Narcolepsy
Adults: 200 mg/day P.O. as a single dose in morning

Dosage adjustment

- Severe hepatic impairment

Contraindications

- Hypersensitivity to drug

Precautions

Use cautiously in:

- recent myocardial infarction, unstable angina, severe hepatic impairment, hyperthyroidism, hypertension, glaucoma, anxiety
- history of left ventricular hypertrophy, ischemic ECG changes, chest pain,

arrhythmias, or mitral valve prolapse with previous CNS stimulant use
• history of psychosis
• drug abuse
• pregnant or breastfeeding patients
• children (safety and efficacy not established).

Administration
• Give without food (food delays drug absorption).

Route	Onset	Peak	Duration
P.O.	Unknown	2-4 hr	Unknown

Adverse reactions
CNS: headache, dizziness, nervousness, insomnia, depression, anxiety, amnesia, tremor, emotional lability
CV: hypertension, chest pain, vasodilation, hypotension, syncope, **arrhythmias**
EENT: abnormal vision, amblyopia, epistaxis, rhinitis, pharyngitis
GI: nausea, vomiting, diarrhea, dry mouth, anorexia
GU: abnormal urine, urinary retention, albuminuria, abnormal ejaculation
Hematologic: eosinophilia
Metabolic: hyperglycemia
Musculoskeletal: joint disorders, neck pain and rigidity
Respiratory: lung disorder, dyspnea, **asthma**
Skin: dry skin
Other: fever, chills, herpes simplex infection

Interactions
Drug-drug. *Carbamazepine, phenobarbital, rifampin, other CYP3A4 inducers:* decreased modafinil blood level
Cyclosporine, theophylline: decreased blood levels of these drugs
Diazepam, phenytoin, propranolol, tricyclic antidepressants, warfarin: increased blood levels of these drugs
Hormonal contraceptives: decreased contraceptive efficacy
Itraconazole, ketoconazole, other CYP3A4 inhibitors: increased modafinil blood level
Methylphenidate: delayed modafinil absorption
Drug-diagnostic tests. *Aspartate aminotransferase, eosinophils, gamma-glutamyl transferase, glucose:* increased levels
Hepatic enzymes: abnormal levels

Patient monitoring
• Monitor respiratory and cardiovascular status, including vital signs and ECG.
• Monitor neurologic status, including mood, motor function, cognition, and emotional lability.
• Monitor blood glucose level in diabetic patient.
• Monitor patient carefully if he's also receiving MAO inhibitors. (However, interaction studies with MAO inhibitors haven't been done.)

Patient teaching
• Tell patient he may take with or without food, but that food may delay drug absorption up to 1 hour.
◀ Advise patient to immediately report chest pain, irregular heart beats, light-headedness, or fainting.
• Caution patient to avoid driving and other hazardous activities until he knows how drug affects concentration, vision, motor function, and alertness.
• Instruct female patient to use reliable nonhormonal contraception during and for 1 month after therapy.
• Tell diabetic patient to monitor blood glucose level closely and stay alert for hyperglycemia.
• As appropriate, review all other significant and life-threatening adverse reactions and interactions, especially those related to the drugs and tests mentioned above.

m

moexipril hydrochloride
Univasc

Pharmacologic class: Angiotensin-converting enzyme (ACE) inhibitor
Therapeutic class: Antihypertensive
Pregnancy risk category C (first trimester), ***D*** (second and third trimesters)

Action
Inhibits conversion of angiotensin I to the vasoconstrictor angiotensin II, inactivates bradykinin and other vasodilatory prostaglandins, increases plasma renin levels, and reduces aldosterone levels. Net effect is systemic vasodilation.

Availability
Tablets: 7.5 mg, 15 mg

Indications and dosages
➢ Hypertension
Adults: 7.5 mg P.O. daily 1 hour before a meal; may increase if blood pressure control is inadequate. Range is 7.5 mg to 30 mg/day in one or two divided doses given 1 hour before a meal.

Dosage adjustment
- Renal impairment
- Concurrent diuretic therapy

Contraindications
- Hypersensitivity to drug
- Angioedema secondary to ACE inhibitor use

Precautions
Use cautiously in:
- renal or hepatic impairment, hypovolemia, hyponatremia, aortic stenosis or hypertrophic cardiomyopathy, cardiac or cerebrovascular insufficiency
- family history of angioedema
- concurrent diuretic therapy
- black patients
- elderly patients
- pregnant or breastfeeding patients
- children (safety not established).

Administration
- Give 1 hour before meals (food reduces drug absorption).
- Adjust dosage, as ordered, according to blood pressure response.

Route	Onset	Peak	Duration
P.O.	30 min	6 hr	Up to 24 hr

Adverse reactions
CNS: dizziness, fatigue
CV: chest pain, peripheral edema
EENT: pharyngitis, sinusitis
GI: nausea, diarrhea
GU: urinary frequency
Metabolic: hyperkalemia
Musculoskeletal: myalgia
Respiratory: upper respiratory infection, increased cough
Skin: rash, flushing, angioedema
Other: fever, flulike symptoms, hypersensitivity reaction

Interactions
Drug-drug. *Allopurinol:* increased risk of hypersensitivity reaction
Antacids: decreased moexipril absorption
Antihypertensives, general anesthetics, nitrates, phenothiazines: additive hypotension
Cyclosporine, indomethacin, potassium-sparing diuretics, potassium supplements, salt substitutes: hyperkalemia
Digoxin, lithium: increased blood levels of these drugs
Diuretics: excessive hypotension
Nonsteroidal anti-inflammatory drugs: blunted antihypertensive response
Drug-diagnostic tests. *Alanine aminotransferase, alkaline phosphatase, aspartate aminotransferase, bilirubin, blood urea nitrogen, creatinine, potassium:* increased levels

Antinuclear antibody: positive titer
Sodium: decreased level
Drug-food. *Salt substitutes containing potassium:* hyperkalemia
Drug-behaviors. *Acute alcohol ingestion:* additive hypotension

Patient monitoring

- Monitor vital signs and neurologic and cardiovascular status.
- Assess respiratory status, staying alert for persistent dry cough.
- Evaluate for allergic reactions and angioedema.
- Know that moexipril monotherapy is less effective in black patients, who may need additional concurrent antihypertensives.

Patient teaching

- Instruct patient to take 1 hour before a meal.
- Tell patient to report persistent dry cough and signs or symptoms of infection (especially upper respiratory infection).
- Advise patient to change position slowly (especially during first few days of therapy), to minimize hypotension and dizziness.
- Instruct patient to limit foods high in potassium and avoid salt substitutes containing potassium.
- As appropriate, review all other significant and life-threatening adverse reactions and interactions, especially those related to the drugs, tests, foods, and behaviors mentioned above.

montelukast sodium

Singulair

Pharmacologic class: Leukotriene receptor antagonist
Therapeutic class: Antiasthmatic
Pregnancy risk category B

Action

Blocks action of leukotrienes, decreasing smooth muscle contractions and edema in bronchial airways and preventing inflammation and bronchospasm

Availability

Oral granules: 4-mg base/packet
Tablets: 10 mg
Tablets (chewable): 4 mg, 5 mg

Indications and dosages

➤ Long-term asthma management
Adults and children ages 15 and older: 10-mg tablet P.O. daily in evening
Children ages 6 to 14: 5-mg chewable tablet P.O. daily in evening
Children ages 2 to 5: 4-mg chewable tablet or one 4-mg packet oral granules P.O. daily in evening
Children ages 12 to 23 months: 4-mg packet oral granules P.O. daily in evening

Off-label use

- Chronic urticaria

Contraindications

- Hypersensitivity to drug or its components
- Status asthmaticus

Precautions

Use cautiously in:

- acute asthma attack, hepatic impairment, phenylketonuria
- pregnant or breastfeeding patients

m

• children younger than age 1 (safety not established).

Administration

• Give with or without food. If desired, mix granules with applesauce or ice cream.

Route	Onset	Peak	Duration
P.O.	Unknown	3-4 hr	Unknown
P.O. (chewable)	Unknown	2-2.5 hr	Unknown
P.O. (granules)	Unknown	Unknown	Unknown

Adverse reactions

CNS: fatigue, headache, dizziness, asthenia
EENT: nasal congestion, otitis and sinusitis (in children)
GI: abdominal pain; nausea and diarrhea (in children); dyspepsia; infectious gastroenteritis
Respiratory: cough
Skin: rash
Other: dental pain, influenza, fever

Interactions

Drug-drug. *CYP450 inducers (such as phenobarbital, rifampin):* decreased montelukast effects
Drug-diagnostic tests. *Alanine aminotransferase, aspartate aminotransferase, eosinophils:* increased levels

Patient monitoring

• Assess eosinophil count.
• Monitor temperature. Watch for fever and other signs and symptoms of infection.

Patient teaching

• Advise patient to take drug once daily in evening.
• Inform patient he may sprinkle granules onto soft food and take immediately, but must not dissolve in liquid.
• Tell patient drug is for preventive use only, not for treatment of acute asthma attacks.
• Caution patient to avoid driving and other hazardous activities, because drug causes dizziness.
• Tell patient to minimize GI upset by eating small, frequent servings of food and drinking plenty of fluids.
• As appropriate, review all other significant adverse reactions and interactions, especially those related to the drugs and tests mentioned above.

moricizine hydrochloride

Ethmozine

Pharmacologic class: Sodium channel blocker
Therapeutic class: Antiarrhythmic (class IA)
Pregnancy risk category B

Action

Prolongs PR interval and QRS duration by blocking sodium influx across myocardial cell membrane, thereby decreasing myocardial irritability and preventing arrhythmias

Availability

Tablets: 200 mg, 250 mg, 300 mg

Indications and dosages

➤ Life-threatening ventricular arrhythmias, including sustained ventricular tachycardia
Adults: 600 to 900 mg/day P.O. q 8 hours in divided doses. Adjust by 150 mg/day q 3 days as needed and tolerated.

Dosage adjustment

• Hepatic or renal impairment

Contraindications

• Hypersensitivity to drug
• Cardiogenic shock
• Heart block

Precautions

Use cautiously in:
- severe renal or hepatic impairment, heart failure, coronary artery disease, sick sinus syndrome, electrolyte disturbances
- pregnant or breastfeeding patients
- children (safety not established).

Administration

- Administer with meals.
- Know that some patients tolerate dosing every 12 hours. Assess closely for increased dizziness and nausea.

Route	Onset	Peak	Duration
P.O.	1 hr	0.5-2 hr	10-24 hr

Adverse reactions

CNS: dizziness, fatigue, headache, nervousness, weakness, paresthesia, sleep disorders, **cerebrovascular events**
CV: chest pain, palpitations, hypotension, hypertension, **thrombophlebitis, arrhythmias, heart failure**
EENT: blurred vision
GI: nausea, vomiting, diarrhea, dyspepsia, dry mouth
Musculoskeletal: pain
Respiratory: dyspnea
Skin: sweating
Other: drug fever

Interactions

Drug-drug. *Cimetidine:* increased moricizine blood level
Digoxin: prolonged PR interval
Theophylline: decreased theophylline blood level

Patient monitoring

- Assess baseline ECG; monitor periodically during therapy.
- Monitor vital signs. Watch for drug-induced fever, hypotension, and rebound hypertension.
- Monitor patient's weight and fluid intake and output.
- Assess cardiovascular and neurologic status carefully.

Patient teaching

- Instruct patient to take with meals to minimize GI upset.
- Advise patient to take exactly as prescribed and not to double the dose. Tell him he may take missed dose up to 6 hours after previous dose.
- 🔊 Caution patient not to stop taking drug suddenly. Dosage must be tapered gradually.
- 🔊 Teach patient to recognize and immediately report signs and symptoms of heart failure, irregular heart beats, and cerebrovascular events.
- Caution patient to avoid driving and other hazardous activities until he knows how drug affects concentration and alertness.
- As appropriate, review all other significant and life-threatening adverse reactions and interactions, especially those related to the drugs mentioned above.

morphine hydrochloride

Dolora✤, Morphitec✤

morphine sulfate

Astramorph PF, Avinza, DepoDur, Duramorph, Epimorph✤, Infumorph, Kadian, Morphine H.P.✤, MS Contin, MSIR, Statex✤

Pharmacologic class: Opioid agonist
Therapeutic class: Opioid analgesic
Controlled substance schedule II
Pregnancy risk category C

Action

Interacts with opioid receptor sites, primarily in limbic system, thalamus, and spinal cord. This interaction alters neurotransmitter release, altering perception of and tolerance for pain.

Availability

morphine hydrochloride

Rectal suppositories: 20 mg, 30 mg
Syrup: 1 mg/ml, 5 mg/ml, 10 mg/ml, 20 mg/ml, 50 mg/ml
Tablets: 10 mg, 20 mg, 40 mg, 60 mg

morphine sulfate

Capsules: 15 mg, 30 mg
Capsules (extended-release): 30 mg, 60 mg, 90 mg, 120 mg
Capsules (sustained-release): 10 mg, 20 mg, 30 mg, 50 mg, 60 mg, 100 mg
Oral solution: 2 mg/ml, 4 mg/ml, 20 mg/ml (concentrate), 10 mg/5 ml, 20 mg/5 ml, 100 mg/5 ml
Rectal suppositories: 5 mg, 10 mg, 20 mg, 30 mg
Solution for epidural injection (extended-release, liposomal): 10 mg/ml, 15 mg/1.5 ml, 20 mg/2-ml vials
Solution for epidural or intrathecal use (preservative free, for continuous microinfusion device): 10 mg/ml and 25 mg/ml in 20-ml vials
Solution for epidural or I.V. injection (preservative-free): 0.5 mg/ml, 1 mg/ml
Solution for I.M., I.V., or subcutaneous injection: 1 mg/ml, 2 mg/ml, 4 mg/ml, 5 mg/ml, 8 mg/ml, 10 mg/ml, 15 mg/ml, 25 mg/ml, 50 mg/ml
Solution for I.V. injection (for patient-controlled analgesia [PCA] device): 1 mg/ml, 2 mg/ml, 3 mg/ml, 5 mg/ml
Tablets: 15 mg, 30 mg
Tablets (controlled-release, sustained-release): 15 mg, 30 mg, 60 mg, 100 mg, 200 mg
Tablets (soluble): 10 mg, 15 mg, 30 mg

Indications and dosages

➢ Severe to moderate pain

Oral use—

Adults: 5 to 30 mg P.O. (immediate-release) q 4 hours p.r.n. Or 20 mg P.O. (controlled-release, Kadian) once or twice daily p.r.n. Or 200 mg P.O. (MS Contin) in opioid-tolerant patients who require daily morphine-equivalent dosages above 400 mg.

I.M. or subcutaneous use—

Adults: 5 to 20 mg/70 kg I.M. or subcutaneously q 4 hours p.r.n.

I.V. use—

Adults: 2 to 10 mg/70 kg I.V. p.r.n. given slowly over 4 to 5 minutes. As a continuous I.V. infusion, 0.1 to 1 mg/ml in dextrose 5% in water delivered by controlled-infusion device.

Rectal use—

Adults: 10 to 30 mg P.R. q 4 hours p.r.n.

Epidural use—

Adults: Initially 5 mg (Astramorph PF, Duramorph) injected in lumbar region (may relieve pain up to 24 hours). If response isn't adequate within 1 hour, carefully give incremental doses of 1 to 2 mg p.r.n., up to 10 mg/24 hours. For continuous epidural infusion, 2 to 4 mg/24 hours. For epidural injection (DepoDur) before orthopedic leg surgery, recommended dosage is 15 mg; before lower abdominal or pelvic surgery, 10 to 15 mg. For cesarean section after umbilical cord clamping, recommended dosage is 10 mg.

Intrathecal use—

Adults: Usual intrathecal dosage is one-tenth of epidural dosage; 0.2 to 1 mg as a single injection in lumbar area may relieve pain up to 24 hours.

Dosage adjustment

- Adults weighing less than 50 kg (110 lb)
- Elderly patients
- Children

Contraindications

- Hypersensitivity to drug, tartrazine, bisulfites, or alcohol
- Acute bronchial asthma
- Upper airway obstruction
- Respiratory depression
- GI obstruction, paralytic ileus

Precautions

Use cautiously in:

- head trauma; increased intracranial pressure; severe renal, hepatic, or pulmonary disease; hypothyroidism; adrenal insufficiency; prostatic hypertrophy
- elderly or debilitated patients
- pregnant or breastfeeding patients.

Administration

- For best response, give at pain onset.
- Give oral form with food or milk to minimize GI upset.
- If desired, crush immediate-release form and mix with food or fluids.
- Don't crush or break extended-release form; remind patient to swallow it whole.
- If desired, open sustained-release capsules (Kadian) and sprinkle entire contents onto small amount of food (such as applesauce). Have patient consume mixture immediately without chewing, crushing, or dissolving pellets.
- When giving by direct I.V., dilute in at least 5 ml of sterile water for injection or normal saline solution. Give 2.5 to 10 mg over 4 to 5 minutes.
- For continuous I.V. infusion, use infusion pump or PCA pump. Titrate dosage to provide adequate pain relief.
- Don't use parenteral form if it's cloudy or contains visible particulates.

Route	Onset	Peak	Duration
P.O.	Unknown	60-120 min	4-5 hr
P.O. (extended)	Unknown	Unknown	8-24 hr
I.V.	Rapid	20 min	4-5 hr
I.M.	10-30 min	30-60 min	4-5 hr
Subcut.	20 min	50-90 min	4-5 hr
Epidural	6-30 min	Unknown	Up to 24 hr
Epidural (ext., liposomal)	Unknown	Unknown	Unknown
Intrathecal	Rapid (min)	Unknown	Up to 24 hr
P.R.	Unknown	20-60 min	4-5 hr

Adverse reactions

CNS: confusion, sedation, dizziness, dysphoria, euphoria, floating feeling, hallucinations, headache, nightmares
CV: hypotension, bradycardia
EENT: blurred vision, diplopia, miosis
GI: nausea, vomiting, constipation, dry mouth
GU: urinary retention
Respiratory: apnea, respiratory depression, respiratory arrest
Skin: flushing, itching, sweating
Other: physical or psychological drug dependence, drug tolerance

Interactions

Drug-drug. *Antihistamines, barbiturates, clomipramine, sedative-hypnotics, tricyclic antidepressants:* additive CNS depression
Buprenorphine, butorphanol, dezocine, nalbuphine, pentazocine: decreased analgesia
Cimetidine: decreased morphine metabolism and increased effects
MAO inhibitors: severe, unpredictable reactions
Mixed opioid agonist-antagonists: precipitation of withdrawal symptoms in physically dependent patients
Warfarin: increased anticoagulant effect
Drug-diagnostic tests. *Amylase, lipase:* increased levels
Drug-herbs. *Chamomile, hops, kava, skullcap, valerian:* increased CNS depression
Drug-behaviors. *Alcohol use:* increased CNS depression

Patient monitoring

- Monitor vital signs. Contact prescriber if respiratory rate is 10 breaths/minutes or less.
- Assess pain character, location, and intensity.
- Monitor fluid intake and output. Stay alert for urinary retention.

m

• Monitor bowel elimination pattern. If constipation occurs, intervene as appropriate.
• Assess neurologic status. Implement safety measures as needed to prevent injury.
• Evaluate patient for signs and symptoms of physical or psychological dependence. Be watchful for drug hoarding.

Patient teaching

• Tell patient he may crush immediate-release form and mix with food or fluids.
• Advise patient not to crush or break extended-release form. Instruct him to swallow it whole.
• Tell patient he may open sustained-release capsule (Kadian), sprinkle entire contents of capsule onto a small amount of food (such as applesauce), and consume immediately. Stress importance of not chewing, crushing, or dissolving pellets.
• Advise patient to take drug at the first sign of pain, because continuous dosing is more effective than p.r.n. dosing.
Clinical alert: Tell patient and caregiver that drug may cause respiratory depression. Instruct them to immediately report respiratory rate of 10 breaths/minute or less.
• Inform patient that drug may cause constipation or urinary retention. Encourage high-fiber diet and high fluid intake.
• Stress importance of taking drug only as prescribed. Point out that drug may cause psychological or physical dependence.
• Caution patient to avoid driving and other hazardous activities until he knows how drug affects concentration, vision, and alertness.
• Teach patient and caregiver about appropriate safety measures to prevent injury.
• Caution patient to avoid alcohol and other CNS depressants during and for 24 hours after therapy.
• Advise patient to avoid herbs, which may worsen adverse CNS effects.
• As appropriate, review all other significant and life-threatening adverse reactions and interactions, especially those related to the drugs, tests, herbs, and behaviors mentioned above.

moxifloxacin hydrochloride

Avelox, Vigamox

Pharmacologic class: Fluoroquinolone
Therapeutic class: Anti-infective
Pregnancy risk category C

Action

Selectively inhibits DNA synthesis by disrupting DNA replication and transcription and suppressing protein synthesis, causing bacterial cell death

Availability

Injection (premixed): 400 mg/250-ml bag
Ophthalmic solution: 5% (3 ml in 6-ml bottle)
Tablets: 400 mg

Indications and dosages

➢ Acute bacterial sinusitis
Adults: 400 mg P.O. or I.V. q 24 hours for 10 days
➢ Acute bacterial exacerbation of chronic bronchitis
Adults: 400 mg P.O. or I.V. q 24 hours for 5 days
➢ Community-acquired pneumonia
Adults: 400 mg P.O. or I.V. q 24 hours for 7 to 14 days
➢ Uncomplicated skin and skin-structure infections
Adults: 400 mg P.O. or I.V. q 24 hours for 7 days

➢ Bacterial conjunctivitis
Adults: Instill one drop of ophthalmic solution into affected eye t.i.d. for 7 days.

Contraindications

• Hypersensitivity to drug, its components, or other fluoroquinolones

Precautions

Use cautiously in:
• underlying CNS diseases or disorders, renal impairment, cirrhosis, bradycardia, acute myocardial ischemia, prolonged QTc interval, uncorrected hypokalemia, dialysis
• elderly patients
• pregnant or breastfeeding patients (safety not established except in postexposure inhalation anthrax).
• children younger than age 18 (except in postexposure inhalation anthrax)
• children younger than age 1 (ophthalmic use).

Administration

• Give premixed I.V. dose over 60 minutes. Avoid bolus or rapid infusion.
• Don't mix with other drugs in same I.V. line.
• Know that although milk or yogurt may impair absorption of P.O. moxifloxacin, drug may be given with other calcium products.

Route	Onset	Peak	Duration
P.O.	Within 1 hr	1-3 hr	24 hr
I.V.	Rapid	End of infusion	24 hr
Ophthalmic	Unknown	Unknown	Unknown

Adverse reactions

CNS: dizziness, drowsiness, headache, confusion, light-headedness, insomnia, agitation, hallucinations, acute psychoses, tremor, **seizures**
CV: hypertension, vasodilation, tachycardia, **prolonged QT interval, arrhythmias**
EENT: conjunctivitis; decreased visual acuity; keratitis; eye dryness, discomfort, pain, pruritus, and hyperemia; subconjunctival hemorrhage; tearing; otitis media; pharyngitis; rhinitis (all with ophthalmic solution)
GI: nausea, diarrhea, abdominal pain, **pseudomembranous colitis**
GU: vaginitis
Hematologic: eosinophilia, **thrombocytopenia, leukopenia**
Musculoskeletal: joint pain, tendinitis, tendon rupture
Respiratory: increased cough (with ophthalmic solution)
Skin: rash, photosensitivity, phototoxicity, **Stevens-Johnson syndrome**
Other: altered taste, fever (with ophthalmic solution), phlebitis at I.V. site, superinfection, hypersensitivity reactions including **anaphylaxis**

Interactions

Drug-drug. *Amiodarone, bepridil, disopyramide, erythromycin, pentamidine, phenothiazines, pimozide, procainamide, quinidine, sotalol, tricyclic antidepressants:* increased risk of serious adverse cardiovascular reactions
Antacids, bismuth subsalicylate, iron salts, sucralfate, zinc salts: decreased moxifloxacin absorption
Theophylline: increased theophylline blood level and possible toxicity
Drug-diagnostic tests. *Alanine aminotransferase, alkaline phosphatase, aspartate aminotransferase, bilirubin, lactate dehydrogenase, platelets:* increased levels
Drug-food. *Concurrent tube feedings, milk, yogurt:* impaired absorption of P.O. moxifloxacin
Drug-herbs. *Dong quai, St. John's wort:* phototoxicity
Fennel: decreased moxifloxacin absorption
Drug-behaviors. *Sun exposure:* phototoxicity

m

Patient monitoring

Watch for hypersensitivity reaction (such as anaphylaxis) and other allergic reactions, which may occur after initial dose.
- Monitor cardiovascular and neurologic status closely.
- Stay alert for tendinitis and Achilles tendon rupture.
- Monitor CBC and liver function tests.
- Assess GI status. Report signs or symptoms of pseudomembranous colitis.
- Watch closely for superinfection.

Patient teaching

- Advise patient to take tablets once a day with or without food, 4 hours before or 8 hours after antacids, multivitamins, sucralfate, or preparations containing aluminum, magnesium, iron, or zinc.

Tell patient drug may cause serious allergic reactions even several days after therapy begins. Advise him to stop taking drug and report these reactions immediately.

Urge patient to promptly report tendon pain, diarrhea with blood or pus, and signs and symptoms of superinfection.
- Teach patient how to use eye drops. Caution him to avoid touching applicator tip to eye, finger, or other object.
- Instruct patient being treated for bacterial conjunctivitis not to wear contact lenses.
- Caution patient to avoid driving and other hazardous activities until he knows how drug affects concentration and alertness.
- As appropriate, review all other significant and life-threatening adverse reactions and interactions, especially those related to the drugs, tests, foods, herbs, and behaviors mentioned above.

mupirocin (pseudomonic acid, pseudomonic acid A)

Bactroban, Bactroban Nasal 2%

Pharmacologic class: Dermatologic agent
Therapeutic class: Anti-infective, topical
Pregnancy risk category B

Action

Inhibits bacterial protein and RNA synthesis by reversibly and specifically binding to bacterial isoleucyl-transfer RNA synthetase. Bactericidal.

Availability

Intranasal ointment: 2.15%
Topical cream: 2%
Topical ointment: 2%

Indications and dosages

➢ Impetigo
Adults and children ages 2 months to 16 years: Apply a small amount of ointment topically t.i.d. for 3 to 5 days. Reevaluate if no response.
➢ Infected traumatic skin lesions
Adults and children ages 3 months to 16 years: Apply a small amount of cream topically t.i.d. for 10 days.
➢ Nasal colonization of methicillin-resistant *Streptococcus aureus*
Adults and children ages 12 and older: Apply intranasal ointment (half of single-use tube to each nostril) topically to anterior nares b.i.d. for 5 days.

Contraindications

- Hypersensitivity to drug or its components

Precautions

Use cautiously in:
- moderate or severe renal impairment (with large doses)

- breastfeeding patients
- children younger than age 12 (intranasal ointment), younger than age 3 months (cream), or younger than age 2 months (ointment).

Administration

- After intranasal application, press nares together repeatedly to distribute drug.
- Avoid contact with eyes.
- Discontinue use if sensitization or severe local irritation occurs.
- If desired, cover affected area with gauze dressing after applying cream or ointment.
- Don't use intranasal form with any other nasal spray.
- Don't use Bactroban ointment on mucosal surfaces. Use Bactroban Nasal (mupirocin calcium ointment) intranasally.
- Know that although mupirocin isn't absorbed systemically, polyethylene glycol (its water-miscible ointment base) may be absorbed from open wounds and damaged skin and may be excreted by kidney.

Route	Onset	Peak	Duration
Topical, intranasal	Not systemically absorbed		

Adverse reactions

CNS: headache (with intranasal use)
EENT: rhinitis, nasal stinging or burning, pharyngitis (all with intranasal use)
GI: mouth and lip sores
Skin: pruritus (with intranasal use); dry skin, rash, redness, stinging or pain, secondary wound infection
Other: taste disorders (with intranasal use)

Interactions

None significant

Patient monitoring

- Monitor for drug efficacy.

Patient teaching

- Instruct patient to wash affected area with soap and water and dry it thoroughly, then apply small amount of drug to area and rub in gently. If desired, tell him to apply gauze dressing.
- Advise patient to complete entire course of therapy, even if symptoms disappear. Tell him to try not to miss doses.
- If patient misses a dose, tell him to apply dose as soon as he remembers. However, if it's almost time for next dose, advise him to skip missed dose and resume regular dosing schedule.
- Advise patient to contact prescriber if skin infection doesn't improve within 3 to 5 days or if it worsens.
- Caution patient not to apply drug to eye or mucous membranes (except nasal form for intranasal use).
- As appropriate, review all other significant adverse reactions.

muromonab-CD3

Orthoclone OKT3

Pharmacologic class: Murine monoclonal antibody
Therapeutic class: Immunosuppressant
Pregnancy risk category C

Action

Binds to and blocks function of T lymphocytes responsible for antigen recognition, thereby reversing graft rejection

Availability

Injection: 1 mg/1 ml in 5-ml ampules

Indications and dosages

➢ Acute allograft rejection in kidney transplant patients; steroid-resistant acute allograft rejection in heart and liver transplant patients
Adults and children weighing more

than 30 kg (66 lb): 5 mg/day I.V. for 10 to 14 days
Children weighing 30 kg (66 lb) or less: 2.5 mg/day I.V. for 10 to 14 days

Contraindications
- Hypersensitivity to drug or other murine products
- Uncompensated heart failure
- Uncontrolled hypertension
- Predisposition to or history of seizures
- Antimouse antibody titer of 1:1000 or higher
- Pregnancy or breastfeeding

Precautions
Use cautiously in:
- fever
- children younger than age 2.

Administration
- In kidney transplant patients, know that therapy should start as soon as acute kidney rejection is diagnosed. In heart and liver transplant patients, therapy should start when physician determines that steroid therapy hasn't reversed allograft rejection.

Clinical alert: Know that drug must be given in facility equipped and staffed to treat cardiopulmonary arrest.
- For I.V. bolus injection, draw solution into syringe through low-protein-binding 0.2- or 0.22-micron filter. Discard filter and attach needle-free adapter.
- Administer bolus over less than 1 minute.
- Give antipyretics to decrease fever and corticosteroids to reduce allergic response, as prescribed.

Route	Onset	Peak	Duration
I.V.	Immediate	Unknown	1 wk

Adverse reactions
CNS: fatigue, headache, weakness, tremors, hallucinations, **aseptic meningitis, cerebral edema, seizures, encephalopathy**
CV: chest pain, hypertension, hypotension, **heart failure, tachycardia, cardiac arrest, shock**
EENT: vision loss, blurred vision, conjunctivitis, photophobia, tinnitus, otitis media
GI: nausea, vomiting, diarrhea
GU: oliguria, anuria
Respiratory: dyspnea, wheezing, **severe pulmonary edema, adult respiratory distress syndrome (ARDS)**
Skin: flushing
Other: fever, chills, flulike symptoms, infection, **anaphylaxis, cytokine release syndrome**

Interactions
Drug-drug. *Indomethacin:* increased muromonab blood level, encephalopathy and other adverse CNS effects
Live-virus vaccines: increased viral replication and effects
Other immunosuppressants: increased risk of infection
Drug-diagnostic tests. *Blood urea nitrogen, creatinine:* increased levels
Drug-herbs. *Astragalus, echinacea, melatonin:* interference with immunosuppressant effect

Patient monitoring
- Evaluate vital signs and cardiovascular status. Monitor ECG closely.

Clinical alert: Stay alert for signs and symptoms of cytokine release syndrome, including fever up to 41.6° C (107° F), chills, rigor, nausea, vomiting, abdominal pain, diarrhea, malaise, joint and muscle pain, headache, and tremors.

Clinical alert: Be aware that most adverse reactions occur within 30 minutes to 6 hours of first dose.
- Monitor temperature closely. Stay alert for fever and other signs and symptoms of infection.

Clinical alert: Assess neurologic status and respiratory status closely. Evaluate for evidence of aseptic meningitis, encephalopathy, cerebral edema, pulmonary edema, and ARDS.

Patient teaching

- Inform patient that drug can cause serious adverse reactions. Reassure him that he will be monitored closely and will receive interventions to relieve these reactions. Teach him which signs and symptoms to report immediately.
- Reassure patient that adverse reactions will subside as treatment progresses.
- Advise female patient to avoid becoming pregnant or breastfeeding during therapy.
- As appropriate, review all other significant and life-threatening adverse reactions and interactions, especially those related to the drugs, tests, and herbs mentioned above.

mycophenolate mofetil
CellCept

mycophenolate mofetil hydrochloride
CellCept Intravenous

mycophenolate sodium
Myfortic

Pharmacologic class: Mycophenolic acid derivative

Therapeutic class: Immunosuppressant

Pregnancy risk category C

Action

Inhibits binding of interleukin (IL)-1 to IL-1 receptors, preventing proliferation and differentiation of activated B and T cells. Binds to intracellular proteins to prevent T-cell activation, suppressing immune responses.

Availability

Capsules: 250 mg
Injection: 500 mg/vial
Oral suspension: 200 mg/ml (after constitution)
Tablets: 500 mg
Tablets (delayed-release): 180 mg, 360 mg

Indications and dosages

➢ To prevent organ rejection in patients receiving allogeneic kidney transplants

Adults: 1 g P.O. or I.V. b.i.d. or 720 mg P.O. b.i.d. (delayed-release), given with corticosteroids and cyclosporine

Children: 400 mg/m^2 P.O. b.i.d. (delayed-release), up to a maximum of 720 mg b.i.d; or 600 mg/m^2 P.O. b.i.d., up to a maximum daily dosage of 2 g/10 ml (oral suspension). Given with corticosteroids and cyclosporine.

➢ To prevent organ rejection in patients receiving allogeneic heart transplants

Adults: 1.5 g P.O. or I.V. b.i.d., given with corticosteroids and cyclosporine. May start I.V. therapy less than 24 hours after transplantation; switch to P.O. dosing when tolerated.

➢ To prevent organ rejection in patients receiving allogeneic liver transplants

Adults: 1.5 g b.i.d. P.O. or 1 g I.V. b.i.d., given with corticosteroids and cyclosporine

Dosage adjustment

- Severe chronic renal impairment
- Neutropenia

Contraindications

- Hypersensitivity to drug or its components, mycophenolic acid, or polysorbate 80 (I.V. form)

Precautions

Use cautiously in:

- lymphoma, cancer, neutropenia, renal disease, or GI disorders

m

• elderly patients
• pregnant or breastfeeding patients
• children (indicated for kidney transplant only).

Administration

• Give P.O. form at least 1 hour before or 2 hours after meals. To enhance absorption, don't give with other drugs.
• Give delayed-released tablets whole. Don't let patient crush or chew them.
• Know that pharmacist should mix oral solution before dispensing.
🔊 Be aware that drug is teratogenic. Avoid inhaling powder in capsules or letting powder contact skin, mucous membranes, or eyes. If contact occurs, wash skin thoroughly with soap and water or flush eyes with water.
• Know that delayed-release tablets aren't interchangeable with immediate-release tablets, capsules, or oral suspension.
• For I.V. use, reconstitute with dextrose 5% in water and dilute to 6 mg/ml. Administer over 2 hours.
🔊 Don't give by rapid I.V. push or bolus.

Route	Onset	Peak	Duration
P.O.	Unknown	30-75 min	7.5-18 hr
P.O. (delayed, suspension)	Unknown	Unknown	Unknown
I.V.	Unknown	Unknown	10-17 hr

Adverse reactions

CNS: headache, dizziness, insomnia, asthenia, tremor
CV: chest pain, hypertension, peripheral edema
EENT: pharyngitis, oral moniliasis
GI: nausea, vomiting, diarrhea, constipation, abdominal pain, dyspepsia, **GI hemorrhage**
GU: urinary tract infection, hematuria, **renal tubular necrosis**
Hematologic: anemia, hypochromic anemia, **leukocytosis, leukopenia, thrombocytopenia**
Metabolic: hypophosphatemia, hyperglycemia, hypokalemia, **hyperkalemia**
Musculoskeletal: back pain
Respiratory: dyspnea, cough, bronchitis, pneumonia
Skin: acne, rash
Other: pain, fever, opportunistic infections, **fatal infections, sepsis, lymphoma and other cancers** (especially of skin)

Interactions

Drug-drug. *Acyclovir, ganciclovir, other drugs that undergo renal tubular secretion:* increased risk of toxicity from either drug
Antacids containing aluminum or magnesium: decreased mycophenolate absorption
Cholestyramine: reduced mycophenolate bioavailability
Hormonal contraceptives: reduced contraceptive efficacy
Phenytoin, theophylline: increased blood levels of both drugs
Probenecid, salicylates: increased mycophenolate blood level
Drug-diagnostic tests. *Cholesterol:* increased level
Drug-herbs. *Astragalus, echinacea, melatonin:* interference with immunosuppressant effect

Patient monitoring

• Monitor CBC with white cell differential, electrolyte levels, lipid panel, blood chemistry, and liver function tests frequently.
• Evaluate vital signs. Assess cardiovascular and respiratory status carefully. Watch for signs and symptoms of bronchitis and pneumonia.
🔊 Assess all body systems carefully for signs and symptoms of infection.
🔊 Monitor patient closely for bleeding tendency.

Patient teaching

• Advise patient to take oral drug at least 1 hour before or 2 hours after meals. Tell him not to crush, break, or chew tablets, not to open or chew capsules, and not to take with other drugs.

Clinical alert: If capsule breaks, tell patient not to inhale powder or let it contact skin, mucous membranes, or eyes. If contact occurs, tell him to wash skin thoroughly with soap and water or flush eyes with water.

Clinical alert: Instruct patient to take his temperature and promptly report fever or other signs or symptoms of infection. Tell him to immediately report unusual bleeding or bruising.

- Caution patient to avoid driving and other hazardous activities until he knows how drug affects concentration and alertness.
- Instruct patient to avoid crowds and people with known infections.
- Advise patient not to take herbs without consulting prescriber.
- Tell patient to avoid live-virus vaccines.

Clinical alert: Instruct patient to avoid excessive exposure to sunlight and ultraviolet light, because of increased risk of skin cancer.

Clinical alert: Tell female patient to use abstinence or two other contraceptive methods during and for 6 weeks after therapy (even if she has a history of infertility). Urge her to report suspected pregnancy immediately.

- As appropriate, review all other significant and life-threatening adverse reactions and interactions, especially those related to the drugs, tests, and herbs mentioned above.

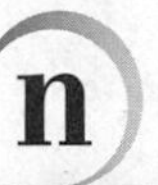

nabumetone

Gen-Nabumetone*, Relafen

Pharmacologic class: Nonsteroidal anti-inflammatory drug (NSAID)
Therapeutic class: Antiarthritic
Pregnancy risk category C (first and second trimesters), ***D*** (third trimester)

Action

Unknown. Thought to stimulate anti-inflammatory response and block pain impulses by inhibiting cyclooxygenase, an enzyme needed for prostaglandin synthesis.

Availability

Tablets: 500 mg, 750 mg

Indications and dosages

➢ Rheumatoid arthritis; osteoarthritis

Adults: 1,000 mg/day P.O. as a single dose or in two divided doses; may increase up to 2,000 mg/day

Contraindications

- Hypersensitivity to drug
- Active GI bleeding or ulcer disease
- History of aspirin- or NSAID-induced asthma, urticaria, or other allergic-type reaction
- Concurrent use of other NSAIDs
- Pregnancy (third trimester)

Precautions

Use cautiously in:

- severe cardiovascular, renal, or hepatic disease
- history of ulcer disease
- pregnant (first or second trimester) or breastfeeding patients
- children (safety and efficacy not established).

Administration

• Give with food or milk to increase absorption.
• In chronic therapy, use lowest effective dosage.

Route	Onset	Peak	Duration
P.O.	1-2 hr	5 hr	12-24 hr

Adverse reactions

CNS: dizziness, drowsiness, fatigue, headache, insomnia, malaise, nervousness
CV: vasculitis
EENT: abnormal vision, tinnitus
GI: nausea, vomiting, diarrhea, constipation, abdominal pain, dyspepsia, flatulence, stomatitis, dry mouth, **GI bleeding**
Skin: pruritus, rash, **angioedema**
Other: edema, fluid retention, allergic reactions including **anaphylaxis**

Interactions

Drug-drug. *Acetaminophen:* increased risk of adverse renal reactions (with chronic nabumetone use)
Anticoagulants, cefamandole, cefoperazone, cefotetan, clopidogrel, eptifibatide, plicamycin, thrombolytics, ticlopidine, tirofiban, valproic acid: increased risk of bleeding
Antihypertensives, diuretics: decreased nabumetone efficacy
Antineoplastics: increased risk of adverse hematologic reactions
Aspirin, corticosteroids, other NSAIDs, potassium supplements: additive adverse GI effects
Cyclosporine: increased risk of renal toxicity
Insulins, oral hypoglycemics: increased hypoglycemic effect
Methotrexate: increased risk of methotrexate toxicity

Patient monitoring

🔊 Watch closely for signs and symptoms of angioedema, anaphylaxis, or other hypersensitivity reactions (including hives, swelling, shortness of breath, and abdominal pain).
• Monitor GI status. Report nutritional deficiencies.
• Assess vital signs.
• Monitor fluid intake and output.

Patient teaching

• Tell patient he may crush tablet if he can't swallow it whole.
• To minimize GI upset, advise patient to take drug with food; eat small, frequent servings of healthy food; and drink plenty of fluids.
• Advise patient to continue taking drug for entire duration prescribed.
🔊 Teach patient to recognize and immediately report signs and symptoms of hypersensitivity reaction and angioedema (hives, swelling, shortness of breath, abdominal pain).
• Caution patient to avoid driving and other hazardous activities until he knows how drug affects concentration, vision, strength, and alertness.
• Advise patient not to drink alcohol. Tell him to avoid aspirin, ibuprofen, and over-the-counter preparations (unless prescribed).
• Caution female patient not to take drug, especially during third trimester.
• As appropriate, review all other significant and life-threatening adverse reactions and interactions, especially those related to the drugs mentioned above.

nadolol

Apo-Nadolol✱, Corgard, Novo-Nadolol✱, Syn-Nadolol✱

Pharmacologic class: Beta-adrenergic blocker (nonselective)
Therapeutic class: Antianginal, antihypertensive
Pregnancy risk category C

Action
Blocks stimulation of $beta_1$- and $beta_2$-adrenergic receptor sites, decreasing cardiac output and thereby slowing heart rate and reducing blood pressure

Availability
Tablets: 20 mg, 40 mg, 80 mg, 120 mg, 160 mg

Indications and dosages
➢ Angina pectoris
Adults: Initially, 40 mg P.O. daily; may increase by 40 to 80 mg q 3 to 7 days p.r.n., up to a maximum of 240 mg/day
➢ Hypertension
Adults: Initially, 40 mg P.O. daily; may increase by 40 to 80 mg q 7 days p.r.n., up to 320 mg/day

Dosage adjustment
- Renal impairment

Off-label uses
- Hyperthyroidism
- Migraine headache
- Parkinson's tremor

Contraindications
- Hypersensitivity to drug or other beta-adrenergic blockers
- Pulmonary edema or cardiogenic shock
- Sinus bradycardia or heart block
- Heart failure (unless secondary to tachyarrhythmia treatable with beta blockers)
- Bronchial asthma (including severe chronic obstructive pulmonary disease)

Precautions
Use cautiously in:
- renal or hepatic impairment, pulmonary disease, diabetes mellitus, thyrotoxicosis
- history of severe allergic reactions
- elderly patients
- pregnant or breastfeeding patients
- children (safety not established).

Administration
- Give with or without food.
- Be aware that drug may be given alone or with diuretic for hypertension.

Route	Onset	Peak	Duration
P.O.	5 days	3-4 hr	24 hr

Adverse reactions
CNS: dizziness, fatigue, paresthesia, behavior changes, sedation
CV: bradycardia, peripheral vascular insufficiency (Raynaud's phenomenon), **heart failure**
EENT: blurred vision, dry eyes, nasal congestion
GI: nausea, constipation, diarrhea, abdominal discomfort or bloating, indigestion, anorexia
Respiratory: bronchospasm
Skin: rash

Interactions
Drug-drug. *Amphetamines, ephedrine, epinephrine, norepinephrine, phenylephrine, pseudoephedrine:* severe vasoconstriction and bradycardia
Antihypertensives, nitrates: additive hypotension
Clonidine: increased hypotension and bradycardia
Digoxin: additive bradycardia
Diltiazem, general anesthetics, phenytoin (I.V.), verapamil: additive myocardial depression
Insulins, oral hypoglycemics: altered glycemic control
Nonsteroidal anti-inflammatory drugs: decreased antihypertensive action
Thyroid hormones: decreased nadolol efficacy
Drug-behaviors. *Acute alcohol ingestion:* additive hypotension
Cocaine use: severe vasoconstriction, bradycardia

n

Patient monitoring

- Monitor vital signs and peripheral circulation. Notify prescriber of heart rate below 55 beats/minute.
- Assess for signs and symptoms of heart failure or bronchospasm.

Patient teaching

- Advise patient to take drug with meals and a bedtime snack to minimize GI upset.
- Teach patient how to measure pulse and blood pressure; tell him when to notify prescriber.
- Instruct patient to avoid over-the-counter products containing stimulants, such as some cold and flu remedies and nasal decongestants.
- Tell diabetic patient and family that drug may mask hypoglycemia symptoms. Advise patient to monitor urine or blood glucose regularly.
- Caution patient to avoid driving and other hazardous activities until he knows how drug affects concentration and alertness.
- As appropriate, review all other significant and life-threatening adverse reactions and interactions, especially those related to the drugs and behaviors mentioned above.

nafarelin acetate

Synarel

Pharmacologic class: Gonadotropin-releasing hormone (GnRH)

Therapeutic class: Hormone

Pregnancy risk category X

Action

Inhibits secretion of gonadotropin, a luteinizing hormone (LH)-releasing hormone. Initially increases pituitary production of LH and follicle-stimulating hormone (FSH), which ultimately leads to deactivation of testicular and ovarian functions.

Availability

Nasal spray: 2 mg/ml in 10-ml bottle (200 mcg/spray)

Indications and dosages

➢ Endometriosis

Adults: One spray (200 mcg) intranasally in one nostril in morning and one spray in other nostril in evening (400 mcg/day). May increase to one spray in each nostril in morning and evening (800 mcg/day).

➢ Central precocious puberty

Children: Two sprays in each nostril in morning and evening (1,600 mcg/day). May increase up to 1,800 mcg/day (three sprays in alternating nostrils t.i.d.).

Contraindications

- Hypersensitivity to GnRH, its analogs, or sorbitol
- Undiagnosed abnormal vaginal bleeding
- Pregnancy or breastfeeding

Precautions

Use cautiously in:

- rhinitis, ovarian cysts, major risk factors for bone density loss (such as chronic alcoholism or chronic corticosteroid use).

Administration

- Make sure patient isn't pregnant before starting therapy.
- For endometriosis, start therapy on day 2 to day 4 of menstrual period.
- If patient needs topical decongestant, wait at least 2 hours after nafarelin dose before giving.
- Know that retreatment for endometriosis isn't recommended.

Route	Onset	Peak	Duration
Intranasal	Within 4 wk	3-4 wk	3-6 mo

Adverse reactions

CNS: emotional lability, headache, depression, insomnia
CV: chest pain
EENT: nasal irritation, rhinitis
GU: vaginal dryness, bleeding, or discharge; menses cessation; transient breast enlargement; decreased libido
Musculoskeletal: reduced bone density, myalgia
Respiratory: dyspnea
Skin: urticaria, rash, pruritus, acne, oily skin, hirsutism, transient pubic hair increase
Other: weight changes, hot flashes, edema, body odor, hypersensitivity reaction

Interactions

Drug-drug. *Topical nasal decongestants:* reduced nafarelin absorption

Patient monitoring

- Monitor patient for emotional lability or depression.
- Assess nasal mucosa for erosion.
- Monitor vital signs. Weigh patient regularly; report edema.
- Stay alert for adverse hormonal effects, including hot flashes, menses cessation followed by breakthrough bleeding, hirsutism, acne, decreased libido, and vaginal dryness.

Patient teaching

- Instruct patient to complete entire course of therapy. Advise her to keep enough of drug on hand to prevent interruption.
- Inform patient that regular menstruation should cease after 4 to 6 weeks of therapy but that breakthrough bleeding may still occur.
- Tell patient ovulation may still occur. Instruct her to use barrier contraception during therapy and to report suspected pregnancy.
- Caution patient not to breastfeed.
- Teach patient about adverse hormonal effects. Identify which signs and symptoms to report.
- Inform patient that drug may cause emotional changes or depression. Advise her to report these to prescriber.
- As appropriate, review all other significant adverse reactions and interactions, especially those related to the drugs mentioned above.

nafcillin sodium

Pharmacologic class: Penicillinase-resistant penicillin
Therapeutic class: Anti-infective
Pregnancy risk category B

Action

Inhibits cell-wall synthesis during microorganism multiplication; resists inactivation by staphylococcal penicillinase. Bactericidal.

Availability

I.V. infusion (piggyback): 1 g, 2 g

Indications and dosages

➢ Systemic infections caused by penicillinase-producing staphylococci
Adults: 500 mg I.V. q 4 hours; for more severe infections, 1 g I.V. q 4 hours. Duration depends on type and severity of infection.

Dosage adjustment

- Children

Contraindications

- Hypersensitivity to drug or other penicillins

Precautions

Use cautiously in:

- cephalosporin hypersensitivity
- renal disorders, GI distress

n

• pregnant or breastfeeding patients
• children.

Administration

• Ask patient about penicillin allergy before giving.
• Reconstitute with normal saline solution, dextrose 5% in water (D_5W), dextrose 10% in water, half D_5W/normal saline solution, or half D_5W/lactated Ringer's solution. Administer over 30 to 60 minutes. Don't mix with other drugs in same solution.

Route	Onset	Peak	Duration
I.V.	Immediate	15 min	4 hr

Adverse reactions

CNS: lethargy, hallucinations, anxiety, depression, twitching, **coma, seizures**
CV: thrombophlebitis
GI: nausea, vomiting, diarrhea
Hematologic: anemia, **bone marrow depression, granulocytopenia**
Skin: angioedema
Other: superinfection, vein irritation, hypersensitivity reactions including **serum sickness** and **anaphylaxis**

Interactions

Drug-drug. *Aminoglycosides:* synergistic effects
Cyclosporine: subtherapeutic cyclosporine blood level
Hormonal contraceptives: decreased contraceptive efficacy
Probenecid: increased nafcillin blood level
Rifampin: antagonism (dose-dependent)
Warfarin: increased risk of bleeding
Drug-diagnostic tests. *Granulocytes, neutrophils, platelets:* decreased counts
Drug-herbs. *Khat:* delayed and reduced nafcillin absorption

Patient monitoring

Assess for signs and symptoms of hypersensitivity reaction (including anaphylaxis, serum sickness, and angioedema), which may occur several days after therapy begins.
Monitor neurologic status. Stay alert for seizures, depression, and hallucinations.
• Evaluate CBC with white cell differential.
• In prolonged therapy, assess for superinfection.

Patient teaching

• Instruct patient to complete entire course of therapy even if symptoms disappear.
Teach patient to recognize and immediately report signs and symptoms of hypersensitivity reactions (including serum sickness and angioedema) as well as bleeding and easy bruising.
• Teach patient about signs and symptoms of superinfection. Instruct him to report these promptly.
• Caution patient to avoid driving and other hazardous activities until he knows how drug affects alertness and motor function.
• As appropriate, review all other significant and life-threatening adverse reactions and interactions, especially those related to the drugs, tests, and herbs mentioned above.

nalbuphine hydrochloride

Nubain

Pharmacologic class: Opioid agonist-antagonist
Therapeutic class: Analgesic, adjunct to anesthesia
Pregnancy risk category C

Action

Binds to opiate receptors in CNS, inhibiting ascending pain pathways. This inhibition alters perception of and response to painful stimuli.

Availability
Injection: 10 mg/ml, 20 mg/ml

Indications and dosages
➢ Moderate to severe pain
Adults: 10 mg/70 kg I.V., I.M., or subcutaneously q 3 to 6 hours p.r.n., up to 160 mg/day. Maximum for single dose is 20 mg.
➢ Adjunct to balanced anesthesia
Adults: 0.3 mg to 3 mg/kg I.V. over 10 to 15 minutes, followed by maintenance dose of 0.25 mg to 0.50 mg/kg I.V. in single doses p.r.n.

Contraindications
- Hypersensitivity to drug

Precautions
Use cautiously in:
- increased intracranial pressure, head trauma, myocardial infarction, severe heart disease, respiratory depression, renal or hepatic disease, impaired ventilation, hypothyroidism, adrenal insufficiency, prostatic hypertrophy, emotional instability, alcoholism
- history of substance abuse or dependence
- pregnant or breastfeeding patients
- children.

Administration
Make sure emergency resuscitation equipment and naloxone (antidote) are available before starting therapy.
- For I.M. use, inject deep into large muscle mass; rotate injection sites.
- When giving I.V. for pain, infuse undiluted over 2 to 3 minutes into vein or I.V. line with compatible solution (such as dextrose 5% in water, normal saline solution, or lactated Ringer's solution).

Route	Onset	Peak	Duration
I.V.	2-3 min	30 min	3-6 hr
I.M.	15 min	1 hr	3-6 hr
Subcut.	15 min	Unknown	3-6 hr

Adverse reactions
CNS: dizziness, sedation, headache, vertigo
CV: hypertension, hypotension, tachycardia, bradycardia
EENT: miosis
GI: nausea, vomiting, dry mouth
Respiratory: dyspnea, **respiratory depression**
Skin: sweating, clammy skin
Other: hypersensitivity reactions including **anaphylaxis**

Interactions
Drug-drug. *CNS depressants (including general anesthetics, MAO inhibitors, sedative-hypnotics, tranquilizers, tricyclic antidepressants):* additive CNS effects
Drug-diagnostic tests. *Amylase, lipase:* increased levels
Drug-herbs. *Chamomile, hops, kava, skullcap, valerian:* increased CNS depression
Drug-behaviors. *Alcohol use:* additive CNS and respiratory depression

Patient monitoring
- Monitor vital signs. Watch for respiratory depression and heart rate changes.
- Evaluate patient for CNS changes. Institute safety measures as needed to prevent injury.

Watch for hypersensitivity reactions, including anaphylaxis.

Patient teaching
- Instruct patient to change position slowly and carefully to avoid dizziness from sudden blood pressure decrease.
- Tell patient to avoid CNS depressants (including alcohol, sedative-hypnotics, and some herbs) for at least 24 hours after taking nalbuphine.
- Advise patient to consult prescriber before taking herbs.
- Caution patient to avoid driving and other hazardous activities until he knows how drug affects concentration, vision, and alertness.

n

• As appropriate, review all other significant and life-threatening adverse reactions and interactions, especially those related to the drugs, tests, herbs, and behaviors mentioned above.

nalidixic acid
NegGram

Pharmacologic class: Quinolone antibiotic

Therapeutic class: Urinary tract anti-infective

Pregnancy risk category B

Action
Interferes with DNA and RNA synthesis in susceptible gram-negative bacteria. Bactericidal.

Availability
Oral suspension: 250 mg/5 ml
Tablets: 250 mg, 500 mg, 1 g

Indications and dosages
➢ Urinary tract infections (UTIs) caused by susceptible gram-negative bacteria

Adults: Initially, 1 g P.O. q.i.d. for 1 to 2 weeks. In prolonged therapy, dosage may be reduced to 2 g/day.
Children ages 3 months to 12 years: 55 mg/kg (25 mg/lb) daily P.O. in four equally divided doses. In prolonged therapy, dosage may be reduced to 33 mg/kg (15 mg/lb) daily.

Contraindications
• Hypersensitivity to drug
• Seizure disorder

Precautions
Use cautiously in:
• renal or hepatic disease, G6PD deficiency, cerebral arteriosclerosis, CNS damage
• elderly patients
• pregnant or breastfeeding patients
• prepubertal children.

Administration
• Give with food or milk to avoid GI upset.

Route	Onset	Peak	Duration
P.O.	Variable	1-2 hr	Unknown

Adverse reactions
CNS: drowsiness, weakness, headache, dizziness, malaise, vertigo, syncope, excitement, hallucinations, confusion, depression, insomnia, **seizures**
EENT: blurred vision, light sensitivity, decreased visual acuity, diplopia, altered color perception
GI: nausea, vomiting, diarrhea, abdominal pain
Hematologic: eosinophilia
Skin: rash, urticaria, pruritus, photosensitivity, **angioedema, Stevens-Johnson syndrome**
Other: fever, chills, **anaphylaxis**

Interactions
Drug-drug. *Antacids:* decreased nalidixic acid absorption
Nitrofurantoin: decreased nalidixic acid effects
Oral anticoagulant: increased anticoagulant effects
Drug-diagnostic tests. *Urinary vanillylmandelic acid, urine 17-ketogenic steroids, urine 17-ketosteroids:* false increases
Urine glucose tests using cupric sulfate reagents (such as Benedict's test): false-positive reaction
Drug-food. *Caffeine-containing foods and beverages:* increased stimulation
Drug-herbs. *Dong quai, St. John's wort:* photosensitivity

Patient monitoring
• Monitor clinical response. If no improvement occurs, repeat culture and sensitivity tests.

• Assess neurologic and nutritional status carefully.
• Watch for GI signs and symptoms.
Clinical alert: Monitor for hypersensitivity reactions, including anaphylaxis and angioedema.

Patient teaching

• Instruct patient to take with food to minimize GI upset.
Clinical alert: Teach patient to recognize and immediately report serious adverse effects, including CNS changes and angioedema.
• Advise patient to minimize GI upset by eating small, frequent servings of food and drinking plenty of fluids.
• Caution patient to avoid driving and other hazardous activities until he knows how drug affects concentration and alertness.
• As appropriate, review all other significant and life-threatening adverse reactions and interactions, especially those related to the drugs, tests, foods, and herbs mentioned above.

naproxen

Apo-Naproxen✱, EC-Naprosyn, Naprosyn, Naprosyn-E✱, Naprosyn SR✱, Novo-Naprox✱

naproxen sodium

Aleve, Anaprox, Anaprox DS, Apo-Napro-Na✱, Apo-Napro-Na DS✱, Naprelan, Novo-Naprox Sodium✱, Novo-Naprox Sodium DS✱, Synflex✱

Pharmacologic class: Nonsteroidal anti-inflammatory drug (NSAID)
Therapeutic class: Nonopioid analgesic, antipyretic, anti-inflammatory
Pregnancy risk category B (first and second trimesters), ***D*** (third trimester)

Action

Unknown. Thought to inhibit prostaglandin synthesis.

Availability

naproxen
Oral suspension: 125 mg/5 ml
Suppositories: 500 mg
Tablets: 125 mg, 250 mg, 375 mg, 500 mg
Tablets (controlled-release): 375 mg, 500 mg
Tablets (delayed-release): 250 mg, 375 mg, 500 mg
Tablets (extended-release): 750 mg
naproxen sodium
Caplets, tablets: 220 mg, 275 mg, 550 mg

Indications and dosages

➢ Pain; osteoarthritis; ankylosing spondylitis; dysmenorrhea; bursitis; acute tendinitis
Adults: 250 to 500 mg (naproxen) P.O. b.i.d. (up to 1.5 g/day); 375 to 500 mg (naproxen delayed-release) P.O. t.i.d.; 250 mg, 375 mg, or 500 mg (naproxen oral suspension) P.O. b.i.d.; 275 to 550 mg (naproxen sodium) P.O. b.i.d. (up to 1.65 g/day); or 750 or 1,000 mg/day (naproxen controlled-release) P.O., not to exceed 1,500 mg/day
Children: 10 mg/kg P.O. daily in two divided doses (naproxen only)
➢ Mild to moderate pain; primary dysmenorrhea
Adults: Initially, 500 mg (naproxen) P.O., followed by 250 mg q 6 to 8 hours p.r.n., to a maximum of 1.25 g/day. Or initially, 550 mg (naproxen sodium) P.O., followed by 275 mg q 6 to 8 hours p.r.n., to a maximum of 1,375 mg/day. Or 1,000 mg/day (naproxen controlled-release) P.O., to a maximum of 1,500 mg/day for a limited time; then no more than 1,000 mg/day.
➢ Gout
Adults: Initially, 750 mg (naproxen) P.O., followed by 250 mg q 8 hours; or

initially, 825 mg (naproxen sodium) P.O., followed by 275 mg q 8 hours. Or 1,000 to 1,500 mg (naproxen controlled-release) P.O. once on day 1, followed by 1,000 mg daily.

Contraindications

- Hypersensitivity to drug or other NSAIDs
- Active GI bleeding or ulcer disease
- Asthma
- Pregnancy (third trimester)

Precautions

Use cautiously in:

- severe cardiovascular, renal, or hepatic disease
- history of ulcer disease
- chronic alcohol use or abuse
- pregnant (first and second trimesters) or breastfeeding patients
- children younger than age 2 (safety not established).

Administration

- Give with food or milk to avoid GI upset.

Route	Onset	Peak	Duration
P.O. (analgesia)	1 hr	2-4 hr	8-12 hr
P.O. (anti-inflamm.)	14 days	2-4 wk	Unknown

Adverse reactions

CNS: dizziness, drowsiness, headache, vertigo, light-headedness
CV: palpitations, tachycardia
EENT: visual disturbances, tinnitus, auditory disturbances
GI: nausea, diarrhea, constipation, heartburn, abdominal pain, stomatitis, **GI bleeding**
Skin: rash, pruritus, skin eruptions, sweating, photosensitivity
Other: thirst, edema, allergic reactions including **anaphylaxis**

Interactions

Drug-drug. *Acetaminophen (chronic use), cyclosporine:* increased risk of adverse renal effects
Anticoagulants, thrombolytics: increased anticoagulant effect
Antihypertensives, cefamandole, cefoperazone, cefotetan, diuretics, eptifibatide: decreased response
Antineoplastics, methotrexate: increased risk of nephrotoxicity
Aspirin: decreased naproxen efficacy
Aspirin, corticosteroids, other NSAIDs: additive adverse GI effects
Clopidogrel, plicamycin, ticlopidine, valproic acid: increased risk of bleeding
Insulin, oral hypoglycemics: increased risk of hypoglycemia
Lithium: increased lithium blood level and risk of nephrotoxicity
Other photosensitizing agents: increased risk of photosensitivity
Probenecid: increased naproxen blood level, increased risk of toxicity
Drug-diagnostic tests. *Alanine aminotransferase, alkaline phosphatase, aspartate aminotransferase, blood urea nitrogen, creatinine, lactate dehydrogenase, potassium:* increased levels
Bleeding time: prolonged for up to 4 days after therapy ends
Creatinine clearance, glucose, hematocrit, hemoglobin, leukocytes, platelets: decreased values
Urine 5-hydroxy-indoleacetic acid, urine steroids: test interference
Drug-herbs. *Anise, arnica, chamomile, clove, dong quai, fenugreek, feverfew, garlic, ginger, ginkgo, ginseng, licorice:* increased anticoagulant effect, increased risk of bleeding

Patient monitoring

- Monitor GI status. Stay alert for signs and symptoms of GI bleeding.
- In long-term use, assess CBC with white cell differential and coagulation studies, and monitor for visual and hearing impairment.

• Monitor cardiovascular status for tachycardia, palpitations, and edema.
• Monitor blood glucose level closely in diabetic patients.

Patient teaching

• Tell patient to take with food or milk followed by 8 oz of water, and to stay upright for 30 minutes afterward.
• Inform patient that he may crush or break regular tablets but must swallow extended-, delayed-, or controlled-release form whole.
• Tell patient that drug's full therapeutic effect may take up to 2 weeks.
• Caution patient not to exceed recommended dosage.
• Advise patient to use sunscreen to prevent photosensitivity reaction.
• Instruct patient not to take over-the-counter medications unless prescribed.
• Tell patient to consult prescriber before taking herbs.
• Caution pregnant patient not to take drug, especially during third trimester.
• As appropriate, review all other significant and life-threatening adverse reactions and interactions, especially those related to the drugs, tests, and herbs mentioned above.

naratriptan hydrochloride

Amerge

Pharmacologic class: Selective 5-hydroxytryptamine$_1$ (5-HT$_1$) agonist
Therapeutic class: Vascular headache suppressant, antimigraine drug
Pregnancy risk category C

Action

Binds with specific 5-HT$_1$ receptors in intracranial blood vessels and sensory trigeminal nerves, leading to vasoconstriction and migraine relief

Availability

Tablets: 1 mg, 2.5 mg

Indications and dosages

➢ Migraine headache
Adults: 1 or 2.5 mg P.O. as single dose; may repeat in 4 hours. Don't exceed 5 mg in 24 hours; don't use to treat more than four headaches per month.

Dosage adjustment

• Mild to moderate renal or hepatic impairment

Contraindications

• Hypersensitivity to drug or its components
• Hemiplegic or basilar headaches
• Severe renal, cardiovascular or hepatic impairment
• History of cerebrovascular or peripheral vascular conditions
• Ischemic bowel disease
• Uncontrolled hypertension
• Use of ergot-type drugs (such as dihydroergotamine) and other 5-HT$_1$ agonists within 24 hours
• MAO inhibitor use within past 14 days

Precautions

Use cautiously in:
• mild to moderate renal or hepatic impairment, cardiovascular risk factors
• elderly patients (not recommended)
• pregnant or breastfeeding patients
• children (safety not established).

Administration

• Know that drug does not prevent migraine.
• Give only if patient's cardiovascular status has been evaluated and determined to be safe, and if first dose can be given under supervision.

Route	Onset	Peak	Duration
P.O.	30-60 min	2-3 hr	Up to 24 hr

n

Adverse reactions

CNS: dizziness, drowsiness, malaise, fatigue, paresthesia
CV: coronary artery vasospasm, myocardial infarction, ventricular fibrillation or tachycardia
GI: nausea, vomiting
Other: pain or pressure sensation in throat or neck

Interactions

Drug-drug. *Ergot-type compounds (dihydroergotamine, methysergide):* prolonged vasospastic reaction
Hormonal contraceptives: increased naratriptan blood level and effects
MAO inhibitors: increased systemic exposure to naratriptan, increased risk of adverse reactions
Selective serotonin reuptake inhibitors: weakness, hyperreflexia, incoordination
Sibutramine: serotonin syndrome
Drug-herbs. *S-adenosylmethionine (SAM-e), St. John's wort:* increased risk of adverse serotonergic effects
Drug-behaviors. *Cigarette smoking:* increased naratriptan metabolism

Patient monitoring

- Maintain especially close monitoring in patients with cardiovascular risk factors (such as hypertension, hypercholesterolemia, obesity, diabetes mellitus, cigarette smoking, strong family history), postmenopausal women, and men older than age 40.
- Assess vital signs and ECG.
- Monitor neurologic status closely. Institute safety measures as needed to prevent injury.

Patient teaching

- Tell patient to take at first sign of headache.
- Advise patient to take second dose (if approved) at least 4 hours after first dose if headache has not gone away completely or has returned.
- Caution patient not to take more than two tablets in a 24-hour period.
- Advise patient to avoid driving and other hazardous activities until he knows how drug affects concentration and alertness.
- Tell patient to avoid cigarette smoking and to discuss herb use with prescriber.
- As appropriate, review all other significant and life-threatening adverse reactions and interactions, especially those related to the drugs, herbs, and behaviors mentioned above.

nateglinide

Starlix

Pharmacologic class: Amino acid derivative
Therapeutic class: Hypoglycemic
Pregnancy risk category C

Action

Decreases blood glucose level by stimulating insulin secretion from pancreatic beta cells; interacts with calcium and potassium channels in pancreas

Availability

Tablets: 60 mg, 120 mg

Indications and dosages

➤ To decrease glucose levels in type 2 (non-insulin-dependent) diabetes mellitus not adequately controlled by diet and exercise
Adults: 120 mg P.O. t.i.d. up to 30 minutes before meals, or 60 mg P.O. t.i.d. if patient is near glycosylated hemoglobin (HbA1c) goal

Contraindications

- Hypersensitivity to drug or its components
- Diabetic ketoacidosis
- Type 1 (insulin-dependent) diabetes mellitus

Precautions

Use cautiously in:
• renal or hepatic impairment, adrenal or pituitary insufficiency
• elderly or malnourished patients
• pregnant or breastfeeding patients.

Administration

• Give 30 minutes before meals. If meal is missed, don't give dose.
• Know that drug may be given alone or with metformin.

Route	Onset	Peak	Duration
P.O.	Rapid	Within 1 hr	4 hr

Adverse reactions

CNS: dizziness
GI: diarrhea
Metabolic: hypoglycemia
Musculoskeletal: back pain, joint pain
Respiratory: upper respiratory tract infection, bronchitis, coughing
Other: flulike symptoms, trauma

Interactions

Drug-drug. *Beta-adrenergic blockers, MAO inhibitors, nonsteroidal anti-inflammatory drugs, salicylates:* increased hypoglycemic effect
Corticosteroids, sympathomimetics, thiazides, thyroid products: reduced hypoglycemic effect
Drug-diagnostic tests. *Glucose:* decreased level

Patient monitoring

• Monitor blood glucose and HbA1c levels.
• Assess pulmonary status for bronchitis, upper respiratory infection, and flulike signs and symptoms.
• Monitor musculoskeletal status. Check for back pain and arthropathy.
• Note GI complaints, and identify nutritional deficiencies.

Patient teaching

• Instruct patient to take dose up to 30 minutes before each main meal.
• Advise patient not to skip a meal. If he does, tell him to also skip accompanying nateglinide dose, to prevent hypoglycemia.
• Teach patient how to monitor blood and urine for glucose and ketones, as prescribed.
• Instruct patient to report adverse CNS effects and signs and symptoms of respiratory infection.
• Caution patient to avoid driving and other hazardous activities until he knows how drug affects sensation and balance.
• As appropriate, review all other significant and life-threatening adverse reactions and interactions, especially those related to the drugs and tests mentioned above.

nedocromil sodium

Tilade

Pharmacologic class: Mast cell stabilizer
Therapeutic class: Antiasthmatic
Pregnancy risk category B

Action

Blocks allergen-triggered release of histamine and slow-releasing substance of anaphylaxis from mast cells, decreasing overall allergic response and inflammatory reaction

Availability

Aerosol for inhalation: 1.75 mg/spray in 16.2-g canister

Indications and dosages

➢ Maintenance therapy in mild to moderate bronchial asthma
Adults and children ages 6 and older: Two inhalations (1.75 mg/spray) two to four times daily

Contraindications
• Hypersensitivity to drug or its components

Precautions
Use cautiously in:
• acute asthma attack
• pregnant or breastfeeding patients
• children younger than age 6 (safety not established).

Administration
• Know that drug isn't indicated for bronchospasm reversal in acute asthma attack.
Stop drug immediately if bronchospasm occurs.
• Be aware that therapeutic response may take up to 4 weeks.

Route	Onset	Peak	Duration
Inhalation	Unknown	30 min	3.5 hr

Adverse reactions
CNS: headache
CV: chest pain
EENT: conjunctivitis, rhinitis, sinusitis, pharyngitis
GI: nausea, diarrhea, abdominal pain
Respiratory: cough, upper respiratory tract infection, increased sputum, bronchitis, dyspnea, **worsening of bronchial asthma, bronchospasm**
Other: unpleasant taste, viral infection, hypersensitivity reactions including **anaphylaxis**

Interactions
None significant

Patient monitoring
• Monitor pulmonary function tests.
• Assess respiratory status frequently.
Watch for increasing bronchospasm and anaphylaxis.

Patient teaching
• Advise patient to expectorate mucus from airway before using inhaler.
• Provide instructions on proper inhalation technique.
• Encourage patient to use spacer as needed to achieve therapeutic dosage.
• Tell patient to gargle and sip water after inhalation, to reduce mouth irritation.
• Inform patient that therapeutic response may take up to 4 weeks.
• Inform patient that drug should be used only for asthma prevention and not as rescue inhaler in emergencies.
• As appropriate, review all other significant and life-threatening adverse reactions.

nefazodone hydrochloride

Pharmacologic class: Phenylpiperazine
Therapeutic class: Antidepressant
Pregnancy risk category C

Action
Potentiates effects of norepinephrine and serotonin by blocking synaptic reuptake in nerve cells and disrupting $alpha_1$-adrenergic receptors

Availability
Tablets: 50 mg, 100 mg, 150 mg, 200 mg, 250 mg

Indications and dosages
➤ Major depression
Adults: Initially, 100 mg P.O. b.i.d. May increase weekly up to 600 mg/day in two divided doses.

Dosage adjustment
• Elderly patients

Contraindications
• Hypersensitivity to drug, its components, or other phenylpiperazines
• Active hepatic disease, baseline transaminase elevation, or previous

drug withdrawal necessitated by hepatic damage
- MAO inhibitor use within past 14 days
- Concurrent cisapride (not available in U.S.), pimozide, carbamazepine, or triazolam therapy

Precautions
Use cautiously in:
- cardiovascular or cerebrovascular disease
- history of suicide attempt, drug abuse, or mania
- elderly patients
- pregnant or breastfeeding patients
- children younger than age 18 (safety not established).

Administration
- Give with food or milk if GI upset occurs.
- Know that tablets may be crushed.

Don't give concurrently with cisapride, pimozide, carbamazepine, or triazolam.

Don't give within 14 days of MAO inhibitors.

Route	Onset	Peak	Duration
P.O.	Days-wks	Few wks	Unknown

Adverse reactions
CNS: dizziness, asthenia, agitation, light-headedness, insomnia, drowsiness, confusion, weakness, headache, impaired memory, poor concentration, paresthesia, psychomotor retardation, tremor, **suicidal behavior or ideation (especially in child or adolescent)**
CV: hypotension, orthostatic hypotension, peripheral edema
EENT: abnormal or blurred vision, eye pain, tinnitus, pharyngitis
GI: nausea, vomiting, diarrhea, constipation, dyspepsia, dry mouth
GU: urinary frequency or retention, urinary tract infection
Hepatic: hepatotoxicity, hepatic failure
Respiratory: increased cough
Skin: rash, pruritus
Other: increased appetite, thirst, infection, chills, fever, flulike symptoms

Interactions
Drug-drug. *Alprazolam, triazolam:* increased blood level and effects of these drugs
Antihypertensives, nitrates: additive hypotension
Carbamazepine, cisapride, pimozide: increased nefazodone blood level, leading to toxicity
CNS depressants (including antihistamines, opioids, sedative-hypnotics): additive CNS depression
Digoxin: increased digoxin blood level
HMG-CoA reductase inhibitors: increased risk of myopathy
MAO inhibitors: potentially fatal reactions (hyperpyrexia, excitation, seizures, delirium, coma)
Drug-diagnostic tests. *CBC, cholesterol, glucose, hematocrit:* decreased levels
Hepatic enzymes: increased levels
Drug-herbs. *Chamomile, hops, kava, skullcap, valerian:* increased CNS depression
S-adenosylmethionine (SAM-e), St. John's wort: increased risk of adverse serotonergic effects, including serotonin syndrome
Drug-behaviors. *Acute alcohol ingestion:* additive hypotension
Alcohol use: increased CNS depression

Patient monitoring
- Monitor vital signs with patient lying down, sitting, and standing. Notify prescriber if blood pressure drops 20 mm Hg.
- Assess CBC.

Monitor liver function tests frequently. Notify prescriber of abnormal results.
- Closely monitor neurologic status.

n

• Evaluate patient for withdrawal symptoms (which may occur if therapy stops abruptly).
Clinical alert: Monitor closely for increasing depression and suicidal ideation (especially in child or adolescent).

Patient teaching

• Advise patient to take with food or milk to minimize GI upset.
• Tell patient to crush drug if he can't swallow it whole.
• Inform patient that therapeutic response may take up to 4 weeks. Encourage him to keep taking drug as prescribed.
Clinical alert: Tell patient drug may cause adverse CNS effects. Advise him to report significant mood changes (especially depression or suicidal thoughts). Caution parent to report these problems in child or adolescent.
Clinical alert: Instruct patient to immediately report unusual tiredness, yellowing of skin or eyes, nausea, or anorexia.
• Instruct patient to rise slowly and carefully, to avoid dizziness from temporary blood pressure drop.
• Tell patient to avoid alcohol and to consult prescriber before taking herbs.
Clinical alert: Instruct patient not to stop taking drug abruptly. Dosage must be tapered.
• As appropriate, review all other significant and life-threatening adverse reactions and interactions, especially those related to the drugs, tests, herbs, and behaviors mentioned above.

nelfinavir mesylate

Viracept

Pharmacologic class: Protease inhibitor
Therapeutic class: Antiretroviral
Pregnancy risk category B

Action

Inhibits action of human immunodeficiency virus (HIV) protease and prevents cleavage of viral polyproteins, resulting in production of immature, noninfectious virus

Availability

Oral powder: 50 mg/1 g powder (1 g powder/level scoopful)
Tablets: 250 mg, 625 mg

Indications and dosages

➢ HIV infection
Adults and children older than age 13: 750 mg P.O. t.i.d. or 1,250 mg b.i.d., given with other antiretrovirals
Children ages 2 to 13: 20 to 30 mg/kg P.O. t.i.d., given with a meal or light snack

Contraindications

• Hypersensitivity to drug or its components
• Concurrent use of astemizole, cisapride (not available in U.S.), amiodarone, dihydroergotamine, ergotamine, midazolam, quinidine, rifampin, terfenadine, or triazolam

Precautions

Use cautiously in:
• hemophilia, diabetes mellitus, hepatic impairment
• phenylketonuria (oral powder contains phenylalanine)
• breastfeeding patients.

Administration

• Give tablets with food.
• For adult who can't swallow tablets whole, crush and mix in food or dissolve in small amount of water. Have patient consume mixture immediately, or refrigerate for up to 6 hours.
• For child who can't swallow tablets, mix oral powder with small amount of water, formula, or milk. Have child consume mixture immediately, or refrigerate for up to 6 hours.

• Don't mix powder with water in its original container.
• Don't mix powder with acidic juice (combination produces bitter taste).
Don't give concurrently with amiodarone, astemizole, cisapride, dihydroergotamine, ergotamine, midazolam, quinidine, rifampin, terfenadine, or triazolam.

Route	Onset	Peak	Duration
P.O.	Rapid	2-4 hr	8 hr

Adverse reactions

CNS: anxiety, depression, dizziness, drowsiness, emotional lability, headache, hyperkinesia, insomnia, malaise, migraine headache, sleep disorders, weakness, myasthenia, paresthesia, **suicidal ideation, seizures**
EENT: acute iritis, rhinitis, sinusitis, pharyngitis
GI: nausea, diarrhea, abdominal pain, flatulence
GU: nephrolithiasis, sexual dysfunction
Hematologic: anemia, **leukopenia, thrombocytopenia**
Metabolic: dehydration, hyperuricemia, **hypoglycemia**
Musculoskeletal: joint pain, arthritis, back pain, myalgia, myopathy
Respiratory: dyspnea, **bronchospasm**
Skin: pruritus, rash, sweating, fungal dermatitis, folliculitis, urticaria
Other: fever, body fat redistribution, allergic reactions

Interactions

Drug-drug. *Amiodarone, dihydroergotamine, ergotamine, midazolam, quinidine, triazolam:* excessive sedation, vasoconstriction, serious arrhythmias
Carbamazepine, phenobarbital, phenytoin, rifampin: decreased nelfinavir blood level and efficacy
Hormonal contraceptives: decreased contraceptive blood level and efficacy
Rifabutin: decreased rifabutin metabolism and effects
Drug-diagnostic tests. *Lipids:* increased levels
Drug-food. *Most foods:* enhanced drug absorption
Drug-herbs. *St. John's wort:* decreased nelfinavir blood level and efficacy

Patient monitoring

Watch for signs and symptoms of depression and suicidal ideation.
• Evaluate neurologic status closely, particularly for seizures and sensorimotor dysfunction.
• Assess CBC, lipid panel, uric acid level, and HIV-specific tests.
• Watch for secondary infections, particularly fungal and EENT infections.

Patient teaching

• Advise patient to take with a meal or snack. Inform him that he may mix oral powder with nonacidic fluids.
• Tell patient he may take missed dose up to 1 hour before next scheduled dose.
Instruct patient to report depression or suicidal thoughts.
• Tell patient that drug may predispose him to other infections, especially fungal and EENT infections. Advise him to avoid crowds and to wash hands often and thoroughly.
• Tell patient with phenylketonuria (or caregiver) that powder contains phenylalanine.
• Instruct female patient to use reliable barrier contraception.
• Advise female patient not to breastfeed, because breast milk may transfer HIV to infant.
• Caution patient to avoid driving and other hazardous activities until he knows how drug affects concentration, vision, strength, and alertness.
• As appropriate, review all other significant and life-threatening adverse reactions and interactions, especially those related to the drugs, tests, foods, and herbs mentioned above.

n

neomycin sulfate

Mycifradin, Neo-Fradin, Neo-Tabs

Pharmacologic class: Aminoglycoside
Therapeutic class: Anti-infective
Pregnancy risk category D

Action

Interferes with bacterial protein synthesis by binding to 30S ribosomal subunit, causing misreading of genetic code. Inaccurate peptide sequence then forms in protein chain, causing bacterial death.

Availability

Ointment: 0.5%
Oral solution: 125 mg/5 ml
Tablets: 500 mg

Indications and dosages

➢ Preoperative intestinal antisepsis
Adults: 1 g P.O. q hour for four doses, then 1 g q 4 hours for 24 hours or 1 g at 19 hours, 18 hours, and 9 hours before surgery
➢ Hepatic encephalopathy
Adults: 4 to 12 g/day P.O. in divided doses
➢ Superficial bacterial infections
Adults: Apply ointment topically one to five times daily.

Contraindications

- Hypersensitivity to drug or other aminoglycosides
- Intestinal obstruction

Precautions

Use cautiously in:
- renal impairment, neuromuscular diseases (such as myasthenia gravis), hearing impairment
- obese patients
- elderly patients
- pregnant or breastfeeding patients
- children under age 18 (safety not established).

Administration

- Give preoperative dose before bowel surgery, after cathartic administration, as ordered.

Route	Onset	Peak	Duration
P.O.	Variable	1-4 hr	Unknown
Topical	Unknown	Unknown	Unknown

Adverse reactions

CNS: neuromuscular blockade
EENT: ototoxicity (with prolonged, high-dose use)
GI: nausea, vomiting, diarrhea, malabsorption syndrome
GU: nephrotoxicity (with prolonged, high-dose use)
Other: superinfection

Interactions

Drug-drug. *Acyclovir, amphotericin B, cephalosporin, cisplatin, other aminoglycosides, vancomycin:* increased risk of ototoxicity and nephrotoxicity
Digoxin: decreased digoxin absorption
Dimenhydrinate: masking of ototoxicity symptoms
Oral anticoagulants: increased anticoagulant effect
Potent loop diuretics: increased risk of ototoxicity

Patient monitoring

- Assess for neuromuscular blockade, ototoxicity, and nephrotoxicity.
- Monitor kidney function tests.

Patient teaching

- Instruct patient to drink plenty of water.
- Tell patient to complete full course of therapy.
- Inform patient that drug may cause muscle weakness.
- Instruct patient to report hearing problems and change in urination pattern.

• Caution patient to avoid driving and other hazardous activities until he knows how drug affects neuromuscular status.
• Tell patient he'll undergo frequent blood testing during therapy.
• As appropriate, review all other significant and life-threatening adverse reactions and interactions, especially those related to the drugs mentioned above.

neostigmine bromide
Prostigmin

neostigmine methylsulfate
PMS-Neostigmine Methylsulfate✦, Prostigmin

Pharmacologic class: Anticholinesterase
Therapeutic class: Muscle stimulant
Pregnancy risk category C

Action
Inhibits enzyme acetylcholinesterase, leading to increased acetylcholine concentration at synapse and prolonged acetylcholine effects. Exerts direct cholinomimetic effect on skeletal muscle.

Availability
Injection (methylsulfate): 2 mg/ml, 1 mg/ml, 0.5 mg/ml, 0.25 mg/ml
Tablets (bromide): 15 mg

Indications and dosages
➢ Myasthenia gravis
Adults: 15 mg/day P.O.; may increase p.r.n. up to 375 mg/day; average dosage is 150 mg/day. Or 1 ml of 1:2,000 solution (0.5 mg) subcutaneously or I.M. based on response and tolerance.
➢ Postoperative abdominal distention and bladder atony
Adults: 0.5 to 1 mg I.M. or subcutaneously. If given for urinary retention and no response occurs within 1 hour, catheterize patient as ordered and repeat dose q 3 hours for five doses.
➢ Antidote for nondepolarizing neuromuscular blockers
Adults: 0.5 to 2.5 mg I.V.; repeat p.r.n. up to 5 mg. Precede initial dose with 0.6 to 1.2 mg atropine sulfate I.V., as ordered.

Contraindications
• Hypersensitivity to cholinergics or bromide
• Mechanical obstruction of GI or urinary tract
• Peritonitis

Precautions
Use cautiously in:
• asthma, peptic ulcer, bradycardia, arrhythmias, recent coronary occlusion, vagotonia, hyperthyroidism, seizure disorder
• pregnant or breastfeeding patients.

Administration
Before giving, ensure that atropine sulfate is available to treat cholinergic crisis.
• Know that atropine may be combined with usual neostigmine dose to decrease risk of adverse reactions.
• Give oral form 1 hour before or 2 hours after a meal.
• Administer I.V. dose undiluted directly into vein or I.V. line. Give 0.5-mg dose slowly over 1 minute.
Keep resuscitation equipment nearby.

Route	Onset	Peak	Duration
P.O.	45-75 min	1-2 hr	2-4 hr
I.V.	4-8 min	1-2 hr	2-4 hr
I.M., subcut.	20-30 min	1-2 hr	2-4 hr

Adverse reactions

CNS: dizziness, headache, drowsiness, asthenia, **loss of consciousness**
CV: hypotension, tachycardia, bradycardia, **atrioventricular (AV) block, cardiac arrest**
EENT: vision changes, lacrimation, miosis
GI: nausea, vomiting, diarrhea, abdominal cramping, flatulence, increased peristalsis
GU: urinary frequency
Musculoskeletal: muscle cramps, spasms, and fasciculations; joint pain
Respiratory: dyspnea, **bronchospasm, respiratory depression, respiratory arrest, laryngospasm**
Skin: rash, urticaria, flushing
Other: anaphylaxis

Interactions

Drug-drug. *Aminoglycosides, anticholinergics, atropine, corticosteroids, local and general anesthetics:* reversal of anticholinergic effects
Cholinergics: additive toxicity
Kanamycin, neomycin, streptomycin: increased neuromuscular blockade
Succinylcholine: potentiation of neuromuscular blockade, prolonged respiratory depression

Patient monitoring

Monitor vital signs. Assess patient for hypotension, bradycardia or tachycardia, AV block, and evidence of impending cardiac arrest.
- Evaluate respiratory and neurologic status.

Patient teaching

- Instruct patient to take tablets 1 hour before or 2 hours after meals.

Tell patient drug may alter his respiratory and cardiac status. Teach him to recognize and immediately report warning signs.
- Caution patient to avoid driving and other hazardous activities until he knows how drug affects concentration, vision, muscle function, and alertness.
- As appropriate, review all other significant and life-threatening adverse reactions and interactions, especially those related to the drugs mentioned above.

nesiritide

Natrecor

Pharmacologic class: Human B-type natriuretic peptide
Therapeutic class: Vasodilator
Pregnancy risk category C

Action

Binds to receptors on vascular smooth muscle and endothelial cells, causing smooth muscle relaxation and vasodilation. As a result, systemic and pulmonary pressures decrease and diuresis occurs.

Availability

Injection: 1.5 mg in single-use vials

Indications and dosages

➢ Acutely decompensated heart failure in patients who have dyspnea at rest or with minimal activity
Adults: 2 mcg/kg I.V. bolus, followed by continuous I.V. infusion of 0.01 mcg/kg/minute

Contraindications

- Hypersensitivity to drug or its components
- Systolic pressure below 90 mm Hg
- Primary therapy for cardiogenic shock

Precautions

Use cautiously in:
- restrictive or obstructive cardiomyopathy, constrictive pericarditis, peri-

cardial tamponade, renal dysfunction, hypotension
• pregnant or breastfeeding patients.

Administration

Clinical alert: Know that nesiritide is a high-alert drug.
• For I.V. use, prime tubing before connecting to patient. Withdraw bolus and infuse over 60 seconds into I.V. port of tubing. Follow immediately with constant infusion delivering 0.01 mcg/kg/minute.
• Know that drug should be mixed and infused in dextrose 5% in water, normal saline solution, or dextrose in half-normal saline solution.
Clinical alert: Don't mix with other drug solutions. Always administer through separate line.
• Know that nesiritide therapy beyond 48 hours has not been studied.

Route	Onset	Peak	Duration
I.V.	Immediate	15 min	Unknown

Adverse reactions

CNS: dizziness, headache, insomnia, anxiety
CV: hypotension, angina pectoris, bradycardia, ventricular extrasystole, **ventricular tachycardia**
GI: nausea, vomiting, abdominal pain
Musculoskeletal: leg cramps, back pain
Respiratory: cough, hemoptysis, **apnea**
Other: injection site reactions

Interactions

Drug-drug. *Angiotensin-converting enzyme inhibitors, nitrates:* increased hypotension
Bumetanide, enalaprilat, ethacrynate sodium, furosemide, heparin, hydralazine, insulin: physical and chemical incompatibility with nesiritide
Drug-diagnostic tests. *Hematocrit, hemoglobin:* decreased values

Patient monitoring

• Monitor vital signs and pulmonary artery wedge pressure continuously during and for several hours after infusion.
• Assess cardiovascular status closely.

Patient teaching

• Tell patient he'll be monitored closely during and for several hours after infusion.
• Inform patient that drug may cause serious adverse effects. Reassure him that he'll receive appropriate interventions to relieve symptoms.
• Instruct patient to report chest pain, dizziness, palpitations, and other uncomfortable symptoms.
• As appropriate, review all other significant and life-threatening adverse reactions and interactions, especially those related to the drugs and tests mentioned above.

nevirapine

Viramune

Pharmacologic class: Nonnucleoside reverse transcriptase inhibitor
Therapeutic class: Antiretroviral
Pregnancy risk category C

Action

Inhibits human immunodeficiency virus (HIV) nonnucleoside reverse transcriptase by binding directly to reverse transcriptase and blocking RNA-dependent and DNA-dependent polymerase activity

Availability

Oral suspension: 50 mg/5 ml
Tablets: 200 mg

Indications and dosages

➢ Adjunctive treatment of HIV-1 infection in patients showing deterioration

Adults: 200 mg P.O. daily for 14 days, then 200 mg P.O. b.i.d., given with a nucleoside analogue. Total daily dosage is 400 mg.
Children ages 8 and older: 4 mg/kg P.O. daily for 14 days, followed by 4 mg/kg b.i.d. Total daily dosage is 400 mg.
Children ages 2 months to 8 years: 4 mg/kg P.O. daily for 14 days, followed by 7 mg/kg b.i.d. Total daily dosage is 400 mg.

Dosage adjustment

- Hepatic impairment
- Chronic hemodialysis

Off-label uses

- Prophylaxis of maternal-fetal HIV transmission

Contraindications

- Hypersensitivity to drug or its components

Precautions

Use cautiously in:
- impaired renal or hepatic function
- pregnant or breastfeeding patients
- children.

Administration

- Give with or without food.

Route	Onset	Peak	Duration
P.O.	Unknown	4 hr	Unknown

Adverse reactions

CNS: paresthesia, headache, malaise, fatigue
GI: nausea, diarrhea, abdominal pain
Hematologic: agranulocytosis
Hepatic: hepatitis, hepatotoxicity, hepatic failure
Musculoskeletal: myalgia, pain
Skin: rash, blistering, toxic epidermal necrolysis, **Stevens-Johnson syndrome**
Other: fever

Interactions

Drug-drug. *Drugs extensively metabolized by CYP3A-P450, hormonal contraceptives, protease inhibitors:* decreased blood levels of these drugs
Prednisone: increased risk of rash
Rifabutin, rifamycin: decreased nevirapine blood level
Drug-diagnostic tests. *Alanine aminotransferase, aspartate aminotransferase, bilirubin, gamma-glutamyltransferase:* increased levels
Hemoglobin, neutrophils: decreased levels
Drug-herbs. *St. John's wort:* decreased nevirapine blood level

Patient monitoring

[Clinical alert] Check closely for rash (which may be first sign of Stevens-Johnson syndrome), especially during first 6 months of therapy.
- Monitor patient's weight, temperature, and chest X-ray periodically.
- Assess patient's appetite and energy and physical activity levels.
- Monitor liver function tests and CBC with white cell differential.

Patient teaching

- Tell patient he may take with or without food.
- Instruct patient to take missed dose as soon as he remembers. But if it's almost time for next dose, tell him to skip missed dose. Caution him not to double the dose.
- Inform female patient that hormonal contraceptives, implants, or shots may be ineffective during nevirapine therapy. Urge her to use alternative birth-control method.

[Clinical alert] Teach patient to recognize and immediately report rash, easy bruising or bleeding, and signs and symptoms of hepatotoxicity.

• Inform patient that nevirapine won't cure HIV or prevent its transmission.
• Caution female not to breastfeed, because breast milk may transfer HIV to infant.
• As appropriate, review all other significant and life-threatening adverse reactions and interactions, especially those related to the drugs, tests, and herbs mentioned above.

nicardipine

Cardene, Cardene IV, Cardene SR

Pharmacologic class: Calcium channel blocker
Therapeutic class: Antianginal, antihypertensive
Pregnancy risk category C

Action

Inhibits calcium transport into myocardial and vascular smooth muscle cells, causing cardiac output and myocardial contractions to decrease

Availability

Capsules: 20 mg, 30 mg
Capsules (sustained-release): 30 mg, 45 mg, 60 mg
Injection: 2.5 mg/ml in 10-ml ampules

Indications and dosages

➢ Chronic stable angina, given alone or with beta-adrenergic blockers
Adults: Titrate dosage individually, starting with 20 to 40 mg P.O. (immediate-release) t.i.d. Wait at least 3 days before increasing dosage.
➢ Hypertension, given alone or other antihypertensives
Adults: Titrate dosage individually, starting with 20 mg P.O. (immediate release) t.i.d. Wait at least 3 days before increasing dosage. Dosage range is 20 to 40 mg P.O. t.i.d. Patient may be switched to sustained-release capsules at nearest equivalent daily dosage of immediate-release capsules, starting with 30 mg P.O. b.i.d. Effective range is 30 to 60 mg/day.
➢ Short-term treatment of hypertension when oral therapy isn't feasible or desirable
Adults: Continuous I.V. infusion of 0.5 mg/hour (equal to 20 mg P.O. q 8 hours), or 1.2 mg/hour (equal to 30 mg P.O. q 8 hours), or 2.2 mg/hour (equal to 40 mg P.O. q 8 hours)

Off-label uses

• Raynaud's disease
• Heart failure
• Migraine

Contraindications

• Hypersensitivity to drug
• Advanced aortic stenosis

Precautions

Use cautiously in:
• hepatic or mild renal impairment
• hypotension, heart failure, significant left ventricular dysfunction
• pheochromocytoma
• pregnant or breastfeeding patients (safety not established)
• children younger than age 18 (safety not established).

Administration

• Give immediate-release capsules without regard to meals; if GI upset occurs, give with meals. Don't give with grapefruit or grapefruit juice.
• Don't open, crush, break, or let patient chew sustained-release capsules. Give with meals, but not with high-fat meals, grapefruit, or grapefruit juice.
• For I.V. use, dilute each 25-mg ampule with 240 ml of compatible I.V. fluid (such as dextrose 5% in water, normal saline solution, dextrose 5% with normal saline solution, or half-normal saline solution) to a concentration of 0.1 mg/ml.

n

Don't dilute with sodium bicarbonate 5% or lactated Ringer's injection (incompatible).
- Don't mix with furosemide, heparin, or thiopental.

Give by slow I.V. infusion. Titrate dosage to blood pressure response.

Route	Onset	Peak	Duration
P.O.	20 min	0.5-2 hr	8 hr
P.O. (sustained)	Unknown	Unknown	12 hr
I.V.	Few min	45 min	Unknown

Adverse reactions

CNS: dizziness, headache, asthenia, drowsiness, paresthesia
CV: hypotension, peripheral edema, chest pain, increased angina, palpitations, tachycardia
GI: nausea, dyspepsia, dry mouth
Musculoskeletal: myalgia
Skin: flushing

Interactions

Drug-drug. *Cimetidine:* increased nifedipine blood level
Cyclosporine: increased cyclosporine blood level
Fentanyl anesthesia: increased hypotension
Drug-food. *Grapefruit, grapefruit juice:* increased drug blood level and effects
High-fat meal (sustained-release form): decreased drug blood level
Drug-herbs. *Ephedra (ma huang), yohimbine:* antagonism of drug's antihypertensive effect
St. John's wort: decreased nifedipine blood level
Drug-behaviors. *Alcohol use:* additive hypotension, increased drowsiness or dizziness

Patient monitoring

- Assess vital signs and cardiovascular status.
- Monitor fluid intake and output. Assess for signs and symptoms of heart failure.

Patient teaching

- Tell patient he may take immediate-release capsules without regard to meals. If GI upset occurs, advise him to take them with food, but not with grapefruit or grapefruit juice.
- Tell patient not to open, crush, break, or chew sustained-release capsules. Instruct him to take them with meals, but not with high-fat meals, grapefruit, or grapefruit juice.
- Tell patient to monitor blood pressure and report abnormal findings.

Advise patient to immediately report chest pain or blood pressure drop.
- Instruct patient to consult prescriber before drinking alcohol or taking herbs or over-the-counter drugs (especially cold remedies).
- As appropriate, review all other significant adverse reactions and interactions, especially those related to the drugs, foods, herbs, and behaviors mentioned above.

nicotine

nicotine inhaler
Nicotrol Inhaler

nicotine nasal spray
Nicotrol NS

nicotine polacrilex
Nicorette

nicotine transdermal system
Clear Nicoderm CQ, Habitrol, Nicoderm CQ, Nicotrol

Pharmacologic class: Cholinergic
Therapeutic class: Smoking deterrent
Pregnancy risk category C (gum), ***D*** (inhalation, nasal, transdermal)

Action

Supplies nicotine during controlled withdrawal from cigarette smoking. Binds selectively to nicotinic-cholinergic receptors in central and peripheral nervous systems, autonomic ganglia, adrenal medulla, and neuromuscular junction. At low doses, has a stimulating effect; at high doses, a reward effect.

Availability

Chewing gum: 2 mg, 4 mg
Inhalation: 42 cartridges/system, each containing 10 mg nicotine (delivers 4 mg)
Nasal spray: 10 mg/ml (0.5 mg/spray) in 10-ml bottles (100 doses)
Transdermal patch: 7 mg/day, 11 mg/day, 14 mg/day, 15 mg/day, 21 mg/day, 22 mg/day

Indications and dosages

➢ Adjunctive therapy (with behavior modification) for nicotine withdrawal
Transdermal system—
Adults: 21 mg/day transdermally (Habitrol) for 4 to 8 weeks, then 14 mg/day for 2 to 4 weeks, then 7 mg/day for 2 to 4 weeks, for a total of 8 to 16 weeks; patient must wear system 24 hours/day. Or 21 mg/day transdermally (Nicoderm CQ) for 6 weeks, then 14 mg/day for 2 weeks, then 7 mg/day for 2 weeks, for a total of 10 weeks; patient must wear system 24 hours/day. Or 15 mg/day transdermally (one Nicotrol patch) for 6 weeks; patient must wear system 16 hours/day, removing it at bedtime.
Adults, adolescents, and children weighing less than 45 kg (100 lb) who smoke fewer than 10 cigarettes daily or have underlying cardiovascular disease: 14 mg/day transdermally (Habitrol) for 4 to 8 weeks, then 7 mg/day for 2 to 4 weeks, for a total of 6 to 8 weeks; patient must wear system 24 hours/day. Or 14 mg/day transdermally (Nicoderm CQ) for 6 weeks, then 7 mg/day for 2 weeks, for a total of 8 weeks; patient must wear system 24 hours/day.
Nasal spray—
Adults: One spray intranasally in each nostril once or twice per hour, up to five times per hour or 40 times per day, for no longer than 6 months
Inhalation—
Adults: For optimal response, at least six cartridges inhaled daily for first 3 to 6 weeks, to a maximum of 16 cartridges daily for up to 12 weeks. Patient self-titrates dosage to required nicotine level (usually 6 to 16 cartridges daily), followed by gradual withdrawal over 6 to 12 weeks.
Chewing gum—
Adults: Use as needed depending on smoking urge or chewing rate, or use on fixed schedule q 1 to 2 hours. Initial requirement may range from 18 to 48 mg/day, not to exceed 60 mg/day.

Contraindications

- Hypersensitivity to drug or its components or to menthol (inhaler only)
- Allergy to adhesive (transdermal forms only)

n

Precautions

Use cautiously in:

- cardiovascular disease, hypertension, bronchospastic disease, diabetes mellitus, pheochromocytoma, peripheral vascular disease, hyperthyroidism, peptic ulcer disease, hepatic disease
- immediately after myocardial infarction, severe arrhythmia, or severe or worsening angina (use not recommended)
- skin disorders (transdermal form)
- dental disorders, esophagitis, pharyngitis, stomatitis (gum form)
- females of childbearing age
- pregnant or breastfeeding patients.
- children under age 18 (safety and efficacy not established).

Administration

• Apply patch when patient awakens and remove patch (as prescribed) at same time each day.
• Administer nasal spray regularly during first week, to help patient get used to irritant effects.
• With inhalation use, give at least six cartridges daily for first 3 to 6 weeks.
• Encourage patient to titrate dosage to level required, followed by gradual withdrawal.

Route	Onset	Peak	Duration
Gum	Rapid	15-30 min	Unknown
Inhalation	Rapid	15 min	Unknown
Nasal spray	Rapid	4-15 min	Unknown
Transdermal (Habitrol)	Rapid	6-12 hr	Unknown
Transdermal (Nicoderm CQ)	Rapid	2-4 hr	Unknown

Adverse reactions

CNS: headache, dizziness, drowsiness, poor concentration, nervousness, weakness, paresthesia, insomnia, abnormal dreams
CV: chest pain, hypertension, tachycardia, **atrial fibrillation**
EENT: sinusitis; pharyngitis (with gum); mouth and throat irritation (with inhaler); nasopharyngeal irritation, rhinitis, sneezing, watering eyes, eye irritation (with nasal spray)
GI: nausea, vomiting, diarrhea, constipation, abdominal pain, dry mouth, dyspepsia; increased salivation, sore mouth (with gum)
GU: dysmenorrhea
Musculoskeletal: joint pain, back pain, myalgia; jaw ache (with gum)
Respiratory: increased cough (with nasal spray or inhaler), **bronchospasm**
Skin: burning at patch site, erythema, pruritus, cutaneous hypersensitivity, rash, sweating (all with transdermal patch)
Other: abnormal taste, increased appetite (with gum), allergy, hiccups

Interactions

Drug-drug. *Acetaminophen, adrenergic antagonists (such as prazosin, labetalol), clozapine, furosemide, imipramine, oxazepam, pentazocine, propranolol and other beta-adrenergic blockers, theophylline:* increased effects of these drugs
Bupropion: treatment-emergent hypertension
Insulin: decreased insulin requirement
Isoproterenol, phenylephrine: increased requirements for these drugs
Propoxyphene: decreased nicotine metabolism
Drug-food. *Caffeine-containing foods and beverages:* increased nicotine effects
Drug-behaviors. *Cigarette smoking:* increased nicotine metabolism and effects

Patient monitoring

• Assess for signs and symptoms of nicotine withdrawal (irritability, drowsiness, fatigue, headache).
🔊 Watch for bronchospasm and evidence of nicotine toxicity (nausea, vomiting, diarrhea, increased salivation, headache, dizziness, visual disturbances).

Patient teaching

🔊 Caution patient against any type of smoking during therapy. Urge him to immediately report chest tightness or difficulty breathing.
• If patient uses gum, advise him to chew one piece whenever nicotine craving occurs. Instruct him to chew it slowly until he feels a tingling sensation, then store it between cheek and gum until tingling disappears.
• Instruct patient to apply transdermal patch to clean, dry skin of upper arm or torso when he awakens; to keep it in place when showering, bathing, or swimming; and to remove it at same time each day.
• If patient uses nasal spray, instruct him to tilt head back slightly when

spraying. Remind him not to sniff, swallow, or inhale through nose.

- If patient uses inhalation form, teach him to puff continuously for 20 minutes and to use at least six cartridges daily for first 3 to 6 weeks.
- As appropriate, review all significant and life-threatening adverse reactions and interactions, especially those related to the drugs, foods, and behaviors mentioned above.

nifedipine

Adalat, Adalat CC, Adalat PA✱, Adalat XL✱, Apo-Nifed✱, Gen-Nifedical✱, Nifedical XL, Novo-Nifedin✱, Nu-Nifed, Procardia, Procardia XL

Pharmacologic class: Calcium channel blocker

Therapeutic class: Antianginal, antihypertensive

Pregnancy risk category C

Action

Inhibits calcium transport into myocardial and vascular smooth muscle cells, suppressing contractions. Dilates main coronary arteries and arterioles and inhibits coronary artery spasm, increasing oxygen delivery to heart and decreasing frequency and severity of angina attacks.

Availability

Capsules: 5 mg, 10 mg, 20 mg
Tablets (extended-release): 10 mg, 20 mg, 30 mg, 60 mg, 90 mg

Indications and dosages

➢ Vasospastic (Prinzmetal's) angina; chronic stable angina

Adults: Initially, 10 mg P.O. (immediate-release) t.i.d. titrated over 7 to 14 days; usual effective range is 10 to 20 mg t.i.d., not to exceed 180 mg/day. Patient may be switched to extended-release at nearest equivalent of immediate-release daily dosage (for instance, 30-mg immediate-release dose may be switched to 90-mg extended-release dose). Total extended-release dosage should not exceed 90 mg/day.

➢ Hypertension

Adults: 30 to 60 mg/day P.O. (extended-release only) titrated over 7 to 14 days to a maximum of 120 mg/day

Off-label uses

- Aortic regurgitation
- Heart failure
- Migraine
- Prevention of labor

Contraindications

- Hypersensitivity to drug

Precautions

Use cautiously in:

- chronic renal insufficiency
- hypotension, aortic stenosis, heart failure, significant left ventricular dysfunction (especially when used with beta-adrenergic blockers), peripheral edema
- elderly patients
- pregnant or breastfeeding patients (safety not established)
- children (safety not established).

Administration

- Give immediate-release form with or without food. If GI upset occurs, give with meals, but never with grapefruit or grapefruit juice.
- Don't crush or break extended-release tablet. Make sure patient swallows it whole. Give on empty stomach, and not with grapefruit or grapefruit juice.
- Know that Procardia XL and Adalat CC are not equivalent because of their pharmacokinetic differences.

• Be aware that only extended-release tablets are used to treat hypertension.

Route	Onset	Peak	Duration
P.O.	20 min	Unknown	6-8 hr
P.O. (Adalat PA)	Unknown	4 hr	12 hr
P.O. (Adalat CC, PA, XL)	Unknown	6 hr	24 hr

Adverse reactions

CNS: headache, dizziness, fatigue, asthenia, paresthesia, vertigo
CV: peripheral edema, chest pain, hypotension
EENT: epistaxis, rhinitis
GI: nausea, constipation
GU: urinary frequency, erectile dysfunction
Musculoskeletal: leg cramps
Skin: flushing, rash

Interactions

Drug-drug. *Beta-adrenergic blockers:* increased risk of heart failure, severe hypotension, or angina exacerbation
Cimetidine: increased nifedipine blood level
Coumarin anticoagulants: increased prothrombin time
Digoxin: increased risk of digoxin toxicity
Quinidine: decreased quinidine blood level
Drug-diagnostic tests. *Antinuclear antibody, direct Coombs' test:* false-positive results
Drug-food. *Grapefruit, grapefruit juice:* increased nifedipine blood level and effects
Drug-herbs. *Ephedra (ma huang), yohimbine:* antagonism of nifedipine effect
Ginkgo, ginseng: increased nifedipine blood level
St. John's wort: decreased nifedipine blood level
Drug-behaviors. *Alcohol use:* additive hypotension

Patient monitoring

• Monitor vital signs and cardiovascular status. Stay alert for chest pain and edema.
• Watch for rash.

Patient teaching

• Tell patient he may take immediate-release form with or without meals. If GI upset occurs, tell him to take it with meals, but never with grapefruit or grapefruit juice.
• Caution patient not to crush or break extended-release tablets. Tell him to swallow them whole. Advise him to take on empty stomach, and not with grapefruit or grapefruit juice.
• Inform patient that angina attacks may occur 30 minutes after a dose. Explain that these attacks usually are temporary and don't mean that drug should be withdrawn.
[Clinical alert] Tell patient to report rash immediately.
• Caution patient to avoid driving and other hazardous activities until he knows how drug affects concentration, balance, and alertness.
• Instruct patient to consult prescriber before taking herbs or over-the-counter drugs (especially cold remedies).
• As appropriate, review all other significant adverse reactions and interactions, especially those related to the drugs, tests, foods, herbs, and behaviors mentioned above.

nilutamide

Anandron✦, Nilandron

Pharmacologic class: Antiandrogen
Therapeutic class: Antineoplastic
Pregnancy risk category C

Action
Inhibits testosterone uptake in target tissue, preventing normal androgenic response and arresting tumor growth in androgen-sensitive tissue

Availability
Tablets: 50 mg, 150 mg

Indications and dosages
➢ Metastatic prostate cancer (used with surgical castration)
Adults: 300 mg/day P.O. for 30 days, starting on day of or day after surgery; then 150 mg/day P.O.

Contraindications
• Hypersensitivity to drug or its components
• Severe hepatic or respiratory insufficiency

Precautions
Use cautiously in:
• renal impairment.

Administration
• Give with or without food.
• Start therapy on same day as or day after surgical castration.

Route	Onset	Peak	Duration
P.O.	Rapid	Days	Wks

Adverse reactions
CNS: dizziness, depression, hyperesthesia, insomnia
CV: hypertension, peripheral edema, **heart failure**
EENT: abnormal vision, impaired dark and light adaptation, chromatopsia
GI: nausea, vomiting, constipation, dyspepsia, anorexia
GU: hematuria, nocturia, urinary tract infection, gynecomastia, testicular atrophy, decreased libido, erectile dysfunction
Hematologic: anemia, **aplastic anemia**
Hepatic: hepatitis
Respiratory: dyspnea, upper respiratory infection, **interstitial pneumonia**
Other: flulike symptoms, pain, fever, hot flushes, alcohol intolerance

Interactions
Drug-drug. *Phenytoin, theophylline, vitamin K:* increased risk of toxicity from these drugs
Drug-diagnostic tests. *Alanine aminotransferase, aspartate aminotransferase:* increased levels
Drug-behaviors. *Alcohol use:* disulfiram-like reaction

Patient monitoring
• Check for signs and symptoms of hepatitis. Monitor liver function tests.
• Monitor CBC.
• Assess fluid intake and output and weight. Watch for signs and symptoms of heart failure.
• Monitor respiratory status, including chest X-rays.

Patient teaching
• Advise patient he may take with or without food.
• Tell patient therapy will start on day of or day after surgical castration.
• Caution patient not to stop taking drug without consulting prescriber.
• Instruct patient to weigh himself daily and report sudden increases.
Advise patient to report new onset or worsening of dyspnea as well as signs and symptoms of hepatotoxicity, such as nausea, vomiting, abdominal pain, unusual tiredness, or yellowing of skin or eyes.
• Advise patient to avoid alcohol during therapy, because serious adverse reactions may occur.
• Tell patient drug may impair his adaptation to darkness and light, which may cause difficulty driving at night or through tunnels.
• As appropriate, review all other significant and life-threatening adverse

n

reactions and interactions, especially those related to the drugs, test, and behaviors mentioned above.

nimodipine

Nimotop

Pharmacologic class: Calcium channel blocker

Therapeutic class: Cerebral vasodilator

Pregnancy risk category C

Action

Inhibits calcium transport into vascular smooth muscle cells, suppressing contractions; also dilates coronary and cerebral arteries

Availability

Capsules: 30 mg

Indications and dosages

➢ Subarachnoid hemorrhage

Adults: 60 mg P.O. q 4 hours for 21 days. Therapy should start within 96 hours of subarachnoid hemorrhage.

Dosage adjustment

- Hepatic impairment

Contraindications

None

Precautions

Use cautiously in:

- hepatic impairment, hypotension
- elderly patients
- pregnant or breastfeeding patients (safety not established)
- children (safety not established).

Administration

- Give at least 1 hour before or 2 hours after meals. Don't let patient consume grapefruit or grapefruit juice within 1 hour before or 2 hours after dose.
- If patient can't swallow capsule, puncture it with sterile needle and empty contents into syringe. Administer through nasogastric tube, then flush with normal saline solution (30 ml).

Route	Onset	Peak	Duration
P.O.	Unknown	1 hr	4 hr

Adverse reactions

CNS: headache, depression

CV: hypotension, peripheral edema, ECG abnormalities, bradycardia, tachycardia

GI: nausea, diarrhea, abdominal discomfort

Musculoskeletal: muscle cramps

Respiratory: dyspnea

Skin: acne, flushing, rash

Interactions

Drug-drug. *Other calcium channel blockers:* enhanced cardiovascular effects

Drug-diagnostic tests. *Liver function tests:* abnormal results

Drug-food. *Any food:* decreased drug blood level and effects

Grapefruit juice, grapefruit juice: increased drug blood level and effects

Drug-herbs. *Ephedra (ma huang), yohimbine:* antagonism of nimodipine effects

St. John's wort: decreased drug blood level

Drug-behaviors. *Alcohol use:* increased hypotension

Patient monitoring

- Monitor weight and fluid intake and output. Stay alert for fluid retention.
- Assess neurologic status and mood, watching for signs of depression.
- Check vital signs and ECG.

Patient teaching

- Tell patient to complete full course of therapy (21 days).
- Advise patient to take on an empty stomach 1 hour before or 2 hours after

a meal. Instruct him to not to consume grapefruit or grapefruit juice within 1 hour before or 2 hours after taking drug.
• Tell patient to report irregular heartbeat, shortness of breath, rash, or swollen hands or feet.
• Instruct patient to minimize GI upset by eating small, frequent meals.
• Advise patient to weigh himself daily and report sudden weight gain.
• As appropriate, review all other significant adverse reactions and interactions, especially those related to the drugs, tests, foods, herbs, and behaviors mentioned above.

nisoldipine

Sular

Pharmacologic class: Calcium channel blocker
Therapeutic class: Antihypertensive
Pregnancy risk category C

Action

Suppresses calcium transport into vascular smooth muscle cells. This suppression inhibits vasoconstriction and dilates coronary arteries, improving myocardial oxygen uptake.

Availability

Tablets (extended-release): 10 mg, 20 mg, 30 mg, 40 mg

Indications and dosages

➢ Hypertension
Adults: Initially, 20 mg P.O. daily as a single dose; may increase by 10 mg daily q 7 days, up to 60 mg daily. Usual range is 20 to 40 mg daily.

Contraindications

• Hypersensitivity to drug or dihydropyridine calcium channel blockers

Precautions

Use cautiously in:
• heart failure and left ventricular dysfunction, hepatic impairment, renal disease, coronary artery disease, hypotension
• concurrent phenytoin use
• elderly patients
• pregnant or breastfeeding patients
• children (safety not established).

Administration

• Give with meals, but not with high-fat meals, grapefruit, or grapefruit juice.
• Don't crush or break extended-release tablets. Make sure patient swallows them whole.
• Know that drug may be given alone or with other antihypertensives.

Route	Onset	Peak	Duration
P.O.	Unknown	6-12 hr	24 hr

Adverse reactions

CNS: headache, dizziness
CV: peripheral edema, chest pain, vasodilation, hypotension, palpitations
EENT: pharyngitis, sinusitis
GI: nausea
Skin: rash

Interactions

Drug-drug. *Cimetidine:* increased nisoldipine blood level
Phenytoin, other CYP3A4 inducers: decreased nisoldipine blood level and efficacy
Drug-food. *Grapefruit juice:* significantly increased drug blood level and effects
High-fat meal: decreased drug blood level
Drug-herbs. *Ephedra (ma huang), yohimbine:* antagonism of nimodipine effects
St. John's wort: decreased nimodipine blood level

n

Drug-behaviors. *Alcohol use:* increased hypotensive effects

Patient monitoring
- Check vital signs and ECG.
- Monitor fluid intake and output. Watch for peripheral edema.

Patient teaching
- Tell patient to swallow extended-release tablets whole and not to crush or break them.
- Advise patient to take with food, but not high-fat food. Recommend small, frequent meals.
- Instruct patient to avoid high-fat meals, alcohol, grapefruit, and grapefruit juice.
- Tell patient to immediately report irregular heart beat, shortness of breath, swelling, pronounced dizziness, rash, or chest pain.
- As appropriate, review all other significant adverse reactions and interactions, especially those related to the drugs, foods, herbs, and behaviors mentioned above.

nitrofurantoin
Apo-Nitrofurantoin✤, Furadantin

nitrofurantoin macrocrystals
Macrobid, Macrodantin

Pharmacologic class: 5-nitrofuran derivative

Therapeutic class: Anti-infective, urinary tract anti-infective

Pregnancy risk category B

Action
Inhibits bacterial enzymes required for normal cell activity at low concentrations; inhibits normal cell-wall synthesis at high concentrations

Availability
Capsules: 25 mg, 50 mg, 100 mg (macrocrystals)
Capsules (extended-release): 100 mg (macrocrystals)
Oral suspension: 25 mg/5 ml
Tablets: 50 mg, 100 mg (macrocrystals)

Indications and dosages
➢ Active urinary tract infections (UTIs)
Adults: 50 to 100 mg P.O. q.i.d. or 100 mg q 12 hours (extended-release), continued for 1 week, or for 3 days after urine becomes sterile
Children older than 1 month: 5 to 7 mg/kg/day P.O. in four divided doses, continued for 1 week, or for 3 days after urine becomes sterile
➢ Chronic suppression of UTIs
Adults: 50 to 100 mg P.O. at bedtime
Children: 1 mg/kg/day P.O. in one or two divided doses

Contraindications
- Hypersensitivity to drug or parabens (oral suspension)
- Oliguria, anuria, or significant renal impairment
- Pregnancy near term (38 to 42 weeks' gestation), imminent labor onset, labor and delivery
- Infants younger than 1 month

Precautions
Use cautiously in:
- diabetes mellitus, renal impairment
- blacks and patients of Mediterranean or near-Eastern descent (because of possible G6PD deficiency)
- elderly or debilitated patients
- pregnant (to week 32) or breastfeeding patients.

Administration
- As appropriate, obtain specimens for repeat urine culture and sensitivity tests before therapy.
- To avoid GI upset and increase drug bioavailability, give with food or milk.

Route	Onset	Peak	Duration
P.O.	Unknown	30 min	6-12 hr

Adverse reactions

CNS: dizziness, drowsiness, headache, asthenia, peripheral neuropathy, vertigo
CV: chest pain
EENT: nystagmus
GI: nausea, vomiting, diarrhea, abdominal pain, anorexia, parotitis, pancreatitis
Hematologic: eosinophilia, **agranulocytosis, thrombocytopenia, leukopenia, granulocytopenia, G6PD deficiency anemia, hemolytic anemia, megaloblastic anemia**
Hepatic: hepatitis, hepatic necrosis
Musculoskeletal: arthralgia, myalgia
Respiratory: asthma attacks, pulmonary hypersensitivity reactions including **diffuse interstitial pneumonitis** (with prolonged therapy)
Skin: rash, exfoliative dermatitis, alopecia, pruritus, urticaria, angioedema, photosensitivity, **Stevens-Johnson syndrome**
Other: drug fever, chills, superinfection (limited to urinary tract), hypersensitivity reactions including **anaphylaxis, lupus-like syndrome**

Interactions

Drug-drug. *Anticholinergics:* increased nitrofurantoin absorption and bioavailability
Drugs that can cause pulmonary toxicity: increased risk of pneumonitis
Hepatotoxic drugs: increased risk of hepatotoxicity
Magnesium salts: decreased nitrofurantoin absorption
Neurotoxic drugs: increased risk of neurotoxicity
Uricosurics (such as probenecid): decreased renal clearance and increased blood level of nitrofurantoin
Drug-diagnostic tests. *Alanine aminotransferase, alkaline phosphatase, aspartate aminotransferase, bilirubin, blood urea nitrogen, creatinine:* increased levels
Granulocytes, platelets, hemoglobin: decreased levels
Urine glucose tests using Benedict's reagent or Fehling's solution: false-positive results
Drug-food. *Any food:* increased drug bioavailability

Patient monitoring

- Monitor patient's response to therapy. Assess urine culture and sensitivity tests.

🔊 Watch for and immediately report peripheral neuropathy.

🔊 Assess respiratory status. Watch for signs and symptoms of serious pulmonary hypersensitivity reaction.

🔊 Monitor CBC and liver function tests closely. Stay alert for evidence of hematologic and hepatic disorders.

- Evaluate patient for rash.

Patient teaching

- Instruct patient to take with food or milk at regular intervals around the clock.
- Advise patient to complete entire course of therapy.
- Tell patient not to take magnesium-containing drugs (such as antacids) during therapy.
- Caution patient not to drive or perform other hazardous activities until he knows how drug affects vision, concentration, and alertness.

🔊 Tell patient to immediately report fever, chills, cough, chest pain, difficulty breathing, rash, bleeding or easy bruising, dark urine, yellowing of skin or eyes, numbness or tingling of fingers or toes, or intolerable GI distress.

- Advise female patient to avoid taking drug during pregnancy, especially near term.
- As appropriate, review all other significant and life-threatening adverse reactions and interactions, especially

n

those related to the drugs, tests, and foods mentioned above.

nitroglycerin

Deponit, Minitran, Nitro-Dur, Notroject✱, Nitrolingual, Nitrostat

Pharmacologic class: Nitrate
Therapeutic class: Antianginal
Pregnancy risk category C

Action

Inhibits calcium transport into myocardial and vascular smooth muscle cells, suppressing contractions. Dilates main coronary arteries and arterioles, inhibits coronary artery spasm, increases oxygen delivery to heart, and reduces frequency and severity of angina attacks.

Availability

Capsules (extended-release): 2.5 mg, 6.5 mg, 9 mg
Injection: 0.5 mg/ml, 5 mg/ml
Ointment (transdermal): 2%
Solution for injection: 25 mg/250 ml, 50 mg/250 ml, 50 mg/500 ml, 100 mg/250 ml, 200 mg/500 ml
Spray (translingual): 0.4 mg/spray in 14.5-g canister (200 doses)
Tablets (buccal, extended-release): 1 mg, 2 mg, 3 mg, 5 mg
Tablets (extended-release): 2.6 mg, 6.5 mg, 9 mg
Tablets (sublingual): 0.3 mg, 0.4 mg, 0.6 mg
Transdermal system (patch): 0.1 mg/hour, 0.2 mg/hour, 0.3 mg/hour, 0.4 mg/hour, 0.6 mg/hour, 0.8 mg/hour

Indications and dosages

➢ Management and prophylaxis of angina pectoris
Adults: For acute angina attack, 0.3 to 0.6 mg S.L., repeated q 5 minutes for 15 minutes p.r.n.; or one to two translingual sprays, repeated q 5 minutes for 15 minutes p.r.n. For long-term or prophylactic use, 1-mg extended-release buccal tablet q 5 hours, with dosage and frequency increased p.r.n.; or 2.5 to 9 mg (extended-release tablets) P.O. q 8 to 12 hours; or 1.3 to 6.5 mg (extended-release capsules) P.O. q 8 to 12 hours.

➢ Hypertension during surgery; adjunct in heart failure
Adults: 5 mcg/minute I.V., increased by 5 mcg/minute q 3 to 5 minutes up to 20 mcg/minute, then increased by 10 to 20 mcg/minute q 3 to 5 minutes (dosage based on hemodynamic parameters)

➢ Heart failure associated with acute myocardial infarction (MI)
Adults: 12.5 to 25 mcg I.V., then a continuous infusion of 10 to 20 mcg/minute q 5 to 10 minutes; increase by 5 to 10 mcg/minute q 5 to 10 minutes as needed to a maximum of 200 mcg/minute.

Contraindications

- Hypersensitivity to drug, other organic nitrates, nitrites, or adhesives (transdermal form)
- Angle-closure glaucoma
- Orthostatic hypotension
- Hypotension or uncorrected hypovolemia (I.V. form)
- Early MI (S.L. form)
- Increased intracranial pressure (as from head trauma or cerebral hemorrhage)
- Severe anemia
- Pericardial tamponade or constrictive pericarditis
- Concurrent sildenafil therapy

Precautions

Use cautiously in:
- severe renal or hepatic impairment, glaucoma, hypertrophic cardiomyopathy

- hypovolemia, normal or decreased pulmonary capillary wedge pressure (with I.V. use)
- alcohol intolerance (with large I.V. doses)
- pregnant or breastfeeding patients
- children (safety not established).

Administration

- Administer tablets and capsules with water. Don't crush, break, or let patient chew them.
- For S.L. use, administer under tongue or in buccal pouch; instruct patient not to swallow tablet. For acute angina, give at pain onset. For angina prophylaxis, give before activities that may cause anginal pain.
- For translingual use, spray directly onto oral mucosa. Don't let patient inhale spray. Give at pain onset and as needed prophylactically before activities that trigger angina.
- For transdermal use, apply system to skin site with little hair and movement. Don't apply to distal extremities. Rotate application sites to avoid irritation and sensitization.
- Apply transdermal ointment to skin by spreading prescribed amount over 6" × 6" area (using an applicator, not your fingers). Cover area with plastic wrap and tape. Rotate sites to reduce risk of irritation and inflammation.

Know that solution for injection is a concentrate. Dilute with dextrose 5% in water or normal saline solution before giving by I.V. infusion.

Don't mix solution for injection with other drugs, and don't give by direct I.V. injection.

- Be aware that solution for injection is affected by type of infusion set used and that dosage is based on use of conventional PVC tubing. When using nonabsorbent tubing, reduce dosage.
- For I.V. use, administer with infusion pump. Increase dosage in increments of 5 mcg/minute every 3 to 5 minutes p.r.n. to achieve desired blood pressure response. Once achieved, reduce dosage and lengthen dosage adjustment intervals.

Don't give concurrently with sildenafil (may cause life-threatening hypotension).

Route	Onset	Peak	Duration
P.O. (extended)	40-60 min	Unknown	8-12 hr
I.V.	Immediate	Unknown	Several min
Buccal (extended)	Unknown	Unknown	5 hr
S.L.	1-3 min	Unknown	30-60 min
Transdermal (ointment)	20-60 min	Unknown	4-8 hr
Transdermal (patch)	40-60 min	Unknown	8-24 hr
Translingual	2-4 min	Unknown	30-60 min

Adverse reactions

CNS: dizziness, headache
CV: hypotension, syncope
Hematologic: methemoglobinemia
Skin: contact dermatitis (with transdermal or ointment use), rash, exfoliative dermatitis, flushing

Interactions

Drug-drug. *Antihypertensives, beta-adrenergic blockers, calcium channel blockers, haloperidol, phenothiazines:* additive hypotension
Drugs with anticholinergic properties (antihistamines, phenothiazines, tricyclic antidepressants): decreased absorption of lingual, S.L., or buccal nitroglycerin
Sildenafil: increased risk of potentially fatal hypotension
Drug-diagnostic tests. *Cholesterol:* false elevation

Methemoglobin: significant levels (with excessive doses)
Urine catecholamines, urine vanillylmandelic acid: increased levels
Drug-behaviors. *Alcohol use, acute alcohol ingestion:* increased risk of potentially fatal hypotension

Patient monitoring

🔊 With I.V. use, monitor blood pressure frequently. Titrate dosage to obtain desired results.
- With transdermal use, check for rash or skin irritation.
- Monitor patient for angina relief.

Patient teaching

- Instruct patient to place S.L. tablet directly under tongue and hold it there as it dissolves. Caution him not to chew or swallow tablet.
- Tell patient to use drug before physical activities that may cause angina.
- Instruct patient to take drug at pain onset and repeat every 5 minutes for three doses. If pain doesn't subside, advise him to seek medical attention.
- Tell patient not to chew or crush sustained-release tablets.
- Advise patient to apply correct amount of ointment using applicator. Caution him to avoid rubbing site. Instruct him to cover ointment with plastic wrap and tape it, to wash hands after placement, and to rotate sites.
- Advise patient to consult prescriber or pharmacist before changing brands of transdermal system. Different brands may have different drug concentrations.
- As appropriate, review all significant and life-threatening adverse reactions and interactions, especially those related to the drugs, tests, and behaviors mentioned above.

nitroprusside sodium

Nipride✤, Nitropress

Pharmacologic class: Vasodilator
Therapeutic class: Antihypertensive
Pregnancy risk category C

Action

Interferes with calcium influx and intracellular activation of calcium, causing peripheral vasodilation and direct blood pressure decrease

Availability

Injection: 50 mg/vial in 2 ml- and 5-ml vials

Indications and dosages

➢ Hypertensive emergencies; controlled hypotension during anesthesia
Adults and children: 0.3 to 10 mcg/kg/minute I.V., titrated to response

Dosage adjustment

- Hepatic insufficiency
- Renal impairment
- Elderly patients

Contraindications

- Hypertension caused by aortic coarctation or atrioventricular shunting
- Acute heart failure caused by reduced peripheral vascular resistance
- Congenital (Leber's) optic atrophy, tobacco amblyopia
- Inadequate cerebral circulation
- Moribund patients

Precautions

Use cautiously in:
- hepatic or renal disease, fluid and electrolyte imbalances, hypothyroidism
- elderly patients
- pregnant or breastfeeding patients
- children.

Administration

Be aware that nitroprusside is a high-alert drug.

Give only in settings with trained personnel and continuous blood pressure monitoring equipment.

- Dilute 50 mg in 2 to 3 ml of dextrose 5% in water (D_5W); then dilute in 250 to 1,000 ml of D_5W.
- Administer with microdrip regulator, infusion pump, or other device that allows precise flow rate measurement.
- Wrap infusion solution in aluminum foil or other opaque material to protect it from light.

Route	Onset	Peak	Duration
I.V.	1-2 min	1-10 min	10 min

Adverse reactions

CNS: increased intracranial pressure
CV: ECG changes, bradycardia, tachycardia, **marked hypotension**
GI: ileus
Hematologic: decreased platelet aggregation, **methemoglobinemia**
Metabolic: hypothyroidism
Skin: rash, flushing
Other: pain, irritation, and venous streaking at injection site; too-rapid blood pressure decrease (causing apprehension, restlessness, palpitations, retrosternal discomfort, nausea, retching, abdominal pain, diaphoresis, headache, dizziness, muscle twitching); **thiocynate or cyanide toxicity** (initially, tinnitus, miosis, and hyperreflexia) at blood level of 60 mg/L; **severe cyanide toxicity** (air hunger, confusion, **lactic acidosis, death**) at level of 200 mg/L

Interactions

Drug-drug. *Enflurane, ganglionic blockers, halothane, negative inotropic drugs, volatile liquid anesthetics:* severe hypotension
Drug-diagnostic tests. *Creatinine:* increased level
Methemoglobin: hemoglobin sequestration as methemoglobin

Patient monitoring

Measure blood pressure frequently (preferably with continuous arterial line) to detect rapid drop.

- Monitor injection site closely to avoid extravasation. Use central line whenever possible. Ensure that infusion rate is precisely controlled to prevent too-rapid infusion.
- Obtain baseline ECG and monitor for changes.

Watch for signs and symptoms of cyanide toxicity (lactic acidosis, dyspnea, headache, vomiting, confusion, and loss of consciousness).

Patient teaching

- Tell patient he'll be closely monitored during therapy.

Instruct patient to immediately report headache, nausea, or pain at injection site.

- As appropriate, review all other significant and life-threatening adverse reactions and interactions, especially those related to the drugs and tests mentioned above.

n

nizatidine

Axid, Axid AR

Pharmacologic class: Histamine$_2$ (H_2)-receptor antagonist
Therapeutic class: Antiulcer drug
Pregnancy risk category B

Action

Inhibits histamine action at H_2-receptor sites in gastric parietal cells, reducing gastric acid secretion and pepsin production

Availability

Capsules: 150 mg, 300 mg
Oral solution: 15 mg/ml
Tablets: 75 mg

Indications and dosages

➢ Active duodenal ulcer

Adults: 300 mg P.O. daily at bedtime or 150 mg b.i.d. for up to 8 weeks

➢ Maintenance of healed duodenal ulcers

Adults and children ages 12 and older: 150 mg P.O. daily at bedtime for up to 1 year

➢ Esophagitis and associated heartburn caused by gastroesophageal reflux disease (GERD)

Adults: 150 mg P.O. b.i.d. for up to 12 weeks

➢ Active benign gastric ulcer

Adults: 150 mg P.O. b.i.d. or 300 mg P.O. once daily at bedtime

➢ Erosive esophagitis; GERD

Children ages 12 and older: 150 mg P.O. b.i.d. for up to 8 weeks

Dosage adjustment

- Moderate to severe renal impairment
- Elderly patients

Contraindications

- Hypersensitivity to drug or other H_2-receptor antagonists

Precautions

Use cautiously in:

- mild renal impairment
- elderly patients
- pregnant or breastfeeding patients
- children younger than age 12 (safety and efficacy not established).

Administration

- Give with or without food.
- If patient is to take drug twice daily, give one dose in morning and one at bedtime.

Route	Onset	Peak	Duration
P.O.	Unknown	0.5-3 hr	8-12 hr

Adverse reactions

CNS: dizziness, drowsiness, headache, anxiety, nervousness, insomnia, abnormal dreams, asthenia
CV: chest pain
EENT: amblyopia, sinusitis, rhinitis, pharyngitis
GI: nausea, vomiting, diarrhea, constipation, dyspepsia, abdominal pain, flatulence, anorexia, dry mouth
Hematologic: anemia
Musculoskeletal: back pain, myalgia
Respiratory: cough
Skin: rash, pruritus
Other: tooth disorder, infection, fever, pain

Interactions

Drug-drug. *Salicylates (high doses):* increased salicylate blood level
Drug-diagnostic tests. *Alanine aminotransferase, alkaline phosphatase, aspartate aminotransferase:* elevated levels
Urobilinogen tests using Multistix: false-positive result
Drug-herbs. *Pennyroyal:* altered rate of herbal metabolite formation

Patient monitoring

- Monitor liver and renal function tests.
- Check temperature; watch for fever and other signs and symptoms of infection.

Patient teaching

- Advise patient to take once-daily dose at bedtime with or without food, or twice-daily doses in morning and at bedtime.
- Instruct patient to take exactly as prescribed. Caution him not to take other OTC drugs (especially aspirin).
- Tell patient to report signs and symptoms of infection.
- Caution patient to avoid driving and other hazardous activities until he knows how drug affects concentration and alertness.
- As appropriate, review all other significant adverse reactions and interactions, especially those related to the drugs, tests, and herbs mentioned above.

norelgestromin/ethinyl estradiol

Ortho Evra

Pharmacologic class: Estrogen
Therapeutic class: Hormone
Pregnancy risk category X

Action

Suppresses gonadotropin and inhibits ovulation by causing changes in cervical mucus and endometrium, thereby preventing egg implantation

Availability

Transdermal patch: 6 mg norelgestromin and 0.75 mg ethinyl estradiol (releases 150 mcg norelgestromin and 20 mcg ethinyl estradiol q 24 hours)

Indications and dosages

➢ To prevent pregnancy

Adults: Apply patch on day 1 of menstrual cycle (or first Sunday after period begins). Change patch weekly thereafter for 3 weeks (on same day each week), and then remove patch for fourth week. Repeat q month.

Contraindications

- Hypersensitivity to drug or its components
- Undiagnosed vaginal bleeding
- Breast or reproductive system cancer
- Thromboembolism, history of thromboembolic disease
- Coronary artery disease
- Valvular heart disease with complications
- Severe hypertension, diabetes with vascular involvement
- Cerebrovascular disease
- Headache with focal neurologic symptoms
- Cholestatic jaundice of pregnancy, jaundice with previous hormonal contraceptive use
- Acute or chronic hepatic disease with abnormal liver function tests
- Hepatic adenomas or carcinomas
- Major surgery with prolonged immobilization
- Pregnancy or breastfeeding

Precautions

Use cautiously in:

- cardiovascular disease, severe hepatic or renal disease, asthma, bone disease, migraine, lipid disorders, fibrocystic breasts, increased risk for endometrial cancer, sexually transmitted diseases
- family history of breast or genital tract cancer
- abnormal mammogram.

Administration

- Apply patch to clean, dry, intact skin on buttock, abdomen, upper torso, or upper outer arm.
- Change patch on same day each week (except for fourth week, when patch is removed).

Route	Onset	Peak	Duration
Transdermal	Rapid	2 days	Unknown

Adverse reactions

CNS: headache, dizziness, lethargy, depression, emotional lability, **increased risk of cerebrovascular accident**
CV: edema, hypertension, **myocardial infarction, thromboembolism**
EENT: contact lens intolerance, worsening of myopia or astigmatism
GI: nausea, vomiting, jaundice, abdominal cramps, bloating, anorexia, gallbladder disease, **pancreatitis**
GU: amenorrhea, dysmenorrhea, breakthrough bleeding, cervical erosion, vaginal candidiasis, breast tenderness, breast enlargement or secretion, menstrual cramps, libido loss, **increased risk of breast or endometrial cancer**

n

Hepatic: cholestatic jaundice, **hepatic adenoma**
Metabolic: hyperglycemia, hypercalcemia, sodium and water retention
Musculoskeletal: leg cramps
Respiratory: upper respiratory infection, **pulmonary embolism**
Skin: acne, oily skin, increased pigmentation, urticaria, patch site reaction
Other: increased appetite, weight changes

Interactions

Drug-drug. *Acetaminophen, ascorbic acid, atorvastatin, miconazole (vaginal capsules):* increased ethinyl estradiol blood level
Antibiotics, barbiturates, carbamazepine, fosphenytoin, phenobarbital, phenytoin, rifampin: decreased contraceptive efficacy
Corticosteroids: enhanced corticosteroid effects
Cyclosporine: increased risk of cyclosporine toxicity
CYP3A4 inhibitors (such as ketoconazole, itraconazole): increased hormone level
Dantrolene, other hepatotoxic drugs: increased risk of hepatotoxicity
Insulin, oral hypoglycemics, warfarin: altered requirements for these drugs
Protease inhibitors: increased contraceptive metabolism
Tamoxifen: interference with tamoxifen effects
Drug-diagnostic tests. *Antithrombin III, folate, low-density lipoproteins, pyridoxine, total cholesterol, urine pregnanediol:* decreased levels
Cortisol; factors VII, VIII, IX, and X; glucose; high-density lipoproteins; phospholipids; prolactin; prothrombin; sodium; triglycerides: increased levels
Metyrapone test: false decrease
Thyroid function tests: false interpretation
Drug-food. *Caffeine:* increased blood caffeine level
Drug-herbs. *Black cohosh:* increased adverse drug effects
Red clover: interference with hormonal therapy
Saw palmetto: antiestrogenic effects
St. John's wort: decreased drug blood level and effects
Drug-behaviors. *Smoking (15 or more cigarettes daily):* increased risk of adverse cardiovascular reactions

Patient monitoring

- Evaluate menstrual pattern.

🔈 Monitor blood pressure. Watch for signs and symptoms of thromboembolic disease (swelling or warmth in calf, sudden chest pain, shortness of breath).

- Check blood glucose level in diabetic patient.

Patient teaching

- Instruct patient to start using patch on first day of menstrual period or on first Sunday after period starts. Advise her to use calendar to keep track of which day each week to change patch.
- Tell patient to remove patch during fourth week of each cycle. Explain that she will have bleeding that week.
- Advise patient to check daily to ensure that patch is attached firmly to skin. Explain that if patch is detached for 1 day or less, she should try to reattach it more firmly. If patch is detached for more than 1 day or for an unknown length of time, she should start with new patch and new calendar.
- Instruct patient to use alternative contraception during first week of patch use.

🔈 Inform patient that smoking while using patch increases risk of thromboembolic disease and other serious cardiovascular reactions. Stress importance of not smoking. Tell her to immediately report swelling or warmth in calf, chest pain, or shortness of breath.

- As appropriate, review all other significant and life-threatening adverse

reactions and interactions, especially those related to the drugs, tests, foods, herbs, and behaviors mentioned above.

norepinephrine bitartrate
Levophed

Pharmacologic class: Sympathomimetic
Therapeutic class: Alpha- and beta-adrenergic agonist, cardiac stimulant, vasopressor
Pregnancy risk category C

Action
Stimulates $beta_1$ and $alpha_1$ receptors in sympathetic nervous system, causing vasoconstriction, increased blood pressure, enhanced contractility, and decreased heart rate

Availability
Injection: 1 mg/ml

Indications and dosages
➤ Severe hypotension
Adults: 8 to 12 mcg/minute I.V.; then titrate based on blood pressure response. For maintenance, 2 to 4 mcg/minute.

Contraindications
- Concurrent cyclopropane or halothane anesthesia
- Hypotension caused by blood volume deficit (except in emergencies until blood volume replacement is completed), profound hypoxia or hypercarbia
- Mesenteric or peripheral vascular thrombosis

Precautions
Use cautiously in:
- sulfite sensitivity (some products), especially in asthmatic patients
- arterial embolism, cardiac disease, peripheral vascular disease, hypertension, hyperthyroidism
- patients receiving MAO inhibitors or tricyclic antidepressants concurrently
- elderly patients
- pregnant or breastfeeding patients
- children (safety and efficacy not established).

Administration
- Mix with dextrose 5% in water or dextrose 5% in normal saline solution.
- Inspect solution to make sure it's clear and colorless. Don't infuse if it's brown or pink.
- Administer through infusion pump. Titrate infusion rate to achieve and maintain low-normal systolic blood pressure (80 to 100 mm Hg).
- Continue infusion until adequate blood pressure and tissue perfusion persist without drug therapy.
- Gradually titrate dosage downward.
- To avoid extravasation, administer only into large vein (antecubital) or through central line. Don't use femoral vein in patients who are elderly or have occlusive vascular disorders.

🔊 To prevent delivery of large drug concentrations, avoid line stasis and flushing.

Route	Onset	Peak	Duration
I.V.	Immediate	Immediate	1-2 min after infusion ends

Adverse reactions
CNS: headache, anxiety
CV: bradycardia, **severe hypertension, arrhythmias**
Respiratory: respiratory difficulty
Skin: irritation with extravasation, necrosis
Other: ischemic injury

Interactions
Drug-drug. *Alpha-adrenergic blockers:* antagonism of norepinephrine effects

Antihistamines, ergot alkaloids, guanethidine, MAO inhibitors, oxytocin, tricyclic antidepressants: severe hypertension
Bretylium, inhalation anesthetics: increased risk of arrhythmias

Patient monitoring

◀ Check blood pressure every 2 minutes until desired pressure is achieved. Recheck every 5 minutes for duration of infusion.
• Maintain continuous ECG monitoring and blood pressure monitoring.
◀ Be aware that headache may signal extreme hypertension and overdose.
• Monitor infusion site for extravasation.
◀ Watch for signs and symptoms of peripheral vascular insufficiency (decreased capillary refill, pale to cyanotic to black skin color).
◀ Never leave patient unattended during infusion.

Patient teaching

• When patient is alert, explain why he's receiving drug.
• Reassure patient he'll be monitored continuously until he's stable.

norethindrone acetate

Aygestin

Pharmacologic class: Progesterone, hormone
Therapeutic class: Progestin
Pregnancy risk category X

Action

Inhibits pituitary gonadotropin secretion, suppressing follicular maturation and ovulation and stimulating mammary tissue growth

Availability

Tablets: 5 mg

Indications and dosages

➢ Endometriosis
Adults: 5 mg P.O. daily for 2 weeks, increased in increments of 2.5 mg/day q 2 weeks until 15 mg daily is reached
➢ Amenorrhea; abnormal uterine bleeding
Adults: 2.5 to 10 mg P.O. daily starting on day 5 of menstrual cycle

Contraindications

• Hypersensitivity to drug
• Severe hepatic disease
• Thromboembolic disorders
• Breast or reproductive tract cancer
• Undiagnosed vaginal bleeding
• Missed abortion
• Pregnancy

Precautions

Use cautiously in:
• hypertension, blood dyscrasias, bone marrow disease, hepatic or renal disease, gallbladder disease, heart failure, diabetes mellitus, depression, migraine, asthma, seizure disorder
• family history of breast or reproductive tract cancer
• breastfeeding patients.

Administration

• Give with or without food.
• Know therapy may continue for 6 to 9 months or until breakthrough bleeding necessitates a temporary halt.

Route	Onset	Peak	Duration
P.O.	Variable	Unknown	24 hr

Adverse reactions

CNS: migraine, depression, insomnia, drowsiness
EENT: retinal vascular lesions, sudden partial or complete vision loss, proptosis, diplopia, **papilledema**
GI: nausea
GU: breakthrough bleeding, menstrual flow changes, amenorrhea, changes in cervical erosion and secretions, breast tenderness and secretion

Hepatic: cholestatic jaundice
Metabolic: fluid retention, decreased glucose tolerance
Skin: rash, urticaria, acne, hirsutism, chloasma
Other: edema, weight gain or loss, fever

Interactions

Drug-drug. *Hepatic enzyme-inducing drugs (such as carbamazepine, phenobarbital, phenytoin, rifampin):* decreased norethindrone efficacy
Drug-diagnostic tests. *Alkaline phosphatase; amino acids; factors VII, VIII, IX, and X; nitrogen; pregnanediol:* increased levels
Gamma-glutamyltransferase, high-density lipoproteins: decreased levels
Drug-herbs. *Cola nut, guarana, yerba maté:* increased CNS stimulation
St. John's wort: decreased contraceptive efficacy
Drug-behaviors. *Smoking:* risk of serious cardiovascular reactions

Patient monitoring

- Monitor pretreatment and annual physical exams to check blood pressure, breasts, abdomen, pelvic organs, and Pap smear results.
- (Clinical alert) Assess for signs and symptoms of depression, especially in patients with history of depression. Stop giving drug if significant depression recurs.
- Check blood glucose level in diabetic patients.

Patient teaching

- Instruct patient to avoid pregnancy or to discontinue drug if she gets pregnant (may cause serious fetal anomalies or fetal death).
- (Clinical alert) Advise patient to discontinue drug and consult prescriber if she experiences sudden partial or complete vision loss.
- If patient's receiving drug to treat amenorrhea, tell her to mark administration days on calendar.
- Tell diabetic patient to monitor blood glucose level closely and to watch for hyperglycemia.
- Instruct patient to report breakthrough bleeding, spotting, change in menstrual flow, or amenorrhea.
- Caution patient not to smoke during therapy.
- As appropriate, review all other significant and life-threatening adverse reactions and interactions, especially those related to the drugs, tests, herbs, and behaviors mentioned above.

norfloxacin

Chibroxin, Noroxin

Pharmacologic class: Fluoroquinolone
Therapeutic class: Anti-infective
Pregnancy risk category C

Action

Inhibits bacterial DNA synthesis by blocking DNA gyrase in susceptible gram-negative and gram-positive aerobic and anaerobic bacteria

Availability

Ophthalmic solution: 0.3% in 5-ml bottle
Tablets: 400 mg

Indications and dosages

➢ Urinary tract infections (UTIs) caused by *Escherichia coli, Klebsiella pneumoniae,* or *Proteus mirabilis*
Adults: 400 mg P.O. q 12 hours for 3 days
➢ UTIs caused by all organisms except *E. coli, K. pneumoniae,* and *P. mirabilis*
Adults: 400 mg P.O. q 12 hours for 7 to 10 days. For complicated UTIs, may give for up to 21 days.
➢ Gonorrhea
Adults: 800 mg P.O. as a single dose

➢ Prostatitis caused by *E. coli*
Adults: 400 mg P.O. q 12 hours for 28 days
➢ Conjunctivitis caused by susceptible organisms
Adults and children ages 1 and older: One or two drops of ophthalmic solution instilled into affected eye(s) q.i.d. for up to 7 days. Depending on infection severity, first-day dosage may be one or two drops q 2 hours while awake.

Dosage adjustment

- Renal impairment

Contraindications

- Hypersensitivity to drug
- History of tendinitis or tendon rupture with fluoroquinolone use

Precautions

Use cautiously in:
- CNS diseases or disorders, renal impairment, cirrhosis, bradycardia, acute myocardial ischemia
- elderly patients
- pregnant or breastfeeding patients (safety not established except in post-exposure inhalation or cutaneous anthrax).
- children younger than age 18 (except with ophthalmic solution).

Administration

- Give with glass of water 1 hour before or 2 hours after a meal.
- Don't give antacids within 2 hours of norfloxacin.

Route	Onset	Peak	Duration
P.O.	Rapid	2-3 hr	12 hr
Ophthalmic	Unknown	Unknown	Unknown

Adverse reactions

CNS: dizziness, light-headedness, drowsiness, headache, asthenia, insomnia, agitation, confusion, acute psychoses, hallucinations, tremors, **increased intracranial pressure, seizures**
CV: vasodilation, **QT prolongation, arrhythmias**
EENT: eye burning and discomfort, conjunctival hyperemia, corneal deposits, photophobia (all with ophthalmic use)
GI: nausea, diarrhea, abdominal pain, **pancreatitis, pseudomembranous colitis**
GU: interstitial cystitis, vaginitis
Hematologic: leukopenia
Hepatic: hepatitis
Metabolic: hyperglycemia, **hypoglycemia**
Musculoskeletal: tendinitis, tendon rupture
Skin: rash, hyperhidrosis, photosensitivity, phototoxicity, **Stevens-Johnson syndrome**
Other: altered taste, hypersensitivity reactions including **anaphylaxis**

Interactions

Drug-drug. *Antacids, bismuth, iron salts, subsalicylate, sucralfate, zinc salts:* decreased norfloxacin absorption
Antineoplastics: decreased norfloxacin blood level
Cimetidine: interference with norfloxacin elimination
Corticosteroids: increased risk of tendon rupture
Nitrofurantoin: antagonism of norfloxacin's antibacterial effects in GU tract
Other fluoroquinolones: increased risk of nephrotoxicity
Probenecid: decreased renal elimination of norfloxacin
Theophylline: increased theophylline blood level, greater risk of toxicity
Warfarin: increased anticoagulant effect
Drug-diagnostic tests. *Alanine aminotransferase, alkaline phosphatase, aspartate aminotransferase, bilirubin, eosinophils, lactate dehydrogenase, platelets:* increased levels
Hemoglobin, hematocrit: decreased values

Drug-food. *Caffeine:* decreased hepatic metabolism of caffeine
Milk or yogurt (consumed alone): impaired drug absorption
Tube feedings: impaired drug absorption
Drug-herbs. *Dong quai, St. John's wort:* phototoxicity
Fennel: decreased drug absorption
Drug-behaviors. *Sun exposure:* phototoxicity

Patient monitoring

- Monitor vital signs and cardiovascular status.
- Check fluid intake and output. Keep patient well-hydrated.
- Assess patient's response to therapy. Obtain specimens for repeat culture and sensitivity tests if he relapses or doesn't improve.
- Monitor renal function.

Patient teaching

- Tell patient to take on empty stomach with full glass of water, 1 hour before or 2 hours after a meal.
- If patient needs antacid for GI upset, instruct him not to take it within 2 hours of norfloxacin.

Advise patient to promptly report rash, severe GI problems, or weakness.

- Caution patient to avoid driving and other hazardous activities until he knows how drug affects concentration and alertness.
- Teach patient ways to counteract photosensitivity, such as by wearing sunglasses and avoiding excessive exposure to bright light.
- Teach patient how to use eye drops. Caution him not to touch dropper tip to any surface (including eye).
- As appropriate, review all other significant and life-threatening adverse reactions and interactions, especially those related to the drugs, tests, foods, herbs, and behaviors mentioned above.

norgestrel

Ovrette

Pharmacologic class: Estrogen
Therapeutic class: Contraceptive
Pregnancy risk category X

Action

Suppresses gonadotropin and inhibits ovulation by causing endometrial changes that prevent implantation of egg

Availability

Tablets: 0.075 mg

Indications and dosages

➢ To prevent pregnancy
Adults: 1 tablet P.O. daily

Contraindications

- Thromboembolism
- Undiagnosed vaginal bleeding
- Breast or reproductive organ cancer
- Cerebrovascular or coronary artery disease
- Cholestatic jaundice or hepatic disease
- Pregnancy or breastfeeding

Precautions

Use cautiously in:

- underlying cardiovascular disease, severe hepatic or renal disease, asthma, bone disease, migraine, seizures, lipid disorders, diabetes, fibrocystic breasts, sexually transmitted diseases
- increased risk of endometrial cancer
- family history of breast or reproductive tract cancer
- cigarette smokers.

Administration

- Give daily at same time, starting on first day of menstrual period.

n

Route	Onset	Peak	Duration
P.O.	Unknown	Unknown	24 hr

Adverse reactions

CNS: headache, dizziness, lethargy, depression, emotional lability, **increased risk of cerebrovascular accident, seizures**
CV: edema, hypertension, **myocardial infarction, thromboembolism**
EENT: worsening of myopia or astigmatism, contact lens intolerance
GI: nausea, vomiting, jaundice, abdominal cramps, bloating, anorexia, gallbladder disease, **pancreatitis**
GU: amenorrhea, dysmenorrhea, breakthrough bleeding, cervical erosion, vaginal candidiasis, breast tenderness, breast enlargement or secretion, libido loss, **increased risk of breast and endometrial cancer**
Hepatic: cholestatic jaundice, **hepatic adenoma**
Metabolic: hyperglycemia, hypercalcemia, sodium and water retention
Musculoskeletal: leg cramps
Respiratory: pulmonary embolism
Skin: acne, oily skin, increased pigmentation, urticaria
Other: increased appetite, weight changes

Interactions

Drug-drug. *Acetaminophen:* decreased acetaminophen blood level
Antibiotics, barbiturates, carbamazepine, fosphenytoin, phenobarbital, phenytoin, rifampin: decreased norgestrel efficacy
Corticosteroids: enhanced corticosteroid effects
Cyclosporine: increased risk of cyclosporine toxicity
Dantrolene, other hepatotoxic drugs: increased risk of hepatotoxicity
Insulin, oral hypoglycemics, warfarin: altered requirements for these drugs
Miconazole (vaginal capsules): increased norgestrel blood level
Protease inhibitors: increased norgestrel metabolism
Tamoxifen: interference with tamoxifen effects
Drug-diagnostic tests. *Antithrombin III, folate, low-density lipoproteins, pyridoxine, total cholesterol, urine pregnanediol:* decreased values
Cortisol; factors VII, VIII, IX, and X; glucose; high-density lipoproteins; phospholipids; prolactin; prothrombin; sodium; triglycerides: increased levels
Metyrapone test: false decrease
Thyroid function tests: false interpretation
Drug-food. *Caffeine:* increased blood caffeine level
Drug-herbs. *Black cohosh:* increased adverse reactions to norgestrel
Red clover: interference with norgestrel therapy
Saw palmetto: antiestrogenic effects
St. John's wort: decreased drug blood level and effects
Drug-behaviors. *Smoking:* increased risk of adverse cardiovascular reactions

Patient monitoring

- Check vital signs and cardiovascular status.

Watch for signs and symptoms of thromboembolic disease (leg pain, swelling, shortness of breath).

Patient teaching

- Tell patient to take at bedtime or with a meal, to help establish a daily routine.
- Caution patient that taking drug during pregnancy can cause serious fetal anomalies.

Instruct patient to immediately report calf swelling or warmth, chest pain, shortness of breath, sudden severe headache, bleeding, or spotting.

- Caution patient to avoid driving and other hazardous activities until she knows how drug affects concentration and alertness.

• As appropriate, review all other significant and life-threatening adverse reactions and interactions, especially those related to the drugs, tests, foods, herbs, and behaviors mentioned above.

nortriptyline hydrochloride

Aventyl, Norventyl✤, Pamelor, PMS-Nortriptyline✤

Pharmacologic class: Tricyclic compound
Therapeutic class: Antidepressant
Pregnancy risk category D

Action

Increases serotonin and norepinephrine release by blocking their reuptake by presynaptic neurons; also possesses anticholinergic properties

Availability

Capsules: 10 mg, 25 mg, 50 mg, 75 mg
Oral solution: 10 mg/5 ml

Indications and dosages

➢ Depression
Adults: 25 mg P.O. t.i.d. or q.i.d., up to a maximum of 150 mg daily

Dosage adjustment

• Elderly patients
• Adolescents

Off-label uses

• Postherpetic neuralgia
• Neurologic pain

Contraindications

• Hypersensitivity to drug or dibenzazepines
• Acute recovery phase of myocardial infarction
• MAO inhibitor use within past 14 days

Precautions

Use cautiously in:
• asthma, cardiovascular disease, cardiac or hepatic disease, hyperthyroidism, increased intraocular pressure, angle-closure glaucoma, urinary retention, severe depression
• history of seizures
• elderly patients (especially elderly men with prostatic hyperplasia)
• pregnant or breastfeeding patients
• children (use not recommended).

Administration

• Give as prescribed, either in divided doses three or four times daily or as single dose at bedtime.
• Administer with meals or snack to minimize stomach upset.
Clinical alert: Don't give within 14 days of MAO inhibitors.

Route	Onset	Peak	Duration
P.O.	2-3 wk	6 wk	Unknown

Adverse reactions

CNS: dizziness, drowsiness, fatigue, headache, lethargy, insomnia, agitation, confusion, extrapyramidal reactions, hallucinations, **seizures, suicidal behavior or ideation** (especially in child or adolescent)
CV: hypotension, ECG changes, palpitations, **heart block, arrhythmias, myocardial infarction, cerebrovascular accident**
EENT: blurred vision, dry eyes
GI: nausea, constipation, anorexia, dry mouth, **paralytic ileus**
GU: urinary retention, gynecomastia
Hematologic: blood dyscrasias
Hepatic: jaundice, **hepatotoxicity**
Skin: photosensitivity
Other: unpleasant taste, weight gain

Interactions

Drug-drug. *Anticholinergics, anticholinergic-like drugs (including antidepressants, antihistamines, atropine, disopyramide, haloperidol, phenothia-*

zines, quinidine): additive anticholinergic effects
Antihypertensives: poor therapeutic response to antihypertensives
Antithyroid drugs: increased risk of agranulocytosis
Cimetidine, fluoxetine, hormonal contraceptives: increased nortriptyline blood level and possible toxicity
Clonidine: hypertensive crisis
CNS depressants (including antihistamines, opioids, sedative-hypnotics): additive CNS depression
Decongestants, vasoconstrictors: additive adrenergic effects
MAO inhibitors: hypertension, hyperpyrexia, seizures, death
Drug-diagnostic tests. *Alkaline phosphatase, bilirubin:* increased levels
Glucose: increased or decreased level
Drug-herbs. *Angel's trumpet, belladonna, henbane, jimson weed, scopolia:* increased anticholinergic effects
Chamomile, hops, kava, skullcap, scopolia, valerian: increased CNS depression
St. John's wort: decreased drug blood level and efficacy
Drug-behaviors. *Alcohol use:* increased drowsiness, impaired motor skills

Patient monitoring

- Check vital signs and ECG.
- Monitor bladder and bowel function. Stay alert for urine retention and constipation.
- Assess neurologic status and document mood swings.
- Monitor liver function tests.

Watch for suicidal tendency, especially in child or adolescent.

Patient teaching

- Explain that drug's full effect may take 4 weeks.
- Tell patient drug may cause drowsiness or dizziness, but these effects should subside within a few weeks.

Advise patient (and family as appropriate) to immediately report worsening depression or suicidal ideation, especially in child or adolescent.

- Caution patient to avoid driving and other hazardous activities until he knows how drug affects him.
- Tell patient to avoid alcohol and to consult prescriber before using herbs.
- As appropriate, review all other significant and life-threatening adverse reactions and interactions, especially those related to the drugs, tests, herbs, and behaviors mentioned above.

nystatin

Mycostatin, Nadostine✤, Nilstat, Nyaderm, Nystex, Nystop, Pedi-Dri, PMS-Nystatin✤

Pharmacologic class: Antifungal
Therapeutic class: Anti-infective
Pregnancy risk category A

Action

Interferes with fungal cell-wall synthesis, inhibiting formation of ergo sterols, increasing cell-wall permeability, and causing osmotic instability

Availability

Cream: 100,000 units/g
Ointment: 100,000 units/g
Powder: 100,000 units/g
Suspension: 100,000 units/ml
Tablets: 500,000 units
Troches: 200,000 units
Vaginal tablets: 100,000 units

Indications and dosages

➤ Candidiasis (topical use)
Adults and children: Apply cream, ointment, or powder two or three times daily until healing is complete.
➤ Oral candidiasis
Adults: 400,000 to 600,000 units (suspension) P.O. q.i.d. Have patient gargle

and then swallow half of dose in each side of mouth.
Infants: 200,000 units (suspension) P.O. q.i.d. Use half of dose in each side of mouth.
Newborn and premature infants: 100,000 units (suspension) P.O. q.i.d. Use half of dose in each side of mouth.
➢ GI infections
Adults: 500,000 to 1 million units (one to two tablets) P.O. t.i.d. Continue for 48 hours after desired response occurs.
➢ Vaginal candidiasis
Adults: 100,000 units (one vaginal tablet) intravaginally daily for 2 weeks, or 100,000- to 500,000-unit applicatorful (cream) intravaginally once or twice daily for 2 weeks

Contraindications
• Hypersensitivity to drug or its components

Precautions
Use cautiously in:
• renal or hepatic disease, achlorhydria
• pregnant or breastfeeding patients
• children younger than age 2.

Administration
• Give oral suspension by placing half of dose in each side of patient's mouth. Instruct patient to hold suspension in mouth, swish it around, or gargle for several minutes before swallowing it.
• To prepare oral solution from powder, add one-eighth teaspoon to 120 ml of water and stir well. Give immediately.
• Advise patient to let troche dissolve slowly and completely in mouth. Tell her not to chew or swallow it whole.
• Know that nystatin vaginal tablets can be given orally to treat oral candidiasis.
• To apply cream, ointment, or powder, gently and thoroughly massage preparation into skin.
• Use applicator provided for vaginal administration.

Route	Onset	Peak	Duration
P.O., topical, vaginal	Unknown	Unknown	Unknown

Adverse reactions
GI: nausea, vomiting, diarrhea, GI distress, oral irritation
GU: vulvovaginal irritation (with intravaginal form)
Skin: pruritus, rash

Interactions
Drug-drug. *Topical corticosteroids:* increased corticosteroid absorption
Drug-behaviors. *Latex contraceptive use:* damage to contraceptive (with intravaginal use)

Patient monitoring
• If patient takes oral tablets, inspect oral mucous membranes for irritation.
• With topical use, monitor affected area for increase in redness, swelling, or irritation.

Patient teaching
• Advise patient to continue taking for at least 48 hours after symptoms resolve.
• Instruct patient to let lozenge dissolve slowly in mouth. Tell her not to chew or swallow it.
• If patient misses a dose, tell her to take dose as soon as possible and then resume her regular dosing schedule.
• Inform patient that diabetes mellitus, reinfection by sexual partner, tight-fitting pantyhose, and use of antibiotics, hormonal contraceptives, or corticosteroids predispose her to vaginal infection. Urge her to wear cotton underwear.
• Tell female patient to practice careful hygiene in affected areas.
• Instruct patient using vaginal tablets to wash applicator thoroughly after each use.

n

• Tell patient to continue therapy during menstruation.
• As appropriate, review all significant adverse reactions and interactions, especially those related to the drugs and behaviors mentioned above.

octreotide acetate

Sandostatin, Sandostatin LAR Depot

Pharmacologic class: Somatostatin analog
Therapeutic class: Antidiarrheal
Pregnancy risk category B

Action

Suppresses secretion of serotonin, serotonin metabolites, and gastrohepatic peptides, increasing fluid and electrolyte absorption from GI tract. Also suppresses growth hormone, insulin, and glucagon.

Availability

Depot injection: 10 mg, 20 mg, 30 mg
Injection: 0.05 mg/ml, 0.1 mg/ml, and 0.5 mg/ml in 1-ml ampules; 0.2 mg/ml and 1 mg/ml in 5-ml vials

Indications and dosages

➢ Diarrhea and flushing associated with carcinoid tumors
Adults: 100 to 600 mcg (Sandostatin) subcutaneously or I.V. daily in two to four divided doses for 2 weeks. Then, depending on response, 20 mg (LAR Depot) I.M. q 4 weeks for 2 months.
➢ Diarrhea caused by vasoactive intestinal peptide tumors (VIPomas)
Adults: 200 to 300 mcg (Sandostatin) subcutaneously or I.V. daily in two to four divided doses for 2 weeks. Then, depending on response, 20 mg (LAR Depot) I.M. q 2 weeks for 2 months.
➢ Acromegaly
Adults: 50 to 100 mcg (Sandostatin) subcutaneously or I.V. two or three times daily. Then, depending on response, 20 mg (LAR Depot) I.M. q 4 weeks for 3 months. Then adjust based on growth hormone levels.

Dosage adjustment

• Renal impairment

Off-label uses

• Dumping syndrome (postprandial hypotension)
• GI and pancreatic fistulas
• Variceal bleeding

Contraindications

• Hypersensitivity to drug or its components

Precautions

Use cautiously in:
• gallbladder disease, renal impairment, hyperglycemia or hypoglycemia, fat malabsorption
• pregnant or breastfeeding patients
• children.

Administration

• When giving subcutaneously, rotate administration site with each injection.
Clinical alert: Don't give LAR Depot I.V.
• Mix I.M. solution and inject deep into gluteal muscle over 3 minutes. Don't use deltoid.
• For I.V. administration, dilute in 50 to 200 ml of dextrose 5% in water or normal saline solution. Infuse over 15 to 30 minutes.
• Know that octreotide suppression test and octreotide scintigraphy may be done to determine if drug will aid carcinoid tumor treatment.
• Drug may be kept at room temperature for 2 weeks. Refrigerate ampules.

Route	Onset	Peak	Duration
Subcut., I.V.	Unknown	0.4 hr	Up to 12 hr
I.M.	Unknown	2 wk	Up to 4 wk

Adverse reactions
CNS: dizziness, drowsiness, fatigue, headache, weakness
CV: edema, bradycardia, conduction abnormalities, **arrhythmias**
EENT: vision disturbances
GI: nausea, vomiting, diarrhea, abdominal pain, cholelithiasis, fat malabsorption
Skin: flushing
Metabolic: hypothyroidism, hyperglycemia, **hypoglycemia**
Other: injection site pain

Interactions
Drug-drug. *Cyclosporine:* reduced cyclosporine blood level
Insulin, oral hypoglycemics: altered requirements for these drugs
Orally administered drugs: altered absorption of these drugs
Drug-diagnostic tests. *Glucose:* increased or decreased level
Hepatic enzymes: slightly increased levels
Schilling's test: abnormal results
Thyroxine, vitamin B_{12}: decreased levels
Drug-food. *Fats:* altered octreotide absorption

Patient monitoring
- Assess bowel sounds and stool frequency and consistency.
- Monitor vital signs and fluid intake and output. Stay alert for dehydration or edema.
- Evaluate diabetic patient for hypoglycemia or hyperglycemia.

Patient teaching
- Tell patient being treated for carcinoid tumor to keep track of number of daily stools or flushing episodes.
- Instruct patient to weigh himself daily and report significant changes.
- If patient will use drug at home, teach correct methods for injection, storage, and needle disposal.
- Caution patient to avoid driving and other hazardous activities until he knows how drug affects concentration, vision, and alertness.
- As appropriate, review all other significant and life-threatening adverse reactions and interactions, especially those related to the drugs, tests, and foods mentioned above.

ofloxacin
Floxin, Ocuflox

Pharmacologic class: Fluoroquinolone
Therapeutic class: Anti-infective
Pregnancy risk category C

Action
Inhibits bacterial DNA synthesis by inhibiting DNA gyrase in susceptible bacteria

Availability
Injection: 40 mg/ml
Ophthalmic solution: 3 mg/ml (0.3%)
Otic solution: 0.3%
Premixed injection: 200 mg/50 ml, 400 mg/100 ml
Tablets: 200 mg, 300 mg, 400 mg

Indications and dosages
➢ Prostatitis caused by *Escherichia coli*
Adults: 300 mg P.O. or I.V. q 12 hours for 6 weeks
➢ Complicated urinary tract infections caused by *E. coli, Klebsiella pneumoniae,* or *Proteus mirabilis*
Adults: 200 mg P.O. or I.V. q 12 hours for 10 days
➢ Uncomplicated cystitis caused by *E. coli* or *K. pneumoniae*
Adults: 200 mg P.O. or I.V. q 12 hours for 3 days

O

➢ Acute uncomplicated urethral and cervical gonorrhea
Adults: 400 mg P.O. or I.V. as a single dose
➢ Nongonococcal cervicitis or urethritis caused by *Chlamydia trachomatis*; mixed infections of cervix or urethra caused by *C. trachomatis* or *Neisseria gonorrhoeae*
Adults: 300 mg P.O. or I.V. q 12 hours for 7 days
➢ Acute bacterial exacerbation of chronic bronchitis, community-acquired pneumonia, and uncomplicated skin and skin-structure infections caused by susceptible organisms
Adults: 400 mg P.O. or I.V. q 12 hours for 10 days
➢ Acute pelvic inflammatory disease
Adults: 400 mg P.O. or I.V. q 12 hours for 10 to 14 days
➢ Bacterial conjunctivitis
Adults and children ages 1 and older: One to two drops of ophthalmic solution in affected eye q 2 to 4 hours on days 1 and 2; then one to two drops q.i.d. on days 3 through 7
➢ Corneal ulcers
Adults: One to two drops of ophthalmic solution in affected eye q 30 minutes while awake on days 1 and 2, then one to two drops q hour while awake on days 3 to 7, then one to two drops q.i.d. while awake on days 7 to 9
➢ Otitis externa
Adults and children ages 13 and older: 10 drops of otic solution into affected ear daily for 7 days
➢ Chronic suppurative otitis media with perforated tympanic membrane
Adults and children ages 12 and older: 10 drops of otic solution into affected ear b.i.d. for 14 days

Dosage adjustment
- Renal impairment
- Severe hepatic impairment

Contraindications
- Hypersensitivity to drug or other fluoroquinolones

Precautions
Use cautiously in:
- underlying CNS disease, renal impairment, cirrhosis, bradycardia, acute myocardial ischemia
- history of tendinitis or tendon rupture with fluoroquinolone use
- dialysis patients
- elderly patients
- pregnant or breastfeeding patients (safety not established except in postexposure inhalation or cutaneous anthrax).
- children younger than age 18 (except in postexposure inhalation or cutaneous anthrax and in ophthalmic and otic use).

Administration
- For intermittent I.V. infusion, dilute to a concentration of 4 mg/ml using normal saline solution, dextrose 5% in water (D_5W), dextrose 5% in normal saline solution, or dextrose 5% in lactated Ringer's solution. Infuse slowly over at least 60 minutes.
- Don't give zinc- or iron-containing drugs within 2 hours of ofloxacin.

Route	Onset	Peak	Duration
P.O.	Rapid	1-2 hr	12 hr
I.V.	Rapid	End of infusion	12 hr
Ophthalmic, otic	Unknown	Unknown	Unknown

Adverse reactions
CNS: dizziness, drowsiness, headache, light-headedness, insomnia, acute psychoses, agitation, confusion, tremors, hallucinations, **increased intracranial pressure, seizures**
CV: chest pain, vasodilation
GI: nausea, diarrhea, constipation, abdominal pain, **pseudomembranous colitis**

GU: interstitial cystitis, vaginitis
Hematologic: eosinophilia, **leukopenia**
Musculoskeletal: tendinitis, tendon rupture, joint pain, back pain
Skin: rash, photosensitivity, phototoxicity, **Stevens-Johnson syndrome**
Other: altered taste, superinfection, phlebitis at I.V. site, hypersensitivity reactions including **anaphylaxis**

Interactions

Drug-drug. *Amiodarone, bepridil, disopyramide, erythromycin, pentamidine, phenothiazines, pimozide, procainamide, quinidine, sotalol, tricyclic antidepressants:* increased risk of serious adverse cardiovascular reactions
Antacids, bismuth subsalicylate, iron or zinc salts, sucralfate: decreased ofloxacin absorption
Corticosteroids: increased risk of tendon rupture
Probenecid: decreased renal elimination of ofloxacin
Theophylline: increased theophylline blood level and possible toxicity
Warfarin: increased warfarin effects
Drug-diagnostic tests. *Alanine aminotransferase, aspartate aminotransferase, platelets:* increased levels
Hemoglobin, hematocrit: decreased values
Drug-food. *Milk or yogurt (consumed alone), tube feedings:* impaired drug absorption
Drug-herbs. *Fennel:* decreased drug absorption
Dong quai, St. John's wort: phototoxicity
Drug-behaviors. *Sun exposure:* phototoxicity

Patient monitoring

- Assess patient for signs and symptoms of superinfection.
- Inspect for rash. Check for signs and symptoms of hypersensitivity reaction.
- Watch for fever with diarrhea, diarrhea containing pus, or severe, persistent diarrhea.
- Evaluate neurologic status closely.

Patient teaching

- Encourage patient to maintain fluid intake of at least 1,500 ml daily to prevent crystalluria.
- Inform patient being treated for gonorrhea that partners must be treated.

[Clinical alert] Tell patient to immediately report fever and diarrhea, especially if stool contains blood, pus, or mucus. Caution him not to treat diarrhea without consulting prescriber.

[Clinical alert] Instruct patient to immediately report rash or tendon pain or inflammation.

- Instruct patient not to take iron- or zinc-containing drugs or antacids within 2 hours of ofloxacin.
- Teach patient ways to counteract photosensitivity, such as by wearing sunglasses and avoiding excessive exposure to bright light.
- Teach patient how to use eye or ear drops. Caution him not to touch dropper tip to any surface (including eye or ear).
- As appropriate, review all other significant and life-threatening adverse reactions and interactions, especially those related to the drugs, tests, foods, herbs, and behaviors mentioned above.

O

olanzapine

Zyprexa, Zyprexa IntraMuscular, Zyprexa Zydis

Pharmacologic class: Thienobenzodiazepine

Therapeutic class: Antipsychotic

Pregnancy risk category C

Action

Unknown. Thought to antagonize dopamine and serotonin type 2 in CNS. Also antagonizes muscarinic receptors in respiratory tract, causing cholinergic activation.

Availability

Solution for injection: 10-mg vials
Tablets: 2.5 mg, 5 mg, 7.5 mg, 10 mg, 15 mg, 20 mg
Tablets (orally disintegrating): 5 mg, 10 mg, 15 mg, 20 mg

Indications and dosages

➢ Schizophrenia
Adults: Initially, 5 to 10 mg P.O. daily; may increase q week by 5 mg/day (not to exceed 20 mg/day)
➢ Psychotic disorders, including acute manic episodes
Adults: Initially, 10 to 15 mg P.O. daily; may increase q 24 hours by 5 mg/day (not to exceed 20 mg/day). Or 10 mg I.M.; maximum dosage is three 10-mg doses given I.M. 2 to 4 hours apart.
➢ Maintenance treatment of bipolar disorder
Adults: 12.5 mg P.O. daily

Dosage adjustment

- Elderly or debilitated patients
- Patients predisposed to hypotensive reactions

Off-label uses

- Borderline personality disorder (with oral use)

Contraindications

- Hypersensitivity to drug

Precautions

Use cautiously in:
- hepatic impairment, cardiovascular or cerebrovascular disease, diabetes mellitus, prostatic hypertrophy, angle-closure glaucoma, phenylketonuria (with orally disintegrating tablets)
- history of seizures, paralytic ileus, or suicide attempt
- elderly patients
- pregnant or breastfeeding patients
- children younger than age 18 (safety not established).

Administration

- Give without regard to meals.
- To remove orally disintegrating tablet from package, peel back foil; don't push tablet through foil.
- Reconstitute for I.M. injection with 2.1 ml of sterile water for injection only, into single-packaged vial.
- After reconstitution, withdraw total contents of vial for 10-mg dose; 1.5 ml for 7.5-mg dose; 1 ml for 5-mg dose, or 0.5 ml for 2.5-mg dose.
- Use solution for I.M. injection within 1 hour of reconstitution.
- Don't combine in syringe with diazepam, lorazepam, or haloperidol.
- Be aware that total daily dosages above 30 mg P.O. or 10 mg I.M. given more often than 2 hours after initial dose and 4 hours after second dose aren't recommended.

Route	Onset	Peak	Duration
P.O.	Unknown	6 hr	Unknown
I.M.	Rapid	15-45 min	Unknown

Adverse reactions

CNS: dizziness, headache, weakness, fatigue, restlessness, sedation, insomnia, mood changes, agitation, personality disorder, impaired speech, tardive dyskinesia, dystonia, tremor, extrapyramidal effects, **neuroleptic malignant syndrome, coma**
CV: orthostatic hypotension, chest pain, tachycardia
EENT: amblyopia, rhinitis, pharyngitis
GI: nausea, constipation, abdominal pain, increased salivation, dry mouth
GU: urinary incontinence, urinary tract infection
Hematologic: leukopenia
Metabolic: goiter, increased thirst, **severe hyperglycemia**
Musculoskeletal: hypertonia, joint pain
Respiratory: cough, dyspnea
Skin: ecchymosis, photosensitivity
Other: increased appetite, weight gain

or loss, fever, flulike symptoms, impaired body temperature regulation, **death**

Interactions

Drug-drug. *Antihypertensives:* additive hypotension
Carbamazepine, omeprazole, rifampin: decreased olanzapine effects
CNS depressants: additive CNS depression
Dopamine agonists, levodopa: antagonism of these drugs' effects
Drug-diagnostic tests. *Alanine aminotransferase, alkaline phosphatase, aspartate aminotransferase, bilirubin, glucose, creatinine phosphokinase, gamma-glutamyltransferase:* elevated levels
Platelets: decreased count
Drug-behaviors. *Alcohol use:* additive CNS depression
Smoking: increased drug clearance
Sun exposure: increased risk of photosensitivity

Patient monitoring

- Assess patient's mental status during therapy.
- Monitor vital signs during dosage adjustment periods.
- Make sure patient takes drug and doesn't hoard it.

🔊 Watch for signs and symptoms of neuroleptic malignant syndrome (fever, respiratory distress, tachycardia, seizures, diaphoresis, hypertension or hypotension, tiredness, severe muscle stiffness, loss of bladder control).

- Evaluate patient for onset of akathisia, tardive dyskinesia, and extrapyramidal effects.

🔊 Watch for signs of increasing depression.

🔊 Monitor blood glucose level closely, especially in patient with diabetes mellitus. Severe hyperglycemia, coma, and death may occur.

- Watch for orthostatic hypotension before I.M. injection. Keep patient recumbent if drowsiness or dizziness follows injection.

Patient teaching

- Tell patient he may take without regard to meals.
- Instruct patient to remove orally disintegrating tablet from package by peeling back foil—not by pushing tablet through foil. Instruct him to remove tablet from foil using dry hands, and place entire tablet in mouth. Tell him tablet will disintegrate with or without liquid.
- Tell patient drug may cause extrapyramidal symptoms, akathisia, and tardive dyskinesia leading to involuntary movements, tremors, rigidity, muscle contractions, and restlessness.

🔊 Caution patient with diabetes mellitus to monitor blood glucose closely.

- Tell patient to move slowly when sitting up or standing to avoid dizziness. Advise him to dangle legs briefly before getting out of bed.
- Advise patient to avoid smoking, alcohol, or other CNS depressants.
- Tell patient to exercise in moderation and to avoid overly hot baths and showers, because drug impairs body temperature regulation.
- Caution patient to avoid driving and other hazardous activities until he knows how drug affects concentration and alertness.
- As appropriate, review all other significant and life-threatening adverse reactions and interactions, especially those related to the drugs, tests, and behaviors mentioned above.

O

olmesartan medoxomil

Benicar

Pharmacologic class: Angiotensin II type 1-receptor antagonist
Therapeutic class: Antihypertensive
Pregnancy risk category C (first trimester), ***D*** (second and third trimesters)

Action

Selectively blocks binding of angiotensin II to specific tissue receptors in vascular smooth muscle and adrenal gland. This action blocks vasoconstrictive effects of renin-angiotensin system as well as aldosterone release, thereby reducing blood pressure and possibly preventing vascular remodeling related to arteriosclerosis.

Availability

Tablets: 5 mg, 20 mg, 40 mg

Indications and dosages

➢ Hypertension

Adults: 20 mg P.O. once daily; may titrate to 40 mg daily after 2 weeks, if needed

Dosage adjustment

- Volume depletion

Contraindications

- Hypersensitivity to drug or its components

Precautions

Use cautiously in:

- hepatic disease, renal dysfunction, hypovolemia, sodium depletion
- elderly patients
- pregnant patients (first trimester; not recommended in second and third trimesters)
- breastfeeding patients
- children (safety and efficacy not established).

Administration

- Give with or without food.
- Know that drug may be used alone or with other antihypertensives.

Route	Onset	Peak	Duration
P.O.	Variable	1-2 hr	Unknown

Adverse reactions

CNS: fatigue, dizziness, headache, insomnia
CV: orthostatic hypotension, chest pain, peripheral edema, syncope, tachycardia
EENT: sinusitis, rhinitis, pharyngitis
GI: nausea, diarrhea, constipation, abdominal pain, dry mouth
GU: hematuria
Hematologic: hyperglycemia
Musculoskeletal: back pain, arthritis, muscle weakness
Respiratory: upper respiratory infection symptoms, bronchitis, cough
Skin: dry skin, rash, inflammation, pruritus, alopecia, angioedema
Other: dental pain, flulike symptoms

Interactions

Drug-diagnostic tests. *Triglycerides:* increased level
Drug-herbs. *Ephedra (ma huang):* antagonism of antihypertensive effect

Patient monitoring

- Monitor vital signs and cardiovascular status. Stay alert for orthostatic hypotension, syncope, and peripheral edema.
- Check temperature and watch for signs and symptoms of flu and other infections (especially respiratory and EENT infections).
- Watch for angioedema.
- In volume-depleted patient, monitor blood pressure carefully after initial dose. Transient blood pressure drop may occur.

Patient teaching

• Tell patient to take at same time each day, with or without food.
• Advise patient to promptly report signs and symptoms of infection, particularly respiratory symptoms.
• Inform patient that when he begins therapy, inadequate fluid intake, excessive perspiration, vomiting, or diarrhea may cause blood pressure to drop. Tell him to change position slowly to avoid dizziness or fainting.
• Caution patient to avoid driving and other hazardous activities until he knows how drug affects concentration and alertness.
Tell female patient to notify prescriber immediately if she suspects pregnancy.
• As appropriate, review all other significant adverse reactions and interactions, especially those related to the tests and herbs mentioned above.

olsalazine sodium

Dipentum

Pharmacologic class: Salicylate
Therapeutic class: Anti-inflammatory
Pregnancy risk category C

Action

Unknown. Converts to active form, mesalamine, which blocks cyclooxygenase and inhibits prostaglandin production in colon.

Availability

Capsules: 250 mg

Indications and dosages

➢ Ulcerative colitis in patients who can't tolerate sulfasalazine
Adults: 500 mg P.O. b.i.d.

Contraindications

• Hypersensitivity to drug or other salicylates

Precautions

Use cautiously in:
• hepatic or renal impairment, severe allergy, bronchial asthma
• pregnant or breastfeeding patients
• children younger than age 14.

Administration

• Give with meals to reduce GI irritation.

Route	Onset	Peak	Duration
P.O.	Variable	60 min	Unknown

Adverse reactions

CNS: headache, fatigue, depression, vertigo
GI: nausea, vomiting, diarrhea, abdominal pain, cramps, dyspepsia, bloating, stomatitis
Musculoskeletal: joint pain
Respiratory: upper respiratory infection
Skin: rash, itching

O

Interactions

Drug-drug. *Anticoagulants, coumarin derivatives:* prolonged prothrombin time, increased International Normalized Ratio
Drug-food. *Any food:* decreased GI irritation

Patient monitoring

• Monitor neurologic status. Stay alert for depression.
• Assess GI symptoms. Encourage adequate fluid intake to avoid dehydration.
• Monitor urinalysis, blood urea nitrogen, and creatinine in patients with renal impairment.

Patient teaching

• Instruct patient to take with food and to continue taking drug even after symptoms improve.

• Tell patient to eat appropriate foods in small, frequent servings to minimize GI upset.
• Advise patient to contact prescriber if symptoms worsen or don't improve after 1 to 2 months of therapy.
• Tell patient he may require periodic proctoscopy and sigmoidoscopy to determine response to drug.
• Caution patient to avoid driving and other hazardous activities until he knows how drug affects mood and wakefulness.
• As appropriate, review all significant adverse reactions and interactions, especially those related to the drugs and foods mentioned above.

omalizumab

Xolair

Pharmacologic class: Recombinant DNA-derived immunoglobulin G subclass 1 (IgG1) monoclonal antibody

Therapeutic class: Monoclonal antibody

Pregnancy risk category B

Action

Inhibits binding of IgE to high-affinity IgE receptors on surface of mast cells and basophils

Availability

Powder for injection: 150 mg/vial

Indications and dosages

➢ Persistent asthma in patients with positive skin tests or in vitro reactivity to perennial allergens whose symptoms aren't adequately controlled by inhaled corticosteroids

Adults and adolescents ages 12 and older: 150 to 375 mg subcutaneously q 2 to 4 weeks, with dosing frequency determined by serum IgE level and weight

Dosage adjustment

• Significant weight change

Contraindications

• Hypersensitivity to drug

Precautions

Use cautiously in:
• elderly patients
• pregnant or breastfeeding patients
• children younger than age 12.

Administration

Clinical alert: Be aware that omalizumab isn't a rescue drug and isn't intended for acute asthma attacks or status asthmaticus.
Clinical alert: Don't discontinue abruptly.
• Don't administer more than 150 mg per injection site.
• Prepare injection only with sterile water for injection.

Route	Onset	Peak	Duration
Subcut.	Unknown	7-8 days	Unknown

Adverse reactions

CNS: headache, fatigue, dizziness
EENT: sinusitis, pharyngitis, earache
Musculoskeletal: arthralgia, fracture, leg or arm pain
Respiratory: upper respiratory infection
Skin: pruritus, dermatitis
Other: injection-site reaction, viral infection, pain, **cancer, anaphylaxis**

Interactions

Drug-diagnostic tests. *Serum IgE:* elevated level

Patient monitoring

Clinical alert: Monitor patient for severe hypersensitivity reactions, including anaphylaxis.
Clinical alert: Watch for signs and symptoms of cancer (rare).

Patient teaching

🔊 Tell patient to take exactly as prescribed and not to change dosage or stop drug abruptly (unless hypersensitivity reaction occurs).

🔊 Instruct patient to discontinue drug and notify prescriber immediately at first sign of hypersensitivity reaction, such as rash, hives, or itching.

- Inform patient that asthma symptoms may not improve immediately after starting drug.
- Tell patient drug isn't intended for acute asthma attacks.
- As appropriate, review all other significant and life-threatening adverse reactions and interactions, especially those related to the tests mentioned above.

omeprazole

Losec*, Prilosec, Prilosec OTC, Zegerid

Pharmacologic class: Proton pump inhibitor
Therapeutic class: Antiulcer drug
Pregnancy risk category C

Action

Reduces gastric acid secretion and increases gastric mucus and bicarbonate production, creating protective coating on gastric mucosa and easing discomfort from excess gastric acid

Availability

Capsules (delayed-release): 10 mg, 20 mg, 40 mg
Powder for oral suspension: 20 mg
Tablets (delayed-release): 20 mg

Indications and dosages

➢ Gastroesophageal reflux disease
Adults: 20 mg P.O. (capsules, powder) daily for 4 weeks

➢ Erosive esophagitis
Adults: 20 mg P.O. (capsules, powder) daily for 4 to 8 weeks

➢ Short-term treatment of active duodenal ulcer
Adults: 20 mg P.O. (capsules, powder) daily for 4 weeks. Some patients may need 4 additional weeks of therapy.

➢ To reduce risk of duodenal ulcers caused by *Helicobacter pylori*
Adults: 40 mg P.O. (capsules) daily in morning, given with clarithromycin t.i.d. for 2 weeks; then 20 mg daily for 2 weeks

➢ Gastric ulcers
Adults: 40 mg P.O. (capsules) daily for 4 to 8 weeks

➢ Pathologic hypersecretory conditions, including Zollinger-Ellison syndrome
Adults: Initially, 60 mg P.O. (capsules) daily; may increase up to 120 mg t.i.d. Divide daily dosages above 80 mg.

➢ Frequent heartburn (two or more episodes a week)
Adults ages 18 and older: 20 mg P.O. (OTC tablets) daily for 14 days

Off-label uses

- Posterior laryngitis
- To enhance pancreatin efficacy in treating steatorrhea in cystic fibrosis patients

Contraindications

- Hypersensitivity to drug or its components

Precautions

Use cautiously in:
- hepatic disease
- pregnant or breastfeeding patients
- children (safety not established).

Administration

- Give 30 to 60 minutes before a meal, preferably in morning.
- If desired, give concurrently with antacids.

O

• Know that if patient has ulcer at start of therapy, treatment may be extended.
• When giving through nasogastric tube, use powder for oral suspension, or separate capsule and mix pellets with water. Agitate syringe while injecting. After administration, flush with 30 to 60 ml of water.
• Don't crush capsules.
• Be aware that symptomatic response doesn't rule out gastric cancer.

Route	Onset	Peak	Duration
P.O.	Within 1 hr	Within 2 hr	72-96 hr
P.O. (delayed)	Unknown	10-90 min	Unknown

Adverse reactions
CNS: dizziness, headache, asthenia
GI: nausea, vomiting, diarrhea, constipation, abdominal pain
Musculoskeletal: back pain
Respiratory: cough, upper respiratory tract infection
Skin: rash

Interactions
Drug-drug. *Ampicillin, cyanocobalamin, iron salts, ketoconazole:* reduced absorption of these drugs
Clarithromycin: increased omeprazole blood level
Diazepam, phenytoin, warfarin: prolonged elimination and increased effects of these drugs
Digoxin: increased digoxin absorption and blood level, possible digoxin toxicity
Drugs metabolized by CYP450 system: competitive metabolism
Drug-diagnostic tests. *Alanine phosphatase, alkaline aminotransferase, aspartate aminotransferase, bilirubin:* increased levels
Gastrin: increased level during first 1 to 2 weeks of therapy

Patient monitoring
• Assess vital signs.
• Check for abdominal pain, emesis, diarrhea, or constipation.
• Evaluate fluid intake and output.
• Watch for elevated liver function test results (rare).

Patient teaching
• Tell patient to take 30 to 60 minutes before a meal, preferably in morning.
• Instruct patient to swallow capsules or tablets whole and not to chew or crush them. If he can't swallow capsule, tell him he may open it, carefully sprinkle and mix entire contents into 1 tbsp of cool applesauce, and swallow immediately with glass of water.
• Inform patient taking OTC delayed-release tablets for heartburn that full effect may take 1 to 4 days. Advise him not to take tablets for more than 14 days without consulting healthcare professional.
• Caution patient to avoid driving and other hazardous activities until he knows how drug affects concentration and alertness.
• As appropriate, review all other significant adverse reactions and interactions, especially those related to the drugs and tests mentioned above.

ondansetron hydrochloride
Zofran, Zofran ODT, Zofran Preservative Free

Pharmacologic class: Serotonin type 3 ($5\text{-}HT_3$) antagonist
Therapeutic class: Antiemetic
Pregnancy risk category B

Action
Blocks serotonin at $5\text{-}HT_3$ receptor sites in vagal nerve terminals by disrupting CNS chemoreceptor trigger zone

Availability

Injection: 2 mg/ml in 2- and 20-ml vials
Injection (premixed): 32 mg/50 ml single-dose containers
Injection USP (preservative-free): 2 mg/ml in 2-ml single-dose vials
Oral solution: 4 mg/5 ml
Tablets: 4 mg, 8 mg, 24 mg
Tablets (orally disintegrating): 4 mg, 8 mg

Indications and dosages

➢ To prevent nausea and vomiting caused by moderately emetogenic chemotherapy
Adults and children older than age 12: 8 mg (tablet) or 10 ml (oral solution) P.O. b.i.d.; give first dose 30 minutes before chemotherapy and repeat dose 8 hours later. Give 8 mg (tablet) or 10 ml (oral solution) P.O. q 12 hours for 1 to 2 days after chemotherapy ends.
Children ages 4 to 11: 4 mg (tablet) or 5 ml (oral solution) P.O. q 8 hours; give first dose 30 minutes before chemotherapy and repeat dose 4 and 8 hours later. Give 4 mg (tablet) or 5 ml (oral solution) P.O. q 8 hours for 1 to 2 days after chemotherapy ends.
➢ To prevent nausea and vomiting caused by highly emetogenic chemotherapy
Adults and children older than age 12: 32 mg I.V. as a single dose infused over 15 minutes, starting 30 minutes before chemotherapy; or three 0.15-mg/kg doses I.V., with first dose infused over 15 minutes, starting 30 minutes before chemotherapy and repeated 4 hours and 8 hours later.
➢ To prevent nausea and vomiting caused by radiation
Adults and children older than age 12: 8 mg (tablet) or 10 ml (oral solution) P.O. 1 to 2 hours before radiation and repeated q 8 hours, depending on radiation type, location, and extent
➢ Prevention and treatment of postoperative nausea and vomiting
Adults and children older than age 12: 16 mg (tablet) or 20 ml (oral solution) P.O. 1 hour before anesthesia induction, or 4 mg I.V. or I.M. before anesthesia or postoperatively
Children ages 2 to 12 weighing more than 40 kg (88 lb): 4 mg I.V. before anesthesia or postoperatively
Children ages 2 to 12 weighing less than 40 kg (88 lb): 0.1 mg/kg I.V. before anesthesia or postoperatively

Dosage adjustment

- Hepatic impairment

Contraindications

- Hypersensitivity to drug

Precautions

Use cautiously in:
- hepatic disease
- phenylketonuria (with orally disintegrating tablets)
- pregnant or breastfeeding patients
- children younger than age 12.

Administration

- Give first dose before emetogenic event.
- Remove orally disintegrating tablet by peeling back foil with dry hands; don't push tablet through foil backing. After removing, place tablet on patient's tongue, where it will dissolve within seconds. Tell patient to swallow saliva.
- Give undiluted when administering I.M. before anesthesia induction.
- Give undiluted by direct I.V. immediately before anesthesia induction, or postoperatively if nausea and vomiting occur. Administer slowly, over at least 30 seconds (preferably over 2 to 5 minutes).
- For intermittent I.V. infusion, dilute in 50 ml of dextrose 5% in water (D_5W) and normal saline solution or

D_5W and half-normal saline solution. Infuse over 15 minutes.
• When giving I.V., don't use flexible plastic container in series connection.

Route	Onset	Peak	Duration
P.O., I.V.	Rapid	15-30 min	4-8 hr
I.M.	Rapid	40 min	Unknown

Adverse reactions

CNS: headache, dizziness, malaise, drowsiness, fatigue, weakness, extrapyramidal reactions
CV: chest pain, hypotension
GI: constipation, diarrhea, abdominal pain, dry mouth
GU: urinary retention
Respiratory: bronchospasm
Skin: rash
Other: pain at injection site, shivering, **anaphylaxis**

Interactions

Drug-drug. *Drugs that alter hepatic enzyme activity:* altered pharmacokinetics of ondansetron
Drug-diagnostic tests. *Alanine aminotransferase, aspartate aminotransferase, bilirubin:* transient elevations

Patient monitoring

• Monitor GI status.
• Assess for extrapyramidal reactions.
• Check vital signs. Watch for hypotension and bronchospasm.
• Monitor fluid intake and output. Stay alert for urinary retention.

Patient teaching

• Tell patient to remove orally disintegrating tablet by peeling back foil with dry hands—not by pushing tablet through foil backing. Instruct him to place tablet on tongue, where it will dissolve within seconds, and then to swallow saliva.
Clinical alert: Instruct patient to immediately report extrapyramidal symptoms or allergic reaction.
• Inform patient with phenylketonuria (or caregiver) that powder contains phenylalanine.
• Caution patient to avoid driving and other hazardous activities until he knows how drug affects concentration and alertness.
• As appropriate, review all other significant and life-threatening adverse reactions and interactions, especially those related to the drugs and tests mentioned above.

orlistat

Xenical

Pharmacologic class: GI lipase inhibitor
Therapeutic class: Weight control drug
Pregnancy risk category B

Action

Inhibits absorption of dietary fats in stomach and small intestine

Availability

Capsules: 120 mg

Indications and dosages

➢ Obesity management (in conjunction with reduced-calorie diet); to reduce risk of regaining after weight loss
Adults: 120 mg P.O. t.i.d. with each meal containing fat

Contraindications

• Hypersensitivity to drug or its components
• Chronic malabsorption syndrome or cholestasis

Precautions

Use cautiously in:
• hypothyroidism, nephrolithiasis, diabetes mellitus, clinically significant GI disease, fat-soluble vitamin deficiencies
• history of bulimia or anorexia nervosa

• pregnant or breastfeeding patients
• children.

Administration

• Know that organic causes of obesity should be ruled out before therapy starts.
• Give three times daily with a meal, or up to 1 hour after a meal.
• If patient misses a meal or eats a fat-free meal, omit dose.
• Know that orlistat therapy is frequently combined with psychotherapy.

Route	Onset	Peak	Duration
P.O.	Unknown	8 hr	48-72 hr

Adverse reactions

CNS: dizziness, headache, fatigue, insomnia, depression, anxiety
EENT: ear, nose, and throat symptoms
GI: fecal urgency, flatus with discharge, oily or increased bowel movements, oily spotting, fecal incontinence
GU: urinary tract infection (UTI), vaginitis, menstrual irregularities
Musculoskeletal: back pain, arthritis, myalgia, tendinitis
Respiratory: upper or lower respiratory infection
Skin: dry skin, rash
Other: dental pain, tooth disorder, influenza

Interactions

Drug-drug. *Beta-carotene, fat-soluble vitamins:* reduced vitamin absorption
Cyclosporine: reduced cyclosporine blood level
Pravastatin: increased lipid-lowering effects

Patient monitoring

• Watch for signs and symptoms of UTI, respiratory infection, and EENT disorders.
• Monitor patient for weight loss.
• Evaluate patient's diet for appropriate caloric intake.

Patient teaching

• Instruct patient to take with meals as directed. Tell him he may omit a dose if he misses a meal or eats a fat-free meal.
• Advise patient to consume reduced-calorie diet and to spread daily fat intake over three main meals.
• Inform patient that drug predisposes him to EENT, respiratory, and urinary infections. Instruct him to promptly report signs and symptoms.
• Tell patient about common adverse GI reactions, including problems controlling bowel movements. If significant GI upset occurs, encourage him to consult prescriber about taking psyllium at bedtime or with each dose.
• Advise patient to ask prescriber if he should take a daily multivitamin containing vitamins D, E, K, and beta-carotene at least 2 hours before or after orlistat.
• As appropriate, review all other significant adverse reactions and interactions, especially those related to the drugs mentioned above.

oseltamivir phosphate

Tamiflu

Pharmacologic class: Viral neuroaminidase inhibitor
Therapeutic class: Antiviral
Pregnancy risk category C

Action

Inhibits influenza virus neuraminidase, altering viral particle aggregation and decreasing viral release from infected cells

Availability

Capsules: 75 mg
Powder for oral suspension: 12 mg/ml

Indications and dosages

➢ To prevent influenza type A

Adults and children older than age 13: 75 mg P.O. daily for more than 7 days, starting within 2 days of exposure

➢ Treatment of influenza type A

Adults and children older than age 13: 75 mg P.O. b.i.d. for 5 days, starting within 2 days of symptom onset

Children ages 1 and older who weigh more than 40 kg (88 lb): 75 mg P.O. b.i.d. for 5 days, starting within 2 days of symptom onset

Children ages 1 and older who weigh more than 23 kg and up to 40 kg (51 to 88 lb): 60 mg P.O. b.i.d. for 5 days, starting within 2 days of symptom onset

Children ages 1 year and older who weigh more than 15 kg and up to 23 kg (33 to 51 lb): 45 mg P.O. b.i.d. for 5 days, starting within 2 days of symptom onset

Children ages 1 and older who weigh less than 15 kg (33 lb): 30 mg P.O. b.i.d. for 5 days, starting within 2 days of symptom onset

Dosage adjustment

- Renal impairment

Contraindications

- Hypersensitivity to drug or its components

Precautions

Use cautiously in:

- chronic cardiac or renal disease, respiratory disorders
- elderly patients
- pregnant or breastfeeding patients.

Administration

- For flu treatment, give first dose at onset of symptoms. For flu prevention, give within 2 days of exposure.

Route	Onset	Peak	Duration
P.O.	Variable	2.5	6 hr

Adverse reactions

CNS: headache, dizziness, fatigue, insomnia

GI: nausea, vomiting, diarrhea

Respiratory: cough, bronchitis

Interactions

None significant

Patient monitoring

- Monitor respiratory status. Watch for signs and symptoms of secondary infection.

Patient teaching

- Instruct patient to take as soon as flu symptoms occur and to complete entire course of therapy.
- Advise patient to take with food or milk to minimize GI irritation.
- Tell patient to prepare oral solution by adding water to powder and shaking well.
- Caution patient not to share drug with others, even if they have similar symptoms.
- Instruct patient to consult prescriber before taking other drugs.
- As appropriate, review all other significant adverse reactions.

oxacillin sodium

Bactocil

Pharmacologic class: Penicillinase-resistant penicillin

Therapeutic class: Broad-spectrum anti-infective

Pregnancy risk category B

Action

Interferes with bacterial cell-wall synthesis during multiplication of susceptible organisms; shows minimal immunosuppressant activity

Availability

Capsules: 250 mg, 500 mg
Injection: 250 mg, 500 mg, 1 g, 2 g, 4 g
I.V. infusion: 1 g, 2 g
Oral solution: 250 mg/5 ml

Indications and dosages

➢ Systemic infections caused by penicillinase-producing staphylococci
Adults and children weighing more than 40 kg (88 lb): For mild to moderate infections, 250 mg to 500 mg I.M. or I.V. q 4 to 6 hours, with follow-up therapy of 500 mg P.O. q 4 to 6 hours. For severe infections, 1g I.M. or I.V. q 4 to 6 hours, with follow-up therapy of 1g P.O. q 4 to 6 hours.
Children weighing less than 40 kg (88 lb): For mild to moderate infections, 50 mg/kg I.M. or I.V. q 6 hours, with follow-up therapy of 50 mg/kg P.O. q 6 hours. For severe infections, 100 mg/kg I.M. or I.V. q 4 to 6 hours, with follow-up therapy of 100 mg/kg P.O. q 4 to 6 hours.
Premature infants and neonates: 25 mg/kg/day I.M. or I.V.

Contraindications

- Hypersensitivity to drug or other penicillins

Precautions

Use cautiously in:
- renal disorders
- pregnant or breastfeeding patients
- neonates.

Administration

- Give oral form on empty stomach 1 hour before or 2 hours after meals.
- For I.M. use, reconstitute to a dilution of 250 mg/1.5 ml sterile water, and inject deep into muscle.
- For I.V. use, infuse slowly to prevent vein irritation.

Route	Onset	Peak	Duration
P.O.	Unknown	0.5-2 hr	Unknown
I.V.	Immediate	Immediate	Unknown
I.M.	Unknown	0.5 hr	Unknown

Adverse reactions

CNS: depression, agitation, confusion, anxiety, hallucinations, lethargy, twitching, neuropathy, neuromuscular irritability, **seizures, coma**
CV: thrombophlebitis
GI: nausea, vomiting, diarrhea, abdominal pain, enterocolitis, oral lesions, **pseudomembranous colitis**
GU: proteinuria, hematuria, vaginitis, moniliasis, **oliguria, glomerulonephritis**
Hematologic: anemia, eosinophilia, **hemolytic anemia, thrombocytopenia, neutropenia, granulocytopenia, increased bleeding, bone marrow depression**
Hepatic: hepatotoxicity
Other: overgrowth of nonsusceptible organisms, hypersensitivity reaction, **anaphylaxis, serum sickness**

O

Interactions

Drug-drug. *Aminoglycosides:* aminoglycoside inactivation
Aspirin, disulfiram, probenecid: increased oxacillin blood level, increased bone marrow depression
Hormonal contraceptives: decreased contraceptive efficacy
Rifampin, tetracyclines: decreased antimicrobial activity
Drug-diagnostic tests. *Alanine aminotransferase, alkaline phosphatase, aspartate aminotransferase, eosinophils, low-density lipoproteins:* increased levels
Granulocytes, hemoglobin, neutrophils, platelets: decreased levels
Drug-herbs. *Khat:* delayed drug absorption

Patient monitoring

- Stay alert for severe anaphylaxis.
- Watch for signs and symptoms of in-

fection. Obtain specimens for repeat cultures if therapeutic effects don't occur.

🔊 Monitor CBC with white cell differential. Watch for signs and symptoms of blood dyscrasias.

🔊 Assess neurologic status carefully. Stay alert for seizures or impending coma.

- Check bowel movements for severe persistent diarrhea (with or without fever) and pus in stool.

Patient teaching

- Advise patient to take oral form on empty stomach 1 hour before or 2 hours after meals.
- Tell patient to complete entire course of therapy even if he feels better.

🔊 Instruct patient to immediately report rash, easy bruising or bleeding, difficulty breathing, nausea, unusual fatigue, yellowing of skin or eyes, severe diarrhea, or black or furry tongue.

- Caution patient to avoid driving and other hazardous activities until he knows how drug affects concentration and alertness.
- As appropriate, review all other significant and life-threatening adverse reactions and interactions, especially those related to the drugs, tests, and herbs mentioned above.

oxaliplatin

Eloxitan

Pharmacologic class: Alkylator
Therapeutic class: Antineoplastic
Pregnancy risk category D

Action

Unclear. Thought to form reactive platinum complexes that inhibit DNA synthesis through formation of interstrand and intrastrand cross-linking of DNA molecules. Cell-cycle-phase nonspecific.

Availability

Powder for injection: 50 mg, 100 mg in single-use vials

Indications and dosages

➢ Metastatic cancer of colon or rectum, given with 5-fluorouracil (5-FU) and leucovorin

Adults: On day 1, 85 mg/m² oxaliplatin I.V. infusion and 200 mg/m² leucovorin; give both drugs simultaneously over 2 hours, followed by 400 mg/m² I.V. bolus of 5-FU over 2 to 4 minutes, then 600 mg/m² 5-FU I.V. as 22-hour continuous infusion. On day two, 200 mg/m² leucovorin I.V. infusion over 2 hours, followed by 400 mg/m² 5-FU I.V. bolus over 2 to 4 minutes, then 600 mg/m² 5-FU I.V. as 22-hour continuous infusion.

Contraindications

- Hypersensitivity to drug or platinum products

Precautions

Use cautiously in:

- thrombocytopenia
- radiation therapy
- recent pneumococcal or smallpox vaccination
- elderly patients
- pregnant or breastfeeding patients
- children.

Administration

🔊 Follow facility policy for preparing, handling, and administering mutagenic, teratogenic, and carcinogenic drugs.

- Premedicate patient with antiemetics, as prescribed.
- Reconstitute with sterile water or dextrose 5% in water (D_5W)—never with normal saline solution or other solutions containing chloride.

• Further dilute reconstituted drug in 250 to 500 ml of D_5W.
• Infuse over 2 hours simultaneously with leucovorin, but in a separate I.V. bag.
• Don't use administration sets or needles that contain aluminum.
Clinical alert: Be aware of importance of using leucovorin rescue with this drug.
Clinical alert: Avoid extravasation, which may cause necrosis and other severe reactions.
• Know that treatment cycles are usually repeated every 2 weeks.

Route	Onset	Peak	Duration
I.V.	Unknown	Unknown	Unknown

Adverse reactions

CNS: headache, dizziness, fatigue, insomnia, peripheral neuropathy
CV: cardiac abnormalities
EENT: decreased visual acuity, hearing loss, tinnitus, rhinitis, pharyngitis
GI: severe nausea, vomiting, diarrhea, constipation, dyspepsia, gastroesophageal reflux, mucositis, flatulence, stomatitis, anorexia
GU: hematuria, dysuria
Hematologic: anemia, **thrombocytopenia, leukopenia, pancytopenia, neutropenia, hemolytic uremic syndrome**
Metabolic: hypokalemia
Respiratory: dyspnea, cough, upper respiratory infection, **pulmonary fibrosis**
Skin: alopecia, rash, flushing, extravasation, redness, swelling, angioedema
Other: weight loss, increased cold sensitivity, pain at injection site, **anaphylaxis**

Interactions

Drug-drug. *Aminoglycosides, loop diuretics:* increased risk of nephrotoxicity
Aspirin, nonsteroidal anti-inflammatory drugs: increased risk of bleeding
Live-virus vaccines: decreased antibody response to vaccine
Myelosuppressants: increased bone marrow depression
Drug-diagnostic tests. *Alanine aminotransferase, aspartate aminotransferase, bilirubin, creatinine:* increased levels
Hemoglobin, neutrophils, platelets, white blood cells: decreased levels
Drug-behaviors. *Alcohol use:* increased risk of bleeding

Patient monitoring

Clinical alert: Monitor I.V. site frequently to avoid extravasation.
• Monitor CBC, blood chemistry, and kidney and liver function tests before each treatment cycle.
Clinical alert: Watch closely for blood dyscrasias, hemolytic uremic syndrome, serious pulmonary problems, and anaphylaxis.
• Conduct complete neurologic exam before and after each dose.
• Monitor vital signs and ECG. Evaluate cardiovascular and respiratory status closely.
• Assess patient's comfort level. Keep him warm during infusion to minimize neurologic effects.
• Watch for signs and symptoms of toxicity (paresthesia, nausea, vomiting).

Patient teaching

• Inform patient that chemotherapy drugs can cause many adverse effects.
• Tell patient he'll receive drug from trained healthcare professionals in hospital setting.
Clinical alert: Instruct patient to inform nurse immediately if drug contacts his skin, eyes, or mouth.
• Advise patient to notify nurse if pain or redness occurs at I.V. site.
• Instruct patient to stay warm and avoid iced drinks to minimize neurologic symptoms.
Clinical alert: Tell patient to report itching, hives, swelling of hands or face, chest tightness, difficulty breathing, unsteadiness, severe diarrhea or vomiting, or tingling sensation in hands, arms, legs, or feet.

O

• As appropriate, review all other significant and life-threatening adverse reactions and interactions, especially those related to the drugs, tests, and behaviors mentioned above.

oxandrolone

Oxandrin

Pharmacologic class: Hormone
Therapeutic class: Anabolic steroid
Controlled substance schedule III
Pregnancy risk category X

Action

Promotes body-tissue building process, reverses catabolic or tissue-depleting processes, and increases hemoglobin and red cell mass. Also has androgenic and anabolic properties.

Availability

Tablets: 2.5 mg, 10 mg

Indications and dosages

➢ To promote weight gain; to relieve bone pain accompanying osteoporosis
Adults: 2.5 mg P.O. two to four times daily, to a maximum of 20 mg/day, usually for 2 to 4 weeks. Repeat intermittently p.r.n.
Children: Total daily dosage of 0.1 mg/kg P.O. or less

Off-label uses

• Alcoholic hepatitis

Contraindications

• Hypersensitivity to anabolic steroids
• Nephrotic phase of nephritis
• Women with breast cancer and hypercalcemia
• Men with prostate or breast cancer
• Pregnancy

Precautions

Use cautiously in:
• renal, hepatic, or cardiac impairment; benign prostatic hypertrophy; pituitary insufficiency; myocardial infarction
• breastfeeding patients.

Administration

• Verify that patient isn't pregnant before giving.
• Give with food or meals if GI upset occurs.

Route	Onset	Peak	Duration
P.O.	Slow	Unknown	Unknown

Adverse reactions

CNS: insomnia, excitation, toxic confusion
GI: nausea, vomiting, diarrhea, abdominal fullness, burning sensation of tongue, anorexia, **intra-abdominal hemorrhage**
GU: increased risk of prostatic hypertrophy, virilization, phallic enlargement in prepubertal boys, inhibited testicular function in postpubertal males, gynecomastia, priapism, epididymitis, libido changes, clitoral enlargement, menstrual irregularities
Hematologic: iron deficiencies
Hepatic: hepatotoxicity, peliosis hepatitis, hepatic cell tumor
Metabolic: fluid retention, hypercalcemia
Musculoskeletal: ankle swelling, premature epiphyseal closure in children
Skin: acne, increased skin pigmentation, hirsutism and male-pattern baldness in women
Other: chills, hoarseness, deepening of voice in women

Interactions

Drug-drug. *Anticoagulants:* potentiation of anticoagulant action
Insulin, oral hypoglycemics: decreased requirements for these drugs

Drug-diagnostic tests. *Creatinine, creatinine clearance:* increased values
Cholesterol, lipids: altered levels
Glucose tolerance tests: altered results
Thyroid function: decreased values

Patient monitoring

- Assess patient for edema and need for diuretic therapy.
- Monitor periodic liver function tests and electrolyte levels.
- Assess periodic cholesterol levels in patients at increased risk for coronary artery disease.
- Monitor diabetic patients carefully (drug may alter glucose tolerance).

Patient teaching

- Tell patient to take with food or meals.
- Inform patient that drug shouldn't be taken to increase muscle strength; it doesn't enhance athletic ability and can cause serious side effects.
- Advise diabetic patient to monitor urine or blood glucose carefully and report abnormal levels.
- Instruct patient to report ankle swelling, skin color changes, severe nausea or vomiting, unusual body hair growth, acne, and menstrual changes.
- Advise female patient not to take drug if she is or plans to become pregnant.
- As appropriate, review all other significant and life-threatening adverse reactions and interactions, especially those related to the drugs and tests mentioned above.

oxaprozin

Daypro

oxaprozin potassium

Daypro ALTA

Pharmacologic class: Propionic acid derivative, nonsteroidal anti-inflammatory drug (NSAID)

Therapeutic class: Anti-inflammatory, analgesic

Pregnancy risk category C (first and second trimesters), ***D*** (third trimester)

Action

Unclear. Thought to inhibit prostaglandin synthesis by blocking cyclooxygenase (COX-2), thereby reducing inflammation

Availability

Tablets: 600 mg
Caplets: 600 mg

Indications and dosages

➢ Rheumatoid arthritis; osteoarthritis
Adults: 1,200 mg daily in two to three divided doses. Maximum daily dosage is 1,800 mg (1,200 mg for potassium form).

Dosage adjustment

- Mild disease
- Renal impairment
- Low body weight

Contraindications

- Hypersensitivity to drug
- Concurrent use of other NSAIDs (including aspirin)
- Active GI bleeding or ulcer disease

Precautions

Use cautiously in:

- severe cardiovascular or hepatic disease, renal impairment

• history of ulcer disease
• pregnant or breastfeeding patients
• children (safety not established).

Administration

• Give with food or after meals if GI upset occurs.
• Use lowest effective dosage to minimize adverse reactions.

Route	Onset	Peak	Duration
P.O.	Unknown	3-5 hr	Unknown

Adverse reactions

CNS: dizziness, fatigue, headache, agitation, anxiety, confusion, depression, insomnia, malaise, paresthesia, tremor
CV: edema, vasculitis, blood pressure changes
EENT: abnormal vision, tinnitus
GI: nausea, vomiting, diarrhea, constipation, abdominal pain, gastritis, dyspepsia, duodenal ulcer, flatulence, stomatitis, dry mouth, anorexia, **GI bleeding**
GU: albuminuria, azotemia, **interstitial nephritis, acute renal failure**
Hematologic: anemia
Hepatic: cholestatic jaundice, **hepatitis**
Respiratory: dyspnea, **hypersensitivity pneumonitis**
Skin: rash, pruritus, diaphoresis, photosensitivity, angioedema, **Stevens-Johnson syndrome**
Other: appetite and weight increases, allergic reactions including **anaphylaxis**

Interactions

Drug-drug. *Alcohol, aspirin and other NSAIDs, corticosteroids, potassium supplements:* additive adverse GI effects and toxicity
Anticoagulants, cefamandole, cefoperazone, cefotetan, clopidogrel, eptifibatide, plicamycin, thrombolytics, ticlopidine, tirofiban, vitamin A: increased risk of bleeding
Antineoplastics: increased risk of adverse hematologic reactions
Insulin, oral hypoglycemics: increased hypoglycemic effects of these drugs
Methotrexate: increased risk of methotrexate toxicity
Drug-diagnostic tests. *Alanine aminotransferase, alkaline phosphatase, aspartate aminotransferase, blood urea nitrogen, creatinine, lactate dehydrogenase, potassium:* increased levels
Bleeding time: prolonged (for up to 2 weeks after drug discontinuation)
Creatinine clearance, glucose, hemoglobin, hematocrit, platelets, white blood cells: decreased levels
Liver function tests: abnormal results
Drug-herbs. *Alfalfa, anise, arnica, astragalus, bilberry, black currant seed oil, bladderwrack, bogbean, boldo (with fenugreek), borage oil, buchu, capsaicin, cat's claw, celery, chamomile, chapparal, chincona bark, clove, clove oil, dandelion, dong quai, evening primrose oil, fenugreek, feverfew, garlic, ginger, ginkgo, ginseng, guggul, licorice, papaya extract, red clover, rhubarb, safflower oil, skullcap, tan-shen:* increased anticoagulant effect and bleeding risk

Patient monitoring

• Monitor kidney and liver function tests, coagulation studies, and CBC.
🔊 Watch for signs and symptoms of acute renal failure, nephritis, hepatitis, bleeding tendency, and anemia.
• Monitor hearing and vision, including results of eye exams.
🔊 Watch for and promptly report rash or swelling.
• Assess respiratory status closely. Stay alert for dyspnea and pneumonitis.

Patient teaching

• Instruct patient to take with food or meal.
• Inform patient that many common over-the-counter drugs (including acetaminophen, aspirin, and other NSAIDs) and herbal preparations increase drug's adverse effects. Tell him

to consult prescriber before taking these products.

Instruct patient to immediately report rash, unusual tiredness, yellowing of skin or eyes, easy bruising or bleeding, change in urination pattern, weight gain, arm or leg swelling, vision changes, and black or tarry stools.

- Advise patient to minimize GI upset by eating small, frequent servings of food and drinking plenty of fluids.
- Caution patient to avoid driving and other hazardous activities until he knows how drug affects concentration and alertness.
- Advise patient on long-term therapy to have periodic eye exams.
- As appropriate, review all other significant and life-threatening adverse reactions and interactions, especially those related to the drugs, tests, and herbs mentioned above.

oxazepam

Apo-Oxazepam✱, Novoxapam✱, Serax

Pharmacologic class: Benzodiazepine

Therapeutic class: Anxiolytic, sedative-hypnotic

Controlled substance schedule IV

Pregnancy risk category D

Action

Suppresses CNS stimulation at limbic and subcortical levels by potentiating effects of gamma-aminobutyrate, an inhibitory neurotransmitter. This suppression reduces anxiety and diminishes alcohol withdrawal symptoms.

Availability

Capsules: 10 mg, 15 mg, 30 mg
Tablets: 15 mg

Indications and dosages

➢ Mild to moderate anxiety

Adults: 10 to 15 mg P.O. three to four times daily

➢ Severe anxiety; alcohol withdrawal symptoms

Adults: 15 to 30 mg P.O. three to four times daily

Dosage adjustment

- Elderly patients

Off-label uses

- Insomnia

Contraindications

- Hypersensitivity to drug or tartrazine (some products)

Precautions

Use cautiously in:

- hepatic dysfunction, severe chronic obstructive pulmonary disease, myasthenia gravis, CNS depression, uncontrolled severe pain
- history of suicide attempt or drug abuse
- concurrent use of other benzodiazepines
- elderly or debilitated patients
- pregnant or breastfeeding patients.

Administration

- Administer with or without food.
- Taper dosage after long-term therapy.

Route	Onset	Peak	Duration
P.O.	45-90 min	3 hr	6-12 hr

Adverse reactions

CNS: dizziness, drowsiness, headache, confusion, poor memory, hangover effect, slurred speech, depression, paradoxical stimulation

CV: orthostatic hypotension, hypotension, ECG changes, tachycardia

EENT: blurred vision, mydriasis, tinnitus

GI: nausea, vomiting, constipation, diarrhea

O

GU: urinary retention, urinary incontinence
Hematologic: leukopenia
Hepatic: jaundice, **hepatitis**
Respiratory: respiratory depression
Skin: rash, dermatitis, itching
Other: physical and psychological drug dependence, drug tolerance, withdrawal symptoms

Interactions

Drug-drug. *Azole antifungals:* increased oxazepam blood level, greater risk of toxicity
Hormonal contraceptives, phenytoin: decreased oxazepam efficacy
Levodopa: decreased levodopa efficacy
Other CNS depressants (including antidepressants, antihistamines, other benzodiazepines, sedative-hypnotics, opioids): additive CNS depression
Theophylline: decreased sedative effect of oxazepam
Drug-diagnostic tests. *Alanine aminotransferase, alkaline phosphatase, aspartate aminotransferase, lactate dehydrogenase:* increased levels
Hematocrit, thyroid uptake of sodium iodide ^{123}I and ^{131}I, white blood cells: decreased values
Drug-food. *Cabbage:* decreased drug blood level
Drug-herbs. *Chamomile, hops, kava, valerian, skullcap:* increased CNS depression
Drug-behaviors. *Alcohol use:* increased CNS depression

Patient monitoring

🔊 Monitor liver function tests and watch for signs and symptoms of hepatitis.
• Check vital signs. Stay alert for respiratory depression, orthostatic hypotension, and tachycardia.
• Monitor neurologic status. As needed, take measures to prevent injury.
• Watch for signs and symptoms of psychological or physical dependence.
• When tapering, watch for withdrawal symptoms.

Patient teaching

• Tell patient he may take with or without meals, but should avoid cabbage.
• Advise patient to take exactly as prescribed. Tell him drug can cause dependence, and emphasize importance of following tapering instructions to avoid withdrawal symptoms.
🔊 Urge patient to immediately report unusual tiredness, nausea, appetite loss, or yellowing of skin or eyes.
• Tell patient to change position slowly to avoid blood pressure decrease.
• Instruct patient to report severe dizziness, weakness, persistent drowsiness, palpitations, or visual changes.
• Advise patient not to drink alcohol.
• Caution patient to avoid driving and other hazardous activities until he knows how drug affects vision, cognition, and balance.
• As appropriate, review all other significant and life-threatening adverse reactions and interactions, especially those related to the drugs, tests, foods, herbs, and behaviors mentioned above.

oxcarbazepine

Trileptal

Pharmacologic class: Carboxamide derivative
Therapeutic class: Anticonvulsant
Pregnancy risk category C

Action

Blocks sodium channels in neural membranes, stabilizing hyperexcitable states and inhibiting neuronal firing and impulse transmission in brain

Availability
Oral suspension: 300 mg/5-ml bottle
Tablets: 150 mg, 300 mg, 600 mg

Indications and dosages
➤ Adjunctive therapy for partial seizures
Adults: 300 mg P.O. b.i.d. May increase by up to 600 mg/day q week, to a maximum of 1,200 mg/day.
Children ages 4 to 16: Initially, 8 to 10 mg/kg/day P.O. to a maximum of 600 mg/day
➤ Conversion to monotherapy for partial seizures
Adults: 300 mg P.O. b.i.d. May increase by 600 mg/day at weekly intervals over 2 to 4 weeks, to a maximum of 2,400 mg/day
Children ages 4 to 16: Initially, 8 to 10 mg/kg/day P.O. given in two divided doses, increased to a maximum of 10 mg/kg/day
➤ Initiation of monotherapy
Adults: 300 mg P.O. b.i.d., increased by 300 mg/day P.O. q 3 days up to 1,200 mg/day
Children ages 4 to 16: Initially, 8 to 10 mg/kg/day P.O. given in two divided doses; increase by 5 mg/kg q 3 days to a maximum of 1,200 mg/day

Dosage adjustment
• Renal impairment

Contraindications
• Hypersensitivity to drug or its components

Precautions
Use cautiously in:
• renal impairment
• pregnant or breastfeeding patients
• children younger than age 4 (safety not established).

Administration
• Administer twice daily with or without food.
• Shake oral suspension well. If desired, mix in small glass of water.

Route	Onset	Peak	Duration
P.O.	Unknown	Unknown	Unknown

Adverse reactions
CNS: dizziness, vertigo, drowsiness, fatigue, headache, ataxia, tremor, emotional lability
EENT: abnormal vision, diplopia, nystagmus, rhinitis
GI: nausea, vomiting, diarrhea, constipation, abdominal pain, dyspepsia
Metabolic: hyponatremia
Skin: acne, rash
Other: thirst, allergic reactions, edema, lymphadenopathy

Interactions
Drug-drug. *Carbamazepine, valproic acid, verapamil:* decreased oxcarbazepine blood level
CNS depressants (including antidepressants, antihistamines, opioids, sedative-hypnotics): additive CNS depression
Felodipine, hormonal contraceptives: decreased blood levels of these drugs
Phenobarbital: decreased oxcarbazepine and increased phenobarbital blood levels
Phenytoin: increased phenytoin blood level
Drug-diagnostic tests. *Sodium:* decreased level
Drug-behaviors. *Alcohol use:* additive CNS depression

Patient monitoring
• Monitor neurologic status closely for changes in cognition, mood, wakefulness, balance, and gait.
• Check sodium level. Watch for signs and symptoms of hyponatremia.

Patient teaching
• Instruct patient to take at same time each day, with or without food.
• Tell patient to report vision changes and significant neurologic changes.

O

• Advise patient to have periodic eye exams.
• Tell female patient that drug makes hormonal contraceptives less effective.
• Inform patient that he may need frequent tests to check drug blood levels.
• Tell patient not to drink alcohol.
• Caution patient to avoid driving and other hazardous activities until he knows how drug affects him.
• As appropriate, review all significant adverse reactions and interactions, especially those related to the drugs, tests, and behaviors mentioned above.

oxybutynin
Oxytrol

oxybutynin chloride
Ditropan, Ditropan XL

Pharmacologic class: Anticholinergic
Therapeutic class: Urinary tract antispasmodic
Pregnancy risk category B

Action
Inhibits acetylcholine action at postganglionic receptors, relaxing smooth muscle lining of GU tract and preventing bladder irritability

Availability
Syrup: 5 mg/5 ml
Tablets: 5 mg
Tablets (extended-release): 5 mg, 10 mg, 15 mg
Transdermal system (patch): 39 cm^2/36 mg

Indications and dosages
➤ Frequent urination, urinary urgency or incontinence, and nocturia caused by neurogenic bladder; overactive bladder
Adults: 5 mg P.O. two to three times daily (not to exceed 5 mg q.i.d.); or 5 to 15 mg P.O. once daily (extended-release); or one 3.9 mg/day transdermal system applied twice weekly
Children older than age 5: 5 mg P.O. b.i.d., to a maximum of 5 mg t.i.d.

Dosage adjustment
• Elderly patients

Contraindications
• Hypersensitivity to drug
• Glaucoma
• Intestinal obstruction, severe colitis, atony, paralytic ileus, megacolon, or hemorrhage
• Obstructive uropathy, urinary retention
• Myasthenia gravis
• Acute hemorrhage with shock

Precautions
Use cautiously in:
• cardiovascular disease, hyperthyroidism, GI disease
• elderly patients
• pregnant or breastfeeding patients
• children younger than age 5 (safety not established).

Administration
• Give without regard to food.
• Don't crush or break tablets.

Route	Onset	Peak	Duration
P.O.	30-60 min	3-6 hr	6-10 hr
P.O. (extended)	30-60 min	3-6 hr	Up to 24 hr
Transdermal	24-48 hr	48-96 hr	96 hr after removal

Adverse reactions
CNS: dizziness, drowsiness, hallucinations, insomnia, weakness, anxiety, restlessness, headache
CV: palpitations, hypotension, tachycardia
EENT: blurred vision, cycloplegia, increased intraocular pressure, mydriasis, photophobia

GI: nausea, vomiting, diarrhea, constipation, bloating, dry mouth
GU: urinary hesitancy, urinary retention, erectile dysfunction, suppressed lactation
Metabolic: hyperthermia
Skin: decreased sweating, urticaria
Other: allergic reactions, fever, hot flashes

Interactions

Drug-drug. *Anticholinergics, anticholinergic-like drugs (including amantadine, antidepressants, disopyramide, haloperidol, phenothiazines):* additive anticholinergic effects
Atenolol: increased atenolol absorption
CNS depressants (including antidepressants, antihistamines, opioids, sedative-hypnotics): additive CNS depression
Digoxin: increased digoxin blood level (with extended-release oxybutynin)
Haloperidol: decreased haloperidol blood level, tardive dyskinesia, worsening of schizophrenia
Levodopa: decreased levodopa efficacy
Nitrofurantoin: increased nitrofurantoin blood level, greater risk of toxicity
Drug-herbs. *Angel's trumpet, jimsonweed, scopolia:* increased anticholinergic effects
Drug-behaviors. *Alcohol use:* additive CNS depression

Patient monitoring

- Monitor vital signs and temperature. Watch for hypotension, fever, and tachycardia.
- Evaluate patient's vision.
- Assess results of cystometric studies. Stay alert for urinary retention.

Patient teaching

- Tell patient he may take with or without food. Caution him not to crush, break, or chew extended-release tablets.
- Instruct patient to apply transdermal patch to dry, intact skin on abdomen, hip, or buttock. Tell him to use a new skin area with each new system and not to reapply new patch to same site within 7 days. Caution him not to cut or puncture patch.
- Tell patient to report blurred vision, fever, skin rash, nausea, or vomiting.
- Advise patient he'll need to undergo periodic bladder exams.
- Caution patient to avoid driving and other hazardous activities if drug causes drowsiness or blurred vision.
- As appropriate, review all other significant adverse reactions and interactions, especially those related to the drugs, herbs, and behaviors mentioned above.

oxycodone hydrochloride

Endocodone, OxyContin, Roxicodone, Supeudol✱

Pharmacologic class: Opioid agonist
Therapeutic class: Narcotic analgesic
Controlled substance schedule II
Pregnancy risk category B

O

Action

Unknown. Thought to interact with opioid receptor sites primarily in limbic system, thalamus, and spinal cord, blocking transmission of pain impulses.

Availability

Capsules (immediate-release): 5 mg
Solution (oral): 5 mg/5 ml
Solution (oral concentrate): 20 mg/ml
Tablets: 5 mg
Tablets (controlled-release): 10 mg, 20 mg, 40 mg, 80 mg, 160 mg
Tablets (immediate-release): 15 mg, 30 mg

Indications and dosages

➢ Moderate to severe pain
Adults: 5 mg P.O. q 6 hours p.r.n., increased gradually to 10 to 30 mg q 6 hours p.r.n.

➢ Moderate or severe pain when continuous around-the-clock analgesia is needed
Adults: 10 mg P.O. (controlled-release) q 12 hours. For patients already taking opioids, use total oral oxycodone daily equianalgesic dosage and then round down to closest tablet strength. For breakthrough pain, give supplemental immediate-release doses.

Dosage adjustment

- Hepatic disease
- Renal impairment
- Debilitated or opioid-naive patients

Off-label uses

- Postherpetic neuralgia (controlled-release form)

Contraindications

- Hypersensitivity to drug
- Paralytic ileus
- When opioids are contraindicated (as in respiratory depression, severe bronchial asthma, hypercarbia)

Precautions

Use cautiously in:

- head trauma; increased intracranial pressure (ICP); severe renal, hepatic, or pulmonary disease; hypothyroidism; adrenal insufficiency; urethral stricture; undiagnosed abdominal pain or prostatic hyperplasia; extensive burns; alcoholism
- history of substance abuse
- prolonged or high-dose therapy
- elderly or debilitated patients
- labor and delivery
- pregnant or breastfeeding patients.
- children younger than age 18.

Administration

- Be aware that drug has high abuse potential.
- Know that controlled-release OxyContin isn't indicated for p.r.n. pain control but is reserved for patients who need continuous, around-the-clock analgesia.
- Be aware that 80-mg and 160-mg controlled-release tablets are for opioid-tolerant patients only.

🔊 Never break, crush, or let patient chew controlled-release forms. Otherwise, rapid release and absorption of potentially fatal dose may occur.

- Add concentrated solution to juice, applesauce, pudding, or other semisolid food immediately before giving.
- When discontinuing, taper dosage gradually to prevent withdrawal symptoms.

Route	Onset	Peak	Duration
P.O.	15-30 min	1 hr	4-6 hr
P.O. (controlled)	Unknown	24-36 hr	>12 hr

Adverse reactions

CNS: dizziness, asthenia, drowsiness, euphoria, light-headedness, insomnia, confusion, anxiety, twitching, abnormal dreams and thoughts
CV: orthostatic hypotension, **circulatory depression, bradycardia, shock**
GI: nausea, vomiting, constipation, diarrhea, ileus, abdominal pain, dyspepsia, gastritis, anorexia
GU: urinary retention
Respiratory: apnea, respiratory depression, respiratory arrest
Skin: pruritus, sweating
Other: chills, fever, hiccups, physical and psychological drug dependence

Interactions

Drug-drug. *Antihistamines, sedative-hypnotics:* additive CNS depression
Barbiturates, protease inhibitors: increased respiratory and CNS depression
Opioid agonist-antagonists: precipitation of opioid withdrawal in physically dependent patients
Drug-diagnostic tests. *Amylase, lipase:* increased levels

Drug-behaviors. *Alcohol use:* additive CNS depression

Patient monitoring

🔊 Monitor vital signs and respiratory status. Withhold drug in significant respiratory or CNS depression.
- Assess patient's pain level frequently.
- Monitor bowel and bladder function.
- Assess patient for anxiety, twitching, and other CNS symptoms.
- Closely monitor head-trauma patient. Drug may increase ICP while masking signs and symptoms.
- Carefully assess patient with acute abdominal pain. Drug may obscure diagnosis.
- Stay alert for drug hoarding, tolerance, and dependence.

Patient teaching

🔊 Caution patient not to break, crush, chew, or dissolve controlled-release tablets. Warn him that doing so may cause rapid drug release and absorption (possibly fatal).
- Tell patient taking controlled-release form not to drive for 3 to 4 days after dosage increase, after consuming even a single alcoholic beverage, or if also taking antihistamines or other drugs that cause drowsiness.

🔊 Instruct patient to promptly report adverse reactions, especially difficulty breathing or slow pulse.
- Advise patient not to drink alcohol.
- Tell patient not to be alarmed if tablets appear in stools; drug has already been absorbed.
- Advise ambulatory patient to change position slowly, to avoid dizziness from orthostatic hypotension.
- Instruct patient to consult prescriber before taking other drugs.
- Caution patient to avoid driving and other hazardous activities, because drug may cause drowsiness or dizziness.
- As appropriate, review all other significant and life-threatening adverse reactions and interactions, especially those related to the drugs, tests, and behaviors mentioned above.

oxymorphone hydrochloride

Numorphan

Pharmacologic class: Opioid agonist
Therapeutic class: Narcotic analgesic
Controlled substance schedule II
Pregnancy risk category C

Action

Unknown. Thought to interact with opioid receptor sites primarily in limbic system, thalamus, and spinal cord, blocking pain impulse transmission.

Availability

Injection: 1 mg/ml, 1.5 mg/ml
Suppositories: 5 mg

Indications and dosages

➢ Moderate to severe pain
Adults: 1 to 1.5 mg I.M. or subcutaneously q 4 to 6 hours p.r.n.; or initially, 0.5 mg I.V., increased cautiously until pain relief is satisfactory; or 5 mg P.R. q 4 to 6 hours p.r.n., increased cautiously until pain relief is satisfactory
➢ To reduce labor pain
Adults: 0.5 to 1 mg I.M.

Contraindications

- Hypersensitivity to drug
- Children younger than age 12

Precautions

Use cautiously in:
- head trauma; increased intracranial pressure; severe renal, hepatic, or pulmonary disease; hypothyroidism; adrenal insufficiency; urethral stricture; undiagnosed abdominal pain or prostatic hyperplasia; extensive burns; alcoholism

O

- history of substance abuse
- prolonged or high-dose therapy
- elderly or debilitated patients
- labor and delivery
- pregnant or breastfeeding patients.

Administration

Keep naloxone available to reverse respiratory depression, if necessary.

- Give I.V. dose by direct injection over 2 to 3 minutes.

Route	Onset	Peak	Duration
I.V.	5-10 min	30-60 min	3-6 hr
I.M., subcut.	10-15 min	30-60 min	3-6 hr
P.R.	15-30 min	1-2 hr	3-6 hr

Adverse reactions

CNS: headache, drowsiness, confusion, dysphoria, euphoria, dizziness, hallucinations, lethargy, impaired mental and physical performance, depression, restlessness, insomnia, paradoxical stimulation, **seizures**

CV: hypotension, orthostatic hypotension, palpitations, **bradycardia, tachycardia**

EENT: blurred vision, miosis, diplopia, visual disturbances, tinnitus

GI: nausea, vomiting, constipation, biliary tract spasm, cramps, dry mouth, anorexia, **paralytic ileus, toxic megacolon**

GU: urinary hesitancy or retention, urethral spasm, antidiuretic effect

Respiratory: suppressed cough reflex, **atelectasis, respiratory depression, allergic bronchospastic reaction, allergic laryngeal edema or laryngospasm, apnea**

Skin: rash, urticaria, pruritus, facial flushing, diaphoresis

Other: physical or psychological drug dependence, drug tolerance, allergic reaction, injection site reaction

Interactions

Drug-drug. *Antihistamines (first-generation), antipsychotics, barbiturates, general anesthetics, MAO inhibitors, sedative-hypnotics, skeletal muscle relaxants, tricyclic antidepressants:* increased risk of respiratory depression

Drug-diagnostic tests. *Amylase, lipase:* increased levels

Drug-behaviors. *Alcohol use or abuse, opiate abuse:* increased risk of respiratory depression

Patient monitoring

Closely monitor respiratory status. Stay alert for respiratory depression and allergic responses affecting bronchi and larynx.

- Monitor vital signs and ECG.
- With prolonged use, watch for signs and symptoms of drug dependence.
- Assess neurologic status carefully. Institute protective measures as needed.

Patient teaching

Instruct patient to immediately report seizures or difficulty breathing.

- Tell patient to rise slowly when changing position, to avoid dizziness from blood pressure decrease.
- Advise patient to avoid alcohol.
- Caution patient not to drive or perform other hazardous activities.
- Tell patient not to stop taking drug suddenly after several weeks, because withdrawal symptoms may occur.
- As appropriate, review all other significant and life-threatening adverse reactions and interactions, especially those related to the drugs, tests, and behaviors mentioned above.

oxytocin

Pitocin, Syntocinon

Pharmacologic class: Posterior pituitary hormone

Therapeutic class: Uterine-active agent

Pregnancy risk category NR

Action
Unknown. Thought to directly stimulate smooth muscle contractions in uterus and cervix.

Availability
Injection: 10 units/ml ampule or vial

Indications and dosages
➢ To induce or stimulate labor
Adults: Initially, 1-ml ampule (10 units) in compatible I.V. solution infused at 1 to 2 milliunits/minute (0.001 to 0.002 units/minute). Increase rate in increments of 1 to 2 milliunits/minute q 15 to 30 minutes until acceptable contraction pattern is established.
➢ To control postpartum bleeding
Adults: 10 to 40 units in compatible I.V. solution infused at rate adequate to control bleeding; or 10 units I.M. after placenta delivery
➢ Incomplete abortion
Adults: 10 units in compatible I.V. solution infused at 10 to 20 milliunits/minute (0.01 to 0.02 units/minute)

Off-label uses
- Antepartal fetal heart rate testing
- Breast enlargement

Contraindications
- Hypersensitivity to drug
- Cephalopelvic disproportion
- Fetal distress when delivery is not imminent
- Prolonged use in uterine inertia or severe toxemia
- Hypertonic or hyperactive uterine pattern
- Unfavorable fetal position or presentation that's undeliverable without conversion
- Labor induction or augmentation when vaginal delivery is contraindicated (as in invasive cervical cancer, active genital herpes, or total placenta previa)

Precautions
Use cautiously in:
- previous cervical or uterine surgery, history of uterine sepsis
- breastfeeding patients.

Administration
- Reconstitute by adding 1 ml (10 units) to 1,000 ml of normal saline solution, lactated Ringer's solution, or dextrose 5% in water.

Clinical alert: Don't give by I.V. bolus injection.
- Infuse I.V. using controlled-infusion device.
- Be aware that drug isn't routinely given I.M.
- Know that drug should be given only to inpatients at critical care facilities when prescriber is immediately available.

Route	Onset	Peak	Duration
I.V.	Immediate	40 min	1 hr
I.M.	3-5 min	40 min	2-3 hr

Adverse reactions
CNS: seizures, coma, neonatal brain damage, subarachnoid hemorrhage
CV: premature ventricular contractions, **arrhythmias, neonatal bradycardia**
GI: nausea, vomiting
GU: postpartal hemorrhage; pelvic hematoma; uterine hypertonicity, spasm, or tetanic contraction; abruptio placentae; uterine rupture (with excessive doses)
Hematologic: afibrinogenemia
Hepatic: neonatal jaundice
Other: hypersensitivity reactions including **anaphylaxis, low 5-minute Apgar score (neonate)**

Interactions
Drug-drug. *Sympathomimetics:* postpartal hypertension
Thiopental anesthetics: delayed anesthesia induction

Vasoconstrictors: severe hypertension (when given within 3 to 4 hours of oxytocin)
Drug-herbs. *Ephedra (ma huang):* increased hypertension

Patient monitoring

◀ Continuously monitor contractions, fetal and maternal heart rate, and maternal blood pressure and ECG. Discontinue infusion if uterine hyperactivity occurs.
◀ Monitor patient extremely closely during first and second stages of labor because of risk of cervical laceration, uterine rupture, and maternal and fetal death.
- When giving drug to control postpartal bleeding, monitor and record vaginal bleeding.
- Assess fluid intake and output. Watch for signs and symptoms of water intoxication.

Patient teaching

- Inform patient about risks and benefits of oxytocin-induced labor.

◀ Teach patient to recognize and immediately report adverse drug effects.

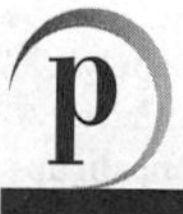

paclitaxel

Onxol, Taxol

Pharmacologic class: Antimicrotubule agent
Therapeutic class: Antineoplastic
Pregnancy risk category D

Action

Stabilizes cellular microtubules to prevent depolymerization. This action inhibits microtubule network (essential for vital interphase and mitotic cellular functions) and induces abnormal microtubule arrays or bundles throughout cell cycle and during mitosis.

Availability

Concentrate for injection: 30 mg/5-ml vial, 100 mg/16.7-ml vial, 300 mg/50-ml vial

Indications and dosages

➢ Advanced ovarian cancer
Adults: As first-line therapy, 175 mg/m² I.V. over 3 hours q 3 weeks, or 135 mg/m² I.V. over 24 hours q 3 weeks, followed by cisplatin. After failure of first-line therapy, 135 mg/m² I.V. or 175 mg/m² I.V. over 3 hours q 3 weeks.
➢ Breast cancer after failure of combination chemotherapy
Adults: As adjuvant treatment for node-positive breast cancer, 175 mg/m² I.V. over 3 hours q 3 weeks for four courses given sequentially with doxorubicin combination chemotherapy. After chemotherapy failure for metastatic disease or relapse within 6 months of adjuvant therapy, 175 mg/m² I.V. over 3 hours q 3 weeks.
➢ Non-small-cell lung cancer
Adults: 135 mg/m² I.V. over 24 hours q 3 weeks, followed by cisplatin
➢ AIDS-related Kaposi's sarcoma
Adults: 135 mg/m² I.V. over 3 hours q 3 weeks, or 100 mg/m² I.V. over 3 hours q 2 weeks

Dosage adjustment

- Advanced human immunodeficiency virus infection (when used for Kaposi's sarcoma)

Off-label uses

- Advanced head and neck cancer
- Small-cell lung cancer
- Upper GI tract adenocarcinoma
- Non-Hodgkin's lymphoma
- Pancreatic cancer
- Polycystic kidney disease

Contraindications
- Hypersensitivity to drug or castor oil
- Solid tumors when baseline neutrophil count is below 1,500 cells/mm^3
- AIDS-related Kaposi's sarcoma when baseline neutrophil count is below 1,000 cells/mm^3

Precautions
Use cautiously in:
- severe hepatic impairment, active infection, decreased bone marrow reserve, chronic debilitating illness
- patients with childbearing potential
- breastfeeding patients (not recommended)
- children (safety not established).

Administration
🔊 Follow facility protocol for handling chemotherapeutic drugs and preparing solutions.
- Dilute in dextrose 5% in water, normal saline solution, or dextrose 5% in lactated Ringer's solution per manufacturer's guidelines.
- Inspect solution for particles. Administer through polyethylene-lined administration set attached to 0.22-micron in-line filter.
- To prevent severe hypersensitivity reaction, premedicate with dexamethasone 20 mg 12 and 6 hours before infusion, as prescribed. Also give diphenhydramine 50 mg I.V., plus either cimetidine 300 mg or ranitidine 50 mg I.V. 30 to 60 minutes before paclitaxel.

🔊 Keep epinephrine available. If severe hypersensitivity reaction occurs, stop infusion immediately and give epinephrine, I.V. fluids, and additional antihistamine and corticosteroid doses, as indicated and prescribed.

Route	Onset	Peak	Duration
I.V.	Unknown	Unknown	Unknown

Adverse reactions
CNS: peripheral neuropathy
CV: hypotension, hypertension, syncope, abnormal ECG, bradycardia, **venous thrombosis**
GI: nausea, vomiting, diarrhea, stomatitis, mucositis
Hematologic: anemia, **leukopenia, neutropenia, bleeding, thrombocytopenia**
Musculoskeletal: joint pain, myalgia
Skin: alopecia, radiation reactions
Other: infection, injection site reaction, hypersensitivity reactions including **anaphylaxis**

Interactions
Drug-drug. *Carbamazepine, phenobarbital:* decreased paclitaxel blood level and efficacy
Cisplatin: increased bone marrow depression (when paclitaxel dose follows cisplatin dose)
Cyclosporine, diazepam, doxorubicin, felodipine, ketoconazole, midazolam: inhibited paclitaxel metabolism and greater risk of toxicity
Doxorubicin: increased doxorubicin blood level and toxicity
Live-virus vaccines: decreased antibody response to vaccine, increased risk of adverse reactions
Other antineoplastics: increased risk of bone marrow depression
Drug-diagnostic tests. *Liver function tests:* abnormal results
Triglycerides: increased levels

Patient monitoring
🔊 Watch closely for hypersensitivity reaction.
- Monitor heart rate and blood pressure.
- Assess infusion site for local effects and extravasation, especially during prolonged infusion.

🔊 Monitor CBC, including platelet count. If neutropenia develops, monitor patient for infection; if thrombocy-

p

topenia develops, watch for signs and symptoms of bleeding.
• If patient has preexisting cardiac conduction abnormality, maintain continuous cardiac monitoring.

Patient teaching

• Instruct neutropenic patient to minimize infection risk by avoiding crowds, plants, and fresh fruits and vegetables.
• Tell thrombocytopenic patient to avoid activities that can cause injury. Advise him to use soft toothbrush and electric razor.
Clinical alert: Advise patient to promptly report signs and symptoms of infection, bleeding, or peripheral neuropathy (such as numbness and tingling of feet and hands).
• Tell patient to promptly report pain or burning at injection site.
• Explain that temporary hair loss may occur.
• As appropriate, review all other significant and life-threatening adverse reactions and interactions, especially those related to the drugs and tests mentioned above.

palivizumab

Synagis

Pharmacologic class: Monoclonal antibody
Therapeutic class: Immunologic agent
Pregnancy risk category C

Action

Neutralizes and suppresses activity of syncytial virus in respiratory tract, inhibiting respiratory syncytial virus (RSV) replication

Availability

Injection: 50 mg, 100-mg vial

Indications and dosages

➢ To prevent serious lower respiratory disease caused by RSV in high-risk children
Children: 15 mg/kg I.M. q month throughout RSV season

Contraindications

• Hypersensitivity to drug or its components

Precautions

Use cautiously in:
• thrombocytopenia, coagulation disorders, established RSV infection.

Administration

Clinical alert: Keep epinephrine 1:1,000 available in case anaphylaxis occurs. (However, drug isn't known to cause anaphylaxis.)
• Dilute in sterile water for injection. Gently swirl for 30 seconds to avoid foaming.
• Keep reconstituted solution at room temperature for at least 20 minutes before administering. Give within 6 hours of reconstitution.
• Inject I.M. into anterolateral thigh. Avoid gluteal injection, which may damage sciatic nerve.

Route	Onset	Peak	Duration
I.M.	Unknown	Unknown	Unknown

Adverse reactions

CNS: nervousness, pain
EENT: conjunctivitis, otitis media, rhinitis, pharyngitis, sinusitis
GI: vomiting, diarrhea, gastroenteritis, oral moniliasis
Hematologic: anemia
Respiratory: upper respiratory tract infection, cough, wheezing, dyspnea, bronchiolitis, bronchitis, pneumonia, croup, **asthma, apnea**
Skin: rash, fungal dermatitis, eczema
Other: hernia, pain, fever, injection site reaction, viral infection, flulike symptoms, failure to thrive

Interactions

Drug-diagnostic tests. *Alanine aminotransferase, aspartate aminotransferase:* increased levels
Hemoglobin: decreased level

Patient monitoring

Watch closely for signs and symptoms of anaphylaxis immediately after dosing.
• Assess for signs and symptoms of infection, particularly EENT and respiratory infection.
• Monitor liver function tests and CBC.
• Assess patient's weight and hydration status.

Patient teaching

• Tell parent that monthly injections are necessary during RSV season (November through April).
• Inform parent that drug may cause GI symptoms and failure to thrive. Provide dietary consultation as needed.
Caution parent that EENT and respiratory infections may follow administration. Advise parent to contact prescriber immediately if child has fever or other signs or symptoms of infection.
• As appropriate, review all other significant and life-threatening adverse reactions and interactions, especially those related to the tests mentioned above.

palonosetron hydrochloride

Aloxi

Pharmacologic class: Selective serotonin subtype 3 ($5\text{-}HT_3$) receptor antagonist
Therapeutic class: Antiemetic
Pregnancy risk category B

Action

Selectively binds to and antagonizes $5\text{-}HT_3$ receptors on vagal nerve terminals and in chemoreceptor trigger zone. This action blocks serotonin release, reducing the vomiting reflex.

Availability

Solution: 0.25 mg (free base) in 5-ml vial

Indications and dosages

➢ To prevent nausea and vomiting caused by cancer chemotherapy
Adults: 0.25 mg I.V. as a single dose 30 minutes before chemotherapy. Repeated doses within 7 days aren't recommended.

Contraindications

• Hypersensitivity to drug or its components

Precautions

Use cautiously in:
• hypersensitivity to other $5\text{-}HT_3$ receptor antagonists
• diabetes mellitus, hepatic dysfunction
• pregnant or breastfeeding patients
• children.

Administration

• Flush I.V. line with normal saline solution before and after giving.
• Deliver into I.V. line over 30 seconds. Don't mix with other drugs.

Route	Onset	Peak	Duration
I.V.	Unknown	Unknown	Unknown

Adverse reactions

CNS: headache, fatigue, insomnia, dizziness, anxiety
CV: hypotension, vein discoloration and distention, nonsustained tachycardia, bradycardia
GI: constipation, diarrhea, abdominal pain, anorexia
GU: glycosuria

Metabolic: fluctuating electrolyte levels, hyperglycemia, **metabolic acidosis, hyperkalemia**
Musculoskeletal: joint pain
Other: fever, flulike symptoms

Interactions

Drug-diagnostic tests: *Alanine aminotransferase, aspartate aminotransferase, bilirubin, blood and urine glucose, potassium:* increased levels

Patient monitoring

- Monitor vital signs and ECG. Watch closely for tachycardia, bradycardia, and hypotension.
- Watch electrolyte levels for fluctuations (especially hyperkalemia and metabolic acidosis).
- Evaluate temperature. Stay alert for flulike symptoms.
- Closely monitor blood and urine glucose levels in diabetic patients. Stay alert for hyperglycemia.

Patient teaching

- Explain that drug helps prevent nausea and vomiting caused by chemotherapy.
- Teach patient to recognize and report signs and symptoms of hyperkalemia and metabolic acidosis.
- Advise patient to report flulike symptoms.
- Instruct diabetic patient to closely watch blood and urine glucose levels.
- As appropriate, review all other significant and life-threatening adverse reactions and interactions, especially those related to the tests mentioned above.

pamidronate disodium

Aredia

Pharmacologic class: Bisphosphonate, hypocalcemic
Therapeutic class: Bone resorption inhibitor
Pregnancy risk category C

Action

Inhibits normal and abnormal bone resorption and decreases calcium levels

Availability

Injection: 30 mg/vial, 90 mg/vial

Indications and dosages

➢ Hypercalcemia caused by cancer
Adults: For moderate hypercalcemia, 60 to 90 mg as a single-dose I.V. infusion over 2 to 24 hours. For severe hypercalcemia, 90 mg as a single-dose I.V. infusion over 2 to 24 hours.
➢ Osteolytic lesions caused by multiple myeloma
Adults: 90 mg I.V. as a 4-hour infusion q month
➢ Osteolytic bone metastases of breast cancer
Adults: 90 mg I.V. as a 2-hour infusion q 3 to 4 weeks
➢ Paget's disease
Adults: 30 mg I.V. daily as a 4-hour infusion for 3 days

Contraindications

- Hypersensitivity to drug, its components, or other bisphosphonates

Precautions

Use cautiously in:
- renal impairment
- pregnant or breastfeeding patients
- children (safety not established).

Administration

- Hydrate patient with saline solution as needed before starting therapy.
- Because of risk of renal failure, give no more than 90 mg in single doses.

◀ Reconstitute vial using 10 ml of sterile water for injection. When completely dissolved, dilute in 250 to 1,000 ml of half-normal or normal saline solution or dextrose 5% in water.

◀ Don't mix with solutions containing calcium, such as lactated Ringer's solution.

- Administer in I.V. line separate from all other drugs and fluids.

Route	Onset	Peak	Duration
I.V.	Unknown	Unknown	Unknown

Adverse reactions

CNS: anxiety, headache, insomnia, psychosis, drowsiness, weakness
CV: hypertension, syncope, tachycardia, **atrial flutter, arrhythmias, heart failure**
EENT: sinusitis
GI: nausea, vomiting, diarrhea, abdominal pain, constipation, dyspepsia, stomatitis, anorexia, **GI hemorrhage**
GU: urinary tract infection
Hematologic: anemia, **neutropenia, leukopenia, granulocytopenia, thrombocytopenia**
Metabolic: hypothyroidism
Musculoskeletal: bone pain, joint pain, myalgia
Respiratory: crackles, coughing, dyspnea, upper respiratory infection, **pleural effusion**
Other: fever, generalized pain, injection site reaction

Interactions

Drug-diagnostic tests. *Creatinine:* increased level
Electrolytes, hemoglobin, magnesium, phosphorus, platelets, potassium, red blood cells, white blood cells: decreased levels

Patient monitoring

- Monitor hydration status carefully.
- Monitor vital signs and ECG. Evaluate cardiovascular and respiratory status closely.
- Assess hematologic studies and creatinine level before each treatment course.
- Assess electrolyte levels, especially calcium, magnesium, and phosphorus.
- Closely monitor fluid intake and output. Watch for signs and symptoms of urinary tract infection.

Patient teaching

- Instruct patient to weigh himself regularly and report sudden gains.

◀ Advise patient to promptly report significant respiratory problems, peripheral edema, or GI bleeding.

◀ Inform patient that drug lowers resistance to some infections. Tell him to immediately report fever and other signs and symptoms of infection.

- Explain importance of undergoing laboratory tests before, during, and after therapy.
- Caution patient to avoid driving and other hazardous activities until he knows how drug affects concentration, cognition, and alertness.
- Tell patient to minimize GI upset by eating small, frequent servings of food and drinking plenty of fluids.
- As appropriate, review all other significant and life-threatening adverse reactions and interactions, especially those related to the tests mentioned above.

pantoprazole sodium

Protonix, Protonix IV

Pharmacologic class: Proton pump inhibitor
Therapeutic class: GI agent
Pregnancy risk category B

p

Action
Reduces gastric acid secretion and increases gastric mucus and bicarbonate production, creating protective coating on gastric mucosa

Availability
Powder for injection (freeze-dried): 40 mg/vial
Tablets (delayed-release): 20 mg, 40 mg

Indications and dosages
➢ Erosive esophagitis caused by gastroesophageal reflux disease (GERD)
Adults: 40 mg I.V. daily for 7 to 10 days or 40 mg P.O. daily for 8 weeks. May repeat P.O. course for 8 additional weeks.
➢ Erosive esophagitis
Adults: 40 mg P.O. daily
➢ Pathologic hypersecretory conditions
Adults: Initially, 40 mg P.O. b.i.d., increased as needed to maximum of 240 mg P.O. daily; some patients may need up to 2 years of therapy. Alternatively, 80 mg I.V. q 12 hours, to a maximum of 240 mg/day (80 mg q 8 hours).

Contraindications
• Hypersensitivity to drug

Precautions
Use cautiously in:
• severe hepatic disease
• pregnant or breastfeeding patients
• children.

Administration
• For I.V. administration, use in-line filter provided. If Y-site is used, place filter below Y-site closest to patient.
• Dilute I.V. form with 10 ml of normal saline solution; further dilute in dextrose 5% in water, normal saline solution, or lactated Ringer's solution, as directed. Give over 15 minutes at a rate no faster than 3 mg/minute.
• Don't give I.V. form with other I.V. solutions.
• Know that I.V. form is indicated for short-term treatment of GERD in patients with history of erosive esophagitis as alternative to P.O. therapy.

Route	Onset	Peak	Duration
P.O.	Rapid	2.5 hr	>24 hr
I.V.	Rapid	Unknown	>24 hr

Adverse reactions
CNS: dizziness, headache
CV: chest pain
EENT: rhinitis
GI: vomiting, diarrhea, abdominal pain, dyspepsia
Metabolic: hyperglycemia
Skin: rash, pruritus
Other: injection site reaction

Interactions
Drug-drug. *Ampicillin, cyanocobalamin, digoxin, iron salts, ketoconazole:* delayed absorption of these drugs
Clarithromycin, diazepam, flurazepam, phenytoin, triazolam: increased pantoprazole blood level
Sucralfate: delayed pantoprazole absorption
Warfarin: increased bleeding
Drug-diagnostic tests. *Aspartate aminotransferase, glucose:* increased levels
Tetrahydrocannabinol test: false-positive result

Patient monitoring
• Assess for symptomatic improvement.
• Monitor blood glucose level in diabetic patient.

Patient teaching
• Tell patient to swallow delayed-release tablets whole without crushing, chewing, or splitting.
• Tell patient he may take tablets with or without food.
• Explain that antacids don't affect drug absorption.

• Instruct diabetic patients to monitor blood glucose level carefully and stay alert for signs and symptoms of hyperglycemia.
• As appropriate, review all other significant adverse reactions and interactions, especially those related to the drugs and tests mentioned above.

paroxetine hydrochloride

Paxil, Paxil CR

Pharmacologic class: Selective serotonin reuptake inhibitor (SSRI)
Therapeutic class: Antidepressant, anxiolytic
Pregnancy risk category C

Action

Unknown. Thought to inhibit neuronal reuptake of serotonin in CNS.

Availability

Oral suspension: 10 mg/5 ml in 250-ml bottles
Tablets: 10 mg, 20 mg, 30 mg, 40 mg
Tablets (controlled-release): 12.5 mg, 25 mg, 37.5 mg

Indications and dosages

➢ Major depressive disorder
Adults: Initially, 20 mg/day P.O. (immediate-release) as a single dose; may increase as needed by 10 mg/day at weekly intervals (range is 20 to 50 mg); daily dosages of approximately 30 mg may maintain efficacy for up to 1 year. Or initially, 25 mg P.O. (controlled-release) daily; may increase by 12.5 mg/day at weekly intervals, up to 62.5 mg/day.
➢ Obsessive-compulsive disorder
Adults: Initially, 20 mg/day P.O. (immediate-release); increase as needed by 10 mg/day at weekly intervals, up to 60 mg P.O. (range is 20 to 60 mg/day).
➢ Panic disorder
Adults: Initially, 10 mg/day P.O. (immediate-release); may increase by 10 mg/day at weekly intervals, up to 40 mg P.O. (range is 10 to 60 mg/day); maximum dosage is 60 mg/day. Or initially, 12.5 mg/day P.O. (controlled-release); may increase by 12.5 mg/day at weekly intervals, to a maximum of 75 mg/day.
➢ Social anxiety disorder
Adults: 20 to 60 mg P.O. (immediate-release) daily; however, dosages greater than 20 mg/day may not provide added benefit. Recommended initial dosage (controlled-release) is 12.5 mg/day P.O., with range of 12.5 to 37.5 mg/day. Make any dosage increases if needed in increments of 12.5 mg/day at intervals of at least 1 week, to a maximum of 37.5 mg/day.
➢ Posttraumatic stress disorder
Adults: Initially, 20 mg/day P.O.; range is 20 to 50 mg/day. Make any dosage increases if needed in increments of 10 mg/day at intervals of at least 1 week. For maintenance, adjust to lowest effective dosage.
➢ Generalized anxiety disorder
Adults: Initially, 20 mg/day P.O.; range is 20 to 50 mg/day; however, dosages greater than 20 mg/day may not provide added benefit. Make any dosage increases if needed in increments of 10 mg/day at intervals of at least 1 week.
➢ Premenstrual dysphoric disorder
Adults: 12.5 to 25 mg/day P.O. (controlled-release) daily. May give either daily throughout menstrual cycle or only during luteal phase cycle (per prescriber). Make any dosage changes if needed at intervals of at least 1 week.

Dosage adjustment

• Hepatic impairment, severe renal impairment
• Elderly or debilitated patients

Contraindications

• Hypersensitivity to drug

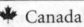

p

• MAO inhibitor use within past 14 days
• Concurrent thioridazine use

Precautions

Use cautiously in:
• severe renal or hepatic impairment
• history of seizures, mania, or suicide attempt
• increased risk of suicide attempt, hyponatremia, or abnormal bleeding
• elderly or debilitated patients
• pregnant or breastfeeding patients
• children (safety not established).

Administration

• Give with or without food.
• Give controlled-release tablets whole. Make sure patient doesn't chew or crush them.
Don't give to patients receiving MAO inhibitors or thioridazine.
• Reassess patient periodically to gauge need for continued therapy.

Route	Onset	Peak	Duration
P.O.	Unknown	2-8 hr	Unknown
P.O. (controlled)	Unknown	6-10 hr	Unknown

Adverse reactions

CNS: anxiety, agitation, dizziness, drowsiness, asthenia, vascular headache, confusion, hangover, depression, paresthesia, tremor, twitching, myoclonus, amnesia, insomnia, abnormal dreams, **cerebral ischemia, suicidal behavior or ideation** (especially in child or adolescent)
CV: chest pain, hypertension, hypotension, palpitations, orthostatic hypotension, angina pectoris, ventricular or supraventricular extrasystoles, tachycardia, bradycardia, **thrombophlebitis, myocardial ischemia**
EENT: blurred vision, rhinitis, dry mouth
GI: nausea, vomiting, diarrhea, constipation, abdominal pain, dyspepsia, flatulence
GU: urinary frequency, urinary disorders, urinary tract infection, genital disorders, ejaculatory disturbance, decreased libido
Musculoskeletal: back pain, myalgia, myasthenia, myopathy, joint pain
Respiratory: cough, bronchitis, respiratory disorders
Skin: sweating, pruritus, pallor, rash, photosensitivity
Other: chills, edema, appetite and weight changes, accidental injury

Interactions

Drug-drug. *Cimetidine:* increased paroxetine blood level
Digoxin: decreased digoxin efficacy
Drugs metabolized by liver (such as amitriptyline, class IC antiarrhythmics, desipramine): decreased metabolism and increased effects of these drugs
5-hydroxytryptamine receptor agonists (such as frovatriptan, naratriptan, rizatriptan): weakness, hyperreflexia, incoordination
MAO inhibitors: potentially fatal reactions (hyperthermia, rigidity, myoclonus, autonomic instability, fluctuating vital signs, extreme agitation, delirium, coma)
Phenobarbital, phenytoin: decreased paroxetine efficacy
Theophylline: increased risk of theophylline toxicity
Thioridazine: increased thioridazine blood level, serious ventricular arrhythmias, sudden death
Tryptophan: headache, nausea, sweating, dizziness
Warfarin: increased risk of bleeding (without altering prothrombin time)
Drug-diagnostic tests. *Alkaline phosphatase, bilirubin, glucose:* increased levels
5-hydroxyindole acetic acid, vanillylmandelic acid: decreased levels
Urinary catecholamines: false increases
Drug-herbs. *S-adenosylmethionine (SAM-e), St. John's wort:* increased risk

of adverse serotonergic effects, including serotonin syndrome

Patient monitoring

- Check for signs and symptoms of toxicity, including drowsiness, nausea, tremor, tachycardia, confusion, and dizziness.
- Assess vital signs and cardiovascular status.

Monitor neurologic status. Watch closely for depression and suicidal behavior and ideation (especially in child or adolescent).

- Evaluate respiratory status. Stay alert for signs and symptoms of infection.

Patient teaching

- Tell patient to swallow controlled-release tablets whole without chewing or crushing them.

Describe signs and symptoms of drug toxicity. Tell patient to report these immediately.

Teach patient or caregiver to recognize and immediately report signs of suicidal intent or expressions of suicidal ideation (especially in child or adolescent).

- Tell patient to continue to take drug even if he feels better. Caution him not to stop therapy abruptly.
- Advise patient to consult prescriber before taking other prescription drugs or over-the-counter preparations.
- Caution patient to avoid driving and other hazardous activities until he knows how drug affects him.
- As appropriate, review all other significant and life-threatening adverse reactions and interactions, especially those related to the drugs, tests, and herbs mentioned above.

pegaspargase (PEG-L-asparaginase)

Oncaspar

Pharmacologic class: Enzyme
Therapeutic class: Antineoplastic
Pregnancy risk category C

Action

Stimulates production of effector proteins, such as serum neopterin and 2', 5' oligodenylate synthetase; raises body temperature and reversibly lowers white blood cell and platelet counts

Availability

Injection: 750 international units/ml, 5-ml vial in phosphate-buffered saline solution

Indications and dosages

➢ Acute lymphoblastic leukemia

Adults and children with body surface area (BSA) greater than 0.6 m²: 2,500 international units/m² I.M. or I.V. q 14 days

Adults and children with BSA less than 0.6 m²: 82.5 international units/m² I.M. or I.V. q 14 days

Contraindications

- Hypersensitivity or previous serious allergic reaction (such as generalized urticaria, bronchospasm, laryngeal edema, hypotension) to drug
- Pancreatitis or history of pancreatitis
- Previous hemorrhagic events related to L-asparaginase therapy

Precautions

Use cautiously in:

- renal or hepatic disease, CNS disorders
- concurrent use of hepatotoxic agents, anticoagulants, aspirin or other non-

p

steroidal anti-inflammatory drugs (NSAIDs)
• pregnant or breastfeeding patients.

Administration

◀ Follow facility protocol for handling, preparing, and disposing of chemotherapeutic drugs.
◀ Avoid inhaling vapors and contact with skin or mucous membranes.
◀ Keep resuscitation equipment, epinephrine, oxygen, steroids, and antihistamines readily available.
• Know that I.M. route is preferred because it's less likely to cause hepatotoxicity, coagulopathy, and GI or renal disorders. For single I.M. injection, don't exceed volume of 2 ml.
• For I.V. use, dilute in 100 ml of normal saline solution or dextrose 5% in water. Infuse over 1 to 2 hours.
◀ Don't freeze; freezing inactivates drug.

Route	Onset	Peak	Duration
I.V.	Unknown	72-96 hr	2 wk
I.M.	Unknown	Unknown	Unknown

Adverse reactions

CNS: dizziness, headache, confusion, hallucinations, emotional lability, drowsiness, neuritis, Parkinson-like syndrome, malaise, **coma, seizures**
CV: hypertension, hypotension, chest pain, peripheral edema, tachycardia, **endocarditis**
GI: nausea, vomiting, diarrhea, constipation, abdominal pain, flatulence, anorexia, **pancreatitis**
GU: glycosuria, polyuria, urinary frequency, hematuria
Hematologic: hemolytic anemia, leukopenia, pancytopenia, thrombocytopenia, disseminated intravascular coagulation
Hepatic: jaundice, fatty liver deposits, **hepatotoxicity, hepatomegaly**
Metabolic: hypoproteinemia, hyperuricemia, hyperammonemia, hyponatremia, hyperglycemia, **hypoglycemia**
Respiratory: dyspnea, cough, **bronchospasm**
Skin: rash, urticaria, pruritus, night sweats, alopecia
Other: increased appetite and thirst, weight loss, chills, fever, injection site reaction, facial or lip edema, hypersensitivity reactions including **anaphylaxis, septic shock**

Interactions

Drug-drug. *Aspirin, dipyridamole, heparin, NSAIDs, warfarin:* increased risk of bleeding or thrombosis
Methotrexate: decreased methotrexate action
Drug-diagnostic tests. *Amylase, blood urea nitrogen, creatinine, lipase, uric acid:* increased levels
Glucose: increased or decreased level
Liver function tests: abnormal results
Lymphoblasts: decreased count
Plasma proteins: altered levels

Patient monitoring

◀ Watch for anaphylaxis and other hypersensitivity reactions, especially during first hour of therapy.
• Monitor CBC (including platelet count); fibrinogen; prothrombin and partial thromboplastin times; International Normalized Ratio; and serum amylase, lipase, and uric acid levels.
◀ Assess neurologic status. Stay alert for decreased level of consciousness and evidence of impending seizure.
• Check for signs and symptoms of bleeding, infection, and hyperglycemia.
• Monitor heart rate, blood pressure, respiratory rate, temperature, and fluid intake and output.

Patient teaching

◀ Teach patient to recognize and immediately report signs and symptoms of hypersensitivity reactions, bleeding, infection, and other adverse reactions.
• Tell patient drug is likely to cause reversible hair loss.

• Stress importance of undergoing follow-up laboratory tests.
• Advise patient to avoid situations that increase risk for infection.
• Instruct patient to consult prescriber before taking other prescription drugs or over-the-counter preparations.
• As appropriate, review all other significant and life-threatening adverse reactions and interactions, especially those related to the drugs and tests mentioned above.

pegfilgrastim

Neulasta

Pharmacologic class: Granulocytic colony stimulating factor
Therapeutic class: Hematopoietic drug
Pregnancy risk category C

Action

Binds to specific cell-surface receptors on hematopoietic cells, stimulating their proliferation and differentiation in bone marrow

Availability

Injection: 6 mg/0.6 ml in prefilled syringes

Indications and dosages

➢ To reduce risk of infection in nonmyeloid cancer patients who are receiving myelosuppressive drugs
Adults: 6 mg subcutaneously as a single dose once per chemotherapy cycle

Contraindications

• Hypersensitivity to drug, *Escherichia coli*-derived proteins, filgrastim, or other drug components

Precautions

Use cautiously in:
• myeloid cancers, sickle cell disease
• patients undergoing chemotherapy or radiation
• pregnant or breastfeeding patients
• children (safety and efficacy not established).

Administration

• Inspect solution for particles; discard if particles or discoloration appear.
• Don't give 14 days before to 24 hours after administration of cytotoxic chemotherapy.

Route	Onset	Peak	Duration
Subcut.	Variable	Variable	Variable

Adverse reactions

CNS: headache, weakness, fatigue, dizziness, insomnia
CV: peripheral edema
GI: nausea, vomiting, diarrhea, abdominal pain, dyspepsia, stomatitis, **splenic rupture**
Hematologic: leukocytosis, granulocytopenia
Musculoskeletal: bone pain, myalgia, joint pain
Respiratory: adult respiratory distress syndrome (ARDS) in septic patients
Skin: alopecia, mucositis
Other: taste perversion, allergic reaction, increased pain, fever, neutropenic fever, **aggravation of sickle cell disease**

Interactions

Drug-drug. *Lithium:* potentiation of neutrophil release
Drug-diagnostic tests. *Alkaline phosphatase, lactate dehydrogenase, uric acid:* increased levels

Patient monitoring

🔊 Assess for signs and symptoms of impending splenic rupture, such as left upper abdominal quadrant or shoulder pain and splenic enlargement.
• Monitor vital signs and temperature.

P

Watch for signs and symptoms of sepsis, ARDS, and neutropenic fever.
• Monitor CBC, uric acid level, and liver function tests.

Patient teaching

• Teach patient or caregiver how to administer injection and dispose of syringes at home, if appropriate.
Teach patient to recognize and immediately report respiratory distress or signs and symptoms of splenic rupture.
• Caution patient to avoid driving and other hazardous activities until he knows how drug affects concentration and alertness.
• Advise patient to minimize GI upset by eating small, frequent servings of food and drinking plenty of fluids.
• Instruct patient to have follow-up laboratory tests as needed.
• As appropriate, review all other significant and life-threatening adverse reactions and interactions, especially those related to the drugs and tests mentioned above.

peginterferon alfa-2a

Pegasys

Pharmacologic class: Interferon

Therapeutic class: Biological response modifier

Pregnancy risk category C

Action

Unclear. Thought to bind to specific cell-surface receptors, suppressing cell proliferation and viral replication. Also increases effector protein levels and reduces white blood cell (WBC) and platelet counts.

Availability

Injection: 180-mcg/ml vial

Indications and dosages

➢ Chronic hepatitis C virus infection

Adults: 180 mcg subcutaneously q week for 48 weeks. If poorly tolerated, reduce to 135 mcg weekly; some patients may need reduction to 90 mcg.

Dosage adjustment

• Neutrophil count less than 750 cells/mm^3 or platelet count less than 50,000 cells/mm^3
• Hepatic disease
• End-stage renal disease requiring dialysis
• Serious adverse reactions

Off-label uses

• Renal cell carcinoma

Contraindications

• Hypersensitivity to drug
• Autoimmune hepatitis
• Decompensated hepatic disease
• Infants and neonates (due to benzyl alcohol content)

Precautions

Use cautiously in:
• thyroid disorders; bone marrow depression; hepatic, renal, or cardiac disease; pancreatitis; autoimmune disorders; pulmonary disorders; colitis; ophthalmic disorders; depression
• elderly patients
• pregnant or breastfeeding patients
• children younger than age 18.

Administration

• Keep refrigerated. Before giving, roll vial between palms for 1 minute to warm; don't shake. Protect solution from light.
• Don't use if solution is cloudy or contains visible particles.
• Administer undiluted in abdomen or thigh by subcutaneous injection.
• Know that drug may be used alone or with ribavirin.

Route	Onset	Peak	Duration
Subcut.	Gradual	72-96 hr	Unknown

Adverse reactions

CNS: dizziness, vertigo, insomnia, fatigue, rigors, poor memory and concentration, asthenia, depression, irritability, anxiety, peripheral neuropathy, mood changes, **suicidal ideation**
CV: hypertension, chest pain, **supraventricular arrhythmias, myocardial infarction**
EENT: vision loss, blurred vision, retinal artery or vein thrombosis, retinal hemorrhage, optic neuritis, retinopathy, **papilledema**
GI: nausea, vomiting, diarrhea, abdominal pain, dry mouth, anorexia, **GI tract bleeding, ulcerative and hemorrhagic colitis, pancreatitis**
Hematologic: anemia, **leukopenia, thrombocytopenia, neutropenia**
Metabolic: diabetes mellitus, aggravated hypothyroidism or hyperthyroidism
Musculoskeletal: myalgia, back pain, joint pain
Respiratory: pneumonia, **interstitial pneumonitis, bronchoconstriction, respiratory failure**
Skin: alopecia, pruritus, diaphoresis, rash, dermatitis, dry skin, eczema
Other: weight loss, flulike symptoms, injection-site reaction, pain, **autoimmune phenomena, severe and possibly fatal bacterial infections, severe hypersensitivity reactions including angioedema and anaphylaxis**

Interactions

Drug-drug. *Theophylline:* increased theophylline blood level
Drug-diagnostic tests. *Absolute neutrophil count, hematocrit, hemoglobin, platelets, WBCs:* decreased values
Alanine aminotransferase: transient increase
Glucose, thyroid function tests: decreased or increased levels
Triglycerides: increased levels

Patient monitoring

◀ Assess cardiac and pulmonary status closely. Watch for evidence of infections and hypersensitivity reactions, including anaphylaxis.
- Before therapy begins, assess CBC (including platelet count), blood glucose level, and thyroid, kidney, and liver function tests. Continue to monitor at 1, 2, 4, 6, and 8 weeks and then every 4 weeks during therapy (more often if abnormalities occur). Monitor thyroid function tests every 12 weeks.

◀ Monitor for development of diabetes mellitus, hypothyroidism, and hyperthyroidism.
◀ If serious adverse reaction occurs, discontinue drug or adjust dosage until reaction abates, as prescribed. If reaction persists or recurs despite adequate dosage adjustment, discontinue drug.

Patient teaching

- Teach patient or caregiver how to administer injection subcutaneously in thigh or abdomen and how to dispose of equipment properly, if appropriate.

◀ Advise patient to promptly report rash, bleeding, bloody stools, infection symptoms (such as fever), decreased vision, chest pain, severe stomach or lower back pain, shortness of breath, depression, or suicidal thoughts.
- Instruct patient to administer drug exactly as prescribed. If he misses a dose but remembers it within 2 days, tell him to take missed dose as soon as possible; if more than 2 days have elapsed, tell him to contact prescriber.
- Caution patient not to switch brands without prescriber's approval.
- Instruct patient to have periodic eye exams.
- Advise female patient of childbearing age to avoid pregnancy and use two birth control methods before, during, and up to 6 months after therapy. Instruct male patient to use condoms.
- As appropriate, review all other significant and life-threatening adverse

p

reactions and interactions, especially those related to the drugs and tests mentioned above.

peginterferon alfa-2b

PEG-Intron

Pharmacologic class: Immunomodulator
Therapeutic class: Immunologic agent
Pregnancy risk category C (monotherapy), ***X*** (when given with ribavirin)

Action

Binds to specific cell-surface membrane receptors, causing suppression of cell proliferation, enhanced phagocytic macrophage activity, and inhibition of viral replication

Availability

Powder for injection with diluent: 50 mcg/0.5-ml vial, 80 mcg/0.5-ml vial, 120 mcg/0.5-ml vial, 150 mcg/0.5-ml vial (Redipen)

Indications and dosages

➢ Chronic hepatitis C virus infection (HCV)

Adults ages 18 and older: For monotherapy, 1 mcg/kg/week subcutaneously for 1 year. When given with ribavirin, 1.5 mcg/kg/week subcutaneously.

Dosage adjustment

- Serious adverse reactions

Contraindications

- Hypersensitivity to drug or its components
- Autoimmune hepatitis
- Decompensated hepatic damage

Precautions

Use cautiously in:

- human immunodeficiency virus, hepatitis B infection
- patients who have failed other interferon alfa therapy
- patients who develop neutralizing antibodies
- organ transplant recipients
- elderly patients
- pregnant or breastfeeding patients
- children.

Administration

- Reconstitute by holding dual-chamber glass cartridge upright with dose button down and pressing two halves of pen together until you hear an audible click. Then gently invert (don't shake) pen to mix solution.
- Discard solution if it is discolored or cloudy or contains particulates.
- To administer, hold pen upright, attach supplied needle, and select appropriate dosage by pulling back on dosing button until dark bands are visible. Then turn button until dark band aligns with correct dose.
- Use reconstituted solution immediately.

Route	Onset	Peak	Duration
Subcut.	Unknown	15-44 hr	Unknown

Adverse reactions

CNS: fatigue, headache, malaise, asthenia, dizziness, insomnia, depression, anxiety, emotional lability, irritability, poor concentration, agitation, nervousness, rigors, **suicidal behavior, suicidal or homicidal ideation**
CV: hypotension, tachycardia, chest pain, angina pectoris, **arrhythmias, cardiomyopathy, myocardial infarction**
EENT: vision decrease or loss, retinal artery or vein thrombosis, retinal hemorrhage, cotton-wool spots in visual field, rhinitis, sinusitis, pharyngitis
GI: nausea; vomiting; diarrhea; constipation; abdominal pain; dyspepsia; right upper abdominal quadrant pain; anorexia; dry mouth; **ulcerative, hem-**

orrhagic, or ischemic colitis; pancreatitis
GU: menstrual disorder
Hematologic: neutropenia, thrombocytopenia
Hepatic: hepatomegaly
Metabolic: aggravated hypothyroidism or hyperthyroidism
Musculoskeletal: myalgia, arthralgia, musculoskeletal pain
Respiratory: dyspnea, pneumonia, bronchiolitis obliterans, cough, **sarcoidosis, pulmonary infiltrates, interstitial pneumonitis, bronchoconstriction**
Skin: rash, dry skin, pruritus, sweating, flushing, alopecia
Other: exacerbation or development of autoimmune disorders, injection-site reaction, fever, viral or fungal infection, **systemic lupus erythematosus, severe hypersensitivity reactions including angioedema and anaphylaxis**

Interactions

Drug-diagnostic tests. *Bilirubin, triglycerides, uric acid:* increased levels
Glucose, thyroid function tests: decreased or increased levels
Hemoglobin, neutrophils, platelets, white blood cells: decreased levels

Patient monitoring

- Before therapy begins, assess CBC (including platelet count); blood glucose level, and thyroid, kidney, and liver function tests. Continue to monitor at weeks 2, 4, 8, and 12 and then every 6 weeks during therapy (more often if abnormalities occur). Monitor thyroid function tests every 12 weeks.

🔊 Assess cardiac and pulmonary status closely. Watch for signs and symptoms of infection and hypersensitivity reactions, including anaphylaxis.

🔊 Monitor neurologic status. Stay alert for such behavioral changes as irritability, anxiety, depression, and homicidal or suicidal ideation.

🔊 If serious adverse reaction occurs, know that drug will be discontinued or dosages adjusted accordingly.

- Monitor patient for development of diabetes mellitus, hypothyroidism, or hyperthyroidism.
- Be aware that if HCV level remains high after 6 months, drug should be discontinued.

Patient teaching

- Tell patient to take exactly as prescribed. If he misses a dose but remembers it within 2 days, instruct him to take it as soon as possible. However, if more than 2 days have elapsed, advise him to contact prescriber.
- Teach patient or caregiver how to administer injection subcutaneously into thigh or abdomen, if appropriate, and how to properly dispose of equipment.

🔊 Advise patient to stop drug and promptly report infection symptoms, such as high fever, easy bruising or bleeding, decreased vision, chest pain, shortness of breath, severe stomach or lower back pain, depression, or suicidal or homicidal thoughts.

- Urge patient to have periodic eye exams.
- Instruct female patient of childbearing age to avoid pregnancy and to use two birth control methods before, during, and up to 6 months after therapy. Instruct male patient to use condoms.
- As appropriate, review all other significant and life-threatening adverse reactions and interactions, especially those related to the tests mentioned above.

pegvisomant
Somavert

Pharmacologic class: Growth hormone (GH) receptor antagonist
Therapeutic class: GH analog
Pregnancy risk category B

Action
Selectively binds to GH receptors on cell surfaces, where it blocks binding of endogenous GH and interferes with GH signal transduction. This action decreases blood levels of insulin-like growth factor-1 (IGF-1) and other GH-responsive serum proteins.

Availability
Solution: 10-mg, 15-mg, and 20-mg vials

Indications and dosages
➢ Acromegaly
Adults: Initial subcutaneous loading dose of 40 mg, followed by 10 mg/day subcutaneously. May adjust in 5-mg increments after serum IGF-1 measurement q 4 to 6 weeks; don't exceed maximum daily maintenance dosage of 30 mg.

Contraindications
• Hypersensitivity to drug, its components, or latex (in vial stopper)

Precautions
Use cautiously in:
• GH-excreting tumors, diabetes mellitus, hepatic dysfunction
• pregnant or breastfeeding patients
• children.

Administration
• Reconstitute in vial with 1 ml of sterile water for injection.
• Roll vial gently between palms to mix; don't shake. Withdraw prescribed dosage and administer subcutaneously.

Route	Onset	Peak	Duration
Subcut.	Unknown	Unknown	24 hr

Adverse reactions
CNS: dizziness, paresthesia
CV: chest pain, hypertension, peripheral edema
EENT: sinusitis
GI: nausea, diarrhea, abdominal pain
Musculoskeletal: back pain
Other: infection, pain, injection site reaction, accidental injury, flulike symptoms

Interactions
Drug-drug. *Insulin, oral hypoglycemics:* decreased insulin sensitivity, reduced requirements for these drugs
Opioids: increased pegvisomant requirement
Drug-diagnostic tests. *GH assays:* interference with GH measurement
Liver function tests: abnormal results
Drug-behaviors. *Opioid addiction:* increased pegvisomant requirement

Patient monitoring
• Assess liver function tests; watch for signs and symptoms of hepatic dysfunction.
• Monitor serum IGF-1 level. If appropriate, discuss dosage adjustments with prescriber.
• Monitor vital signs; check for hypertension, chest pain, and peripheral edema.
• Measure temperature. Watch for signs and symptoms of infection, especially sinusitis or flulike symptoms.
• Assess blood glucose level closely in diabetic patient. Notify prescriber of significant decrease.

Patient teaching

- Teach patient proper technique for reconstituting and administering drug subcutaneously.

Clinical alert: Instruct patient to immediately report chest pain, peripheral edema, or signs or symptoms of infection.

- Caution patient to avoid driving and other hazardous activities until he knows how drug affects him.
- Teach diabetic patient to monitor blood glucose level closely and report significant decrease.

Clinical alert: Instruct patient to report yellowing of skin or eyes and other signs and symptoms of hepatic dysfunction. Tell him he'll undergo frequent liver function tests.

- As appropriate, review all other significant adverse reactions and interactions, especially those related to the drugs, tests, and behaviors mentioned above.

pemoline

Cylert, PemADD, PemADD CT

Pharmacologic class: CNS stimulant
Therapeutic class: Analeptic
Controlled substance schedule IV
Pregnancy risk category B

Action

Unknown. May act by blocking dopaminergic mechanism at cerebral cortex and subcortical structures and by stimulating CNS and respiratory system.

Availability

Tablets: 18.75 mg, 37.5 mg, 75 mg
Tablets (chewable): 37.5 mg

Indications and dosages

➢ Attention deficit hyperactivity disorder

Children ages 6 and older: Initially, 37.5 mg/day P.O. as a single morning dose; may increase by 18.75 mg at weekly intervals until optimal response occurs. Range is 56.25 to 75 mg/day; don't exceed 112.5 mg/day.

Off-label uses

- Narcolepsy
- Fatigue
- Excessive daytime sleepiness

Contraindications

- Hypersensitivity to drug
- Hepatic impairment

Precautions

Use cautiously in:

- tics, psychosis, emotional instability, drug abuse
- history of seizure disorders
- pregnant or breastfeeding patients (safety not established)
- children younger than age 6.

Administration

- Give in morning to minimize insomnia.
- Administer with food if GI upset occurs.

Route	Onset	Peak	Duration
P.O.	Unknown	2-4 hr	Unknown

Adverse reactions

CNS: headache, irritability, insomnia, depression, nervousness, drowsiness, dyskinetic movements, Tourette syndrome, hallucinations, **seizures**
CV: tachycardia
EENT: abnormal oculomotor function, nystagmus, oculogyric crisis
GI: nausea, diarrhea, abdominal pain, anorexia
Hematologic: aplastic anemia
Hepatic: jaundice, **hepatic failure, hepatitis**
Metabolic: growth suppression
Skin: rash, sweating
Other: fever, weight loss

Interactions

Drug-drug. *Anticonvulsants:* lowered seizure threshold
Other CNS stimulants: additive CNS stimulation
Drug-diagnostic tests. *Acid phosphatase, alanine aminotransferase, alkaline phosphatase, aspartate aminotransferase, lactate dehydrogenase:* increased levels

Patient monitoring

- Assess neurologic function. Watch for seizures, tics, depression, and dyskinetic movements.
- Monitor CBC and liver function tests frequently. Watch for signs and symptoms of hepatic dysfunction.
- Check for symptomatic improvement, which should occur by week 3.
- Assess patient's height and weight. (Long-term therapy may cause growth abnormalities.)

Patient teaching

- Tell patient and parents that drug should be taken in morning to minimize insomnia. Recommend taking it with food if it causes GI upset.
- Inform patient and parents about drug's risks and benefits. Stress importance of immediately reporting signs or symptoms of liver problems, such as malaise, yellowing of skin or eyes, anorexia, and GI complaints.
- Teach patient and parents to recognize and promptly report adverse CNS effects.
- Advise patient and parents of need for periodic eye exams.
- Explain that patient should have follow-up laboratory tests to monitor hepatic function.
- As appropriate, review all other significant and life-threatening adverse reactions and interactions, especially those related to the drugs and tests mentioned above.

penicillin G benzathine

Bicillin L-A, Megacillin✦, Permapen

Pharmacologic class: Penicillin
Therapeutic class: Anti-infective
Pregnancy risk category B

Action

Inhibits biosynthesis of cell-wall mucopeptide; kills penicillin-susceptible bacteria during active multiplication stage

Availability

Suspension for I.M. injection: 600,000 units/ml in 1-, 2-, and 4-ml prefilled syringes

Indications and dosages

➢ Upper respiratory infections
Adults: 1.2 million units I.M. as a single dose
Children weighing 27 kg (60) or more: 900,000 units I.M. as a single dose
Infants and children weighing less than 27 kg (60 lb): 300,000 to 600,000 units I.M. as a single dose
➢ Early syphilis (primary, secondary, or latent)
Adults: 2.4 million units I.M. as a single dose
Children: 50,000 units/kg I.M. as a single dose, increased as needed up to adult dosage
➢ Congenital syphilis
Children younger than age 2: 50,000 units/kg I.M. as a single dose
➢ Late (tertiary) syphilis and neurosyphilis
Adults: 2.4 million units I.M. q week for up to 3 weeks, after aqueous penicillin G or procaine penicillin therapy
➢ Gummas and cardiovascular syphilis
Adults: 2.4 million units I.M. q week for 3 weeks

➢ Yaws, bejel, and pinta
Adults: 1.2 million units I.M. as a single dose
➢ Prophylaxis of rheumatic fever and glomerulonephritis
Adults: After acute attack, 1.2 million units I.M. q month or 600,000 units q 2 weeks

Contraindications

- Hypersensitivity to penicillins, beta-lactamase inhibitors (piperacillin/tazobactam), or benzathine

Precautions

Use cautiously in:

- severe renal insufficiency, significant allergies, asthma
- pregnant or breastfeeding patients.

Administration

- Before giving, ask patient about allergy to penicillin, beta-lactamase inhibitors, and benzathine. Be aware that cross-sensitivity to cephalosporins and imipenem also may occur.
- Inject deep I.M. into upper outer quadrant of buttock in adult or mid-lateral thigh in infant or small child. Don't inject into gluteal muscle in child younger than age 2. Rotate injection sites with repeated doses.
- If using prefilled syringes, follow manufacturer's instructions carefully.

🔊 Keep epinephrine and emergency equipment at hand in case of anaphylaxis.

- Be aware that Hoigne's syndrome (transient bizarre behavior and neurologic reactions) may immediately follow I.M. injection.
- Know that in syphilis treatment, Jarisch-Hersheimer reaction (fever, chills, headache, sweating, malaise, hypotension or hypertension) may occur 2 to 12 hours after therapy begins and usually subsides within 24 hours.

Route	Onset	Peak	Duration
I.M.	Delayed	Dose dependent	Dose dependent

Adverse reactions

CNS: headache, lethargy, hallucinations, anxiety, neuropathy, fatigue, nervousness, tremors, euphoria, asthenia, Hoigne's syndrome, **cerebrovascular accident, seizures, coma**
CV: hypotension, pulmonary hypertension, vasodilation, vasovagal reaction, syncope, palpitations, tachycardia, **cardiac arrest, pulmonary embolism**
EENT: blurred vision, vision loss, laryngeal edema
GI: nausea, vomiting, diarrhea, epigastric distress, abdominal pain, colitis, blood in stool, glossitis, **pseudomembranous colitis**
GU: hematuria, proteinuria, urogenic bladder, erectile dysfunction, priapism, nephropathy, **renal failure**
Hematologic: hemolytic anemia, leukopenia, thrombocytopenia
Metabolic: hypernatremia, **hyperkalemia**
Respiratory: dyspnea, hypoxia, **apnea, pulmonary embolism**
Skin: rash, urticaria, sweating
Other: fever, superinfection, injection site reactions and pain, Jarisch-Hersheimer reaction, **anaphylaxis, serum sickness**

Interactions

Drug-drug. *Aspirin, probenecid:* increased penicillin blood level
Erythromycins, tetracyclines: decreased antimicrobial activity of penicillin
Hormonal contraceptives: decreased contraceptive efficacy
Drug-diagnostic tests. *Alanine aminotransferase, blood urea nitrogen, creatinine, eosinophils, granulocytes, hemoglobin, platelets, potassium, white blood cells:* increased levels
Direct Coombs' test: positive result

p

Sodium: decreased level
Urine glucose, urine protein: false-positive results

Patient monitoring

◀ Watch closely for anaphylaxis and serum sickness.
- In long-term therapy, monitor electrolyte levels and CBC with white cell differential; watch for electrolyte imbalances and blood dyscrasias.
- Assess neurologic status, especially for seizures and decreasing level of consciousness.

◀ Watch for evidence of superinfection and pseudomembranous colitis.

Patient teaching

◀ Teach patient to recognize anaphylaxis symptoms and to contact emergency medical services immediately if these occur.

◀ Tell patient drug may cause diarrhea. Instruct him to immediately report severe, persistent diarrhea, and fever.
- Urge patient to complete entire course of therapy as prescribed, even after symptoms improve.
- Advise patient to contact prescriber if infection symptoms get worse.
- Tell female patient that drug may make hormonal contraceptives ineffective. Advise her to use barrier birth control if she wishes to avoid pregnancy.
- As appropriate, review all other significant and life-threatening adverse reactions and interactions, especially those related to the drugs and tests mentioned above.

penicillin G potassium

Pfizerpen

Pharmacologic class: Penicillin
Therapeutic class: Anti-infective
Pregnancy risk category B

Action

Inhibits biosynthesis of cell-wall mucopeptide; bactericidal against penicillin-susceptible microorganisms during active multiplication stage

Availability

Powder for injection: 1 million, 5 million, and 20 million units/vial
Premixed (frozen) solution for injection: 1 million, 2 million, and 3 million units/50 ml

Indications and dosages

➢ Meningococcal meningitis

Adults: 1 to 2 million units I.M. q 2 hours or 20 to 30 million units/day by continuous I.V. infusion for 14 days, or until afebrile for 7 days

➢ Meningitis caused by susceptible pneumococcal or meningococcal strains

Children: 250,000 units/kg/day in equally divided doses I.M. or by continuous I.V. infusion q 4 hours for 7 to 14 days (depending on causative organism)

Infants older than 7 days: 200,000 to 300,000 units/kg/day I.V. in divided doses q 6 hours

Infants less than 7 days old: 100,000 to 150,000 units/kg/day I.V. in divided doses q 12 hours

➢ Actinomycosis

Adults: 1 to 6 million units/day I.M. or I.V. for cervicofacial infections; 10 to 20 million units/day I.V. q 4 to 6 hours for 6 weeks for thoracic and abdominal infections

➢ Clostridial infections

Adults: 20 million units/day I.M. or I.V. infusion q 4 to 6 hours, given with antitoxin therapy

➢ Fusospirochetal infections

Adults: 5 to 10 million units/day I.M. or 200,000 to 500,000 units I.V. infusion q 4 to 6 hours

➢ Rat bite fever; Haverhill fever

Adults: 12 to 20 million units/day I.M.

or I.V. infusion q 4 to 6 hours for 3 or 4 weeks
➢ *Pasteurella* infections
Adults: 4 to 6 million units/day I.M. or I.V. infusion q 4 to 6 hours for 2 weeks
➢ Erysipeloid endocarditis
Adults: 12 to 20 million units/day I.M. or I.V. infusion q 4 to 6 hours for 4 to 6 weeks
➢ Diphtheria (as adjunctive therapy with antitoxin to prevent carrier state)
Adults: 2 to 3 million units/day I.M. or I.V. infusion in divided doses q 4 to 6 hours for 10 to 12 days
➢ Anthrax
Adults: At least 5 million units/day I.M. or I.V. infusion
➢ Serious streptococcal infections
Adults: 5 to 24 million units/day I.M. or I.V. infusion in divided doses q 4 to 6 hours
➢ Neurosyphilis
Adults: 18 to 24 million units/day I.V. (given in doses of 3 to 4 million units q 4 hours) for 10 to 14 days
➢ *Listeria* infections
Adults: 15 to 20 million units/day I.M. or I.V. infusion q 4 to 6 hours for 2 weeks in meningitis or 4 weeks in endocarditis
➢ Disseminated gonococcal infections
Adults: 10 million units/day I.V. (3 to 4 million units q 4 hours) for 10 to 14 days

Off-label uses

- Lyme disease
- Predental prophylaxis against bacterial endocarditis

Contraindications

- Hypersensitivity to penicillins or beta-lactamase inhibitors (piperacillin/tazobactam)

Precautions

Use cautiously in:
- severe renal insufficiency, significant allergies, asthma
- pregnant or breastfeeding patients.

Administration

- Before giving, ask patient about allergy to penicillin, beta-lactamase inhibitors, or benzathine. Know that cross-sensitivity to imipenem and cephalosporins also may occur.

🔈 Keep epinephrine and emergency equipment at hand in case anaphylaxis occurs.

- For I.V. use, dilute in sterile water for injection, normal saline solution, or dextrose 5% in water (D_5W). For continuous infusion, further dilute in 1 to 2 L of compatible solution and infuse over 24 hours. For intermittent infusion, further dilute in 50 or 100 ml of normal saline solution or D_5W; administer over 1 to 2 hours in adults or 15 to 30 minutes in children and infants.
- Know that drug also may be given by intrapleural or intrathecal route.
- Be aware that in syphilis treatment, Jarisch-Hersheimer reaction (fever, chills, headache, sweating, malaise, hypotension or hypertension) may occur 2 to 12 hours after therapy starts and usually subsides within 24 hours.

Route	Onset	Peak	Duration
I.M.	Rapid	15-30 min	4-6 hr
I.V.	Rapid	End of infusion	4-6 hr

P

Adverse reactions

CNS: hyperreflexia, neuropathy, **coma, seizures**
CV: arrhythmias, cardiac arrest, heart failure (with high I.V. doses)
GI: nausea, vomiting, diarrhea, epigastric distress, abdominal pain, colitis, blood in stool, glossitis, **pseudomembranous colitis**
GU: nephropathy
Hematologic: hemolytic anemia, leukopenia, thrombocytopenia
Metabolic: hyperkalemia (with high-dose, continuous I.V. infusion)
Skin: rash, urticaria, exfoliative dermatitis

Other: pain at I.M. injection site, phlebitis at I.V. site, Jarisch-Hersheimer reaction, superinfection, **anaphylaxis, serum sickness**

Interactions

Drug-drug. *Aspirin, probenecid:* increased penicillin blood level
Erythromycins, tetracyclines: decreased antimicrobial activity of penicillin
Hormonal contraceptives: decreased contraceptive efficacy
Drug-diagnostic tests. *Alanine aminotransferase, eosinophils, granulocytes, hemoglobin, platelets, potassium, white blood cells:* increased levels
Direct Coombs' test: positive result
Sodium: decreased level
Urine glucose, urine protein: false-positive results

Patient monitoring

🔊 Watch closely for signs and symptoms of anaphylaxis and serum sickness.
• In long-term therapy, monitor electrolyte levels and CBC with white cell differential; watch for electrolyte imbalances and blood dyscrasias.
• Closely monitor neurologic status, especially for seizures and decreasing level of consciousness.
🔊 Stay alert for signs and symptoms of superinfection and pseudomembranous colitis.

Patient teaching

🔊 Teach patient to recognize signs and symptoms of anaphylaxis. Tell him to contact emergency medical services immediately if these occur.
🔊 Tell patient drug may cause diarrhea. Instruct him to immediately report severe, persistent diarrhea and fever.
• Urge patient to complete entire course of therapy as prescribed, even after symptoms improve.
• Tell patient to contact prescriber if infection symptoms worsen.
• Inform female patient that drug may make hormonal contraceptives ineffective. Advise her to use barrier birth-control method if she wishes to avoid pregnancy.
• As appropriate, review all other significant and life-threatening adverse reactions and interactions, especially those related to the drugs and tests mentioned above.

penicillin G procaine

Ayercillin✤, Crysticillin-AS✤, Wycillin

Pharmacologic class: Penicillin
Therapeutic class: Anti-infective
Pregnancy risk category B

Action

Inhibits biosynthesis of cell-wall mucopeptide; bactericidal against penicillin-susceptible microorganisms during active multiplication stage

Availability

Suspension for I.M. injection: 600,000 units/ml vial, 1.2 million units/2-ml vial, 2.4 million units/4-ml vial, 3 million units/10-ml vial

Indications and dosages

➤ Anthrax; bacterial endocarditis; erysipeloid and fusospirochetal infections; group A streptococcal infections; moderately severe, uncomplicated pneumococcal pneumonia and staphylococcal infections; rat-bite fever
Adults: 600,000 to 1 million units/day I.M.
➤ Diphtheria
Adults: 300,000 to 600,000 units/day I.M. given with antitoxin for 14 days. For carrier state, 300,000 units/day I.M. for 10 days.
➤ Syphilis; yaws; bejel; pinta
Adults and children older than age 12: 600,000 units/day I.M. for 8 days; for

late infections, continue for 10 to 15 days. For neurosyphilis, 2.4 million units/day I.M. for 10 to 14 days, given with probenecid.

➢ Congenital syphilis
Children: 50,000 units/kg I.M. daily for at least 10 days

➢ Uncomplicated gonorrhea
Adults: 4.8 million units/day I.M., divided into at least two doses and two sites at one visit, with P.O. probenecid given 30 minutes before injection

Off-label uses

- Lyme disease
- Predental prophylaxis against bacterial endocarditis

Contraindications

- Hypersensitivity to penicillins, beta-lactamase inhibitors (piperacillin/tazobactam), or procaine

Precautions

Use cautiously in:

- severe renal insufficiency, significant allergies, asthma
- pregnant or breastfeeding patients
- neonates.

Administration

- Before giving, ask patient about allergy to penicillin, beta-lactamase inhibitors, or benzathine. Know that cross-sensitivity to imipenem and cephalosporins may occur.

Keep epinephrine and emergency equipment at hand in case anaphylaxis occurs.

- In adults, inject I.M. deep into upper outer aspect of buttock.
- In infants and small children, inject at a slow, steady rate into midlateral aspect of thigh.
- Be aware that Hoigne's syndrome (transient bizarre behavior and neurologic reactions) may immediately follow I.M. injection.
- Know that in syphilis treatment, Jarisch-Hersheimer reaction (fever, chills, headache, sweating, malaise, hypotension or hypertension) may occur 2 to 12 hours after therapy starts and usually subsides within 24 hours.

Route	Onset	Peak	Duration
I.M.	Delayed	1-3 hr	24 hr

Adverse reactions

CNS: lethargy, hallucinations, anxiety, depression, twitching, Hoigne's syndrome, **seizures, coma**
EENT: laryngeal edema
GI: nausea, vomiting, diarrhea, epigastric distress, abdominal pain, colitis, blood in stool, glossitis, **pseudomembranous colitis**
GU: interstitial nephritis
Hematologic: increased bleeding, hemolytic anemia, bone marrow depression, leukopenia, thrombocytopenia, granulocytopenia
Skin: rash, urticaria
Other: pain at I.M. injection site, fever, superinfection, Jarisch-Hersheimer reaction, sterile abscess, procaine toxicity, **anaphylaxis, serum sickness**

Interactions

Drug-drug. *Aspirin, probenecid:* increased penicillin blood level
Erythromycins, tetracyclines: decreased antimicrobial activity of penicillin
Hormonal contraceptives: decreased contraceptive efficacy
Drug-diagnostic tests. *Alanine aminotransferase, eosinophils, granulocytes, hemoglobin, platelets, potassium, white blood cells:* increased levels
Direct Coombs' test: positive result
Sodium: decreased level
Urine glucose, urine protein: false-positive results

Patient monitoring

Watch closely for signs and symptoms of anaphylaxis and serum sickness.

- In long-term therapy, monitor electrolyte levels and CBC with white cell

differential. Watch for electrolyte imbalances and blood dyscrasias.
• Assess neurologic status, especially for seizures and decreasing level of consciousness.
🔊 Monitor patient for signs and symptoms of superinfection and pseudomembranous colitis.

Patient teaching

🔊 Teach patient to recognize signs and symptoms of anaphylaxis. Tell him to contact emergency medical services immediately if these occur.
🔊 Tell patient drug may cause diarrhea. Instruct him to immediately report severe, persistent diarrhea and fever.
• Stress importance of completing entire course of therapy as prescribed, even after symptoms improve.
• Advise patient to contact prescriber if infection symptoms worsen.
• Tell female patient that drug may make hormonal contraceptives ineffective. Encourage her to use barrier birth-control method if she wishes to avoid pregnancy.
• As appropriate, review all other significant and life-threatening adverse reactions and interactions, especially those related to the drugs and tests mentioned above.

penicillin V potassium

Apo-Pen VK✤, Nadopen-V✤, Novo-Pen-VK✤, Pen-Vee, Pen-Vee K, PVF K✤, Veetids

Pharmacologic class: Penicillin
Therapeutic class: Anti-infective
Pregnancy risk category B

Action

Inhibits biosynthesis of cell-wall mucopeptide; bactericidal against penicillin-susceptible microorganisms during active multiplication stage

Availability

Oral solution: 200,000 units (125 mg)/5 ml, 400,000 units (250 mg)/5 ml
Tablets: 400,000 units (250 mg), 800,000 units (500 mg)

Indications and dosages

➢ Upper respiratory streptococcal infections, including scarlet fever and mild erysipelas
Adults and children ages 12 and older: 125 to 250 mg P.O. q 6 to 8 hours for 10 days
Children younger than age 12: 25 to 50 mg/kg/day P.O. in divided doses q 6 hours for 10 days
➢ Pneumococcal respiratory infections, including otitis media
Adults and children ages 12 and older: 250 to 500 mg P.O. q 6 hours until afebrile for at least 2 days
➢ Skin and soft-tissue staphylococcal infections; fusospirochetosis (Vincent's infection) of oropharynx
Adults and children ages 12 and older: 250 to 500 mg P.O. q 6 to 8 hours
➢ To prevent recurrence of rheumatic fever or chorea
Adults and children ages 12 and older: 125 to 250 mg P.O. b.i.d. on a continuing basis

Off-label uses

• Prophylaxis of *Streptococcus pneumoniae* septicemia in children with sickle cell anemia or splenectomy
• Early Lyme disease
• Actinomycosis
• Preexposure prophylaxis of anthrax
• Prophylaxis of bacterial endocarditis for dental procedures

Contraindications

• Hypersensitivity to penicillins or beta-lactamase inhibitors (piperacillin/tazobactam)

Precautions

Use cautiously in:

- severe renal insufficiency
- pregnant or breastfeeding patients.

Administration

- Before giving, ask patient about allergies to penicillin, beta-lactamase inhibitors, or benzathine. Know that cross-sensitivity to imipenem and cephalosporins may occur.

🔊 Keep epinephrine and emergency equipment at hand in case anaphylaxis occurs.

- Give with water 1 hour before or 2 hours after meals. Don't give with fruit juice or carbonated beverages.

Route	Onset	Peak	Duration
P.O.	Unknown	1 hr	6 hr

Adverse reactions

CNS: lethargy, hallucinations, anxiety, depression, twitching, **seizures, coma**
GI: nausea, vomiting, diarrhea, epigastric distress, abdominal pain, colitis, blood in stool, glossitis, **pseudomembranous colitis**
GU: interstitial nephritis
Hematologic: anemia, **hemolytic anemia, increased bleeding, leukopenia, granulocytopenia, bone marrow depression, thrombocytopenia, thrombocytopenic purpura**
Metabolic: hypokalemia, **hyperkalemia, metabolic alkalosis**
Skin: rash, urticaria
Other: fever, superinfection, **anaphylaxis, serum sickness**

Interactions

Drug-drug. *Aspirin, probenecid:* increased penicillin blood level
Erythromycins, tetracyclines: decreased antimicrobial activity of penicillin
Hormonal contraceptives: decreased contraceptive efficacy
Drug-diagnostic tests. *Alanine aminotransferase, eosinophils, granulocytes, hemoglobin, platelets:* increased levels
Albumin, lymphocytes, protein, sodium, uric acid, white blood cells: decreased levels
Direct Coombs' test: positive result
Potassium: increased or decreased level
Urine glucose, urine protein: false-positive results
Drug-herbs. *Khat:* delayed and reduced penicillin absorption

Patient monitoring

🔊 Watch for signs and symptoms of anaphylaxis and serum sickness.

- In long-term therapy, monitor electrolyte levels and CBC with white cell differential; watch for electrolyte imbalances and blood dyscrasias.
- Assess neurologic status, especially for seizures and decreasing level of consciousness.

🔊 Monitor patient closely for signs and symptoms of superinfection and pseudomembranous colitis.

Patient teaching

- Instruct patient to take with water 1 hour before or 2 hours after meals. Tell him not to take with fruit juice or carbonated beverages.

🔊 Teach patient to recognize anaphylaxis symptoms. Tell him to immediately contact emergency medical services if these occur.

- Instruct patient to report signs and symptoms of superinfection.
- Advise patient to contact prescriber if infection symptoms get worse.

🔊 Tell patient drug may cause diarrhea. Instruct him to immediately report severe, persistent diarrhea and fever.

- Instruct patient to complete entire course of therapy as prescribed, even after symptoms improve.
- Tell female patient drug may make hormonal contraceptives ineffective. Advise her to use barrier birth-control method if she wishes to avoid pregnancy.

p

• As appropriate, review all other significant and life-threatening adverse reactions and interactions, especially those related to the drugs, tests, and herbs mentioned above.

pentamidine isethionate

NebuPent, Pentacarinat✦, Pentam 300, Pneumopent✦

Pharmacologic class: Antiprotozoal
Therapeutic class: Anti-infective
Pregnancy risk category C

Action

Unknown. May interfere with nuclear metabolism and synthesis of DNA, RNA, and proteins.

Availability

Aerosol: 300 mg
Injection: 300 mg/vial

Indications and dosages

➢ *Pneumocystis jiroveci* pneumonia
Adults and children ages 5 and older: 4 mg/kg I.V. or deep I.M. daily for 14 days
➢ To prevent *P. jiroveci* pneumonia in high-risk patients with human immunodeficiency virus
Adults: 300 mg by inhalation once q 4 weeks using Respigard II nebulizer

Off-label uses

• Trypanosomiasis
• Visceral leishmaniasis

Contraindications

• History of anaphylaxis from pentamidine or diamidine compounds (inhalation only)
(*Note:* No absolute contraindications exist for patients with *P. jiroveci.*)

Precautions

Use cautiously in:
• anemia, blood dyscrasias, hepatic or renal disease, hypoglycemia, diabetes mellitus, ventricular tachycardia, hypocalcemia, hypertension, hypotension
• pregnant or breastfeeding patients
• children (safety and efficacy of inhalation solution not established).

Administration

• For I.V. infusion, dilute 300 mg-vial with sterile water for injection. Withdraw prescribed dosage, then dilute further in 50 to 250 ml of dextrose 5% in water; infuse over 60 to 120 minutes.
• For I.M. use, dilute 300 mg-vial with 3 ml of sterile water for injection. Withdraw prescribed dosage; administer deep I.M. using Z-track method.
• Keep patient supine during I.M. or I.V. administration to minimize hypotension.
• For inhalation, dilute in 6 ml of sterile water and administer through nebulizer at a flow rate of 6 L/minute from 50-psi compressed air source. Don't mix inhalation solution with other drugs.

Route	Onset	Peak	Duration
I.V.	Unknown	1 hr	Unknown
I.M., inhalation	Unknown	0.5 hr	Unknown

Adverse reactions

CNS: headache, disorientation, hallucinations, dizziness, confusion, fatigue, neuralgia
CV: chest pain, ECG abnormalities, syncope, vasodilation, vasculitis, phlebitis, hypertension, palpitations, **arrhythmias, severe hypotension**
EENT: pharyngitis
GI: nausea, vomiting, diarrhea, abdominal pain, anorexia, **acute pancreatitis**
Hematologic: anemia, **leukopenia, thrombocytopenia**

Metabolic: hypocalcemia, hyperglycemia, **hypoglycemia, hyperkalemia**
Musculoskeletal: myalgia
Respiratory: cough, dyspnea, congestion, **pneumothorax, bronchospasm**
Skin: rash, night sweats, urticaria, sterile abscess or induration at injection site
Other: metallic or bad taste, fever, chills, pain at injection site or elsewhere, edema, allergic reactions

Interactions

Drug-diagnostic tests. *Blood urea nitrogen, creatinine, liver function tests, potassium:* increased values
Calcium, hemoglobin, hematocrit, platelets, white blood cells: decreased levels
ECG: alterations
Glucose: increased or decreased level

Patient monitoring

🔊 Closely monitor blood pressure and blood glucose. Watch for arrhythmias and evidence of pulmonary infection, blood dyscrasias, and pancreatitis during and after I.M. or I.V. administration, until patient is stable. (Severe, life-threatening reactions may occur.)
- Assess I.V. site closely during and after I.V. administration. Know that sterile abscess, pain, or induration may occur at injection site.
- Evaluate neurologic status.
- Monitor CBC (including platelet count), calcium and potassium levels, and kidney and liver function tests.

Patient teaching

- Explain purpose of therapy. Stress importance of completing entire course of treatment.

🔊 Teach patient to recognize and immediately report serious cardiovascular and neurologic reactions, abdominal pain, and easy bruising or bleeding.
- Teach patient how to use aerosol.
- Tell patient to notify prescriber if infection worsens.
- Advise patient to minimize GI upset by eating small, frequent servings of food and drinking plenty of fluids.
- Caution patient to avoid driving and other hazardous activities until he knows how drug affects concentration and alertness.
- As appropriate, review all other significant and life-threatening adverse reactions and interactions, especially those related to the tests mentioned above.

pentazocine hydrochloride
Talwin

pentazocine hydrochloride and acetaminophen
Talacen

pentazocine hydrochloride and naloxone hydrochloride
Talwin Nx

Pharmacologic class: Opioid agonist-antagonist
Therapeutic class: Opioid analgesic, adjunct to anesthesia
Controlled substance schedule IV
Pregnancy risk category C

Action

Unknown. Thought to interact with opioid receptor sites primarily in limbic system, thalamus, and spinal cord, blocking transmission of pain impulses.

Availability

Injection: 30 mg/ml (as lactate salt)
Tablets: 50 mg pentazocine and 0.5 mg naloxone (Talwin NX); 25 mg pentazocine and 650 mg acetaminophen (Talacen)

Indications and dosages

➢ Moderate to severe pain; preoperative or preanesthetic medication; adjunct to surgical anesthesia
Adults: 30 mg subcutaneously, I.M., or I.V. q 3 to 4 hours (not to exceed 60 mg/dose subcutaneously or I.M., or 30 mg/dose I.V.). Maximum daily dosage is 360 mg.

➢ Moderate to severe pain
Adults: Initially, one tablet (Talwin Nx) q 3 to 4 hours, increased to two tablets p.r.n., up to a maximum of 12 tablets daily

➢ Mild to moderate pain
Adults: One tablet (Talacen) P.O. q 4 hours; up to a maximum of six tablets daily

➢ Labor
Adults: 20 mg I.V. for two or three doses at 2- to 3-hour intervals, or 30 mg I.M. as a single dose

Contraindications

• Hypersensitivity to drug, acetaminophen, or naloxone (with oral form)

Precautions

Use cautiously in:

• head trauma, increased intracranial pressure, respiratory conditions, adrenal insufficiency, seizure disorder, acute CNS manifestations, hepatic impairment, acute myocardial infarction, alcohol or narcotic use
• sulfite sensitivity (Talacen)
• history of drug abuse
• pregnant or breastfeeding patients
• children (safety not established).

Administration

• Administer each 5-mg I.V. dose by slow direct infusion over 1 minute, with patient lying supine.
• Use subcutaneous route only when necessary (may cause tissue damage).

Route	Onset	Peak	Duration
P.O. (Talwin NX)	15-30 min	1-3 hr	3 hr
P.O. (Talacen)	15-30 min	60-90 min	3 hr
I.V.	12-30 min	Unknown	3 hr
I.M., subcut.	15-20 min	15-60 min	3 hr

Adverse reactions

CNS: dizziness, drowsiness, euphoria, hallucinations, headache, sedation, dysphoria, insomnia, unusual dreams, weakness, depression, irritability, excitement, tremor, paresthesia
CV: hypertension, hypotension, syncope, tachycardia, **circulatory depression, shock**
EENT: blurred vision, diplopia, nystagmus, miosis (with high doses), tinnitus
GI: nausea, vomiting, constipation, diarrhea, dry mouth, ileus, cramps, abdominal distress, anorexia
GU: urinary retention, altered rate and strength of labor contractions
Hematologic: thrombocytopenia purpura (with Talacen)
Respiratory: dyspnea, transient apnea in neonates whose mothers received pentazocine during labor, **respiratory depression**
Skin: clammy skin, diaphoresis, rash, urticaria, nodules, cutaneous depression, skin and subcutaneous sclerosis, dermatitis, pruritus, flushing
Other: altered taste, chills, soft-tissue induration, stinging on injection, facial edema, physical or psychological drug dependence, drug tolerance, **anaphylaxis**

Interactions

Drug-drug. *Barbiturates, first-generation (sedating) antihistamines, other sedating drugs:* additive CNS depression
MAO inhibitors: unpredictable reactions
Opioids: decreased analgesic effects

Drug-diagnostic tests. *Amylase, lipase:* increased levels
Granulocytes, white blood cells: reduced counts
Drug-herbs. *Chamomile, hops, kava, skullcap, valerian:* increased CNS depression
Drug-behaviors. *Alcohol use:* increased CNS depression

Patient monitoring

Monitor vital signs. Watch closely for evidence of shock, dyspnea, and circulatory or respiratory depression.
- Monitor drug efficacy.
- In prolonged use, assess for signs and symptoms of drug dependence.

Patient teaching

Tell patient receiving Talacen or Talwin NX that drug is for oral use only. Life-threatening reactions may result from misusing drug by injection.
- Inform patient that withdrawal symptoms may occur if he stops taking drug suddenly after prolonged use.
- Urge patient to avoid alcohol.
- Advise patient to consult prescriber before taking other prescription drugs or over-the-counter preparations.
- Caution patient to avoid driving and other hazardous activities until he knows how drug affects him.
- Advise patient to have periodic eye exams.
- As appropriate, review all other significant and life-threatening adverse reactions and interactions, especially those related to the drugs, tests, herbs, and behaviors mentioned above.

pentobarbital sodium

Nembutal Sodium

Pharmacologic class: Barbiturate
Therapeutic class: Sedative-hypnotic, anticonvulsant
Controlled substance schedule II
Pregnancy risk category D

Action

Depresses sensory cortex, decreases motor activity, and alters cerebellar function; may interfere with nerve impulse transmission in brain

Availability

Capsules: 100 mg
Elixir: 20 mg/5 ml
Injection: 50 mg/ml in 2-ml prefilled syringes
Suppositories: 30 mg, 120 mg, 200 mg

Indications and dosages

➢ Sedation

Adults: 20 to 30 mg P.O. three to four times daily. Alternatively, 120 to 200 mg P.R as a single dose.
Children: 2 to 6 mg/kg P.O. daily in divided doses; maximum of 100 mg/dose daily.
Alternatively, for P.R. dosing—
Children ages 12 to 14 weighing 36.4 to 50 kg (80 to 110 lb): 60 or 120 mg P.R.
Children ages 5 to 12 weighing 18.2 to 36.4 kg (40 to 80 lb): 60 mg P.R.
Children ages 1 to 4 weighing 9 to 18.2 kg (20 to 40 lb): 30 or 60 mg P.R.
Children ages 2 months to 1 year weighing 4.5 to 9 kg (10 to 20 lb): 30 mg P.R.

➢ Preoperative sedation

Adults: Initially, 100 mg P.O., 150 to 200 mg I.M., or 100 mg I.V.

➢ Seizures

Adults: Initially, 100 mg. I.V.; may give

P

additional doses after 1 minute. Maximum dosage is 500 mg.
Children: Initially, 50 mg. I.V.; may give additional doses until desired response occurs. Don't exceed 100 mg/dose.

Contraindications

- Hypersensitivity to drug or other barbiturates
- Nephritis (with large doses)
- Severe hepatic impairment
- Severe respiratory disease with dyspnea or obstruction
- Manifest or latent porphyria
- History of sedative-hypnotic abuse
- Subcutaneous or intra-arterial administration

Precautions

Use cautiously in:

- hepatic or renal impairment, increased risk for suicide, alcohol use
- history of drug addiction
- labor and delivery
- elderly or debilitated patients.

Administration

🔊 When giving I.V., make sure resuscitation equipment is available.

- Give I.V. by direct injection no faster than 50 mg/minute.
- Inject I.M. deep into large muscle mass.

🔊 Don't give by subcutaneous or intra-arterial routes, because severe reactions (such as tissue necrosis and gangrene) may occur.

- Know that drug is for short-term use only, losing efficacy after about 2 weeks.
- Be aware that rectal suppositories are used when P.O. or parenteral administration isn't undesirable.
- Don't divide rectal suppositories.

Route	Onset	Peak	Duration
P.O.	15-60 min	3-4 hr	3-4 hr
I.V.	Immediate	1 min	3-4 hr
I.M.	10-25 min	Unknown	3-4 hr
Rectal	20-60 min	Unknown	3-4 hr

Adverse reactions

CNS: drowsiness, agitation, confusion, hyperkinesia, ataxia, nightmares, nervousness, hallucinations, insomnia, anxiety, abnormal thinking
CV: hypotension, syncope, **bradycardia** (all with I.V. use)
GI: nausea, vomiting, constipation
Hepatic: hepatic damage
Musculoskeletal: joint pain, myalgia, neuralgia
Respiratory: laryngospasm (with I.V. use), **bronchospasm, respiratory depression**
Skin: rash, urticaria, exfoliative dermatitis
Other: phlebitis at I.V. site, physical or psychological drug dependence, fever, hypersensitivity reactions including angioedema

Interactions

Drug-drug. *Acetaminophen:* increased risk of hepatotoxicity
Activated charcoal: decreased pentobarbital absorption
Anticoagulants, beta-adrenergic blockers (except timolol), carbamazepine, clonazepam, corticosteroids, digoxin, doxorubicin, doxycycline, felodipine, fenoprofen, griseofulvin, hormonal contraceptives, metronidazole, quinidine, theophylline, verapamil: decreased efficacy of these drugs
Antihistamines (first-generation), opioids, other sedative-hypnotics: additive CNS depression
Chloramphenicol, hydantoins, narcotics: increased or decreased effects of either drug
Divalproex, MAO inhibitors, valproic

acid: decreased pentobarbital metabolism, increased sedation
Rifampin: increased pentobarbital metabolism and decreased effects
Drug-diagnostic tests. *Sulfobromophthalein:* false increase
Drug-herbs. *Chamomile, hops, kava, valerian, or skullcap:* increased CNS depression
St. John's wort: decreased pentobarbital effects
Drug-behaviors. *Alcohol use:* increased sedation, additive CNS depression

Patient monitoring

Closely monitor blood pressure and heart and respiratory rates. Watch for evidence of respiratory depression.
- Monitor neurologic status before and during therapy.
- Assess CBC and kidney and liver function tests.
- In long-term therapy, monitor patient for signs of drug dependence.

Patient teaching

- Instruct patient to take exactly as prescribed.
- Tell patient that increasing dosage without prescriber's approval may lead to dependence.
- Advise patient to avoid other CNS depressants, alcohol, and herbs.
- Caution patient to avoid driving and other hazardous activities.
- Advise patient taking hormonal contraceptives to use alternate birth-control method during therapy.
- As appropriate, review all other significant and life-threatening adverse reactions and interactions, especially those related to the drugs, tests, herbs, and behaviors mentioned above.

pentostatin

Nipent

Pharmacologic class: Antimetabolite
Therapeutic class: Antineoplastic
Pregnancy risk category D

Action

Unknown. Thought to inhibit adenosine deaminase, thereby increasing levels of deoxyadenosine triphosphate in cells, blocking DNA synthesis, and inhibiting ribonucleotide reductase.

Availability

Powder for injection: 10-mg vials

Indications and dosages

➢ Hairy cell leukemia
Adults: 4 mg/m^2 I.V. every other week

Contraindications

- Hypersensitivity to drug

Precautions

Use cautiously in:
- renal disease, bone marrow depression
- pregnant or breastfeeding patients
- children.

Administration

- Before giving, hydrate patient with 500 to 1,000 ml of dextrose 5% and normal saline solution (or its equivalent). After administering, give 500 ml of dextrose 5% in water (D_5W) or its equivalent.

Follow facility protocol for handling, administering, and disposing of chemotherapeutic drugs.
- Give by direct I.V. bolus injection or dilute with 25 to 50 ml of D_5W or normal saline solution; infuse over 20 to 30 minutes.

P

Route	Onset	Peak	Duration
I.V.	Unknown	Unknown	Unknown

Adverse reactions

CNS: headache, malaise, anxiety, confusion, depression, dizziness, insomnia, nervousness, paresthesia, drowsiness, abnormal thinking, fatigue, asthenia, hallucinations, hostility, amnesia
CV: peripheral edema, cellulitis, vasculitis, hypotension, angina, tachycardia, bradycardia, phlebitis, **thrombophlebitis, cardiac arrest, heart failure, hemorrhage, ventricular asystole, pericardial effusion, sinus arrest**
EENT: abnormal vision, nonreactive pupils, photophobia, retinopathy, eye pain, conjunctivitis, dry or watery eyes, hearing loss, tinnitus, ear pain, epistaxis, pharyngitis, rhinitis
GI: nausea, vomiting, diarrhea, constipation, dyspepsia, abdominal pain, ileus, flatulence, stomatitis, glossitis, anorexia
GU: amenorrhea, breast lump, erectile dysfunction, decreased libido, renal calculi, **renal dysfunction, renal insufficiency, renal failure**
Hematologic: ecchymosis, anemia, **hemolytic anemia, agranulocytosis, aplastic anemia, leukopenia, thrombocytopenia**
Metabolic: hyperuricemia, hypercalcemia, hyponatremia
Musculoskeletal: myalgia, joint pain
Respiratory: cough, dyspnea, respiratory tract infection, **pulmonary embolism**
Skin: rash, eczema, petechiae, dry skin, pruritus, skin disorder, furunculosis, acne, alopecia, diaphoresis, photosensitivity
Other: unusual taste, gingivitis, fever, chills, pain, facial edema, lymphadenopathy, herpes simplex or herpes zoster infection, flulike symptoms, viral or bacterial infection, allergic reaction, **sepsis, neoplasm**

Interactions

Drug-drug. *Allopurinol:* hypersensitivity vasculitis
Carmustine, cyclophosphamide, etoposide: potentially fatal acute pulmonary edema and hypotension
Fludarabine: severe or fatal pulmonary toxicity
Vidarabine: increased risk and severity of adverse reactions
Drug-diagnostic tests. *Calcium, liver function tests, serum uric acid:* increased values
Granulocytes, platelets, sodium, white blood cells: decreased levels

Patient monitoring

Monitor CBC (including platelet count). Watch for evidence of blood dyscrasias.
• Assess kidney and liver function tests. Stay alert for evidence of organ dysfunction.
• Monitor temperature. Watch for signs and symptoms of bacterial and viral infection.
• Closely monitor vital signs and ECG, particularly for life-threatening arrhythmias, heart failure, and pulmonary edema.

Patient teaching

Tell patient drug lowers resistance to infection. Instruct him to avoid crowds and to immediately report fever, cough, sore throat, and other infection symptoms.
• Advise patient to minimize GI upset by eating small, frequent servings of food and drinking plenty of fluids.
• Instruct female patient of childbearing age to avoid pregnancy during drug therapy and to seek medical advice before becoming pregnant.
• Caution patient to avoid driving and other hazardous activities until he knows how drug affects concentration and alertness.
• As appropriate, review all other significant and life-threatening adverse

reactions and interactions, especially those related to the drugs and tests mentioned above.

pentoxifylline

Trental

Pharmacologic class: Hemorrheologic, xanthine derivative

Therapeutic class: Hematologic agent

Pregnancy risk category C

Action

Unknown. Thought to enhance blood flow to the circulatory system by increasing vasoconstriction and oxygen concentrations.

Availability

Tablets (controlled-release, extended-release): 400 mg

Indications and dosages

➢ Intermittent claudication

Adults: 400 mg t.i.d. If adverse reactions occur, decrease to 400 mg b.i.d.

Dosage adjustment

- Renal impairment

Off-label uses

- Diabetic angiopathies and neuropathies
- Transient ischemic attacks
- Severe idiopathic recurrent aphthous stomatitis
- Raynaud's phenomenon

Contraindications

- Hypersensitivity to drug or methylxanthines (such as caffeine, theophylline, theobromine)
- Recent cerebral or retinal hemorrhage

Precautions

Use cautiously in:

- patients at risk for bleeding
- pregnant or breastfeeding patients
- children (safety not established).

Administration

- Give with meals to minimize GI distress.
- Make sure patient swallows tablets whole without crushing, breaking, or chewing.

Route	Onset	Peak	Duration
P.O.	Variable	2-4 hr	8 hr

Adverse reactions

CNS: agitation, dizziness, drowsiness, headache, insomnia, nervousness, tremor, anxiety, confusion, malaise

CV: angina, edema, hypotension, **arrhythmias**

EENT: blurred vision, epistaxis, laryngitis, nasal congestion, sore throat

GI: nausea, vomiting, constipation, diarrhea, abdominal discomfort, belching, bloating, dyspepsia, flatus, cholecystitis, dry mouth, excessive salivation, anorexia

Hematologic: leukopenia

Respiratory: dyspnea

Skin: rash, urticaria, pruritus, brittle fingernails, flushing, angioedema

Other: bad taste, weight changes, thirst, flulike symptoms, lymphadenopathy

Interactions

Drug-drug. *Anticoagulants, nonsteroidal anti-inflammatory drugs (NSAIDs):* increased risk of bleeding

Antihypertensives: additive hypotension

Theobromide, theophylline: increased risk of theophylline toxicity

Drug-herbs. *Anise, arnica, asafetida, chamomile, clove, dong quai, fenugreek, feverfew, garlic, ginger, ginkgo, ginseng, licorice:* increased risk of bleeding

Drug-behaviors. *Smoking:* decreased pentoxifylline efficacy

P

Patient monitoring

- Monitor vital signs and cardiovascular status. Watch for arrhythmias, angina, edema, and hypotension.
- Frequently monitor prothrombin time and International Normalized Ratio in patients receiving warfarin concurrently.
- Assess theophylline level in patients receiving theophylline-containing drugs concurrently.

Patient teaching

- Instruct patient to take with meals and to swallow tablets whole without crushing, breaking, or chewing.

Inform patient that drug can cause serious adverse effects. Instruct him to immediately report chest pain, swelling, and flulike symptoms.

- Tell patient smoking may make drug less effective and that many over-the-counter preparations (including aspirin, NSAIDs, and herbs) increase risk of bleeding.
- As appropriate, review all other significant and life-threatening adverse reactions and interactions, especially those related to the drugs, herbs, and behaviors mentioned above.

perindopril erbumine

Aceon

Pharmacologic class: Angiotensin-converting enzyme (ACE) inhibitor

Therapeutic class: Antihypertensive

Pregnancy risk category C (first trimester), ***D*** (second and third trimesters)

Action

Inhibits conversion of angiotensin I to angiotensin II (a potent vasoconstrictor). This effect leads to decreased plasma angiotensin II, reduced vasoconstriction, enhanced plasma renin activity, and decreased aldosterone activity.

Availability

Tablets: 2 mg, 4 mg, 8 mg

Indications and dosages

➢ Essential hypertension

Adults: 4 mg P.O. daily; may titrate upward to 16 mg/day, given as a single dose or in two divided doses. (Start with 2 to 4 mg/day in patients receiving diuretics.)

Dosage adjustment

- Renal impairment
- Elderly patients

Off-label uses

- Heart failure
- Diabetic nephropathy

Contraindications

- Hypersensitivity to drug or other ACE inhibitors
- Angioedema during previous ACE inhibitor use
- Pregnancy

Precautions

Use cautiously in:

- hepatic failure, renal impairment, renal artery stenosis, hyperkalemia, cough
- black patients with hypertension
- breastfeeding patients
- children (safety not established).

Administration

- Give without regard to food.

Know that drug (especially first dose) may cause angioedema. Keep epinephrine and antihistamines at hand in case of airway obstruction.

- For elderly patient, titrate dosage upward very slowly.
- Know that drug may be given alone or with other drugs.

Route	Onset	Peak	Duration
P.O.	1 hr	3-7 hr	12-24 hr

Adverse reactions

CNS: dizziness, fatigue, headache, insomnia, sleep disorder, weakness, asthenia, drowsiness, vertigo, depression, paresthesia
CV: hypotension, angina pectoris, palpitations, chest pain, abnormal ECG, tachycardia
EENT: ear infection, sinusitis, rhinitis, pharyngitis
GI: nausea, vomiting, diarrhea, abdominal pain, flatulence
GU: proteinuria, urinary tract infection, erectile or other male sexual dysfunction, decreased libido, menstrual disorder
Metabolic: hyperkalemia
Musculoskeletal: back, arm, leg, neck, or joint pain; hypertonia; myalgia; arthritis
Respiratory: cough, upper respiratory infection
Skin: rash, **angioedema**
Other: fever, viral infection, edema

Interactions

Drug-drug. *Antacids:* decreased perindopril absorption
Antihypertensives, general anesthetics, nitrates, phenothiazines: additive hypotension
Cyclosporine, heparin, indomethacin, potassium-sparing diuretics, potassium supplements: hyperkalemia
Diuretics: excessive hypotension
Lithium: increased lithium toxicity
Nonsteroidal anti-inflammatory drugs: blunted antihypertensive response
Drug-diagnostic tests. *Alanine aminotransferase, aspartate aminotransferase, blood urea nitrogen, creatinine, potassium, triglycerides:* increased levels
Hematocrit, hemoglobin: decreased values
Drug-food. *Salt substitutes containing potassium:* hyperkalemia
Drug-herbs. *Capsaicin:* cough
Drug-behaviors. *Acute alcohol ingestion:* additive hypotension

Patient monitoring

- Assess blood pressure. Be aware that dosage increases or concomitant diuretic use may cause severe hypotension.

[Clinical alert] Watch for angioedema, especially after first dose.

- Stay alert for signs and symptoms of infection, particularly EENT and respiratory infections.
- Monitor potassium level. Watch for signs and symptoms of hyperkalemia.
- Monitor liver and kidney function tests before and during therapy.

[Clinical alert] In black patients, watch closely for angioedema and monitor drug efficacy. Monotherapy may be less effective in these patients.

Patient teaching

- Tell patient to take at same time each day, with or without food.

[Clinical alert] Instruct patient to stop using drug and contact prescriber immediately if hoarseness or difficulty swallowing or breathing occurs.

- Tell patient to avoid excessive perspiration or decreased fluid intake, which may cause symptomatic blood pressure drop. Inform him that vomiting or diarrhea also may lower blood pressure.
- Tell patient to report signs and symptoms of infection.
- Advise patient not to use potassium-containing salt substitutes.

[Clinical alert] Caution female patient of childbearing age to contact prescriber immediately if she suspects pregnancy.

- As appropriate, review all other significant and life-threatening adverse reactions and interactions, especially those related to the drugs, tests, foods, herbs, and behaviors mentioned above.

P

perphenazine

Apo-Perphenazine✤, Phenazine✤, Trilafon

Pharmacologic class: Phenothiazine, dopaminergic antagonist

Therapeutic class: Antipsychotic, antiemetic

Pregnancy risk category NR

Action

Unknown. Thought to antagonize dopamine and serotonin type 2 in CNS. Also antagonizes muscarinic receptors in respiratory tract, causing cholinergic activation.

Availability

Injection: 5 mg/ml
Oral concentrate: 16 mg/5 ml
Tablets: 2 mg, 4 mg, 8 mg, 16 mg

Indications and dosages

➢ Schizophrenia in nonhospitalized patients

Adults and children older than age 12: Initially, 4 to 8 mg P.O. t.i.d.

➢ Schizophrenia in hospitalized patients

Adults and children older than age 12: Initially, 8 to 16 mg P.O. two to four times daily, increased p.r.n.; avoid dosages greater than 64 mg daily. Or 5 to 10 mg by deep I.M. injection q 6 hours p.r.n., not to exceed 30 mg/day.

➢ Severe nausea and vomiting

Adults: 8 to 16 mg P.O. daily in divided doses, to a maximum of 24 mg; or 5 to 10 mg by deep I.M. injection p.r.n.; or up to 5 mg I.V. by slow injection or infusion.

Off-label uses

• Intractable hiccups

Contraindications

• Hypersensitivity to drug, its components, or related compounds
• Blood dyscrasias
• Bone marrow depression
• Hepatic damage
• Subcortical damage
• Coma
• Concurrent use of high-dose CNS depressants

Precautions

Use cautiously in:
• respiratory disorders, hepatic or renal dysfunction, breast cancer, alcohol withdrawal symptoms, suicidal tendency, surgery
• patients taking CNS depressants or anticholinergics
• elderly patients
• pregnant or breastfeeding patients
• children younger than age 12.

Administration

• Give oral forms with food to avoid GI upset.
• Dilute oral solution in water or fruit juice just before giving; use at least 60 ml of diluent for each 5 ml of solution.
• Avoid contact with oral or injection solution; contact dermatitis may occur.
• Administer I.M injection deep into upper outer aspect of buttocks. Massage site to prevent abscess.
• Know that I.V. route is rarely indicated and should be used only in recumbent hospitalized patients. For I.V. use, dilute with normal saline solution to a concentration of 0.5 mg/ml; give slowly (no more than 1 mg q 2 minutes). I.V. dose shouldn't exceed 5 mg.
• Replace parenteral therapy with oral therapy as soon as possible.

Route	Onset	Peak	Duration
P.O.	Variable	1-3 hours	Unknown
I.M., I.V.	5-10 min	1-2 hr	6 hr

Adverse reactions

CNS: drowsiness, dizziness, insomnia, vertigo, headache, hyperactivity, nocturnal confusion, bizarre dreams, tremor, ataxia, slurring, exacerbation of psychotic symptoms, paranoid reactions, parkinsonism, dystonias, akathisia, tardive dyskinesia, hyperreflexia, cerebrospinal fluid abnormality, catatonic-like state, paradoxical stimulation, **seizures, neuroleptic malignant syndrome**
CV: hypotension, orthostatic hypotension, hypertension, peripheral edema, ECG changes, tachycardia, bradycardia, **cardiac arrest, heart failure**
EENT: glaucoma, blurred vision, miosis, mydriasis, corneal and lens deposits, pigmentary retinopathy, oculogyric crisis, photophobia, nasal congestion, dysphagia
GI: nausea, vomiting, diarrhea, constipation, obstipation, abnormal tongue color or movement, dry mouth, anorexia, **adynamic ileus**
GU: dark urine, urinary retention, urinary frequency, urinary incontinence, bladder paralysis, galactorrhea, lactation, breast enlargement, menstrual irregularities, inhibited ejaculation, libido changes
Hematologic: hemolytic anemia, leukopenia, agranulocytosis, thrombocytopenic purpura
Hepatic: jaundice, biliary stasis
Metabolic: hyponatremia, glycosuria, hyperglycemia, **hypoglycemia, syndrome of inappropriate antidiuretic hormone secretion, pituitary tumor**
Musculoskeletal: numbness and aching of arms and legs
Respiratory: dyspnea, suppressed cough reflex, **asthma, bronchospasm, laryngospasm, laryngeal edema**
Skin: urticaria, pallor, erythema, eczema, pruritus, perspiration, pigmentation changes, photosensitivity, angioedema, exfoliative dermatitis
Other: increased appetite, weight gain, fever, systemic lupus erythematosus-like syndrome, pain at I.M. injection site, hypersensitivity reactions including **anaphylactoid reaction**

Interactions

Drug-drug. *Anticholinergics:* increased risk of adverse anticholinergic reactions
CNS depressants: increased perphenazine effects, increased adverse CNS reactions
Tricyclic antidepressants: increased perphenazine blood level, greater risk of adverse reactions
Drug-diagnostic tests. *Eosinophils, liver function tests:* increased values
Glucose: increased or decreased level
Granulocytes, hemoglobin, platelets, sodium, white blood cells: decreased levels
Pregnancy test: false-positive result
Drug-herbs. *Kava:* dystonic reactions
St. John's wort: photosensitivity
Yohimbe: yohimbe toxicity
Drug-behaviors. *Alcohol use:* increased CNS depression
Sun exposure: increased risk of photosensitivity reaction

Patient monitoring

[Clinical alert] Watch for anaphylactoid reaction and angioedema. Monitor neurologic status; stay alert for signs and symptoms of neuroleptic malignant syndrome (high fever, unstable blood pressure, stupor, muscle rigidity, autonomic dysfunction), parkinsonian symptoms, and catatonic-like state.
- Assess blood pressure and heart rate continuously during I.V. use. Monitor cardiovascular status and vital signs periodically.

[Clinical alert] Evaluate respiratory status, especially for dyspnea and airway spasm.
[Clinical alert] Monitor CBC, glucose level, and liver function tests. Watch for evidence of blood dyscrasias.

Patient teaching

- Explain importance of combining drug therapy with psychotherapy.

P

• Tell patient to take exactly as prescribed and to report adverse reactions promptly.
• Instruct patient to avoid sun exposure and to wear sunscreen outdoors to prevent photosensitivity reaction.
• Advise patient to consult prescriber before taking other prescription drugs or over-the-counter preparations.
• Caution patient to avoid driving and other hazardous activities until he knows how drug affects him.
• Instruct patient to avoid alcohol, smoking, caffeine, and herbs.
• As appropriate, review all other significant and life-threatening adverse reactions and interactions, especially those related to the drugs, tests, herbs, and behaviors mentioned above.

phenazopyridine hydrochloride

Azo-Standard, Baridium, Geridium, Phenazo✦, Prodium, Pyridiate, Pyridium, Urogesic, UTI Relief

Pharmacologic class: Nonopioid analgesic
Therapeutic class: Urinary analgesic
Pregnancy risk category B

Action

Unknown. Thought to act locally on urinary tract mucosa to produce analgesic or anesthetic effects, relieving urinary burning, urgency, and frequency.

Availability

Tablets: 95 mg, 97.2 mg, 100 mg, 200 mg

Indications and dosages

➢ Pain caused by lower urinary tract irritation
Adults: 200 mg P.O. t.i.d.
Children: 12 mg/kg P.O. daily in three divided doses

Contraindications

• Hypersensitivity to drug
• Renal insufficiency

Precautions

Use cautiously in:
• hepatitis
• pregnant or breastfeeding patients
• children younger than age 12.

Administration

• Give with or after meals.
• Discontinue after 2 days, as prescribed, when administering with antibiotics.

Route	Onset	Peak	Duration
P.O.	Unknown	Unknown	6-8 hr

Adverse reactions

CNS: headache
EENT: contact lens staining
GI: GI disturbances
GU: bright orange urine, **renal toxicity**
Hepatic: hepatotoxicity
Hematologic: hemolytic anemia, methemoglobinemia
Skin: rash, pruritus
Other: anaphylactoid-like reaction

Interactions

Drug-diagnostic tests. *Bilirubin, glucose, ketones, protein, steroids:* interference with urine tests based on spectrophotometry or color reactions

Patient monitoring

• Monitor patient for symptomatic improvement of urinary tract infection (UTI).
• Assess follow-up urine culture after antibiotic therapy ends.
Clinical alert: Monitor for yellowing of skin or sclera. This change may indicate drug accumulation caused by impaired renal excretion, warranting drug withdrawal.

Patient teaching

- Explain drug therapy and measures to help prevent UTI recurrence.
- Tell patient drug may discolor urine and tears and may stain clothing and contact lenses.

Advise patient to contact prescriber promptly if symptoms don't improve or if skin or eyes become yellow.

- As appropriate, review all other significant and life-threatening adverse reactions and interactions, especially those related to the tests mentioned above.

phenelzine sulfate

Nardil

Pharmacologic class: MAO inhibitor
Therapeutic class: Antidepressant
Pregnancy risk category C

Action

Nonselectively inhibits metabolism of MAO, an enzyme that increases accumulation of endogenous epinephrine, norepinephrine, and serotonin in CNS

Availability

Tablets: 15 mg

Indications and dosages

➢ Atypical or neurotic depression
Adults: Initially, 15 mg P.O. t.i.d.; may increase rapidly to at least 60 mg/day, then 90 mg/day if needed for adequate response. Then reduce slowly to a maintenance dosage as low as 15 mg/day.

Contraindications

- Hypersensitivity to drug
- Pheochromocytoma
- Heart failure or other cardiovascular disease
- Abnormal liver function tests, history of hepatic disease
- History of headache
- Concurrent use of sympathomimetics, guanethidine, dextromethorphan, CNS depressants, buspirone, or serotonergic drugs

Precautions

Use cautiously in:

- hyperthyroidism, seizure disorders, hypotension, hypomania, diabetes mellitus, hepatic complications, myocardial ischemia
- patients switching from other MAO inhibitors
- suicidal or drug-dependent patients
- elderly patients
- pregnant or breastfeeding patients
- children younger than age 16.

Administration

If hypertensive crisis occurs, discontinue drug immediately and give phentolamine 5 mg I.V. slowly as ordered.

Ask patient about other drugs he's using; MAO inhibitors can cause dangerous interactions with many drugs.

Route	Onset	Peak	Duration
P.O.	Unknown	2-6 hr	Variable

Adverse reactions

CNS: dizziness, headache, drowsiness, hyperreflexia, hypersomnia, tremors, fatigue, insomnia, palilalia, euphoria, paresthesia, ataxia, manic reaction, acute anxiety reaction, schizophrenia precipitation, **shock-like coma, seizures, toxic delirium**, **suicidal behavior or ideation** (especially in child or adolescent)
CV: orthostatic hypotension, edema, **hypertensive crisis, arrhythmias**
EENT: blurred vision, glaucoma, nystagmus
GI: nausea, vomiting, diarrhea, constipation, GI disturbances, epigastric or abdominal pain, dry mouth

GU: urinary retention, sexual disturbances
Hematologic: leukopenia
Hepatic: jaundice, **fatal progressive necrotizing hepatocellular disease**
Metabolic: hypernatremia, hypermetabolic syndrome
Musculoskeletal: muscle twitching
Skin: pruritus, rash, sweating
Other: weight changes, fever, lupus-like syndrome, edema

Interactions

Drug-drug. *Amphetamines, CNS depressants, dextromethorphan, dibenzazepine derivatives, other MAO inhibitors, serotonergic agents (such as fluoxetine, paroxetine), tryptophan:* hypertensive crisis, seizures, fever, diaphoresis, excitation, delirium, tremor, coma, circulatory collapse
Antidepressants, buspirone: hypertension
Antihypertensives, beta-adrenergic blockers, thiazide diuretics: increased hypotensive effect
Epinephrine, guanadrel, guanethidine, norepinephrine, reserpine, vasoconstrictors: hypertensive crisis
Insulin, oral hypoglycemics: additive hypoglycemia
Drug-diagnostic tests. *Sodium, transaminases:* increased levels
White blood cells: decreased count
Drug-food. *Aged, pickled, fermented, or smoked foods; wine; alcohol-free wine and beer; broad bean pods; cheese (except cottage and cream cheese); excessive amounts of chocolate or caffeine; dry sausage (including hard salami, pepperoni, and Lebanon bologna); foods containing L-tryptophan (such as dairy foods, soy, poultry, and meat); liver; spoiled or improperly refrigerated, handled, or stored protein-rich foods; yeast extract; yogurt:* hypertensive crisis
Drug-herbs. *Ephedra (ma huang), L-tryptophan:* hypertensive crisis
Drug-behaviors. *Alcohol use:* hypertensive crisis

Patient monitoring

- Monitor blood pressure. Drug may cause orthostatic hypotension or hypertensive crisis.
- Assess patient for symptomatic improvement.
- Monitor CBC, liver function tests, and blood glucose level before and during therapy.
- Watch for increasing depression, suicide attempt, or suicidal ideation (especially in child or adolescent).

Patient teaching

- Explain importance of taking drug exactly as prescribed.
- Tell patient to discontinue drug at least 10 days before elective surgery.
- Stress importance of avoiding alcohol, certain foods and beverages, prescription drugs, and over-the-counter preparations during and for 14 days after therapy. Ask pharmacist to provide patient with complete list of foods to avoid.

[Clinical alert] Instruct patient to immediately report occipital headache, palpitations, stiff neck, nausea, sweating, dilated pupils, and photophobia (indications of hypertensive crisis).

[Clinical alert] Advise patient or caregiver to immediately report increasing depression, suicide attempt, or suicidal ideation (especially in child or adolescent).

[Clinical alert] Tell patient to immediately report nausea, unusual tiredness, yellowing of skin or eyes, or irregular heart beats.

- Advise patient to rise slowly to avoid dizziness.
- Caution patient to avoid driving and other hazardous activities until he knows how drug affects concentration, vision, and alertness.
- As appropriate, review all other significant and life-threatening adverse reactions and interactions, especially those related to the drugs, tests, foods, herbs, and behaviors mentioned above.

phenobarbital
Luminal, Solfoton

phenobarbital sodium
Luminal Sodium

Pharmacologic class: Barbiturate
Therapeutic class: Anxiolytic, anticonvulsant, sedative-hypnotic
Controlled substance schedule IV
Pregnancy risk category D

Action
Interferes with gamma-aminobutyric acid receptors, blocking nerve impulse transmission in CNS, which reduces motor activity and raises seizure threshold

Availability
Capsules: 16 mg
Elixir: 15 mg/5 ml, 20 mg/5 ml
Injection: 30 mg/ml and 60 mg/ml in 1-ml prefilled syringes; 65 mg/ml in 1-ml vials; 130 mg/ml in 1-ml prefilled syringes, 1-ml vials, and 1-ml ampules
Tablets: 15 mg, 16 mg, 30 mg, 60 mg, 90 mg, 100 mg

Indications and dosages
➢ Tonic-clonic (grand mal) and partial seizures; febrile seizures in children
Adults: 60 to 100 mg/day P.O. as a single dose or in two or three divided doses; or initially, 100 to 320 mg I.V. p.r.n. (a total of 600 mg I.V. in a 24-hour period).
Infants and children: Loading dose of 15 to 20 mg/kg P.O. (produces drug blood level of 20 mcg/ml shortly after dosing). To achieve therapeutic blood level (10 to 25 mcg/ml), children usually need higher dosage/kg than adults. Follow loading dose with 3 to 6 mg/kg/day P.O. Alternatively, 4 to 6 mg/kg/day I.M. or I.V. for 7 to 10 days to achieve blood level of 10 to 15 mcg/ml.
➢ Status epilepticus
Adults: 200 to 320 mg I.M. or I.V., repeated q 6 hours p.r.n.
Children: 15 to 20 mg/kg I.V. given over 10 to 15 minutes
➢ Sedation or hypnotic effect
Adults: For sedation, 30 to 120 mg/day P.O. or 30 to 120 mg/day I.M. or I.V. in two or three divided doses. As a hypnotic, 100 to 200 mg P.O. or 100 to 320 mg I.M. or I.V. at bedtime. Don't exceed 400 mg in a 24-hour period.
➢ Preoperative sedation
Adults: 100 to 200 mg I.M. 60 to 90 minutes before surgery
Children: 1 to 3 mg/kg I.M. or I.V., as prescribed.

Dosage adjustment
- Impaired hepatic or renal function
- Elderly or debilitated patients

Off-label uses
- Prevention and treatment of hyperbilirubinemia

Contraindications
- Hypersensitivity to drug or other barbiturates
- Manifest or latent porphyria
- Nephritis (with large doses)
- Severe respiratory disease with dyspnea or obstruction
- History of sedative-hypnotic abuse
- Subcutaneous or intra-arterial administration

Precautions
Use cautiously in:
- hepatic dysfunction, renal impairment, seizure disorder, fever, hyperthyroidism, diabetes mellitus, severe anemia, pulmonary or cardiac disease
- history of suicide attempt or drug abuse
- chronic phenobarbital use
- elderly or debilitated patients

p

- pregnant or breastfeeding patients
- children younger than age 6.

Administration

- Inject I.M. deep into large muscle mass; limit volume to 5 ml.

◀ Give I.V. no faster than 60 mg/minute. Keep resuscitation equipment at hand.

- Stop injection immediately if patient complains of pain or if circulation at injection site diminishes (indicating inadvertent intra-arterial injection).

◀ Don't give by subcutaneous route; severe reactions (such as pain and tissue necrosis) may occur.

◀ Know that when given I.V. for status epilepticus, drug may take 15 minutes to attain peak blood level in brain. If injected continuously until seizures stop, drug brain level would keep rising and could exceed that required to control seizures. To avoid barbiturate-induced depression, use minimal amount required and wait for anticonvulsant effect to occur before giving second dose.

- Use parenteral route only when patient can't receive drug P.O.
- Know that drug is intended only for short-term use, losing efficacy after about 2 weeks.

Route	Onset	Peak	Duration
P.O.	30-60 min	Unknown	10-16 hr
I.V.	5 min	30 min	10-16 hr
I.M.	10-30 min	Unknown	10-16 hr

Adverse reactions

CNS: headache, dizziness, anxiety, depression, drowsiness, excitation, delirium, lethargy, agitation, confusion, hyperkinesia, ataxia, vertigo, nightmares, nervousness, paradoxical stimulation, abnormal thinking, hallucinations, insomnia, CNS depression
CV: hypotension, syncope, **bradycardia** (with I.V. use)
GI: nausea, vomiting, constipation
Hematologic: megaloblastic anemia
Hepatic: hepatic damage
Musculoskeletal: joint pain, myalgia
Respiratory: hypoventilation, **laryngospasm, bronchospasm, apnea** (with I.V. use); **respiratory depression**
Skin: rash, urticaria, exfoliative dermatitis, **Stevens-Johnson syndrome**
Other: phlebitis at I.V. site, drug dependence, hypersensitivity reactions including angioedema

Interactions

Drug-drug. *Acetaminophen:* increased risk of hepatotoxicity
Activated charcoal: decreased phenobarbital absorption
Anticoagulants, beta-adrenergic blockers (except timolol), carbamazepine, clonazepam, corticosteroids, digoxin, doxorubicin, doxycycline, felodipine, fenoprofen, griseofulvin, hormonal contraceptives, metronidazole, quinidine, theophylline, verapamil: decreased efficacy of these drugs
Chloramphenicol, hydantoins, narcotics: increased or decreased effects of either drug
Cyclophosphamide: increased risk of hematologic toxicity
Divalproex, MAO inhibitors, valproic acid: decreased phenobarbital metabolism, increased sedative effect
Other CNS depressants (including first-generation antihistamines, opioids, other sedative-hypnotics): additive CNS depression
Rifampin: increased phenobarbital metabolism and decreased effects
Drug-diagnostic tests. *Bilirubin:* decreased level in neonates and patients with seizure disorders or congenital nonhemolytic unconjugated hyperbilirubinemia
Drug-herbs. *Chamomile, hops, kava, skullcap, valerian:* increased CNS depression
St. John's wort: decreased drug effects
Drug-behaviors. *Alcohol use:* additive CNS effects

Patient monitoring

- Monitor vital signs; watch for bradycardia and hypotension.

🔊 In patients with seizure disorders, know that drug withdrawal may cause status epilepticus.

- Assess neurologic status. Institute safety measures as needed.

🔊 Closely monitor respiratory status, especially for respiratory depression and airway spasm.

- Monitor phenobarbital blood level, CBC, and kidney and liver function tests.
- Watch for signs of drug dependence.

Patient teaching

🔊 Instruct patient to promptly report rash, facial and lip edema, syncope, dyspnea, or depression.

🔊 Stress importance of taking exactly as prescribed, with or without food. Caution patient not to stop therapy abruptly, especially if he's taking drug for seizures.

- Tell patient that prolonged use may lead to dependence.
- Instruct patient to seek medical advice before taking other prescription or over-the-counter drugs.
- Caution patient to avoid driving and other hazardous activities until he knows how drug affect him.
- Advise patient to avoid herbs, alcohol, and other CNS depressants.
- Instruct patient taking hormonal contraceptives to use alternate birth-control method.
- As appropriate, review all other significant and life-threatening adverse reactions and interactions, especially those related to the drugs, tests, herbs, and behaviors mentioned above.

phentolamine mesylate

Regitine, Rogitine✱

Pharmacologic class: Alpha-adrenergic blocker

Therapeutic class: Diagnostic agent, antihypertensive agent in pheochromocytoma

Pregnancy risk category C

Action

Competitively blocks postsynaptic (alpha$_1$) and presynaptic (alpha$_2$) adrenergic receptors. Acts on arterial tree and venous bed, reducing total peripheral resistance and lowering venous return to heart.

Availability

Powder for injection: 5 mg

Indications and dosages

➢ To prevent or control hypertensive episodes before or during pheochromocytomectomy

Adults: 5 mg I.V. or I.M. 1 to 2 hours before surgery, then 5 mg I.V. during surgery as indicated

Children: 1 mg I.V. or I.M. 1 to 2 hours before surgery, then 1 mg I.V. during surgery as indicated

➢ To aid pheochromocytoma diagnosis

Adults: 2.5 or 5 mg (in 1 ml of sterile water) by I.V. injection; record blood pressure q 30 seconds for 3 minutes, then q minute for next 7 minutes. Or 5 mg (in 1 ml sterile water) I.M.; record blood pressure q 5 minutes for 30 to 45 minutes.

➢ To prevent or treat dermal necrosis after norepinephrine extravasation

Adults: For prevention, add 10 mg to each liter of I.V. solution containing norepinephrine. For treatment, inject 5 to 10 mg in 10 ml of normal saline so-

P

lution into extravasated area within 12 hours.

Off-label uses

- Hypertensive crisis caused by MAO inhibitors
- Rebound hypertension caused by withdrawal of clonidine, propranolol, or other antihypertensives
- Erectile dysfunction (given with papaverine)

Contraindications

- Hypersensitivity to drug
- Coronary artery disease
- Myocardial infarction (MI) or history of MI
- Coronary insufficiency
- Angina

Precautions

Use cautiously in:

- patients receiving cardiac glycosides concurrently
- pregnant or breastfeeding patients.

Administration

- Reconstitute powder by diluting with 1 ml of sterile water for injection.
- For pheochromocytoma diagnosis, withhold sedatives, analgesics, and nonessential drugs for 24 to 72 hours before test (until hypertension returns). Keep patient supine until blood pressure stabilizes; then rapidly inject drug I.V. Maximum effect usually occurs within 2 minutes of dosing.

Route	Onset	Peak	Duration
I.V., I.M.	Immediate	Unknown	Brief

Adverse reactions

CNS: weakness, dizziness
CV: tachycardia, acute and prolonged hypotension, orthostatic hypotension, **arrhythmias**
EENT: nasal congestion
GI: nausea, vomiting, diarrhea
Skin: flushing

Interactions

Drug-drug. *Ephedrine, epinephrine:* antagonism of these drugs' effects
Drug-herbs. *Ephedra (ma huang):* antagonism of vasoconstrictive effects

Patient monitoring

- When using for norepinephrine extravasation, monitor injection site closely and assess blood pressure, heart rate, and respiratory rate.
- For pheochromocytoma diagnosis, monitor blood pressure. In pheochromocytoma, systolic and diastolic pressures drop immediately and steeply. Monitor and record blood pressure immediately after injection, at 30-second intervals for first 3 minutes, and at 1-minute intervals for next 7 minutes. Systolic decrease of 60 mmHg and diastolic decrease of 25 mmHg within 2 minutes after I.V. administration indicates a positive reaction for pheochromocytoma.

Patient teaching

- Explain drug administration procedure.
- [Clinical alert] Instruct patient to promptly report adverse reactions. Assure him he'll be monitored closely.
- Tell patient to withhold other drugs (especially sedatives and analgesics) for at least 24 hours before pheochromocytoma testing, if appropriate.
- As appropriate, review all other significant and life-threatening adverse reactions and interactions, especially those related to the drugs and herbs mentioned above.

phenylephrine hydrochloride

Afrin Children's Pump Mist, AH-Chew D, Coricidin, Dioephrine✱, Neo-Synephrine, Rhinall, Vicks Sinex Ultra Fine Mist

Pharmacologic class: Sympathomimetic, alpha-adrenergic agonist

Therapeutic class: Vasopressor, nasal decongestant, ophthalmic vasoconstrictor

Pregnancy risk category C

Action

Stimulates alpha-adrenergic receptors, increasing blood pressure and causing pronounced vasoconstriction in skin, mucous membranes, and mucosa. Produces mydriasis by contracting pupillary dilator muscle.

Availability

Injection: 10 mg/ml
Nasal solution: 0.125%, 0.25%, 0.5%, 1%
Ophthalmic solution: 0.12%, 2.5%, 10%
Tablets (chewable): 10 mg

Indications and dosages

➢ Mild to moderate hypotension
Adults: 1 to 10 mg subcutaneously or I.M.; don't exceed an initial dosage of 5 mg.

➢ Severe hypotension and shock
Adults: 0.1 to 0.18 mg/minute I.V. infusion. For maintenance infusion, 40 to 60 mcg/minute.

➢ To prevent hypotension during spinal anesthesia
Adults: 2 to 3 mg subcutaneously or I.M. 3 to 4 minutes before spinal anesthetic is injected

➢ Hypotensive emergency during spinal anesthesia
Adults: 0.2 mg I.V., up to a maximum of 0.5 mg/dose

➢ To prolong spinal anesthesia
Adults: 2 to 5 mg added to anesthetic solution (prolongs spinal block by up to 50%)

➢ Vasoconstrictor for regional anesthesia
Adults: 1 mg of phenylephrine added to every 20 ml of local anesthetic solution

➢ Paroxysmal supraventricular tachycardia
Adults: 0.5 mg by rapid I.V. injection, not to exceed initial dosage of 0.5 mg. Subsequent dosages (determined by blood pressure) shouldn't exceed preceding dosage by more than 0.1 to 0.2 mg; maximum dosage is 1 mg.

➢ Nasal congestion
Adults: One or two sprays of 0.25% or 0.5% nasal solution in each nostril q 3 to 4 hours p.r.n.; severe congestion may warrant 1% solution. Or 10 to 20 mg P.O. (chewable tablets) q 4 hours.

➢ Vasoconstriction and pupil dilation
Adults: After topical anesthetic is applied, instill one drop of 2.5% ophthalmic solution into lacrimal sac; repeat 1 hour later.

➢ Uveitis
Adults: Instill one drop of 2.5% or 10% ophthalmic solution to upper surface of cornea. May repeat up to three times p.r.n.

➢ Open-angle glaucoma
Adults: Instill one drop of 10% ophthalmic solution to upper surface of cornea as often as necessary.

➢ For wide pupil dilation before intraocular surgery
Adults: Instill 2.5% or 10% ophthalmic solution, as prescribed, into lacrimal sac 30 to 60 minutes before surgery.

➢ Refraction
Adults: Before procedure, instill one drop of 2.5% ophthalmic solution

P

combined with a rapid-acting cycloplegic into lacrimal sac, as prescribed.
Children: Before procedure, instill one drop of 2.5% ophthalmic solution into lacrimal sac 5 minutes after cycloplegic administration, as prescribed.
➢ Provocative test for angle-closure glaucoma
Adults: 2.5% ophthalmic solution applied to dilate pupil, with intraocular pressure (IOP) measured before application and after dilation. IOP rise of 3 to 5 mm Hg suggests angle block in patients with glaucoma; however, negative response doesn't rule out glaucoma from other causes.
➢ Retinoscopy (shadow test)
Adults: 2.5% ophthalmic solution
➢ Blanching test
Adults: Instill one to two drops of 2.5% ophthalmic solution into affected eye.
➢ Decongestant to relieve minor eye irritation
Adults: Instill one or two drops of 0.12% ophthalmic solution into eye(s) up to q.i.d. p.r.n.

Dosage adjustment

- Hyperthyroidism
- Cardiac disease
- Elderly patients

Contraindications

- Hypersensitivity to drug or its components
- Severe hypertension
- Ventricular tachycardia
- Angle-closure glaucoma
- Aneurysm (10% ophthalmic solution)
- During intraocular surgery when corneal epithelial barrier has been disturbed (ophthalmic solution)
- Elderly patients with severe arteriosclerotic or cerebrovascular disease
- Some low-birth-weight infants

Precautions

Use cautiously in:

- sulfite sensitivity (some products)
- hyperthyroidism, partial heart block, bradycardia, hypertension, cardiac disease, arteriosclerosis, unstable vasomotor syndrome
- type 1 (insulin-dependent) diabetes mellitus, hypertension, hyperthyroidism, arteriosclerosis or other cardiac disease (10% ophthalmic solution)
- within 21 days of MAO inhibitors (2.5% or 10% ophthalmic solution)
- elderly patients
- pregnant or breastfeeding patients.

Administration

- In emergencies, drug may be given by direct I.V. injection. Dilute 1 ml of solution containing 10 mg/ml with 9 ml of sterile water for injection.

🔊 For I.V. infusion, dilute 10 mg in 500 ml of dextrose 5% in water or normal saline solution; titrate dosage until blood pressure is slightly below patient's normal level or until maximum dosage is reached. Infuse I.V. in large vein (preferably through central venous catheter) using infusion pump. After condition stabilizes, taper dosage gradually; don't withdraw abruptly. Avoid extravasation.

🔊 Be aware that systemic absorption of ophthalmic solution during pupil dilation in patients with angle-closure glaucoma may trigger asthma attack.

- As ordered, apply a drop of suitable topical anesthetic before instilling ophthalmic solution, to prevent pain and drug dilution (caused by excessive lacrimation induced by pain).

🔊 Compress lacrimal sac for 1 minute after instilling 10% ophthalmic solution, to avoid excessive systemic absorption (which could cause serious cardiovascular problems, especially in elderly patients).

- Be aware that patients with heavily pigmented irides may require larger ophthalmic doses for diagnostic procedures.

Route	Onset	Peak	Duration
P.O.	Unknown	Unknown	Unknown
I.V.	Immediate	Unknown	15-20 min
I.M., subcut.	10-15 min	Unknown	0.5-2 hr
Nasal	15-20 min	Unknown	0.5-4 hr
Ophth. (0.12%)	Rapid	Unknown	30 min-4 hr
Ophth. (2.5%)	Rapid	15-60 min	3 hr
Ophth. (10%)	Rapid	10-60 min	6 hr

Adverse reactions

CNS: headache, weakness, anxiety, restlessness, tremor, light-headedness, dizziness, drowsiness, insomnia, hallucinations, nervousness, restlessness, giddiness, prolonged psychosis, orofacial dystonia
CV: hypertension, palpitations, tachycardia, bradycardia, **arrhythmias**
EENT: with ophthalmic solution—transient pigment floaters in aqueous humor; rebound miosis; rebound hyperemia (with prolonged use); light sensitivity; photophobia; blurred vision; allergic conjunctivitis; eye burning, stinging, and irritation; transient epithelial keratitis; decreased IOP; with nasal solution—rebound congestion, burning, stinging, sneezing, dryness, local irritation
GI: nausea, vomiting, gastric irritation, anorexia
GU: urinary retention (in males with prostatitis)
Hematologic: leukopenia, agranulocytosis, thrombocytopenia
Musculoskeletal: brow ache (with ophthalmic solution)
Respiratory: asthmatic episodes
Skin: sweating, rash, urticaria, contact dermatitis, necrosis and sloughing (with extravasation at I.V. site)

Interactions

Drug-drug. *Beta-adrenergic blockers:* blocked cardiostimulatory effects of phenylephrine
Bretylium, sympathomimetics: serious arrhythmias
Furazolidone: excessive hypertension
Guanethidine, methyldopa: decreased antihypertensive effects
Halogenated hydrocarbon anesthetics: serious arrhythmias
MAO inhibitors: severe headache, hypertension, hyperpyrexia
Oxytocics, tricyclic antidepressants: increased pressor response
Drug-diagnostic tests. *Tonometry:* false-normal readings (with ophthalmic form)
Drug-behaviors. *Sun exposure:* photophobia

Patient monitoring

- Monitor ECG continuously during I.V. administration; monitor blood pressure every 5 to 15 minutes until it stabilizes, then every 30 to 60 minutes.
- Monitor central venous pressure and fluid intake and output. Keep in mind that drug doesn't eliminate need for fluid resuscitation.
- Assess CBC; watch for evidence of blood dyscrasias.
- Monitor I.V. site; extravasation can cause tissue damage.
- Assess for symptomatic improvement in patients using nasal form.

Monitor for adverse reactions, particularly life-threatening asthmatic episodes.

Patient teaching

- Tell patient to take exactly as directed and not to exceed recommended dosage.
- Advise patient using nasal solution that dropper, inhaler, or spray dispenser shouldn't be used by more than one person. Teach proper instillation technique: Instill nasal solution into dependent nostril with head down and

P

in lateral position. Stay in this position for 5 minutes; then instill solution in other nostril in same manner. Advise patient to rinse container tip with hot water after each use. Instruct him to discontinue use and contact prescriber if symptoms don't improve after 3 days. Tell him not to use for more than 3 days and to contact prescriber if symptoms persist.

• Teach proper technique for instilling eye drops. Stress importance of compressing lacrimal sac after instilling, to decrease systemic drug absorption. Tell patient that ophthalmic solution may cause light sensitivity lasting several hours. Inform elderly patient that he may see transient floaters 40 to 45 minutes after administration.

• As appropriate, review all other significant and life-threatening adverse reactions and interactions, especially those related to the drugs, tests, and behaviors mentioned above.

phenytoin (diphenylhydantoin)

Dilantin-125, Dilantin Infatabs

phenytoin sodium (diphenylhydantoin sodium)

Dilantin Kapseals, Diphenylan✦, Phenytek✦

Pharmacologic class: Hydantoin derivative

Therapeutic class: Anticonvulsant

Pregnancy risk category D

Action

Thought to limit seizure activity by promoting sodium efflux from neurons in motor cortex and reducing activity in brainstem centers responsible for tonic phase of tonic-clonic seizures

Availability

Capsules (prompt-release): 30 mg, 100 mg
Capsules (extended-release): 30 mg, 100 mg
Injection: 50 mg/ml in 2- and 5-ml ampules
Oral suspension: 30 mg/5 ml, 125 mg/5 ml
Tablets (chewable): 50 mg

Indications and dosages

➤ Status epilepticus

Adults: Loading dose of 10 to 15 mg/kg by slow I.V., then a maintenance dosage of 100 mg P.O. or I.V. q 6 to 8 hours

Neonates and children: Loading dose of 15 to 20 mg/kg I.V. in divided doses of 5 to 10 mg/kg

➤ Generalized tonic-clonic (grand mal) and complex partial (psychomotor, temporal lobe) seizures

Adults: Loading dose of 1 g P.O. (extended-release) in three divided doses (400 mg, 300 mg, and 300 mg) at 2-hour intervals in hospitalized patients requiring rapid steady-state serum levels (when I.V. route isn't desired). Maintenance dosing usually starts 24 hours after loading dose. Patients who haven't had previous treatment usually start at 100 mg (125 mg suspension) P.O. t.i.d., adjusted as needed to a maximum of 600 mg (625 mg suspension) P.O. daily. Alternatively, if divided doses control seizures, one daily dose of 300 mg P.O. (extended-release phenytoin sodium).

Children: Initially, 5 mg/kg/day P.O. in two or three equally divided doses; maintenance dosage individualized and given in two to three divided doses (not to exceed 300 mg/day).

➢ To prevent seizures during neurosurgery
Adults: 100 to 200 mg I.M. at 4-hour intervals

Off-label uses

- Arrhythmias
- Severe preeclampsia
- Trigeminal neuralgia
- Recessive dystrophic epidermolysis bullosa, junctional epidermolysis bullosa

Contraindications

- Hypersensitivity to drug
- Sinus bradycardia, sinoatrial block, second- or third-degree atrioventricular block, Adams-Stokes syndrome

Precautions

Use cautiously in:

- hepatic disease, diabetes mellitus, skin rash
- pregnant or breastfeeding patients (safety not established).

Administration

- Before I.V. use, check designated line for patency and flush with normal saline solution. Deliver no faster than 50 mg/minute for adults or 1 to 3 mg/kg/minute in children and neonates; then flush with normal saline solution. Avoid extravasation (can cause severe tissue damage).

🔊 Don't administer I.V. into dorsal hand veins, because purple glove syndrome may occur.

- When giving oral solution through nasogastric tube, dilute dose with sterile water or normal saline solution; after administration, flush tube with at least 20 ml of diluent.
- Withhold enteral feedings for at least 1 hour before and 1 hour after oral administration.
- Give I.M. only as last resort (may cause pain and reduce drug absorption).
- Know that patients with history of renal or hepatic disease should not receive P.O. loading dose.

Route	Onset	Peak	Duration
P.O.	Unknown	3 hr	6-12 hr
P.O. (extended)	Unknown	4-12 hr	12-36 hr
I.V.	Unknown	Rapid	12-24 hr
I.M.	Unknown	Erratic	12-24 hr

Adverse reactions

CNS: headache, fatigue, dizziness, drowsiness, weakness, depression, ataxia, slurred speech, confusion, agitation, dysarthria, dyskinesia, extrapyramidal symptoms, insomnia, irritability, twitching, nervousness, numbness, psychotic disturbances, tremor, CNS depression (with I.V. use), **coma**
CV: vasodilation, edema, chest pain, **tachycardia, hypotension** (increased with I.V. use), **cardiovascular collapse** (with I.V. use)
EENT: diplopia, amblyopia, nystagmus, visual field defect, eye pain, conjunctivitis, photophobia, mydriasis, hearing loss, tinnitus, ear pain, epistaxis, rhinitis, sinusitis, pharyngitis
GI: nausea, vomiting, diarrhea, constipation, lip enlargement, dry mouth
GU: pink, red, or reddish-brown urine; gynecomastia; Peyronie's disease
Hepatic: jaundice, **toxic hepatitis, hepatic damage**
Hematologic: macrocytosis, simple anemia, **megaloblastic anemia, monocytosis, leukocytosis, hemolytic anemia, thrombocytopenia, agranulocytosis, granulocytopenia, leukopenia, pancytopenia**
Metabolic: hypocalcemia, diabetes insipidus, hyperglycemia
Musculoskeletal: back pain, pelvic pain, osteomalacia
Respiratory: dyspnea, increased cough and sputum, pneumonia, hyperventilation, hypoxia, hemoptysis, bronchitis, **apnea, asthma, aspiration pneumo-**

P

nia, pulmonary fibrosis, atelectasis, pneumothorax
Skin: rash, pruritus, bruising, exfoliative dermatitis, hypertrichosis, hirsutism, alopecia, **Stevens-Johnson syndrome**
Other: gingival hyperplasia, altered taste, fever, lymphadenopathy, weight gain or loss, injection site reaction, coarsened facial features, lupus erythematosus syndrome, allergic reactions

Interactions

Drug-drug. *Acetaminophen, amiodarone, carbamazepine, cardiac glycosides, corticosteroids, dicumarol, disopyramide, doxycycline, estrogens, haloperidol, hormonal contraceptives, methadone, metapyrone, mexiletine, quinidine, theophylline, valproic acid:* increased metabolism and decreased effects of these drugs
Activated charcoal, antacids, sucralfate: decreased phenytoin absorption
Allopurinol, amiodarone, benzodiazepines, chloramphenicol, chlorpheniramine, cimetidine, disulfiram, fluconazole, ibuprofen, isoniazid, metronidazole, miconazole, omeprazole, phenacemide, phenothiazines, phenylbutazone, salicylates, succinimides, sulfonamides, tricyclic antidepressants, trimethoprim, valproic acid: increased phenytoin effects
Antineoplastics, barbiturates, carbamazepine, diazoxide, folic acid, influenza vaccine, loxapine, nitrofurantoin, pyridoxine, rifampin, theophylline: decreased phenytoin effects
Cyclosporine, dopamine, furosemide, levodopa, levonorgestrel, mebendazole, muscle relaxants, nondepolarizing phenothiazines, sulfonylureas: decreased effects of these drugs
Drug-diagnostic tests. *Alkaline phosphatase, eosinophils, gamma-glutamyltransferase, glucose:* increased levels
Dexamethasone (1-mg) suppression test, metyrapone test: interference with test results
Free thyroxine, serum thyroxine: decreased levels
Drug-food. *Enteral tube feedings:* decreased phenytoin absorption
Folic acid: decreased folic acid absorption
Drug-behaviors. *Acute alcohol ingestion:* increased phenytoin blood level
Chronic alcohol ingestion: decreased phenytoin blood level

Patient monitoring

- Assess blood pressure, ECG, and heart rate, especially during I.V. loading dose. Watch for adverse reactions.
- Monitor phenytoin blood level; therapeutic range is 10 to 20 mcg/ml.
- Evaluate CBC and kidney and liver function tests.
- Closely monitor prothrombin time and Internationalized Normal Ratio in patients receiving warfarin concurrently.
- Monitor drug efficacy.

Patient teaching

- Explain drug therapy, need for follow-up tests, and importance of taking drug exactly as prescribed.
- Caution patient not to stop therapy abruptly.
- Advise patient to avoid alcohol.

Instruct patient to report rash immediately.

- Inform patient that drug may discolor urine.
- Tell female patient drug may make hormonal contraceptives ineffective.
- Instruct patient to practice good dental hygiene to minimize gingival hyperplasia.
- Encourage patient to seek medical advice before taking over-the-counter preparations.
- As appropriate, review all other significant and life-threatening adverse reactions and interactions, especially those related to the drugs, tests, foods, and behaviors mentioned above.

pimecrolimus
Elidel

Pharmacologic class: Dermatologic agent
Therapeutic class: Immunomodulator
Pregnancy risk category C

Action
Unknown. Thought to inhibit T-cell activation by blocking transcription of early cytokines. Also blocks release of inflammatory cytokines and mediators from mast cells after stimulation by antigen/immunoglobin E.

Availability
Cream: 1%

Indications and dosages
➤ Mild to moderate atopic dermatitis
Adults and children ages 2 and older: Apply 1% cream topically b.i.d. to clean, dry, affected area.

Contraindications
- Hypersensitivity to drug or its components

Precautions
Use cautiously in:
- eczema herpeticum (Kaposi's varicelliform eruption), varicella zoster (chickenpox or shingles), herpes simplex infection, lymphadenopathy, mononucleosis, acute infectious Netherton's syndrome, skin infections or papilloma, warts, immunocompromised state
- concurrent use of CYP3A inhibitors
- pregnant or breastfeeding patients
- children younger than age 2 (safety not established).

Administration
- Apply thin layer to affected area.
- Don't use with occlusive dressing (may increase systemic absorption).

Route	Onset	Peak	Duration
Topical	Not systemically absorbed		

Adverse reactions
CNS: headache
EENT: sinus congestion, rhinorrhea
GI: nausea, vomiting, diarrhea, gastritis
Respiratory: upper respiratory tract infection
Skin: pruritus, application-site reaction or discomfort
Other: pyrexia, increased risk of viral or bacterial infections

Interactions
Drug-drug. *CYP3A inhibitors (such as calcium channel blockers, cimetidine, erythromycin):* inhibition of action by hepatic enzymes that eliminate pimecrolimus
Drug-behaviors. *Sunbathing:* possible increased risk of skin cancer

Patient monitoring
- Reevaluate at 6 weeks if lesions haven't healed.
- Discontinue therapy, as prescribed, if disease resolves.

Patient teaching
- Tell patient to apply to clean, dry skin and to wash hands afterward (unless hands are being treated).
- Caution patient not to use occlusive dressings.
- Tell patient drug may cause local reaction, such as a feeling of warmth or burning sensation. Advise him to contact prescriber if reaction is severe or lasts more than 1 week.
- Advise patient to apply missed dose as soon as possible. If it's almost time for next dose, tell him to skip missed dose and resume regular schedule.

• Tell patient to avoid natural or artificial sunlight and to use adequate sunblock on skin and lips.
• Instruct patient to contact prescriber if no improvement occurs after 6 weeks or if condition worsens.
• As appropriate, review all other significant adverse reactions and interactions, especially those related to the drugs and behaviors mentioned above.

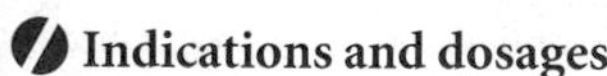

pimozide

Orap

Pharmacologic class: Diphenylbutylpiperidine
Therapeutic class: Antipsychotic
Pregnancy risk category C

Action

Unclear. Thought to relieve tics by blocking dopaminergic receptors on neurons in CNS.

Availability

Tablets: 1 mg, 2 mg

Indications and dosages

➢ Motor and phonic tics in Tourette's syndrome
Adults: Initially, 1 to 2 mg P.O. daily in divided doses, increased every other day p.r.n. For maintenance, 0.2 mg/kg/day or 10 mg/day (whichever is smaller).

Contraindications

• Hypersensitivity to drug
• Severe toxic CNS depression
• Congenital long-QT syndrome
• History of arrhythmias
• Concurrent use of itraconazole, ketoconazole, macrolide antibiotics, protease inhibitors, nefazodone, or other drugs that prolong QT interval or cause motor and phonic tics
• Simple tics or tics other than those associated with Tourette syndrome

Precautions

Use cautiously in:
• history of seizures, cardiovascular disorders, hepatic or renal dysfunction, ECG abnormalities
• disorders that could be aggravated by adverse anticholinergic effects
• pregnant or breastfeeding patients
• children younger than age 12.

Administration

• Give with or without food.
• To minimize daytime sedation, give entire daily dose at bedtime.

Route	Onset	Peak	Duration
P.O.	Unknown	6-8 hr	Unknown

Adverse reactions

CNS: drowsiness, headache, dizziness, insomnia, akathisia, rigidity, speech disorder, handwriting changes, sedation, depression, excitement, nervousness, abnormal dreams, hyperkinesia, tardive dyskinesia, parkinsonian-like symptoms, tremor, **neuroleptic malignant syndrome**
CV: abnormal ECG, hypotension, orthostatic hypotension, hypertension, palpitations, chest pain, tachycardia, **prolonged QT interval**
EENT: visual disturbance, perception of spots before eyes, decreased visual accommodation
GI: nausea, vomiting, diarrhea, constipation, eructation, dysphagia, excessive salivation, dry mouth
GU: urinary frequency, menstrual disorder, breast secretions, erectile dysfunction, libido loss
Musculoskeletal: muscle cramps or tightness, stooped posture, torticollis
Skin: rash, skin irritation, sweating, photosensitivity
Other: taste changes, thirst, appetite changes, weight gain or loss

Interactions

Drug-drug. *Amphetamines, methylphenidate, pemoline:* tics
Antiarrhythmics, azole antifungals, macrolide antibiotics, phenothiazines, protease inhibitors, tricyclic antidepressants: ECG abnormalities
Anticholinergics: increased anticholinergic effects
CNS depressants: additive CNS depression
Drug-diagnostic tests. *ECG:* abnormalities
Drug-food. *Grapefruit juice:* inhibited pimozide metabolism
Drug-behaviors. *Alcohol use:* increased CNS depression

Patient monitoring

◀ Assess neurologic status, especially for signs and symptoms of neuroleptic malignant syndrome (high fever, stupor, sweating, unstable blood pressure, muscle rigidity, and autonomic dysfunction) and parkinsonian-like symptoms.
- Monitor for tardive dyskinesia, even after drug therapy ends.
- Assess vital signs and ECG. Stay alert for prolonged QT interval, hypertension, or orthostatic hypotension.

Patient teaching

- Tell patient he may take with or without food but not with grapefruit juice.
- Caution patient not to stop taking suddenly. Dosage must be tapered.

◀ Teach patient to recognize and immediately report signs and symptoms of neuroleptic malignant syndrome and tardive dyskinesia. Tell patient tardive dyskinesia may develop long after drug therapy ends.
- Instruct patient to rise slowly and carefully, because blood pressure may drop if he stands up suddenly.
- Advise patient that drug may cause erectile dysfunction and libido loss. Encourage him to discuss these problems with prescriber.
- Tell patient drug may cause appetite changes. Encourage good nutrition.
- Inform patient that drug may cause vision changes and photosensitivity, which he should report.
- Instruct patient not to drink alcohol or grapefruit juice while taking drug.
- Caution patient to avoid driving and other hazardous activities until he knows how drug affects concentration, vision, and alertness.
- As appropriate, review all other significant and life-threatening adverse reactions and interactions, especially those related to the drugs, tests, foods, and behaviors mentioned above.

pindolol

Apo-Pindol✤, Novo-Pindol✤, Nu-Pindol✤, Visken

Pharmacologic class: Beta-adrenergic blocker (nonselective)
Therapeutic class: Antihypertensive
Pregnancy risk category B

Action

Competes with beta-adrenergic agonists for receptor sites, inhibiting both $beta_1$ (myocardial) and $beta_2$ (respiratory) sites

Availability

Tablets: 5 mg, 10 mg

Indications and dosages

➤ Hypertension
Adults: Initially, 5 mg b.i.d.; may increase by 10 mg/day q 3 to 4 weeks p.r.n. to a maximum of 60 mg/day

Contraindications

- Hypersensitivity to beta-adrenergic blockers
- Overt heart failure
- Cardiogenic shock

P

- Severe bradycardia
- Second- or third-degree heart block
- Bronchial asthma (including severe chronic obstructive pulmonary disease)

Precautions

Use cautiously in:

- renal or hepatic impairment, pulmonary disease, diabetes mellitus, thyrotoxicosis, severe allergic reactions, major surgery
- elderly patients
- pregnant or breastfeeding patients
- children (safety not established).

Administration

- Give with or without food.
- Know that drug may be used alone or with other antihypertensives.

Route	Onset	Peak	Duration
P.O.	Rapid	1 hr	8-15 hr

Adverse reactions

CNS: dizziness, drowsiness, lethargy, weakness, anxiety, depression, insomnia, nervousness, paresthesia
CV: orthostatic hypotension, peripheral vasoconstriction, chest pain, palpitations, tachycardia, bradycardia, **heart failure**
EENT: blurred vision, dry eyes
GI: nausea, vomiting, constipation, diarrhea
GU: erectile dysfunction, decreased libido
Musculoskeletal: joint pain, back pain, muscle cramps
Metabolic: hyperglycemia, **hypoglycemia**
Respiratory: wheezing, dyspnea, **bronchospasm**
Skin: itching, rash
Other: drug-induced lupus syndrome, edema, cold extremities

Interactions

Drug-drug. *Amphetamines, ephedrine, epinephrine, norepinephrine, phenylephrine, pseudoephedrine:* excessive hypertension and bradycardia
Beta-adrenergic bronchodilators, theophylline: decreased theophylline antagonism or antagonism of both drugs
Catecholamine-depleting drugs (such as reserpine): additive beta blockade
Insulin, oral hypoglycemics: altered efficacy of these drugs
Nonsteroidal anti-inflammatory drugs: decreased antihypertensive action
Other antihypertensives, nitrates: additive hypotension
Thyroid preparations: decreased pindolol efficacy
Drug-diagnostic tests. *Alanine aminotransferase, alkaline phosphatase, aspartate aminotransferase, lactate dehydrogenase, uric acid:* increased levels
Glucose: increased or decreased level
Drug-herbs. *Cocaine, ephedra (ma huang):* unopposed alpha-adrenergic stimulation

Patient monitoring

- Monitor apical heart rate. Withhold drug and notify prescriber if rate is below 60 beats/minute.
- Closely monitor ECG, vital signs, and cardiovascular status. Stay alert for signs and symptoms of heart failure.
- Assess respiratory status, especially for wheezing and dyspnea.
- Monitor blood glucose level in patients with diabetes. (Drug may mask signs and symptoms of hypoglycemia.)

Patient teaching

- Instruct patient to take at same time each day, with or without food.

[Clinical alert] Caution patient that stopping drug abruptly may worsen angina or cause severe cardiac problems.

- Advise patient to rise slowly from a lying or sitting position, to avoid dizziness from sudden blood pressure drop.

[Clinical alert] Instruct patient to report signs and symptoms of heart failure (such as swelling in legs and shortness of breath

when lying down) or other breathing difficulties.
• Advise diabetic patient to monitor blood glucose level closely.
• As appropriate, review all other significant and life-threatening adverse reactions and interactions, especially those related to the drugs, tests, and herbs mentioned above.

pioglitazone hydrochloride

Actos

Pharmacologic class: Thiazolidinedione

Therapeutic class: Hypoglycemic

Pregnancy risk category C

Action

Enhances insulin sensitivity in muscle and adipose tissue; inhibits hepatic gluconeogenesis

Availability

Tablets: 15 mg, 30 mg, 45 mg

Indications and dosages

➤ Adjunct to diet and exercise to improve glycemic control in type 2 (non-insulin-dependent) diabetes mellitus

Adults: 15 to 30 mg/day; may increase to 45 mg/day if needed

Contraindications

• Hypersensitivity to drug, its components, or rosiglitazone

Precautions

Use cautiously in:
• edema, hepatic impairment
• female patients of childbearing age
• pregnant or breastfeeding patients
• children (safety and efficacy not established).

Administration

• Give with or without food.
• Know that drug may be used with sulfonylureas, metformin, or insulin when combination of diet, exercise, and monotherapy doesn't achieve adequate glycemic control.

Route	Onset	Peak	Duration
P.O.	30 min	2 hr	24 hr

Adverse reactions

CNS: headache
EENT: sinusitis, pharyngitis
Hematologic: anemia
Metabolic: aggravation of diabetes mellitus, **hypoglycemia, hyperglycemia**
Musculoskeletal: myalgia
Respiratory: upper respiratory infection
Other: tooth disorders, pain, edema

Interactions

Drug-drug. *Hormonal contraceptives:* decreased contraceptive efficacy
Ketoconazole: increased pioglitazone effects
Drug-diagnostic tests. *Creatine kinase:* transient increase
Hematocrit, hemoglobin: decreased values (usually during first 4 to 12 weeks of therapy)
Drug-herbs. *Chromium, coenzyme Q10, fenugreek:* additive hypoglycemic effects
Glucosamine: poor glycemic control

Patient monitoring

• Assess patient's weight and compliance with diet and exercise program.
• Monitor liver function tests before and during therapy.
• Monitor glycosylated hemoglobin, hemoglobin, hematocrit, and blood glucose levels.
• Assess for signs and symptoms of hypoglycemia or hyperglycemia.

p

Patient teaching

- Instruct patient to take exactly as prescribed. Tell him he may take drug without regard to food.
- Tell patient drug may increase his risk for EENT and respiratory infections. Instruct him to contact prescriber if symptoms occur.

Advise patient to immediately report unexplained nausea, vomiting, abdominal pain, fatigue, anorexia, dark urine, fever, trauma, infection, rapid weight gain, edema, or shortness of breath.

- Tell premenopausal anovulatory patient that drug may cause ovulation. Recommend use of reliable contraception.
- Advise female of childbearing age to contact prescriber promptly if pregnancy occurs.
- As appropriate, review all other significant and life-threatening adverse reactions and interactions, especially those related to the drugs, tests, and herbs mentioned above.

piperacillin sodium

Pipracil

Pharmacologic class: Penicillin (extended-spectrum)

Therapeutic class: Anti-infective

Pregnancy risk category B

Action

Inhibits bacterial cell-wall synthesis during active multiplication stage, resulting in cell death

Availability

Injection: 2 g, 3 g, 4 g, 40 g

Indications and dosages

➢ To prevent infection during abdominal and vaginal surgery

Adults: For intra-abdominal surgery, 2 g I.V. just before surgery, followed by 2 g during surgery, then 2 g q 6 hours postoperatively for no more than 24 hours. For vaginal hysterectomy, 2 g I.V. just before surgery, followed by 2 g at 6 hours and 2 g at 12 hours after the initial dose. In cesarean delivery, 2 g I.V. after umbilical cord is clamped, followed by 2 g at 4 hours and 2 g at 8 hours after the initial dose. In abdominal hysterectomy, 2 g I.V. just before surgery, followed by 2 g on return to recovery room and 2 g 6 hours later.

➢ Serious infections

Adults: 12 to 18 g/day I.V. in divided doses q 4 to 6 hours

➢ Complicated urinary tract infection (UTI)

Adults: 8 to 16 g/day I.V. in divided doses q 6 to 8 hours

➢ Uncomplicated UTI or community-acquired pneumonia

Adults: 6 to 8 g/day I.M. or I.V. in divided doses q 6 to 12 hours

➢ Uncomplicated gonorrhea

Adults: 2 g I.M. as a single dose, with 1 g probenecid P.O. given 30 minutes before piperacillin injection

Dosage adjustment

- Renal impairment
- Elderly patients
- Children

Contraindications

- Hypersensitivity to penicillin or cephalosporins

Precautions

Use cautiously in:

- uremia, hypokalemia, cystic fibrosis, bleeding tendencies, drug allergies, sodium restriction
- pregnant or breastfeeding patients
- children younger than age 12.

Administration

• Ask patient about allergy to penicillin and cephalosporins before administering.
Keep epinephrine and emergency equipment available.
• For I.M. use, dilute in sterile water for injection or normal saline solution, to yield a final concentration of 400 mg/ml. Limit dosage to 2 g. Preferably, inject into upper outer buttock area.
• For intermittent I.V. infusion, dilute reconstituted solution in 50 ml of dextrose 5% in water, normal saline solution, dextrose 5% in normal saline solution, or lactated Ringer's solution. Infuse over 20 to 30 minutes.
• When giving I.V. bolus, inject reconstituted solution over 3 to 5 minutes.
• Don't mix with aminoglycosides in syringe or infusion container; doing so inactivates aminoglycoside.

Route	Onset	Peak	Duration
I.V.	Immediate	Immediate	Dose dependent
I.M.	Unknown	30-50 min	Dose dependent

Adverse reactions

CNS: headache, dizziness, fatigue, **seizures**
CV: thrombophlebitis, deep-vein thrombosis
GI: nausea, vomiting, constipation, diarrhea, bloody diarrhea, **pseudomembranous colitis**
Hematologic: hematoma, eosinophilia, **neutropenia, leukopenia, thrombocytopenia**
Hepatic: cholestatic hepatitis
Metabolic: hypokalemia, hypernatremia, sodium overload
Skin: rash, erythema, induration, bruising, **erythema multiforme, Stevens-Johnson syndrome**
Other: pain, superinfection, **anaphylaxis**

Interactions

Drug-drug. *Aminoglycosides:* aminoglycoside inactivation
Aspirin, probenecid: increased piperacillin blood level
Hormonal contraceptives: decreased contraceptive efficacy
Methotrexate: increased risk of methotrexate toxicity
Tetracyclines: decreased piperacillin efficacy
Vecuronium: prolonged neuromuscular blockade
Drug-diagnostic tests. *Bilirubin, blood urea nitrogen, creatinine, eosinophils, hepatic enzymes:* increased values
Coombs' test (with I.V. piperacillin): false-positive result
Granulocytes, hemoglobin, platelets, white blood cells: decreased levels

Patient monitoring

Monitor for signs and symptoms of anaphylaxis or superinfection.
Be aware that high doses may cause seizures.
Watch for signs and symptoms of thrombophlebitis and deep-vein thrombosis.
• Assess drug efficacy. Obtain repeat cultures after therapy ends.
Monitor potassium level and CBC with white cell differential. Check for blood dyscrasias and hypokalemia.
Assess for signs and symptoms of erythema multiforme (sore throat, rash, cough, iris lesions, mouth sores, cough, fever). Report early signs before condition can progress to Stevens-Johnson syndrome.

Patient teaching

• Stress importance of completing entire course of therapy.
Instruct patient to immediately report allergic reactions, rash, or severe diarrhea.
• Instruct patient to contact prescriber if signs and symptoms of infection worsen or if new symptoms develop.

p

• Advise female patient taking hormonal contraceptives to use alternate birth-control method.
• As appropriate, review all other significant and life-threatening adverse reactions and interactions, especially those related to the drugs and tests mentioned above.

piperacillin sodium and tazobactam sodium

Zosyn

Pharmacologic class: Penicillin (extended-spectrum), beta-lactamase inhibitor
Therapeutic class: Anti-infective
Pregnancy risk category B

Action

Piperacillin inhibits bacterial cell-wall synthesis, resulting in cell death. Tazobactam increases piperacillin efficacy.

Availability

Powder for injection: 2 g piperacillin and 0.25 g tazobactam/vial, 3 g piperacillin and 0.375 g tazobactam/vial, 4 g piperacillin and 0.5 g tazobactam/vial

Indications and dosages

➢ Community-acquired pneumonia; ruptured appendix; peritonitis; pelvic inflammatory disease; skin and skin-structure infections
Adults and children older than age 12: 3.375 g (3 g piperacillin and 0.375 g tazobactam) I.V. q 6 hours for 7 to 10 days
➢ Nosocomial pneumonia
Adults and children ages 12 and older: 3.375 g (3 g piperacillin and 0.375 g tazobactam) I.V. over 30 minutes q 4 hours for 7 to 14 days, given with an aminoglycoside

Dosage adjustment

• Renal impairment

Contraindications

• Hypersensitivity to penicillins, cephalosporins, imipenems, or beta-lactamase inhibitors
• Neonates

Precautions

Use cautiously in:
• heart failure, renal insufficiency (in children), seizures, bleeding disorders, uremia, hypokalemia, cystic fibrosis
• patients with sodium restrictions
• pregnant or breastfeeding patients.
• children younger than age 12 (safety and efficacy not established).

Administration

• Ask patient about allergy to penicillins, cephalosporins, imipenems, or beta-lactamase inhibitors before giving.
• Dilute each gram with 5 ml of diluent, such as sterile or bacteriostatic water for injection, normal saline solution for injection, dextrose 5% in water, dextrose 5% in normal saline solution for injection, or 6% dextran in normal saline solution. Don't use lactated Ringer's solution.
• Shake vial until drug dissolves. Dilute again to a final volume of 50 ml; infuse over 30 minutes.
• Don't mix with other drugs. If possible, stop primary infusion while piperacillin infuses.
• Don't mix in same container with aminoglycosides, which are chemically incompatible with piperacillin.

Route	Onset	Peak	Duration
I.V.	Immediate	Immediate	Unknown

Adverse reactions

CNS: headache, insomnia, agitation, dizziness, anxiety, lethargy, hallucinations, depression, twitching, **coma, seizures**

CV: hypertension, chest pain, tachycardia
EENT: rhinitis, glossitis
GI: nausea, vomiting, diarrhea, constipation, dyspepsia, abdominal pain, **pseudomembranous colitis**
GU: proteinuria, hematuria, vaginal candidiasis, vaginitis, **oliguria, interstitial nephritis, glomerulonephritis**
Hematologic: anemia, **increased bleeding, bone marrow depression, leukopenia, thrombocytopenia**
Metabolic: hypokalemia, hypernatremia
Respiratory: dyspnea
Skin: rash, pruritus
Other: fever; pain, edema, inflammation, or phlebitis at I.V. site; superinfection; hypersensitivity reactions including **serum sickness and anaphylaxis**

Interactions

Drug-drug. *Aminoglycosides:* aminoglycoside inactivation
Aspirin, probenecid: increased piperacillin blood level
Hormonal contraceptives: decreased contraceptive efficacy
Methotrexate: increased risk of methotrexate toxicity
Tetracyclines: decreased piperacillin efficacy
Vecuronium: prolonged neuromuscular blockade
Drug-diagnostic tests. *Coombs' test, urine glucose tests using copper reduction method (Clinitest, Benedict's or Fehling's solution), urine protein:* false-positive results
Eosinophils: increased count
Granulocytes, hemoglobin, platelets, white blood cells: decreased levels

Patient monitoring

- Assess neurologic status, especially for seizures.
- Monitor vital signs and fluid intake and output.
- Evaluate electrolyte levels, CBC with white cell differential, and culture and sensitivity tests. Watch for evidence of hypokalemia and blood dyscrasias.
- In patients receiving high doses or prolonged therapy, monitor for signs and symptoms of bacterial or fungal superinfection and pseudomembranous colitis.
- Monitor patient's dietary sodium intake (drug has high sodium content).

[Clinical alert] Immediately report rash, hives, severe diarrhea, black tongue, sore throat, fever, or unusual bleeding or bruising.

Patient teaching

- Tell patient to monitor urinary output and report significant changes.
- Instruct patient to report unusual pain, redness, swelling, or other changes at infusion site.
- As appropriate, review all other significant and life-threatening adverse reactions and interactions, especially those related to the drugs and tests mentioned above.

P

pirbuterol acetate

Maxair Autohaler

Pharmacologic class: Beta-adrenergic agonist
Therapeutic class: Bronchodilator
Pregnancy risk category C

Action

Increases production of cyclic adenosine monophosphate at beta-adrenergic receptors, producing bronchodilation and inhibiting histamine release. Primarily selective for $beta_2$-adrenergic (pulmonary) receptors, with minimal effect on $beta_1$-adrenergic (cardiac) receptors.

Availability

Inhalation aerosol: 200 mcg/spray (up to 400 inhalations/14.0-g canister)

Indications and dosages

➢ Reversible airway disease

Adults and children older than age 12: One or two inhalations q 4 to 6 hours (not to exceed 12 inhalations/day)

Contraindications

• Hypersensitivity to drug, adrenergic amines, or fluorocarbons

Precautions

Use cautiously in:

• cardiac disease, hypertension, hyperthyroidism, diabetes mellitus, glaucoma, hypokalemia
• elderly patients
• pregnant (near term) or breastfeeding patients
• children younger than age 12 (safety not established).

Administration

• If patient also uses a corticosteroid inhaler, give pirbuterol first, then wait 5 minutes before giving steroid.

Route	Onset	Peak	Duration
Inhalation	Within 5 min	1.5 hr	6-8 hr

Adverse reactions

CNS: headache, nervousness, restlessness, tremor, insomnia
CV: angina, hypertension, tachycardia, **arrhythmias**
GI: nausea, vomiting
Metabolic: hyperglycemia
Respiratory: paradoxical bronchospasm

Interactions

Drug-drug. *Beta-adrenergic blockers:* negation of pirbuterol's therapeutic effects
Diuretics: hypokalemia, exacerbation of ECG changes
MAO inhibitors: hypertensive crisis
Other adrenergics: additive adverse adrenergic effects
Drug-diagnostic tests. *Glucose:* increased level
Drug-food. *Caffeine-containing foods and beverages:* increased stimulant effect
Drug-herbs. *Caffeine-containing herbs (such as cola nut, guarana, yerba maté), ephedra (ma huang):* increased stimulant effect

Patient monitoring

Be aware that excessive use may lead to tolerance and paradoxical bronchospasm.
• Monitor respiratory status before and after administering. Note improvements.
• Assess dosage and dosing frequency needed to control symptoms. Notify prescriber if patient needs higher dosage to control symptoms.
• Assess vital signs and cardiovascular status. Stay alert for angina, hypertension, and arrhythmias.
• Monitor patient for worsening bronchospasm after administration.

Patient teaching

• Teach patient how to use metered-dose inhaler or autoinhaler.
• Instruct patient to wait at least 2 minutes between inhalations.
• If patient also uses inhaled corticosteroid, tell him to use pirbuterol first and then wait 5 minutes before using steroid.
• Advise patient to contact prescriber if he needs higher or more frequent doses to control symptoms.
• Teach patient to recognize signs and symptoms of bronchospasm. Advise him to notify prescriber if these worsen after he takes drug.
• Tell patient that herbs containing ephedra or caffeine may increase stimulant effects, such as nervousness and tremors.

• As appropriate, review all other significant and life-threatening adverse reactions and interactions, especially those related to the drugs, tests, foods, and herbs mentioned above.

piroxicam

Apo-Piroxicam✤, Feldene, Novo-Pirocam✤, Nu-Pirox✤

Pharmacologic class: Oxicam derivative, nonsteroidal anti-inflammatory drug (NSAID)
Therapeutic class: Analgesic, anti-inflammatory, antipyretic
Pregnancy risk category C (first and second trimesters), ***D*** (third trimester)

Action

Inhibits cyclooxygenase (an enzyme needed for prostaglandin synthesis), stimulating anti-inflammatory response and blocking pain impulses

Availability

Capsules: 10 mg, 20 mg

Indications and dosages

➢ Inflammatory disorders (such as arthritis)
Adults: 20 mg P.O. daily as a single dose or in two divided doses

Dosage adjustment

• Hepatic or renal impairment
• Elderly patients

Off-label uses

• Dysmenorrhea
• Ankylosing spondylitis
• Gout

Contraindications

• Hypersensitivity to drug or other NSAIDs (including aspirin)
• Active GI bleeding or ulcer disease
• Third trimester of pregnancy

Precautions

Use cautiously in:
• renal impairment, severe cardiovascular or hepatic disease
• history of ulcer disease
• pregnant patients in first or second trimester
• breastfeeding patients (not recommended)
• children (safety not established).

Administration

• Give with milk, antacids, or food to minimize GI upset.

Route	Onset	Peak	Duration
P.O. (analgesia)	1 hr	Unknown	48-72 hr
P.O. (anti-inflam.)	7-12 days	2-3 wk	Unknown

Adverse reactions

CNS: headache, drowsiness, dizziness
CV: edema, hypertension, vasculitis, tachycardia, **arrhythmias**
EENT: blurred vision, tinnitus
GI: nausea, vomiting, diarrhea, constipation, abdominal pain, flatulence, dyspepsia, anorexia, **severe GI bleeding**
GU: proteinuria, **renal failure**
Hematologic: anemia, **blood dyscrasias**
Hepatic: jaundice, **hepatitis**
Skin: rash
Other: allergic reactions including **anaphylaxis**

Interactions

Drug-drug. *Acetaminophen (chronic use), cyclosporine, gold compounds:* increased risk of adverse renal reactions
Anticoagulants, cefamandole, cefoperazone, cefotetan, clopidogrel, eptifibatide, heparin, plicamycin, thrombolytics, ticlopidine, tirofiban, valproic acid, vitamin A: increased risk of bleeding
Antineoplastics: increased risk of hematologic toxicity

Aspirin: decreased piroxicam blood level and efficacy
Corticosteroids, other NSAIDs: additive adverse GI reactions
Diuretics, other antihypertensives: decreased response to these drugs
Insulin, oral hypoglycemics: increased risk of hypoglycemia
Lithium: increased lithium blood level and risk of toxicity
Probenecid: increased piroxicam blood level and risk of toxicity
Drug-diagnostic tests. *Alanine aminotransferase, alkaline phosphatase, aspartate aminotransferase, blood urea nitrogen, creatinine, electrolytes, lactate dehydrogenase:* increased levels
Bleeding time: prolonged
Hematocrit, hemoglobin, platelets, white blood cells: decreased levels
Liver function tests: abnormal results
Drug-herbs. *Alfalfa, anise, arnica, astragalus, bilberry, black currant seed oil, bladderwrack, bogbean, boldo, borage oil, buchu, capsaicin, cat's claw, celery, chaparral, cinchona bark, clove oil, coenzyme Q10, dandelion, danshen, dong quai, evening primrose oil, fenugreek, feverfew, garlic, ginger, ginkgo, guggul, papaya extract, red clover, rhubarb, safflower oil, skullcap, St. John's wort:* increased anticoagulant effect, greater bleeding risk

Patient monitoring

- Monitor vital signs and cardiovascular status. Stay alert for hypertension and arrhythmias.
- Monitor kidney and liver function tests, hearing, and CBC.

Watch for signs and symptoms of drug-induced hepatitis and GI toxicity, including ulcers and bleeding.

- Monitor for signs and symptoms of infection, which drug may mask.

Patient teaching

- Advise patient to take with milk, antacids, or food to minimize GI upset.
- Tell patient drug may mask signs and symptoms of infection. Instruct him to contact prescriber if he suspects he has an infection.

Teach patient to recognize and immediately report signs and symptoms of allergic reaction or GI bleeding.

- Inform patient that many herbs increase the risk of GI bleeding. Caution him not to use herbs without prescriber's approval.
- Instruct patient to drink plenty of fluids and to report decreased urination.
- Caution patient to avoid driving and other hazardous activities until he knows how drug affects concentration and alertness.
- Tell female patient to inform prescriber if she is pregnant or breastfeeding.
- As appropriate, review all other significant and life-threatening adverse reactions and interactions, especially those related to the drugs, tests, and herbs mentioned above.

plasma protein fraction

Plasmanate, Plasma-Plex, Plasmatein, Protenate

Pharmacologic class: Human plasma protein
Therapeutic class: Plasma expander
Pregnancy risk category C

Action

Maintains plasma colloid osmotic pressure, enhancing movement of fluid from interstitial tissues into circulatory system and thereby regulating blood volume

Availability

Solution for injection: 5% in 50-ml, 250-ml, and 500-ml vials

Indications and dosages

➢ Hypovolemic shock

Adults: Initially, 250 to 500 ml by I.V. infusion, up to a maximum of 10 ml/minute

Infants and young children: 20 to 30 ml/kg (10 to 15 ml/lb) I.V. infused at a rate slower than 10 ml/minute. May repeat dose if needed.

➢ Hypoproteinemia

Adults: 1,000 to 1,500 ml daily by I.V. infusion, up to a maximum of 8 ml/minute

Contraindications

- Hypersensitivity to drug or albumin
- Heart failure
- Severe anemia
- Normal or increased intravascular volume
- During cardiopulmonary bypass

Precautions

Use cautiously in:

- hepatic or renal impairment, reduced cardiac reserve, decreased sodium intake
- pregnant patients.

Administration

- Ensure that patient is adequately hydrated before administering.
- Know that dosage and infusion rate depend on patient's condition and response to drug.
- Don't infuse through same I.V. line with solutions containing amino acids or alcohol.
- Don't use infusion that has been frozen or contains visible sediment.
- Infuse at a site distant from infection or trauma, usually at a rate no faster than 8 to 10 ml/minute.

Be aware that rapid infusion (especially in normovolemic patient) may cause vascular overload, dyspnea, and pulmonary edema.

- Monitor blood pressure. Slow infusion rate if hypotension occurs.

Route	Onset	Peak	Duration
I.V.	Immediate	Immediate	Unknown

Adverse reactions

CNS: headache, paresthesia

CV: hypotension, tachycardia, **vascular overload and heart failure** (with rapid I.V. infusion)

GI: nausea, vomiting, increased salivation

Respiratory: dyspnea, **pulmonary edema** (with rapid I.V. infusion)

Skin: rash, flushing

Other: fever, chills

Interactions

Drug-diagnostic tests. *Alkaline phosphatase:* false increase

Patient monitoring

Assess for signs and symptoms of vascular overload, including heart failure and pulmonary edema.

- Monitor vital signs hourly. Expect a gradual return to normal during and after drug therapy.
- Monitor fluid intake and output.

Patient teaching

- Instruct patient to report difficulty breathing.
- Tell patient drug may cause headache, nausea, and vomiting. Advise him to report these problems.
- Inform patient that he'll undergo regular blood tests.
- As appropriate, review all other significant and life-threatening adverse reactions and interactions, especially those related to the tests mentioned above.

plicamycin (mithramycin)

Mithracin

Pharmacologic class: Crystalline compound produced by *Streptomyces plicatus*

Therapeutic class: Antibiotic antineoplastic

Pregnancy risk category X

Action

Unknown. Thought to form complex that causes cross-linking of DNA strands, inhibiting cellular RNA and enzymatic RNA synthesis.

Availability

Injection: 2.5-mg vials

Indications and dosages

➢ Testicular cancer

Adults: 25 to 30 mcg/kg/day I.V. over 4 to 6 hours for 8 to 10 days, unless significant adverse effects or toxicity occur. Treatment course exceeding 10 daily doses not recommended.

➢ Hypercalcemia and hypercalciuria related to advanced cancer

Adults: 25 mcg/kg/day I.V. over 4 to 6 hours for 3 to 4 days; may repeat weekly until adequate response occurs

Dosage adjustment

- Renal failure

Contraindications

- Hypersensitivity to drug
- Thrombocytopenia, thrombocytopathy
- Bone marrow depression
- Coagulation disorders or increased risk of bleeding
- Females of childbearing potential
- Pregnancy or breastfeeding

Precautions

Use cautiously in:

- renal or hepatic disease, electrolyte imbalances.

Administration

◀ Follow facility policy for preparing, handling, and administering carcinogenic, mutagenic, or teratogenic drugs. Don't let drug touch skin or mucous membranes.

- Give antiemetic before plicamycin, as prescribed, to reduce nausea and vomiting.
- Dilute with 4.9 ml of sterile water for injection. Shake vial to dissolve.
- Further dilute in 1,000 ml of dextrose 5% in water or normal saline solution.
- Infuse I.V. over 4 to 6 hours. Discard unused portion.

Route	Onset	Peak	Duration
I.V.	1-2 days	3 days	3-15 days

Adverse reactions

CNS: headache, malaise, drowsiness, asthenia, lethargy, depression

CV: phlebitis

GI: nausea, vomiting, diarrhea, stomatitis, anorexia

GU: proteinuria

Hematologic: leukopenia, thrombocytopenia, bleeding syndrome

Hepatic: mild and reversible hepatotoxicity

Metabolic: hypokalemia, hypocalcemia, hypophosphatemia

Skin: facial flushing; rash; pain, redness, or swelling at injection site; cellulitis with extravasation

Other: fever

Interactions

Drug-drug. *Other antineoplastics:* increased plicamycin toxicity

Drug-diagnostic tests. *Blood urea nitrogen, creatinine, hepatic enzymes:* increased levels

Calcium, phosphate, potassium, platelets, white blood cells (WBCs): decreased levels
Drug-herbs. *Anise, arnica, chamomile, clove, dong quai, fenugreek, garlic, ginger, ginkgo, ginseng, licorice:* increased risk of bleeding
Chaparral, comfrey, eucalyptus, germander, jin bu huan, kava, pennyroyal, skullcap, valerian: increased risk of hepatotoxicity

Patient monitoring

Watch closely for bleeding syndrome, which usually starts with epistaxis and progresses quickly.
- Monitor liver function tests, electrolyte levels, platelet and WBC counts, and prothrombin time. Notify prescriber of platelet count less than 150,000/mm^3, WBC count less than 4,000/mm^3, or prothrombin time greater than 4 seconds longer than control.

Assess for indications of sudden drop in calcium level, such as Chvostek's sign, muscle cramps, carpopedal spasm, or tetany.
- Monitor I.V. site closely to avoid extravasation.

Patient teaching

Teach patient to recognize and immediately report easy bruising, bleeding, and hypocalcemia. Inform him that nosebleed may be first sign of a bleeding problem.
- Instruct patient to report unusual pain, redness, swelling, or other changes at infusion site.
- Caution female of childbearing age to avoid pregnancy during therapy. Advise her to report suspected pregnancy right away.
- Instruct patient to avoid herbs, because many herbs increase the risk of liver damage.
- As appropriate, review all other significant and life-threatening adverse reactions and interactions, especially those related to the drugs, tests, and herbs mentioned above.

poractant alfa

Curosurf

Pharmacologic class: Porcine lung extract
Therapeutic class: Exogenous pulmonary agent
Pregnancy risk category NR

Action

Stabilizes and expands alveoli by reducing their surface tension and replenishing surfactant, preventing alveolar collapse

Availability

Suspension for endotracheal instillation: 120 mg (1.5 ml), 240 mg (3 ml)

Indications and dosages

➢ Respiratory distress syndrome (RDS) in premature infants
Infants: 2.5 ml/kg birth weight endotracheally, with half of dose instilled into each bronchus; up to two subsequent doses of 1.25 ml/kg birth weight at 12-hour intervals may be needed. Maximum dosage is 5 ml/kg (initial dose plus two subsequent doses).

Off-label uses

- Adult RDS caused by viral pneumonia or near-drowning
- Infants with human immunodeficiency virus accompanied by *Pneumocystis jiroveci* pneumonia

Contraindications

None

Precautions

Use cautiously in:
- bradycardia, crackles, infection
- family history of pork allergy.

Administration

Clinical alert: Know that drug should be given only by clinicians experienced in intubation, ventilatory management, and resuscitation of neonates, because it can rapidly affect oxygenation and pulmonary function.

- Give first dose as soon as possible after RDS diagnosis, when patient's on ventilator.
- Be aware that drug is meant for endotracheal use only.
- Before use, slowly warm vial to room temperature and gently turn upside-down to ensure uniform suspension. Don't shake.
- Using large-gauge needle, withdraw entire contents of vial into 3-ml or 5-ml syringe. Attach precut, 8-cm #5 French catheter to syringe. Fill catheter with drug; discard excess drug through catheter so that only prescribed dose remains in syringe.
- Before giving, verify proper placement and patency of endotracheal tube. Make sure catheter doesn't extend beyond endotracheal tube.

Route	Onset	Peak	Duration
Intratracheal	Immediate	3 hr	Unknown

Adverse reactions

CV: transient hypotension and bradycardia

Respiratory: transient endotracheal tube blockage, decreased oxygen saturation, airway obstruction

Interactions

None significant

Patient monitoring

- Monitor vital signs and ECG. Watch for hypotension and bradycardia.

Clinical alert: Assess closely for endotracheal tube blockage and proper ventilation.

Patient teaching

- Reassure parents that infant will be monitored closely.

porfimer sodium

Photofrin

Pharmacologic class: Photosensitizing agent

Therapeutic class: Antineoplastic

Pregnancy risk category C

Action

Exerts photosensitizing action by damaging cancer cells through propagation of radical reactions; subsequent laser light photoactivation produces cytotoxic reaction in affected tissues

Availability

Injection (cake or freeze-dried powder): 75 mg/vial

Indications and dosages

➢ Obstructive esophageal cancer; obstructive endobronchial non-small-cell lung cancer

Adults: 2 mg/kg I.V. over 3 to 5 minutes, followed 40 to 50 hours later by laser light illumination. Second laser light application may be given 96 to 120 hours after injection. A total of three courses may be given, separated by at least 30 days.

Contraindications

- Hypersensitivity to porphyrins
- Porphyria
- Bronchoesophageal or tracheoesophageal fistula, tumor erosion into major blood vessels, and other conditions that rule out photodynamic therapy

Precautions

Use cautiously in:

- esophageal varices, endobronchial tumors in sites where treatment-induced inflammation could block main airway

- elderly patients
- pregnant or breastfeeding patients
- children (safety not established).

Administration

Know that drug should be given by slow I.V. push over 3 to 5 minutes only by clinicians trained in photodynamic therapy.

- Reconstitute with 31.8 ml of 5% dextrose injection or normal saline solution injection. Shake well until dissolved. Use immediately.
- Don't mix with other drugs in same syringe.

Take care to prevent extravasation. If extravasation occurs, protect area from light.

Don't let drug contact skin or eyes. Wear rubber gloves and eye protection. If contact occurs, avoid bright light, which could cause photosensitivity reaction.

Route	Onset	Peak	Duration
I.V.	30-40 hr	Unknown	Up to 90 days

Adverse reactions

CNS: anxiety, confusion, insomnia, asthenia
CV: hypotension, hypertension, chest pain, tachycardia, sick sinus syndrome, **heart failure, atrial fibrillation, myocardial infarction**
EENT: diplopia, photophobia, pharyngitis
GI: nausea, vomiting, diarrhea, constipation, abdominal pain, gastric ulcer, dyspepsia, melena, hematemesis, dysphagia, eructation, esophagitis, anorexia, **esophageal edema, esophageal tumor bleeding, esophageal stricture, esophageal perforation, peritonitis**
GU: urinary tract infection, candidiasis
Hematologic: anemia
Hepatic: jaundice
Metabolic: dehydration
Musculoskeletal: back pain
Respiratory: cough, dyspnea, bronchitis, pneumonia, stridor, **respiratory insufficiency or failure, bronchospasm, tracheoesophageal fistula, laryngotracheal edema, pleural effusion, pulmonary edema**
Skin: photosensitivity, local inflammatory response
Other: substernal or general pain, edema, weight loss, fever, surgical complications

Interactions

Drug-drug. *Glucocorticoids:* decreased efficacy of photodynamic therapy
Other photosensitizing drugs (fluoroquinolones, griseofulvin, phenothiazines, sulfonamides, sulfonylureas, tetracyclines, thiazide diuretics): increased photosensitivity
Drug-diagnostic tests. *Hemoglobin:* decreased level
Drug-behaviors. *Sun exposure:* increased risk of photosensitivity

Patient monitoring

Monitor for signs and symptoms of esophageal obstruction.

Assess vital signs and cardiovascular status. Watch for evidence of cardiac complications.

Monitor respiratory status, especially for difficulty breathing.

- Evaluate nutritional and hydration status.
- Watch for photosensitivity reaction. Protect patient's skin and eyes from direct sunlight and bright indoor light.

Patient teaching

Tell patient to immediately report difficulty breathing or swallowing.

- Emphasize importance of avoiding sun exposure for at least 30 days (or even up to 90 days or more) after therapy ends. Instruct patient to wear dark sunglasses with average white light transmittance below 4%.
- Inform patient that conventional ultraviolet sunscreens don't prevent photosensitivity reactions caused by drug.

P

• As appropriate, review all other significant and life-threatening adverse reactions and interactions, especially those related to the drugs, tests, and behaviors mentioned above.

potassium acetate

Pharmacologic class: Mineral, electrolyte

Therapeutic class: Electrolyte replacement, nutritional supplement

Pregnancy risk category C

Action

Maintains acid-base balance, isotonicity, and electrophysiologic balance throughout body tissues; crucial to nerve impulse transmission and contraction of cardiac, skeletal, and smooth muscle. Also essential for normal renal function and carbohydrate metabolism.

Availability

Concentrate for injection: 2 mEq/ml in 20-, 50-, and 100-ml vials; 4 mEq/ml in 50-ml vials

Indications and dosages

➢ To prevent or treat potassium depletion; diabetic acidosis; metabolic alkalosis; arrhythmias; periodic paralysis attacks; hyperadrenocorticism; primary aldosteronism; healing phase of burns or scalds; overmedication with adrenocorticoids, testosterone, or corticotropin

Adults: Dosage highly individualized. For potassium level above 2.5 mEq/L, give 40 mEq/L as additive to I.V. infusion at a maximum rate of 10 mEq/hour; maximum daily dosage is 200 mEq. For potassium level less than 2 mEq/L, give 80 mEq/L as additive to I.V. infusion at a maximum rate of 40 mEq/ hour (with cardiac monitoring); maximum daily dosage is 400 mEq.

Children: Dosage highly individualized; up to 3 mEq/kg or 40 mEq/m²/day as additive to I.V. infusion.

Contraindications

• Acute dehydration
• Heat cramps
• Hyperkalemia
• Hyperkalemic familial periodic paralysis
• Severe renal impairment
• Severe hemolytic reactions
• Untreated Addison's disease
• Severe tissue trauma
• Concurrent use of potassium-sparing diuretics, angiotensin-converting enzyme (ACE) inhibitors, or salt substitutes containing potassium

Precautions

Use cautiously in:
• cardiac disease, renal impairment, diabetes mellitus, hypomagnesemia
• pregnant or breastfeeding patients
• children (safety and efficacy not established).

Administration

• Make sure patient is well hydrated and urinating before starting therapy.

Give only as additive to I.V. infusion. Never give by I.V. push or I.M. route, and never give undiluted. Use peripheral line with maximum rate of 40 mEq/hour (with cardiac monitoring).

To ensure that potassium is well mixed in compatible solution, don't add potassium to I.V. bottle in hanging position.

Dilute in compatible I.V. solution. Administer slowly to reduce risk of fatal hyperkalemia.

• Know that maximum infusion rate without cardiac monitoring is 20 mEq/hour. Infusion rates above 20 mEq/hour necessitate cardiac monitoring.

- If patient complains of burning with I.V. administration, decrease flow rate.
- Be aware that potassium preparations are not interchangeable.
- Know that dosages are expressed in mEq of potassium and that potassium acetate contains 10.2 mEq/g.

Route	Onset	Peak	Duration
I.V.	Rapid	End of infusion	Unknown

Adverse reactions

CNS: confusion, unusual fatigue, restlessness, asthenia, flaccid paralysis, paresthesia, absent reflexes
CV: ECG changes, hypotension, **arrhythmias, heart block, cardiac arrest**
GI: nausea, vomiting, diarrhea, abdominal discomfort, flatulence
Metabolic: hyperkalemia
Musculoskeletal: weakness and heaviness of legs
Respiratory: respiratory paralysis
Other: irritation at I.V. site

Interactions

Drug-drug. *ACE inhibitors, potassium-sparing diuretics, other potassium-containing preparations:* increased risk of hyperkalemia
Drug-diagnostic tests. *Potassium:* increased level
Drug-food. *Salt substitutes containing potassium:* increased risk of hyperkalemia
Drug-herbs. *Dandelion:* increased risk of hyperkalemia
Licorice: decreased response to potassium

Patient monitoring

- Monitor renal function, fluid intake and output, and potassium, creatinine, and blood urea nitrogen levels.
- [Clinical alert] Know that potassium is contraindicated in severe renal impairment and must be used with extreme caution (if at all) in patients with any degree of renal impairment, because of risk of life-threatening hyperkalemia.
- Assess vital signs and ECG. Watch for arrhythmias.
- Evaluate patient's neurologic status. Stay alert for neurologic complications.
- Monitor I.V. site for irritation.

Patient teaching

- Instruct patient to report unusual pain, redness, swelling, or other reactions at infusion site.
- Advise patient to report nausea, vomiting, confusion, numbness and tingling, unusual tiredness or weakness, or heavy feeling in legs.
- Instruct patient to avoid salt substitutes.
- As appropriate, review all other significant and life-threatening adverse reactions and interactions, especially those related to the drugs, tests, foods, and herbs mentioned above.

potassium bicarbonate

K+Care ET

Pharmacologic class: Mineral, electrolyte
Therapeutic class: Electrolyte replacement, nutritional supplement
Pregnancy risk category C

Action

Maintains acid-base balance, isotonicity, and electrophysiologic balance throughout body tissues; crucial to nerve impulse transmission and contraction of cardiac, skeletal, and smooth muscle. Also essential for normal renal function and carbohydrate metabolism.

Availability

Tablets for effervescent oral solution: 25 mEq

P

Indications and dosages

➤ To prevent potassium depletion
Adults: Dosage highly individualized. Usual dosage is 25 mEq/day P.O. in divided doses.

➤ To treat potassium depletion
Adults: 50 to 100 mEq/day P.O. in divided doses, not to exceed a maximum daily dosage of 150 mEq

Contraindications

- Hypersensitivity to tartrazine or alcohol (with some products)
- Acute dehydration
- Heat cramps
- Hyperkalemia
- Hyperkalemic familial periodic paralysis
- Severe renal impairment
- Severe hemolytic reaction
- Severe tissue trauma
- Untreated Addison's disease
- Concurrent use of potassium-sparing diuretics, angiotensin-converting enzyme (ACE) inhibitors, or salt substitutes containing potassium

Precautions

Use cautiously in:
- cardiac disease, renal impairment, diabetes mellitus, hypomagnesemia
- pregnant or breastfeeding patients
- children (safety and efficacy not established).

Administration

- Ensure that patient is adequately hydrated and urinating before starting therapy.
- Give with meals and a full glass of water or juice to minimize GI upset.
- Be aware that potassium preparations aren't interchangeable.
- Know that dosages are expressed in mEq of potassium and that potassium bicarbonate contains 10 mEq potassium/g.

Route	Onset	Peak	Duration
P.O.	Unknown	1-2 hr	Unknown

Adverse reactions

CNS: confusion, unusual fatigue, restlessness, asthenia, flaccid paralysis, paresthesia
CV: ECG changes, hypotension, **heart block, arrhythmias, cardiac arrest**
GI: nausea, vomiting, diarrhea, abdominal discomfort, flatulence
Metabolic: hyperkalemia
Musculoskeletal: weakness and heaviness of legs

Interactions

Drug-drug. *ACE inhibitors, potassium-sparing diuretics, other potassium-containing preparations:* increased risk of hyperkalemia
Drug-diagnostic tests. *Potassium:* increased level
Drug-food. *Salt substitutes containing potassium:* increased risk of hyperkalemia
Drug-herbs. *Dandelion:* increased risk of hyperkalemia
Licorice: decreased response to potassium

Patient monitoring

- Monitor renal function, fluid intake and output, and potassium, creatinine, and blood urea nitrogen levels.

[Clinical alert] Be aware that potassium is contraindicated in patients with severe renal impairment and must be used with extreme caution (if at all) in patients with any degree of renal impairment, because of risk of life-threatening hyperkalemia.

- Assess vital signs. Check ECG for arrhythmias.
- Monitor neurologic status. Stay alert for neurologic complications.

Patient teaching

- Instruct patient to dissolve tablets thoroughly in 4 to 8 oz of cold water or juice and to sip solution over 5 to 10 minutes with a meal.

• Advise patient to minimize GI upset by eating small, frequent servings of food and drinking plenty of fluids.
• Tell patient to report nausea, vomiting, confusion, numbness and tingling, unusual tiredness or weakness, or a heavy feeling in legs.
• Instruct patient to avoid salt substitutes.
• As appropriate, review all other significant and life-threatening adverse reactions and interactions, especially those related to the drugs, tests, foods, and herbs mentioned above.

potassium chloride

Apo-K✱, K+ 8, K+ 10, Klor-Con, K-Med✱, K-Tab, Micro-K, Micro-K Extencaps, Slow-K

Pharmacologic class: Mineral, electrolyte

Therapeutic class: Electrolyte replacement, nutritional supplement

Pregnancy risk category C

Action

Maintains acid-base balance, isotonicity, and electrophysiologic balance throughout body tissues; crucial to nerve impulse transmission and contraction of cardiac, skeletal, and smooth muscle. Also essential for normal renal function and carbohydrate metabolism.

Availability

Capsules (extended-release): 8 mEq, 10 mEq
Powder for oral solution: 20 mEq, 25 mEq
Parenteral injection (concentrate): 2 mEq/ml
Parenteral solution: 0.1 mEq/ml, 0.2 mEq/ml, 0.3 mEq/ml, 0.4 mEq/ml
Potassium chloride in 5% dextrose injection: 10 mEq/L, 20 mEq/L, 30 mEq/L, 40 mEq/L
Potassium chloride in 0.9% sodium chloride injection: 20 mEq/L, 40 mEq/L
Potassium chloride in dextrose and lactated Ringer's injection: various strengths
Potassium chloride in dextrose and sodium chloride injection: various strengths
Solution (oral): 6.7 mEq, 10 mEq, 13.3 mEq, 15 mEq, 20 mEq, 30 mEq, 40 mEq
Tablets: 500 mg, 595 mg
Tablets (effervescent): 25 mEq, 50 mEq
Tablets (extended-release): 8 mEq, 10 mEq, 20 mEq
Tablets (extended-release crystals): 10 mEq, 20 mEq
Tablets (extended-release, film coated): 8 mEq, 10 mEq
Tablets (film-coated): 2.5 mEq, 10 mEq

Indications and dosages

➢ To prevent potassium depletion
Adults: Dosage highly individualized. Usual single dosage is 20 mEq/day P.O. in divided doses.
➢ Potassium depletion; diabetic acidosis; metabolic alkalosis; arrhythmias; periodic paralysis attacks; hyperadrenocorticism; primary aldosteronism; healing phase of scalds or burns; overmedication with adrenocorticoids, testosterone, or corticotropin
Adults: Dosage highly individualized. 40 to 100 mEq/day P.O. in divided doses, not to exceed 20 mEq in a single dose. For serum potassium level above 2.5 mEq/L, 40 mEq/L as additive to I.V. infusion at a maximum rate of 10 mEq/hour; maximum daily dosage is 200 mEq. For serum potassium level less than 2 mEq/L, 80 mEq/L as additive to I.V. infusion at a maximum rate of 40 mEq/hour (with cardiac monitoring); maximum daily dosage is 400 mEq.
Children: Dosage highly individualized; give up to 3 mEq/kg or 40 mEq/m^2/day as additive to I.V. infusion.

Contraindications

- Hypersensitivity to tartrazine or alcohol (with some products)
- Acute dehydration
- Heat cramps
- Hyperkalemia
- Hyperkalemic familial periodic paralysis
- Severe renal impairment
- Severe hemolytic reactions
- Severe tissue trauma
- Untreated Addison's disease
- Esophageal compression caused by enlarged left atrium (with wax matrix forms)
- Concurrent use of potassium-sparing diuretics, angiotensin-enzyme converting (ACE) inhibitors, or salt substitutes containing potassium

Precautions

Use cautiously in:

- cardiac disease, renal impairment, diabetes mellitus, hypomagnesemia
- pregnant or breastfeeding patients
- children (safety and efficacy not established).

Administration

◀ Know that I.V. potassium chloride is a high-alert drug.

◀ Give I.V. form as additive by infusion only. Never give undiluted or by I.V. push or I.M. route. Use peripheral line and infuse at a maximum rate of 40 mEq/hour (with cardiac monitoring).

◀ Dilute in compatible I.V. solution per manufacturer's instructions. Administer slowly to reduce risk of fatal hyperkalemia.

◀ To ensure that potassium is well mixed in compatible solution, don't add potassium to I.V. bottle in hanging position.

◀ Be aware that maximum infusion rate without cardiac monitoring is 20 mEq/hour. Rates above 20 mEq/hour require cardiac monitoring.

- Make sure patient is well-hydrated and urinating before starting therapy.
- If patient complains of burning with I.V. administration, decrease flow rate.
- Give P.O. form with meals and a full glass of water or juice, to minimize GI upset.
- Ensure that patient swallows wax-matrix tablets completely, to avoid serious esophageal problems.
- Don't give wax matrix tablets to patients who have swallowing problems or possible esophageal compression.
- Be aware that potassium preparations aren't interchangeable.
- Know that dosages are expressed in mEq of potassium and that potassium chloride contains 13.4 mEq potassium/g.

Route	Onset	Peak	Duration
P.O.	Unknown	1-2 hr	Unknown
I.V.	Rapid	End of infusion	Unknown

Adverse reactions

CNS: confusion, unusual fatigue, restlessness, asthenia, flaccid paralysis, paresthesia, absent reflexes
CV: ECG changes, hypotension, **arrhythmias, heart block, cardiac arrest**
GI: nausea, vomiting, diarrhea, abdominal discomfort, flatulence
Metabolic: hyperkalemia
Musculoskeletal: weakness and heaviness of legs
Respiratory: respiratory paralysis
Other: irritation at I.V. site

Interactions

Drug-drug. *ACE inhibitors, potassium-sparing diuretics, other potassium-containing preparations:* increased risk of hyperkalemia
Drug-diagnostic tests. *Potassium:* increased level
Drug-food. *Salt substitutes containing potassium:* increased risk of hyperkalemia

Drug-herbs. *Dandelion:* increased risk of hyperkalemia
Licorice: decreased response to potassium

Patient monitoring

- Monitor renal function, fluid intake and output, and potassium, creatinine, and blood urea nitrogen levels.
- Assess vital signs and ECG. Stay alert for arrhythmias.
- Monitor neurologic status. Watch for neurologic complications.
- Monitor I.V. site for irritation.

Know that potassium is contraindicated in patients with severe renal impairment and must be used with extreme caution (if at all) in patients with any degree of renal impairment, because of risk of life-threatening hyperkalemia.

Patient teaching

- Instruct patient to mix and dissolve powder completely in 3 to 8 oz of water or juice.
- Tell patient to swallow extended-release capsules whole without crushing or chewing them.
- Instruct patient to take oral form with or just after a meal, with a glass of water or fruit juice.
- Tell patient to sip diluted liquid form over 5 to 10 minutes.
- Advise patient to report nausea, vomiting, confusion, numbness and tingling, unusual fatigue or weakness, or a heavy feeling in legs.
- Tell patient to minimize GI upset by eating frequent, small servings of food and drinking plenty of fluids.
- Inform patient that although wax matrix form may appear in stool, drug has already been absorbed.
- Advise patient not to use salt substitutes.
- As appropriate, review all other significant and life-threatening adverse reactions and interactions, especially those related to the drugs, tests, foods, and herbs mentioned above.

potassium gluconate

Potassium-Rougier✦

Pharmacologic class: Mineral, electrolyte
Therapeutic class: Electrolyte replacement, nutritional supplement
Pregnancy risk category C

Action

Maintains acid-base balance, isotonicity, and electrophysiologic balance throughout body tissues; crucial to nerve impulse transmission and contraction of cardiac, skeletal, and smooth muscle. Also essential for normal renal function and carbohydrate metabolism.

Availability

Elixir: 20 mEq/15 ml
Tablets: 2 mEq, 5 mEq

Indications and dosages

➢ To prevent potassium depletion
Adults: Dosage highly individualized. Usual daily dosage is 20 mEq P.O. in divided doses.

➢ To treat potassium depletion
Adults: 40 to 100 mEq/day P.O. in divided doses, not to exceed 20 mEq in a single dose

Contraindications

- Hypersensitivity to tartrazine or alcohol (with some products)
- Acute dehydration
- Heat cramps
- Hyperkalemia
- Hyperkalemic familial periodic paralysis
- Severe renal impairment
- Severe hemolytic reactions
- Severe tissue trauma

p

- Untreated Addison's disease
- Concurrent use of potassium-sparing diuretics, angiotensin-converting enzyme (ACE) inhibitors, or salt substitutes containing potassium

Precautions

Use cautiously in:
- cardiac disease, renal impairment, diabetes mellitus, hypomagnesemia
- pregnant or breastfeeding patients
- children (safety and efficacy not established).

Administration

- Make sure patient is adequately hydrated and urinating before starting therapy.
- Give with food or meals and a full glass of water or juice to minimize GI upset.
- Be aware that potassium preparations are not interchangeable.
- Know that dosages are expressed in mEq of potassium and that potassium gluconate contains 4.3 mEq/g.

Route	Onset	Peak	Duration
P.O.	Unknown	1-2 hr	Unknown

Adverse reactions

CNS: confusion, unusual tiredness, restlessness, asthenia, flaccid paralysis, paresthesia
CV: ECG changes, hypotension, **arrhythmias, heart block, cardiac arrest**
GI: nausea, vomiting, diarrhea, abdominal discomfort, flatulence
Metabolic: hyperkalemia
Musculoskeletal: weakness and heaviness of legs

Interactions

Drug-drug. *ACE inhibitors, potassium-sparing diuretics, other potassium preparations:* increased risk of hyperkalemia
Drug-diagnostic tests. *Potassium:* increased level
Drug-food. *Salt substitutes containing potassium:* increased risk of hyperkalemia
Drug-herbs. *Dandelion:* increased risk of hyperkalemia
Licorice: decreased response to potassium

Patient monitoring

- Monitor renal function, fluid intake and output, and potassium, creatinine, and blood urea nitrogen levels.
- [Clinical alert] Know that potassium is contraindicated in patients with severe renal impairment and must be used with extreme caution (if at all) in patients with any degree of renal impairment, because of risk of life-threatening hyperkalemia.
- Monitor vital signs and check ECG for arrhythmias.
- Monitor patient's neurologic status for signs or symptoms of complications.

Patient teaching

- Tell patient to take oral form with or just after meals, with a glass of water or fruit juice.
- Instruct patient to dilute liquid form in water or juice and to sip it over 5 to 10 minutes.
- Advise patient to report nausea, vomiting, confusion, numbness and tingling, unusual tiredness or weakness, or a heavy feeling in legs.
- Tell patient to minimize GI upset by eating small, frequent servings of food and drinking plenty of fluids.
- Advise patient not to use salt substitutes.
- As appropriate, review all other significant and life-threatening adverse reactions and interactions, especially those related to the drugs, tests, foods, and herbs mentioned above.

potassium iodide
Pima, Thyro-Block

Pharmacologic class: Iodine, iodide
Therapeutic class: Antithyroid agent, expectorant
Pregnancy risk category D

Action
Rapidly inhibits thyroid hormone release, reduces thyroid vascularity, and decreases thyroid uptake of radioactive iodine after radiation emergencies or administration of radioactive iodine isotopes. As expectorant, thought to increase respiratory tract secretions, thereby decreasing mucus viscosity.

Availability
Saturated solution (SSKI): 1 g potassium iodide/ml in 30- and 240-ml bottles
Solution (strong iodine solution, Lugol's solution): 5% iodine and 10% potassium iodide in 120-ml bottle
Syrup: 325 mg potassium iodide/5 ml
Tablets: 130 mg (available only through state and federal agencies)

Indications and dosages
➢ Preparation for thyroidectomy
Adults and children: One to five drops SSKI P.O. t.i.d. or three to six drops strong iodine solution P.O. t.i.d. for 10 days before surgery
➢ Thyrotoxic crisis
Adults and children: 500 mg P.O. (approximately 10 drops SSKI) q 4 hours or 1 ml P.O. (strong iodine solution) t.i.d., at least 1 hour after initial propylthiouracil or methimazole dose
➢ Radiation protectant in emergencies
Adults older than age 40 with predicted thyroid exposure of 500 centigrays (cGy), adults ages 18 to 40 with predicted exposure of 10 cGy, pregnant or breastfeeding women with predicted exposure of 5 cGy, and adolescents weighing 70 kg (154 lb) or more with predicted exposure of 5 cGy: 130 mg P.O. (tablet)
Children ages 3 to 18 (except adolescents weighing 70 kg [154 lb] or more) with predicted thyroid exposure of 5 cGy: 65 mg P.O. (tablet)
Children ages 1 month to 3 years with predicted thyroid exposure of 5 cGy: 32 mg P.O. (tablet)
Infants from birth to age 1 month with predicted thyroid exposure of 5 cGy: 16 mg P.O. (tablet)
➢ Expectorant
Adults: 300 to 650 mg P.O. (SSKI) three or four times daily, given with at least 6 oz of fluid
Children: 60 to 250 mg P.O. (SSKI) q.i.d., given with at least 6 oz of fluid

Off-label uses
- Lymphocutaneous sporotrichosis

Contraindications
- Hypersensitivity to iodine, shellfish, or bisulfites (with some products)
- Hypothyroidism
- Renal impairment
- Acute bronchitis
- Addison's disease
- Acute dehydration
- Heat cramps
- Hyperkalemia
- Tuberculosis
- Iodism
- Concurrent use of potassium-containing drugs, potassium-sparing diuretics, or salt substitutes containing potassium

Precautions
Use cautiously in:
- cystic fibrosis, adolescent acne, hypocomplementemic vasculitis, goiter, autoimmune thyroid disease
- pregnant or breastfeeding patients
- children.

p

Administration

• Dilute saturated solution with at least 6 oz of water.

Clinical alert: Don't give concurrently with other potassium-containing drugs or potassium-sparing diuretics, because of increased risk of hyperkalemia, arrhythmias, and cardiac arrest.

• Know that U.S. government stockpiles potassium iodide 130-mg tablets for emergency use.

• When giving to very young children or patients who can't swallow tablets, crush tablet, dissolve in 20 ml of water, and add 20 ml of selected beverage (such as orange juice).

• Be aware that potassium iodide use as expectorant has been largely replaced by safer and more effective drugs.

Route	Onset	Peak	Duration
P.O.	24 hr	10-15 days	Variable

Adverse reactions

CNS: confusion; unusual fatigue; paresthesia, pain, or weakness in hands or feet

Metabolic: thyroid hyperplasia, goiter (with prolonged use), thyroid adenoma, severe hypothyroidism, **hyperkalemia, iodism** (with large doses or prolonged use)

Musculoskeletal: weakness and heaviness of legs

Other: tooth discoloration (with strong iodide solution), hypersensitivity reactions including angioedema, fever, cutaneous and mucosal hemorrhage, serum sickness–like reaction

Interactions

Drug-drug. *Lithium, other thyroid drugs:* additive hypothyroidism

Potassium-sparing diuretics, other potassium preparations: increased risk of hyperkalemia, arrhythmias, and cardiac arrest

Drug-diagnostic tests. *Radionuclide thyroid imaging:* altered test results

Thyroid uptake of ^{131}I, ^{123}I, *sodium pertechnetate Tc 99m:* decreased uptake

Drug-food. *Salt substitutes containing potassium:* increased risk of hyperkalemia

Patient monitoring

Clinical alert: In long-term use, check for signs and symptoms of iodism (metallic taste, sore teeth and gums, sore throat, burning of mouth and throat, coldlike symptoms, severe headache, productive cough, GI irritation, diarrhea, angioedema, rash, fever, and cutaneous or mucosal hemorrhage). Discontinue drug immediately if these occur.

• Monitor potassium level; watch for signs and symptoms of potassium toxicity.

• Assess ECG, renal function, fluid intake and output, and creatinine and blood urea nitrogen levels.

• Monitor thyroid function tests. Watch for evidence of hypothyroidism or hyperthyroidism.

Patient teaching

• Tell patient to dilute in at least 6 oz of water or juice and to take with meals.

• Advise patient to sip strong iodine solution through a straw to help prevent tooth discoloration.

Clinical alert: Teach patient to recognize and immediately report signs and symptoms of iodism and potassium toxicity.

• Instruct patient to minimize GI upset by eating small, frequent servings of food and drinking plenty of fluids.

• Inform patient that many salt substitutes are high in potassium. Advise him not to use these without prescriber's approval.

• Caution patient not to take drug if she is pregnant or breastfeeding (except in emergency use).

• As appropriate, review all other significant and life-threatening adverse reactions and interactions, especially those related to the drugs, tests, and foods mentioned above.

pramipexole dihydrochloride

Mirapex

Pharmacologic class: Non-ergot dopamine agonist
Therapeutic class: Antidyskinetic
Pregnancy risk category C

Action

Unknown. May directly stimulate postsynaptic dopamine receptors in corpus striatum (unlike levodopa, which may increase brain's dopamine concentration).

Availability

Tablets: 0.125 mg, 0.25 mg, 0.5 mg, 1 mg, 1.5 mg

Indications and dosages

➢ Idiopathic Parkinson's disease
Adults: Initially, 0.125 mg P.O. t.i.d.; may increase by 0.125 mg q 5 to 7 days over 6 to 7 weeks. Maintenance dosage ranges from 1.5 to 4.5 mg/day in three divided doses.

Dosage adjustment

- Renal impairment

Contraindications

- Hypersensitivity to drug or its components

Precautions

Use cautiously in:
- renal impairment
- elderly patients
- pregnant or breastfeeding patients
- children (safety not established).

Administration

- Don't give at same time as other CNS depressants.
- Don't stop therapy abruptly. Taper dosage over 1 week.

Route	Onset	Peak	Duration
P.O.	Unknown	2 hr	8 hr

Adverse reactions

CNS: headache, dizziness, drowsiness, hallucinations, asthenia, confusion, dyskinesia, insomnia, hypertonia, unsteadiness, sleep attacks, abnormal dreams, amnesia
CV: orthostatic hypotension
GI: nausea, constipation, dyspepsia, dry mouth
GU: urinary frequency, erectile dysfunction
Musculoskeletal: leg cramps
Respiratory: fibrotic complications (such as retroperitoneal fibrosis, pulmonary infiltrates, pleural effusion or thickening)
Other: accidental injury, edema

Interactions

Drug-drug. *Cimetidine:* increased pramipexole blood level
Dopamine antagonists (such as butyrophenones, metoclopramide, phenothiazines, thioxanthenes): decreased pramipexole efficacy
Levodopa: increased risk of hallucinations and dyskinesia

Patient monitoring

- Evaluate patient for therapeutic and adverse effects.
- Assess blood pressure; watch for orthostatic hypotension.
- Monitor neurologic status, especially for sleep attacks and extrapyramidal symptoms.
- Watch closely for pulmonary complications.

Patient teaching

- Instruct patient to take drug with food if it causes nausea. Tell him not to take at same time as other CNS depressants.

• Advise patient to report respiratory problems, dyskinesia, hallucinations, and sleep attacks.
• Tell patient drug may cause erectile dysfunction. Encourage him to discuss this effect with prescriber.
• Inform patient and family that drug's neurologic and motor effects increase risk of accidental injury. Teach them ways to prevent injury.
• Tell patient to move slowly when sitting up or standing, to avoid dizziness from sudden blood pressure decrease.
• As appropriate, review all other significant and life-threatening adverse reactions and interactions, especially those related to the drugs mentioned above.

pravastatin sodium

Pravachol

Pharmacologic class: HMG-CoA reductase inhibitor
Therapeutic class: Antilipemic
Pregnancy risk category X

Action

Inhibits HMG-CoA reductase, an enzyme that catalyzes cholesterol synthesis pathway. This action decreases cholesterol, triglyceride, apolipoprotein B, and low-density lipoprotein (LDL) levels and increases high-density lipoprotein levels.

Availability

Tablets: 10 mg, 20 mg, 40 mg, 80 mg

Indications and dosages

➢ Adjunct to diet to control levels of total cholesterol, LDL, triglycerides, and apolipoprotein B in primary hypercholesterolemia, mixed dyslipidemia (including Fredrickson types IIa and IIb), primary dysbetalipoproteinemia (Fredrickson type III), and hypertriglyceridemia (including Fredrickson type IV); primary and secondary prevention of cardiovascular events

Adults: 10 to 80 mg P.O. daily. Usual dosage is 40 mg/day.
Children ages 5 to 13: 20 mg daily

Contraindications

• Hypersensitivity to drug or other HMG-CoA reductase inhibitors
• Active hepatic disease or unexplained, persistent transaminase elevations
• Pregnancy, breastfeeding, females of childbearing age

Precautions

Use cautiously in:
• renal impairment; severe hypotension or hypertension; severe acute infection; severe metabolic, endocrine, or electrolyte disorders; uncontrolled seizures; visual disturbances; myopathy; major surgery; trauma; alcoholism
• history of hepatic disease
• concurrent use of gemfibrozil or azole antifungals
• children under age 18 (safety not established).

Administration

• If patient's also receiving bile-acid resin, give pravastatin at bedtime, at least 4 hours after resin.

Route	Onset	Peak	Duration
P.O.	Unknown	Unknown	Unknown

Adverse reactions

CNS: headache, malaise, fatigue, dizziness, insomnia, anxiety, depression, tremor, vertigo, memory loss, peripheral nerve palsy, paresthesia, peripheral neuropathy, asthenia
EENT: impaired extraocular eye movements, cataract progression, ophthalmoplegia, dry eyes
GI: nausea, vomiting, diarrhea, constipation, abdominal or biliary pain, flat-

ulence, dyspepsia, heartburn, anorexia, **pancreatitis**
GU: decreased libido, erectile dysfunction, gynecomastia
Hematologic: anemia, **thrombocytopenia, leukopenia**
Hepatic: jaundice, cholestatic jaundice, fatty liver changes, **hepatoma, hepatic necrosis, hepatitis**
Musculoskeletal: joint pain, myalgia, myositis, **rhabdomyolysis**
Respiratory: dyspnea
Skin: nodules, skin discoloration, alopecia, dry skin, pruritus, rash, urticaria, nail changes, photosensitivity
Other: altered taste, localized pain, rare hypersensitivity reactions (including polymyalgia rheumatica, arthritis, dermatomyositis, vasculitis, purpura, positive antinuclear antibody, eosinophilia, fever, chills, flushing, **hemolytic anemia, epidermal necrolysis, erythema multiforme, Stevens-Johnson syndrome, angioedema, lupus erythematosus–like reaction, and anaphylaxis**)

Interactions

Drug-drug. *Antacids, colestipol:* decreased pravastatin blood level
Azole antifungals, cyclosporine, erythromycin, gemfibrozil, niacin, other HMG-CoA reductase inhibitors: increased risk of myopathy
Drug-diagnostic tests. *Alanine aminotransferase, aspartate aminotransferase, creatine kinase, creatinine phosphokinase:* increased levels
Drug-herbs. *Chaparral, comfrey, eucalyptus, germander, jin bu huan, kava, pennyroyal, skullcap, valerian:* increased risk of hepatotoxicity
Red yeast rice: increased risk of adverse drug reactions

Patient monitoring

- Watch for signs and symptoms of allergic reaction.
- Monitor vital signs and cardiovascular status.

🔊 Evaluate liver function tests before starting therapy, 6 to 12 weeks later, and at least semiannually thereafter. Also monitor lipid levels, and watch for evidence of hepatic disorders (rare).

🔊 Assess creatine kinase level if patient has muscle pain or is receiving other drugs associated with myopathy.

- Monitor for signs and symptoms of rhabdomyolysis (rare).

Patient teaching

- Caution patient not to take with antacids.

🔊 Teach patient to recognize and immediately report signs and symptoms of allergic response and other adverse reactions, especially myositis.

- Tell patient drug may cause headache and musculoskeletal pain. Encourage him to discuss activity recommendations and pain management with prescriber.

🔊 Advise patient to promptly report unusual fatigue, yellowing of skin or eyes, and unexplained muscle pain, tenderness, or weakness.

- Advise female of childbearing age to notify prescriber of suspected pregnancy. Caution her not to breastfeed during therapy.
- Tell male patient that drug may cause erectile dysfunction and abnormal ejaculation. Suggest that he discuss these issues with prescriber.
- Caution patient to avoid driving and other hazardous activities until he knows how drug affects concentration, alertness, and vision.
- As appropriate, review all other significant and life-threatening adverse reactions and interactions, especially those related to the drugs, tests, and herbs mentioned above.

prazosin hydrochloride

Minipress, Minipress XL

Pharmacologic class: Alpha$_1$-adrenergic blocker (peripherally acting)
Therapeutic class: Antihypertensive
Pregnancy risk category C

Action

Induces peripheral vasodilation by blocking postsynaptic alpha$_1$-adrenergic receptors, thereby lowering blood pressure. Decreases smooth muscle contractions of prostatic capsule and relaxes smooth muscles in bladder neck and prostate.

Availability

Capsules: 1 mg, 2 mg, 5 mg

Indications and dosages

➢ Hypertension

Adults: Initially, 1 mg P.O. two or three times daily for 3 days, with first dose at bedtime; increase gradually to a maintenance dosage of 6 to 15 mg/day given in two or three divided doses.

Off-label uses

- Benign prostatic hypertrophy

Contraindications

- Hypersensitivity to drug or other quinazoline alpha$_1$-adrenergic blockers

Precautions

Use cautiously in:

- renal insufficiency, angina pectoris, hepatic impairment
- patients receiving diuretics concurrently
- pregnant or breastfeeding patients
- children (safety not established).

Administration

- Give test dose of 1 mg at bedtime to prevent first-dose syncope.
- Don't stop therapy suddenly. Dosage must be tapered.

Route	Onset	Peak	Duration
P.O.	2 hr	2-4 hr	10 hr

Adverse reactions

CNS: dizziness, headache, asthenia, drowsiness, depression, syncope
CV: first-dose orthostatic hypotension, palpitations, angina
EENT: blurred vision, nasal congestion, epistaxis
GI: nausea, vomiting, diarrhea, abdominal cramps, dry mouth
GU: erectile dysfunction, priapism
Musculoskeletal: joint and bone pain, myalgia
Other: edema

Interactions

Drug-drug. *Antihypertensives, nitrates:* additive hypotension
Nonsteroidal anti-inflammatory drugs: decreased antihypertensive effect
Drug-diagnostic tests. *Pheochromocytoma screening test:* false-positive result
Sodium, urinary vanillylmandelic acid: increased levels
Drug-herbs. *Ephedra (ma huang):* acute hypertension

Patient monitoring

- After first dose, observe closely for hypotension and syncope.
- Monitor blood pressure and pulse. Watch for orthostatic hypotension.

Patient teaching

- Caution patient not to stop therapy suddenly. Dosage must be tapered.
- Tell patient drug may cause headache, muscle aches, or bone pain. Encourage him to discuss activity recommendations and pain management with prescriber.

- Inform patient that drug may cause sexual dysfunction. Advise him to discuss this issue with prescriber.
- Instruct patient to move slowly when sitting up or standing, to avoid dizziness from sudden blood pressure decrease.
- As appropriate, review all other significant adverse reactions and interactions, especially those related to the drugs, tests, and herbs mentioned above.

prednisolone
Prelone

prednisolone acetate
Econopred Plus Ophthalmic, Pred Forte Ophthalmic, Pred Mild Ophthalmic

prednisolone sodium phosphate
Inflamase Mild Ophthalmic, Orapred, Pediapred

prednisolone tebutate

Pharmacologic class: Corticosteroid (intermediate-acting)

Therapeutic class: Anti-inflammatory, immunosuppressant

Pregnancy risk category C

Action
Exerts potent anti-inflammatory (glucocorticoid) and weak sodium-retaining (mineralocorticoid) activity. Glucocorticoid activity causes profound and varied metabolic effects.

Availability
Oral solution: 5 mg/ml
Suspension for injection (acetate): 25 mg/ml, 40 mg/ml, 50 mg/ml
Suspension for injection (tebutate): 20 mg/ml
Suspension (ophthalmic): 0.12%, 0.125%, 1%
Syrup: 5 mg/5 ml, 15 mg/5 ml
Tablets: 5 mg

Indications and dosages
➢ Severe inflammation; immunosuppression
Adults: Dosage individualized based on diagnosis, severity of condition, and response. Usual dosage ranges from 5 to 60 mg P.O. (prednisolone) daily in two to four divided doses, or 4 to 60 mg I.M. (acetate) daily in divided doses, or 5 to 50 mg P.O. (sodium phosphate) daily in divided doses.
➢ Short-term adjunctive therapy for severe inflammation
Adults: 20 to 30 mg (tebutate) injected into large joints or bursae, 8 to 10 mg injected into small joints, 4 to 10 mg injected into tendon sheaths, or 10 to 20 mg injected into ganglia
➢ Acute exacerbation of multiple sclerosis
Adults: 200 mg P.O. daily for 1 week, followed by 80 mg every other day for 1 month
➢ Refractory bronchial asthma
Children: 1 to 2 mg/kg/day (sodium phosphate) as a single dose or in divided doses; may continue for 3 to 10 days or until symptoms resolve or patient achieves peak expiratory flow rate of 80% of personal best
➢ Nephrotic syndrome in children
Children: 60 mg/m^2 P.O. (sodium phosphate solution) daily in three divided doses for 4 weeks, then 4 weeks of alternate-day therapy at single doses of 40 mg/m^2
➢ Steroid-responsive inflammatory eye conditions
Adults: In severe cases, initially one to two drops (acetate or sodium phosphate) instilled into conjunctival sac q hour during day and q 2 hours at night. In mild or moderate inflammation or

P

in severe cases that respond favorably, one to two drops q 3 to 12 hours.

Contraindications

- Hypersensitivity to drug, other corticosteroids, alcohol, bisulfite, or tartrazine (with some products)
- Systemic fungal infections
- Active untreated infections (except in selected patients with meningitis)
- Acute superficial herpes simplex, keratitis, fungal or viral eye diseases, tuberculosis of eye, or after uncomplicated removal of superficial corneal foreign body (ophthalmic use)
- Idiopathic thrombocytopenic purpura (with I.M. use)
- Live-virus vaccines (with immunosuppressive prednisolone dosages)

Precautions

Use cautiously in:

- diabetes mellitus, glaucoma, renal or hepatic disease, hypothyroidism, cirrhosis, diverticulitis, nonspecific ulcerative colitis, recent intestinal anastomoses, inflammatory bowel disease, thromboembolic disorders, seizures, myasthenia gravis, heart failure, hypertension, osteoporosis, ocular herpes simplex, immunosuppression, emotional instability
- pregnant or breastfeeding patients
- children younger than age 6.

Administration

◀ Be aware that prednisolone has many different formulations, which may be given by various routes: P.O., I.M., intralesional, intra-articular, soft tissue, or ophthalmic. Before administering, make sure prescribed formulation can be given by prescribed route.

- Inject I.M. form deep into gluteal muscle. Rotate injection sites.
- Avoid subcutaneous injection.

◀ In systemic therapy, don't discontinue drug abruptly, even if inhaled steroid is added.

- Know that additional corticosteroids are needed during stress or trauma.

Route	Onset	Peak	Duration
P.O. (prednisolone, sod. phos.)	Unknown	1-2 hr	1.25-1.5 days
I.M. (acetate)	Slow	Unknown	Unknown
Intrales., soft tissue, intra-artic.	Slow	Unknown	Prolonged
Ophth. (acetate, sod. phos.)	Unknown	Unknown	Unknown

Adverse reactions

CNS: headache, nervousness, depression, euphoria, personality changes, psychosis, vertigo, paresthesia, insomnia, restlessness, **increased intracranial pressure, seizures, meningitis**
CV: hypotension, hypertension, vasculitis, **thrombophlebitis, thromboembolism, fat embolism, arrhythmias, heart failure, shock**
EENT: cataracts, glaucoma, visual disturbances, exacerbation of ocular infection, secondary ocular infections, globe perforation at corneal or scleral thinning site, transient stinging or burning of eyes, dry eyes, corneal ulcers, mydriasis (all with ophthalmic use); posterior subcapsular cataracts (especially in children), glaucoma, nasal irritation and congestion, rebound congestion, sneezing, epistaxis, nasopharyngeal and oropharyngeal fungal infections, perforated nasal septum, anosmia, dysphonia, hoarseness, throat irritation (with long-term use)
GI: nausea, vomiting, abdominal distention, rectal bleeding, dry mouth, esophageal candidiasis, esophageal ulcer, **pancreatitis, peptic ulcer**
GU: amenorrhea, irregular menses
Hematologic: purpura
Metabolic: sodium and fluid retention, hypokalemia, hypocalcemia, hyper-

glycemia, decreased carbohydrate tolerance, growth retardation (in children), diabetes mellitus, cushingoid effects (with long-term use), **hypothalamic-pituitary-adrenal suppression** (with systemic use longer than 5 days), **adrenal suppression** (with high-dose, long-term use)
Musculoskeletal: muscle weakness or atrophy, myalgia, myopathy, osteoporosis, aseptic joint necrosis, spontaneous fractures (with long-term use), osteonecrosis, tendon rupture
Respiratory: cough, wheezing, **bronchospasm**
Skin: rash, pruritus, contact dermatitis, acne, striae, poor wound healing, thin fragile skin, bruising, hirsutism, petechiae, subcutaneous fat atrophy, urticaria, angioedema
Other: bad taste; increased or decreased appetite; aggravation or masking of infections; weight gain (with long-term use); facial edema; pain, burning, and atrophy at injection site; hypersensitivity reaction

Interactions

Drug-drug. *Amphotericin B, mezlocillin, piperacillin, thiazide and loop diuretics, ticarcillin:* additive hypokalemia
Anticholinesterase drugs: decreased anticholinesterase effect (when prednisolone is used for myasthenia gravis)
Aspirin, other nonsteroidal anti-inflammatory drugs: increased risk of GI discomfort and bleeding
Cardiac glycosides: increased risk of digitalis toxicity due to hypokalemia
Cyclosporine: therapeutic benefits in organ transplant recipients, but with increased risk of toxicity
Erythromycin, indinavir, itraconazole, ketoconazole, ritonavir, saquinavir: increased prednisolone blood level and effects
Hormonal contraceptives: impaired metabolism and increased effects of prednisolone
Isoniazid: decreased isoniazid blood level
Live-virus vaccines: decreased antibody response to vaccine, increased risk of adverse effects
Oral anticoagulants: reduced anticoagulant requirement, opposition to anticoagulant action
Phenobarbital, phenytoin, rifampin: decreased prednisolone efficacy
Salicylates: reduced salicylate blood level
Somatrem: inhibition of somatrem's growth-promoting effects
Theophylline: altered pharmacologic effects of either drug
Drug-diagnostic tests. *Calcium, potassium, thyroid* ^{131}*I uptake, thyroxine, triiodothyronine:* decreased levels
Cholesterol, glucose: increased levels
Nitroblue tetrazolium test for bacterial infection: false-negative result
Drug-herbs. *Alfalfa:* activation of quiescent systemic lupus erythematosus
Echinacea: increased immune-stimulating effects
Ephedra (ma huang): decreased drug blood level
Ginseng: potentiation of immunomodulating effect
Licorice: prolonged drug activity
Drug-behaviors. *Alcohol use:* increased risk of gastric irritation and GI ulcers

Patient monitoring

- Monitor weight, blood pressure, and electrolyte levels.
- Watch for cushingoid effects (moon face, central obesity, buffalo hump, hair thinning, high blood pressure, frequent infections).
- [Clinical alert] Assess patient for depression and psychosis.
- Monitor blood glucose level carefully in diabetic patient.
- Evaluate for signs and symptoms of infection, which drug may mask or exacerbate.
- [Clinical alert] Monitor for signs and symptoms of early adrenal insufficiency (fatigue,

p

weakness, joint pain, fever, anorexia, shortness of breath, dizziness, syncope).
• Assess musculoskeletal status for joint, tendon, and muscle pain.

Patient teaching

• Tell patient to take oral dose with food or milk to reduce GI upset.
🔊 Teach patient to recognize and immediately report cushingoid effects and signs and symptoms of early adrenal insufficiency.
🔊 Advise patient and significant other to immediately report depression or psychosis.
• Explain that drug increases risk of infection. Instruct patient to contact prescriber at first sign of infection.
🔊 Caution patient not to suddenly stop drug (including ophthalmic forms). Instruct him to discuss any changes in therapy with prescriber.
🔊 Tell patient to immediately report bleeding or joint, muscle, tendon, or abdominal pain.
• Inform patient that he may need higher dosage during periods of stress. Encourage him to wear or carry medical identification stating this.
• Tell patient to avoid vaccinations during therapy. Mention that others in household shouldn't receive oral polio vaccine because they could pass poliovirus to him.
• Caution patient not to take over-the-counter drugs or herbs during therapy.
• Teach patient how to use eye drops. Caution him not to touch dropper tip to eye or any other surface.
• As appropriate, review all other significant and life-threatening adverse reactions and interactions, especially those related to the drugs, tests, herbs, and behaviors mentioned above.

prednisone

Apo-Prednisone🍁, Deltasone, Winpred🍁

Pharmacologic class: Corticosteroid (intermediate acting)
Therapeutic class: Anti-inflammatory, immunosuppressant
Pregnancy risk category C

Action

Decreases inflammation by reversing increased cell capillary permeability and inhibiting migration of polymorphonuclear leukocytes. Suppresses immune system by reducing lymphatic activity.

Availability

Oral solution: 5 mg/ml, 5 mg/5 ml
Syrup: 5 mg/5 ml
Tablets: 1 mg, 2.5 mg, 5 mg, 10 mg, 20 mg, 50 mg

Indications and dosages

➢ Severe inflammation; immunosuppression
Adults: Dosage individualized based on diagnosis, severity of condition, and response. Usual dosage is 5 to 60 mg P.O. daily as a single dose or in divided doses.
➢ Acute exacerbation of multiple sclerosis
Adults: 200 mg P.O. daily for 1 week, then 80 mg every other day for 1 month
➢ Adjunctive therapy for *Pneumocystis jiroveci* pneumonia in AIDS patients
Adults: 40 mg P.O. b.i.d. for 5 days, then 40 mg once daily for 5 days, then 20 mg once daily for 11 days

Contraindications

• Hypersensitivity to drug, other corticosteroids, alcohol, bisulfite, or tartrazine (with some products)

• Systemic fungal infections
• Live-virus vaccines (with immunosuppressant doses)
• Active untreated infections (except in selected meningitis patients)

Precautions

Use cautiously in:
• diabetes mellitus, glaucoma, renal or hepatic disease, hypothyroidism, cirrhosis, diverticulitis, nonspecific ulcerative colitis, recent intestinal anastomoses, inflammatory bowel disease, thromboembolic disorders, seizures, myasthenia gravis, heart failure, hypertension, osteoporosis, hypothyroidism, ocular herpes simplex, immunosuppression, emotional instability
• pregnant or breastfeeding patients
• children under age 6.

Administration

• Give with food or milk to reduce GI upset.
• Administer once-daily dose early in morning.

Route	Onset	Peak	Duration
P.O.	Unknown	1-2 hr	1.25-1.5 days

Adverse reactions

CNS: headache, nervousness, depression, euphoria, personality changes, psychosis, vertigo, paresthesia, insomnia, restlessness, **seizures, meningitis, increased intracranial pressure**
CV: hypotension, hypertension, vasculitis, **heart failure, thrombophlebitis, thromboembolism, fat embolism, arrhythmias, shock**
EENT: posterior subcapsular cataracts (especially in children), glaucoma, nasal irritation and congestion, rebound congestion, sneezing, epistaxis, nasopharyngeal and oropharyngeal fungal infections, perforated nasal septum, anosmia, dysphonia, hoarseness, throat irritation (all with long-term use)
GI: nausea, vomiting, abdominal distention, rectal bleeding, esophageal candidiasis, dry mouth, esophageal ulcer, **pancreatitis, peptic ulcer**
GU: amenorrhea, irregular menses
Hematologic: purpura
Metabolic: sodium and fluid retention, hypokalemia, hypocalcemia, hyperglycemia, decreased carbohydrate tolerance, diabetes mellitus, growth retardation (in children), cushingoid effects (with long-term use), **hypothalamic-pituitary-adrenal suppression** (with systemic use longer than 5 days), **adrenal suppression** (with high-dose, long-term use)
Musculoskeletal: muscle weakness or atrophy, myalgia, myopathy, osteoporosis, aseptic joint necrosis, spontaneous fractures (with long-term use), osteonecrosis, tendon rupture
Respiratory: cough, wheezing, **bronchospasm**
Skin: rash, pruritus, contact dermatitis, acne, striae, poor wound healing, hirsutism, thin fragile skin, petechiae, bruising, subcutaneous fat atrophy, urticaria, angioedema
Other: bad taste, increased or decreased appetite, weight gain (with long-term use), facial edema, aggravation or masking of infections, hypersensitivity reaction

Interactions

Drug-drug. *Amphotericin B, mezlocillin, piperacillin, thiazide and loop diuretics, ticarcillin:* additive hypokalemia
Aspirin, other nonsteroidal anti-inflammatory drugs: increased risk of GI discomfort and bleeding
Cardiac glycosides: increased risk of digitalis toxicity due to hypokalemia
Cyclosporine: therapeutic benefits in organ transplant recipients, but with increased risk of toxicity
Erythromycin, indinavir, itraconazole, ketoconazole, ritonavir, saquinavir: in-

creased prednisone blood level and effects
Hormonal contraceptives: impaired metabolism and increased effects of prednisone
Isoniazid: decreased isoniazid blood level
Live-virus vaccines: decreased antibody response to vaccine, increase risk of adverse effects
Oral anticoagulants: reduced anticoagulant requirements, opposition to anticoagulant action
Phenobarbital, phenytoin, rifampin: decreased prednisone efficacy
Salicylates: reduced salicylate blood level
Somatrem: inhibition of somatrem's growth-promoting effects
Theophylline: altered pharmacologic effects of either drug
Drug-diagnostic tests. *Calcium, potassium, thyroid ^{131}I uptake, thyroxine, triiodothyronine:* decreased levels
Cholesterol, glucose: increased levels
Nitroblue tetrazolium test for bacterial infection: false-negative result
Drug-herbs. *Alfalfa:* activation of quiescent systemic lupus erythematosus
Echinacea: increased immune-stimulating effects
Ephedra (ma huang): decreased drug blood level
Ginseng: potentiation of immunomodulating effect
Licorice: prolonged drug activity
Drug-behaviors. *Alcohol use:* increased risk of gastric irritation and GI ulcers

Patient monitoring

- Monitor weight, blood pressure, and electrolyte levels.
- Watch for cushingoid effects (moon face, central obesity, buffalo hump, hair thinning, high blood pressure, frequent infections).
- ◀ Check for signs and symptoms of depression and psychosis.
- Assess blood glucose level carefully in diabetic patient.
- Monitor patient for signs and symptoms of infection, which drug may mask or exacerbate.
- ◀ Assess for early indications of adrenal insufficiency (fatigue, weakness, joint pain, fever, appetite loss, shortness of breath, dizziness, syncope).
- Monitor musculoskeletal status for joint, tendon, and muscle pain.

Patient teaching

- Tell patient to take with food or milk to reduce GI upset.
- ◀ Teach patient to recognize and immediately report signs and symptoms of early adrenal insufficiency and cushingoid effects.
- ◀ Inform patient that drug increases his risk of infection. Instruct him to contact prescriber at first sign of infection.
- ◀ Caution patient not to stop drug suddenly. Advise him to discuss any changes in therapy with prescriber.
- ◀ Tell patient to immediately report bleeding or joint, muscle, tendon, or abdominal pain.
- ◀ Advise patient or significant other to immediately report depression or psychosis.
- Caution patient not to take herbs or over-the-counter drugs during therapy.
- Instruct patient to avoid vaccinations during therapy. Tell him that others in household shouldn't receive oral polio vaccine because they could pass poliovirus to him.
- Tell patient he may need higher dosage during periods of stress. Encourage him to wear or carry medical identification stating this.
- As appropriate, review all other significant and life-threatening adverse reactions and interactions, especially those related to the drugs, tests, herbs, and behaviors mentioned above.

primaquine phosphate

Pharmacologic class: 8-aminoquinoline compound

Therapeutic class: Antimalarial

Pregnancy risk category C

Action

Unknown. Thought to disrupt parasitic mitochondria and bind to native DNA, leading to structural changes that disrupt metabolic processes and to inhibition of gametocyte and erythrocyte forms. Destroys some gametocytes and makes others incapable of undergoing maturation division.

Availability

Tablets: 26.3 mg (15 mg base)

Indications and dosages

➢ To prevent or treat relapse of malaria caused by *Plasmodium vivax*

Adults: 15 mg base P.O. daily for 14 days

Children: 0.3 mg base/kg/day P.O. for 14 days, to a maximum of 15 mg base daily

Off-label uses

• *Pneumocystis jiroveci* pneumonia

Contraindications

• Hypersensitivity to drug
• Concurrent use of quinacrine, other hemolytic drugs, or myelosuppressants
• Bone marrow depression
• Systemic disease with history of or tendency to granulocytopenia (such as lupus erythematosus or rheumatoid arthritis)

Precautions

Use cautiously in:

• porphyria, methemoglobinemia, methemoglobin reductase deficiency, hemolytic anemia in G6PD deficiency (particularly in Blacks, Asians, and persons of Mediterranean descent), iodine deficiency, anemia
• pregnant patients.

Administration

Clinical alert: Before giving, check prescription to see if dosage is written as mg or mg base.

• Start therapy during last 2 weeks of suppression course with chloroquine or comparable drug, or after suppression course ends.

Route	Onset	Peak	Duration
P.O.	Unknown	1-3 hr	Unknown

Adverse reactions

CNS: headache, dizziness, asthenia

CV: hypertension

EENT: blurred vision, difficulty focusing

GI: nausea, vomiting, diarrhea, constipation, abdominal pain, epigastric distress

Hematologic: mild anemia, **leukocytosis, hemolytic anemia, methemoglobinemia**

Skin: pruritus, skin eruptions, pallor

Interactions

Drug-drug. *Aluminum and magnesium salts:* decreased GI absorption of primaquine

Quinacrine: increased risk of primaquine toxicity

Drug-diagnostic tests. *Hemoglobin, red blood cells:* decreased levels

White blood cells: increased or decreased count

Patient monitoring

Clinical alert: Monitor CBC. Watch for evidence of blood dyscrasias or hemolytic reaction (dark urine, chills, fever, chest pain, bluish skin). Stop drug and notify prescriber at once if these occur.

• Monitor blood pressure.

Patient teaching

- Advise patient to take with food to minimize GI upset.

🔊 Teach patient to recognize and immediately report signs and symptoms of hemolytic reactions.

- Caution patient to avoid driving and other hazardous activities until he knows how drug affects concentration, vision, and alertness.
- Instruct patient to complete entire course of therapy as prescribed, even after symptoms improve.
- As appropriate, review all other significant and life-threatening adverse reactions and interactions, especially those related to the drugs and tests mentioned above.

primidone

Apo-Primidone✱, Mysoline, PMS-Primidone✱, Sertan✱

Pharmacologic class: Barbiturate
Therapeutic class: Anticonvulsant
Pregnancy risk category NR

Action

Unknown. May raise seizure threshold by decreasing neuronal firing after being converted to phenobarbital.

Availability

Suspension: 250 mg/5 ml
Tablets: 50 mg, 250 mg

Indications and dosages

➢ Grand mal, psychomotor, or focal epileptic seizures

Adults and children ages 8 and older: Initially, 100 to 125 mg P.O. at bedtime on days 1 to 3, then 100 to 125 mg P.O. b.i.d. on days 4 to 6, then 100 to 125 mg P.O. t.i.d. on days 7 to 9, followed by a maintenance dosage of 250 mg P.O. three or four times daily

Children younger than age 8: Initially, 50 mg P.O. at bedtime on days 1 to 3, then 50 mg P.O. b.i.d. on days 4 to 6, then 100 mg P.O. b.i.d. on days 7 to 9. For maintenance, 125 to 250 mg t.i.d. or 10 to 25 mg/kg/day in divided doses.

Dosage adjustment

- Renal impairment

Off-label uses

- Benign familial (essential) tremor

Contraindications

- Hypersensitivity to drug or phenobarbital
- Porphyria

Precautions

Use cautiously in:

- hepatic, renal, or chronic obstructive pulmonary disease
- pregnant or breastfeeding patients
- hyperactive children.

Administration

- Don't change brands. Bioequivalency problems have occurred.

🔊 Don't stop therapy suddenly. Dosage must be tapered.

- Know that drug may be given alone or with other anticonvulsants.

Route	Onset	Peak	Duration
P.O.	Unknown	3-4 hr	Unknown

Adverse reactions

CNS: headache, dizziness, stimulation, drowsiness, sedation, confusion, hallucinations, psychosis, ataxia, vertigo, hyperirritability, emotional disturbances, paranoid symptoms, **coma**
EENT: diplopia, nystagmus, eyelid edema
GI: nausea, vomiting, anorexia
GU: erectile dysfunction
Hematologic: megaloblastic anemia, thrombocytopenia
Skin: flushing, rash

Interactions

Drug-drug. *Acetazolamide, succinimide:* decreased primidone blood level
Carbamazepine: decreased primidone blood level, increased carbamazepine blood level
Hydantoins, isoniazid, nicotinamide: increased primidone blood level
Drug-diagnostic tests. *Hemoglobin, platelets:* decreased levels
Liver function tests: altered results

Patient monitoring

- Monitor primidone and phenobarbital blood levels.
- Monitor CBC and blood chemistry. Watch for evidence of blood dyscrasias.
- Assess neurologic status regularly. Stay alert for excessive drowsiness and emotional status changes.

Patient teaching

🔊 Caution patient not to discontinue therapy suddenly. Advise him to discuss dosage changes with prescriber.

🔊 Instruct patient to immediately report unusual bleeding, bruising, or rash.

- Tell patient drug may cause sexual dysfunction. Advise him to discuss this issue with prescriber.
- Caution patient to avoid driving and other hazardous activities until he knows how drug affects concentration, vision, and alertness.
- As appropriate, review all other significant and life-threatening adverse reactions and interactions, especially those related to the drugs and tests mentioned above.

probenecid

Benemid, Benuryl✱, Probalan

Pharmacologic class: Sulfonamide-derived uricosuric
Therapeutic class: Antigout drug, tubular blocking agent
Pregnancy risk category B

Action

Promotes uric acid excretion from kidney by blocking tubular reabsorption; also inhibits tubular secretion of weak organic acids (most penicillins and cephalosporins, some beta-lactams)

Availability

Tablets: 0.5 g

Indications and dosages

➢ Hyperuricemia caused by gout
Adults and children weighing more than 50 kg (110 lb): After acute gout attack subsides, 250 mg P.O. b.i.d. for 1 week, then 500 mg b.i.d.; may increase by 500 mg/day q 4 weeks (not to exceed 3 g/day)

➢ To prolong action or increase blood level of penicillins or cephalosporins
Adults: 500 mg P.O. q.i.d.
Children ages 2 to 14: Initially, 25 mg/kg or 0.7 g/m^2, then a maintenance dosage of 40 mg/kg/day or 1.2 g/m^2 in four divided doses

➢ Gonorrhea
Adults: 1 g P.O. as a single dose given with or immediately before prescribed ampicillin dose

Dosage adjustment

- Renal impairment

Off-label uses

- Hyperuricemia secondary to thiazide therapy

p

Contraindications

- Hypersensitivity to drug
- Acute gout attack
- Uric acid calculi
- Blood dyscrasias
- Concurrent salicylate use
- Concurrent penicillin use in patients with renal impairment
- Children younger than age 2

Precautions

Use cautiously in:

- peptic ulcer, renal impairment
- pregnant or breastfeeding patients.

Administration

Don't give until acute gout attack subsides.

- Ensure high fluid intake and alkaline urine during therapy.

Route	Onset	Peak	Duration
P.O.	30 min	2-4 hr	8 hr

Adverse reactions

CNS: headache, dizziness
GI: nausea, vomiting, diarrhea, abdominal pain, anorexia
GU: urinary frequency, uric acid calculi, renal colic, **nephrotic syndrome**
Hematologic: anemia, **hemolytic anemia, aplastic anemia**
Hepatic: hepatitis, hepatic necrosis
Metabolic: gout exacerbation
Musculoskeletal: costovertebral pain
Skin: flushing, rash, pruritus
Other: sore gums, fever, hypersensitivity reactions including **anaphylaxis**

Interactions

Drug-drug. *Acyclovir, allopurinol, barbiturates, cephalosporins, pantothenic acid, penicillins:* increased blood levels of these drugs, enhanced uric acid–reducing effect of probenecid
Benzodiazepines: faster onset and prolonged effects of these drugs
Clofibrate: increased clofibrate blood level
Dapsone: accumulation of dapsone and its metabolites
Dyphylline: increased half-life and decreased clearance of dyphylline
Methotrexate, nonsteroidal anti-inflammatory drugs, rifampin, sulfonamides: increased blood levels, therapeutic effects, and toxicity of these drugs
Oral hypoglycemics: increased half-life and effects of these drugs
Penicillamine: increased pharmacologic effect of penicillamine
Salicylates: decreased probenecid or salicylate activity
Thiopental: extended anesthetic effect of thiopental
Zidovudine: increased risk of zidovudine toxicity
Drug-diagnostic tests. *Urine glucose tests using copper reduction method (such as Clinitest):* false-positive result

Patient monitoring

- Monitor kidney and liver function tests, CBC, and blood urea nitrogen level.
- Assess fluid intake and output to ensure good hydration and reduce urinary side effects.
- During first 6 to 12 months of therapy, monitor pattern and severity of acute gout attacks to assess need for additional anti-inflammatory drugs.

Patient teaching

- Advise patient to take with food or milk to minimize GI upset.
- Teach patient about causes of gout and proper use of drug. Stress that he must wait until acute attack subsides and then take drug regularly to prevent further attacks.
- Tell patient drug may exacerbate acute gout attacks for first 6 to 12 months, necessitating colchicine or other anti-inflammatory drug for 3 to 6 months.
- Instruct patient to drink 2 to 3 liters of fluids daily.

• Tell patient with gout to limit foods high in purine (such as anchovies, organ meats, and legumes).
• Instruct diabetic patient to test urine glucose level during therapy.
• As appropriate, review all other significant and life-threatening adverse reactions and interactions, especially those related to the drugs and tests mentioned above.

procainamide hydrochloride

Apo-Procainamide✱, Procanbid, Pronestyl, Pronestyl-SR✱

Pharmacologic class: Membrane stabilizer
Therapeutic class: Antiarrhythmic (class IA)
Pregnancy risk category C

Action

Decreases myocardial excitability by inhibiting conduction velocity. Also depresses myocardial contractility.

Availability

Capsules: 250 mg, 375 mg, 500 mg
Injection: 100 mg/ml, 500 mg/ml
Tablets: 250 mg, 375 mg, 500 mg
Tablets (extended-release): 250 mg, 500 mg, 750 mg, 1,000 mg

Indications and dosages

➤ Life-threatening ventricular arrhythmias

Adults: 100 mg by slow I.V. push at a rate of 50 mg/minute, repeated q 5 minutes until arrhythmia subsides, up to a maximum advisable dosage of 1 g. Alternatively, loading dose of 500 to 600 mg by I.V. infusion over 25 to 30 minutes. With either I.V. method, maximum loading dose is 1 g. When arrhythmia subsides, give continuous I.V. infusion of 2 to 6 mg/minute. Or 50 mg/kg I.M. in divided doses q 3 to 6 hours until patient can tolerate P.O. therapy.

For long-term maintenance, usual dosage is 50 mg/kg (extended-release) P.O. daily in equally divided doses q 6 hours. Or 50 mg/kg/day P.O. (prompt-release) in divided doses at 3-, 4-, or 6-hour intervals.

Dosage adjustment

• Renal impairment

Contraindications

• Hypersensitivity to drug, tartrazine, procaine, or sulfites
• Complete heart block
• Torsades de pointes
• Lupus erythematosus

Precautions

Use cautiously in:
• procaine hypersensitivity, renal impairment, ischemic heart disease, heart failure, first-degree heart block, atypical ventricular tachycardia, myasthenia gravis, systemic lupus erythematosus, cytopenia
• patients receiving other antiarrhythmics concurrently
• pregnant or breastfeeding patients
• children.

Administration

🔊 Ask patient about procaine sensitivity before giving; cross-sensitivity may occur.
• Don't crush tablets.
• For I.V. use, dilute with dextrose 5% in water.
• Administer I.V. doses with patient in supine position to avoid hypotensive effects.
• When giving by I.V. infusion, use infusion pump to ensure that drug infuses at 50 mg/minute or less.
🔊 Don't leave patient's bedside during I.V. administration.

p

Route	Onset	Peak	Duration
P.O.	Unknown	90-120 min	Unknown
I.V.	Immediate	Immediate	Unknown
I.M.	10-30 min	15-60 min	Unknown

Adverse reactions

CNS: headache, dizziness, confusion, psychosis, restlessness, asthenia, depression, neuropathy, **seizures**
CV: hypotension, bradycardia, **atrioventricular block, ventricular fibrillation, ventricular asystole, cardiovascular collapse, cardiac arrest**
GI: nausea, vomiting, diarrhea, anorexia
Hematologic: hemolytic anemia, agranulocytosis, thrombocytopenia, neutropenia
Skin: rash, urticaria, pruritus, flushing
Other: bitter taste, lupuslike syndrome, edema

Interactions

Drug-drug. *Amiodarone:* increased procainamide blood level and risk of toxicity
Anticholinesterase drugs: decreased anticholinesterase effects
Antihypertensives: additive hypotension
Beta-adrenergic blockers, cimetidine, ranitidine, trimethoprim: increased procainamide blood level
Lidocaine: additive cardiodepressant action, conduction abnormalities
Neuromuscular blockers: increased skeletal muscle relaxation
Other antiarrhythmics: additive or antagonistic effects, additive toxicity
Trimethoprim: increased pharmacologic effect of procainamide
Drug-herbs. *Henbane:* increased anticholinergic activity
Jimsonweed: adverse cardiovascular effects
Licorice: prolonged QT interval
Drug-behaviors. *Alcohol use:* altered drug blood level

Patient monitoring

🔈 When giving I.V., stay at patient's bedside and monitor blood pressure and ECG continuously.
🔈 If ECG shows prolonged QT interval and QRS complexes, heart block, or worsening arrhythmia, stop drug therapy, run rhythm strip, and contact prescriber immediately.
- Assess blood levels of procainamide and *N*-acetylprocainamide (drug's active metabolite).

🔈 Monitor electrolyte levels, CBC, and antinuclear antibody titers. Watch for signs and symptoms of blood dyscrasias.
- Evaluate patient for signs and symptoms of lupuslike syndrome.

Patient teaching

- Tell patient not to crush tablets.

🔈 Advise patient to immediately report cardiovascular symptoms or bleeding tendency.
- Emphasize importance of taking exactly as prescribed. Advise patient to use alarm clock to help him remember to take nighttime doses.
- Advise patient to avoid alcohol.
- Instruct patient not to take herbal remedies unless prescriber approves.
- As appropriate, review all other significant and life-threatening adverse reactions and interactions, especially those related to the drugs, herbs, and behaviors mentioned above.

procarbazine hydrochloride

Matulane, Natulan🍁

Pharmacologic class: Alkylating agent
Therapeutic class: Antineoplastic
Pregnancy risk category D

Action
Thought to inhibit DNA, RNA, and protein synthesis, resulting in death of rapidly dividing cells. Also inhibits MAO.

Availability
Capsules: 50 mg

Indications and dosages
➢ Hodgkin's disease

Adults: 2 to 4 mg/kg P.O. daily as a single dose or in divided doses for 1 week, then 4 to 6 mg/kg P.O. daily until white blood cell (WBC) count is less than 4,000/mm^3 or platelet count is less than 100,000/mm^3, or until desired response occurs. With desired response, give maintenance dosage of 1 to 2 mg/kg P.O. daily (rounded off to nearest 50 mg). As component of MOPP (mechlorethamine, vincristine, procarbazine, prednisone) regimen for advanced Hodgkin's disease, usual dosage is 100 mg/m^2 P.O. daily on days 1 to 14 of 28-day cycle.

Children: Dosage highly individualized. Usual dosage is 50 mg/m^2 P.O. daily for first week, then 100 mg/m^2 P.O. daily until leukopenia, thrombocytopenia, or desired response occurs. With desired response, maintenance dosage is 50 mg/m^2 P.O. daily.

Off-label uses
- Brain tumor
- Lymphoma

Contraindications
- Hypersensitivity to drug
- Inadequate bone marrow reserve

Precautions
Use cautiously in:
- infection, chronic debilitating illness, headache, hepatic or renal impairment, cardiovascular disease, heart failure, diarrhea, stomatitis, pheochromocytoma, psychiatric illness, alcoholism
- patients who have undergone radiation therapy or received other chemotherapy drugs within previous month
- elderly patients
- pregnant or breastfeeding patients
- females of childbearing age.

Administration
- Weigh patient; know that dosages are based on weight. However, use caution in patients with edema or ascites.

Route	Onset	Peak	Duration
P.O.	Rapid	1 hr	Unknown

Adverse reactions
CNS: confusion, dizziness, drowsiness, hallucinations, headache, mania, depression, nightmares, psychosis, syncope, tremor, neuropathy, paresthesia, **seizures**

CV: edema, hypotension, tachycardia

EENT: nystagmus, photophobia, retinal hemorrhage

GI: nausea, vomiting, diarrhea, dysphagia, ascites, stomatitis, dry mouth, anorexia

GU: gonadal suppression, gynecomastia

Hematologic: anemia, **leukopenia, thrombocytopenia**

Hepatic: hepatic dysfunction

Respiratory: cough, **pleural effusion**

Skin: alopecia, photosensitivity, pruritus, rash

Interactions
Drug-drug. *Digoxin:* decreased digoxin blood level

Levodopa: flushing, hypertension

Opioids: deep coma, death

Sympathomimetics (indirect-acting): abrupt, life-threatening hypertension

Tricyclic antidepressants: severe toxicity and fatal reactions (including blood pressure fluctuations, seizures, and coma)

Drug-diagnostic tests. *Hematocrit, hemoglobin, platelets, reticulocytes, WBCs:* decreased levels

P

Drug-food. *Caffeine-containing foods and beverages:* hypertension, arrhythmias
Tyramine-containing foods and beverages: life-threatening hypertension
Drug-behaviors. *Alcohol use:* disulfiram-like reaction

Patient monitoring

• Monitor vital signs and nutritional status.
• Assess fluid intake and output. Watch for evidence of fluid overload.
🔊 Monitor neurologic status for seizures, paresthesia, neuropathy, and confusion. Discontinue drug and notify prescriber if these occur.
🔊 Monitor CBC and platelet count. Discontinue drug and contact prescriber if WBC count falls below 4,000/mm^3 or platelet count falls below 100,000/mm^3.
🔊 Evaluate patient's concurrent drug use to ensure that he isn't receiving other drugs that could cause potentially fatal interactions.
🔊 Check for diarrhea. Discontinue drug and contact prescriber if patient has frequent bowel movements or watery stools.
• Monitor blood urea nitrogen level, liver and kidney function tests, and urinalysis.
🔊 Discontinue drug at first sign of hypersensitivity, stomatitis, diarrhea, or bleeding.

Patient teaching

• Instruct patient to avoid caffeine-containing foods and beverages.
🔊 Tell patient to avoid foods and beverages containing tyramine (such as cheese, Chianti wine, tea, coffee, cola, and bananas).
• Advise patient to avoid alcohol.
• Tell female of childbearing age to discuss contraception with prescriber.
• As appropriate, review all other significant and life-threatening adverse reactions and interactions, especially those related to the drugs, tests, foods, and behaviors mentioned above.

prochlorperazine
Compazine, Stemetil✱

prochlorperazine edisylate
Compazine

prochlorperazine maleate
Compazine, Compazine Spansule, Stemetil✱

Pharmacologic class: Phenothiazine
Therapeutic class: Antiemetic, antipsychotic, anxiolytic
Pregnancy risk category C

Action

Exerts anticholinergic, CNS depressant, and antihistaminic effects. Depresses release of hypothalamic and hypophyseal hormones, decreases sensitivity of middle-ear labyrinth, and reduces conduction in vestibular-cerebellar pathways.

Availability

Capsules (extended-release, maleate): 10 mg, 15 mg, 30 mg
Injection (edisylate): 5 mg/ml
Oral solution (edisylate): 5 mg/5 ml
Suppositories: 2.5 mg, 5 mg, 25 mg
Tablets: 5 mg, 10 mg, 25 mg

Indications and dosages

➢ Nausea
Adults: 5 to 10 mg P.O. three to four times daily or 15 mg P.O. once daily or 10 mg P.O. (extended-release) b.i.d., up to 40 mg/day. Or 2.5 to 10 mg I.V., not to exceed 40 mg/day.
Children weighing 18 to 38 kg (40 to 85 lb): 2.5 mg P.O. or P.R. t.i.d. or 5 mg P.O. or P.R. b.i.d., not to exceed 15 mg/day

Children weighing 13.6 to 17.7 kg (30 to 39 lb): 2.5 mg P.O. or P.R. two or three times daily, not to exceed 10 mg/day
Children weighing 9 to 13 kg (20 to 29 lb): 2.5 mg P.O. or P.R. daily to b.i.d., not to exceed 7.5 mg/day
➢ Nausea and vomiting related to surgery
Adults: 5 to 10 mg I.V. 15 to 30 minutes before anesthesia induction, repeated once if necessary; or 5 to 10 mg I.M. 1 to 2 hours before anesthesia induction, repeated once in 30 minutes if necessary
➢ Schizophrenia
Adults and children older than age 12: For mild symptoms, 5 to 10 mg P.O. three to four times daily; for moderate to severe symptoms in hospitalized or supervised patients, 10 mg P.O. three to four times daily, increased p.r.n. q 2 to 3 days to 50 to 75 mg P.O. daily or up to 150 mg/day as tolerated p.r.n. for more severely disturbed patients. Or 10 to 20 mg I.M.; may repeat q 2 to 4 hours for up to four doses p.r.n.
Children ages 2 to 12: Initially, 2.5 mg P.O. or P.R. two or three times daily (maximum of 10 mg on day 1); then increase based on response. Don't exceed 25 mg/day for children ages 6 to 12 or 20 mg/day for children ages 2 to 5.
➢ Anxiety
Adults and children older than age 12: 5 mg P.O. three to four times daily; or 15 mg P.O. (extended-release) once daily or 10 mg P.O. (extended-release) q 12 hours; up to 20 mg/day for a maximum of 12 weeks

Off-label uses
- Migraine

Contraindications
- Hypersensitivity to drug or other phenothiazines
- Coma
- Concurrent use of large amounts of CNS depressants
- Pediatric surgery
- Children younger than age 2 or weighing less than 9 kg (20 lb)

Precautions
Use cautiously in:
- cardiovascular or hepatic disease, glaucoma, seizures
- anticipated exposure to extreme heat
- children with acute illness.

Administration
- For I.V. infusion, dilute 20 mg in 1 L of compatible I.V. solution, such as normal saline solution.
- Don't mix in same syringe with other drugs.
- Know that injection solution may cause contact dermatitis. Don't get it on hands or clothing.

🔊 Give I.V. by slow infusion only. Don't give as bolus.
- Know that I.M. injection is not preferred because it can cause local irritation. However, if I.M. route is prescribed, inject deep into upper outer quadrant of gluteal area.
- Don't give by subcutaneous route.
- After desired response, switch to P.O. form as prescribed.
- When infusing I.V., watch for hypotension. Keep patient supine for 30 minutes after infusion.

Route	Onset	Peak	Duration
P.O.	30-40 min	Unknown	3-4 hr
P.O. (extended)	30-40 min	Unknown	10-12 hr
I.V.	Rapid (min)	10-30 min	3-4 hr
I.M.	10-20 min	10-30 min	3-4 hr
P.R.	60 min	Unknown	3-4 hr

Adverse reactions
CNS: sedation, extrapyramidal reactions, tardive dyskinesia, **neuroleptic malignant syndrome**
CV: orthostatic hypotension, ECG changes, tachycardia

EENT: blurred vision, lens opacities, pigmentary retinopathy, dry eyes
GI: constipation, ileus, dry mouth, anorexia
GU: pink or reddish-brown urine, urinary retention, galactorrhea
Hematologic: agranulocytosis, leukopenia
Hepatic: cholestatic jaundice, **hepatitis**
Metabolic: hyperthermia
Skin: photosensitivity, pigmentation changes, rash
Other: allergic reactions

Interactions

Drug-drug. *Anticonvulsants:* reduced seizure threshold
Antineoplastics: masking of antineoplastic toxicity
CNS depressants (including antihistamines, anticholinergics, opioids, other phenothiazines, sedative-hypnotics): additive CNS depression
Guanethidine: inhibition of antihypertensive effects
Oral anticoagulants: decreased anticoagulant effect
Phenytoin: increased or decreased phenytoin blood level
Propranolol: increased blood levels of both drugs
Thiazide diuretics: increased risk of orthostatic hypotension
Drug-diagnostic tests. *Liver function tests:* abnormal results
Phenylketonuria test: false-positive result
Drug-herbs. *Betel nut:* increased risk of extrapyramidal reactions
Evening primrose oil: increased risk of seizures
Kava: increased risk of drug-related adverse reactions
Drug-behaviors. *Alcohol use:* additive CNS depression

Patient monitoring

Monitor neurologic status, especially for signs and symptoms of neuroleptic malignant syndrome (high fever, sweating, unstable blood pressure, stupor, muscle rigidity, and autonomic dysfunction).
- In long-term therapy, assess for other adverse CNS effects, including extrapyramidal symptoms and tardive dyskinesia.
- Monitor patient closely if he's receiving drug for nausea and vomiting associated with chemotherapy, because it may mask symptoms of chemotherapy toxicity.
- Evaluate CBC and liver function tests.

Patient teaching

- Instruct patient to dilute oral solution with tomato or fruit juice, milk, coffee, soda, tea, water, or soup.

Teach patient to recognize and immediately report signs and symptoms of an allergic reaction or neuroleptic malignant syndrome.
- Inform patient about drug's other CNS effects. Tell him to contact prescriber if these occur.
- Caution patient to avoid driving and other hazardous activities until he knows how drug affects concentration, vision, alertness, and motor skills.
- Tell patient drug may turn urine pink or reddish brown.
- As appropriate, review all other significant and life-threatening adverse reactions and interactions, especially those related to the drugs, tests, herbs, and behaviors mentioned above.

progesterone

Crinone, Progesterone Injection, Prometrium

Pharmacologic class: Progestin
Therapeutic class: Hormone
Pregnancy risk category B (oral), ***D*** (injection), ***NR*** (vaginal)

Action

Suppresses ovulation by altering the vaginal epithelium, relaxing uterine smooth muscle, and promoting mammary tissue growth. Also inhibits pituitary activity and causes withdrawal bleeding in presence of estrogen.

Availability

Injection (in sesame or peanut oil with benzyl alcohol): 50 mg/ml in 10-ml vials
Micronized capsules (oral) in peanut oil: 100 mg, 200 mg
Micronized vaginal gel: 4%, 8%

Indications and dosages

➢ Secondary amenorrhea
Adults: 400 mg/day P.O. in evening for 10 days, or 5 to 10 mg/day I.M. for 6 to 8 days, given 8 to 10 days before expected menstrual period. Or 45 mg (one applicatorful of 4% gel) vaginally once every other day for up to six doses; may increase to 90 mg (one applicatorful of 8% gel) once every other day for up to six doses.
➢ Dysfunctional uterine bleeding
Adults: 5 to 10 mg I.M. daily for 6 days
➢ To prevent postmenopausal estrogen-induced endometrial hyperplasia
Adults: 200 mg/day P.O. at bedtime for 14 days on days 8 to 21 of 28-day cycle or on days 12 to 25 of 30-day cycle. If patient currently receives estrogen 1.25 mg/day, 300 mg progesterone in two divided doses (100 mg 2 hours after breakfast and 200 mg at bedtime); further adjustment may be required.
➢ Corpus luteum insufficiency; assisted reproduction technology
Adults: For luteal-phase support, 90 mg (one applicatorful of 8% gel) vaginally once daily. For in vitro fertilization, 90 mg (one applicatorful of 8% gel) vaginally once daily, starting within 24 hours of embryo transfer and continued through day 30 after transfer; if pregnancy occurs, treatment may continue for up to 12 weeks. For partial or complete ovarian failure, 90 mg (one applicatorful of 8% gel) vaginally b.i.d. while patient undergoes donor oocyte transfer; if pregnancy occurs, treatment may last up to 12 weeks.

Contraindications

- Hypersensitivity to drug, peanuts (injection, micronized capsules), or sesame (injection)
- Thromboembolic disease
- Cerebrovascular disease
- Severe hepatic disease
- Porphyria
- Breast or reproductive system cancer
- Missed abortion
- Undiagnosed vaginal bleeding
- Diagnosis of pregnancy

Precautions

Use cautiously in:
- renal or cardiovascular disease, seizure disorders, fluid retention, diabetes mellitus, asthma, migraine, depression
- history of hepatic disease
- breastfeeding patients.

P

Administration

- Before first dose, make sure patient has read package insert regarding adverse effects. Reinforce written information with oral review.

🔊 Before first I.M. dose, ask if patient has allergy to peanuts or sesame. Before giving micronized capsules, ask about peanut allergy.
- Inject I.M. dose deep into muscle. Rotate injection sites.

Route	Onset	Peak	Duration
P.O.	Unknown	2-4 hr	Unknown
I.M., vaginal	Unknown	Unknown	Unknown

Adverse reactions

CNS: depression, emotional lability, **cerebrovascular accident**

CV: thrombophlebitis, thromboembolism
EENT: retinal thrombosis
GI: abdominal cramps
GU: amenorrhea, breakthrough bleeding, spotting, cervical erosions, breast tenderness, menstrual flow changes, galactorrhea
Hepatic: hepatitis
Respiratory: pulmonary embolism
Skin: melasma, rash, angioedema
Other: gingival bleeding, weight gain or loss, hypersensitivity reactions including **anaphylaxis**

Interactions

Drug-drug. *Conjugated estrogens:* increased levels of both drugs
Drug-diagnostic tests. *Alkaline phosphatase, amino acids, low-density lipoproteins:* increased levels
Chloride and sodium excretion: reduced (with high doses)
High-density lipoproteins: decreased level
Pregnanediol excretion: reduced
Thyroid function tests: altered results
Drug-herbs. *Red clover:* interference with drug effects
Drug-behaviors. *Smoking:* increased risk of thromboembolic effects

Patient monitoring

Watch for evidence of thromboembolic disorders, including cerebrovascular accident, pulmonary embolism, diplopia, proptosis, or sudden partial or complete vision loss (may signal retinal thrombosis). If these occur, discontinue drug and notify prescriber immediately.

Assess for emotional lability and depression.

Patient teaching

Teach patient to recognize and immediately report signs and symptoms of thromboembolic disorders.

Instruct patient and significant other to stay alert for and immediately report depression.

- Advise patient to monitor weight regularly and report significant changes.
- Tell female patient that drug may cause menstrual abnormalities.
- Advise female patient to discuss breastfeeding with prescriber before taking drug.

Instruct patient to immediately report possible pregnancy.

- Tell patient that smoking increases thromboembolism risk. Encourage her to stop smoking if she smokes.
- As appropriate, review all other significant and life-threatening adverse reactions and interactions, especially those related to the drugs, tests, herbs, and behaviors mentioned above.

promethazine hydrochloride

Phenergan, Promethacon, Promethegan

Pharmacologic class: Phenothiazine (nonselective)
Therapeutic class: Antihistamine, antiemetic, sedative-hypnotic
Pregnancy risk category C

Action

Blocks effects but not release of histamine and exerts strong alpha-adrenergic effect. Also inhibits chemoreceptor trigger zone in medulla and alters dopamine effects by indirectly reducing reticular stimulation in CNS.

Availability

Injection: 25 mg/ml and 50 mg/ml in 1-ml ampules and 1- and 10-ml vials
Suppositories: 12.5 mg, 25 mg, 50 mg
Syrup: 6.25 mg/5 ml
Tablets: 12.5 mg, 25 mg, 50 mg

Indications and dosages

➢ Type 1 hypersensitivity reaction

Adults: 25 mg P.O. or P.R. at bedtime or 12.5 mg P.O. before meals and at bedtime. Or 25 mg I.M. or I.V.; may repeat in 2 hours.

Children older than age 2: 25 mg P.O. or P.R. at bedtime or 6.25 to 12.5 mg P.O. t.i.d.

➢ Motion sickness

Adults: Initially, 25 mg P.O. or P.R. 30 to 60 minutes before traveling; may repeat 8 to 12 hours later if needed. On successive travel days, 25 mg P.O. or P.R. b.i.d. (on arising and before evening meal).

Children older than age 2: 12.5 to 25 mg P.O. or P.R. b.i.d.

➢ Sedation

Adults: 25 to 50 mg P.O., I.M., I.V., or P.R. at bedtime

Children older than age 2: 12.5 to 25 mg P.O. or P.R. at bedtime

➢ Adjunct to preoperative or postoperative analgesia

Adults: 25 to 50 mg P.O., P.R., I.M., or I.V. given with appropriately reduced dosage of narcotic or barbiturate and required dosage of belladonna alkaloid

Children older than age 2: 0.5 mg/lb P.O., P.R., I.M., or I.V., given with appropriately reduced dosage of narcotic or barbiturate and required dosage of belladonna alkaloid

➢ Nausea

Adults: 25 mg P.O. or P.R.; may repeat doses of 12.5 to 25 mg P.O. or P.R. q 4 to 6 hours p.r.n. Or 12.5 to 25 mg I.M. or I.V.; may repeat q 4 hours p.r.n.

Children older than age 2: 25 mg or 0.5 mg/lb P.O. or P.R.; may repeat doses of 12.5 to 25 mg P.O. or P.R. q 4 to 6 hours p.r.n. May give I.M. or I.V. as no more than half of adult dosage. Know that drug should not be given if cause of vomiting is unknown.

Contraindications

- Hypersensitivity to drug
- Previous idiosyncratic reaction to phenothiazines
- Asthma, chronic obstructive pulmonary disease, sleep apnea
- Coma

Precautions

Use cautiously in:

- cardiovascular or hepatic disease, seizures, bone marrow depression, narrow-angle glaucoma, prostatic hypertrophy, stenosing peptic ulcer, pyloroduodenal or bladder neck obstruction
- CNS depression caused by narcotics, barbiturates, general anesthesia, tranquilizers, or alcohol
- pregnant or breastfeeding patients
- children younger than age 2 (safety and efficacy not established).

Administration

- Don't give I.V. at concentrations greater than 25 mg/ml or faster than 25 mg/minute.
- Use light-resistant covering for I.V. drug.

🔈 Inject I.M. deep into large muscle. Don't give by subcutaneous route.

Route	Onset	Peak	Duration
P.O., I.M., P.R.	20 min	Unknown	4-12 hr
I.V.	3-5 min	Unknown	4-12 hr

Adverse reactions

CNS: confusion, disorientation, fatigue, marked drowsiness, sedation, dizziness, extrapyramidal reactions, insomnia, nervousness, **neuroleptic malignant syndrome**

CV: hypertension, hypotension, bradycardia, tachycardia

EENT: blurred vision, diplopia, tinnitus

GI: constipation, dry mouth

Hematologic: blood dyscrasias

Hepatic: cholestatic jaundice

Respiratory: respiratory depression

Skin: photosensitivity, rash

Other: hypersensitivity reaction

P

Interactions

Drug-drug. *Anticholinergics:* additive anticholinergic effects
CNS depressants: additive CNS depression
Epinephrine: reversal of epinephrine's vasopressor effects
MAO inhibitors: increased extrapyramidal effects
Drug-diagnostic tests. *Glucose:* increased level
Granulocytes, platelets, white blood cells: decreased counts
Pregnancy test: false-positive or false-negative result
Skin tests using allergen extracts: false-negative results
Drug-herbs. *Betel nut:* increased risk of extrapyramidal reactions
Evening primrose oil: increased risk of seizures
Kava: increased risk of adverse drug effects
Drug-behaviors. *Alcohol use:* additive CNS depression
Sun exposure: increased risk of photosensitivity

Patient monitoring

Monitor neurologic status. Stay alert for signs and symptoms of neuroleptic malignant syndrome (high fever, sweating, unstable blood pressure, stupor, muscle rigidity, and autonomic dysfunction).
• In long-term therapy, assess for other adverse CNS effects, including extrapyramidal reactions.
• Monitor CBC and liver function tests.

Patient teaching

Teach patient to recognize and immediately report signs and symptoms of hypersensitivity reaction or neuroleptic malignant syndrome.
• Tell patient about drug's other significant neurologic effects. Instruct him to contact prescriber if these occur.
• Caution patient to avoid driving and other hazardous activities until he knows how drug affects concentration, vision, alertness, and motor skills.
• As appropriate, review all other significant and life-threatening adverse reactions and interactions, especially those related to the drugs, tests, herbs, and behaviors mentioned above.

propafenone hydrochloride

Rythmol

Pharmacologic class: Direct membrane stabilizer
Therapeutic class: Antiarrhythmic (class IC)
Pregnancy risk category C

Action

Slows conduction velocity in atrioventricular (AV) node, decreases automaticity, and increases ratio of effective refractory period to action potential duration; also has mild beta-adrenergic blocking properties

Availability

Tablets: 150 mg, 225 mg, 300 mg

Indications and dosages

➤ Life-threatening ventricular arrhythmias; paroxysmal atrial fibrillation or flutter; paroxysmal supraventricular tachycardia
Adults: Dosage highly individualized based on response and tolerance. Initially, 150 mg P.O. q 8 hours (450 mg/day); may increase after 3 to 4 days to 225 mg P.O. q 8 hours (675 mg/day) or, if necessary, up to 300 mg P.O. q 8 hours (900 mg/day). Don't exceed 900 mg/day P.O.

Dosage adjustment

• Hepatic disease
• Supraventricular tachycardia, ar-

rhythmias associated with Wolff-Parkinson-White syndrome
• Elderly patients

Contraindications
• Hypersensitivity to drug
• Sick-sinus syndrome, sinoatrial or AV block (unless patient has artificial pacemaker)
• Cardiogenic shock
• Bradycardia
• Uncontrolled heart failure
• Marked hypotension
• Bronchospastic disorders
• Electrolyte imbalances

Precautions
Use cautiously in:
• hepatic or renal impairment, myasthenia gravis
• pregnant or breastfeeding patients
• children.

Administration
• Give with food (but not with grapefruit juice) in three divided doses daily, once every 8 hours.

Route	Onset	Peak	Duration
P.O.	Variable	3.5 hr	Unknown

Adverse reactions
CNS: headache, dizziness, drowsiness, syncope, vertigo, confusion, asthenia, speech disturbances, memory loss, ataxia, paresthesia, anxiety, abnormal dreams, insomnia, tremor
CV: palpitations, angina, chest pain, hypotension, bradycardia, premature ventricular contractions, **first-degree AV block, supraventricular or ventricular arrhythmias, heart failure, atrial fibrillation, intraventricular conduction delay**
EENT: blurred vision, tinnitus
GI: nausea, vomiting, diarrhea, constipation, dyspepsia, abdominal pain or cramps, flatulence, dry mouth, anorexia
GU: reversible disorders of spermatogenesis
Hematologic: purpura, **hemolytic anemia, leukopenia, agranulocytosis, thrombocytopenia, neutropenia**
Hepatic: cholestasis, **abnormal hepatic function**
Musculoskeletal: muscle weakness, myalgia, leg cramps, myasthenia gravis exacerbation
Respiratory: dyspnea
Skin: rash, alopecia, diaphoresis
Other: altered taste, edema

Interactions
Drug-drug. *Beta-adrenergic blockers:* increased blood level and effects of beta-adrenergic blockers metabolized by liver
Cimetidine: increased propafenone blood level
Cyclosporine, desipramine, digoxin, theophylline, warfarin: increased blood levels of these drugs
Quinidine: delayed propafenone metabolism
Rifampin: decreased blood level and antiarrhythmic efficacy of propafenone
Drug-diagnostic tests. *Antinuclear antibody:* positive titer
Bleeding time: prolonged
Creatine kinase, glucose: increased levels
Granulocytes, white blood cells: decreased counts
Drug-herbs. *Aloe, buckthorn, cascara sagrada, senna pod or leaf:* increased antiarrhythmic action, decreased potassium level

Patient monitoring
• Monitor ECG and vital signs.
• Evaluate neurologic status. Stay alert for decreasing level of consciousness.
🔊 Monitor CBC and liver function tests. Watch for evidence of blood dyscrasias and abnormal hepatic function.
• Monitor respiratory status for dyspnea.

Patient teaching

- Tell patient which cardiac, neurologic, and respiratory adverse effects to report immediately.
- Instruct patient to immediately report unusual bleeding or bruising.
- Caution patient to avoid driving and other hazardous activities until he knows how drug affects concentration, vision, and alertness.
- As appropriate, review all other significant and life-threatening adverse reactions and interactions, especially those related to the drugs, tests, and herbs mentioned above.

propantheline bromide

Pro-Banthine, Propanthel✦

Pharmacologic class: Parasympatholytic

Therapeutic class: Anticholinergic, antimuscarinic, antispasmodic

Pregnancy risk category C

Action

Prevents muscarinic action of acetylcholine at postganglionic parasympathetic neuroeffector sites, relaxing GI tract and blocking gastric acid secretion

Availability

Tablets: 7.5 mg, 15 mg

Indications and dosages

➢ Peptic ulcer

Adults: 15 mg P.O. 30 minutes before each meal and 30 mg at bedtime, for a total of four daily doses

Adults of small stature: 7.5 mg P.O. t.i.d. before each meal

Dosage adjustment

- Mild peptic ulcer symptoms
- Elderly patients

Off-label uses

- Neurogenic bladder
- Urinary incontinence
- Antisecretory and antispasmodic effects

Contraindications

- Hypersensitivity to drug or other anticholinergics
- Angle-closure glaucoma
- Unstable cardiovascular adjustment in acute hemorrhage
- GI tract obstruction
- GI atony in elderly or debilitated patients
- Toxic megacolon, severe ulcerative colitis
- GU tract obstruction
- Myasthenia gravis

Precautions

Use cautiously in:

- heart failure, hypertension, arrhythmias, coronary artery disease, hepatic disease, hiatal hernia, chronic lung disease in debilitated patients, hyperthyroidism, autonomic neuropathy
- elderly patients
- pregnant or breastfeeding patients
- children.

Administration

- Give 30 minutes before meals and at bedtime—except in adults of small stature, who should receive doses three times daily before meals.

Route	Onset	Peak	Duration
P.O.	30-60 min	2-6 hr	6 hr

Adverse reactions

CNS: confusion, stimulation, headache, insomnia, dizziness, anxiety, asthenia, hallucinations

CV: palpitations, orthostatic hypotension, tachycardia

EENT: blurred vision, photophobia, mydriasis, cycloplegia, increased intraocular pressure, nasal congestion

GI: nausea, vomiting, constipation,

heartburn, dysphagia, bloating, gastroesophageal reflux disease (GERD), dry mouth, **paralytic ileus**
GU: urinary hesitancy or retention, erectile dysfunction, suppressed lactation
Skin: rash, urticaria, pruritus, anhidrosis
Other: taste loss, fever, heat prostration, allergic reaction

Interactions

Drug-drug. *Amantadine:* increased propantheline effects
Atenolol: increased pharmacologic effects of atenolol
Phenothiazines: decreased antipsychotic efficacy of phenothiazines, increased adverse effects of propantheline
Tricyclic antidepressants: increased anticholinergic effects
Drug-herbs. *Henbane, jimsonweed, scopolia:* increased anticholinergic effects

Patient monitoring

- Monitor vital signs. Watch for orthostatic hypotension.
- Assess patient for sensory and neurologic impairment.

Patient teaching

- Tell patient drug may inhibit sweating and make him susceptible to heat prostration. Teach him effective ways to maintain normal body temperature.
- Describe drug's adverse anticholinergic effects. Recommend appropriate measures to minimize these.
- Advise patient to report GERD symptoms.
- Tell male patient drug may cause erectile dysfunction. Encourage him to discuss this problem with prescriber.
- Caution patient to avoid driving and other hazardous activities until he knows how drug affects concentration, vision, and alertness.
- Instruct patient to move slowly when sitting up or standing, to avoid dizziness from sudden blood pressure decrease.
- As appropriate, review all other significant and life-threatening adverse reactions and interactions, especially those related to the drugs and herbs mentioned above.

propoxyphene hydrochloride

Darvon

propoxyphene napsylate

Darvon-N

Pharmacologic class: Opioid-like agonist
Therapeutic class: Nonopioid analgesic
Controlled substance schedule IV
Pregnancy risk category C

Action

Alters perception of and emotional response to pain by binding with opiate receptors in brain, causing CNS depression

Availability

propoxyphene hydrochloride
Capsules: 65 mg
propoxyphene napsylate
Tablets: 100 mg

Indications and dosages

➢ Mild to moderate pain
Adults: 65 mg (hydrochloride) P.O. q 4 hours or 100 mg (napsylate) P.O. q 4 hours as needed. Don't exceed 390 mg/day hydrochloride or 600 mg/day napsylate.

Dosage adjustment

- Hepatic or renal impairment
- Elderly or debilitated patients

P

Contraindications

- Hypersensitivity to drug or its components
- Suicidal or substance abuse–prone patients

Precautions

Use cautiously in:

- head trauma; increased intracranial pressure; severe renal, hepatic, or pulmonary disease; hypothyroidism; adrenal insufficiency; prostatic hypertrophy; undiagnosed abdominal pain; alcoholism
- patients receiving MAO inhibitors
- elderly or debilitated patients
- pregnant or breastfeeding patients
- children.

Administration

- Give with milk or food to reduce GI upset.
- Be aware that 100 mg propoxyphene napsylate is equivalent to 65 mg propoxyphene hydrochloride.

Route	Onset	Peak	Duration
P.O.	15-60 min	2-3 hr	4-6 hr

Adverse reactions

CNS: dizziness, headache, dysphoria, euphoria, insomnia, paradoxical excitement, asthenia, sedation
CV: hypotension
EENT: blurred vision
GI: nausea, vomiting, constipation, abdominal pain
Skin: rash
Other: physical or psychological drug dependence, drug tolerance

Interactions

Drug-drug. *Antidepressants, sedative-hypnotics:* additive CNS depression
Buprenorphine, dezocine, nalbuphine, pentazocine: decreased analgesic effect
MAO inhibitors: unpredictable and potentially fatal effects
Partial-antagonist opioid analgesics: precipitation of withdrawal in physically dependent patients
Drug-diagnostic tests. *Alanine aminotransferase, alkaline phosphatase, aspartate aminotransferase:* altered levels
Drug-herbs. *Chamomile, hops, kava, skullcap, valerian:* increased CNS depression
Drug-behaviors. *Alcohol use:* increased CNS depression
Smoking: increased metabolism and decreased analgesic efficacy of propoxyphene

Patient monitoring

- Assess patient's pain level 30 minutes after giving drug.
- Evaluate CNS effects. As needed, institute measures to prevent injury.
- In long-term therapy, monitor liver function tests and evaluate patient regularly for signs of physical or psychological drug dependence.

Patient teaching

- Advise patient to take with milk or food to minimize GI upset.
- Inform patient that drug may cause physical or psychological dependence. Stress that he should take it only when needed and only as prescribed.
- Tell patient that alcohol use and smoking affect drug blood level. Discourage these habits.
- Caution patient to avoid driving and other hazardous activities until he knows how drug affects concentration, vision, and alertness.
- As appropriate, review all other significant adverse reactions and interactions, especially those related to the drugs, tests, herbs, and behaviors mentioned above.

propranolol hydrochloride

Apo-Propranolol♣, Betachron E-R, Inderal, Inderal LA, Innopran XL, Novopranol♣, PMS Propranolol♣

Pharmacologic class: Beta-adrenergic blocker (nonselective)

Therapeutic class: Antianginal, antiarrhythmic (class II), antihypertensive, vascular headache suppressant

Pregnancy risk category C

Action

Blocks stimulation of beta$_1$-adrenergic (myocardial) and beta$_2$-adrenergic (pulmonary, vascular, and uterine) receptor sites. This action decreases cardiac output, slows heart rate, and reduces blood pressure.

Availability

Capsules (extended-release, sustained-release): 60 mg, 80 mg, 120 mg, 160 mg
Injection: 1 mg/ml
Oral solution: 4 mg/ml, 8 mg/ml, 80 mg/ml
Tablets: 10 mg, 20 mg, 40 mg, 60 mg, 90 mg

Indications and dosages

➢ Angina pectoris
Adults: 80 to 320 mg P.O. daily in three to four divided doses or 160 mg (extended- or sustained-release) P.O. daily; maximum daily dosage is 320 mg.

➢ Hypertension
Adults: 40 mg P.O. b.i.d. or 80 mg (extended- or sustained-release) P.O. daily. Maximum daily dosage is 640 mg; usual maintenance dosage is 120 to 240 mg/day.

➢ Prophylaxis after myocardial infarction
Adults: 180 to 240 mg P.O. daily in three to four divided doses; maximum daily dosage is 240 mg.

➢ Hypertrophic subaortic stenosis
Adults: 20 to 40 mg P.O. three to four times daily (before meals and at bedtime) or 80 to 160 mg (extended- or sustained-release) P.O. daily

➢ Adjunctive therapy in pheochromocytoma
Adults: 60 mg P.O. daily in divided doses for 3 days, given after primary therapy with alpha-adrenergic blocker

➢ To prevent migraine or vascular headache
Adults: 80 mg P.O. (extended- or sustained-release) daily; may increase as needed up to 240 mg/day. Effective range is 160 mg to 240 mg/day.

➢ Essential tremor
Adults: 40 mg P.O. b.i.d.; if necessary, 240 mg to 320 mg/day. Maximum daily dosage is 320 mg.

➢ Arrhythmias
Adults: 10 to 30 mg P.O. (tablets or oral solution) three or four times daily

➢ Life-threatening arrhythmias; arrhythmias occurring during anesthesia
Adults: 1 to 3 mg slow I.V. injection. If necessary, give second dose after 2 minutes and additional doses at intervals of no less than 4 hours until desired response occurs.

p

Contraindications

- Hypersensitivity to drug, its components, or other beta-adrenergic blockers
- Uncompensated heart failure
- Cardiogenic shock
- Sinus bradycardia, heart block greater than first degree
- Bronchospastic disease

Precautions

Use cautiously in:

- renal or hepatic impairment, sinus node dysfunction, pulmonary disease, diabetes mellitus, hyperthyroidism, Raynaud's syndrome, hypertensive emergencies, myasthenia gravis

- concurrent thioridazine use
- history of severe allergic reactions
- elderly patients
- pregnant or breastfeeding patients
- children (safety not established).

Administration

🔈 Take apical pulse for 1 full minute. Withhold dose and notify prescriber if patient has bradycardia or tachycardia.
🔈 Be aware that I.V. use is usually reserved for arrhythmias that are life-threatening or occur during anesthesia.
- Inject I.V. dose directly into large vein or into tubing of compatible I.V. solution (dextrose 5% in water, normal or half-normal saline solution, or lactated Ringer's solution).
- Don't give as continuous I.V. infusion.
- For intermittent I.V. infusion, dilute with normal saline solution and infuse in 0.1- to 0.2-mg increments over 10 to 15 minutes.

🔈 Keep I.V. isoproterenol, atropine, or glucagon at hand in case of emergency.
🔈 Don't stop giving drug suddenly. Dosage must be tapered.

Route	Onset	Peak	Duration
P.O.	30 min	60-90 min	6-12 hr
P.O. (extended, sustained)	Unknown	6 hr	24 hr
I.V.	Immediate	1 min	4-6 hr

Adverse reactions

CNS: fatigue, asthenia, anxiety, dizziness, drowsiness, insomnia, memory loss, depression, mental status changes, nervousness, paresthesia, nightmares
CV: peripheral vasoconstriction, orthostatic hypotension, bradycardia, **arrhythmias, heart failure, myocardial infarction and sudden death** (with abrupt withdrawal in angina therapy)
EENT: blurred vision, dry eyes, nasal congestion, rhinitis, sore throat
GI: nausea, vomiting, diarrhea, constipation, dry mouth
GU: erectile dysfunction, decreased libido
Hematologic: purpura, **thrombocytopenic purpura**
Metabolic: fluid retention, hyperglycemia, **hypoglycemia** (increased in children), **thyrotoxicosis** (with abrupt withdrawal in hypertension therapy)
Musculoskeletal: joint pain, back pain, myalgia, muscle cramps
Respiratory: wheezing, **bronchospasm, pulmonary edema**
Skin: pruritus, rash
Other: fever

Interactions

Drug-drug. *Antacids (aluminum-based):* decreased propranolol absorption
Anticholinergics, tricyclic antidepressants: antagonism of cardiac beta-adrenergic blocking effect
Chlorpromazine: additive hypotension
Cimetidine: increased propranolol blood level and risk of toxicity
Digoxin: additive bradycardia
Diuretics, other antihypertensives: increased hypotensive effect
Glucagon, isoproterenol: antagonism of propranolol's effects
Insulin, oral hypoglycemics: impaired glucose tolerance, increased risk of hypoglycemia
Neuromuscular blockers: increased neuromuscular blockade (with high propranolol doses)
Nonsteroidal anti-inflammatory drugs: decreased hypotensive effect
Theophylline: decreased theophylline clearance, antagonism of theophylline's bronchodilating effect
Thioridazine: increased thioridazine blood level, leading to prolonged QT interval
Drug-diagnostic tests. *Alkaline phosphatase, blood urea nitrogen, eosinophils, lactate dehydrogenase, serum*

transaminases, triiodothyronine: increased levels
Glucose: decreased or increased level
Platelets, thyroxine: decreased levels
Drug-behaviors. *Acute alcohol ingestion:* additive hypotension

Patient monitoring

- Monitor vital signs, ECG, and central venous pressure.
- Assess fluid balance. Check for signs and symptoms of heart failure.
- Monitor CBC and liver and thyroid function tests.
- Watch closely for signs and symptoms of hypoglycemia, which drug may mask.
- Monitor blood glucose level in diabetic patient, to identify need for altered insulin or oral hypoglycemic dosage. Be aware that in labile diabetes, hypoglycemia may be accompanied by steep blood pressure rise.

Patient teaching

- Advise patient to take with meals at same time every day to minimize GI upset.

Caution patient not to stop taking drug suddenly. Tell him dosage must be tapered.

- Tell patient to monitor pulse and to promptly report bradycardia or tachycardia.
- Inform patient that drug may cause muscle aches or bone pain. Advise him to discuss activity recommendations and pain management with prescriber.
- Caution patient to avoid driving and other hazardous activities until he knows how drug affects concentration, vision, and alertness.
- As appropriate, review all other significant and life-threatening adverse reactions and interactions, especially those related to the drugs, tests, and behaviors mentioned above.

propylthiouracil (PTU)

Propyl-Thyracil✽

Pharmacologic class: Thioamide derivative
Therapeutic class: Antithyroid agent
Pregnancy risk category D

Action

Directly interferes with thyroid synthesis by preventing iodine from combining with thyroglobulin, leading to decreased thyroid hormone levels

Availability

Tablets: 50 mg

Indications and dosages

➢ Hyperthyroidism
Adults: Initially, 300 to 450 mg P.O. daily in equally divided doses q 8 hours; for maintenance, 100 to 150 mg P.O. daily.
➢ Thyrotoxic crisis
Adults: 200 mg P.O. q 4 to 6 hours during first 24 hours, then a maintenance dosage of 100 to 150 mg P.O. daily

Contraindications

- Hypersensitivity to drug
- Pregnancy and breastfeeding

Precautions

Use cautiously in:
- decreased bone marrow reserve.

Administration

- Give with meals to reduce GI upset.

Route	Onset	Peak	Duration
P.O.	Unknown	1-1.5 hr	Unknown

Adverse reactions

CNS: drowsiness, headache, vertigo, neuritis, paresthesia

GI: nausea, vomiting, diarrhea, epigastric distress
Hematologic: agranulocytosis, leukopenia, thrombocytopenia
Hepatic: jaundice, **hepatic necrosis**
Metabolic: hypothyroidism
Musculoskeletal: joint pain, myalgia
Skin: rash, urticaria, pruritus, skin discoloration, alopecia, cutaneous vasculitis
Other: taste loss, fever, lymphadenopathy, parotitis, edema

Interactions

Drug-drug. *Anticoagulants:* potentiation of anticoagulant effect
Drug-diagnostic tests. *Alanine aminotransferase, alkaline phosphatase, aspartate aminotransferase, bilirubin, lactate dehydrogenase:* increased levels
Granulocytes, platelets: decreased levels
Prothrombin time: prolonged

Patient monitoring

- Monitor CBC and liver and thyroid function tests.
- Assess for signs and symptoms of hypothyroidism (cold intolerance, nonpitting edema, fatigue, weight gain, and depression).

◀ Monitor for severe rash, fever, or enlarged cervical lymph nodes. If present, stop therapy and notify prescriber.

Patient teaching

- Instruct patient to take with meals to reduce GI upset.
- Teach patient to recognize and report signs and symptoms of hypothyroidism and jaundice.
- Advise patient to discuss iodine intake (as in iodized salt and shellfish) with prescriber.
- Tell patient to avoid over-the-counter cold remedies that contain iodine.
- Caution patient to avoid driving and other hazardous activities until he knows how drug affects concentration and alertness.
- Advise female patient of childbearing age to discuss pregnancy or breastfeeding with prescriber before taking.
- As appropriate, review all other significant and life-threatening adverse reactions and interactions, especially those related to the drugs and tests mentioned above.

pseudoephedrine hydrochloride

Allermed, Cenafed, Children's Congestion Relief, Decofed, DeFed-60, Dimetapp Decongestant Pediatric Drops, Dorcol Children's Decongestant Liquid, Efidac/24, Genaphed, Halofed, PediaCare Infants' Oral Decongestant Drops, Pedia Relief, Pseudo, Pseudo-Gest, Robidrine✤, Seudotabs, Simply Stuffy, Sudafed, Sudafed Children's Nasal Decongestant, Sudafed 12 Hour, Suphedrin, Triaminic AM Decongestant Formula, Triaminic Infant Oral Decongestant Drops✤

pseudoephedrine sulfate

Drixoral Nasal Decongestant, Drixoral Non-Drowsy Formula

Pharmacologic class: Sympathomimetic

Therapeutic class: Decongestant (systemic)

Pregnancy risk category C

Action

Stimulates alpha-adrenergic receptors, causing vasoconstriction of respiratory tract; relaxes bronchial smooth muscle through $beta_2$-adrenergic stimulation

Availability

pseudoephedrine hydrochloride
Capsules: 60 mg
Capsules (extended-release): 120 mg, 240 mg
Capsules (soft gel): 30 mg
Oral solution: 15 mg/5 ml, 30 mg/5 ml
Syrup: 30 mg/5 ml
Tablets: 30 mg, 60 mg
Tablets (chewable): 15 mg
Tablets (extended-release): 120 mg, 240 mg
pseudoephedrine sulfate
Tablets (extended-release, film-coated): 120 mg

Indications and dosages

➢ Nasal, sinus, or eustachian tube congestion
Adults and children ages 12 and older: 60 mg P.O. q 4 to 6 hours p.r.n. (not to exceed 240 mg/day); or 120 mg (extended-release) q 12 hours or 240 mg (extended-release) q 24 hours

Contraindications

- Hypersensitivity to drug or other sympathomimetics
- Alcohol intolerance (with some liquid products)
- Hypertension
- Severe coronary artery disease
- MAO inhibitor use within past 14 days
- Children younger than age 12 (extended-release forms)

Precautions

Use cautiously in:
- hyperthyroidism, diabetes mellitus, prostatic hypertrophy, ischemic heart disease, glaucoma
- elderly patients (more sensitive to drug's CNS effects)
- pregnant or breastfeeding patients.

Administration

- Give at least 2 hours before bedtime to minimize insomnia.

Route	Onset	Peak	Duration
P.O.	30 min	Unknown	4-8 hr
P.O. (extended)	60 min	Unknown	12 hr

Adverse reactions

CNS: anxiety, nervousness, dizziness, drowsiness, excitability, fear, hallucinations, headache, insomnia, restlessness, asthenia, **seizures**
CV: palpitations, hypertension, tachycardia, **cardiovascular collapse**
GI: anorexia, dry mouth
GU: dysuria
Respiratory: respiratory difficulty

Interactions

Drug-drug. *Beta-adrenergic blockers:* increased pressor effects of pseudoephedrine
MAO inhibitors: hypertensive crisis
Mecamylamine, methyldopa, reserpine: decreased antihypertensive effect of these drugs
Other sympathomimetics: additive effects, greater risk of toxicity
Drug-food. *Foods that acidify urine:* decreased drug efficacy
Foods that alkalize urine: increased drug efficacy

Patient monitoring

- Monitor vital signs.
- Assess neurologic and cardiovascular status regularly.

Patient teaching

- Advise patient to take at least 2 hours before bedtime to reduce insomnia.
- Tell patient not to crush or break extended-release tablets or capsules.
- Advise patient to discontinue use and consult prescriber if he experiences nervousness, dizziness, or insomnia.
- Tell patient to consult prescriber before taking other over-the-counter products.
- Caution patient to avoid driving and other hazardous activities until he

P

knows how drug affects concentration and alertness.
• As appropriate, review all other significant and life-threatening adverse reactions and interactions, especially those related to the drugs and foods mentioned above.

psyllium

Alramucil, Fiberall, Genfiber, Hydrocil Instant, Karacil ♣, Konsyl, Maalox Daily Fiber Therapy, Metamucil, Metamucil Orange Flavor, Metamucil Sugar Free, Modane Bulk, Mylanta Natural Fiber Supplement, Perdiem, Prodiem Plain ♣, Reguloid Natural, Reguloid Natural Sugar Free, Reguloid Orange, Reguloid Orange Sugar Free, Restore, Restore Sugar Free, Serutan, Syllact, V-Lax

Pharmacologic class: Psyllium colloid
Therapeutic class: Bulk-forming laxative
Pregnancy risk category B

Action

Stimulates lining of colon, increasing peristalsis and water absorption of stool and promoting evacuation

Availability

Chewable pieces: 1.7 g/piece, 3.4 g/piece
Granules: 2.5 g/tsp, 4.03 g/tsp
Powder: 3.3 g/tsp, 3.4 g/tsp, 3.5 g/tsp, 4.94 g/tsp
Powder (effervescent): 3.4 g/packet, 3.7 g/packet
Wafers: 3.4 g/wafer

Indications and dosages

➢ Chronic constipation; ulcerative colitis; irritable bowel syndrome

Adults and children ages 12 and older: 30 g daily in divided doses of 2.5 to 7.5 g/dose P.O. in 8 oz of water or juice

Contraindications

• Hypersensitivity to drug
• Intestinal obstruction
• Abdominal pain or other appendicitis symptoms
• Fecal impaction

Precautions

Use cautiously in:
• phenylketonuria
• pregnant patients.

Administration

• Mix powder with 8 oz of cold liquid (such as orange juice) to mask taste.
• Give diluted drug immediately after mixing, before it congeals. Follow with another glass of fluid.

Route	Onset	Peak	Duration
P.O.	12-24 hr	3 days	Variable

Adverse reactions

GI: nausea; vomiting; diarrhea (with excessive use); abdominal cramps with severe constipation; anorexia; **esophageal, gastric, small-intestine, or rectal obstruction** (with dry form)
Respiratory: asthma (rare)
Other: severe allergic reactions including **anaphylaxis**

Interactions

None significant

Patient monitoring

• Monitor patient's bowel movements.
• Check for signs and symptoms of severe (but rare) allergic reactions, such as anaphylaxis and asthma.

Patient teaching

• Tell patient to dissolve in 8 oz of cold beverage and drink immediately, followed by another glass of liquid.

• Caution patient not to take without dissolving in liquid.
• Instruct patient to take after meals if drug decreases his appetite.
• Tell patient drug usually causes bowel movement within 12 to 24 hours but may take as long as 3 days.
Instruct patient to immediately stop taking drug and notify prescriber if signs and symptoms of allergic reaction occur.
• Advise diabetic patient to use sugar-free drug form.
• Instruct patient with phenylketonuria to avoid forms containing phenylalanine.
• As appropriate, review all other significant and life-threatening adverse reactions.

pyrantel pamoate

Antiminth, Combantrin✱, Pin-Rid, Pin-X, Reese's Pinworm

Pharmacologic class: Pyrimidine derivative
Therapeutic class: Anthelmintic
Pregnancy risk category C

Action

Stimulates ganglionic receptors in worm, paralyzing it; worm is then expelled through normal peristalsis.

Availability

Capsules: 180 mg
Liquid: 50 mg/ml
Oral suspension: 50 mg/ml, 144 mg/ml

Indications and dosages

➢ Pinworm (enterobiasis); roundworm (ascariasis)
Adults and children older than age 2: 11 mg/kg P.O. as a single dose (maximum of 1 g/day), repeated in 2 weeks

Contraindications

• Hypersensitivity to drug

Precautions

Use cautiously in:
• malnutrition, dehydration, hepatic disease, seizure disorder
• *Trichostrongylus* infection
• pregnant or breastfeeding patients
• children younger than age 2.

Administration

• Shake suspension well.
• Give all forms without regard to food, milk, or juice intake.

Route	Onset	Peak	Duration
P.O.	Slow	1-3 hr	Unknown

Adverse reactions

CNS: dizziness, headache, drowsiness, insomnia, asthenia
GI: nausea, vomiting, diarrhea, abdominal cramps, gastralgia, anorexia
Skin: rash
Other: fever

Interactions

Drug-drug. *Piperazine:* antagonism of both drugs' effects
Drug-diagnostic tests. *Aspartate aminotransferase:* transient increase

Patient monitoring

• Monitor for rash and fever.

Patient teaching

• Tell patient to shake suspension well. Inform him that he may take it with or without food, juice, or milk.
• Instruct patient to report rash or fever.
• If pinworm is suspected, tell patient that everyone in household should be treated.
• Advise patient to practice strict hygiene to prevent reinfection.
• Caution patient to avoid driving and other hazardous activities until he

P

knows how drug affects concentration and alertness.

• As appropriate, review all other significant adverse reactions and interactions, especially those related to the drugs and tests mentioned above.

pyrazinamide

PMS Pyrazinamide✤, Tebrazid✤

Pharmacologic class: Niacinamide derivative

Therapeutic class: Antitubercular

Pregnancy risk category C

Action

Unknown. Thought to exert bacteriostatic activity.

Availability

Tablets: 500 mg

Indications and dosages

➣ Tuberculosis

Adults and children: 15 to 30 mg/kg/day P.O., not to exceed 2 g/day; or 50 to 70 mg/kg P.O. twice weekly, up to a maximum of 4 g/dose; or 50 to 70 mg/kg/dose P.O. three times weekly, up to a maximum of 3 g/dose

Dosage adjustment

• Renal impairment

Contraindications

• Hypersensitivity to drug
• Severe hepatic disease
• Acute gout

Precautions

Use cautiously in:

• renal failure, diabetes mellitus, porphyria, chronic gout, history of gout
• pregnant or breastfeeding patients
• children younger than age 13.

Administration

• Give with other antituberculars, as prescribed, to reduce risk of resistant organisms.
• Be aware that drug therapy may last 6 months or longer.

Route	Onset	Peak	Duration
P.O.	Rapid	2 hr	Unknown

Adverse reactions

CNS: headache
GI: nausea, vomiting, diarrhea, peptic ulcer, abdominal cramps, anorexia
GU: dysuria, increased uric acid secretion
Hematologic: hemolytic anemia
Hepatic: hepatotoxicity
Metabolic: hyperuricemia, gout
Musculoskeletal: joint pain
Skin: urticaria, photosensitivity

Interactions

Drug-drug. *Ethionamide:* increased risk of hepatotoxicity
Probenecid: decreased probenecid efficacy (possibly precipitating gout)
Drug-diagnostic tests. *Acetest or Ketostix urine test:* false interpretation
Liver function tests: abnormal results
Uric acid: increased level

Patient monitoring

• Monitor CBC, uric acid level, and liver and kidney function tests.
• Assess for signs and symptoms of gout, hepatic failure, and hemolytic anemia.
Discontinue at first sign of hepatic impairment or hyperuricemia accompanied by acute gouty arthritis.

Patient teaching

• Advise patient to take regularly with other antituberculars, as prescribed.
Teach patient to recognize and immediately report signs and symptoms of gout and liver impairment.
• As appropriate, review all other significant and life-threatening adverse

reactions and interactions, especially those related to the drugs and tests mentioned above.

pyridostigmine bromide

Mestinon, Mestinon-SR✱, Mestinon Timespans, Regonol

Pharmacologic class: Anticholinesterase

Therapeutic class: Muscle stimulant, antimyasthenic

Pregnancy risk category C

Action

Prevents acetylcholine destruction, resulting in stronger contractions of muscles weakened by myasthenia gravis or curare-like neuromuscular blockers

Availability

Injection: 5 mg/ml
Syrup: 60 mg/5 ml
Tablets: 60 mg
Tablets (extended-release): 180 mg

Indications and dosages

➢ Myasthenia gravis

Adults: 600 mg P.O. given over 24 hours, with doses spaced for maximum symptom relief. For myasthenic crisis, 2 mg or 1/30 of oral dose I.M. or very slow I.V. q 2 to 3 hours.

➢ Postoperative reversal of nondepolarizing neuromuscular blockers

Adults: 10 to 20 mg slow I.V. injection (range is 0.1 to 0.25 mg/kg) with or immediately after 0.6 to 1.2 mg atropine sulfate I.V.

Dosage adjustment

- Renal impairment
- Seizure disorders

Off-label uses

- Myasthenia gravis in children
- Constipation in patients with Parkinson's disease
- Nerve agent prophylaxis

Contraindications

- Hypersensitivity to drug or bromides
- Mechanical intestinal or urinary tract obstruction

Precautions

Use cautiously in:
- seizure disorders, bronchial asthma, coronary occlusion, arrhythmias, bradycardia, hyperthyroidism, peptic ulcer, vagotonia, cholinergic crisis
- pregnant or breastfeeding patients
- children (safety and efficacy not established).

Administration

- Don't exceed I.V. injection rate of 1 mg/minute.
- Don't give concurrently with other anticholinesterase drugs.
- Have atropine available for use in emergencies.

Route	Onset	Peak	Duration
P.O.	20-30 min	Unknown	Unknown
P.O. (extended)	30-60 min	Unknown	6-12 hr
I.V.	2-5 min	Unknown	2-4 hr
I.M.	<15 min	Unknown	2-4 hr

Adverse reactions

CNS: headache, dysarthria, dysphoria, drowsiness, dizziness, headache, syncope, **loss of consciousness, seizures**
CV: decreased cardiac output leading to hypotension, bradycardia, nodal rhythm, **atrioventricular block, cardiac arrest, arrhythmias**
EENT: diplopia, lacrimation, miosis, spasm of accommodation, conjunctival hyperemia
GI: nausea, vomiting, diarrhea, abdominal cramps, increased peristalsis, flatu-

P

lence dysphagia, increased salivation
GU: urinary frequency, urgency, or incontinence
Musculoskeletal: muscle weakness, fasciculations, and cramps; joint pain
Respiratory: increased pharyngeal and tracheobronchial secretions, dyspnea, **central respiratory paralysis, respiratory muscle paralysis, laryngospasm, bronchospasm, bronchiolar constriction**
Skin: diaphoresis, flushing, rash, urticaria
Other: thrombophlebitis at I.V. site, cholinergic crisis, anaphylaxis

Interactions

Drug-drug. *Aminoglycosides:* potentiation of neuromuscular blockade
Anesthetics (general and local), antiarrhythmics: decreased anticholinesterase effects
Atropine, belladonna derivatives: suppression of parasympathomimetic GI symptoms (leaving only fasciculations and voluntary muscle paralysis as signs of anticholinesterase overdose)
Corticosteroids: decreased anticholinesterase effects; after corticosteroid withdrawal, increased anticholinesterase effects
Ganglionic blockers (such as mecamylamine): increased anticholinesterase effects
Magnesium: antagonism of beneficial anticholinesterase effects
Nondepolarizing neuromuscular blockers (atropine, pancuronium, tubocurarine): antagonism of neuromuscular blockade and reversal of muscle relaxation after surgery (with parenteral pyridostigmine)
Other anticholinesterase drugs: in patients with myasthenia gravis, symptoms of anticholinesterase overdose that mimic underdose, causing patient's condition to worsen
Succinylcholine: increased and prolonged neuromuscular blockade (including respiratory depression)

Patient monitoring

- Assess patient's response to each dose.
- Monitor vital signs, ECG, and cardiovascular and respiratory status.

Assess for signs and symptoms of overdose, which indicate cholinergic crisis.

Patient teaching

- If patient is using syrup, advise him to pour it over ice.
- Instruct patient using extended-release tablets not to crush them.

Teach patient to recognize and promptly report signs and symptoms of overdose, including muscle fasciculations, sweating, excessive salivation, and constricted pupils.

- Tell patient drug may cause headache and muscle cramps. Encourage him to discuss activity recommendations and pain management with prescriber.
- Advise patient to monitor and report his response to ongoing therapy so that optimal dosage can be determined.
- As appropriate, review all other significant and life-threatening adverse reactions and interactions, especially those related to the drugs mentioned above.

pyrimethamine

Daraprim

Pharmacologic class: Folic acid antagonist
Therapeutic class: Antiprotozoal, antimalarial
Pregnancy risk category C

Action

Inhibits reduction of dihydrofolic acid to tetrahydrofolic acid (folinic acid) by binding to and reversibly inhibiting dihydrofolate reductase

Availability

Tablets: 25 mg

Indications and dosages

➢ To control plasmodia transmission and suppress susceptible strains

Adults and children ages 10 and older: 25 mg P.O. daily for 2 days, given with a sulfonamide

➢ Toxoplasmosis

Adults: Initially, 50 to 75 mg P.O. daily for 1 to 3 weeks, given with a sulfonamide. Depending on response and tolerance, reduce dosages of both drugs by 50% and continue therapy for 4 to 5 more weeks.

Children: 1 mg/kg P.O. daily in two equally divided doses for 2 to 4 days, then reduced to 0.5 mg/kg/day for approximately 1 month. Alternatively, 2 mg/kg (up to 100 mg) P.O. daily in two equally divided doses for 3 days, then 1 mg/kg (up to 25 mg) in two equally divided doses for 4 weeks, given with sulfadiazine for 4 weeks.

➢ Prophylaxis of malaria caused by susceptible plasmodia strains

Adults and children older than age 10: 25 mg P.O. weekly

Children ages 4 to 10: 12.5 mg P.O. weekly

Infants and children younger than age 4: 6.25 mg P.O. weekly

Off-label uses

- Isosporiasis
- Prophylaxis of *Pneumocystis jiroveci* pneumonia

Contraindications

- Hypersensitivity to drug
- Megaloblastic anemia caused by folate deficiency
- Concurrent folate antagonist therapy

Precautions

Use cautiously in:

- anemia, bone marrow depression, hepatic or renal impairment, G6PD deficiency
- history of seizures
- patients more than 16 weeks pregnant
- breastfeeding patients.

Administration

- Administer with meals.
- When giving tablets to young children, crush them and administer as oral suspension in water, cherry syrup, or sweetened solution.
- Know that because of worldwide resistance to pyrimethamine, its use alone to prevent or treat acute malaria is no longer recommended.
- Be aware that fixed combination of pyrimethamine and sulfadoxine is available and has been used for uncomplicated mild to moderate malaria caused by chloroquine-resistant *Plasmodium falciparum* and for presumptive self-treatment by travelers.

Route	Onset	Peak	Duration
P.O.	Unknown	2-6 hr	2 wk

Adverse reactions

CNS: headache, light-headedness, insomnia, malaise, depression, **seizures**

CV: arrhythmias

EENT: dry throat

GI: nausea, vomiting, diarrhea, anorexia, atrophic glossitis

GU: hematuria

Hematologic: megaloblastic anemia, leukopenia, pancytopenia, thrombocytopenia

Metabolic: hyperphenylalaninemia

Respiratory: pulmonary eosinophilia

Skin: pigmentation changes, dermatitis, erythema multiforme, **toxic epidermal necrolysis, Stevens-Johnson syndrome**

Other: fever, **anaphylaxis**

Interactions

Drug-drug. *Lorazepam:* hepatotoxicity

Myelosuppressants (including antineoplastics): increased risk of bone marrow depression

Drug-diagnostic tests. *Platelets, white blood cells:* decreased counts

Patient monitoring

- Monitor CBC. Watch for evidence of blood dyscrasias.
- Assess for signs and symptoms of folic acid deficiency.
- Closely monitor neurologic and cardiovascular status. Stay alert for seizures and arrhythmias.

◀ Watch for evidence of erythema multiforme, including sore throat, cough, mouth sores, rash, iritic lesions, and fever. Report early signs before condition can progress to Stevens-Johnson syndrome.

Patient teaching

- Advise patient to take with meals.

◀ Tell patient to discontinue drug and contact prescriber at first sign of rash.

- Caution patient to avoid driving and other hazardous activities until he knows how drug affects concentration and alertness.
- As appropriate, review all other significant and life-threatening adverse reactions and interactions, especially those related to the drugs and tests mentioned above.

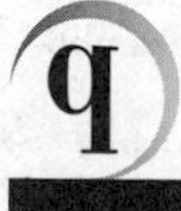

quetiapine fumarate

Seroquel

Pharmacologic class: Dibenzothiazepine derivative

Therapeutic class: Atypical antipsychotic

Pregnancy risk category C

Action

Unknown. Antipsychotic effects may occur through antagonism of dopamine D_2 and serotonin 5-HT_2 receptors. Other effects may result partly from antagonism of other receptors, such as histamine H_1 and alpha$_1$-adrenergic receptors.

Availability

Tablets: 25 mg, 100 mg, 200 mg, 300 mg

Indications and dosages

➤ Schizophrenia

Adults: Initially, 25 mg P.O. b.i.d., increased by 25 to 50 mg given two to three times daily as tolerated over 3 days, up to 300 to 400 mg/day in two to three divided doses by day 4 (not to exceed 800 mg/day)

➤ Acute manic episodes associated with bipolar I disorder

Adults: 100 mg on day 1, 200 mg on day 2, 300 mg on day 3, 400 mg on day 4, up to 600 mg on day 5, and up to 800 mg on day 6. Maximum daily dosage is 800 mg. May be given as monotherapy or as adjunctive therapy with lithium or divalproex.

Dosage adjustment

- Hepatic impairment
- History of hypotensive reactions
- Elderly or debilitated patients

Off-label uses

- Bipolar disorder
- Mania
- Obsessive-compulsive disorder
- Posttraumatic stress disorder
- Psychosis related to Parkinson's disease

Contraindications

- Hypersensitivity to drug or its components

Precautions

Use cautiously in:

- hepatic impairment, cardiovascular or cerebrovascular disease, dehydration, hypovolemia, Alzheimer's dementia, hypothyroidism
- history of seizures, suicide attempt, or hypotensive reactions
- elderly or debilitated patients
- pregnant patients
- children (safety not established).

Administration

- Give with or without food.

Don't confuse Seroquel with Serzone (an antidepressant).

Route	Onset	Peak	Duration
P.O.	Rapid	1.5 hr	8-12 hr

Adverse reactions

CNS: dizziness, sedation, cognitive impairment, extrapyramidal symptoms, tardive dyskinesia, **neuroleptic malignant syndrome, seizures**
CV: palpitations, peripheral edema, orthostatic hypotension
EENT: ear pain, rhinitis, pharyngitis
GI: constipation, dyspepsia, dry mouth, anorexia
Hematologic: leukopenia
Respiratory: cough, dyspnea
Skin: diaphoresis
Other: weight gain, flulike symptoms

Interactions

Drug-drug. *Antihistamines, opioids, sedative-hypnotics, other CNS depressants:* additive CNS depression
Antihypertensives: increased risk of hypotension
Barbiturates, carbamazepine, corticosteroids, phenytoin, rifampin, thioridazine: increased clearance and decreased efficacy of quetiapine
Dopamine agonists, levodopa: antagonism of these drugs' effects
Erythromycin, fluconazole, itraconazole, ketoconazole, other CYP450-3A4 inhibitors: increased quetiapine effects
Drug-diagnostic tests. *Alanine aminotransferase, aspartate aminotransferase:* asymptomatic elevations
Total cholesterol, triglycerides: increased levels
Urine tricyclic antidepressant assay: false-positive screen
White blood cells: decreased count
Drug-behaviors. *Alcohol use:* increased CNS effects

Patient monitoring

Monitor neurologic status, especially for signs and symptoms of tardive dyskinesia or neuroleptic malignant syndrome.

- Monitor blood pressure for orthostatic hypertension.

Patient teaching

- Tell patient he can take with or without food.

Teach patient to recognize and immediately report signs and symptoms of neuroleptic malignant syndrome (such as high fever, sweating, unstable blood pressure, stupor, muscle rigidity, and tardive dyskinesia).

- Instruct patient to move slowly when sitting up or standing, to avoid dizziness from sudden blood pressure decrease.

Tell patient not to stop taking drug abruptly. Tell him dosage must be tapered.

- Caution patient not to drink alcohol.
- Instruct patient to avoid driving and other hazardous activities until he knows how drug affects concentration and alertness.
- As appropriate, review all other significant and life-threatening adverse reactions and interactions, especially those related to the drugs, tests, and behaviors mentioned above.

q

quinapril hydrochloride

Accupril

Pharmacologic class: Angiotensin-converting enzyme (ACE) inhibitor

Therapeutic class: Antihypertensive

Pregnancy risk category C (first trimester), ***D*** (second and third trimesters)

Action

Inhibits conversion of angiotensin I to angiotensin II, a potent vasoconstrictor; decreases cardiac output. Increases plasma renin levels and reduces aldosterone levels, causing systemic vasodilation.

Availability

Tablets: 5 mg, 10 mg, 20 mg, 40 mg

Indications and dosages

➢ Hypertension

Adults: Initially, 10 to 20 mg P.O. daily for patients not receiving diuretics, with subsequent dosages adjusted at 2-week intervals according to blood pressure response at peak (2 to 6 hours) and trough (predose) blood levels; for maintenance, 20 to 80 mg/day as a single dose or in two divided doses. In patients receiving diuretics, discontinue diuretic 2 to 3 days before starting quinapril; if blood pressure isn't controlled, resume diuretic. If diuretic can't be discontinued, start therapy with 5 mg/day quinapril.

➢ Adjunct in heart failure

Adults: Initially, 5 mg P.O. b.i.d., titrated weekly until effective dosage is determined. For maintenance, 20 to 40 mg/day in two evenly divided doses.

Dosage adjustment

- Renal impairment
- Elderly patients

Off-label uses

- Aortic insufficiency
- Atherosclerosis
- Postoperative hypertension
- Myocardial infarction
- Diabetic or nondiabetic neuropathy

Contraindications

- Hypersensitivity to drug or other ACE inhibitors
- Angioedema caused by other ACE inhibitors
- Pregnancy (second and third trimesters)

Precautions

Use cautiously in:

- autoimmune diseases, aortic stenosis, renal artery stenosis, hypertrophic cardiomyopathy, cerebrovascular or cardiac insufficiency, collagen vascular disease, hepatic or renal impairment, hypovolemia, hyponatremia, hypotension, neutropenia, chronic cough, proteinuria, febrile illness
- family history of angioedema
- concurrent immunosuppressant or diuretic therapy
- black patients
- elderly patients
- pregnant (first trimester) or breast-feeding patients
- children (safety not established).

Administration

- Administer with or without food, but not with high-fat meal.
- Know that if quinapril alone doesn't adequately control blood pressure, a diuretic may be added.

Route	Onset	Peak	Duration
P.O.	0.5-1 hr	2-6 hr	Up to 24 hr

Adverse reactions

CNS: dizziness, drowsiness, fatigue, headache, insomnia, depression, vertigo, paresthesia, asthenia, malaise, nervousness, syncope

CV: hypotension, angina pectoris, palpitations, chest pain, tachycardia, **arrhythmias**
EENT: amblyopia, sinusitis, pharyngitis
GI: nausea, vomiting, diarrhea, constipation, abdominal pain, anorexia, dry mouth
GU: erectile dysfunction
Metabolic: hyperkalemia
Musculoskeletal: back pain
Respiratory: cough, dyspnea
Skin: rash, pruritus, alopecia, flushing, diaphoresis, photosensitivity
Other: taste disturbances, fever, viral infections, hypersensitivity reactions including **anaphylaxis**

Interactions

Drug-drug. *Allopurinol:* increased risk of hypersensitivity reactions
Antacids: decreased quinapril absorption
Digoxin, lithium: increased blood levels and risk of toxicity of these drugs
Diuretics, other antihypertensives: increased hypotension
Indomethacin: decreased hypotensive effect of quinapril
Phenothiazines: increased pharmacologic effect of quinapril
Potassium-sparing diuretics, potassium supplements: increased risk of hyperkalemia
Tetracyclines: decreased tetracycline absorption
Drug-diagnostic tests. *Alanine aminotransferase, alkaline phosphatase, aspartate aminotransferase, bilirubin, blood urea nitrogen, creatinine, potassium:* increased levels
Drug-food. *High-fat foods:* decreased rate and extent of drug absorption
Salt substitutes containing potassium: increased risk of hyperkalemia
Drug-herbs. *Capsaicin:* increased incidence of cough
Ephedra (ma huang): decreased drug efficacy, exacerbation of hypertension
Yohimbe: interference with drug's antihypertensive effect
Drug-behaviors. *Alcohol use:* increased hypotension

Patient monitoring

- Monitor vital signs and cardiovascular status. Be sure to ask patient if he's experiencing angina.
- Assess CBC and liver function tests.
- Monitor potassium level. Watch for evidence of hyperkalemia.

Watch closely for signs and symptoms of angioedema, especially in black patients after first dose.

- Assess for dry, nonproductive cough and signs and symptoms of infection.

Patient teaching

- Tell patient he may take with or without food, but not with high-fat meal.

Advise patient to immediately report facial or tongue swelling or difficulty breathing.

- Instruct patient to monitor and record his blood pressure.
- Tell patient to promptly report dry, nonproductive cough and signs and symptoms of infection.
- Instruct patient to move slowly when sitting up or standing, to avoid dizziness or light-headedness from sudden blood pressure decrease.
- Tell patient that excessive fluid loss (as from sweating, vomiting, or diarrhea) and inadequate fluid intake increase the risk of light-headedness (especially in hot weather).
- Caution patient to avoid driving and other hazardous activities until he knows how drug affects concentration and alertness.
- Advise patient to avoid herbal products and salt substitutes containing potassium.
- Tell female patient to notify prescriber of possible pregnancy. Caution her not to breastfeed.
- As appropriate, review all other significant and life-threatening adverse

q

reactions and interactions, especially those related to the drugs, tests, foods, herbs, and behaviors mentioned above.

quinidine gluconate

Quinate✱

quinidine sulfate

Apo-Quinidine✱, Novoquinidin✱

Pharmacologic class: Cinchona alkaloid

Therapeutic class: Antiarrhythmic (class IA), antimalarial

Pregnancy risk category C

Action

Slows conduction and prolongs refractory period, reducing myocardial irritability and interrupting or preventing certain arrhythmias. As an antimalarial, acts primarily as intra-erythrocytic schizonticide.

Availability

quinidine gluconate

Injection: 80 mg/ml

Tablets (extended-release): 324 mg

quinidine sulfate

Tablets: 200 mg, 300 mg

Tablets (extended-release): 300 mg

Indications and dosages

➤ Test dose

Adults: 200 mg sulfate P.O. as a single dose or 200 mg gluconate I.M. to check for idiosyncratic reaction

➤ Premature atrial and ventricular contractions

Adults: 200 to 300 mg sulfate P.O. three to four times daily, or gluconate (extended-release) given as 324 to 660 mg P.O. q 8 to 12 hours

➤ Paroxysmal supraventricular tachycardia (PSVT)

Adults: 400 to 600 mg sulfate P.O. q 2 or 3 hours until arrhythmia ends; or 324 to 660 mg (extended-release) P.O. q 8 to 12 hours. For parenteral use, 400 mg gluconate I.M., repeated q 2 hours if necessary; or 330 mg gluconate I.V. (up to 750 mg) in diluted solution, infused no faster than 1 ml/minute.

➤ To convert atrial fibrillation to sinus rhythm

Adults: 200 mg sulfate P.O. q 2 or 3 hours for five to eight doses, increased daily until sinus rhythm returns or toxic effects occur; maximum daily dosage is 4 g. Or 300 mg sulfate (extended-release) P.O. q 8 to 12 hours, increased cautiously if necessary. Or 324 to 660 mg gluconate (extended-release) P.O. q 8 to 12 hours. For parenteral use, 800 mg gluconate I.V. in diluted solution, infused no faster than 0.25 mg/kg/minute.

➤ Severe, life-threatening *Plasmodium falciparum* malaria

Adults: Loading dose of 10 mg/kg gluconate I.V. diluted in 5 ml/kg of normal saline solution (or 250 ml of normal saline solution in otherwise healthy, 50-kg [110-lb] patient) by continuous infusion over 1 to 2 hours, then a continuous maintenance infusion of 0.02 mg/kg/minute for 72 hours or until parasitemia drops to less than 1% or oral therapy can begin. Or alternative loading dose of 24 mg/kg gluconate I.V. diluted in 250 ml of 0.9% sodium chloride injection by intermittent infusion over 4 hours, followed by maintenance dosage of 12 mg/kg gluconate I.V. at 8-hour intervals, starting 8 hours after loading dose, infused over 4 hours for 7 days or until patient tolerates oral therapy.

Dosage adjustment

- Hepatic insufficiency

Off-label uses

- Myocardial infarction

Contraindications

- Hypersensitivity to drug or related cinchona derivatives
- Thrombocytopenia with previous quinidine therapy
- Myasthenia gravis
- Complete heart block
- Left bundle-branch block or other severe intraventricular conduction defects
- Aberrant ectopic impulses and abnormal rhythm
- History of prolonged QT interval or drug-induced torsades de pointes
- Digoxin toxicity

Precautions

Use cautiously in:

- potassium imbalance, renal or hepatic disease, heart failure, respiratory depression
- elderly patients
- pregnant or breastfeeding patients
- children.

Administration

Clinical alert: Before first dose, assess apical pulse and blood pressure. If patient has bradycardia or tachycardia, withhold dose and contact prescriber.

- If patient has atrial fibrillation, expect to give digoxin, calcium channel blocker, beta-adrenergic blocker, and possibly an anticoagulant before administering quinidine.
- If sinus rhythm isn't restored after patient has received a total of 10 mg/kg quinidine gluconate, other means of cardioversion may be considered.
- Monitor blood pressure and ECG; titrate flow rate to correct arrhythmia.
- When giving large doses, monitor blood pressure and ECG continuously.
- Know that quinidine gluconate is the only parenteral cinchona alkaloid antimalarial commercially available in U.S. Because newer antiarrhythmics have replaced quinidine in many cardiac uses, it may not be readily available and prescribers may not be familiar with its use. For information about availability or use, contact manufacturer at 800-821-0538.

Route	Onset	Peak	Duration
P.O. (extended)	Unknown	3-5 hr	Unknown
P.O. (sulfate)	Unknown	1-3 hr	Unknown
I.V.	Immediate	Immediate	Unknown
I.M.	30-90 sec	Unknown	Unknown

Adverse reactions

CNS: vertigo, headache, ataxia, apprehension, excitement, delirium, syncope, confusion, depression, dementia
CV: ECG changes, hypotension, vasculitis, tachycardia, premature ventricular contractions, paradoxical tachycardia, **ventricular tachycardia, ventricular fibrillation, ventricular flutter, ventricular ectopy, torsades de pointes, complete atrioventricular (AV) block, widened QRS complex, prolonged QT interval, asystole, aggravated heart failure, arterial embolism, vascular collapse**
EENT: diplopia, blurred vision, mydriasis, abnormal color perception, scotoma, photophobia, night blindness, optic neuritis, decreased hearing, tinnitus
GI: nausea, vomiting, diarrhea, abdominal pain, increased salivation, anorexia
GU: lupus nephritis
Hematologic: purpura, **hemolytic anemia, hypothrombinemia, leukocytosis, shift to left in white blood cell differential, neutropenia, thrombocytopenia, thrombocytopenic purpura, agranulocytosis**
Hepatic: hepatotoxicity
Respiratory: acute asthma attack, respiratory arrest
Skin: rash, pruritus, urticaria, photosensitivity, angioedema

q

Other: fever, cinchonism, lupuslike syndrome, hypersensitivity reaction

Interactions

Drug-drug. *Amiodarone:* increased quinidine blood level, causing potentially fatal arrhythmias
Antacids, cimetidine: increased quinidine blood level
Anticholinergics: additive vagolytic effect
Anticoagulants, beta-adrenergic blockers, procainamide, propafenone, tricyclic antidepressants: increased effects of these drugs
Barbiturates, hydantoins, nifedipine, rifampin, sucralfate: decreased therapeutic effect of quinidine
Cardiac glycosides: increased cardiac glycoside blood level, greater risk of toxicity
Cholinergics: decreased quinidine effect (may cause failure to terminate PSVT)
Depolarizing (decamethonium, succinylcholine) and nondepolarizing (tubocurarine, pancuronium) neuromuscular blockers: potentiation of neuromuscular blockade
Diltiazem, verapamil: decreased quinidine clearance, resulting in hypotension, bradycardia, ventricular tachycardia, AV block, or pulmonary edema
Disopyramide: increased disopyramide or decreased quinidine blood level
Potassium, urinary alkalizers: increased blood level and effects of quinidine
Drug-diagnostic tests. *Granulocytes, hemoglobin, platelets:* decreased levels
Creatine kinase, hepatic enzymes: increased levels
Renal function tests: altered results
Drug-food. *Grapefruit juice:* inhibited drug metabolism
Reduced sodium intake: increased quinidine blood level
Drug-herbs. *Jimsonweed:* adverse cardiovascular effects
Licorice: additive effects

Patient monitoring

- Monitor ECG and vital signs closely. Assess for worsening heart failure, especially with I.V. use.
- Assess CBC, kidney and liver function tests and quinidine blood level.
- Watch for signs and symptoms of blood dyscrasias.
- Closely monitor respiratory status. Stay alert for asthma attacks and impending respiratory arrest.
- Monitor for adverse GI effects, which may signify drug toxicity.

Patient teaching

- Advise patient to take with food to reduce GI upset.
- Instruct patient not to crush or chew extended-release tablets.
- Teach patient to recognize and immediately report signs and symptoms of toxicity, including tinnitus, nausea, headache, dizziness, and visual disturbances.
- Caution patient to avoid potassium supplements, licorice, and grapefruit juice. Tell him to maintain constant level of sodium intake.
- Advise patient to consult prescriber before taking herbs.
- As appropriate, review all other significant and life-threatening adverse reactions and interactions, especially those related to the drugs, tests, foods, and herbs mentioned above.

quinine sulfate

Pharmacologic class: Cinchona alkaloid
Therapeutic class: Antimalarial
Pregnancy risk category X

Action

Unknown. Thought to interfere with DNA synthesis by increasing pH in intracellular organelles of susceptible parasites.

Availability

Capsules: 200 mg, 325 mg
Tablets: 260 mg

Indications and dosages

➤ Chloroquine-resistant *Plasmodium falciparum* malaria
Adults: 650 mg P.O. q 8 hours for 3 to 7 days, given with another oral antimalarial
Children: 10 mg/kg P.O. q 8 hours for 7 days, given with another oral antimalarial

Off-label uses

- Nocturnal recumbency leg cramps

Contraindications

- Hypersensitivity to drug or other cinchona alkaloids
- G6PD deficiency
- Optic neuritis
- Tinnitus
- History of blackwater fever or thrombocytopenic purpura
- Pregnancy

Precautions

Use cautiously in:
- myasthenia gravis, recurrent or interrupted malaria therapy
- history of arrhythmias (especially prolonged QT interval), asthma, or heart disease
- breastfeeding patients.

Administration

- Give with or without food.

Route	Onset	Peak	Duration
P.O.	Unknown	1-3 hr	4-11 hr

Adverse reactions

CNS: headache, vertigo, syncope, apprehension, restlessness, excitement, confusion, delirium, dizziness, **seizures**
CV: angina, vasculitis
EENT: diplopia, amblyopia, blurred vision, scotoma, abnormal color perception, photophobia, night blindness, mydriasis, optic atrophy, hearing loss, tinnitus
GI: nausea, vomiting, diarrhea, abdominal cramps, epigastric pain, dysphagia
Hematologic: hemolytic anemia, hypoprothrombinemia, acute hemolysis, thrombocytopenic purpura, agranulocytosis
Hepatic: hepatotoxicity
Metabolic: hypothermia, **hypoglycemia**
Respiratory: asthma
Skin: rash, pruritus, photosensitivity, flushing, diaphoresis
Other: cinchonism, facial edema, hypersensitivity reactions including fever and **hemolytic uremic syndrome**

Interactions

Drug-drug. *Aluminum-containing antacids:* delayed or decreased quinine absorption
Cimetidine: decreased metabolism and increased effects of quinine
Digoxin: increased digoxin blood level
Mefloquine: increased risk of seizures, ECG abnormalities, and cardiac arrest
Neuromuscular blockers: increased effects of these drugs, leading to respiratory difficulty
Rifabutin, rifampin: increased metabolism and decreased effects of quinine
Succinylcholine: delayed succinylcholine metabolism
Urinary alkalizers (such as acetazolamide, sodium bicarbonate): increased quinine blood level and risk of toxicity
Warfarin: increased warfarin effects, increased risk of bleeding
Drug-diagnostic tests. *Urinary 17-ketogenic steroids:* elevated levels

Patient monitoring

Monitor for signs and symptoms of hypersensitivity reaction, including fever and hemolytic uremic syndrome.

q

• Stay alert for signs and symptoms of cinchonism, including tinnitus, headache, nausea, and visual disturbances.
• Assess for bleeding tendency and hepatotoxicity.
• Monitor CBC, liver function tests, and quinine and glucose levels.
• Monitor patient for recumbency leg cramps. After several nights without such cramps, drug may be withdrawn.

Patient teaching

• Tell patient he may take with or without food.
Clinical alert: Teach patient to recognize and immediately report signs and symptoms of cinchonism and hepatotoxicity.
• Instruct patient to report unusual bleeding or bruising.
• Tell female patient to discuss pregnancy or breastfeeding with prescriber before taking drug.
• As appropriate, review all other significant and life-threatening adverse reactions and interactions, especially those related to the drugs and tests mentioned above.

quinupristin and dalfopristin

Synercid

Pharmacologic class: Streptogramin
Therapeutic class: Anti-infective
Pregnancy risk category B

Action

Synergistic effects of drug combination interfere with bacterial cell-wall synthesis by disrupting DNA and RNA transcription

Availability

Injection: 500 mg/10 ml (150 mg quinupristin, 350 mg dalfopristin), 600 mg/10 ml (180 mg quinupristin, 420 mg dalfopristin)

Indications and dosages

➢ Serious or life-threatening infections caused by vancomycin-resistant *Enterococcus faecium*
Adults and adolescents ages 16 and older: 7.5 mg/kg by I.V. infusion over 1 hour q 8 hours
➢ Complicated skin and skin-structure infections caused by *Staphylococcus aureus* (methicillin-susceptible) or *Streptococcus pyogenes*
Adults and adolescents ages 16 and older: 7.5 mg/kg by I.V. infusion over 1 hour q 12 hours for at least 7 days

Dosage adjustment

• Hepatic impairment

Contraindications

• Hypersensitivity to drug or other streptogramins

Precautions

Use cautiously in:
• hepatic impairment
• breastfeeding patients
• children younger than age 16 (safety and efficacy not established).

Administration

Clinical alert: Don't mix with other drugs or saline solution.
• For intermittent infusion through a common I.V. line, flush line with dextrose 5% in water (D_5W) before and after giving drug.
• Add 5 ml of sterile water or D_5W to powdered drug in vial, and swirl gently by hand until powder dissolves; don't shake vial. Solution should be clear.
• Within 30 minutes of first dilution, draw up prescribed dosage and dilute further in D_5W to a final concentration of 2 mg/ml or less.
• Know that if patient has a central venous catheter and is fluid-restricted, drug may be given in 100 ml of D_5W.

• Administer by infusion pump over 60 minutes.
• If significant peripheral vein irritation occurs, dilute in 500 to 750 ml of D_5W.
• Be aware that duration of therapy depends on infection site and severity.

Route	Onset	Peak	Duration
I.V.	Unknown	Unknown	Unknown

Adverse reactions
CNS: headache
CV: thrombophlebitis
GI: nausea, vomiting, diarrhea
Musculoskeletal: joint pain, myalgia
Skin: rash, pruritus
Other: inflammation, pain, or edema at infusion site

Interactions
Drug-drug. *Drugs metabolized by CYP450-3A4 (antiretrovirals; antineoplastics, such as vinca alkaloids, docetaxel, and paclitaxel; astemizole; benzodiazepines; calcium channel blockers; carbamazepine; cisapride; corticosteroids; disopyramide; HMG-CoA reductase inhibitors; immunosuppressants such as cyclosporine and tacrolimus; lidocaine; quinidine; terfenadine):* increased therapeutic and adverse effects of these drugs
Drug-diagnostic tests. *Alanine aminotransferase, aspartate aminotransferase, bilirubin:* increased levels

Patient monitoring
• Monitor closely for infusion site reactions and thrombophlebitis. If these problems occur, consider increasing infusion volume, changing infusion site, or infusing through peripherally inserted central catheter or central venous catheter.
• Assess weight and fluid intake and output to help detect edema.
• Monitor bilirubin level.

Patient teaching
Instruct patient to immediately report pain or redness at infusion site.
• Tell patient to report muscle aches and pains.
• As appropriate, review all other significant and life-threatening adverse reactions and interactions, especially those related to the drugs and tests mentioned above.

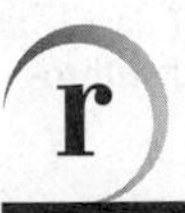

rabeprazole sodium
AcipHex

Pharmacologic class: Proton pump inhibitor
Therapeutic class: Gastric antisecretory agent
Pregnancy risk category B

Action
Reduces gastric acid secretion and increases gastric mucus and bicarbonate production, creating a protective coating on gastric mucosa

Availability
Tablets (delayed-release): 20 mg

Indications and dosages
➢ Erosive or ulcerative gastroesophageal reflux disease (GERD)
Adults: 20 mg P.O. daily for 4 to 8 weeks. If healing doesn't occur within 8 weeks, another 8 weeks of therapy may be considered. Maintenance dosage is 20 mg P.O. daily.
➢ GERD
Adults: 20 mg P.O. daily for 4 weeks. If symptoms don't resolve after 4 weeks,

r

another course of therapy may be considered.

➢ Hypersecretory conditions, including Zollinger-Ellison syndrome

Adults: Initially, 60 mg P.O. daily; adjust dosage as needed up to 100 mg P.O. daily as a single dose or 60 mg P.O. b.i.d. Maximum daily dosage is 120 mg.

➢ Duodenal ulcer

Adults: 20 mg P.O. daily for up to 4 weeks

➢ *Helicobacter pylori* eradication

Adults: 20 mg P.O. b.i.d. for 7 days (given with amoxicillin and clarithromycin)

Off-label uses

- Dyspepsia
- Benign gastric ulcer

Contraindications

- Hypersensitivity to drug, its components, or benzimidazoles

Precautions

Use cautiously in:

- severe hepatic impairment
- pregnant patients
- breastfeeding patients (not recommended)
- children (safety not established).

Administration

- Don't crush or split tablets.
- Give without regard to food.

Route	Onset	Peak	Duration
P.O.	Within 1 hr	Unknown	24 hr

Adverse reactions

CNS: headache

Interactions

Drug-drug. *Gastric pH–dependent drugs (such as digoxin, ketoconazole):* increased or decreased absorption

Warfarin: increased risk of bleeding

Patient monitoring

- Stay alert for symptomatic response, but know that a positive response doesn't rule out gastric cancer.

Patient teaching

- Tell patient he may take with or without food. Instruct him not to crush, chew, or split tablets.
- Caution female patient not to breastfeed during therapy.
- As appropriate, review all significant adverse reactions and interactions, especially those related to the drugs mentioned above.

raloxifene

Evista

Pharmacologic class: Nonsteroidal benzothiophene derivative

Therapeutic class: Selective estrogen receptor modulator, bone resorption inhibitor

Pregnancy risk category X

Action

Binds to estrogen receptors, activating estrogen pathways and increasing bone mineral density. These effects decrease bone resorption and turnover.

Availability

Tablets: 60 mg

Indications and dosages

➢ Osteoporosis in postmenopausal women

Adults: 60 mg P.O. daily

Off-label uses

- Prophylaxis of cardiovascular disease

Contraindications

- Hypersensitivity to drug or its components

- History of thromboembolic events
- Premenopausal women
- Females of childbearing age
- Pregnancy or breastfeeding
- Children

Precautions

Use cautiously in:

- altered lipid metabolism, hepatic dysfunction
- concurrent estrogen therapy (use not recommended)
- immobilized patients and others at increased risk for thromboembolic events.

Administration

- Give with or without food.

Route	Onset	Peak	Duration
P.O.	Unknown	6 hr	Unknown

Adverse reactions

CNS: depression, insomnia, vertigo, syncope, hypoesthesia, migraine, neuralgia
CV: chest pain, peripheral edema, varicose veins, **deep-vein thrombosis, thrombophlebitis**
EENT: conjunctivitis, sinusitis, rhinitis, pharyngitis, laryngitis
GI: nausea, vomiting, diarrhea, abdominal pain dyspepsia, flatulence, gastroenteritis
GU: urinary tract infection or disorder, cystitis, vaginitis, leukorrhea, endometrial disorder, **vaginal hemorrhage**
Musculoskeletal: leg cramps, joint pain, myalgia, arthritis, tendon disorder
Respiratory: cough, pneumonia, bronchitis, **pulmonary embolism**
Skin: rash, diaphoresis
Other: weight gain, hot flashes, infection, pain, flulike symptoms

Interactions

Drug-drug. *Cholestyramine:* reduced raloxifene absorption
Highly protein-bound drugs (such as diazepam, diazoxide, lidocaine): interference with binding of these drugs
Warfarin: decreased prothrombin time
Drug-diagnostic tests. *Albumin, apolipoprotein B, calcium, fibrinogen, inorganic phosphate, low-density lipoproteins, platelets, protein, total cholesterol:* decreased levels
Apolipoprotein A1; corticosteroid-binding, sex steroid–binding, and thyroid-binding globulin: increased levels

Patient monitoring

Watch for thromboembolic events, especially during first 4 months of therapy.

- Stay alert for other adverse effects, particularly leg cramps, other musculoskeletal complaints, and respiratory disorders.
- Assess bone mineral density test results.
- Monitor for unexplained vaginal bleeding.

Patient teaching

- Tell patient she may take with or without food.
- Instruct patient to read package insert before starting drug and then periodically.

Teach patient to recognize and immediately report symptoms of blood clots.

- Instruct patient to stop taking drug 3 days before anticipated period of prolonged immobility, and to restart it only after she regains normal mobility.
- Tell patient that drug may cause hot flashes, but that these are normal effects.
- Advise patient to report unexplained vaginal bleeding or leg cramps.
- As appropriate, review all other significant and life-threatening adverse reactions and interactions, especially those related to the drugs and tests mentioned above.

ramipril

Altace

Pharmacologic class: Angiotensin-converting enzyme (ACE) inhibitor

Therapeutic class: Antihypertensive

Pregnancy risk category C (first trimester), ***D*** (second and third trimesters)

Action

Inhibits conversion of angiotensin I to angiotensin II, a potent vasoconstrictor. Increases plasma renin levels and reduces aldosterone levels, causing systemic vasodilation and decreased cardiac output.

Availability

Capsules: 1.25 mg, 2.5 mg, 5 mg, 10 mg

Indications and dosages

➣ Hypertension

Adults: Initially, 2.5 mg P.O. daily in patients not receiving diuretics; may increase dosage slowly p.r.n. according to response. For maintenance, 2.5 to 20 mg/day P.O. as a single dose or in two equally divided doses. If ramipril alone doesn't control blood pressure, a diuretic may be added.

➣ To reduce the risk of myocardial infarction (MI), cerebrovascular accident, or death from cardiovascular causes

Adults: Initially, 2.5 mg P.O. daily for 1 week, followed by 5 mg P.O. daily for the next 3 weeks, then increased as tolerated to a maintenance dosage of 10 mg P.O. daily. In hypertensive patients and those who've had a recent MI, may divide maintenance dose.

➣ Heart failure after MI

Adults: Initially, 2.5 mg P.O. b.i.d.; may decrease to 1.25 mg b.i.d. if higher dosage causes hypotension. Titrate toward target dosage of 5 mg b.i.d. at 3-week intervals.

Dosage adjustment

- Renal impairment
- Concurrent diuretic use

Off-label uses

- Angina associated with syndrome X
- Atherosclerosis
- Mitral insufficiency
- Renovascular hypertension
- Diabetic or nondiabetic nephropathy
- Erythrocytosis

Contraindications

- Hypersensitivity to drug or other ACE inhibitors
- Angioedema with previous ACE inhibitor use
- Pregnancy (second and third trimesters)

Precautions

Use cautiously in:

- autoimmune diseases, aortic stenosis, hypertrophic cardiomyopathy, cerebrovascular or cardiac insufficiency, collagen vascular disease, febrile illness, hepatic or renal impairment, hypotension, neutropenia, chronic cough, proteinuria, renal artery stenosis
- family history of angioedema
- concurrent immunosuppressant or diuretic therapy
- black patients
- elderly patients
- pregnant (first trimester) or breast-feeding patients
- children (safety not established).

Administration

- If possible, discontinue diuretics 2 to 3 days before ramipril therapy begins to prevent severe hypotension.
- If patient can't swallow capsule, open it and mix contents in water or apple juice or sprinkle in small amount of applesauce.

• Know that drug may be used alone or with other antihypertensives.

Route	Onset	Peak	Duration
P.O.	1-2 hr	2-4 hr	24 hr

Adverse reactions

CNS: dizziness, light-headedness, fatigue, headache, vertigo, asthenia
CV: hypotension, orthostatic hypotension, angina pectoris, tachycardia, **MI, heart failure**
EENT: blurred vision, sinusitis
GI: nausea, vomiting, diarrhea
Hematologic: purpura, **agranulocytosis**
Metabolic: hyperkalemia
Musculoskeletal: muscle cramps
Respiratory: cough, asthma, upper respiratory tract infection, **bronchospasm**
Skin: rash, pruritus, urticaria, photosensitivity, **angioedema, anaphylactoid reactions**
Other: fever

Interactions

Drug-drug. *Allopurinol:* increased risk of hypersensitivity reaction
Antacids: decreased ramipril absorption
Digoxin, lithium: increased blood levels and risk of toxicity from these drugs
Diuretics, other antihypertensives: increased hypotension
Indomethacin: reduced hypotensive effect of ramipril
Phenothiazines: increased pharmacologic effects of ramipril
Potassium-sparing diuretics, potassium supplements: increased risk of hyperkalemia
Tetracyclines: decreased tetracycline absorption
Drug-diagnostic tests. *Alanine aminotransferase, alkaline phosphatase, aspartate aminotransferase, bilirubin, blood urea nitrogen, creatinine, potassium:* increased levels
Drug-food. *Any food:* decreased rate (but not extent) of drug absorption
Salt substitutes containing potassium: increased risk of hyperkalemia
Drug-herbs. *Capsaicin:* increased incidence of cough
Ephedra (ma huang): decreased drug efficacy, exacerbation of hypertension
Yohimbe: interference with drug's antihypertensive effect
Drug-behaviors. *Alcohol use:* increased hypotension

Patient monitoring

• Assess vital signs and cardiovascular status. Ask patient if he's experiencing angina.
• Monitor CBC and liver function tests.
• Closely monitor potassium level. Watch for signs and symptoms of hyperkalemia.
🔊 Stay alert for signs and symptoms of hypersensitivity reactions (including angioedema), especially in black patients after first dose
• Evaluate for dry, nonproductive cough.

Patient teaching

• Tell patient he may take with or without food.
🔊 Instruct patient to immediately report swelling of tongue or face or difficulty breathing.
• Teach patient how to monitor and record blood pressure.
• Tell patient drug may cause dry, nonproductive cough. Instruct him to report this problem if it becomes bothersome.
• Caution patient to avoid driving and other hazardous activities until he knows how drug affects concentration and alertness.
• Advise patient to move slowly when sitting up or standing, to avoid dizziness from sudden blood pressure decrease.

r

• Inform patient that excessive fluid loss (as from sweating, vomiting, or diarrhea) and inadequate fluid intake increase risk of light-headedness (especially in hot weather).
• Tell patient to avoid salt substitutes containing potassium and herbs.
• Advise female patient to tell prescriber if she is pregnant. Caution her not to take drug during third trimester or when breastfeeding.
• As appropriate, review all other significant and life-threatening adverse reactions and interactions, especially those related to the drugs, tests, foods, herbs, and behaviors mentioned above.

ranitidine hydrochloride

Apo-Ranitidine✦, Zantac, Zantac 75, Zantac EFFERdose

Pharmacologic class: Histamine$_2$-receptor antagonist
Therapeutic class: Antiulcer drug
Pregnancy risk category B

Action

Reduces gastric acid secretion and increases gastric mucus and bicarbonate production, creating a protective coating on gastric mucosa

Availability

Capsules (liquid-filled): 150 mg, 300 mg
Solution for injection: 25 mg/ml in 2-, 6-, and 40-ml vials
Solution for injection (pre-mixed): 50 mg/50 ml in 0.45% sodium chloride
Syrup: 15 mg/ml
Tablets: 150 mg, 300 mg
Tablets (effervescent): 150 mg

Indications and dosages

➢ Active duodenal ulcer
Adults: 150 mg or 10 ml P.O. b.i.d., or 300 mg or 20 ml P.O. daily, or 50 mg I.V. or I.M. q 6 to 8 hours
➢ To maintain healing of duodenal ulcers
Adults: 150 mg or 10 ml P.O.
➢ Benign gastric ulcer
Adults: 150 mg or 10 ml P.O. b.i.d. For maintenance, 150 mg or 10 ml P.O. or 50 mg I.V. or I.M. q 6 to 8 hours.
➢ Active duodenal and gastric ulcers
Children ages 1 month to 16 years: 2 to 4 mg/kg/day P.O., up to a maximum of 300 mg/day
➢ To maintain healing of duodenal and gastric ulcers
Children ages 1 month to 16 years: 2 to 4 mg/kg/day P.O., up to a maximum of 150 mg/day
➢ Erosive esophagitis
Adults: 150 mg or 10 ml P.O. q.i.d.
Children ages 1 month to 16 years: 5 to 10 mg/kg P.O. daily in two divided doses
➢ Gastroesophageal reflux disease
Adults: 150 mg or 10 ml P.O. b.i.d.
Children ages 1 month to 16 years: 5 to 10 mg/kg P.O. daily in two divided doses
➢ Pathologic hypersecretory conditions, including Zollinger-Ellison syndrome
Adults: 150 mg or 10 ml P.O. b.i.d., adjusted according to patient's needs. In severe cases, up to 6 g/day may be needed. Continue therapy as long as indicated.
➢ Hospitalized patients with pathologic hypersecretory conditions, including Zollinger-Ellison syndrome; intractable duodenal ulcers; patients who can't receive oral drugs
Adults: 50 mg I.M. q 6 to 8 hours, or 50 mg intermittent I.V. bolus q 6 to 8 hours, or 50 mg intermittent I.V. infusion q 6 to 8 hours.
Children ages 1 month to 16 years: 2 to 4 mg/kg/day I.V. in divided doses q 6 to 8 hours, up to a maximum of 50 mg q 6 to 8 hours

Dosage adjustment
- Renal or hepatic impairment
- Debilitated patients

Off-label uses
- Asthma
- GI hemorrhage
- *Helicobacter pylori* infection
- Short-bowel syndrome
- Immunosuppression reversal
- Psoriasis
- Aspiration pneumonitis prophylaxis

Contraindications
- Hypersensitivity to drug or its components
- Alcohol intolerance (with some oral products)
- History of acute porphyria

Precautions
Use cautiously in:
- renal or hepatic impairment, heart rhythm disturbances, phenylketonuria (effervescent tablets)
- elderly patients
- pregnant or breastfeeding patients.

Administration
- For intermittent I.V. bolus injection, dilute in normal saline solution or other compatible solution to a concentration not exceeding 2.5 mg/ml. Inject no faster than 4 ml/minute (5 minutes).
- For continuous I.V. infusion in patients with Zollinger-Ellison syndrome, add to dextrose 5% in water (D_5W) or other compatible solution; dilute to a concentration not exceeding 2.5 mg/ml, and start infusion at 1 mg/kg/hour. After 4 hours, if measured gastric acid output exceeds 10 mEq/hour or symptoms occur, increase dosage in increments of 0.5 mg/kg/hour, and remeasure acid output.
- Give P.O. doses with or without food. Give once-daily dose at bedtime.
- For intermittent I.V. infusion, dilute in D_5W or other compatible solution to a concentration not exceeding 0.5 mg/ml. Infuse no faster than 7 ml/minute (15 to 20 minutes).
- Be aware that premixed Zantac solution of 50 mg in half-normal saline solution (50 ml) doesn't require dilution. Infuse over 15 to 20 minutes.
- Know that I.V. form may be added to total parenteral nutrition solutions.
- Inject I.M. undiluted deep into large muscle.

Route	Onset	Peak	Duration
P.O.	Unknown	1-3 hr	8-12 hr
I.V., I.M.	Unknown	15 min	8-12 hr

Adverse reactions
CNS: headache, agitation, anxiety
GI: nausea, vomiting, diarrhea, constipation, abdominal discomfort or pain
Hematologic: reversible **granulocytopenia** and **thrombocytopenia**
Hepatic: hepatitis
Skin: rash
Other: pain at I.M. injection site, burning or itching at I.V. site, hypersensitivity reaction

Interactions
Drug-drug. *Antacids:* decreased ranitidine absorption
Propantheline: delayed ranitidine absorption and increased peak blood level
Drug-diagnostic tests. *Creatinine:* slight elevation
Hepatic enzymes: increased levels
Urine protein tests using Multistix: false-negative results
Drug-herbs. *Yerba maté:* decreased drug clearance
Drug-behaviors. *Smoking:* decreased ranitidine effects

Patient monitoring
- Assess vital signs.
- Monitor CBC and liver function tests.

Patient teaching
- Tell patient he may take oral drug with or without food. Advise him to

r

take once-daily prescription drug at bedtime.
- Instruct patient to dissolve EFFER-dose in 6 to 8 oz of water before taking.
- Caution patient to avoid driving and other hazardous activities until he knows how drug affects concentration and alertness.
- Tell patient smoking may decrease drug effects.
- As appropriate, review all other significant and life-threatening adverse reactions and interactions, especially those related to the drugs, tests, herbs, and behaviors mentioned above.

rasburicase

Elitek

Pharmacologic class: Recombinant urate oxidase enzyme

Therapeutic class: Antimetabolite

Pregnancy risk category C

Action

Catalyzes oxidation of uric acid into an inactive soluble metabolite

Availability

Powder for injection: 1.5 mg/vial

Indications and dosages

➤ Chemotherapy-induced hyperuricemia in children with leukemia, lymphoma, or solid-tumor cancers

Children: 0.15 to 0.2 mg/kg by I.V. infusion over 30 minutes as a single daily dose for 5 days. Chemotherapy should begin 4 to 24 hours after first dose.

Off-label uses

- Chemotherapy-induced hyperuricemia in adults with leukemia, lymphoma, or solid-tumor cancers

Contraindications

- Hypersensitivity to drug or its components
- History of anaphylaxis, hemolytic anemia, or methemoglobinemia as a reaction to rasburicase
- G6PD deficiency

Precautions

Use cautiously in:
- pregnant or breastfeeding patients
- children younger than age 2.

Administration

- Know that patients at high risk for G6PD deficiency (those of African or Mediterranean descent) should be screened for this disorder before therapy starts.
- Give 4 to 24 hours before first chemotherapy dose, as ordered.
- Dilute by adding 1-ml vial of diluent provided. Swirl gently; don't shake. Dilute further by injecting diluted dose into infusion bag containing appropriate volume of normal saline solution, to achieve final volume of 50 ml.
- Administer daily by I.V. infusion over 30 minutes.

Don't give as I.V. bolus.
- Don't use I.V. filters.
- Don't mix with other drugs. Use a separate I.V. line, or flush line with 15 ml of normal saline solution before and after infusing rasburicase.
- Know that more than one course of treatment isn't recommended.

Route	Onset	Peak	Duration
I.V.	4 hr	96 hr	Unknown

Adverse reactions

CNS: headache

GI: nausea, vomiting, diarrhea, constipation, abdominal pain

Hematologic: neutropenia, methemoglobinemia, severe hemolysis (in patients with G6PD deficiency)

Respiratory: respiratory distress

Skin: rash

Other: fever, mucositis, hypersensitivity reactions including **anaphylaxis, sepsis**

Interactions

Drug-diagnostic tests. *Neutrophils:* decreased count
Uric acid: interference with measurement (if blood is at room temperature)

Patient monitoring

- Monitor for signs and symptoms of hypersensitivity reaction.
- Assess for respiratory distress and signs and symptoms of infection.
- Monitor CBC and uric acid level frequently.

Watch closely for signs and symptoms of hemolysis, especially in patients of African or Mediterranean descent.

Patient teaching

Teach parents and patient (as appropriate) to recognize and immediately report adverse effects, including hypersensitivity reaction.

Tell parents drug may cause sepsis. Instruct them to monitor child's temperature and immediately report fever and other signs and symptoms of infection.

- As appropriate, review all other significant and life-threatening adverse reactions and interactions, especially those related to the tests mentioned above.

repaglinide

Prandin

Pharmacologic class: Meglitinide
Therapeutic class: Hypoglycemic
Pregnancy risk category C

Action

Inhibits alpha-glucosidases, enzymes that convert oligosaccharides and disaccharides to glucose. This inhibition lowers blood glucose level, especially in postprandial hyperglycemia.

Availability

Tablets: 0.5 mg, 1 mg, 2 mg

Indications and dosages

➤ Adjunct to diet and exercise in type 2 (non-insulin-dependent) diabetes mellitus uncontrolled by diet and exercise alone, or combined with metformin in type 2 diabetes mellitus uncontrolled by diet, exercise, and either repaglinide or metformin alone
Adults: 0.5 to 4 mg P.O. before each meal; may adjust at 1-week intervals based on blood glucose response. Maximum daily dosage is 16 mg.

Contraindications

- Hypersensitivity to drug or its components
- Diabetic ketoacidosis
- Type 1 (insulin-dependent) diabetes mellitus

Precautions

Use cautiously in:
- renal or hepatic impairment; adrenal or pituitary insufficiency; stress caused by infection, fever, trauma, or surgery
- elderly or malnourished patients
- pregnant or breastfeeding patients
- children.

Administration

- Give 15 to 30 minutes before meals. Administer two, three, or four times daily, if needed, to adapt to patient's meal pattern.

Route	Onset	Peak	Duration
P.O.	Within 30 min	60-90 min	<4 hr

Adverse reactions

CNS: headache, paresthesia
CV: angina, chest pain
EENT: sinusitis, rhinitis

r

GI: nausea, vomiting, diarrhea, constipation, dyspepsia
GU: urinary tract infection
Metabolic: hyperglycemia, **hypoglycemia**
Musculoskeletal: joint pain, back pain
Respiratory: upper respiratory infection, bronchitis
Other: tooth disorder, hypersensitivity reaction

Interactions

Drug-drug. *Barbiturates, carbamazepine, rifampin:* decreased repaglinide blood level
Beta-adrenergic blockers, chloramphenicol, MAO inhibitors, nonsteroidal anti-inflammatory drugs, probenecid, sulfonamides, warfarin: potentiation of repaglinide effects
Calcium channel blockers, corticosteroids, estrogens, hormonal contraceptives, isoniazid, phenothiazines, phenytoin, nicotinic acid, sympathomimetics, thyroid preparations: loss of glycemic control
Erythromycin, ketoconazole, miconazole: decreased repaglinide metabolism, increased risk of hypoglycemia
Drug-food. *Any food:* decreased drug bioavailability
Drug-herbs. *Aloe gel (oral), bitter melon, chromium, coenzyme Q10, fenugreek, gymnema sylvestre, psyllium, St. John's wort:* additive hypoglycemic effects
Glucosamine: poor glycemic control

Patient monitoring

- Monitor blood glucose and glycosylated hemoglobin levels.
- Monitor patient's meal pattern. Consult prescriber about adjusting dosage if patient adds or misses a meal.
- Assess for angina, shortness of breath, or other discomforts.
- Watch for signs and symptoms of bronchitis and upper respiratory, urinary, and EENT infections.

Patient teaching

- Tell patient to take 15 to 30 minutes before each meal.
- Instruct patient to monitor blood glucose level carefully. Teach him to recognize signs and symptoms of hypoglycemia and hyperglycemia.
- Advise patient to report signs and symptoms of infection.
- As appropriate, review all other significant and life-threatening adverse reactions and interactions, especially those related to the drugs, foods, and herbs mentioned above.

reteplase, recombinant

Retavase

Pharmacologic class: Tissue plasminogen activator
Therapeutic class: Thrombolytic enzyme
Pregnancy risk category C

Action

Converts plasminogen to plasmin, which in turn breaks down fibrin and fibrinogen, thereby dissolving thrombus

Availability

Injection: Retivase Half-Kit—one vial of 10.4 units (18.1 mg)/vial; Retavase Kit—two vials of 10.4 units (18.1 mg)/vial

Indications and dosages

➢ Acute myocardial infarction
Adults: 10 units by I.V. bolus over 2 minutes, repeated in 30 minutes

Off-label uses

- Pulmonary embolism

Contraindications

- Hypersensitivity to drug or alteplase

- Active internal bleeding
- Bleeding diathesis
- Recent intracranial or intraspinal surgery or trauma
- Intracranial neoplasm
- Arteriovenous malformation or aneurysm
- Severe uncontrolled hypertension
- History of cerebrovascular accident

Precautions

Use cautiously in:

- previous puncture of noncompressible vessels, major surgery, obstetric delivery, organ biopsy, trauma, hypertension, conditions that may cause left-sided heart thrombus (including mitral stenosis), acute pericarditis, subacute bacterial endocarditis, hemostatic defects, diabetic hemorrhagic retinopathy, cerebrovascular disease, severe hepatic or renal dysfunction, septic thrombophlebitis or occluded AV cannula at a seriously infected site, other conditions in which bleeding poses a significant hazard
- concurrent use of oral anticoagulants (such as warfarin)
- patients older than age 75
- pregnant or breastfeeding patients.

Administration

◀⁝ If patient shows signs or symptoms of bleeding or anaphylaxis after first bolus dose, withhold second bolus and contact prescriber immediately.

- Use only diluent supplied (preservative-free sterile water for injection) to reconstitute drug into colorless solution of 1 unit/ml.
- If drug foams, let it sit until foam subsides.
- Don't use solution if it is discolored or contains visible precipitates.
- Don't give with other drugs in same I.V. line. Know that drug is incompatible with heparin.

Route	Onset	Peak	Duration
I.V.	Immediate	End of infusion	Variable

Adverse reactions

CNS: intracranial hemorrhage
CV: arrhythmias, hemorrhage
GI: nausea, vomiting, **GI bleeding**
GU: hematuria
Hematologic: anemia, **bleeding tendency**
Other: fever, bleeding at puncture sites

Interactions

Drug-drug. *Anticoagulants, indomethacin, phenylbutazone, platelet aggregation inhibitors (such as abciximab, aspirin, dipyridamole):* increased risk of bleeding

Drug-diagnostic tests. *Hemoglobin:* decreased level

International Normalized Ratio, partial thromboplastin time, prothrombin time: increased

Drug-herbs. *Ginkgo, many other herbs:* increased risk of bleeding

Patient monitoring

◀⁝ Check closely for signs and symptoms of bleeding in all body systems. Monitor coagulation studies and CBC.

- Monitor ECG for arrhythmias caused by coronary thrombolysis.
- Assess neurologic status to detect early signs and symptoms of intracranial hemorrhage.

Patient teaching

- Teach patient about drug's anticoagulant effect. Review safety measures to avoid injury, which can cause uncontrolled bleeding.

◀⁝ Instruct patient to immediately report signs and symptoms of bleeding problems.

- Tell patient he'll undergo frequent blood testing during therapy.

r

ribavirin

Copegus, Rebetol, Ribasphere, Virazole

Pharmacologic class: Synthetic nucleoside analog
Therapeutic class: Antiviral
Pregnancy risk category X

Action

Unknown. Thought to inhibit RNA and DNA synthesis by depleting nucleotides and blocking replication and maturation of viral cells.

Availability

Capsules: 200 mg
Powder to be reconstituted for inhalation (Virazole): 6 g in 100-ml glass vial
Tablets: 200 mg

Indications and dosages

➢ Chronic hepatitis C infection
Note: Dosage calculated solely on basis of patient's weight.
Adults and children weighing 75 kg (165 lb) or more: 600 mg P.O. q morning and evening, given with interferon alfa-2b
Adults weighing less than 75 kg (165 lb) and children weighing more than 61 kg (134 lb): 400 mg P.O. q morning and 600 mg P.O. q evening, given with interferon alfa-2b
Children weighing 50 to 61 kg (110 to 134 lb): 400 mg P.O. b.i.d., given with interferon alfa-2b
Children weighing 37 to 49 kg (81 to 108 lb): 200 mg P.O. every morning and 400 mg P.O. every evening, given with interferon alfa-2b
Children weighing 25 to 36 kg (55 to 79 lb) : 200 mg P.O. b.i.d., given with interferon alfa-2b

➢ Hospitalized children with severe lower respiratory infection caused by respiratory syncytial virus
Infants and young children: 20 mg/ml by inhalation as a starting solution in Viratek Small Particle Aerosol Generator (SPAG-2) for 12 to 18 hours daily for 3 to 7 days. Give by oxygen hood from SPAG-2 unit to infant who isn't mechanically ventilated.

Dosage adjustment

- Cardiovascular disease
- Chronic obstructive pulmonary disease (COPD)
- Renal impairment
- Hemoglobin below 10 g/dl

Off-label uses

- Influenza A or B
- Pneumonia caused by adenovirus
- Severe lower respiratory tract infection in adults
- Genital herpes
- Hemorrhagic fever

Contraindications

- Hypersensitivity to drug or its components
- Autoimmune hepatitis (oral combination therapy)
- Creatinine clearance below 50 ml/minute
- Significant or unstable cardiac disease
- Hemoglobinopathy (such as sickle cell anemia, thalassemia major)
- Females of childbearing age (inhalation form)
- Pregnancy, pregnant partner of male patient (oral drug)
- Breastfeeding

Precautions

Use cautiously in:
- decompensated hepatic disease, coinfection with hepatitis B or human immunodeficiency virus, COPD

- liver or other transplant recipients
- patients who don't respond to interferon.

Administration

Be aware that oral form must be given with interferon alfa-2b injection.

- Give aerosol by Viratek SPAG-2 only. Don't use other aerosol-generating equipment.
- Dilute powder in sterile water for injection. Don't use solutions with antimicrobial ingredients.
- Know that drug may be given by oral or nasal inhalation.
- Discard solution in SPAG-2 every 24 hours before adding new solution.

Avoid prolonged contact with aerosol, which can cause headache or eye irritation.

Route	Onset	Peak	Duration
Oral	Unknown	Unknown	Unknown
Inhalation	Slow	60-90 min	Unknown

Adverse reactions

CNS: fatigue, headache, nervousness, depression, **suicidal ideation**
CV: hypotension, bradycardia (with inhalation form), **cardiac arrest**
EENT: conjunctivitis, eyelid erythema or rash
GI: nausea, dyspepsia, anorexia, **pancreatitis**
Hematologic: reticulocytosis, hemolytic anemia
Respiratory: bacterial pneumonia, pneumothorax, bronchospasm, pulmonary edema, apnea, worsening respiratory status (with inhalation form)
Skin: rash, pruritus

Interactions

Drug-drug. *Abacavir, didanosine, lamivudine, stavudine, zalcitabine, zidovudine:* potentially fatal lactic acidosis
Stavudine, zidovudine: decreased antiviral activity
Drug-diagnostic tests. *Alanine aminotransferase, aspartate aminotransferase, bilirubin:* increased levels
Hemoglobin: decreased level
Reticulocytes: increased count

Patient monitoring

Carefully monitor patient's respiratory status. Check ventilator often to ensure that drug precipitates don't impede function.

Monitor ECG and vital signs. Watch for hypotension, bradycardia, and other signs of impending cardiac arrest or worsening respiratory condition.

Assess neurologic status. Stay alert for depression and suicidal ideation.

- Monitor liver function tests and CBC with white cell differential.

Patient teaching

- Explain drug delivery system and precautions carefully to patient or to parents of children receiving inhalation form.

Tell patient or parents that drug may cause depression or suicidal thoughts, which should be reported immediately.

Instruct patient or parents to immediately report new or worsening respiratory symptoms.

- Counsel sexually active patients (both males and females) about appropriate birth control. Tell them to use extreme care to avoid pregnancy. Stress importance of using two forms of effective contraception during and for 6 months after treatment (when using oral ribavirin).
- Advise female patient not to breastfeed.
- As appropriate, review all other significant and life-threatening adverse reactions and interactions, especially those related to the drugs and tests mentioned above.

r

rifabutin

Mycobutin

Pharmacologic class: Rifamycin derivative
Therapeutic class: Antimycobacterial
Pregnancy risk category B

Action

Inhibits RNA synthesis by blocking RNA transcription in susceptible organisms (mycobacteria and some gram-positive and gram-negative bacteria)

Availability

Capsules: 150 mg

Indications and dosages

➢ To prevent disseminated *Mycobacterium avium intracellulare* complex in patients with advanced human immunodeficiency virus (HIV) infection
Adults: 300 mg P.O. daily as a single dose or in two divided doses

Off-label uses

- Tuberculosis
- Prophylaxis and treatment of *M. avium intracellulare* in children

Contraindications

- Hypersensitivity to drug
- Active tuberculosis

Precautions

Use cautiously in:
- severe hepatic disease
- pregnant or breastfeeding patients.

Administration

- Give in divided doses twice daily with food to reduce GI upset.

Route	Onset	Peak	Duration
P.O.	Unknown	2-3 hr	>24 hr

Adverse reactions

CNS: headache, asthenia, weakness
CV: pressure sensation in chest
EENT: uveitis; discolored tears, saliva, or sputum
GI: nausea, vomiting, diarrhea, dyspepsia, abdominal pain, eructation, flatulence, discolored feces, anorexia
GU: discolored urine
Hematologic: eosinophilia, **neutropenia, leukopenia, thrombocytopenia**
Musculoskeletal: joint pain, myalgia
Respiratory: dyspnea
Skin: rash, discolored skin or sweat
Other: abnormal taste, fever, flulike symptoms

Interactions

Drug-drug. *Clarithromycin, itraconazole, saquinavir:* reduced blood levels and efficacy of these drugs
Delavirdine: decreased delavirdine blood level, increased rifabutin blood level
Drugs metabolized by liver (such as zidovudine): altered blood levels of these drugs
Hormonal contraceptives: decreased contraceptive efficacy
Indinavir, nelfinavir, ritonavir: increased rifabutin blood level
Drug-diagnostic tests. *Alanine aminotransferase, aspartate aminotransferase, eosinophils:* increased levels
Neutrophils, platelets, white blood cells: decreased counts
Drug-food. *High-fat foods:* delayed drug absorption

Patient monitoring

- Monitor CBC with white cell differential. Watch for signs and symptoms of blood dyscrasias.
- Assess nutritional status.
- Closely monitor vital signs and temperature. Stay alert for dyspnea and flulike symptoms.

Patient teaching

- Advise patient to take twice daily with food (but not high-fat food) if GI upset occurs. To further minimize GI upset, teach him to eat small, frequent servings of healthy food and drink plenty of fluids.
- Instruct patient to take exactly as prescribed, even after symptoms subside.

🔊 Tell patient to immediately report easy bruising or bleeding.

- Tell patient drug may turn tears, urine, and other body fluids reddish or brownish orange. Instruct him not to wear contact lenses during therapy because drug may stain them permanently.
- Inform patient that drug occasionally causes eye inflammation. Instruct him to report symptoms promptly.
- Caution patient to avoid driving and other hazardous activities until effects of drug are known.
- As appropriate, review all other significant and life-threatening adverse reactions and interactions, especially those related to the drugs, tests, and foods mentioned above.

rifampin (rifampicin)

Rifadin, Rimactane, Rofact✱

Pharmacologic class: Rifamycin derivative

Therapeutic class: Antitubercular

Pregnancy risk category C

Action

Inhibits RNA synthesis by blocking RNA transcription in susceptible organisms (mycobacteria and some gram-positive and gram-negative bacteria)

Availability

Capsules: 150 mg, 300 mg
Powder for injection: 600 mg/vial

Indications and dosages

➢ Tuberculosis

Adults: 10 mg/kg/day (up to 600 mg/day) P.O. or I.V. infusion as a single dose

Children: 10 to 20 mg/kg/day (up to 600 mg/day) P.O. or I.V. infusion as a single dose

➢ Asymptomatic *Neisseria meningitidis* carriers

Adults: 600 mg P.O. or I.V. infusion b.i.d. for 2 days

Children ages 1 month and older: 10 mg/kg/day P.O. or I.V. infusion (up to 600 mg/day) q 12 hours for 2 days

Infants younger than 1 month old: 5 mg/kg P.O. or I.V. infusion q 12 hours for 2 days

Off-label uses

- *Mycobacterium avium intracellulare* complex infection
- Brucellosis
- *Haemophilus influenzae* type B
- Severe staphylococcal bone and joint infections
- Prosthetic valve endocarditis caused by coagulase-negative staphylococci
- Leprosy
- Prophylaxis in high-risk close contacts of patients with *N. meningitidis* infections

Contraindications

- Hypersensitivity to drug or other rifamycin derivatives

Precautions

Use cautiously in:

- porphyria
- history of hepatic disease
- concurrent use of other hepatotoxic drugs
- pregnant or breastfeeding patients.

Administration

- Add 10 ml of sterile water to vial to yield a 60-mg/ml solution for I.V. infusion.

• Further dilute in 100 ml of dextrose 5% in water (D_5W) and infuse over 30 minutes, or add to 500 ml of D_5W and infuse over 3 hours.
• Give oral doses with a full glass of water 1 hour before or 2 hours after a meal.
• For an adult who can't swallow capsules or for a young child, mix capsule contents with syrup, shake well, and administer.
• If patient can't receive dextrose, use normal saline solution to dilute. Don't use other I.V. solutions.

Route	Onset	Peak	Duration
P.O.	Rapid	2-4 hr	12-24 hr
I.V.	Rapid	End of infusion	12-24 hr

Adverse reactions

CNS: ataxia, confusion, drowsiness, fatigue, headache, asthenia, psychosis, generalized numbness
EENT: conjunctivitis; discolored tears, saliva, and sputum
GI: nausea, vomiting, diarrhea, abdominal cramps, dyspepsia, epigastric distress, flatulence, discolored feces, anorexia, sore mouth and tongue, **pseudomembranous colitis**
GU: discolored urine
Hematologic: eosinophilia, transient **leukopenia, hemolytic anemia, hemolysis, disseminated intravascular coagulation** (DIC), **thrombocytopenia**
Hepatic: jaundice
Metabolic: hyperuricemia
Musculoskeletal: myalgia, joint pain
Respiratory: dyspnea, wheezing
Skin: flushing, rash, pruritus, discolored sweat, **erythema multiforme, toxic epidermal necrolysis, Stevens-Johnson syndrome**
Other: flulike symptoms, hypersensitivity reactions including vasculitis

Interactions

Drug-drug. *Barbiturates, beta-adrenergic blockers, cardiac glycosides, clarithromycin, clofibrate, cyclosporine, dapsone, diazepam, doxycycline, fluoroquinolones (such as ciprofloxacin), haloperidol, levothyroxine, methadone, progestins, quinine, tacrolimus, theophylline, tricyclic antidepressants, zidovudine:* increased metabolism of these drugs
Chloramphenicol, corticosteroids, disopyramide, efavirenz, estrogens, fluconazole, hormonal contraceptives, itraconazole, ketoconazole, nevirapine, quinidine, opioid analgesics, oral hypoglycemics, phenytoin, quinidine, ritonavir, theophylline, tocainide, verapamil, warfarin: decreased efficacy of these drugs
Delavirdine, indinavir, nelfinavir, saquinavir: decreased blood levels of these drugs
Hepatotoxic drugs (including isoniazid, ketoconazole, pyrazinamide): increased risk of hepatotoxicity
Drug-diagnostic tests. *Alanine aminotransferase, alkaline phosphatase, aspartate aminotransferase, bilirubin, blood urea nitrogen, uric acid:* increased levels
Dexamethasone suppression test: interference with results
Direct Coombs' test: false-positive result
Folate, vitamin B_{12} assay: interference with standard assays
Hemoglobin: decreased value
Liver function tests: abnormal values (transient)
Sulfobromophthalein uptake and excretion test: delayed hepatic uptake and excretion
Drug-behaviors. *Alcohol use:* increased risk of hepatotoxicity

Patient monitoring

• Monitor kidney and liver function tests, CBC, and uric acid level.
Watch for signs and symptoms of bleeding tendency, especially DIC.
• Assess for signs and symptoms of hepatic impairment.

• Monitor bowel movements for diarrhea, which may signal pseudomembranous colitis.

Patient teaching

• Advise patient to take oral dose 1 hour before or 2 hours after meals. If drug causes significant GI upset, instruct him to take it with meals. To further minimize GI upset, teach him to eat small, frequent servings of food and drink plenty of fluids.

Clinical alert: Instruct patient to immediately report easy bruising or bleeding, fever, malaise, appetite loss, nausea, vomiting, or yellowing of skin or eyes.

• Tell patient drug may color his tears, urine, and other body fluids reddish or brownish orange. Instruct him not to wear contact lenses during therapy, because drug may stain them permanently.

• Instruct patient not to drink alcohol.

• Caution patient to avoid driving and other hazardous activities until he knows how drug affects concentration and alertness.

• As appropriate, review all other significant and life-threatening adverse reactions and interactions, especially those related to the drugs, tests, and behaviors mentioned above.

rifapentine

Priftin

Pharmacologic class: Rifamycin derivative

Therapeutic class: Antitubercular

Pregnancy risk category C

Action

Inhibits RNA synthesis by blocking RNA transcription in susceptible organisms (mycobacteria and some gram-positive and gram-negative bacteria)

Availability

Tablets: 150 mg

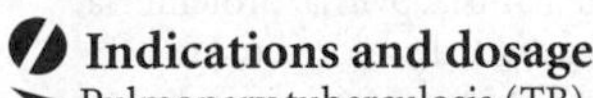

Indications and dosages

➢ Pulmonary tuberculosis (TB)

Adults: *Intensive-phase treatment*—600 mg P.O. twice weekly for 2 months, with doses spaced 72 hours apart; must be given with at least one other antitubercular. *Continuation-phase treatment*—600 mg P.O. once weekly for 4 months, given with another antitubercular.

Off-label uses

• *Mycobacterium avium intracellulare* complex infection

Contraindications

• Hypersensitivity to drug or other rifamycin derivatives

Precautions

Use cautiously in:

• hepatic disorders, porphyria
• concurrent protease inhibitor therapy for human immunodeficiency virus infection
• elderly patients
• pregnant or breastfeeding patients
• children younger than age 12.

Administration

• Know that drug is given with at least one other antitubercular.

• Expect to give drug with pyridoxine to adolescents, malnourished patients, and patients at risk for neuropathy.

Route	Onset	Peak	Duration
P.O.	Slow	5-6 hr	17-18 hr

Adverse reactions

CNS: headache, fatigue, anxiety, dizziness, aggressive behavior

CV: hypertension, peripheral edema

EENT: visual disturbances; discolored tears, sputum, and saliva

GI: nausea, vomiting, diarrhea, dys-

pepsia, esophagitis, gastritis, discolored feces, anorexia, **pancreatitis**
GU: hematuria, pyuria, proteinuria, urinary casts, discolored urine
Hematologic: anemia, thrombocytosis, hematoma, purpura, eosinophilia, **neutropenia, leukopenia**
Hepatic: hepatitis
Metabolic: hyperuricemia, hypovolemia, **hyperkalemia**
Musculoskeletal: gout, arthritis, joint pain
Skin: rash, pruritus, acne, urticaria, discolored skin and sweat
Other: edema

Interactions

Drug-drug. *Amitriptyline, anticoagulants, barbiturates, beta-adrenergic blockers, chloramphenicol, clofibrate, corticosteroids, cyclosporine, dapsone, delavirdine, diazepam, digoxin, diltiazem, disopyramide, doxycycline, fentanyl, fluconazole, fluoroquinolones, haloperidol, hormonal contraceptives, indinavir, itraconazole, ketoconazole, methadone, mexiletine, nelfinavir, nifedipine, nortriptyline, oral hypoglycemics, phenothiazines, progestin, quinidine, quinine, ritonavir, saquinavir, sildenafil, tacrolimus, theophylline, thyroid preparations, tocainide, verapamil, warfarin, zidovudine:* decreased actions of these drugs
Antiretroviral drugs: decreased efficacy of these drugs
Drug-diagnostic tests. *Alanine aminotransferase, alkaline phosphatase, aspartate aminotransferase, bilirubin, eosinophils, lactate dehydrogenase, potassium, uric acid:* increased levels
Folate, vitamin B_{12} assays: interference with standard assays
Hemoglobin, neutrophils, platelets, white blood cells: decreased values

Patient monitoring

• Monitor CBC, uric acid level, and liver function tests. Watch for signs and symptoms of blood dyscrasias and hepatitis.
• Assess vital signs and fluid intake and output. Stay alert for hypertension and edema.
• Closely monitor nutritional status and hydration.

Patient teaching

🔊 Instruct patient to immediately report fever, malaise, appetite loss, nausea, vomiting, or yellowing of skin or eyes.
• Emphasize importance of taking with companion drugs, as prescribed, to prevent growth of resistant TB strains.
• Tell patient drug may color tears, urine, and other body fluids reddish or brownish orange. Instruct him not to wear contact lenses during therapy, because drug may stain them permanently.
• Advise patient to take with meals and to minimize GI upset by eating small, frequent servings of healthy food and drinking plenty of fluids.
• Tell patient to monitor his weight and report sudden gains. Also tell him to report swelling.
🔊 Instruct patient to immediately report rash or unusual bleeding or bruising.
🔊 Caution patient to avoid driving and other hazardous activities until he knows how drug affects concentration, vision, and alertness.
• As appropriate, review all other significant and life-threatening adverse reactions and interactions, especially those related to the drugs and tests mentioned above.

riluzole

Rilutek

Pharmacologic class: Glutamate antagonist

Therapeutic class: Amyotrophic lateral sclerosis (ALS) agent

Pregnancy risk category C

Action

Unknown. Thought to inhibit amino acid accumulation on motor neurons of CNS, improving nerve impulse transmission.

Availability

Tablets: 50 mg

Indications and dosages

➢ ALS

Adults: 50 mg P.O. q 12 hours

Off-label uses

- Cervical dystonia
- Huntington's disease

Contraindications

- Hypersensitivity to drug or its components

Precautions

Use cautiously in:

- hepatic or renal insufficiency, neutropenia, febrile illness
- elderly patients
- female patients and Japanese patients (may have decreased metabolic capacity to eliminate drug)
- pregnant or breastfeeding patients
- children.

Administration

- Give at least 1 hour before or 2 hours after a meal to maximize absorption.

Route	Onset	Peak	Duration
P.O.	Unknown	Unknown	Unknown

Adverse reactions

CNS: headache, dizziness, drowsiness, asthenia, hypertonia, depression, insomnia, malaise, vertigo, circumoral paresthesia

CV: hypertension, orthostatic hypotension, tachycardia, palpitations, peripheral edema, phlebitis, **cardiac arrest**

EENT: rhinitis, sinusitis, oral candidiasis

GI: nausea, vomiting, diarrhea, abdominal pain, dyspepsia, flatulence, stomatitis, dry mouth, anorexia

GU: urinary tract infection, dysuria

Hematologic: neutropenia

Musculoskeletal: back pain, joint pain

Respiratory: decreased lung function, increased cough, pneumonia

Skin: pruritus, eczema, alopecia, exfoliative dermatitis

Other: tooth disorders, weight loss

Interactions

Drug-drug. *Allopurinol, methyldopa, sulfasalazine:* increased risk of hepatotoxicity

CYP450-1A2 inducers (such as omeprazole, rifampin): increased riluzole elimination

CYP450-1A2 inhibitors (such as amitriptyline, phenacetin, quinolones, theophylline): decreased riluzole elimination

Drug-diagnostic tests. *Alanine aminotransferase, aspartate aminotransferase, bilirubin, gamma-glutamyltransferase:* increased levels

Drug-food. *High-fat foods:* decreased riluzole absorption

Drug-behaviors. *Alcohol use:* increased risk of hepatotoxicity

Patient monitoring

- Monitor liver function tests and CBC.
- Assess vital signs and cardiovascular status, particularly for hypertension, orthostatic hypotension, and peripheral edema.

r

• Closely monitor respiratory status for decreased lung function and pneumonia.
• Monitor weight, nutritional status, and hydration.
• Closely monitor females and patients of Japanese origin, who are at increased risk for adverse reactions.

Patient teaching

• Tell patient to take 1 hour before or 2 hours after a meal, at same time each day.
• Instruct patient to take his temperature regularly and report fever.
Teach patient to immediately report arm or leg swelling, difficulty breathing, and other signs of decreased lung function.
• Advise patient to minimize GI upset by eating small, frequent servings of food and drinking plenty of fluids.
• Caution patient to avoid high-fat foods and alcohol.
• Instruct patient to move slowly when sitting up or standing, to avoid dizziness from sudden blood pressure decrease.
• As appropriate, review all other significant and life-threatening adverse reactions and interactions, especially those related to the drugs, tests, foods, and behaviors mentioned above.

rimantadine hydrochloride

Flumadine

Pharmacologic class: Miscellaneous and anticholinergic-like agent
Therapeutic class: Antiviral
Pregnancy risk category C

Action

Prevents nucleic acid uncoating during viral cell replication, preventing penetration in host. Also causes dopamine release from neurons.

Availability

Syrup: 50 mg/5 ml
Tablets: 100 mg

Indications and dosages

➢ Treatment of influenza type A
Adults: 100 mg P.O. b.i.d.
➢ Prophylaxis of influenza type A
Adults and children older than age 10: 100 mg P.O. b.i.d.
Children younger than age 10: 5 mg/kg P.O. daily. Maximum dosage is 150 mg daily.

Dosage adjustment

• Renal or hepatic disease
• Seizure disorders
• Elderly patients

Off-label uses

• Parkinson's disease

Contraindications

• Hypersensitivity to drug or amantadine

Precautions

Use cautiously in:
• history of seizures or renal or hepatic disease
• pregnant or breastfeeding patients
• children younger than age 1.

Administration

• Give several hours before bedtime.
• Start therapy within 48 hours of symptom onset and continue for at least 1 week.

Route	Onset	Peak	Duration
P.O.	Slow	6 hr	Unknown

Adverse reactions

CNS: headache, dizziness, fatigue, depression, insomnia, poor concentration, asthenia, nervousness
CV: hypotension
EENT: tinnitus

GI: nausea, vomiting, diarrhea, abdominal pain, dyspepsia, dry mouth, anorexia
Respiratory: dyspnea
Skin: rash

Interactions

Drug-drug. *Acetaminophen, aspirin:* decreased rimantadine peak blood level
Cimetidine: increased rimantadine blood level

Patient monitoring

- Assess patient's flu symptoms. Notify prescriber if symptoms don't improve within 2 to 3 days.
- Monitor vital signs; watch for hypotension.
- Closely monitor nutritional status and hydration.

Patient teaching

- Advise patient to take several hours before bedtime.
- If patient's taking syrup, tell him to use specially marked oral syringe or measuring device to ensure accurate dose.
- Instruct patient to contact prescriber if symptoms don't improve within 2 to 3 days.
- Caution patient to avoid driving and other hazardous activities until he knows how drug affects concentration, motor function, and alertness.
- As appropriate, review all other significant adverse reactions and interactions, especially those related to the drugs mentioned above.

risedronate sodium

Actonel

Pharmacologic class: Bisphosphonate
Therapeutic class: Calcium regulator
Pregnancy risk category C

Action

Inhibits osteoclast-mediated bone resorption. Also exerts antiresorptive effect, probably by directly inhibiting mature osteoclast activity or indirectly inhibiting osteoblasts.

Availability

Tablets: 5 mg, 30 mg, 35 mg

Indications and dosages

➢ Osteoporosis
Adults: 5 mg P.O. daily. Alternatively for postmenopausal osteoporosis only, 35 mg P.O. weekly.
➢ Paget's disease
Adults: 30 mg P.O. daily for 2 months. If indicated, may retreat with same dosage after post-treatment observation period of at least 2 months.

Off-label uses

- Hypercalcemia of malignancy
- Primary hyperparathyroidism

Contraindications

- Hypersensitivity to drug or other bisphosphonates
- Hypocalcemia
- Inability to stand or sit upright for at least 30 minutes

Precautions

Use cautiously in:
- renal disease, hypotension, upper GI disorders, difficulty swallowing
- pregnant or breastfeeding patients.

Administration

- Give with 6 to 8 oz of water 30 minutes before first food or beverage of day (other than water).

Clinical alert: Make sure patient stays upright for at least 30 minutes after taking.

- Be aware that patient with poor dietary intake may need calcium and vitamin D supplements.
- Give calcium, magnesium, or aluminum supplements or antacids at dif-

r

ferent time of day so they don't interfere with risedronate absorption.

Route	Onset	Peak	Duration
P.O.	Rapid	1 hr	Unknown

Adverse reactions

CNS: headache, anxiety, depression, dizziness, vertigo, syncope, asthenia
CV: hypertension, vasodilation, angina, chest pain, cardiovascular disorder, peripheral edema
EENT: cataract, conjunctivitis, dry eyes, otitis media, rhinitis, sinusitis, pharyngitis
GI: nausea, vomiting, diarrhea, constipation, abdominal pain, dyspepsia, flatulence, gastroenteritis, colitis, esophageal irritation, dry mouth, anorexia
GU: urinary tract infection
Hematologic: anemia
Musculoskeletal: bone, back, or joint pain; bone fracture; bursitis; myalgia; arthritis; leg and muscle cramps
Respiratory: crackles, cough, bronchitis, pneumonia
Skin: rash, pruritus, ecchymosis, **skin cancer**
Other: accidental injury, infection, neck pain, flulike symptoms, allergic reactions, **neoplasm**

Interactions

Drug-drug. *Antacids, aspirin, calcium or magnesium supplements:* decreased risedronate absorption
Nonsteroidal anti-inflammatory drugs, salicylates: increased GI irritation
Drug-diagnostic tests. *Bone-imaging diagnostic agents:* interference with test agents
Calcium, phosphorus: decreased levels
Drug-food. *Any food:* decreased drug absorption

Patient monitoring

- Watch for difficulty swallowing and signs and symptoms of esophageal irritation.
- Assess skin for unusual findings that may indicate skin cancer.

Patient teaching

- Advise patient to read patient information insert before starting therapy.
- ◀ Stress importance of taking with a full glass (6 to 8 oz) of water at least 30 minutes before first food or drink of day and staying upright for at least 30 minutes afterward.
- ◀ Instruct patient to stop taking drug and notify prescriber if she experiences difficulty or pain on swallowing, midline chest pain, or severe, persistent heartburn.
- Tell patient that chewing or sucking tablet may cause mouth irritation.
- Tell patient to report signs and symptoms of colitis.
- If patient must take calcium, magnesium, or aluminum supplements or antacids, tell her to take them at least 2 hours after risedronate.
- Inform patient that drug may cause leg cramps and bone or joint pain. Advise her to discuss these problems with prescriber.
- As appropriate, review all other significant and life-threatening adverse reactions and interactions, especially those related to the drugs, tests, and foods mentioned above.

risperidone

Risperdal, Risperdal Consta, Risperdal M-Tab

Pharmacologic class: Benzisoxazole derivative
Therapeutic class: Antipsychotic
Pregnancy risk category C

Action

Antagonizes $serotonin_2$ and $dopamine_2$ receptors in CNS. Also binds to alpha$_1$- and alpha$_2$-adrenergic receptors and histamine H_1 receptors.

Availability

Oral solution: 1 mg/ml in 30-ml bottles
Tablets: 0.25 mg, 0.5 mg, 1 mg, 2 mg, 3 mg, 4 mg
Tablets (orally disintegrating): 0.5 mg, 1 mg, 2 mg

Indications and dosages

➢ Schizophrenia
Adults: 1 mg P.O. b.i.d., increased by 1 mg b.i.d. as tolerated on days 2 and 3, up to a target dosage of 3 mg b.i.d. by day 3. May adjust in increments or decrements of 1 mg b.i.d. at weekly intervals; usual dosage range is 4 to 8 mg/day. Alternatively, may give as a single daily dose after initial titration. Or 25 mg deep I.M. q 2 weeks.
➢ Bipolar mania
Adults: Initially, 2 to 3 mg/day P.O. May adjust in increments or decrements of 1 mg/day at 24-hour intervals. Range is 1 to 6 mg/day.

Dosage adjustment

- Hepatic or renal impairment
- Elderly or debilitated patients

Off-label uses

- Tourette syndrome

Contraindications

- Hypersensitivity to drug

Precautions

Use cautiously in:
- renal or hepatic impairment, cardiovascular disease, prolonged QT interval, dysphagia, hyperprolactinemia, hypothermia or hyperthermia, Parkinson's disease, phenylketonuria, tardive dyskinesia, previous diagnosis of breast cancer or prolactin-dependent tumors
- history of seizures, drug abuse, or suicide attempt
- elderly or debilitated patients
- pregnant patients
- breastfeeding patients (use not recommended)
- children (safety not established).

Administration

- Record baseline blood pressure before starting therapy.
- For I.M. use, inject deep into buttock; rotate injection sites between buttocks.

Route	Onset	Peak	Duration
P.O.	1-2 wk	Unknown	Up to 6 wk

Adverse reactions

CNS: aggressive behavior, dizziness, drowsiness, extrapyramidal reactions, headache, increased dreams, longer sleep periods, insomnia, sedation, fatigue, nervousness, agitation, anxiety, tardive dyskinesia, hyperkinesia, akathisia, **transient ischemic attack (TIA), cerebrovascular accident (CVA), neuroleptic malignant syndrome**
CV: orthostatic hypotension, chest pain, tachycardia, **arrhythmias**
EENT: vision disturbances, rhinitis, sinusitis, pharyngitis
GI: nausea, vomiting, diarrhea, constipation, abdominal pain, dyspepsia, dry mouth, increased salivation, anorexia
GU: difficulty urinating, polyuria, galactorrhea, dysmenorrhea, menorrhagia, decreased libido
Musculoskeletal: joint or back pain
Respiratory: cough, dyspnea, upper respiratory tract infection
Skin: pruritus, diaphoresis, rash, dry skin, seborrhea, increased pigmentation, photosensitivity
Other: toothache, fever, impaired temperature regulation, weight changes

Interactions

Drug-drug. *Antihistamines, opioids, sedative-hypnotics:* additive CNS depression
Carbamazepine: increased metabolism and decreased efficacy of risperidone

Clozapine: decreased metabolism and increased effects of risperidone
Levodopa, other dopamine agonists: decreased antiparkinsonian effects of these drugs
Drug-behaviors. *Alcohol use:* increased CNS depression
Sun exposure: increased risk of photosensitivity

Patient monitoring

◀ Closely monitor neurologic status, especially for neuroleptic malignant syndrome (high fever, sweating, unstable blood pressure, stupor, muscle rigidity, and autonomic dysfunction), extrapyramidal reactions, TIA, CVA, and tardive dyskinesia.
- Monitor blood pressure, particularly for orthostatic hypotension.
- Assess body temperature. Check for fever and other signs and symptoms of infection.

Patient teaching

- Instruct patient to remove orally disintegrating tablet from blister pack, place on tongue immediately, and swallow as tablet dissolves.
- Tell patient to mix oral solution with water, coffee, orange juice, or low-fat milk. Tell him solution isn't compatible with cola or tea.
- Advise patient to use effective bedtime routine to avoid sleep disorders.

◀ Teach patient to recognize and immediately report signs and symptoms of serious adverse reactions, including tardive dyskinesia and neuroleptic malignant syndrome.
- Instruct patient to move slowly when sitting up or standing, to avoid dizziness from sudden blood pressure decrease.
- Tell patient that excessive fluid loss (as from sweating, vomiting, or diarrhea) and inadequate fluid intake increase risk of light-headedness (especially in hot weather).
- Caution patient to avoid driving and other hazardous activities until he knows how drug affects concentration and alertness.
- Advise female patient to tell prescriber if she is or plans to become pregnant. Caution her not to breastfeed during therapy.
- Advise patient not to drink alcohol.
- As appropriate, review all other significant and life-threatening adverse reactions and interactions, especially those related to the drugs and behaviors mentioned above.

ritonavir

Norvir

Pharmacologic class: Protease inhibitor

Therapeutic class: Antiretroviral

Pregnancy risk category B

Action

Inhibits human immunodeficiency virus (HIV) nonnucleoside reverse transcriptase by binding directly to reverse transcriptase and blocking RNA-dependent and DNA-dependent polymerase activity

Availability

Capsules: 100 mg
Oral solution: 80 mg/ml

Indications and dosages

➢ HIV

Adults: Initially, 300 mg P.O. b.i.d.; increase by 100 mg b.i.d. q 2 to 3 days, up to a usual maintenance dosage of 600 mg b.i.d.
Children ages 2 and older: 400 mg/m^2 b.i.d., not to exceed 600 mg b.i.d. Start with 250 mg/m^2 to minimize nausea.

Off-label uses

- Chronic hepatitis B

Contraindications

• Hypersensitivity to drug or its components
• Concurrent use of astemizole and terfenadine (not available in U.S.), amiodarone, bepridil, cisapride, dihydroergotamine, ergonovine, ergotamine, flecainide, methylergonovine, midazolam, pimozide, propafenone, quinidine, or triazolam

Precautions

Use cautiously in:
• hepatic disease, diabetes mellitus, hemophilia types A and B
• pregnant or breastfeeding patients.

Administration

• Give with meals to increase absorption.
• Mix oral solution with chocolate milk or liquid nutritional supplement to mask taste.
• Know that drug is usually given with other antiretrovirals.
Don't give concurrently with amiodarone, astemizole, bepridil, cisapride, dihydroergotamine, ergonovine, ergotamine, flecainide, methylergonovine, midazolam, pimozide, propafenone, quinidine, terfenadine, or triazolam. Serious interactions may occur.

Route	Onset	Peak	Duration
P.O.	Rapid	2-4 hr	Unknown

Adverse reactions

CNS: headache, dizziness, depression, insomnia, drowsiness, asthenia, paresthesia, syncope, malaise
CV: vasodilation
EENT: pharyngitis
GI: nausea, vomiting, diarrhea, constipation, dyspepsia, flatulence, abdominal pain, anorexia
Musculoskeletal: myalgia
Skin: diaphoresis
Other: abnormal taste, fever, pain

Interactions

Drug-drug. *Amiodarone, bepridil, cisapride, flecainide, midazolam, pimozide, propafenone, quinidine, triazolam:* inhibited metabolism of these drugs, leading to life-threatening reactions (such as arrhythmias, prolonged sedation, and respiratory depression)
Amitriptyline, anticoagulants, atovaquone, carbamazepine, clozapine, cyclosporine, desipramine, diltiazem, disopyramide, divalproex, dofetilide, dronabinol, ethinyl estradiol, lamotrigine, phenytoin, sulfamethoxazole, theophylline, zidovudine: increased risk of toxicity of these drugs
Amprenavir: increased amprenavir blood level
Astemizole, cisapride, encainide: increased risk of arrhythmias
Atorvastatin, cerivastatin, lovastatin, simvastatin, terfenadine: increased blood levels of these drugs, increased risk of rhabdomyolysis
Barbiturates, nevirapine, phenytoin, rifamycins: decreased ritonavir blood level
Bupropion: increased risk of seizures
Clarithromycin, efavirenz: increased blood levels of both drugs
Dihydroergotamine, ergonovine, ergotamine, methylergonovine: ergot toxicity
Fluconazole: increased ritonavir blood level
Drug-diagnostic tests. *Alanine aminotransferase, aspartate aminotransferase, cholesterol, creatine kinase, gamma-glutamyltransferase, triglycerides, uric acid:* increased levels
Hematocrit, hemoglobin, neutrophils, red blood cells, white blood cells: decreased levels
Drug-herbs. *St. John's wort:* decreased ritonavir blood level

Patient monitoring

• Monitor CBC, liver function tests, electrolyte levels, and lipid panel.

r

• Assess neurologic status closely. Stay alert for depression.
• Monitor vital signs and watch for syncope.
• Closely monitor nutritional and hydration status.

Patient teaching
• Advise patient to take with meals to increase absorption.
• Encourage patient to mix oral solution with chocolate milk or liquid nutritional supplement to mask taste.
• Tell patient drug may cause numbness, tingling, weakness, and other CNS effects that increase his injury risk. Urge him to use appropriate safety precautions.
• Instruct patient to report depression.
• Tell female patient not to breastfeed because of risk of serious adverse reactions and possible HIV transmission to infant.
• As appropriate, review all other significant adverse reactions and interactions, especially those related to the drugs, tests, and herbs mentioned above.

rituximab
Rituxan

Pharmacologic class: Murine/human monoclonal antibody
Therapeutic class: Antineoplastic
Pregnancy risk category C

Action
Binds to CD20 antigen on malignant B lymphocytes; recruits immune effector functions to mediate B-cell lysis (possibly through complement-dependent cytotoxicity and antibody-dependent cell-mediated cytotoxicity)

Availability
Injection: 10 mg/ml in 10-ml (100-mg) and 50-ml (500-mg) vials

Indications and dosages
➢ Low-grade or follicular CD20-positive B-cell non-Hodgkin's lymphoma
Adults: Initially, 375 mg/m² by I.V. infusion once weekly for four or eight doses at 50 mg/hour; increase rate by 50 mg/hour q 30 minutes to a maximum of 400 mg/hour. If patient tolerates first infusion, subsequent infusions may begin at 100 mg/hour, then increase by 100 mg/hour q 30 minutes to a maximum of 400 mg/hour as tolerated.

Off-label uses
• Waldenström's macroglobulinemia

Contraindications
• Hypersensitivity to drug, its components, or murine products

Precautions
Use cautiously in:
• history of drug allergy or sensitivity
• previous exposure to murine-based monoclonal antibodies
• high level of circulating malignant cells
• cardiac or pulmonary conditions
• pregnant or breastfeeding patients
• children.

Administration
• Follow facility policy regarding handling, administration, and disposal of chemotherapeutic drugs.
• Premedicate patient with diphenhydramine and acetaminophen, as prescribed.
• Give drug as I.V. infusion.
Never give as I.V. bolus or I.V. push.
• Dilute in dextrose 5% in water (D_5W) or normal saline solution to a

concentration of 1 to 4 mg/ml. Invert bag gently to mix solution; infuse at prescribed rate.

• If hypersensitivity reaction (non-IgE-mediated) or infusion reaction occurs, interrupt or temporarily slow infusion. When symptoms improve, infusion can continue at half of previous rate.

Route	Onset	Peak	Duration
I.V.	Variable	Variable	6-12 mo

Adverse reactions

CNS: dizziness, headache, nervousness, hypertonia, hyperesthesia, insomnia, agitation, malaise, paresthesia, asthenia, fatigue, tremor, rigors
CV: hypotension, hypertension, peripheral edema, chest pain, tachycardia, bradycardia, angina, **arrhythmias**
EENT: conjunctivitis, lacrimation disorders, rhinitis, sinusitis, pharyngitis
GI: nausea, vomiting, diarrhea, constipation, abdominal pain, dyspepsia, anorexia
GU: renal toxicity
Hematologic: anemia, **neutropenia, leukopenia, thrombocytopenia**
Metabolic: hyperglycemia, hypocalcemia
Musculoskeletal: myalgia, back pain
Respiratory: dyspnea, cough, bronchitis, **bronchospasm**
Skin: pruritus, rash, urticaria, flushing, dermatitis, angioedema, **toxic epidermal necrolysis, Stevens-Johnson syndrome**
Other: altered taste, fever, chills, pain at injection site, hypersensitivity reactions including **sepsis, severe infusion reaction**

Interactions

Drug-drug. *Cisplatin:* increased risk of renal failure
Live-virus vaccines: increased risk of infection from vaccine
Drug-diagnostic tests. *Calcium, hemoglobin, neutrophils, platelets, white blood cells:* decreased values
Glucose, lactate dehydrogenase: increased levels

Patient monitoring

• Monitor closely for signs and symptoms of hypersensitivity reaction.
[Clinical alert] Stop drug immediately and notify prescriber if patient develops signs or symptoms of Stevens-Johnson syndrome or other severe mucocutaneous reactions (including severe rash).
[Clinical alert] Monitor pulse and blood pressure throughout I.V. infusion. Stop infusion if hypotension, bronchospasm, or angioedema occurs. Then consult prescriber about restarting infusion at half of previous rate.
[Clinical alert] Monitor ECG throughout infusion. Stop infusion if serious arrhythmia develops.
• Monitor CBC, blood glucose, and electrolyte levels.
• Assess for signs and symptoms of infection, including fever.

Patient teaching

[Clinical alert] Tell patient to immediately report signs and symptoms of hypersensitivity reaction or severe skin reaction.
[Clinical alert] Instruct patient to take his temperature daily and immediately report fever and other signs or symptoms of infection.
[Clinical alert] Instruct patient to immediately report unusual bleeding or bruising.
• Advise patient to minimize GI upset by eating small, frequent servings of food and drinking plenty of fluids.
• As appropriate, review all other significant and life-threatening adverse reactions and interactions, especially those related to the drugs and tests mentioned above.

r

rivastigmine tartrate

Exelon

Pharmacologic class: Cholinesterase inhibitor
Therapeutic class: Anti-Alzheimer's drug
Pregnancy risk category B

Action

Unknown. Thought to enhance cholinergic function by elevating acetylcholine levels in brain through reversible inhibition of its hydrolysis by cholinesterase.

Availability

Capsules: 1.5 mg, 3 mg, 4.5 mg, 6 mg
Oral solution: 2 mg/ml

Indications and dosages

➢ Mild to moderate dementia of Alzheimer's disease

Adults: Initially, 1.5 mg P.O. b.i.d. May increase to 3 mg b.i.d. after 2 weeks; may increase further to 4.5 mg b.i.d. and 6 mg b.i.d., if tolerated, after 2 weeks at previous dosage. Typical effective range is 6 to 12 mg/day, up to a maximum of 12 mg/day.

Off-label uses

- Huntington's disease
- Parkinson's disease

Contraindications

- Hypersensitivity to drug, its components, or carbamate derivatives

Precautions

Use cautiously in:

- renal or hepatic impairment, diabetes mellitus, obstructive pulmonary disease, neurologic conditions that can cause seizures, peptic ulcers, GI bleeding, supraventricular conduction disorders
- patients older than age 85
- pregnant patients.

Administration

- Give with food in morning and evening.

Route	Onset	Peak	Duration
P.O.	Unknown	1 hr	12 hr

Adverse reactions

CNS: depression, dizziness, headache, confusion, insomnia, psychosis, hallucinations, anxiety, tremor, drowsiness, fatigue, syncope, asthenia
CV: chest pain, hypertension, peripheral edema
EENT: rhinitis, pharyngitis
GI: nausea, vomiting, diarrhea, constipation, abdominal pain, flatulence, eructation, dyspepsia, anorexia
GU: urinary tract infection, urinary incontinence
Musculoskeletal: back pain, joint pain, bone fractures
Respiratory: upper respiratory infection, cough, bronchitis
Skin: rash, diaphoresis
Other: weight loss, pain, flulike symptoms

Interactions

Drug-drug. *Anticholinergics:* interference with anticholinergic effects
Cholinergic agonists (such as bethanechol), succinylcholine and similar neuromuscular blockers: synergistic effects
Drug-herbs. *S-adenosylmethionine (SAM-e), St. John's wort:* increased risk of serotonin syndrome
Drug-behaviors. *Nicotine use:* increased drug clearance

Patient monitoring

- Monitor patient's nutritional and hydration status, especially at start of therapy.
- Assess vital signs and cardiovascular status. Stay alert for chest pain and peripheral edema.

• Closely monitor cognitive status, particularly memory. Report significant decline or improvement.
• Assess temperature. Watch for fever and other signs and symptoms of infection.

Patient teaching
• Instruct caregiver to give with food in morning and evening.
• Inform caregiver that drug initially may worsen CNS impairment. Recommend appropriate safety measures.
• Tell caregiver that memory improvement generally is subtle and that drug works by preventing further memory loss.
• Inform caregiver that drug commonly causes nausea, vomiting, decreased appetite, and weight loss, especially at start of therapy.
• Advise caregiver to watch for and report weight loss, dehydration, and signs and symptoms of GI bleeding.
• Tell caregiver that drug interacts with many over-the-counter products and nicotine. Advise him to discuss these products with prescriber before giving to patient.
• As appropriate, review all other significant adverse reactions and interactions, especially those related to the drugs, herbs, and behaviors mentioned above.

rizatriptan benzoate
Maxalt, Maxalt-MLT

Pharmacologic class: Serotonin 5-hydroxytryptamine (5-HT_1) receptor agonist
Therapeutic class: Antimigraine drug
Pregnancy risk category C

Action
Thought to act as agonist at specific 5-HT_1 receptor sites in intracranial vessels, causing vasoconstriction. Also may act on sensory trigeminal nerves, reducing transmission along pain pathways.

Availability
Tablets: 5 mg, 10 mg
Tablets (orally disintegrating): 5 mg, 10 mg

Indications and dosages
➢ Acute migraine
Adults: 5 to 10 mg P.O.; may repeat in 2 hours, not to exceed 30 mg in 24 hours. For patients receiving propranolol concurrently, 5 mg P.O., up to a maximum of three doses in 24 hours.

Contraindications
• Hypersensitivity to drug or its components
• Ischemic heart disease or other significant cardiovascular disease
• Ischemic bowel disease
• Transient ischemic attacks
• Basilar or hemiplegic migraine
• Uncontrolled hypertension
• Use of other 5-HT_1 agonists or ergot-type compounds (dihydroergotamine, methysergide) within 24 hours
• MAO inhibitor use within past 14 days

Precautions
Use cautiously in:
• severe renal impairment (especially in dialysis patients), moderate hepatic impairment, cardiovascular risk factors
• phenylketonuria (PKU) in patients receiving orally disintegrating tablets
• pregnant or breastfeeding patients
• children younger than age 18 (safety not established).

Administration
• Place orally disintegrating tablet on patient's tongue to dissolve. Make sure he swallows it with saliva only. Don't give with beverages.

Don't give within 14 days of MAO inhibitors (may cause serious adverse reactions).

Route	Onset	Peak	Duration
P.O.	30 min	1-1.5 hr	Unknown

Adverse reactions

CNS: headache, dizziness, drowsiness, asthenia, fatigue, paresthesia, decreased mental acuity, euphoria, tremor
CV: chest pain, tightness, heaviness, or pressure
GI: nausea, vomiting, diarrhea, dry mouth
Respiratory: dyspnea
Skin: flushing
Other: neck, throat, or jaw pain, tightness, or pressure; hot flashes; warm or cold sensations

Interactions

Drug-drug. *Ergot or ergot-type compounds (such as dihydroergotamine, methysergide), other 5-HT_1 agonists:* additive vasoactive effects
MAO inhibitors, propranolol: increased rizatriptan blood level, greater risk of adverse effects
Selective serotonin reuptake inhibitors: weakness, hyperreflexia, incoordination
Drug-herbs. *S-adenosylmethionine (SAM-e), St. John's wort:* increased risk of adverse serotonergic effects, including serotonin syndrome

Patient monitoring

- Monitor patient's response to drug. Assess need for repeat doses.
- Assess vital signs and cardiovascular status, especially if patient has cardiovascular risk factors.

Patient teaching

- Teach patient how to use drug. Stress that it's effective only in treating diagnosed migraine—not in preventing migraine or treating other types of headache.
- Advise patient to peel back blister pack of Maxalt-MLT with dry hands and place tablet on tongue. Tell him to swallow drug with saliva only, not beverages.
- Tell patient he may repeat dose in 2 hours if headache recurs, but should take no more than 30 mg in 24 hours.
- Inform patient with PKU that orally disintegrating tablets contain phenylalanine.

Instruct female patient to immediately report possible pregnancy.

- As appropriate, review all other significant adverse reactions and interactions, especially those related to the drugs and herbs mentioned above.

ropinirole hydrochloride

Requip

Pharmacologic class: Dopamine agonist
Therapeutic class: Antidyskinetic
Pregnancy risk category C

Action

Unknown. Thought to stimulate dopamine receptors in brain.

Availability

Tablets: 0.25 mg, 0.5 mg, 1 mg, 2 mg, 3 mg, 4 mg, 5 mg

Indications and dosages

➢ Idiopathic Parkinson's disease
Adults: Initially, 0.25 mg P.O. t.i.d. for 1 week, followed by 0.5 mg P.O. t.i.d. for 1 week, then 0.75 mg t.i.d. for 1 week, and then 1 mg t.i.d. for 1 week. After week 4, may increase by 1.5 mg/day q week, up to 9 mg/day; then may increase further by up to 3 mg/day q week, up to 24 mg/day.

Off-label uses
• Restless leg syndrome

Contraindications
• Hypersensitivity to drug or its components

Precautions
Use cautiously in:
• severe hepatic impairment or cardiovascular disease, bradycardia
• elderly patients
• pregnant patients
• breastfeeding patients (use not recommended).

Administration
• Give with food if drug causes nausea.
• Know that drug withdrawal should occur over 7 days, with frequency reduced to twice-daily dosing for first 4 days and then to once-daily dosing for next 3 days.

Route	Onset	Peak	Duration
P.O.	30-60 min	1-2 hr	16 hr

Adverse reactions
CNS: headache, dizziness, confusion, drowsiness, fatigue, neuralgia, amnesia, hyperesthesia, yawning, dystonia, increased dyskinesia, hyperkinesia, akathisia, hallucinations, abnormal thinking, poor concentration, syncope, vertigo, myoclonus, asthenia, malaise, sleep attacks
CV: orthostatic hypotension, hypertension, palpitations, extrasystole, peripheral edema, peripheral ischemia, chest pain, tachycardia, **atrial fibrillation**
EENT: abnormal vision, rhinitis, sinusitis, pharyngitis
GI: nausea, vomiting, flatulence, abdominal pain, dyspepsia, dry mouth, anorexia
GU: urinary tract infection, decreased libido, erectile dysfunction
Respiratory: bronchitis, dyspnea
Skin: diaphoresis, flushing
Other: viral infection, pain, edema

Interactions
Drug-drug. *Butyrophenones (such as haloperidol), metoclopramide, phenothiazines, thioxanthenes:* decreased ropinirole effects
Ciprofloxacin, estrogens: increased ropinirole effects
Drugs that alter activity of CYP450-1A2 enzyme system: altered ropinirole clearance
Levodopa: increased levodopa effects
Drug-diagnostic tests. *Alkaline phosphatase, blood urea nitrogen:* increased levels
Drug-herbs. *Kava:* decreased ropinirole efficacy

Patient monitoring
• Monitor vital signs, especially for orthostatic hypotension. Assess for peripheral edema.
• Assess neurologic status carefully. Report severe adverse reactions.
• Monitor nutritional and hydration status.

Patient teaching
• Encourage patient to take drug with food if it causes nausea.
• Inform patient (and caregiver, as appropriate) that drug can cause serious CNS reactions; tell him which ones to report. Recommend appropriate safety measures.
• Instruct patient to move slowly when sitting up or standing, to avoid dizziness from sudden blood pressure decrease.
🔈 Caution patient not to stop drug abruptly. Dosage must be tapered.
• Advise patient to report swelling of hands or feet.
• Caution patient to avoid driving and other hazardous activities until he knows how drug affects concentration, vision, and alertness.
• As appropriate, review all other significant and life-threatening adverse reactions and interactions, especially

those related to the drugs, tests, and herbs mentioned above.

rosiglitazone maleate

Avandia

Pharmacologic class: Thiazolidinedione

Therapeutic class: Hypoglycemic

Pregnancy risk category C

Action

Inhibits alpha-glucosidases, enzymes that convert oligosaccharides and disaccharides to glucose. This inhibition lowers blood glucose level, especially in postprandial hyperglycemia.

Availability

Tablets: 2 mg, 4 mg, 8 mg

Indications and dosages

➢ Adjunct to diet and exercise in type 2 (non-insulin-dependent) diabetes mellitus (used alone); given with metformin, insulin, or a sulfonylurea when combination of diet, exercise, and monotherapy with another hypoglycemic drug don't achieve glycemic control

Adults: 4 mg P.O. once daily or 2 mg b.i.d. After 12 weeks, may increase to 8 mg daily or 4 mg b.i.d. if needed.

Off-label uses

- Polycystic ovary syndrome

Contraindications

- Hypersensitivity to drug or its components

Precautions

Use cautiously in:

- diabetic ketoacidosis, type 1 (insulin-dependent) diabetes mellitus (use not recommended)
- edema, heart failure, jaundice, hypertension, hepatic impairment
- NYHA Class III or IV cardiac status
- pregnant patients
- breastfeeding patients (use not recommended)
- children (safety and efficacy not established).

Administration

- Give with or without food.
- Be aware that drug is active only in presence of endogenous insulin and thus is ineffective in diabetic ketoacidosis or type 1 diabetes mellitus.

Route	Onset	Peak	Duration
P.O.	Unknown	Unknown	12-24 hr

Adverse reactions

CNS: fatigue, headache
EENT: sinusitis
GI: diarrhea
Hematologic: anemia
Metabolic: hyperglycemia, **hypoglycemia**
Musculoskeletal: back pain
Respiratory: upper respiratory infection
Other: edema, injury, weight gain

Interactions

Drug-diagnostic tests. *Free fatty acids, high-density lipoproteins, low-density lipoproteins, total cholesterol:* increased levels

Hematocrit, hemoglobin: decreased levels

Drug-herbs. *Aloe, bitter melon, chromium, coenzyme Q10, fenugreek, glucomannan, gymnema sylvestre, psyllium, St. John's wort:* additive hypoglycemic effects

Glucosamine: poor glycemic control

Patient monitoring

- Monitor CBC, lipid panel, blood glucose, and glycosylated hemoglobin levels.

• Monitor patient's weight. Assess for fluid retention, which may lead to heart failure.
• Closely monitor liver function tests; drug may cause hepatotoxicity.

Patient teaching

• Tell patient he may take with or without food.
• Advise patient to monitor blood glucose level regularly and report significant changes.
Inform patient that drug may increase fluid retention, causing or exacerbating heart failure. Encourage him to weigh himself regularly and report sudden weight gain, swelling, or shortness of breath.
• Tell patient he'll undergo regular blood testing during therapy.
• Caution female patient not to breastfeed during therapy.
• As appropriate, review all other significant and life-threatening adverse reactions and interactions, especially those related to the tests and herbs mentioned above.

rosuvastatin calcium

Crestor

Pharmacologic class: HMG-CoA reductase inhibitor
Therapeutic class: Antilipemic
Pregnancy risk category X

Action

Selectively and competitively inhibits HMG-CoA reductase, which catalyzes its conversion to the cholesterol precursor mevalonate and thus limits cholesterol synthesis. This action increases high-density lipoprotein level and decreases low-density lipoprotein (LDL) level.

Availability

Tablets: 5 mg, 10 mg, 20 mg, 40 mg

Indications and dosages

➤ Primary heterozygous hypercholesterolemia; mixed dyslipidemia (Fredrickson types IIa and IIb)
Adults: Initially, 10 mg/day P.O. Patients who need less aggressive cholesterol reduction or have predisposing factors for myopathy may start at 5 mg/day. Patients with marked hypercholesterolemia (LDL above 190 mg/dl) and more aggressive LDL goals may start at 20 mg/day. For maintenance, 5 to 40 mg/day P.O.
➤ Homozygous familial hypercholesterolemia
Adults: 20 mg/day P.O. Maximum recommended dosage is 40 mg/day.
➤ Hypertriglyceridemia (Fredrickson type IV)
Adults: Initially, 10 mg/day P.O. For maintenance, 5 to 40 mg/day P.O.

Contraindications

• Hypersensitivity to drug or its components
• Active hepatic disease or persistent, unexplained hepatic enzyme elevations
• Pregnancy or breastfeeding

Precautions

Use cautiously in:
• predisposing factors for myopathy (such as renal impairment, advanced age, hypothyroidism)
• heavy alcohol use
• history of hepatic disease or hypersensitivity to other HMG-CoA reductase inhibitors (such as fluvastatin, simvastatin)
• patients of Japanese or Chinese descent
• women of childbearing age (except those who are highly unlikely to conceive and have been informed of potential hazards)
• children (safety and efficacy not established).

r

Administration

🔊 Check liver function tests before therapy starts.

- Give with or without food.
- Measure lipid levels within 2 to 4 weeks after therapy starts and after titration.
- Know that drug should be used as adjunct to other lipid-lowering treatments, such as diet.

Route	Onset	Peak	Duration
P.O.	Unknown	3-5 hr	Unknown

Adverse reactions

CNS: headache, dizziness, anxiety, depression, insomnia, hypertonia, paresthesia, asthenia, tremor, vertigo, neuralgia
CV: palpitations, tachycardia, chest pain, angina pectoris, hypertension, vasodilation, peripheral edema
EENT: rhinitis, sinusitis, pharyngitis
GI: nausea, vomiting, diarrhea, constipation, abdominal pain, dyspepsia, flatulence, gastritis, gastroenteritis
GU: urinary tract infection, **acute renal failure**
Hematologic: anemia
Metabolic: hypokalemia, hyperglycemia, **hypoglycemia**
Musculoskeletal: myalgia; myopathy; arthritis; pathologic fractures; back, pelvic, neck, or joint pain; **rhabdomyolysis**
Respiratory: respiratory tract infection, bronchitis, increased cough, dyspnea, pneumonia, **asthma**
Skin: rash, pruritus, bruising
Other: periodontal abscess, flulike symptoms, infection

Interactions

Drug-drug. *Antacids:* decreased rosuvastatin blood level
Cyclosporine, gemfibrozil: increased rosuvastatin bioavailability
Hormonal contraceptives: increased contraceptive blood level
Warfarin: increased International Normalized Ratio
Drug-diagnostic tests. *Alanine aminotransferase (ALT), alkaline phosphatase, aspartate aminotransferase (AST), bilirubin, creatine kinase (CK), glucose:* increased levels
Potassium: decreased level
Thyroid function tests: altered results
Urine protein: present beyond trace
Drug-food. *Caffeine-containing foods and beverages:* increased stimulant effect
Oat bran, pectin: impaired drug absorption
Urine-acidifying foods: increased drug blood level
Drug-herbs. *Caffeine-containing herbs (such as cola nut, yerba maté), ephedra (ma huang):* increased stimulant effect

Patient monitoring

🔊 Monitor CK, creatinine, and urine protein levels closely. Also watch for signs and symptoms of rhabdomyolysis with acute renal failure: CK level above 10 times normal limits, muscle ache or weakness, creatinine elevation, and urine protein level beyond trace, accompanied by hematuria. If these findings occur, withhold drug and notify prescriber immediately.

🔊 Monitor liver function tests 12 weeks after therapy begins, after dosage increases, and at least semiannually thereafter. Reduce dosage or withdraw drug if ALT or AST persists at three times normal levels.

🔊 Temporarily withhold drug in patients with acute, serious conditions predisposing to renal failure caused by rhabdomyolysis (such as sepsis, hypotension, major surgery, trauma, uncontrolled seizures, or severe metabolic, endocrine, and electrolyte disorders).

- Monitor blood glucose, electrolyte levels, and lipid panel.

• Assess vital signs and cardiovascular status, especially for tachycardia and palpitations.
• Monitor for signs and symptoms of respiratory tract infection.
• Stay alert for tremor and asthenia.

Patient teaching

• Tell patient he may take with or without food. If he's using antacids, instruct him to take these 2 hours after rosuvastatin.
• Instruct patient to maintain a standard cholesterol-lowering diet.
Tell patient to immediately report unexplained muscle pain, tenderness, or weakness (particularly if accompanied by malaise or fever).
Caution female patient of childbearing age not to take drug if she is pregnant, plans to become pregnant, or is breastfeeding.
• Teach patient how to check blood or urine glucose level and recognize signs and symptoms of hypoglycemia and hyperglycemia.
• Tell patient that foods, beverages, and preparations containing caffeine or ephedra may increase drug's stimulant effect. Encourage him to limit caffeine intake and avoid ephedra.
• Advise patient against heavy alcohol use, which increases risk of liver disease.
• As appropriate, review all other significant and life-threatening adverse reactions and interactions, especially those related to the drugs, tests, foods, and herbs mentioned above.

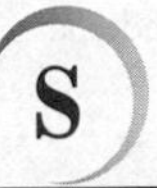

salmeterol xinafoate

Serevent Diskus

Pharmacologic class: $Beta_2$-adrenergic receptor agonist (long-acting)
Therapeutic class: Bronchodilator
Pregnancy risk category C

Action

Stimulates intracellular adenylate cyclase, an enzyme that catalyzes conversion of adenosine triphosphate to cyclic-3', 5'-adenosine monophosphate (cAMP). Increased cAMP levels relax bronchial smooth muscle and inhibit release of mediators of immediate hypersensitivity (especially from mast cells).

Availability

Powder for inhalation using Diskus delivery system: 50 mcg/blister (60 blisters)

Indications and dosages

➢ Maintenance treatment of asthma; prevention of bronchospasm in patients with reversible obstructive airway disease; maintenance treatment of bronchospasm in patients with chronic obstructive pulmonary disease (COPD)
Adults and children older than age 4: 50 mcg (one inhalation) b.i.d. approximately 12 hours apart
➢ Prevention of exercise-induced bronchospasm
Adults and children older than age 4: 50 mcg (one inhalation) 30 to 60 minutes before exercise. Withhold additional doses for at least 12 hours.

Off-label uses

• Cystic fibrosis

S

• High-altitude pulmonary edema
• Atopic asthma

Contraindications

• Hypersensitivity to drug or its components
• Acute asthma attack

Precautions

Use cautiously in:
• cardiovascular disease, diabetes mellitus, hyperthyroidism
• concurrent use of MAO inhibitors or tricyclic antidepressants (extreme caution required)
• pregnant or breastfeeding patients
• children younger than age 4.

Administration

• To use Serevent Diskus, activate device and hold in horizontal position.
• Make sure patient doesn't exhale into device.
• Preferably, give doses 12 hours apart in morning and evening.

Route	Onset	Peak	Duration
Inhalation	10-25 min	3-4 hr	12 hr

Adverse reactions

CNS: headache, nervousness, dizziness, tremor
CV: palpitations, hypertension, tachycardia, **arrhythmias**
GI: nausea, diarrhea, abdominal pain
Metabolic: hyperglycemia, **hypokalemia**
Musculoskeletal: muscle cramps and soreness
Respiratory: paradoxical bronchospasm
Skin: urticaria, angioedema, rash
Other: hypersensitivity reaction

Interactions

Drug-drug. *Beta-adrenergic blockers:* decreased salmeterol efficacy, increased risk of severe bronchospasm in patients with asthma or COPD
Diuretics (except potassium-sparing): increased risk of hypokalemia and ECG changes
MAO inhibitors, tricyclic antidepressants: potentiation of salmeterol's cardiovascular actions
Drug-diagnostic tests. *Glucose:* increased level
Potassium: decreased level
Drug-food. *Caffeine-containing foods and beverages:* increased stimulant effect
Urine-acidifying foods: increased drug blood level
Drug-herbs. *Caffeine-containing herbs (such as cola nut, yerba maté), ephedra (ma huang):* increased stimulant effect

Patient monitoring

• Assess pulmonary status and vital signs.
🔈 Stay alert for signs and symptoms of hypersensitivity reaction, particularly rash, urticaria, angioedema, and paradoxical bronchospasm.

Patient teaching

• Remind patient that drug isn't a rescue bronchodilator and won't give immediate relief in emergency.
• Teach patient proper technique for using inhaler or Diskus. Instruct him not to exhale into device or use a spacer with Diskus.
• Advise patient to keep Diskus dry. Tell him not to rinse, wash, or take it apart.
• Instruct patient to take regular doses 12 hours apart. Tell him to take doses for exercise-induced bronchospasm 30 to 60 minutes before exercising.
• Advise patient to take drug exactly as prescribed and not to exceed one inhalation twice daily.
• Tell patient to consult prescriber if he needs more inhalations than usual.
• Caution patient not to stop taking drug without consulting prescriber.
• As appropriate, review all other significant and life-threatening adverse

reactions and interactions, especially those related to the drugs, tests, foods, and herbs mentioned above.

salsalate

Amigesic, Marthritic, Mono-Gesic, Salflex, Salgesic

Pharmacologic class: Salicylate
Therapeutic class: Nonopioid analgesic, anti-inflammatory
Pregnancy risk category C

Action

Breaks down into salicylic acid, which lowers elevated body temperature by dilating peripheral vessels. Also reduces inflammation and relieves pain, probably by inhibiting prostaglandin synthesis.

Availability

Tablets: 500 mg, 750 mg

Indications and dosages

➢ Rheumatoid arthritis; nonarticular rheumatism; osteoarthritis; polyarthritis
Adults: Initially, 1 g P.O. t.i.d., titrated as needed

Contraindications

- Hypersensitivity to salicylates, other nonsteroidal anti-inflammatory drugs (NSAIDs), or tartrazine
- Hemophilia
- Bleeding ulcers
- Hemorrhagic states
- Blood coagulation defects
- Children and adolescents with viral infections

Precautions

Use cautiously in:

- severe renal disease, hepatic damage, asthma, rhinitis, nasal polyps, hypoprothrombinemia, vitamin K deficiency, chronic alcohol use or abuse
- history of GI bleeding or ulcer disease
- elderly patients
- pregnant (especially during third trimester) or breastfeeding patients.

Administration

- Give with food to minimize GI upset.

Don't administer to children or adolescents with viral infections, because of increased risk of Reye's syndrome.

Route	Onset	Peak	Duration
P.O.	5-30 min	1-3 hr	3-6 hr

Adverse reactions

CNS: drowsiness, dizziness, confusion, headache, stimulation, hallucinations, depression, **seizures, coma**
CV: rapid pulse
EENT: hearing loss, tinnitus, laryngeal edema
GI: nausea, vomiting, dyspepsia, epigastric distress, heartburn, abdominal pain, anorexia, **GI bleeding**
Hematologic: hemolytic anemia, leukopenia, agranulocytosis, thrombocytopenia
Hepatic: hepatitis, hepatotoxicity
Metabolic: hyponatremia, hypokalemia, **hypoglycemia**
Respiratory: wheezing, hyperpnea, **pulmonary edema**
Skin: rash, flushing, urticaria, bruising, angioedema
Other: salicylism, **Reye's syndrome, anaphylaxis**

Interactions

Drug-drug. *Activated charcoal:* decreased salsalate absorption
Angiotensin converting enzyme inhibitors: decreased antihypertensive effect
Antacids, urinary alkalizers: decreased salsalate efficacy

Beta-adrenergic blockers, probenecid, spironolactone, sulfinpyrazone, sulfonylureas: decreased effects of these drugs
Carbonic anhydrase inhibitors: increased risk of salicylism
Cefamandole, clopidogrel, eptifibatide, heparin, oral anticoagulants, plicamycin, thrombolytics, ticlopidine, tirofiban: increased bleeding
Corticosteroids: increased excretion and decreased blood level of salsalate
Insulin, oral hypoglycemics, penicillin, phenytoin, sulfonamide, valproic acid: increased effects of these drugs
Methotrexate: increased methotrexate blood level and risk of toxicity
NSAIDs: decreased NSAID blood level, increased risk of adverse GI effects
Vancomycin: increased risk of ototoxicity
Drug-diagnostic tests. *Activated partial thromboplastin time, bleeding time, prothrombin time:* increased
Alanine aminotransferase, alkaline phosphatase, amylase, aspartate aminotransferase, carbon dioxide, coagulation studies, uric acid, urinary protein: increased levels
Cholesterol, potassium, protein-bound iodine: decreased levels
Erythrocyte survival time: reduced
Pregnancy test, protirelin-induced thyroid-stimulating hormone test, radionuclide thyroid imaging, uric acid, urine catecholamines, urine glucose, urine hydroxyindoleacetic acid, urine ketone tests using ferric chloride method, urine vanillylmandelic acid: interference with test results
Drug-food. *Urine-acidifying foods:* increased salsalate blood level
Drug-herbs. *Anise, arnica, chamomile, clove, fenugreek, feverfew, garlic, ginger, ginkgo, ginseng, horse chestnut, kelp ware, licorice:* increased risk of bleeding
Drug-behaviors. *Alcohol use:* increased risk of GI bleeding

Patient monitoring
- Monitor for signs and symptoms of anaphylaxis.
- Assess hearing and neurologic status.
- Monitor liver function tests, coagulation studies, and electrolyte and glucose levels.
- Assess for bleeding tendency and angioedema.

Patient teaching
🔊 Teach patient to recognize and immediately report signs or symptoms of severe hypersensitivity reaction.
🔊 Caution parents not to give drug to child with symptoms of viral illness.
🔊 Instruct patient to immediately report unusual bleeding or bruising.
- Tell patient that many common herbs increase risk of bleeding. Advise him to consult prescriber before using.
- Caution patient to avoid alcohol, which increases risk of GI bleeding.
- As appropriate, review all other significant and life-threatening adverse reactions and interactions, especially those related to the drugs, tests, foods, herbs, and behaviors mentioned above.

saquinavir
Fortovase

saquinavir mesylate
Invirase

Pharmacologic class: Protease inhibitor
Therapeutic class: Antiretroviral
Pregnancy risk category B

Action
Inhibits human immunodeficiency virus (HIV) protease, preventing cleavage of HIV polyproteins and blocking virus replication and maturation

Availability

saquinavir
Capsules (soft gelatin): 200 mg
saquinavir mesylate
Capsules: 200 mg

Indications and dosages

➢ Advanced HIV infection in selected patients
Adults older than age 16: 1,000 mg P.O. b.i.d. (saquinavir mesylate) given only in combination with ritonavir b.i.d. Or 1,200 mg P.O. t.i.d. (saquinavir). Or 1,000 mg P.O. b.i.d. (saquinavir) given with ritonavir.

Contraindications

- Hypersensitivity to drug or its components
- Concurrent use of antiarrhythmics (amiodarone, bepridil, flecainide, propafenone, quinidine); astemizole, cisapride, or terfenadine (not available in United States); ergot derivatives; midazolam; pimozide; rifampin; or triazolam
- Severe hepatic impairment
- Monotherapy (saquinavir mesylate)

Precautions

Use cautiously in:
- hepatic disease, hemophilia types A and B, diabetes mellitus
- pregnant or breastfeeding patients
- children younger than age 16.

Administration

- Give around the clock without missing doses, within 2 hours of a full meal.
- If prescribed in combination with ritonavir, give both drugs at same time.
- Know that saquinavir mesylate is given only in combination with ritonavir, which inhibits saquinavir mesylate's metabolism and provides saquinavir blood levels at least equal to those achieved with saquinavir.
- Be aware that saquinavir and saquinavir mesylate capsules aren't bioequivalent and therefore aren't interchangeable.
- Clinical alert: Don't give concurrently with antiarrhythmics (amiodarone, bepridil, flecainide, propafenone, quinidine); astemizole, cisapride, terfenadine, ergot derivatives, midazolam, pimozide, rifampin, or triazolam. Life-threatening reactions may occur.

Route	Onset	Peak	Duration
P.O.	Unknown	Unknown	Unknown

Adverse reactions

CNS: headache, dizziness, paresthesia, asthenia, depression, insomnia, anxiety, confusion, ataxia, **seizures, suicidal ideation, intracranial hemorrhage**
CV: chest pain, peripheral vasoconstriction, **thrombophlebitis**
GI: nausea, vomiting, diarrhea, constipation, abdominal pain, flatulence, dyspepsia, buccal mucosal ulcers, pancreatitis
GU: urinary retention, nephrolithiasis, **oliguria, acute renal insufficiency**
Hematologic: hemolytic anemia, pancytopenia, thrombocytopenia, acute myeloblastic leukemia
Hepatic: jaundice, **portal hypertension, exacerbation of chronic hepatic disease** (with grade 4 elevated liver function test results)
Metabolic: hyperglycemia, diabetes mellitus (exacerbation or new onset), hypercalcemia, **hyperkalemia, hypoglycemia**
Musculoskeletal: musculoskeletal pain
Respiratory: bronchitis, cough
Skin: rash, **Stevens-Johnson syndrome**
Other: altered taste, drug fever

Interactions

Drug-drug. *Antiarrhythmics (amiodarone, bepridil, flecainide, propafenone, quinidine), astemizole, cisapride, pimozide, terfenadine:* increased blood levels of these drugs, life-threatening arrhythmias

Benzodiazepines, calcium channel blockers: increased blood levels of these drugs
Carbamazepine, dexamethasone, nevirapine, phenobarbital, phenytoin, rifabutin, rifampin: reduced saquinavir steady-state level
Clarithromycin, indinavir, ketoconazole, nelfinavir, ritonavir: increased saquinavir blood level
Ergot derivatives: elevated blood level of these drugs, life-threatening reactions such as acute ergot toxicity (peripheral vasospasm and ischemia of extremities and other tissues)
HMG-CoA reductase inhibitors: increased risk of myopathy (including rhabdomyolysis)
Midazolam, triazolam: increased risk of life-threatening prolonged or increased sedation or respiratory depression
Nonnucleoside reverse transcriptase inhibitors (delavirdine, nevirapine): increased saquinavir blood level
Sildenafil, tadalafil, tricyclic antidepressants, vardenafil: increased blood levels of these drugs
Warfarin: altered International Normalized Ratio
Drug-diagnostic tests. *Alanine aminotransferase (ALT), amylase, aspartate aminotransferase (AST), bilirubin, calcium, creatinine phosphokinase, potassium:* increased levels
Blood glucose: increased or decreased level
Phosphate: decreased level
Platelets, red blood cells, white blood cells: decreased counts
Drug-food. *Any food:* increased drug absorption
Grapefruit juice: elevated drug blood level, increased pharmacologic and adverse effects
Drug-herbs. *Garlic capsules:* decreased saquinavir blood level
St. John's wort: 50% reduction in saquinavir blood level

Patient monitoring

- Monitor platelet count, CBC, liver function tests, electrolytes, and uric acid and bilirubin levels. Watch for evidence of life-threatening blood dyscrasias and portal hypertension.
- Assess nutritional status and hydration.
- Monitor neurologic status. Stay alert for depression, suicidal ideation, seizures, and signs or symptoms of intracranial hemorrhage.

Patient teaching

- Tell patient to take with food (but not grapefruit juice) or within 2 hours of a full meal. Stress importance of taking doses around the clock on a regular schedule.

◀ Inform patient (and significant other as appropriate) that drug may cause depression and suicidal thoughts, which should be reported immediately.

- Advise patient to notify prescriber if rash occurs.

◀ Teach patient to recognize and immediately report signs and symptoms of liver disorder or bleeding tendency.

- Tell patient drug interacts with many other drugs, causing serious reactions. Advise him to discuss all drug use with prescriber before therapy starts.
- Caution patient to avoid St. John's wort and garlic capsules during therapy.
- Instruct female patient not to breastfeed, because she may transmit drug effects and HIV to infant.
- As appropriate, review all other significant and life-threatening adverse reactions and interactions, especially those related to the drugs, tests, foods, and herbs mentioned above.

sargramostim (GM-CSF)

Leukine

Pharmacologic class: Granulocyte-macrophage colony stimulating factor
Therapeutic class: Hematopoietic agent
Pregnancy risk category C

Action

Stimulates proliferation and differentiation of hematopoietic cells that activate mature granulocytes and macrophages of target cells

Availability

Liquid: 500 mcg/ml
Powder for injection: 250 mcg

Indications and dosages

➢ Post peripheral blood progenitor cell (PBPC) transplantation
Adults: 250 mcg/m²/day I.V. over 24 hours or subcutaneously once daily, starting immediately after progenitor cell infusion

➢ Mobilization of PBPCs into peripheral blood for collection by leukapheresis
Adults: 250 mcg/m²/day I.V. over 24 hours or subcutaneously once daily, continued throughout harvesting

➢ Neutrophil recovery after chemotherapy in acute myelogenous leukemia
Adults: 250 mcg/m²/day I.V. over 4 hours, starting 4 days after completion of chemotherapy induction

➢ Bone-marrow transplantation failure or engraftment delay
Adults: 250 mcg/m²/day as 2-hour I.V. infusion for 14 days. If engraftment doesn't occur, may repeat after 7 days of drug hiatus.

➢ Myeloid reconstitution after autologous or allogeneic bone-marrow transplantation
Adults: 250 mcg/m²/day as a 2-hour I.V. infusion, starting 2 to 4 hours after autologous bone marrow infusion and at least 24 hours after last chemotherapy or radiotherapy dose

Off-label uses

- Crohn's disease
- Melanoma
- Wound healing
- Mucositis
- Stomatitis
- Vaccine adjuvant

Contraindications

- Hypersensitivity to drug, its components, or yeast products
- Excessive leukemic myeloid blasts in bone marrow or peripheral blood (10% or more)
- Within 24 hours before or after chemotherapy or radiation therapy

Precautions

Use cautiously in:
- renal or hepatic insufficiency, fluid retention, pulmonary disorders, pulmonary infiltrates, heart failure, leukocytosis, transient supraventricular arrhythmias
- cancer patients undergoing sargramostim-mobilized PBPC collection
- patients receiving purged bone marrow or previously exposed to intensive chemotherapy or radiation therapy
- pregnant or breastfeeding patients
- children.

S

Administration

Don't give within 24 hours of chemotherapy or radiation therapy.
- Add 1 ml of sterile water to powder for injection by directing water stream against side of vial and swirling vial gently to disperse contents.
- Avoid shaking or agitating solution.
- For a final drug concentration below 10 mcg/ml, add human albumin 0.1% to saline solution; then dilute drug in normal saline solution.

• Infuse as soon as possible after reconstitution, but no more than 6 hours after mixing.
• Don't add other drugs to infusion; don't use in-line filter.

Route	Onset	Peak	Duration
I.V.	Immediate	2 hr	3-6 hr
Subcut.	15 min	1-3 hr	6 hr

Adverse reactions

CNS: malaise, asthenia
CV: peripheral edema, tachycardia, hypotension, transient supraventricular tachycardia, **pericardial effusion**
GI: nausea, vomiting, diarrhea, anorexia, stomatitis, **GI hemorrhage**
GU: urinary tract disorder, **abnormal renal function**
Hematologic: blood dyscrasias, hemorrhage
Hepatic: hepatic damage
Musculoskeletal: joint pain, myalgia, bone pain
Respiratory: dyspnea, lung disorder
Skin: rash, alopecia
Other: fever, chills, sepsis, edema, first-dose reaction (respiratory distress, hypoxia, syncope, tachycardia, hypotension, flushing)

Interactions

Drug-drug. *Corticosteroids, lithium:* potentiation of myeloproliferative effects
Vincristine: severe peripheral neuropathy

Patient monitoring

• Monitor for dyspnea. Halve dosage and contact prescriber if dyspnea occurs.
• Assess CBC with white cell differential. Check for presence of blast cells, and watch for signs and symptoms of blood dyscrasias.
• Closely monitor vital signs and fluid intake and output. Stay alert for signs and symptoms of fluid overload.
• Monitor liver function tests, and watch for evidence of hepatic damage and bleeding (especially GI hemorrhage).

Patient teaching

• Tell patient sargramostim is a powerful drug that can cause significant adverse reactions. Teach him to recognize and report serious reactions at once.
• Instruct patient to immediately report unusual bleeding or bruising or yellowing of skin or eyes.
• Tell patient drug may cause weakness and musculoskeletal pain.
• Inform patient that he'll undergo regular blood testing during therapy.
• As appropriate, review all other significant and life-threatening adverse reactions and interactions, especially those related to the drugs mentioned above.

scopolamine (hyoscine)

Transderm-Scop

scopolamine hydrobromide (hyoscine hydrobromide)

Pharmacologic class: Antimuscarinic, belladonna alkaloid
Therapeutic class: Antiemetic, antivertigo agent, anticholinergic
Pregnancy risk category C

Action

Acts as competitive inhibitor at postganglionic muscarinic receptor sites of parasympathetic nervous system and on smooth muscles that respond to acetylcholine but lack cholinergic innervation. May block cholinergic transmission from vestibular nuclei to higher CNS centers and from reticular formation to vomiting center.

Availability

Injection: 0.3 mg/ml and 1 mg/ml in 1-ml vials, 0.4 mg/ml in 0.5-ml ampules and 1-ml vials, 0.86 mg/ml in 0.5-ml ampules
Tablets: 0.4 mg
Transdermal system (Transderm-Scop): 1.5 mg/patch (releases 0.5 mg scopolamine over 3 days)

Indications and dosages

➢ Excessive GI motility and hypertonia in irritable bowel syndrome, mild dysentery, diverticulitis, pylorospasm, and cardiospasm
Adults: 0.4 to 0.8 mg P.O. daily
➢ Preanesthetic sedation and obstetric amnesia
Adults: 0.3 to 0.6 mg I.M., I.V., or subcutaneously 45 to 60 minutes before anesthesia, usually given with analgesics
➢ Postoperative nausea and vomiting
Adults: One transdermal patch placed behind ear on evening before surgery and kept in place for 24 hours after surgery. For cesarean section, one transdermal patch placed behind ear 1 hour before surgery.
➢ Motion sickness
Adults: One transdermal patch placed behind ear 4 hours before anticipated need, replaced q 3 days if needed

Off-label uses

- Drooling

Contraindications

- Hypersensitivity to scopolamine, other belladonna alkaloids, or barbiturates
- Hypersensitivity to bromides (injection only)
- Angle-closure glaucoma
- Acute hemorrhage
- Myasthenia gravis
- Obstructive uropathy (including prostatic hypertrophy)
- Obstructive GI disease (including paralytic ileus and intestinal atony)
- Reflux esophagitis
- Ulcerative colitis or toxic megacolon
- Hepatic or renal impairment
- Chronic lung disease (with repeated doses)

Precautions

Use cautiously in:
- suspected intestinal obstruction; pulmonary or cardiac disease; tachyarrhythmia or tachycardia; open-angle glaucoma; autonomic neuropathy; hypertension; hyperthyroidism; ileostomy or colostomy
- history of seizures or psychosis
- elderly patients
- pregnant or breastfeeding patients (safety not established)
- children.

Administration

- For I.V. use, give by direct injection at prescribed rate after diluting with sterile water.
- After removing protective strip from transdermal patch, avoid finger contact with exposed adhesive layer to prevent contamination.

Route	Onset	Peak	Duration
P.O., I.M., subcut.	30 min	1 hr	4-6 hr
I.V.	10 min	1 hr	2-4 hr
Transdermal	4 hr	Unknown	72 hr

Adverse reactions

CNS: drowsiness, dizziness, confusion, restlessness, fatigue
CV: tachycardia, palpitations, hypotension, transient heart rate changes
EENT: blurred vision, mydriasis, photophobia, conjunctivitis
GI: constipation, dry mouth
GU: urinary hesitancy or retention
Skin: decreased sweating, rash

S

Interactions

Drug-drug. *Antidepressants, antihistamines, disopyramide, quinidine:* additive anticholinergic effects
Antidepressants, antihistamines, opioid analgesics, sedative-hypnotics: additive CNS depression
Oral drugs: altered absorption of these drugs
Wax-matrix potassium tablets: increased GI mucosal lesions
Drug-herbs. *Angel's trumpet, jimsonweed, scopolia:* increased anticholinergic effects
Drug-behaviors. *Alcohol use:* increased CNS depression

Patient monitoring

- Assess vital signs and neurologic, cardiovascular, and respiratory status.
- Monitor patient for urinary hesitancy or retention.

Patient teaching

- Tell patient transdermal patch is most effective if applied to dry skin behind ear 4 hours before traveling.
- Caution patient to avoid touching exposed adhesive layer of transdermal patch.
- Advise patient to wash and dry hands thoroughly before and after applying patch.
- If patch becomes dislodged, instruct patient to remove it and apply new patch on a different site behind ear.
- Tell patient that using patch for more than 72 hours may cause withdrawal symptoms (headache, nausea, vomiting, dizziness). Advise him to limit use when feasible.
- Inform patient that his eyes may be markedly sensitive to light during patch use. Instruct him to wear sunglasses and use other measures to guard eyes from light.
- Caution patient to avoid alcohol because it may increase CNS depression.
- As appropriate, review all other significant adverse reactions and interactions, especially those related to the drugs, herbs, and behaviors mentioned above.

secobarbital

Seconal

Pharmacologic class: Barbiturate
Therapeutic class: Sedative-hypnotic, preanesthetic
Controlled substance schedule II
Pregnancy risk category D

Action

Depresses sensory cortex, decreases motor activity, alters cerebellar function, and produces drowsiness, sedation, and hypnosis

Availability

Capsules: 100 mg

Indications and dosages

➤ Insomnia
Adults: 100 mg P.O. at bedtime
➤ Preanesthetic sedation
Adults: 200 to 300 mg P.O. 1 to 2 hours before surgery
Children: 2 to 6 mg/kg (maximum of 100 mg) P.O. 1 to 2 hours before surgery

Dosage adjustment

- Renal impairment
- Elderly or debilitated patients

Contraindications

- Hypersensitivity to drug or other barbiturates
- Marked hepatic impairment
- Respiratory disease with obvious dyspnea or obstruction
- History of manifest or latent porphyria

Precautions

Use cautiously in:

- patients with suicidal tendencies or a history of substance abuse
- mild hepatic impairment
- alcohol use
- elderly patients
- labor and delivery
- pregnant or breastfeeding patients.

Administration

- Give with or without food when used for insomnia; give without food when used for preanesthetic sedation.

Route	Onset	Peak	Duration
P.O.	10-15 min	Unknown	3-4 hr

Adverse reactions

CNS: somnolence
CV: bradycardia, hypotension, syncope
Hepatic: hepatic damage
Respiratory: hypoventilation
Skin: exfoliative dermatitis, angioedema
Other: drug dependence or tolerance, hypersensitivity reaction

Interactions

Drug-drug. *Corticosteroids:* enhanced metabolism of these drugs
Doxycycline: shortened doxycycline half-life
Estradiol: increased estradiol metabolism
Griseofulvin (oral): interference with griseofulvin absorption
MAO inhibitors: prolonged barbiturate activity
Oral anticoagulants: decreased anticoagulant response
Other CNS depressants (such as antihistamines, narcotics, tranquilizers): additive CNS depression
Phenytoin: increased or decreased phenytoin blood level
Valproic acid derivatives: increased secobarbital blood level
Drug-herbs. *St. John's wort:* decreased secobarbital blood level
Drug-behaviors. *Alcohol use:* increased sedation, additive CNS depression

Patient monitoring

🔊 Closely monitor blood pressure and heart and respiratory rates. Watch for signs and symptoms of respiratory depression, especially with preoperative use.

- Assess CBC and kidney and liver function tests.
- In long-term therapy, monitor patient for drug dependence.

Patient teaching

- Tell patient to take only as prescribed. Caution him that drug is habit forming.
- Advise patient to avoid alcohol, St. John's wort, and other CNS depressants during drug therapy.
- Caution patient to avoid driving and other hazardous activities.
- Advise patient taking hormonal contraceptives to use alternative birth control method.
- As appropriate, review all other significant and life-threatening adverse reactions and interactions, especially those related to the drugs, herbs, and behaviors mentioned above.

selegiline hydrochloride

Apo-Selegiline✤, Eldepryl, Gen-Selegiline✤, Novo-Selegiline✤, Nu-Selegiline✤, SD Deprenyl✤

Pharmacologic class: MAO inhibitor (type B)
Therapeutic class: Antidyskinetic
Pregnancy risk category C

Action

Unknown. Thought to increase dopaminergic activity by inhibiting MAO type B in nerve cells, increasing dopamine availability to brain cells.

S

Availability
Capsules: 5 mg
Tablets: 5 mg

Indications and dosages
➢ Adjunctive treatment of Parkinson's disease in patients who don't respond to carbidopa-levodopa alone
Adults: 10 mg P.O. daily in divided doses. After 2 to 3 days, attempt to reduce carbidopa-levodopa dosage (typically by 10% to 30%).

Off-label uses
- Initial therapy for Parkinson's disease
- Alzheimer's disease
- Narcolepsy
- Adjunct in schizophrenia

Contraindications
- Hypersensitivity to drug or its components
- Concurrent meperidine therapy

Precautions
Use cautiously in:
- patients receiving tricyclic antidepressants (TCAs), selective serotonin reuptake inhibitors (SSRIs), or opioids concurrently
- elderly patients
- pregnant or breastfeeding patients
- children.

Administration
- Give with breakfast and lunch, but restrict foods high in tyramine (such as aged cheese, red wine, yogurt, and smoked high-protein foods).

Clinical alert: Don't give within 14 days of TCAs or SSRIs (5 weeks for fluoxetine because of its long half-life).

Route	Onset	Peak	Duration
P.O.	Unknown	0.5-2 hr	Unknown

Adverse reactions
CNS: agitation, anxiety, bradykinesia, chorea, confusion, delusions, depression, dizziness, hallucinations, headache, dyskinesias, increased akinetic involuntary movements, insomnia, lethargy, light-headedness, loss of balance, syncope, vivid dreams
CV: orthostatic hypotension, hypertension, new or increased angina, palpitations, **arrhythmias**
GI: nausea, diarrhea, abdominal pain, dry mouth
GU: urinary retention
Musculoskeletal: leg pain, low back pain
Other: generalized aches, weight loss

Interactions
Drug-drug. *Adrenergics:* increased pressor response
Levodopa: increased adverse reactions to levodopa
Meperidine, other opioids: stupor, muscle rigidity, severe agitation, fever, death
Other MAO inhibitors: hypertensive crisis
SSRIs, TCAs: severe mental status changes, CNS toxicity (with possible hyperpyrexia and death)
Drug-food. *Tyramine-rich foods (such as aged cheese, red wine, yogurt, smoked high-protein foods):* hypertensive crisis
Drug-herbs. *Cacao:* vasopressor effects
Ginseng: headache, tremor, mania

Patient monitoring
- Monitor vital signs and cardiovascular status.
- Assess neurologic status and motor function. Institute safety measures as needed to prevent injury.
- Monitor weight and fluid intake and output.
- Monitor CBC and liver and kidney function tests.

Patient teaching
- Tell patient he may take with or without food.
- Instruct patient (and caregiver as appropriate) to monitor neurologic status and motor function and to insti-

tute safety precautions as needed to prevent injury.
- Instruct patient to move slowly when sitting up or standing, to avoid dizziness from sudden blood pressure decrease.
- Tell patient (or caregiver) that drug may cause serious interactions with many drugs. Instruct him to tell all prescribers he's taking it.
- Advise patient to limit foods high in tyramine. Provide a list of these foods.
- As appropriate, review all other significant and life-threatening adverse reactions and interactions, especially those related to the drugs, foods, and herbs mentioned above.

senna, sennosides

Argoral✤, Black Draught, Dr. Caldwell, Dosalax, Ex-Lax Chocolate, Ex-Lax Gentle, Fletcher's Castoria, Maximum Relief Ex-Lax, Nature's Remedy, Senexon, Senna-Gen, Senokot, Senokot Granules, SenokotXTRA, Senolax, X-Prep Liquid✤

Pharmacologic class: Anthraquinone laxative
Therapeutic class: Laxative (stimulant)
Pregnancy risk category C

Action

Causes local irritation in colon, which promotes peristalsis and bowel evacuation. Softens feces by increasing water and electrolytes in large intestine.

Availability

Granules: 15 mg/tsp
Liquid: 8.8 mg/5 ml, 25 mg/5 ml, 33.3 mg/ml (concentrate)
Tablets: 8.6 mg, 10 mg, 15 mg, 17 mg, 25 mg
Tablets (chewable): 15 mg

Indications and dosages

➢ Acute constipation; preparation for bowel examination

Adults and children ages 12 and older: For acute constipation, 12 to 50 mg P.O. daily or b.i.d. For bowel preparation, 105 to 157.5 mg (concentrate) 12 to 14 hours before scheduled procedure.
Children ages 6 to 11: 50% of adult dosage
Children ages 2 to 5: 33% of adult dosage

Contraindications

- Hypersensitivity to drug or its components
- GI bleeding or obstruction
- Suspected appendicitis or undiagnosed abdominal pain
- Acute surgical abdomen
- Fecal impaction
- Inflammatory bowel disease (such as Crohn's disease)

Precautions

Use cautiously in:
- pregnant or breastfeeding patients
- children.

Administration

- Give with a full glass of cold water.
- To prepare patient for bowel examination, give 12 to 14 hours before procedure, followed by a clear liquid diet.

Route	Onset	Peak	Duration
P.O.	6-24 hr	Variable	Variable

Adverse reactions

GI: nausea, vomiting, diarrhea, abdominal cramps, nutrient malabsorption, yellow or yellowish-green feces, loss of normal bowel function (with excessive use), dark pigmentation of rectal mucosa (with long-term use), protein-losing enteropathy
GU: reddish-pink discoloration of alkaline urine, yellowish-brown discoloration of acidic urine

S

Metabolic: electrolyte imbalances (such as hypokalemia)
Other: laxative dependence (with long-term or excessive use)

Interactions

Drug-diagnostic tests. *Calcium, potassium:* decreased levels

Patient monitoring

- Assess bowel movements to determine laxative efficacy.
- In long-term use, monitor fluid balance, nutritional status, and electrolyte levels and watch for laxative dependence.

Patient teaching

- Tell patient using drug for constipation to take at bedtime with a glass of water.
- In long-term use, advise patient to watch for and report signs and symptoms of nutritional deficiencies and fluid and electrolyte imbalance.
- If patient will undergo bowel examination, advise him to take drug 12 to 14 hours before procedure, followed by a clear liquid diet.
- As appropriate, review all other significant adverse reactions and interactions, especially those related to the tests mentioned above.

sertraline hydrochloride

Zoloft

Pharmacologic class: Selective serotonin reuptake inhibitor (SSRI)
Therapeutic class: Antidepressant
Pregnancy risk category C

Action

Inhibits neuronal uptake of serotonin in CNS, potentiating serotonin activity; has little effect on norepinephrine or dopamine uptake

Availability

Oral concentrate: 20 mg/ml
Tablets: 25 mg, 50 mg, 100 mg

Indications and dosages

➢ Depression
Adults: Initially, 50 mg/day P.O. depending on response. May increase at weekly intervals to a maximum of 200 mg/day.
➢ Obsessive-compulsive disorder
Adults and children ages 13 to 17: Initially, 50 mg/day P.O. May increase at weekly intervals to a maximum of 200 mg/day.
Children ages 6 to 12: 25 mg/day P.O.
➢ Panic disorder; social anxiety disorder; posttraumatic stress disorder
Adults: Initially, 25 mg/day P.O. After 1 week, may increase to 50 mg/day; depending on response, may then increase at weekly intervals to a maximum of 200 mg/day.
➢ Premenstrual dysphoric disorder
Adults: Initially, 50 mg/day P.O., either throughout entire menstrual cycle or only during luteal phase. For maintenance, 50 to 150 mg/day.

Off-label uses

- Premature ejaculation

Contraindications

- Hypersensitivity to drug or its components
- MAO inhibitor use within past 14 days
- Concurrent pimozide use
- Concurrent use of disulfiram (oral concentrate)

Precautions

Use cautiously in:

- seizures disorders, severe hepatic or renal impairment, increased risk for suicide
- history of mania
- pregnant or breastfeeding patients
- children.

Administration

• Give as a single dose in morning or evening.

Don't use rubber dropper when giving concentrate to patient with latex allergy.

Don't give concurrently with pimozide or within 14 days of MAO inhibitors.

Route	Onset	Peak	Duration
P.O.	Unknown	4.5-8.5 hr	Unknown

Adverse reactions

CNS: dizziness, drowsiness, fatigue, headache, insomnia, agitation, anxiety, confusion, emotional lability, poor concentration, mania, nervousness, weakness, yawning, tremor, hypertonia, hypoesthesia, paresthesia, **suicidal behavior or ideation** (especially in child or adolescent)
CV: chest pain, palpitations
EENT: vision abnormalities, tinnitus, rhinitis, pharyngitis
GI: nausea, vomiting, diarrhea, constipation, dyspepsia, flatulence, abdominal pain, dry mouth, anorexia
GU: urinary frequency, urinary disorders, sexual dysfunction, menstrual disorders
Musculoskeletal: back pain, myalgia
Skin: diaphoresis, rash
Other: altered taste, increased appetite, fever, thirst, hot flashes

Interactions

Drug-drug. *Adrenergics:* increased adrenergic sensitivity, increased risk of serotonin syndrome
Cimetidine: increased sertraline blood level and effects
Clozapine, most benzodiazepines, phenytoin, tricyclic antidepressants, tolbutamide, warfarin: increased blood levels and effects of these drugs
Disulfiram: disulfiram reaction, indicated by nausea, vomiting, flushing, throbbing headache, diaphoresis, cardiovascular and respiratory reactions (with sertraline oral concentrate)
Drugs metabolized by CYP450-2DC or CYP450-3A4: increased blood levels of these drugs
MAO inhibitors: potentially fatal reactions (hyperthermia, rigidity, myoclonus, autonomic instability)
Pimozide: increased pimozide blood level
Sumatriptan: weakness, hyperreflexia, incoordination
Drug-diagnostic tests. *Alanine aminotransferase, aspartate aminotransferase:* increased levels
Drug-herbs. *S-adenosylmethionine (SAM-e), St. John's wort:* increased risk of serotonergic side effects, including serotonin syndrome
Drug-behaviors. *Alcohol use:* increased CNS effects

Patient monitoring

Monitor patient's mental status carefully. Stay alert for mood changes and indications of suicidal ideation, especially in child or adolescent.

• Evaluate neurologic status regularly. Institute safety measures, as appropriate, to prevent injury.
• Monitor temperature. Watch for fever and other signs or symptoms of infection.

Patient teaching

• Advise patient to take once a day, either in morning or night, with or without food.
• If evening dose causes insomnia, recommend switching to morning dose.
• Instruct patient to mix oral concentrate with 4 oz of recommended liquid only. Advise him to swallow diluted drug immediately after mixing.
• Tell patient using oral concentrate that drug contains alcohol.

Caution patient not to stop taking drug suddenly. Dosage must be tapered.

S

• Inform patient that drug may cause serious interactions with many common drugs. Instruct him to tell all prescribers he's taking it.

Advise patient (and significant other as appropriate) to monitor his mental status carefully and to immediately report increased depression or suicidal thoughts or behavior (especially in child or adolescent).

• Caution patient to avoid driving and other hazardous activities until he knows how drug affects concentration and alertness.

• As appropriate, review all other significant and life-threatening adverse reactions and interactions, especially those related to the drugs, tests, herbs, and behaviors mentioned above.

sildenafil citrate
Viagra

Pharmacologic class: Phosphodiesterase type 5 (PDE5) inhibitor

Therapeutic class: Anti-erectile dysfunction agent

Pregnancy risk category B

Action
Inhibits PDE5, enhancing the effects of nitric oxide released during sexual stimulation. This action inactivates cyclic guanosine monophosphate (cGMP), which then increases cGMP levels in corpus cavernosum. Resulting smooth muscle relaxation promotes increased blood flow and subsequent erection.

Availability
Tablets: 25 mg, 50 mg, 100 mg

Indications and dosages
➢ Erectile dysfunction

Adults: 50 mg P.O., preferably 1 hour before anticipated sexual activity. Range is 25 to 100 mg taken 30 minutes to 4 hours before sexual activity, not to exceed one dose daily.

Dosage adjustment
• Hepatic or renal impairment
• Concurrent use of hepatic isoenzyme inhibitors (such as cimetidine, erythromycin, itraconazole, ketoconazole)
• Elderly patients

Contraindications
• Hypersensitivity to drug
• Concurrent use of nitrates (nitroglycerin, isosorbide mononitrate or dinitrate)

Precautions
Use cautiously in:
• serious cardiovascular disease (such as history of myocardial infarction, cerebrovascular accident, or serious arrhythmia within past 6 months); coronary artery disease (current or previous) with unstable angina; resting blood pressure below 90/50 mm Hg or above 170/110 mm Hg (current or previous); heart failure (current or previous); renal or hepatic impairment (current or previous); bleeding disorder; active peptic ulcer; anatomic penile deformity; retinitis pigmentosa; conditions associated with priapism (sickle cell anemia, multiple myeloma, leukemia)
• history of uncontrolled hypertension or hypotension
• concurrent use of antihypertensives, erythromycin, ketoconazole, itraconazole, or saquinavir
• patients older than age 65.

Administration
Don't give concurrently with nitrates.

• Administer 30 minutes to 4 hours before sexual activity.

Route	Onset	Peak	Duration
P.O.	Within 1 hr	Unknown	Up to 4 hr

Adverse reactions

CNS: headache, dizziness, anxiety, drowsiness, vertigo, **seizures, cerebrovascular hemorrhage, transient ischemic attack**
CV: hypertension, **myocardial infarction (MI), cardiovascular collapse, ventricular arrhythmias, sudden death**
EENT: transient vision loss, blurred or color-tinged vision, increased light sensitivity, ocular redness, retinal bleeding, vitreous detachment or traction, photophobia, nasal congestion
GI: diarrhea, dyspepsia
GU: hematuria, urinary tract infection, priapism
Skin: flushing, rash

Interactions

Drug-drug. *Antihypertensives, nitrates:* increased risk of hypotension
Enzyme inducers, rifampin: reduced sildenafil blood level
Hepatic isoenzyme inhibitors (such as cimetidine, erythromycin, itraconazole, ketoconazole), protease inhibitors (such as indinavir, nelfinavir, ritonavir, saquinavir): increased sildenafil blood level and effects
Drug-food. *High-fat diet:* reduced drug absorption, decreased peak level

Patient monitoring

- Monitor cardiovascular status carefully.
- Evaluate patient's vision.
- Assess for drug efficacy.

Patient teaching

- Advise patient to take 30 minutes to 4 hours before sexual activity.
- Tell patient not to exceed prescribed dosage or take more than one dose daily.

🔊 Instruct patient to stop sexual activity and contact prescriber immediately if chest pain, dizziness, or nausea occurs.

🔊 Teach patient to recognize and immediately report serious cardiac and vision problems.

- Inform patient that drug can cause serious interactions with many common drugs. Instruct him to tell all prescribers he's taking it.

🔊 Caution patient never to take drug with nitrates, because of risk of potentially fatal hypotension.

- Instruct patient to report priapism (persistent, painful erection) or erections lasting more than 4 hours.
- Tell patient that high-fat diet may interfere with drug efficacy.
- Caution patient to avoid driving and other hazardous activities until he knows how drug affects concentration and alertness.
- As appropriate, review all other significant and life-threatening adverse reactions and interactions, especially those related to the drugs and foods mentioned above.

simethicone

Alka-Seltzer Gas Relief Maximum Strength, Gas-X, Gas-X Extra Strength, Genasyme, Maalox Anti-Gas, Maalox Anti-Gas Extra Strength, Maximum Strength Mylanta Gas, Mylanta Gas, Mylicon, Mylicon Infant Drops, Ovol♣, Phazyme, Phazyme Infant Drops

Pharmacologic class: Methylated linear siloxane mixture

Therapeutic class: Antiflatulent, antifoam agent

Pregnancy risk category NR

Action

Causes gas bubbles to coalesce and allows gas to pass through GI tract via belching or passing of flatus. Silicone

S

antifoam spreads on surface of aqueous liquids, forming a film of low surface tension that causes foam bubbles to collapse.

Availability

Capsules: 95 mg, 125 mg
Capsules (liquid-filled): 125 mg, 166 mg
Drops: 40 mg/0.6 ml, 40 mg/1 ml, 95 mg/1.425 ml
Suspension: 40 mg/0.6 ml, 50 mg/5 ml
Tablets: 60 mg, 62.5 mg, 80 mg, 95 mg
Tablets (chewable): 40 mg, 80 mg, 125 mg, 150 mg, 166 mg

Indications and dosages

➢ Excess gas in GI tract after surgery or from air swallowing, dyspepsia, peptic ulcer, or diverticulitis
Adults and children older than age 12: 40 to 125 mg P.O. q.i.d. after meals and at bedtime, up to 500 mg/day
Children ages 2 to 12: 40 mg P.O. q.i.d., up to 240 mg/day
Children younger than age 2: 20 mg P.O. q.i.d.

Contraindications

• Hypersensitivity to drug
• Intestinal perforation or obstruction

Precautions

Use cautiously in:
• abdominal pain of unknown cause (especially when accompanied by fever).

Administration

• Give as needed after meals and at bedtime.

Route	Onset	Peak	Duration
P.O.	Immediate	Unknown	3 hr

Adverse reactions

None significant

Interactions

None significant

Patient monitoring

• Monitor GI status to assess drug efficacy.

Patient teaching

• Tell patient to take after meals and at bedtime as needed.
• Caution patient not to take dose higher than indicated on package unless prescriber approves.

simvastatin

Zocor

Pharmacologic class: HMG-CoA reductase inhibitor
Therapeutic class: Antihyperlipidemic
Pregnancy risk category X

Action

Inhibits hepatic enzyme HMG-CoA reductase, interrupting cholesterol synthesis and low-density lipoprotein (LDL) consumption. Net effect is total cholesterol and serum triglyceride reductions.

Availability

Tablets: 5 mg, 10 mg, 20 mg, 40 mg, 80 mg

Indications and dosages

➢ Coronary artery disease; hyperlipidemia
Adults: 20 to 40 mg P.O. daily in evening, adjusted q 4 weeks based on response. Range is 5 to 80 mg/day.
➢ Hypercholesterolemia
Adults: Initially, 40 mg P.O. daily at bedtime. Alternatively, 80 mg daily divided as 20 mg in morning, 20 mg in afternoon, and 40 mg at bedtime.
Children and adolescents ages 10 to 17: Initially, 10 mg P.O. daily in evening. Range is 10 to 40 mg daily, adjusted at intervals of 4 weeks or longer.

Dosage adjustment
- Severe renal impairment
- Concurrent use of amiodarone, fibrates, niacin, or verapamil
- Elderly patients

Contraindications
- Hypersensitivity to drug or its components
- Active hepatic disease or unexplained persistent serum transaminase elevations
- Pregnancy or breastfeeding

Precautions
Use cautiously in:
- renal impairment; severe acute infection; hypotension; severe metabolic, endocrine, or electrolyte problems; uncontrolled seizures; visual disturbances; myopathy; major surgery; trauma; alcoholism
- history of hepatic disease
- concurrent use of amiodarone, clarithromycin, cyclosporine, digoxin, erythromycin, gemfibrozil and other fibrates, itraconazole, ketoconazole, nefazodone, nicotinic acid, protease inhibitors, verapamil, or warfarin
- cross-sensitivity to other drugs that can affect steroid levels
- females of childbearing age
- children younger than age 18 (safety not established).

Administration
- Check liver function tests before starting therapy.
- Give with evening meal. Don't give with large amounts of grapefruit juice.

Route	Onset	Peak	Duration
P.O.	Unknown	Unknown	Unknown

Adverse reactions
CNS: headache, asthenia
GI: nausea, vomiting, diarrhea, constipation, abdominal pain or cramps, flatulence, dyspepsia
Musculoskeletal: myalgia, **rhabdomyolysis**
Respiratory: upper respiratory infection

Interactions
Drug-drug. *Amiodarone, verapamil:* increased risk of severe myopathy or rhabdomyolysis
Digoxin: increased digoxin blood level and possible toxicity
Other lipid-lowering drugs (such as fibrates, gemfibrozil, nicotinic acid): myopathy
Potent CYP3A4 inhibitors (clarithromycin, cyclosporine, erythromycin, itraconazole, ketoconazole, nefazodone, protease inhibitors): increased risk of severe myopathy or rhabdomyolysis
Propranolol: decreased bioavailability of both drugs
Warfarin: increased anticoagulant effects
Drug-diagnostic tests. *Alanine aminotransferase, aspartate aminotransferase:* increased levels
Drug-food. *Grapefruit juice (more than 1 qt daily):* increased drug blood level, greater risk of adverse reactions
Drug-herbs. *Red yeast rice:* increased risk of adverse reactions
Drug-behaviors. *Alcohol use:* increased risk of hepatotoxicity

Patient monitoring
- ◀ Watch closely for myositis and other adverse musculoskeletal reactions. Know that drug may cause rhabdomyolysis.
- Monitor liver function tests, CBC, and lipid levels.
- In patients receiving warfarin concurrently, closely monitor prothrombin time and International Normalized Ratio.

Patient teaching
- Advise patient to take with evening meal, but not with large amounts of grapefruit juice.

S

• Tell patient drug may take up to 4 weeks to be effective.
Caution patient to stop taking drug and contact prescriber if she suspects she is pregnant.
Teach patient to recognize and report signs and symptoms of myopathy or hepatic disorders.
• Instruct patient to avoid alcohol and red yeast rice.
• As appropriate, review all other significant and life-threatening adverse reactions and interactions, especially those related to the drugs, tests, foods, herbs, and behaviors mentioned above.

sirolimus
Rapamune

Pharmacologic class: Macrocyclic lactone
Therapeutic class: Immunosuppressant
Pregnancy risk category C

Action
Inhibits early activation and proliferation of T lymphocytes and inhibits cell cycle progression at a later stage

Availability
Oral solution: 1 mg/ml
Tablets: 1 mg, 2 mg

Indications and dosages
➣ Prevention of organ rejection in patients with kidney transplants
Adults and adolescents older than age 13 who weigh more than 40 kg (88 lb): Initially, 6 mg P.O. as a single dose as soon as possible after transplantation, then a maintenance dosage of 2 mg P.O. once daily. Usually given with cyclosporine and corticosteroids.

Dosage adjustment
• Mild to moderate hepatic failure

Contraindications
• Hypersensitivity to drug or its components

Precautions
Use cautiously in:
• renal or hepatic disease, cancer, diabetes mellitus, hyperlipidemia, infectious complications
• patients with liver or lung transplants (use not recommended)
• pregnant or breastfeeding patients
• children younger than age 13.

Administration
• Administer consistently either with or without food.
• Use syringe provided to withdraw prescribed amount. Dilute oral solution in a glass or plastic (not Styrofoam) cup containing at least 2 oz of water or orange juice. Don't use other fluids, especially grapefruit juice.
• Swirl cup to mix drug thoroughly; discard syringe. Administer diluted drug right away. Then fill cup with 4 oz of water or orange juice, and have patient drink fluid right away.
If solution touches skin or mucous membranes, immediately wash affected area with soap and water.
• Wait 4 hours after the cyclosporine dose (if prescribed) before giving sirolimus.

Route	Onset	Peak	Duration
P.O.	Unknown	1-3 hr	Unknown

Adverse reactions
CNS: headache, drowsiness, paresthesia, hypoesthesia, hypertonia, hypertonia, emotional lability, dizziness, confusion, syncope, malaise, asthenia, depression, anxiety, tremor, insomnia
CV: hypertension, hypotension, tachycardia, chest pain, edema, palpitations, vasodilation, peripheral edema, peripheral vascular disorders, **thrombo-**

phlebitis, thrombosis, heart failure, atrial fibrillation, hemorrhage
EENT: abnormal vision, cataract, conjunctivitis, hearing loss, ear pain, otitis media, tinnitus, epistaxis, rhinitis, sinusitis, pharyngitis
GI: nausea, vomiting, diarrhea, constipation, abdominal pain, dyspepsia, hernia, enlarged abdomen, ascites, esophagitis, eructation, flatulence, gastritis, gastroenteritis, dysphagia, stomatitis, mouth ulcers, oral candidiasis, anorexia, **peritonitis**
GU: dysuria, nocturia, pyuria, urinary retention, hematuria, albuminuria, urinary frequency or incontinence, urinary tract infection, pelvic pain, kidney or bladder pain, hydronephrosis, erectile dysfunction, scrotal edema, testes disorders, **oliguria, GU tract hemorrhage, renal tubular necrosis, toxic nephropathy**
Hematologic: anemia, bruising, polycythemia, **leukocytosis, thrombocytopenia, leukopenia, thrombotic thrombocytopenia**
Metabolic: glycosuria, hyperglycemia, diabetes mellitus, hypokalemia, hypophosphatemia, hypovolemia, hypercalcemia, dehydration, Cushing's syndrome, **acidosis**
Respiratory: dyspnea, cough, upper respiratory infection, bronchitis, hypoxia, pneumonia, **atelectasis, pleural effusion, pulmonary edema, asthma**
Skin: skin ulcers, skin hypertrophy, pruritus, fungal dermatitis, hirsutism, rash, acne, cellulites, **non-melanoma skin cancer**
Other: gingivitis, gum hyperplasia, weight changes, neck pain, fever, abscess, chills, facial edema, flulike symptoms, infection, lymphadenopathy, abnormal healing, **sepsis, lymphoma**

Interactions

Drug-drug. *Aminoglycosides, amphotericin, other nephrotoxic drugs:* increased risk of nephrotoxicity
Bromocriptine, cimetidine, clarithromycin, danazol, erythromycin, fluconazole, indinavir, itraconazole, metoclopramide, nicardipine, ritonavir, verapamil, other CYP3A4 inhibitors: decreased sirolimus metabolism and increased blood level
Carbamazepine, phenobarbital, phenytoin, rifabutin, rifampin, other CYP3A4 inducers: decreased sirolimus blood level
Cyclosporine, diltiazem: increased sirolimus blood level
Live-virus vaccines: reduced vaccine efficacy
Drug-diagnostic tests. *Blood urea nitrogen, cholesterol, creatinine, hepatic enzymes, lipids, red blood cells:* increased levels
Calcium, glucose, phosphate, white blood cells: increased or decreased levels
Hemoglobin, magnesium, platelets, sodium: decreased levels
Drug-food. *Grapefruit juice:* decreased sirolimus metabolism and increased blood level
Drug-herbs. *Astragalus, echinacea, melatonin, St. John's wort:* decreased sirolimus efficacy

Patient monitoring

- Watch closely for signs and symptoms of infection.
- Monitor renal function tests, lipid panel, electrolyte levels, blood chemistry studies, and sirolimus blood level.
- Evaluate all body systems carefully, especially cardiovascular and renal.
- Assess neurologic status closely. Implement safety precautions as needed to prevent injury.

Patient teaching

- Teach patient correct procedure for taking drug.
- Advise patient to take consistently either with or without food, but not with grapefruit juice.

S

• Instruct patient to wait 4 hours after cyclosporine dose (if prescribed) before taking sirolimus.

🔊 Tell patient to wash affected area with soap and water immediately if drug touches his skin or mucous membranes.

• Inform patient that drug affects almost every body system. Advise him to report significant adverse reactions.

🔊 Advise patient that drug lowers resistance to infection. Instruct him to immediately report fever, cough, breathing problems, sore throat, or other signs and symptoms of infection.

• Caution patient to avoid driving and other hazardous activities until he knows how drug affects concentration and alertness.

🔊 Instruct patient to immediately report unusual bleeding or bruising.

🔊 Advise female patient to use effective contraception before and during therapy and for 12 weeks after discontinuation.

🔊 Caution patient to limit exposure to sunlight and ultraviolet light. Advise him to wear protective clothing and to use sunscreen with a high protection factor to help prevent skin cancer.

• As appropriate, review all other significant and life-threatening adverse reactions and interactions, especially those related to the drugs, tests, foods, and herbs mentioned above.

sodium bicarbonate

Arm & Hammer Baking Soda, Bell/ans, Citrocarbonate, Neut, Soda Mint

Pharmacologic class: Fluid and electrolyte agent

Therapeutic class: Alkalinizer, antacid

Pregnancy risk category C

Action

Restores body's buffering capacity; neutralizes excess acid

Availability

Injection: 4% (2.4 mEq/5 ml), 4.2% (5 mEq/10 ml), 5% (297.5 mEq/500 ml), 7.5% (8.92 mEq/10 ml and 44.6 mEq/50 ml), 8.4% (10 mEq/10 ml and 50 mEq/50 ml)

Oral solution (Citrocarbonate): sodium 30.46 mEq/3.9 g and sodium citrate 1.82 g/3.9 g

Tablets: 325 mg, 650 mg

Indications and dosages

➢ Metabolic acidosis

Adults and children: 2 to 5 mEq/kg by I.V. infusion over 4 to 8 hours. However, dosage highly individualized based on patient's condition and blood pH and carbon dioxide content.

➢ Urinary alkalization

Adults: Initially, 4 g P.O.; then 1 to 2 g P.O. q 4 hours

Children: 1 to 10 mEq/kg/day P.O. in divided doses given q 4 to 6 hours

➢ Renal tubular acidosis

Adults: For distal tubular acidosis, 0.5 to 2 mEq/kg P.O. daily in four to five equal doses. For proximal tubular acidosis, 4 to 10 mEq/kg P.O. daily in divided doses.

➢ Antacid

Adults: 300 mg to 2 g P.O. up to q.i.d., given with a glass of water

Contraindications

• Hypocalcemia
• Metabolic or respiratory alkalosis
• Hypernatremia
• Hypokalemia
• Severe pulmonary edema
• Seizures
• Vomiting resulting in chloride loss
• Diuretic use resulting in hypochloremic alkalosis
• Acute ingestion of mineral acids (with oral form)

Precautions

Use cautiously in:
- renal insufficiency, heart failure, hypertension, peptic ulcer, cirrhosis, toxemia
- pregnant patients.

Administration

- For I.V. use, infuse at prescribed rate using controlled infusion device.

Don't give concurrently with calcium or catecholamines (such as norepinephrine, dobutamine, dopamine). If patient is receiving sodium bicarbonate with any of these drugs, flush I.V. line thoroughly after each dose to prevent contact between drugs.

Route	Onset	Peak	Duration
P.O.	Unknown	Unknown	Unknown
I.V.	Immediate	Immediate	Unknown

Adverse reactions

CNS: headache, irritability, confusion, stimulation, tremors, twitching, hyperreflexia, weakness, **seizures of alkalosis, tetany**
CV: irregular pulse, edema, **cardiac arrest**
GI: gastric distention, belching, flatulence, acid reflux, **paralytic ileus**
GU: renal calculi
Metabolic: hypokalemia, fluid retention, hypernatremia, **hyperosmolarity** (with overdose), **metabolic alkalosis**
Respiratory: slow and shallow respirations, **cyanosis, apnea**
Other: weight gain, pain and inflammation at I.V. site

Interactions

Drug-drug. *Anorexiants, flecainide, mecamylamine, methenamine, quinidine, sympathomimetics:* increased urinary alkalization, decreased renal clearance of these drugs
Chlorpropamide, lithium, methotrexate, salicylates, tetracycline: increased renal clearance and decreased efficacy of these drugs
Enteric-coated tablets: premature gastric release of these drugs
Drug-diagnostic tests. *Lactate, potassium, sodium:* increased levels
Drug-herbs. *Oak bark:* decreased sodium bicarbonate action

Patient monitoring

When giving I.V., closely monitor arterial blood gas results and electrolyte levels.

Stay alert for signs and symptoms of metabolic alkalosis and electrolyte imbalances.

- Monitor fluid intake and output. Assess for fluid overload.

Avoid rapid infusion, which may cause tetany.

- Watch for inflammation at I.V. site.

Patient teaching

- Tell patient using drug as antacid that too much sodium bicarbonate can cause systemic problems. Urge him to use only the amount approved by prescriber.
- Advise patient not to take oral form with milk. Caution him to avoid the herb oak bark.
- Tell patient sodium bicarbonate interferes with action of many common drugs. Instruct him to notify all prescribers if he's taking oral sodium bicarbonate on a regular basis.
- As appropriate, review all other significant and life-threatening adverse reactions and interactions, especially those related to the drugs, tests, and herbs mentioned above.

S

sodium chloride

Minims Sodium Chloride✱, Slo-Salt, Slow Sodium

Pharmacologic class: Electrolyte supplement
Therapeutic class: Sodium replacement
Pregnancy risk category C

Action

Replaces deficiencies of sodium and chloride and maintains these electrolytes at adequate levels

Availability

Injection: 0.45% sodium chloride—25 ml, 50 ml, 150 ml, 250 ml, 500 ml, 1,000 ml; 0.9% sodium chloride—2 ml, 3 ml, 5 ml, 10 ml, 20 ml, 25 ml, 30 ml, 50 ml, 100 ml, 150 ml, 250 ml, 500 ml, 1,000 ml; 3% sodium chloride—500 ml; 5% sodium chloride—500 ml; 14.6% sodium chloride—20 ml, 40 ml, 200 ml; 23.4% sodium chloride—30 ml, 50 ml, 100 ml, 200 ml
Tablets: 650 mg, 1 g, 2.25 g
Tablets (slow-release): 600 mg

Indications and dosages

➢ Water and sodium chloride replacement; metabolic alkalosis; to dilute or dissolve drugs for I.V., I.M., or subcutaneous use; to flush I.V. catheter; as a priming solution in hemodialysis; to initiate or end blood transfusions
Adults: 0.9% sodium chloride (isotonic solution) with dosage individualized
➢ Hydrating solution; hyperosmolar diabetes
Adults: 0.45% sodium chloride (hypotonic solution) with dosage individualized
➢ Rapid fluid and electrolyte replacement in hyponatremia and hypochloremia; severe sodium depletion; drastic body water dilution after excessive water intake
Adults: 3% or 5% sodium chloride (hypertonic solution) with dosage individualized, given by slow I.V. infusion with close monitoring of electrolyte levels
➢ Heat cramps caused by excessive perspiration
Adults: See product label.

Contraindications

- Normal or elevated electrolyte levels (with 3% and 5% solutions)
- Fluid retention

Precautions

Use cautiously in:
- renal impairment, heart failure, edema or sodium retention, hypoproteinemia
- surgical patients.

Administration

◀ Be aware that sodium chloride injection is a high-alert drug.
- Dilute I.V. dose per product label. Infuse slow I.V. to minimize risk of pulmonary edema.

◀ Don't confuse normal saline solution for injection with concentrates meant for use in total parenteral nutrition.
- Avoid salt tablets for heat cramps; they may pass through GI tract undigested, causing vomiting and potassium loss.

Route	Onset	Peak	Duration
P.O.	Unknown	Unknown	Unknown
I.V.	Immediate	Immediate	Unknown

Adverse reactions

CV: edema (when given too rapidly or in excess), **thrombophlebitis, heart failure exacerbation**
Metabolic: fluid and electrolyte disturbances (such as hypernatremia and hyperphosphatemia), **aggravation of ex-**

isting metabolic acidosis (with excessive infusion)
Respiratory: pulmonary edema
Other: pain, swelling, local tenderness, abscess, or tissue necrosis at I.V. site

Interactions

Drug-diagnostic tests. *Phosphate, potassium, sodium:* increased levels

Patient monitoring

- Monitor electrolyte levels and blood chemistry results.

Watch for signs and symptoms of pulmonary edema or worsening heart failure.

- Carefully monitor vital signs, fluid balance, weight, and cardiovascular status.
- Assess injection site closely to help prevent tissue necrosis and thrombophlebitis.

Patient teaching

Teach patient to recognize and immediately report serious adverse reactions, such as breathing problems or swelling.

- Instruct patient to report pain, tenderness, or swelling at injection site.
- As appropriate, review all other significant and life-threatening adverse reactions and interactions, especially those related to the tests mentioned above.

sodium iodide ^{131}I

Iodotope, Sodium Iodide ^{131}I Therapeutic

Pharmacologic class: Radiopharmaceutical
Therapeutic class: Antithyroid drug
Pregnancy risk category X

Action

Incorporated into iodoamino acids in thyroid and deposited in follicular colloid, from where drug is slowly released. Destructive beta particles in follicle act on thyroidal parenchymal cells, minimizing damage to surrounding tissue.

Availability

Iodotope
Capsules: radioactivity ranging from 1 to 130 millicuries (mCi)/capsule at time of calibration
Sodium Iodide ^{131}I Therapeutic
Capsules: radioactivity ranging from 0.75 to 100 mCi/capsule at time of calibration
Oral solution: radioactivity ranging from 3.5 to 150 mCi/vial at time of calibration

Indications and dosages

➤ Thyroid cancer
Adults: Dosage highly individualized. Usual dosage for ablation of normal thyroid tissue is 50 mCi P.O., with subsequent dosages of 100 to 150 mCi P.O.
➤ Hyperthyroidism
Adults: 4 to 10 mCi P.O. (usually achieves remission without destroying thyroid). Toxic nodular goiter may require higher dosages.

Contraindications

- Vomiting and diarrhea
- Known or suspected pregnancy

S

Precautions

Use cautiously in:

- hypersensitivity to sulfites (with some products)
- breastfeeding
- children (safety and efficacy not established).

Administration

Don't administer if you're pregnant.

- Make sure all antithyroid drugs and thyroid preparations are discontinued 7 days before radioactive iodine therapy begins. Otherwise, consult prescriber about giving thyroid-stimulating hormone for 3 days.
- Instruct patient to fast for 12 hours before therapy starts.
- Know that all doses must be measured by suitable radioactivity calibration system immediately before use.
- For female patient of childbearing age, give drug the week of or week after menstruation.
- Be aware that drug rarely is used to treat hyperthyroidism in patients younger than age 30.

Route	Onset	Peak	Duration
P.O.	Unknown	Unknown	Unknown

Adverse reactions

CNS: unusual fatigue
CV: chest pain, tachycardia
EENT: pain on swallowing, sore throat
GI: nausea, vomiting, severe salivary gland inflammation
Hematologic: anemia, **leukopenia, thrombocytopenia, acute leukemia, bone marrow depression, other blood dyscrasias**
Metabolic: hypothyroidism, transient thyroiditis, **acute thyroid crisis**
Respiratory: cough
Skin: temporary hair thinning, rash, hives, urticaria
Other: chromosomal abnormalities, neck tenderness and swelling, lymphedema, increase in clinical symptoms, weight gain, **radiation sickness, death**

Interactions

Drug-drug. *Other antithyroid drugs (such as methimazole), iodine, thyroid agents:* altered uptake of sodium iodide ^{131}I
Drug-diagnostic tests. *Hemoglobin, platelets, white blood cells:* decreased levels
Procedures using contrast media: altered sodium iodide ^{131}I uptake

Patient monitoring

🔊 Monitor patient to make sure he's following full radiation precautions, including proper body fluid disposal.
🔊 If you're pregnant, don't provide care to patient who has received this drug.
- If patient has received drug for thyroid cancer, limit contact with him to 30 minutes per shift on first day. Increase as required to 1 hour on second day and longer on subsequent days.
- Monitor thyroxine and thyroid-stimulating hormone blood levels, along with CBC with white cell differential.
- Assess fluid intake and output 48 hours after administration. Encourage high fluid intake.
- Watch for signs and symptoms of hypothyroidism, including fatigue, cold intolerance, depression, and sudden weight gain.

🔊 Monitor for bleeding tendency and signs and symptoms of radiation sickness (vomiting, dehydration, skin lesions, and fatigue).

Patient teaching

- Instruct patient to fast for 12 hours before therapy starts and to drink as much fluid as possible for 48 hours after administration.

🔊 Teach patient and significant other how to follow full radiation exposure precautions.
🔊 If patient is receiving drug for thyroid cancer, instruct him to avoid contact with small children. Tell him not to sleep in same room with anyone else for 7 days after receiving dose.
🔊 Teach patient to recognize and report signs and symptoms of hypothyroidism and radiation sickness.
🔊 Advise patient to immediately report unusual bleeding or bruising.

• Tell female patient to inform prescriber if she is pregnant or plans to become pregnant. Caution her not to breastfeed during therapy.
• As appropriate, review all other significant and life-threatening adverse reactions and interactions, especially those related to the drugs and tests mentioned above.

sodium phosphates

Fleet Enema, Fleet Pediatric Enema, Fleet Phospho-Soda, Visicol

Pharmacologic class: Phosphoric acid salt
Therapeutic class: Saline laxative
Pregnancy risk category NR

Action

Promote hyperosmotic effect in small intestine and increase water retention, which indirectly stimulates peristalsis

Availability

Enema: 160 mg/ml sodium phosphate and 60 mg/ml dibasic sodium phosphate
Liquid: 2.4 g/5 ml monobasic sodium phosphate and 900 mg/5 ml dibasic sodium phosphate
Tablets: 1.102 g sodium phosphate and 0.398 g dibasic sodium phosphate

Indications and dosages

➢ Bowel evacuation before colonoscopy
Adults: On night before procedure, three tablets P.O. with 240 ml of clear liquid q 15 minutes; repeat dose until patient has received 7.96 g dibasic sodium phosphate and 22.04 g sodium phosphate (20 tablets). On day of procedure, repeat dose 3 to 5 hours before procedure.

➢ Constipation
Adults and children older than age 12: 20- to 30-ml solution mixed with 120 ml cold water P.O., or 60 to 135 ml P.R. as an enema

Contraindications

• Hypertension
• Signs or symptoms of appendicitis (nausea, vomiting, abdominal pain)
• Acute surgical abdomen
• Renal impairment
• Megacolon
• Intestinal obstruction or perforation
• Edema
• Heart failure
• Sodium-restricted diet

Precautions

Use cautiously in:
• anal excoriation or large hemorrhoids
• pregnant patients.

Administration

• Mix oral solution as indicated on label. Have patient drink it right away.

Route	Onset	Peak	Duration
P.O.	0.5-3 hr	Variable	Variable
P.R.	5-10 min	Variable	Variable

Adverse reactions

CV: hypotension, **widened QRS complex, arrhythmias, cardiac arrest**
GI: nausea, diarrhea, cramps
Metabolic: fluid and electrolyte disturbances (such as hypernatremia and hyperphosphatemia)
Other: laxative dependence

Interactions

Drug-diagnostic tests. *Electrolytes:* decreased levels (with prolonged use)
Phosphate, sodium: increased levels

Patient monitoring

• Monitor fluid balance, electrolyte levels, and cardiovascular status if patient is using drug regularly.

• Monitor bowel habits. Watch for indications of laxative dependence.

Patient teaching

• Tell patient to mix oral solution as indicated on label and to drink it right after mixing.
• For enema use, instruct patient (or caregiver as appropriate) to use water-based lubricant to coat tip of applicator bottle.
• Teach patient to recognize and report signs or symptoms of fluid and electrolyte imbalances.
• Inform patient that drug can cause significant cardiovascular and metabolic effects. Instruct him to use it only for short-term therapy.
• Tell patient that long-term use can cause laxative dependence. Encourage him to increase dietary fiber and fluid intake (unless otherwise contraindicated) to help prevent constipation.
• As appropriate, review all other significant and life-threatening adverse reactions and interactions, especially those related to the tests mentioned above.

sodium polystyrene sulfonate

Kayexalate, K-Exit Poudre✤, Kionex, SPS Sodium Polystyrene Sulfonate

Pharmacologic class: Cation exchange resin
Therapeutic class: Potassium-removing resin
Pregnancy risk category C

Action

Exchanges sodium ions for potassium ions in intestine; potassium is then eliminated in feces, which decreases serum potassium level.

Availability

Oral or rectal powder for suspension: 1.25 g/5 ml
Suspension: 15 g/60 ml

Indications and dosages

➢ Hyperkalemia
Adults: 15 g P.O. one to four times daily in water or syrup, or 30 to 50 g P.R. q 6 hours; may instill through nasogastric tube as necessary

Contraindications

• Hypersensitivity to drug
• Severe hyperkalemia
• Hypokalemia or other electrolyte imbalances

Precautions

Use cautiously in:
• renal or heart failure, severe edema, severe hypertension
• pregnant patients.

Administration

• Know that drug may take hours to days to lower serum potassium level. Thus, it shouldn't be used alone to treat severe hyperkalemia.
• For rectal use, mix resin in water or sorbitol only; never use mineral oil. Insert #28F rubber tube 20 cm into sigmoid colon, and tape it in place. Or use indwelling urinary catheter with 30-ml balloon inflated distal to anal sphincter. Keep rectal solution at room temperature; swirl gently while administering. After giving dose, flush tubing with approximately 100 ml of sodium-free fluid; then flush rectum to remove drug residue.
• In elderly patients prone to fecal impaction, give cleansing enema before sodium polystyrene enema.

Route	Onset	Peak	Duration
P.O.	2-12 hr	Unknown	Unknown
P.R.	Unknown	Unknown	Unknown

Adverse reactions

GI: nausea, vomiting, constipation, fecal impaction, gastric irritation, anorexia
Metabolic: hypokalemia, sodium retention, other electrolyte abnormalities

Interactions

Drug-drug. *Antacids, laxatives:* systemic alkalosis
Drug-diagnostic tests. *Calcium, magnesium, potassium:* decreased levels
Sodium: increased level

Patient monitoring

- Monitor electrolyte levels. Watch for signs and symptoms of electrolyte imbalances, particularly sodium overload.
- Monitor bowel movements. Use measures to prevent or correct constipation or diarrhea, as needed.

Patient teaching

- Tell patient drug may cause constipation (or diarrhea, if given with sorbitol). Instruct him to report these problems.
- Teach patient about recommended diet (generally, low in sodium and potassium).
- For oral use, instruct patient to mix only with water, syrup, or sorbitol—never with orange juice.
- Advise patient to refrigerate oral solution to improve taste.
- As appropriate, review all other significant adverse reactions and interactions, especially those related to the drugs and tests mentioned above.

somatropin, recombinant

Genotropin, Humatrope, Norditropin, Nutropin AQ, Nutropin AQ Pen, Nutropin Depot, Saizen, Serostim, Tev-Tropin, Zorbtive

Pharmacologic class: Posterior pituitary hormone
Therapeutic class: Growth hormone (GH)
Pregnancy risk category B (Genotropin, Saizen, Serostim), ***C***

Action

Stimulates linear and skeletal growth, increases number and size of muscle cells, and influences internal organ size

Availability

Genotropin injection: 1.5 mg (about 4 international units/vial), 5.8 mg (about 15 international units/vial), 13.8 mg (about 41.4 international units/vial)
Humatrope injection: 2 mg (about 6 international units/vial), 5 mg (about 15 international units/vial), 6 mg (about 18 international units/vial), 12 mg (about 36 international units/vial), 24 mg (about 72 international units/vial)
Norditropin injection: 4 mg (12 international units/vial), 8 mg (24 international units/vial)
Norditropin injection cartridge: 5 mg/1.5 ml, 10 mg/1.5 ml, 15 mg/1.5 ml
Nutropin AQ injection: 10 mg
Nutropin AQ Pen injection cartridge: 10 mg
Nutropin Depot: 13.5-mg, 18-mg, and 22.5-mg single-use vials; 13.5-mg, 18-mg, and 22.5-mg kits
Nutropin injection: 5 mg (about 15 international units/vial), 10 mg (about 30 international units/vial)
Saizem injection: 5 g (about 15 international units/vial)

S

Serostim injection: 5 mg (about 15 international units/vial), 6 mg (about 18 international units/vial)
Tev-Tropin injection: 5 mg
Zorbtive injection: 8.8 mg in 10-ml vial

Indications and dosages

➢ Growth failure in children with inadequate endogenous GH
Children: 0.16 to 0.24 mg/kg (Genotropin) subcutaneously q week in six or seven divided doses. Or 0.18 mg/kg/week (Humatrope) subcutaneously or I.M., divided equally and given on three alternate days six times weekly (or daily, if epiphyseal closure hasn't occurred). Or 0.024 to 0.034 mg/kg (Norditropin) subcutaneously six or seven times each week using NordiPen injection pen. Or 0.3 mg/kg/week (Nutropin AQ, Nutropin AQ Pen, Tev-Tropin) subcutaneously in equally divided daily doses. Or 0.06 mg/kg (Saizen) subcutaneously or I.M. three times weekly.

➢ Endogenous GH replacement in adults with GH deficiency
Adults: 0.04 mg/kg/week (Genotropin) subcutaneously in six or seven divided doses. Or 0.006 mg/kg/day (Humatrope) subcutaneously. Or initially, no more than 0.006 mg/kg/day (Nutropin AQ, Nutropin AQ Pen, Tev-Tropin) subcutaneously; may increase to a maximum of 0.025 mg/kg daily in patients younger than age 35 or 0.0125 mg/kg/day in patients ages 35 and older. Or 0.005 mg/kg/day (Saizen) subcutaneously; may increase to a maximum of 0.01 mg/kg/day after 4 weeks, depending on patient tolerance.

➢ Short stature related to Turner's syndrome
Children: 0.375 mg/kg/week (Humatrope) subcutaneously, divided into equal doses given on 3 alternate days or daily. Or up to 0.375 mg/kg/week (Nutropin AQ, Nutropin AQ Pen) subcutaneously, divided into equal doses given three or seven times weekly.

➢ Idiopathic short stature (non–GH-deficient) in children whose epiphyses haven't closed
Children: Up to 0.37 mg/kg (Humatrope) subcutaneously q week. Divide dosage and give in equal doses six or seven times weekly.

➢ Growth failure in children with Prader-Willi syndrome
Children: 0.24 mg/kg/week (Genotropin) subcutaneously in six or seven divided doses

➢ Infants born small for gestational age
Children: 0.48 mg/kg/week (Genotropin) subcutaneously in six or seven divided doses

➢ AIDS wasting or cachexia
Adults and children weighing more than 55 kg (121 lb): 6 mg (Serostim) subcutaneously at bedtime
Adults and children weighing 45 to 55 kg (99 to 121 lb): 5 mg (Serostim) subcutaneously at bedtime
Adults and children weighing 35 to 45 kg (77 to 99 lb): 4 mg (Serostim) subcutaneously at bedtime
Adults and children weighing less than 35 kg (77 lb): 0.1 mg/kg/day (Serostim) subcutaneously at bedtime

➢ Growth failure due to chronic renal insufficiency (up to time of kidney transplantation)
Children: Up to 0.35 mg/kg/weekly (Nutropin AQ, Nutropin AQ Pen) subcutaneously, divided into daily doses

➢ Short bowel syndrome in patients receiving specialized nutritional support
Adults: 0.1 mg/kg/day subcutaneously (Zorbtive), to a maximum of 8 mg/day for no more than 4 weeks

Contraindications

- Hypersensitivity to drug, benzyl alcohol, glycerin, or metacresol (with some diluents)
- Active neoplasia

• Acute, critical illness after open-heart surgery, acute respiratory failure, or multiple trauma
• Children with closed epiphyses
• Neonates (Zorbtive)

Precautions

Use cautiously in:
• hypothyroidism
• diabetes mellitus.

Administration

• Reconstitute by injecting supplied diluent through rubber top of vial and aiming liquid stream at side of vial. Swirl vial gently to mix; don't shake.
• Inspect reconstituted solution. Don't use if it has visible particles or is cloudy.
• Keep diluted drug refrigerated; use within 14 days.
• When using prefilled cartridges, follow manufacturer's instructions carefully.
• Know that patients receiving Zorbtive for short bowel syndrome may receive specialized nutritional support as needed.

Route	Onset	Peak	Duration
I.M., subcut.	Unknown	1-5 hr	12-48 hr

Adverse reactions

CNS: headache, weakness
CV: mild and transient edema
GU: hypercalciuria
Hematologic: leukemia
Metabolic: fluid retention, mild hyperglycemia, hypothyroidism, **ketosis**
Musculoskeletal: localized muscle pain, tissue swelling, joint pain
Skin: rash, urticaria
Other: pain, inflammation at injection site

Interactions

Drug-drug. *Androgens, thyroid hormone:* epiphyseal closure
Corticotrophin, corticosteroids: inhibited growth response (with long-term use)
Drug-diagnostic tests. *Alkaline phosphatase, glucose, inorganic phosphorus, parathyroid hormone:* increased levels

Patient monitoring

• Monitor patient's height, X-rays, blood chemistry results, blood glucose level, and thyroid function studies.
Watch for signs and symptoms of leukemia.

Patient teaching

• Advise patient and parents that regular check-ups and blood tests are needed to detect adverse reactions.
• Teach parents how to reconstitute and administer drug. Stress importance of following manufacturer's instructions carefully when using prefilled cartridges.
• Teach parents about proper handling and disposal of syringes, needles, and cartridges.
• As appropriate, review all significant and life-threatening adverse reactions and interactions, especially those related to the drugs and tests mentioned above.

sotalol hydrochloride

Betapace, Betapace AF, Sotacor✤

S

Pharmacologic class: Beta-adrenergic blocker (nonselective)
Therapeutic class: Antiarrhythmic (classes II and III)
Pregnancy risk category B

Action

Blocks stimulation of cardiac $beta_1$-adrenergic and pulmonary, vascular, and uterine $beta_2$-adrenergic receptor sites. This action reduces cardiac output and blood pressure, depresses sinus heart rate, and prolongs refractory period in atria and ventricles.

Availability

Tablets: 80 mg, 120 mg, 160 mg, 240 mg
Tablets (Betapace AF): 80 mg, 120 mg, 160 mg

Indications and dosages

➢ Ventricular arrhythmias
Adults: 80 mg P.O. b.i.d. (Betapace); may increase dosage gradually. For maintenance, 160 to 320 mg/day in two to three divided doses; some patients may require 240 to 320 mg/day in divided doses. For refractory ventricular fibrillation, may increase to 480 to 640 mg/day in divided doses.
➢ Atrial fibrillation or atrial flutter
Adults: 80 mg P.O. b.i.d. (Betapace AF). With careful monitoring, may increase to 120 mg b.i.d. p.r.n., to a maximum of 160 P.O. b.i.d.

Dosage adjustment

• Renal impairment

Contraindications

• Hypersensitivity to drug
• Uncontrolled heart failure
• Bronchial asthma, chronic obstructive pulmonary disease
• Congenital or acquired long-QT syndrome
• Sinus bradycardia, second- or third-degree atrioventricular (AV) block (unless patient has pacemaker)
• Sick sinus syndrome
• Cardiogenic shock
• Hypokalemia
• Creatinine clearance below 40 ml/minute

Precautions

Use cautiously in:
• renal or hepatic impairment, diabetes mellitus, hyperthyroidism
• history of severe allergic reactions
• elderly patients
• pregnant or breastfeeding patients
• children (safety not established).

Administration

• Give 1 hour before or 2 hours after meals or antacids.
• Keep in mind that Betapace and Betapace AF have different indications and are not interchangeable or therapeutically equivalent.

Route	Onset	Peak	Duration
P.O.	Unknown	2-4 hr	8-12 hr

Adverse reactions

CNS: fatigue, weakness, anxiety, dizziness, drowsiness, insomnia, memory loss, depression, mental status changes, nervousness, paresthesia, nightmares
CV: orthostatic hypotension, peripheral vasoconstriction, bradycardia, **arrhythmias, heart failure, AV block**
EENT: blurred vision, dry eyes, nasal stuffiness
GI: nausea, constipation, diarrhea
GU: erectile dysfunction, decreased libido
Metabolic: hyperglycemia, **hypoglycemia**
Musculoskeletal: joint pain, back pain, muscle cramps
Respiratory: wheezing, **bronchospasm**
Skin: itching, rash
Other: lupus syndrome, hypersensitivity reaction

Interactions

Drug-drug. *Amphetamines, ephedrine, epinephrine, norepinephrine, phenylephrine, pseudoephedrine:* unopposed alpha-adrenergic stimulation, causing excessive hypotension and bradycardia
Beta-adrenergic bronchodilators, theophylline: decreased efficacy of these drugs
Calcium channel blockers: increased risk of adverse cardiovascular reactions
Class IA antiarrhythmics (such as amiodarone, quinidine): increased risk of arrhythmias

Clonidine: excessive rebound hypertension with clonidine withdrawal
Ergot alkaloids: peripheral ischemia or gangrene
General anesthetics, phenytoin (I.V.), verapamil: additive myocardial depression
Lidocaine: increased lidocaine blood level, resulting in toxicity
Sulfonylureas: increased hypoglycemic effect
Drug-diagnostic tests. *Antinuclear antibody:* increased titers
Blood urea nitrogen, glucose, lipoproteins, potassium, triglycerides, uric acid: increased levels
Drug-food. *Any food:* decreased drug absorption

Patient monitoring

- Monitor ECG, electrolyte levels, and vital signs closely for first 3 days of therapy.
- Assess patient closely for signs and symptoms of heart failure.
- In long-term use, watch for signs and symptoms of drug-induced lupus syndrome.

Patient teaching

- Tell patient drug may cause significant cardiac effects. Explain need for ECG monitoring during first few days of therapy.

Teach patient to recognize and immediately report signs and symptoms of heart failure and electrolyte imbalances.

- Inform patient that drug can cause serious interactions with many common drugs. Instruct him to tell all prescribers he's taking it.

Teach patient to recognize and promptly report signs and symptoms of drug-induced lupus syndrome.

- Advise patient that drug may cause CNS effects that increase his injury risk. Encourage him to use appropriate safety precautions.
- As appropriate, review all other significant and life-threatening adverse reactions and interactions, especially those related to the drugs, tests, and foods mentioned above.

spironolactone

Aldactone, Novo-spiroton*

Pharmacologic class: Aldosterone inhibitor

Therapeutic class: Potassium-sparing diuretic

Pregnancy risk category D

Action

Inhibits aldosterone effects in distal renal tubule, promoting sodium and water excretion and potassium retention

Availability

Tablets: 25 mg, 50 mg, 100 mg

Indications and dosages

➢ Edema caused by heart failure, hepatic cirrhosis, or nephrotic syndrome
Adults: As sole diuretic, initially 100 mg/day P.O. (range of 25 to 200 mg) in single or divided doses, continued for 5 or more days and then adjusted to optimal therapeutic level
Children: 1 to 3 mg/kg/day P.O. as a single dose or in divided doses
➢ Essential hypertension
Adults: Initially, 50 to 100 mg/day P.O. as a single dose or in divided doses, continued for at least 2 weeks
Children: 1 to 2 mg/kg P.O. b.i.d.
➢ Hypokalemia
Adults: 25 to 100 mg/day P.O.
➢ Diagnosis and treatment of primary hyperaldosteronism
Adults: For diagnosis, 400 mg/day P.O. for 4 days in short test or for 3 to 4 weeks in long test. Resolution of hypokalemia and hypertension confirm

S

diagnosis of primary hyperaldosteronism. Dosages of 100 to 400 mg/day P.O. may be used as a bridge to surgical therapy; in patients unsuitable for this therapy, lowest effective dosage may be used for long-term maintenance.

Off-label uses

• Acne vulgaris
• Familial male precocious puberty (given with other drugs)
• Premenstrual syndrome

Contraindications

• Hypersensitivity to drug
• Anuria
• Acute or chronic renal insufficiency
• Hyperkalemia
• Concurrent use of other potassium-sparing diuretics (such as amiloride, triamterene) or potassium supplements

Precautions

Use cautiously in:
• hepatic dysfunction, diabetes mellitus, fluid and electrolyte imbalances
• elderly or debilitated patients
• pregnant or breastfeeding patients
• children (safety not established).

Administration

• Give single daily dose with breakfast. If two daily doses are prescribed, give second dose with food in mid-afternoon.

Route	Onset	Peak	Duration
P.O.	Unknown	1-2 hr	2-3 days

Adverse reactions

CNS: headache, drowsiness, lethargy, ataxia, confusion
GI: vomiting, diarrhea, cramping, gastritis, GI ulcers, **GI bleeding**
GU: gynecomastia, irregular menses or amenorrhea, postmenopausal bleeding, erectile dysfunction, **breast cancer**
Hematologic: agranulocytosis
Metabolic: hyponatremia, **hyperchloremic metabolic acidosis, hyperkalemia**
Skin: rash, pruritus, hirsutism
Other: deepening of voice, drug fever

Interactions

Drug-drug. *Angiotensin-converting enzyme inhibitors, potassium-sparing diuretics, potassium supplements, other potassium-containing drugs:* increased risk of hyperkalemia
Anticoagulants, heparin: reduced hypoprothrombinemic effects of these drugs
Digoxin: increased digoxin blood level
Salicylates: decreased diuretic effect
Drug-diagnostic tests. *Blood urea nitrogen, potassium:* increased levels
Digoxin assays: false digoxin elevation
Granulocytes: decreased count
Drug-food. *Potassium-containing salt substitutes:* increased risk of hyperkalemia
Drug-herbs. *Licorice:* potassium loss

Patient monitoring

◀ Monitor electrolyte levels (especially potassium). Watch for signs and symptoms of imbalances and metabolic acidosis.
• Monitor weight and fluid intake and output. Stay alert for indications of fluid imbalance.
• Monitor CBC with white cell differential.

Patient teaching

• Tell patient to take daily dose with breakfast. If two daily doses are prescribed, advise him to take second dose with food in mid-afternoon.
• Advise patient to restrict intake of high-potassium foods and to avoid licorice and salt substitutes containing potassium.
• Tell male patient drug may cause breast enlargement.

• Caution patient to avoid driving and other hazardous activities until he knows how drug affects concentration and alertness.
• As appropriate, review all other significant and life-threatening adverse reactions and interactions, especially those related to the drugs, tests, foods, and herbs mentioned above.

stavudine (d4T)
Zerit

Pharmacologic class: Nucleoside reverse transcriptase inhibitor
Therapeutic class: Antiretroviral
Pregnancy risk category C

Action
Inhibits replication of human immunodeficiency virus (HIV) by interfering with the enzyme reverse transcriptase, thereby terminating DNA chain

Availability
Capsules: 15 mg, 20 mg, 30 mg, 40 mg
Powder for oral solution: 1 mg/ml

Indications and dosages
➢ HIV-1 infection
Adults weighing 60 kg (132 lb) or more: 40 mg P.O. q 12 hours
Adults and children weighing less than 60 kg (132 lb): 30 mg P.O. q 12 hours
Children weighing 30 kg (66 lb) or more: 30 mg P.O. q 12 hours
Children 14 days and older who weigh less than 30 kg (66 lb): 1 mg/kg P.O. q 12 hours
Newborns to infants 13 days old: 0.5 mg/kg P.O. q 12 hours

Dosage adjustment
• Renal impairment
• Elderly patients

Contraindications
• Hypersensitivity to drug or its components
• Lactic acidosis
• Hyperlactatemia
• Severe hepatotoxicity

Precautions
Use cautiously in:
• advanced HIV infection, bone marrow depression, renal failure, peripheral neuropathy
• pregnant or breastfeeding patients.

Administration
• Give with or without food.
• Know that drug is usually given with other antiretrovirals.

Route	Onset	Peak	Duration
P.O.	Variable	60-90 min	Unknown

Adverse reactions
CNS: headache, insomnia, peripheral neuropathy
GI: nausea, vomiting, diarrhea, abdominal pain, anorexia, **pancreatitis**
Hematologic: anemia, **leukopenia, thrombocytopenia**
Hepatic: hepatic steatosis, hepatitis, hepatic failure
Metabolic: increased glucose tolerance, **lactic acidosis**
Musculoskeletal: myalgia
Skin: rash
Other: chills, fever, allergic reaction

Interactions
Drug-drug. *Chloramphenicol, dapsone, didanosine, ethambutol, hydralazine, hydroxyurea, lithium, phenytoin, vincristine, zalcitabine:* increased risk of peripheral neuropathy
Doxorubicin, ribavarin, zidovudine: inhibition of stavudine's absorption and metabolism
Myelosuppressants: increased bone marrow depression

S

Drug-diagnostic tests. *Alanine aminotransferase, amylase, aspartate aminotransferase, bilirubin, gamma-glutamyl transferase, lipase:* increased levels
Neutrophils, platelets: decreased counts

Patient monitoring

Monitor closely for signs and symptoms of lactic acidosis. Consult prescriber about drug discontinuation if these occur.
• Watch for and report onset and worsening of peripheral neuropathy.
Monitor CBC. Report evidence of bone marrow depression.
• Monitor liver function tests and blood chemistry results.

Patient teaching

• Tell patient he may take with or without food.
Teach patient to recognize and promptly report signs and symptoms of lactic acidosis (such as fatigue, GI distress, and difficult or rapid breathing).
• Instruct patient to report numbness or tingling in arms, legs, hands, or feet.
• Caution female patient not to breastfeed, because she may transmit drug effects and HIV to infant.
• As appropriate, review all other significant and life-threatening adverse reactions and interactions, especially those related to the drugs and tests mentioned above.

streptokinase

Streptase

Pharmacologic class: Group C beta-hemolytic streptococcal nonenzymatic protein
Therapeutic class: Thrombolytic
Pregnancy risk category C

Action

Converts plasminogen to plasmin, an enzyme that degrades fibrin clots and lyses thrombi and emboli

Availability

Powder for injection: 250,000, 750,000, and 1.5 million international units/vial

Indications and dosages

➢ Acute evolving transmural myocardial infarction
Adults: 1.5 million international units by I.V. infusion over 1 hour as soon as possible after symptom onset. For intracoronary infusion, 20,000 international units by I.V. bolus via coronary catheter, followed by infusion of 2,000 international units/minute over 1 hour (total of 140,000 international units).
➢ Deep-vein thrombosis (DVT)
Adults: Loading dose of 250,000 international units by I.V. infusion over 30 minutes, followed by 100,000 international units/hour I.V. for 72 hours. Begin therapy as soon as possible after thrombotic symptoms begin (preferably within 7 days).
➢ Pulmonary emboli
Adults: Loading dose of 250,000 international units by I.V. infusion over 30 minutes, then 100,000 international units/hour I.V. for 24 hours (or 72 hours if concurrent DVT is suspected). Begin therapy as soon as possible after thrombotic symptoms begin (preferably within 7 days).
➢ Arterial thrombosis or emboli
Adults: Loading dose of 250,000 international units by I.V. infusion over 30 minutes, then 100,000 international units/hour I.V. for 24 to 72 hours. Begin therapy as soon as possible after thrombotic symptoms begin (preferably within 7 days).

Contraindications

• Hypersensitivity to drug or anistreplase

• Cerebrovascular accident, intracranial or intraspinal surgery within past 2 months
• Active internal bleeding
• Intracranial neoplasm
• Severe, uncontrolled hypertension

Precautions

Use cautiously in:
• severe hepatic or renal disease, recent major surgery or trauma, obstetric delivery, acute pericarditis, infectious endocarditis, atrioventricular malformation or aneurysm, suspected thrombus in left side of heart, septic thrombophlebitis or occluded arteriovenous cannula at seriously infected site
• conditions in which bleeding may be hard to manage (such as organ biopsy, peptic ulcer, previous puncture of noncompressible blood vessel)
• history of cerebrovascular disease
• use of drug within past 2 years
• concurrent anticoagulant use
• elderly patients
• pregnant or breastfeeding patients.

Administration

Before giving, make sure hydrocortisone is available to treat allergic reaction and aminocaproic acid is available to treat excessive bleeding.
As ordered, give test dose of 100 international units intradermally to check for hypersensitivity. Wheal-and-flare response within 20 minutes indicates probable allergy.
• To reconstitute, add 5 ml of normal saline solution or dextrose 5% in water to each vial, then dilute again to 45 ml. Roll vial gently between hands; don't shake.
• If necessary, dilute further to 50 ml in plastic container or to 500 ml in glass bottle.
• Don't mix with other drugs or give other drugs through same I.V. line.

Route	Onset	Peak	Duration
I.V.	Immediate	1 hr	4 hr
Intra-coronary	Unknown	Unknown	Unknown

Adverse reactions

CNS: headache, **intracranial hemorrhage**
CV: hypotension, **arrhythmias**
EENT: periorbital swelling
GI: nausea, vomiting, **GI hemorrhage**
GU: hematuria
Hematologic: anemia, **bleeding tendency**
Musculoskeletal: musculoskeletal pain
Respiratory: minor breathing difficulties, **bronchospasm, apnea**
Skin: urticaria, itching, flushing
Other: bleeding at puncture sites, delayed hypersensitivity reaction

Interactions

Drug-drug. *Anticoagulants, aspirin, dipyridamole, indomethacin, phenylbutazone:* increased risk of bleeding
Drug-diagnostic tests. *Hemoglobin:* decreased value
International Normalized Ratio, transaminases: increased values
Partial thromboplastin time (PTT), prothrombin time (PT): prolonged

Patient monitoring

• Monitor vital signs and neurologic status carefully after giving test dose and throughout therapy.
Watch for signs and symptoms of hypersensitivity reaction. Stop drug if these occur.
• Check for bleeding every 15 minutes for first hour, every 30 minutes for next 7 hours, then every 4 hours.
Stop therapy and contact prescriber immediately if excessive bleeding occurs.
• Assess neurologic status closely. Watch for indications of intracranial bleeding.

S

• Handle patient gently and sparingly. If necessary, pad bed rails to prevent injury.
• Monitor pulse rate every hour. Also monitor distal circulation.
• Monitor PTT, PT, plasma thrombin time, hemoglobin, hematocrit, and platelet count.
• Avoid giving I.M. injections during therapy.

Patient teaching

• Tell patient why he's receiving drug.
• Teach patient to recognize and immediately report signs or symptoms of hypersensitivity reaction or excessive bleeding.
• Instruct patient to report unusual bruising or bleeding. Teach him safety measures to avoid bruising and bleeding.
• Advise patient that he'll undergo regular blood testing during therapy.
• As appropriate, review all other significant and life-threatening adverse reactions and interactions, especially those related to the drugs and tests mentioned above.

streptomycin sulfate

Pharmacologic class: Aminoglycoside
Therapeutic class: Anti-infective
Pregnancy risk category D

Action

Binds to 30S ribosomal subunit, inhibiting protein synthesis in bacterial cell, which causes misreading of genetic code and, ultimately, cell death

Availability

Injection: 400 mg/ml in 2.5-ml ampules, 200 mg/ml in 1-g vials

Indications and dosages

➢ Adjunct in tuberculosis and other mycobacterial infections
Adults: 15 mg/kg/day I.M., up to 1 g/day
Children: 20 to 40 mg/kg I.M. daily, up to 1 g/day
➢ Enterococcal or streptococcal infections
Adults: 1 g I.M. b.i.d. for 1 week, then 500 mg I.M. b.i.d. for 1 week. For enterococcal endocarditis, 1 g I.M. b.i.d. given with penicillin for 1 week, then 500 mg I.M. b.i.d. for 4 weeks.
➢ Brucellosis
Adults: 1 g I.M. once or twice daily with tetracycline or doxycycline for 1 week, then once daily for at least 1 more week
➢ Tularemia
Adults: 1 to 2 g I.M. daily in divided doses for 7 to 14 days until patient is afebrile for 5 to 7 days. For tularemia caused by *Francisella tularensis*, 1 g I.M. b.i.d. for 10 days or 7.5 to 10 mg/kg I.M. b.i.d. for 10 to 14 days.
➢ Plague caused by *Yersinis pestis*
Adults: 1 g I.M. b.i.d. for 10 to 14 days

Dosage adjustment

• Renal impairment
• Elderly patients

Off-label uses

• *Mycobacterium avium-intracellulare* complex in AIDS patients

Contraindications

• Hypersensitivity to drug, other aminoglycosides, or bisulfites

Precautions

Use cautiously in:
• renal impairment, hearing impairment, neuromuscular disease (such as myasthenia gravis)
• elderly patients
• pregnant or breastfeeding patients

• infants and neonates (safety not established).

Administration

• Inject I.M. deep into upper outer quadrant of buttock.
• Alternate injection sites.
• Know that drug may be given with other antituberculars.
• Be aware that streptomycin will be withdrawn after several months or when bacteriologic smears are negative and other antituberculars are continued for 1 year.

Route	Onset	Peak	Duration
I.M.	Rapid	30-90 min	Unknown

Adverse reactions

CNS: vertigo, numbness and tingling, peripheral neuropathy, myasthenia gravis–like syndrome, **neuromuscular blockade, seizures**
CV: myocarditis
EENT: amblyopia, ototoxicity
GI: nausea, vomiting
GU: azotemia, **nephrotoxicity**
Hematologic: eosinophilia, **hemolytic anemia, pancytopenia, leukopenia, thrombocytopenia**
Hepatic: hepatic necrosis
Musculoskeletal: muscle weakness, twitching
Respiratory: apnea
Skin: rash, urticaria, exfoliative dermatitis, toxic epidermal necrolysis, angioedema
Other: fever, superinfection, **serum sickness, anaphylaxis**

Interactions

Drug-drug. *Acyclovir, amphotericin B, cephalosporin, cisplatin, potent diuretics, vancomycin:* increased risk of ototoxicity and nephrotoxicity
Depolarizing and nondepolarizing neuromuscular blockers, general anesthetics: potentiation of neuromuscular blockade
Dimenhydrinate: masking of ototoxicity symptoms
Indomethacin: increased streptomycin peak and trough blood levels
Parenteral penicillins (ampicillin, ticarcillin): streptomycin inactivation
Drug-diagnostic tests. *Bilirubin, blood urea nitrogen, creatinine, lactate dehydrogenase, nonprotein nitrogen:* increased levels
Granulocytes, hemoglobin, platelets, white blood cells: decreased levels

Patient monitoring

• Draw blood for peak drug level 1 hour after I.M. injection. Draw blood for trough level just before next dose.
• Monitor liver and kidney function tests. Watch for evidence of hepatotoxicity and nephrotoxicity.
• Monitor temperature. Stay alert for fever and other signs and symptoms of superinfection.
• Assess neurologic status and sensory function carefully. Watch closely for neurotoxicity, neuromuscular blockade, and seizures.
• Assess for signs and symptoms of ototoxicity.
• Monitor CBC. Watch for evidence of blood dyscrasias.

Patient teaching

• Instruct patient to report unusual bleeding or bruising.
Inform patient that drug can be toxic to many body systems. Teach him to recognize and immediately report serious adverse reactions.
Tell patient drug may promote growth of certain organisms. Advise him to immediately report signs and symptoms of superinfection.
• Inform patient that drug may impair cognitive, motor, and sensory function. Advise him to use caution when driving and performing other hazardous activities.
• As appropriate, review all other significant and life-threatening adverse

S

reactions and interactions, especially those related to the drugs and tests mentioned above.

sucralfate

Carafate, Nu-Sucralfate✱, PMS-Sucralfate✱, Sulcrate✱

Pharmacologic class: GI protectant
Therapeutic class: Antiulcer agent
Pregnancy risk category B

Action

Combines with gastric acid to form protective coating on ulcer surface, inhibiting gastric acid secretion, pepsin, and bile salts

Availability

Oral suspension: 500 mg/5 ml
Tablets: 1 g

Indications and dosages

➢ Active duodenal ulcer
Adults: 1 g P.O. q.i.d. 1 hour before meals and at bedtime or 2 g b.i.d. for 4 to 8 weeks. For maintenance, 1 g P.O. b.i.d.

Off-label uses

- Gastroesophageal reflux
- GI symptoms caused by nonsteroidal anti-inflammatory drugs (including aspirin)
- Prevention of stress ulcers and GI bleeding in critically ill patients
- Oral and esophageal ulcers caused by radiation, chemotherapy, or sclerotherapy (oral suspension)

Contraindications

None

Precautions

Use cautiously in:
- renal failure
- pregnant or breastfeeding patients
- children.

Administration

- When giving through nasogastric tube, reconstitute drug and flush tube with water after administration.

Route	Onset	Peak	Duration
P.O.	Unknown	Unknown	6 hr

Adverse reactions

EENT: rhinitis
GI: constipation
Respiratory: respiratory difficulty
Skin: pruritus, rash
Other: facial swelling, hypersensitivity reaction

Interactions

Drug-drug. *Aluminum-containing antacids:* increased total body burden of aluminum
Anticoagulants: decreased hypoprothrombinemic effect
Diclofenac: decreased pharmacologic effects of diclofenac
Digoxin, quinidine: reduced blood levels and efficacy of these drugs
Histamine$_2$-receptor antagonists (such as cimetidine, ranitidine), fluoroquinolones, ketoconazole, tetracyclines, theophylline: decreased bioavailability of these drugs
Levothyroxine, penicillamine: decreased efficacy of these drugs
Phenytoin: decreased phenytoin absorption

Patient monitoring

- Monitor bowel pattern. Report severe, ongoing constipation.
- Assess for rash and itching.

Patient teaching

- Tell patient to take 1 hour before meals and again at bedtime.
- Caution patient not to take within 30 minutes of antacids or other drugs.

• Explain importance of completing entire course of therapy as prescribed, even after pain and other ulcer symptoms improve.
• As appropriate, review all other significant adverse reactions and interactions, especially those related to the drugs mentioned above.

sulfacetamide sodium

AK-Sulf, Bleph-10, Klaron, Ocu-Sul 10, Ocu-Sul 15, Ocu-Sul 30, Sodium Sulamyd

Pharmacologic class: Sulfonamide
Therapeutic class: Anti-infective
Pregnancy risk category C

Action

Inhibits bacterial synthesis of folic acid by preventing condensation of pteridine with aminobenzoic acid through competitive inhibition of dihydropteroate synthetase

Availability

Lotion: 10% in 2-oz and 4-oz bottles
Ointment: 10% in 5-g tubes
Ophthalmic solution: 10%, 15%, and 30% in 5-ml and 15-ml dropper bottles

Indications and dosages

➢ Acne vulgaris
Adults and children ages 12 and older: Apply thin film topically to affected areas b.i.d.
➢ Superficial ocular infections (including conjunctivitis)
Adults and children ages 2 months and older: Initially, apply one to two drops of ophthalmic solution into conjunctival sac of affected eye q 2 to 3 hours, or apply approximately ½" ribbon of ophthalmic ointment into conjunctival sacs of affected eye q 3 to 4 hours and at bedtime. Taper by increasing dosing intervals as condition responds. Usual duration is 7 to 10 days.
➢ Adjunct in trachoma
Adults: Apply two drops of ophthalmic solution into conjunctival sac of affected eye q 2 hours; must be accompanied by systemic sulfonamide therapy.

Contraindications

• Hypersensitivity to drug or other sulfonamides

Precautions

Use cautiously in:
• sulfite allergy
• dry eye syndrome.

Administration

• To avoid contamination, don't touch container tip to eye, eyelid, or any other surface.

Route	Onset	Peak	Duration
Ophth., topical	Unknown	Unknown	Unknown

Adverse reactions

EENT: conjunctival hyperemia, eye burning, stinging, tearing (ophthalmic form)
Skin: local irritation, erythema, itching and edema (topical form), photosensitivity reaction
Other: secondary infections

Interactions

Drug-drug. *Porfimer:* increased severity of photosensitivity reaction, leading to excessive tissue damage
Silver preparations: precipitation

Patient monitoring

• Monitor patient for drug efficacy. Know that drug may be inactivated by purulent exudate.

S

Patient teaching

- Tell patient to apply a thin film of lotion to affected areas, as prescribed.
- Teach patient how to apply ophthalmic form. Instruct him to always wash hands first and to clean eye area of discharge by wiping from inner to outer area before applying.
- As appropriate, review all other significant adverse reactions and interactions, especially those related to the drugs mentioned above.

sulfadiazine

Pharmacologic class: Sulfonamide (intermediate acting)
Therapeutic class: Anti-infective
Pregnancy risk category C

Action

Inhibits formation of bacterial folic acid from para-aminobenzoic acid (PABA), preventing bacterial cell-wall synthesis and exerting a bacteriostatic effect

Availability

Tablets: 500 mg

Indications and dosages

➢ Nocardiosis
Adults: 4 to 8 g P.O. daily in divided doses for at least 6 weeks
➢ Adjunct in toxoplasmosis
Adults: 1 to 1.5 g P.O. daily divided q 6 hours with pyrimethamine for 3 to 4 weeks or until improvement occurs
Children: 100 to 200 mg/kg P.O. daily for 3 to 4 weeks
➢ To prevent relapse of toxoplasmosis in patients with human immunodeficiency virus
Adults and adolescents: 0.5 to 1g P.O. q 6 hours, given with pyrimethamine and leucovorin
Children: 85 to 120 mg/kg P.O. daily in two to four divided doses, given with pyrimethamine and leucovorin
➢ Asymptomatic meningococcal carriers
Adults and children older than age 12: 1g P.O. b.i.d. for 2 days
Children ages 1 to 12: 500 mg P.O. b.i.d. for 2 days
Infants ages 2 to 12 months: 500 mg P.O. daily for 2 days
➢ To prevent recurrent rheumatic fever (as penicillin alternative)
Children weighing 30 kg (66 lb) or more: 1 g P.O. daily
Children weighing less than 30 kg (66 lb): 500 mg P.O. daily

Contraindications

- Hypersensitivity to drug, other sulfonamides, sulfonylureas, thiazides, or loop diuretics
- Porphyria
- Marked renal or hepatic impairment
- Pregnancy at term or when premature birth is possible
- Infants younger than 2 months

Precautions

Use cautiously in:
- urinary obstruction, renal or hepatic disease, bronchial asthma, G6PD deficiency, group A beta-hemolytic streptococcal infections, blood dyscrasias
- history of multiple allergies
- pregnant (before term) or breastfeeding patients.

Administration

- Give with full glass of water. Encourage abundant fluid intake to minimize crystal formation in urine.

Route	Onset	Peak	Duration
P.O.	Unknown	4-6 hr	Unknown

Adverse reactions

CNS: headache, depression, hallucinations, insomnia, drowsiness, vertigo, fatigue, apathy, anxiety, ataxia,

polyneuritis, peripheral neuropathy, **seizures**
CV: allergic myocarditis or pericarditis
EENT: periorbital edema, optic neuritis, transient myopia, tinnitus
GI: nausea, vomiting, abdominal pain, stomatitis, glossitis, anorexia, dry mouth, pancreatitis, **pseudomembranous colitis**
GU: hematuria, proteinuria, **crystalluria, toxic nephrosis with oliguria and anuria, renal failure**
Hematologic: megaloblastic anemia, agranulocytosis, aplastic anemia, thrombocytopenia, leukopenia, hemolytic anemia
Hepatic: jaundice, **hepatitis, hepatocellular necrosis**
Respiratory: shortness of breath, pleuritis, **allergic pneumonitis, pulmonary infiltrates, fibrosing alveolitis**
Skin: generalized skin eruption, urticaria, pruritus, alopecia, local irritation, exfoliative dermatitis, photosensitivity reaction, **epidermal necrolysis, erythema multiforme, Stevens-Johnson syndrome**
Other: chills, drug fever, hypersensitivity reactions including **anaphylaxis, serum sickness, lupus-like syndrome**

Interactions

Drug-drug. *Cyclosporine:* increased nephrotoxicity
Hydantoins: increased hydantoin blood level
Indomethacin, probenecid: increased sulfadiazine blood level
Methenamine: increased risk of crystalluria, causing serious adverse reactions
Methotrexate: increased risk of bone marrow depression
Oral anticoagulants: increased anticoagulant effect
PABA, PABA-derived local anesthetics: inhibited sulfadiazine action
Sulfonylureas: increased risk of hypoglycemia
Thiazide diuretics: increased thrombocytopenic effect
Uricosuric drugs: increased effects of these drugs
Drug-diagnostic tests. *Bilirubin, blood urea nitrogen, creatinine, eosinophils, transaminases:* increased levels
Granulocytes, hemoglobin, platelets, white blood cells: decreased levels
Urine glucose test: false-positive result
Drug-herbs. *Dong quai, St. John's wort:* increased risk of photosensitivity
Drug-behaviors. *Sun exposure:* increased risk of photosensitivity

Patient monitoring

🔊 Monitor CBC with white cell differential. Watch for evidence of blood dyscrasias.
🔊 Stay alert for signs of erythema multiforme. Report early signs before condition can progress to Stevens-Johnson syndrome.
- Monitor patient for signs and symptoms of superinfection, including fever, tachycardia, and chills.

🔊 Monitor liver function tests. Be alert for signs and symptoms of hepatitis.
🔊 Monitor kidney function tests weekly. Evaluate patient's fluid intake, urine output, and urine pH. Promptly report hematuria, oliguria, or anuria.
- Monitor neurologic status. Report seizures, hallucinations, or depression.

Patient teaching

- Tell patient to take on regular schedule as prescribed, along with a full glass of water. Instruct him to drink plenty of fluids to minimize crystal formation in urine.
- Advise patient to complete full course of treatment, even if he feels better after a few days.

🔊 Instruct patient to immediately report signs and symptoms of hypersensitivity, especially rash.
🔊 Tell patient drug can cause blood disorders, GI and liver problems, seri-

S

ous skin reactions, and other infections. Describe key warning signs and symptoms (easy bruising or bleeding, severe diarrhea, unusual tiredness, yellowing of skin or eyes, sore throat, rash, cough, mouth sores, fever). Instruct him to report these right away.

Clinical alert: Advise patient to promptly report scant urine, bloody urine, or inability to urinate.

• Urge patient to contact prescriber if he experiences depression.
• Teach patient effective measures to counteract drug's photosensitivity effect. Tell him that dong quai and St. John's wort increase phototoxicity risk; caution him not to take these herbs during therapy.
• Advise female patient to tell prescriber if she is pregnant. Caution her not to take drug near term or if she is breastfeeding.
• As appropriate, review all other significant and life-threatening adverse reactions and interactions, especially those related to the drugs, tests, herbs, and behaviors mentioned above.

sulfamethoxazole-trimethoprim (co-trimoxazole)

Apo-Sulfatrim♣, Apo-Sulfatrim DS♣, Bactrim, Bactrim DS, Cotrim, Cotrim DS, Novo-Trimel♣, Novo-Trimel DS♣, Nu-Cotrimox♣, Nu-Cotrimox DS♣, Septra, Septra DS, Septra Grape, Sulfamethoprim, Sulfamethoprim-DS, Sulfatrim, Trisulfa♣, Trisulfa DS♣, Trisulfa S Suspension♣

Pharmacologic class: Sulfonamide
Therapeutic class: Anti-infective
Pregnancy risk category C

Action

Sulfamethoxazole inhibits bacterial synthesis of dihydrofolic acid by competing with para-aminobenzoic acid (PABA). Trimethoprim inhibits enzymes of folic acid pathways.

Availability

Injection: 80 mg/ml sulfamethoxazole and 16 mg/ml trimethoprim
Suspension: 200 mg sulfamethoxazole and 40 mg trimethoprim/5 ml
Tablets: 400 mg sulfamethoxazole and 80 mg trimethoprim (single strength); 800 mg sulfamethoxazole and 160 mg trimethoprim (double strength)

Indications and dosages

➢ Urinary tract infections caused by susceptible organisms

Adults: One double-strength tablet or two single-strength tablets or 20 ml suspension P.O. q 12 hours for 10 to 14 days

Children ages 2 months and older: 40 mg/kg sulfamethoxazole and 8 mg/kg trimethoprim P.O. q 12 hours for 10 days

➢ Severe urinary tract infections caused by susceptible organisms

Adults and children ages 2 months and older: 8 to 10 mg/kg (based on trimethoprim component) I.V. q 6, 8, or 12 hours for up to 14 days

➢ Shigellosis caused by susceptible strains of *Shigella flexneri* or *Shigella sonnei*

Adults: One double-strength tablet or two single-strength tablets or 20 ml suspension P.O. q 12 hours for 10 to 14 days. Alternatively, 8 to 10 mg/kg (based on trimethoprim component) I.V. q 6, 8, or 12 hours for 5 days.

Children ages 2 months and older: 40 mg/kg (sulfamethoxazole) and 8 mg/kg (trimethoprim) P.O. q 12 hours for 5 days. Alternatively, 8 to 10 mg/kg (based on trimethoprim component) I.V. q 6, 8, or 12 hours for up to 5 days.

➢ Acute exacerbation of chronic bronchitis caused by susceptible strains of *Streptococcus pneumoniae* or *Haemophilus influenzae*
Adults: One double-strength tablet or two single-strength tablets or 20 ml suspension P.O. q 12 hours for 10 to 14 days
➢ *Pneumocystis jiroveci* pneumonia
Adults and children older than 2 months: 75 to 100 mg/kg (sulfamethoxazole) and 15 to 20 mg/kg (trimethoprim) P.O. daily in equally divided doses q 6 hours for 14 to 21 days. Alternatively, 15 to 20 mg/kg (based on trimethoprim component) I.V. q 6 to 8 hours for up to 14 days.
➢ Prophylaxis of *P. jiroveci* pneumonia
Adults: One double-strength tablet P.O. daily
Children ages 2 months and older: 750 mg/m² (sulfamethoxazole) and 150 mg/m² (trimethoprim) P.O. b.i.d. in equally divided doses on 3 consecutive days each week. Total dosage should not exceed 1,600 mg sulfamethoxazole and 320 mg trimethoprim.
➢ Traveler's diarrhea caused by susceptible strains of enterotoxigenic *Escherichia coli*
Adults: One double-strength tablet or two single-strength tablets or 20 ml suspension q 12 hours for 5 days
➢ Acute otitis media caused by susceptible strains of *S. pneumoniae* or *H. influenzae*
Children ages 2 months and older: 40 mg/kg sulfamethoxazole and 8 mg/kg trimethoprim P.O. q 12 hours for 10 days

Off-label uses
- Granuloma inguinale
- Toxoplasmic encephalitis (as primary prophylaxis)

Dosage adjustment
- Renal impairment

Contraindications
- Hypersensitivity to sulfonamides, trimethoprim, sulfonylureas, thiazides, or loop diuretics
- Porphyria
- Marked renal or hepatic impairment
- Megaloblastic anemia caused by folate deficiency
- Pregnancy at term or when premature birth is possible
- Infants younger than 2 months (except in *P. jiroveci* pneumonia prophylaxis)

Precautions
Use cautiously in:
- urinary obstruction, renal or hepatic disease, bronchial asthma, G6PD deficiency, group A beta-hemolytic streptococcal infection, blood dyscrasias
- history of multiple allergies
- elderly patients
- pregnant (before term) or breastfeeding patients
- children.

Administration
- Dilute each 5 ml of I.V. drug in 125 ml of dextrose 5% in water.
- Infuse I.V. over 60 to 90 minutes. Avoid rapid infusion.
- Don't mix with other drugs or solutions. Don't refrigerate. Use within 6 hours after dilution.

Route	Onset	Peak	Duration
P.O.	Rapid	1-4 hr	Unknown
I.V.	Rapid	1 hr	Unknown

S

Adverse reactions
CNS: headache, depression, hallucinations, insomnia, drowsiness, fatigue, apathy, anxiety, ataxia, vertigo, polyneuritis, peripheral neuropathy, **seizures**
CV: allergic myocarditis or pericarditis
EENT: periorbital edema, optic neuritis, transient myopia, tinnitus

GI: nausea, vomiting, abdominal pain, stomatitis, glossitis, dry mouth, pancreatitis, anorexia, **pseudomembranous colitis**
GU: hematuria, proteinuria, **crystalluria, toxic nephrosis with oliguria and anuria, renal failure**
Hematologic: megaloblastic anemia, agranulocytosis, aplastic anemia, thrombocytopenia, leukopenia, hemolytic anemia
Hepatic: jaundice, **hepatitis, hepatocellular necrosis**
Respiratory: shortness of breath, pleuritis, **allergic pneumonitis, pulmonary infiltrates, fibrosing alveolitis**
Skin: generalized skin eruption, urticaria, pruritus, alopecia, local irritation, exfoliative dermatitis, photosensitivity reaction, **epidermal necrolysis, erythema multiforme, Stevens-Johnson syndrome**
Other: irritation at I.V. site, chills, drug fever, hypersensitivity reactions including **anaphylaxis, serum sickness, lupus-like syndrome**

Interactions

Drug-drug. *Cyclosporine:* increased nephrotoxicity
Dapsone: increased blood levels of both drugs
Hydantoins, zidovudine: increased blood levels of these drugs
Indomethacin, probenecid: increased sulfamethoxazole blood level
Methotrexate: increased risk of bone marrow suppression
Oral anticoagulants: increased anticoagulant effect
PABA, PABA-derived local anesthetics: inhibited sulfamethoxazole action
Sulfonylureas: increased risk of hypoglycemia
Thiazide diuretics: increased thrombocytopenic effects
Uricosuric drugs: increased uricosuric effects
Drug-diagnostic tests. *Bilirubin, blood urea nitrogen, creatinine, eosinophils, transaminases:* increased levels
Granulocytes, hemoglobin, platelets, white blood cells: decreased levels
Urine glucose tests: false-positive results
Drug-herbs. *Dong quai, St. John's wort:* increased risk of photosensitivity
Drug-behaviors. *Sun exposure:* increased risk of photosensitivity

Patient monitoring

Monitor CBC with white cell differential. Watch for evidence of blood dyscrasias.
Stay alert for erythema multiforme. Report early signs before condition can progress to Stevens-Johnson syndrome.
• Monitor patient for signs and symptoms of superinfection, including fever, tachycardia, and chills.
Monitor liver function tests and assess for evidence of hepatitis.
Check kidney function tests weekly. Evaluate patient's fluid intake, urine output, and urine pH. Report hematuria, oliguria, or anuria right away.
• Monitor neurologic status. Report seizures, hallucinations, or depression.

Patient teaching

• Advise patient to take on regular schedule as prescribed, along with a full glass of water. Tell him to drink plenty of fluids to minimize crystal formation in urine.
• If suspension is prescribed, make sure patient has a specially marked measuring spoon or other device so he can measure doses accurately.
• Instruct patient to complete full course of treatment even if he starts to feel better.
Teach patient to recognize and immediately report signs and symptoms of hypersensitivity, especially rash.
Inform patient that drug can cause blood disorders, GI and liver problems,

serious skin reactions, and other infections. Describe key warning signs and symptoms (easy bruising or bleeding, severe diarrhea, unusual tiredness, yellowing of skin or eyes, sore throat, rash, cough, mouth sores, fever). Tell him to report these right away.

Urge patient to promptly report scant or bloody urine or inability to urinate.

- Tell patient to contact prescriber if he develops depression.
- Teach patient effective ways to counteract photosensitivity effect. Advise him that dong quai and St. John's wort increase phototoxicity risk and should be avoided during therapy.
- Advise female patient to inform prescriber if she is pregnant. Tell her not to take drug near term.
- Caution female patient not to breastfeed, because she could pass drug effects to infant.
- As appropriate, review all other significant and life-threatening adverse reactions and interactions, especially those related to the drugs, tests, herbs, and behaviors mentioned above.

sulfasalazine

APO Sulfasalazine♣, Azulfidine, Azulfidine EN-tabs, PMS-Sulfasalazine♣, PMS-Sulfasalazine-E.C.♣, SAS Tab♣, Salazopyrin, Salazopyrin EN-Tabs♣

Pharmacologic class: Sulfonamide

Therapeutic class: Anti-infective, GI tract anti-inflammatory, antirheumatic

Pregnancy risk category B

Action

Unknown. Thought to inhibit prostaglandin synthesis by interfering with secretions in colon and causing local anti-inflammatory action.

Availability

Tablets: 500 mg

Tablets (Azulfidine EN-tabs—delayed-release, enteric-coated): 500 mg

Indications and dosages

➤ Ulcerative colitis

Adults: Initially, 1 to 2 g P.O. daily in equally divided doses q 6 to 8 hours, then 3 to 4 g P.O. daily in equally divided doses q 6 to 8 hours. For maintenance, 500 mg q 6 hours.

Children ages 6 and older: 40 to 60 mg/kg P.O. daily in three to six divided doses. For maintenance, 30 mg/kg P.O. q 6 hours in four divided doses.

➤ Acute rheumatoid arthritis

Adults: Initially, 500 mg to 1 g (delayed-release) P.O. daily for 1 week; then increase by 500 mg/day P.O. q week up to 2 g/day in two divided doses. If no benefit after 12 weeks, increase to 3 g/day given in two divided doses.

➤ Polyarticular-course juvenile rheumatoid arthritis

Children ages 6 and older: 30 to 50 mg/kg P.O. daily in two evenly divided doses. Maximum dosage is 2 g daily.

Off-label uses

- Ankylosing spondylitis
- Crohn's disease
- Psoriatic arthritis

Contraindications

- Hypersensitivity to drug, other sulfonamides, sulfonylureas, thiazides, loop diuretics, or salicylates
- Porphyria
- Marked renal or hepatic impairment
- Urinary tract or intestinal obstruction
- Pregnancy at term or when premature birth is possible
- Children younger than age 2

Precautions

Use cautiously in:

- renal or hepatic disease, bronchial asthma, G6PD deficiency, group A

S

beta-hemolytic streptococcal infections, blood dyscrasias
• history of multiple allergies
• pregnant (before term) or breast-feeding patients
• children (use in systemic-course rheumatoid arthritis not recommended).

Administration
• Give after meals and space doses evenly to reduce GI effects.
• Give with a full glass of water.
• Administer delayed-release tablets whole. Don't let patient crush or chew them.

Route	Onset	Peak	Duration
P.O.	1.5 hr	10 hr	Unknown

Adverse reactions
CNS: headache, depression, hallucinations, insomnia, drowsiness, vertigo, fatigue, apathy, anxiety, ataxia, polyneuritis, peripheral neuropathy, **seizures**
CV: allergic myocarditis or pericarditis
EENT: periorbital edema, optic neuritis, transient myopia, tinnitus
GI: nausea, vomiting, abdominal pain, stomatitis, glossitis, pancreatitis, dry mouth, anorexia, **pseudomembranous colitis**
GU: hematuria, proteinuria, orange-yellow urine, reversible oligospermia, **crystalluria, toxic nephrosis with oliguria and anuria, renal failure**
Hematologic: megaloblastic anemia, agranulocytosis, aplastic anemia, thrombocytopenia, leukopenia, hemolytic anemia
Hepatic: jaundice, **hepatitis, hepatocellular necrosis**
Respiratory: shortness of breath, pleuritis, **cyanosis, allergic pneumonitis, pulmonary infiltrates, fibrosing alveolitis**
Skin: generalized skin eruption, urticaria, pruritus, alopecia, local irritation, orange-yellow skin discoloration, exfoliative dermatitis, photosensitivity reaction, **erythema multiforme, epidermal necrolysis, Stevens-Johnson syndrome**
Other: reversible immunoglobulin suppression, chills, drug fever, hypersensitivity reactions including **anaphylaxis, serum sickness, lupus-like syndrome**

Interactions
Drug-drug. *Cyclosporine:* increased nephrotoxicity
Folic acid: decreased folic acid absorption
Hydantoins: increased hydantoin blood level
Indomethacin, probenecid: increased sulfasalazine blood level
Iron: decreased sulfasalazine absorption
Methenamine: increased risk of crystalluria, causing serious adverse reactions
Methotrexate: increased risk of bone marrow depression
Oral anticoagulants: increased anticoagulant effect
Other anti-infectives: altered sulfasalazine metabolism
Para-aminobenzoic acid (PABA), PABA-derived local anesthetics: inhibited sulfasalazine action
Sulfonylureas: increased risk of hypoglycemia
Thiazide diuretics: increased thrombocytopenic effects
Uricosuric drugs: increased effects of these drugs
Drug-diagnostic tests. *Bilirubin, blood urea nitrogen, creatinine, eosinophils, transaminases:* increased levels
Granulocytes, hemoglobin, platelets, white blood cells: decreased levels
Urine glucose test: false-positive result
Drug-food. *Folic acid, iron:* decreased folic acid or iron absorption

Drug-herbs. *Dong quai, St. John's wort:* increased risk of photosensitivity
Drug-behaviors. *Sun exposure:* increased risk of photosensitivity

Patient monitoring

◀ Monitor CBC with white cell differential. Watch for evidence of blood dyscrasias.
◀ Stay alert for signs of erythema multiforme. Report early signs before condition can progress to Stevens-Johnson syndrome.
- Monitor patient for signs and symptoms of superinfection, including fever, tachycardia, and chills.

◀ Monitor liver function tests; watch for signs and symptoms of hepatitis.
◀ Check kidney function tests weekly. Evaluate patient's fluid intake, urine output, and urine pH. Report hematuria, oliguria, or anuria right away.
- Monitor neurologic status. Report seizures, hallucinations, or depression.
- If patient takes drug for rheumatoid arthritis, monitor therapeutic response 4 to 12 weeks after therapy begins.

Patient teaching

- Tell patient to take on regular schedule as prescribed, along with a full glass of water. Instruct him to drink plenty of fluids to minimize crystal formation in urine.
- Urge patient to complete full course of treatment, even if he feels better after a few days.

◀ Instruct patient to watch for and immediately report signs and symptoms of hypersensitivity reaction, especially rash.
◀ Tell patient drug can cause blood disorders, GI and liver problems, serious skin reactions, and other infections. Describe key warning signs and symptoms (easy bruising or bleeding, severe diarrhea, unusual tiredness, yellowing of skin or eyes, sore throat, rash, cough, mouth sores, fever). Instruct him to report these right away.
◀ Advise patient to promptly report scant or bloody urine or inability to urinate.
- Instruct patient to contact prescriber if he develops depression.
- Teach patient effective ways to counteract photosensitivity effect. Tell him that dong quai and St. John's wort increase phototoxicity risk and should be avoided during therapy.
- Inform patient that drug may discolor skin and body fluids orange-yellow and may permanently stain contact lenses.
- Advise female patient to inform prescriber if she is pregnant. Caution her not to take drug near term or when breastfeeding.
- As appropriate, review all other significant and life-threatening adverse reactions and interactions, especially those related to the drugs, tests, foods, herbs, and behaviors mentioned above.

sulfinpyrazone

Antazone✱, Anturane, Apo-Sulfinpyrazone✱, Novo-Pyrazone✱, Nu-Sulfinpyrazone✱

Pharmacologic class: Pyrazolidine derivative
Therapeutic class: Antigout agent, uricosuric
Pregnancy risk category NR

Action

Blocks uric acid reabsorption in kidney, increasing uric acid excretion. Also decreases platelet adhesion, inhibiting antithrombic effects.

Availability

Capsules: 200 mg
Tablets: 100 mg

 Indications and dosages

➤ Intermittent or chronic gouty arthritis

Adults: 200 to 400 mg P.O. in two divided doses. May increase to a maximum of 800 mg P.O. daily.

Off-label uses

- Inhibition of platelet aggregation
- Mortality reduction after myocardial infarction

Contraindications

- Hypersensitivity to drug or other pyrazolidine derivatives
- Blood dyscrasias
- Active peptic ulcer
- Concurrent salicylate use

Precautions

Use cautiously in:

- history of peptic ulcer or renal calculi
- concurrent use of sulfonamides, sulfonylureas, phenylbutazone, oral anticoagulants, or insulin
- pregnant or breastfeeding patients
- children (safety and efficacy not established).

Administration

- Give on a regular schedule with food, milk, or antacids to reduce GI upset.
- Give with a full glass of water.

Route	Onset	Peak	Duration
P.O.	Unknown	1-2 hr	4-6 hr

Adverse reactions

GI: nausea, vomiting, gastric irritation, dyspepsia, epigastric pain, anorexia
GU: urolithiasis, renal colic
Hematologic: anemia, **leukopenia, agranulocytopenia, thrombocytopenia, aplastic anemia**
Respiratory: bronchoconstriction in patients with aspirin-induced asthma
Skin: rash

Interactions

Drug-drug. *Acetaminophen:* increased risk of hepatotoxicity, reduced therapeutic effects of acetaminophen
Insulin, phenylbutazone, sulfonamide, sulfonylureas: increased effects of these drugs
Niacin, salicylates: reduced uricosuric effect of sulfinpyrazone
Oral anticoagulants: increased anticoagulant effect
Probenecid: inhibited renal excretion of sulfinpyrazone
Theophylline, verapamil: increased clearance of these drugs.
Drug-diagnostic tests. *Blood urea nitrogen (BUN), creatinine, eosinophils:* increased levels
Granulocytes, hemoglobin, platelets, white blood cells: decreased levels
Renal function tests: altered values
Drug-behaviors. *Alcohol use:* decreased sulfinpyrazone efficacy

Patient monitoring

- Monitor intake and output.
- Monitor frequency, severity, and duration of acute gout attacks. Be aware that attacks may increase for first 6 to12 months of therapy.
- Monitor BUN, uric acid level, and renal function tests.
- Assess patient's pain level. Know that sulfinpyrazone doesn't relieve pain or inflammation. Notify prescriber of need for analgesic or anti-inflammatory drug.
- [Clinical alert] Monitor CBC with white cell differential. Watch for signs and symptoms of blood dyscrasias (rare).

Patient teaching

- Advise patient to take as prescribed with food, milk, or antacids to reduce GI effects.
- Encourage patient to drink 10 to 12 glasses of fluid daily.
- Tell patient drug may worsen frequency, severity, and duration of acute

gout attacks for first 6 to12 months. Encourage him to discuss need for analgesic or anti-inflammatory drugs with prescriber.

Advise patient to promptly report unusual bruising or bleeding.

- Caution patient to avoid aspirin and aspirin-containing products during therapy.
- Advise patient not to drink alcohol during therapy.
- Tell patient to avoid foods high in purine (anchovies, sardines, organ meats, legumes), which can trigger gout attacks.
- As appropriate, review all other significant and life-threatening adverse reactions and interactions, especially those related to the drugs, tests, and behaviors mentioned above.

sulfisoxazole

Apo Sulfisoxazole✦, Novo-Soxazole✦, Sosol, Sulfizole✦

sulfisoxazole acetyl

Gantrisin Pediatric Suspension

Pharmacologic class: Sulfonamide (short-acting)

Therapeutic class: Anti-infective

Pregnancy risk category C

Action

Inhibits formation of bacterial folic acid from para-aminobenzoic acid (PABA), preventing bacterial cell-wall synthesis and exerting a bacteriostatic effect

Availability

Suspension: 500 mg/5 ml

Tablets: 500 mg

Indications and dosages

➢ Urinary tract and systemic infections

Adults: Initially, 2 to 4 g P.O.; then 4 to 8 g daily in four to six equally divided doses

Children ages 2 months and older: Initially, 75 mg/kg P.O. or 2 g/m^2, then 150 mg/kg or 4 g/m^2 daily in four to six equally divided doses. Total daily dosage shouldn't exceed 6 g.

Dosage adjustment

- Renal impairment

Contraindications

- Hypersensitivity to drug, other sulfonamides, sulfonylureas, or thiazide or loop diuretics
- Pregnancy at term or when premature birth is possible
- Infant younger than 2 months (except in congenital toxoplasmosis)
- Porphyria

Precautions

Use cautiously in:

- urinary obstruction, renal or hepatic disease, bronchial asthma, G6PD deficiency, group A beta-hemolytic streptococcal infections
- history of multiple allergies
- pregnant (before term) or breast-feeding patients.

Administration

- Give with a full glass of water. Encourage good fluid intake to minimize crystal formation in urine.

Route	Onset	Peak	Duration
P.O.	Unknown	1-4 hr	Unknown

Adverse reactions

CNS: headache, depression, hallucinations, insomnia, drowsiness, vertigo, fatigue, apathy, anxiety, ataxia, polyneuritis, peripheral neuropathy, **seizures**

S

CV: allergic myocarditis or pericarditis
EENT: optic neuritis, transient myopia, periorbital edema, tinnitus
GI: nausea, vomiting, abdominal pain, pancreatitis, stomatitis, glossitis, dry mouth, anorexia, **pseudomembranous colitis**
GU: hematuria, proteinuria, **crystalluria, toxic nephrosis with oliguria and anuria, renal failure**
Hematologic: megaloblastic anemia, agranulocytosis, aplastic anemia, thrombocytopenia, leukopenia, hemolytic anemia
Hepatic: jaundice, **hepatitis, hepatocellular necrosis**
Respiratory: shortness of breath, pleuritis, **allergic pneumonitis, pulmonary infiltrates, fibrosing alveolitis**
Skin: local irritation, urticaria, pruritus, generalized skin eruption, alopecia, exfoliative dermatitis, photosensitivity reaction, **epidermal necrolysis, erythema multiforme, Stevens-Johnson syndrome**
Other: chills, drug fever, hypersensitivity reactions including **anaphylaxis, serum sickness, lupus-like syndrome**

Interactions

Drug-drug. *Cyclosporine:* increased nephrotoxicity
Hydantoins: increased hydantoin blood level
Indomethacin, probenecid: increased sulfisoxazole blood level
Methenamine: increased risk of crystalluria, causing serious adverse reactions
Methotrexate: increased risk of bone marrow depression
Oral anticoagulants: increased anticoagulant effect
PABA, PABA-derived local anesthetics: inhibited sulfisoxazole action
Sulfonylureas: increased risk of hypoglycemia
Thiazide diuretics: increased thrombocytopenic effect
Thiopental, uricosuric drugs: increased effects of these drugs
Drug-diagnostic tests. *Bilirubin, blood urea nitrogen, creatinine, eosinophils, transaminases:* increased levels
Granulocytes, hemoglobin, platelets, white blood cells: decreased levels
Urine glucose test: false-positive result
Drug-herbs. *Dong quai, St. John's wort:* increased risk of photosensitivity
Drug-behaviors. *Sun exposure:* increased risk of photosensitivity

Patient monitoring

🔊 Monitor CBC with white cell differential. Watch for evidence of blood dyscrasias.
🔊 Stay alert for signs of erythema multiforme. Report early signs before condition can progress to Stevens-Johnson syndrome.
• Monitor patient for signs and symptoms of superinfection, including fever, tachycardia, and chills.
🔊 Monitor liver function tests. Be alert for signs and symptoms of hepatitis.
🔊 Check kidney function test results weekly. Evaluate patient's fluid intake, urine output, and urine pH. Report hematuria, oliguria, or anuria right away.
• Monitor neurologic status. Report seizures, hallucinations, or depression.

Patient teaching

• Tell patient to take on regular schedule as prescribed, along with a full glass of water. Advise him to drink plenty of fluids to minimize crystal formation in urine.
• Instruct patient to complete full course of treatment, even if he feels better after a few days.
🔊 Tell patient to watch for and immediately report signs and symptoms of hypersensitivity reaction, especially rash.
🔊 Advise patient that drug can cause blood disorders, GI and liver problems,

serious skin reactions, and other infections. Describe key warning signs and symptoms (easy bruising or bleeding, severe diarrhea, unusual tiredness, yellowing of skin or eyes, sore throat, rash, cough, mouth sores, fever). Tell him to report these right away.
Encourage patient to promptly report scant urine, bloody urine, or inability to urinate.
- Instruct patient to contact prescriber if he develops depression.
- Teach patient effective ways to counteract photosensitivity effect. Tell him that dong quai and St. John's wort increase phototoxicity risk and should be avoided during therapy.
- Advise female patient to inform prescriber if she is pregnant. Caution her not to take drug near term or when breastfeeding.
- As appropriate, review all other significant and life-threatening adverse reactions and interactions, especially those related to the drugs, tests, herbs, and behaviors mentioned above.

sulindac

Apo-Sulin*, Clinoril, Novo-Sundac*, Nu-Sulindac*

Pharmacologic class: Cyclooxygenase-1 (COX-1) enzyme inhibitor

Therapeutic class: Antirheumatic, nonsteroidal anti-inflammatory drug (NSAID)

Pregnancy risk category B (first and second trimesters), ***D*** (third trimester)

Action

Unknown. Thought to inhibit prostaglandin biosynthesis by interfering with activity of the COX-1 enzyme.

Availability

Tablets: 150 mg, 200 mg

Indications and dosages

➤ Rheumatoid arthritis; osteoarthritis; acute gouty arthritis; ankylosing spondylitis; painful shoulder (bursitis or tendinitis)

Adults: 150 to 200 mg P.O. b.i.d. Don't exceed 400 mg/day.

Contraindications

- Hypersensitivity to drug or other NSAIDs (including aspirin)
- Asthma
- Severe renal disease
- Pregnancy (third trimester)

Precautions

Use cautiously in:

- severe cardiovascular, renal, or hepatic disease; bleeding disorders; GI disorders; hyperkalemia
- history of ulcer disease
- concurrent use of other NSAIDs or methotrexate
- pregnant (first and second trimesters) or breastfeeding patients
- children (use not recommended).

Administration

- Give with food, milk, or antacids.

Route	Onset	Peak	Duration
P.O. (analgesic)	Unknown	2 hr	12 hr
P.O. (anti-inflamm.)	Unknown	Unknown	Unknown

Adverse reactions

CNS: dizziness, headache, nervousness
EENT: tinnitus
GI: nausea, vomiting, diarrhea, constipation, abdominal pain or cramps, flatulence, dyspepsia, anorexia, **GI bleeding**
Metabolic: hyperkalemia
Skin: rash, pruritus
Other: edema

S

Interactions

Drug-drug. *Acetaminophen (long-term use), cyclosporine, gold compounds:* increased risk of adverse renal effects
Antacids: decreased blood level and reduced efficacy of sulindac
Anticoagulants, cefamandole, cefoperazone, cefotetan, clopidogrel, eptifibatide, plicamycin, thrombolytics, ticlopidine, tirofiban, valproic acid: increased risk of bleeding
Antihypertensives, diuretics: decreased response to these drugs
Antineoplastics: increased risk of hematologic toxicity
Aspirin: decreased sulindac efficacy
Aspirin, corticosteroids, and other NSAIDs: additive GI adverse reactions
Dimethyl sulfoxide (DMSO): increased risk of peripheral neuropathy, reduced blood levels of sulindac and its metabolite
Insulin, oral hypoglycemics: increased risk of hypoglycemia
Lithium: increased lithium blood level and risk of toxicity
Methotrexate: inhibited renal elimination of methotrexate, increased risk of severe or fatal toxicity
Drug-diagnostic tests. *Potassium:* increased level
Drug-herbs. *Dong quai:* increased risk of bleeding

Patient monitoring

- Monitor liver and kidney function tests in patients on long-term therapy.
- Monitor potassium level and watch for signs and symptoms of hyperkalemia.
- Monitor hearing and vision.

Patient teaching

- Tell patient to take with food, milk, or antacid to reduce GI effects.
- Inform patient that drug increases risk of GI problems, and that ulcers and bleeding can occur without causing symptoms.

Instruct patient to immediately report persistent abdominal pain or black or bloody stools.

- Explain that drug can cause swelling. Tell patient to report swelling or significant weight gain.
- Advise patient to monitor his hearing and report significant changes.
- Tell female patient to inform prescriber if she is pregnant. Caution her not to take drug during last 3 months of pregnancy or when breastfeeding.
- As appropriate, review all other significant and life-threatening adverse reactions and interactions, especially those related to the drugs, tests, and herbs mentioned above.

sumatriptan succinate

Imitrex

Pharmacologic class: Selective 5-hydroxytryptamine$_1$ (5-HT$_1$) agonist
Therapeutic class: Vascular headache suppressant
Pregnancy risk category C

Action

Selectively activates vascular 5-HT$_1$ receptor sites, causing vasoconstriction in intracranial arteries

Availability

Injection: 6 mg/0.5-ml prefilled syringes, 0.6 mg/0.5-ml vials, SELF dose injection kit (containing two prefilled syringes)
Nasal spray: 5 mg in 100-mcl unit dose spray device (package of six), 20 mg in 100-mcl unit dose spray device (package of six)
Tablets: 25 mg, 50 mg, 100 mg

Indications and dosages

➢ Acute migraine

Adults: Initially, 25 mg P.O.; if response inadequate after 2 hours, may give up to 100 mg P.O. If migraine recurs, repeat dose q 2 hours, not to exceed 200 mg/day. Or 6 mg subcutaneously, repeated as needed after 1 hour, not to exceed 12 mg in 24 hours. If P.O. therapy will follow subcutaneous injection, additional P.O. sumatriptan may be given q 2 hours, not to exceed 100 mg/day. Or a single dose of 5, 10, or 20 mg intranasally in one nostril, repeated p.r.n. in 2 hours, not to exceed 40 mg in 24 hours.

Dosage adjustment
• Hepatic impairment

Contraindications
• Hypersensitivity to drug
• Hemiplegic or basilar migraine headache
• Ischemic cardiac, cerebrovascular, or peripheral vascular disease (such as a history of myocardial infarction, stroke, angina, or ischemic bowel)
• Uncontrolled hypertension
• Severe hepatic impairment
• MAO inhibitor use within past 14 days
• Use of other 5-HT_1 agonists, ergotamine-containing drugs, or ergot-type products within past 24 hours

Precautions
Use cautiously in:
• patients with cardiovascular risk factors (hypertension, hypercholesterolemia, smoking, obesity, diabetes, family history of cardiovascular disease, men over age 40, menopausal women)
• elderly patients
• women of childbearing age
• pregnant or breastfeeding patients
• children younger than age 18 (safety not established).

Administration
◀ If patient has risk factors for coronary artery disease, know that first dose should be given in medical setting with emergency equipment at hand.

◀ Don't give within 14 days of MAO inhibitors.

◀ Don't administer within 24 hours of other 5-HT_1 agonists, ergotamine-containing drugs, or ergot-type products.

Route	Onset	Peak	Duration
P.O.	Within 30 min	2-2.5 hr	Unknown
Subcut.	10-20 min	Unknown	Unknown
Intranasal	Unknown	Unknown	Unknown

Adverse reactions
CNS: headache, malaise, dizziness, drowsiness, fatigue, vertigo, anxiety, tight feeling in head, numbness
CV: angina, chest pressure or tightness, transient hypertension, ECG changes, **coronary vasospasm, myocardial infarction**
EENT: vision changes, nasal sinus discomfort, throat discomfort
GI: abdominal discomfort, dysphagia
Musculoskeletal: jaw discomfort, muscle cramps, myalgia, neck pain or stiffness
Skin: flushing; tingling; warm, cool or, burning sensation
Other: injection site reaction, feeling of heaviness or tightness

Interactions
Drug-drug. *Dihydroergotamine, ergotamine, methysergide:* increased risk of vasospastic reaction
Lithium, MAO inhibitors, selective serotonin reuptake inhibitors: weakness, hyperreflexia, incoordination
Drug-herbs. *Horehound:* enhanced serotonergic effects

Patient monitoring
◀ Monitor cardiovascular status closely. Be aware that drug may cause serious and possibly fatal cardiac disorders.

S

• Watch for neurologic and vision changes. Institute safety measures as needed to prevent injury.
• Monitor patient's response to drug. Assess need for repeat doses.
• Watch for injection site reaction, which should subside within 1 hour.

Patient teaching

• Instruct patient to take as soon as possible after migraine onset.
Clinical alert: Teach patient to recognize and immediately report serious cardiovascular reactions.
• Explain proper drug use. Stress that drug is effective only in treating diagnosed migraine, not other headache types. Tell patient it doesn't prevent migraine.
• With subcutaneous use, instruct patient to inject dose using spring-loaded injector system included in package. If headache recurs after dose, tell him he may take a second dose, but should wait at least 1 hour after initial dose and shouldn't exceed two 6-mg injections in a 24-hour period. Instruct him to report injection site reaction that doesn't subside within 1 hour.
• With oral use, tell patient he may take a second dose 2 hours after first dose if migraine recurs. Tell him he may repeat oral doses every 2 hours as needed, up to 200 mg in a 24-hour period.
• With intranasal use, tell patient to spray 5, 10, or 20 mg into one nostril, as prescribed. Tell him he may repeat dose after 2 hours but shouldn't exceed 40 mg in a 24-hour period.
• Advise patient not to use drug for more than four episodes per month.
• Caution patient to avoid driving and other hazardous activities until he knows how drug affects concentration and alertness.
• As appropriate, review all other significant and life-threatening adverse reactions and interactions, especially those related to the drugs and herbs mentioned above.

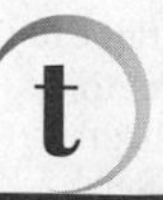

tacrine hydrochloride

Cognex

Pharmacologic class: Cholinergic (cholinesterase inhibitor)

Therapeutic class: Anti-Alzheimer's agent

Pregnancy risk category C

Action

Inhibits acetylcholine breakdown in cerebral cortex, increasing acetylcholine levels

Availability

Capsules: 10 mg, 20 mg, 30 mg, 40 mg

Indications and dosages

➢ Mild to moderate dementia of Alzheimer's disease
Adults: 10 mg P.O. q.i.d. for 4 weeks. If alanine aminotransferase (ALT) level doesn't change, increase to 20 mg q.i.d. As tolerated, increase incrementally at 4-week intervals, up to 160 mg/day (30 to 40 mg P.O. q.i.d.).

Dosage adjustment

• Elevated transaminase levels

Contraindications

• Hypersensitivity to drug or other acridine derivatives
• Jaundice with previous tacrine therapy
• Bilirubin level above 3 mg/dl
• Hypersensitivity symptoms accompanied by transaminase elevations

Precautions

Use cautiously in:
• sick sinus syndrome, bradycardia, hepatic or renal disease, bladder obstruc-

tion, asthma, seizure disorders, prostatic hyperplasia
• history of ulcers or increased risk of GI bleeding (as from concurrent use of nonsteroidal anti-inflammatory drugs)
• pregnant or breastfeeding patients
• children.

Administration

• Preferably, give 1 hour before or 2 hours after meals. However, if GI upset occurs, drug can be given with meals (although food slows its absorption).

Route	Onset	Peak	Duration
P.O.	Unknown	1-2 hr	Unknown

Adverse reactions

CNS: dizziness, headache, confusion, insomnia, tremor, ataxia, drowsiness, anxiety, agitation, depression, hallucinations, hostility, abnormal thinking, fatigue, malaise
CV: hypotension, hypertension, chest pain, peripheral edema
EENT: conjunctivitis, rhinitis, sinusitis, pharyngitis
GI: nausea, vomiting, diarrhea, constipation, dyspepsia, abdominal pain, anorexia
GU: urinary frequency or incontinence, urinary tract infection
Musculoskeletal: back pain, myalgia
Respiratory: upper respiratory infection, cough, bronchitis, pneumonia, dyspnea
Skin: rash, flushing, purpura
Other: chills, fever

Interactions

Drug-drug. *Anticholinergics:* interference with anticholinergic action
Cholinergics (including bethanechol), succinylcholine: synergistic effects
Cimetidine: increased tacrine blood level
Theophylline: increased theophylline blood level, greater risk of toxicity
Drug-diagnostic tests. *Hepatic enzymes:* increased levels
Drug-food. *Any food:* decreased tacrine bioavailability

Patient monitoring

• Monitor neurologic status to assess drug efficacy and determine optimal dosage.
• Check ALT level weekly for first 18 weeks. If level doesn't change markedly by end of this period, monitor level every 3 months. Otherwise, continue weekly monitoring.

Patient teaching

• Tell patient or caregiver that drug should be taken 1 hour before or 2 hours after meals.
• Advise caregiver to monitor patient's neurologic status carefully and to use safety measures at home to prevent injury.
• Recommend small, frequent servings of food and adequate fluid intake to minimize GI upset.
• Explain that drug doesn't change underlying dementia but may improve symptoms or slow further deterioration.
Stress importance of taking drug as prescribed. Caution against sudden dosage decreases or abrupt withdrawal.
• Tell patient or caregiver that if drug is stopped for 4 weeks or longer, dosage adjustment and monitoring schedule should be discussed with prescriber before restarting.
• As appropriate, review all other significant adverse reactions and interactions, especially those related to the drugs, tests, and foods mentioned above.

t

tacrolimus

Prograf

Pharmacologic class: Macrolide
Therapeutic class: Immunosuppressant
Pregnancy risk category C

Action

Unknown. Thought to inhibit T-lymphocyte activation.

Availability

Capsules: 0.5 mg, 1 mg, 5 mg
Injection: 5 mg/ml
Topical ointment: 0.03%, 0.1%

Indications and dosages

➢ Prevention of organ rejection in patients with allogeneic liver transplants
Adults: Initially, 0.1 to 0.15 mg/kg/day P.O. in two divided doses q 12 hours. Alternatively, 0.03 to 0.05 mg/kg/day by continuous I.V. infusion.
Children: 0.15 to 0.2 mg/kg/day P.O. in two divided doses q 12 hours. Alternatively, 0.03 to 0.05 mg/kg/day by continuous I.V. infusion.

➢ Prevention of organ rejection in patients with allogeneic kidney transplants
Adults: Initially, 0.2 mg/kg/day P.O. in two divided doses q 12 hours. Alternatively, 0.03 to 0.05 mg/kg/day by continuous I.V. infusion.

➢ Moderate to severe atopic dermatitis
Adults: 0.03% or 0.1% ointment applied b.i.d. to affected area, continued 1 week after dermatitis symptoms resolve
Children ages 2 and older: 0.03% ointment applied b.i.d. to affected area, continued 1 week after dermatitis symptoms resolve

Dosage adjustment

- Hepatic or renal impairment

Contraindications

- Hypersensitivity to drug or its components (including castor oil derivatives)

Precautions

Use cautiously in:
- severe hepatic disease, renal impairment, diabetes mellitus, hypertension, hyperkalemia, hyperuricemia, lymphoma
- pregnant or breastfeeding patients
- children younger than age 12 (age 2 for ointment use).

Administration

- Give oral form without food.
- Start therapy within 24 hours of kidney transplantation and no earlier than 6 hours after liver transplantation. Switch to oral dosing as soon as tolerated, starting 8 to 12 hours after I.V. dosing ends.

Before giving I.V., ensure that epinephrine 1:1,000 and oxygen are at hand in case of emergency.

- For I.V. use, dilute in normal saline solution or dextrose 5% in water to a concentration of 0.004 to 0.02 mg/ml. Give by infusion only.
- After applying ointment, don't place occlusive dressing or wrapping over affected area.

Route	Onset	Peak	Duration
P.O.	Unknown	1.5-3.5 hr	Unknown
I.V.	Rapid	1-2 hr	Unknown
Ointment	Unknown	Unknown	Unknown

Adverse reactions

CNS: tremor, headache, insomnia, paresthesia, delirium, asthenia, **coma**
CV: hypertension, peripheral edema
GI: nausea, vomiting, diarrhea, constipation, abdominal pain, ascites, anorexia

GU: hematuria, proteinuria, urinary tract infection, albuminuria, abnormal renal function, **oliguria, renal failure**
Hematologic: anemia, **leukocytosis, thrombocytopenia**
Metabolic: hyperglycemia, hypomagnesemia, hypokalemia, **hyperkalemia**
Musculoskeletal: back pain
Respiratory: dyspnea, **pleural effusion, atelectasis**
Skin: burning (with ointment), rash, flushing, pruritus, alopecia, pruritus
Other: pain, fever, chills, **anaphylaxis**

Interactions

Drug-drug. *Bromocriptine, chloramphenicol, cimetidine, clarithromycin, clotrimazole, cyclosporine, danazol, diltiazem, erythromycin, fluconazole, itraconazole, ketoconazole, methylprednisolone, metoclopramide, metronidazole, nicardipine, omeprazole, protease inhibitors, verapamil:* increased tacrolimus blood level
Cyclosporine: increased risk of nephrotoxicity
CYP450 inducers (such as carbamazepine, phenobarbital, phenytoin, rifampin): decreased tacrolimus metabolism
Immunosuppressants (except adrenocorticoids): immunologic oversuppression
Live-virus vaccines: interference with immune response to vaccine
Mycophenolate mofetil: increased mycophenolate blood level
Nephrotoxic drugs (such as aminoglycosides, amphotericin B, cisplatin, cyclosporine): additive or synergistic effects
Drug-diagnostic tests. *Blood urea nitrogen, creatinine, glucose:* increased levels
Hemoglobin, magnesium, platelets, white blood cells: decreased levels
Liver function tests: abnormal values
Potassium: increased or decreased level
Drug-food. *Any food:* inhibited drug absorption
Grapefruit juice: increased drug blood level
Drug-herbs. *Astragalus, echinacea, melatonin:* decreased immunosuppression
St. John's wort: decreased tacrolimus blood level

Patient monitoring

Once I.V. infusion starts, watch closely for signs and symptoms of anaphylaxis.
- Monitor liver and kidney function tests. Watch for signs and symptoms of nephrotoxicity and hepatic dysfunction.
- Assess neurologic status for evidence of neurotoxicity.
- Monitor potassium level closely. Stay alert for signs and symptoms of hyperkalemia.
- Monitor blood glucose. Watch for indications of hyperglycemia.
- Evaluate respiratory status regularly.

Patient teaching

Teach patient to recognize and immediately report serious adverse reactions.
- Tell patient to take oral doses without food.
- Tell diabetic patient to expect increased blood glucose level, which may warrant further antidiabetic therapy. Advise him to monitor glucose level carefully.
- Instruct patient not to place occlusive dressings or wrappings over affected area after applying ointment. Tell him to use drug for 1 week after dermatitis symptoms resolve.
- As appropriate, review all other significant and life-threatening adverse reactions and interactions, especially those related to the drugs, tests, foods, and herbs mentioned above.

t

tadalafil

Cialis

Pharmacologic class: Phosphodiesterase type 5 (PDE5) inhibitor
Therapeutic class: Anti-erectile dysfunction agent
Pregnancy risk category B

Action

Inhibits PDE5, increasing cyclic guanosine monophosphate level and enhancing erectile function

Availability

Tablets: 5 mg, 10 mg, 20 mg

Indications and dosages

➤ Erectile dysfunction

Adults: Initially, 10 mg P.O. before anticipated sexual activity; may increase to 20 mg or decrease to 5 mg based on patient response and tolerance. For most patients, maximum recommended dosing frequency is once daily.

Dosage adjustment

• Mild to moderate hepatic impairment or renal insufficiency

Contraindications

• Hypersensitivity to drug or its components
• Concurrent use of organic nitrates (regularly or intermittently)
• Concurrent use of alpha-adrenergic agonists (except tamsulosin 0.4 mg/day)

Precautions

Use cautiously in:
• cardiac risk that makes sexual activity inadvisable, renal insufficiency, hepatic impairment, left ventricular outflow obstruction, erectile dysfunction whose cause hasn't been evaluated, conditions that increase risk of priapism
• concurrent use of potent CYP450-3A4 inhibitors.

Administration

• Know that patient should take drug (with or without food) before anticipated sexual activity.

Route	Onset	Peak	Duration
P.O.	Rapid	30 min-6 hr	Up to 36 hr

Adverse reactions

CNS: headache, fatigue, dizziness, insomnia, hyperesthesia, paresthesia, drowsiness, vertigo, asthenia
CV: angina pectoris, chest pain, hypertension, hypotension, orthostatic hypotension, palpitations, syncope, tachycardia, **myocardial infarction**
EENT: blurred vision, color vision changes, conjunctivitis, eye pain, increased lacrimation, eyelid swelling, epistaxis, nasal congestion, pharyngitis
GI: nausea, vomiting, diarrhea, dyspepsia, esophagitis, gastroesophageal reflux, gastritis, upper abdominal pain, dysphagia, dry mouth
GU: increased or spontaneous erection
Musculoskeletal: myalgia; back, neck, limb, and joint pain
Respiratory: dyspnea
Skin: pruritus, rash, sweating
Other: facial edema, pain

Interactions

Drug-drug. *Alpha-adrenergic blockers (except tamsulosin 0.4 mg/day):* marked blood pressure decrease
Angiotensin receptor blockers, enalapril, metoprolol: decreased blood pressure
CYP450-3A4 inducers (such as carbamazepine, phenobarbital, phenytoin, rifampin): decreased tadalafil blood level
CYP450-3A4 inhibitors (such as erythromycin, itraconazole, ketoconazole, ritonavir): increased tadalafil blood level

Theophylline: slight increase in heart rate

Drug-diagnostic tests. *Alanine aminotransferase, alkaline phosphatase, aspartate aminotransferase, lactate dehydrogenase, uric acid:* increased levels

Drug-food. *Grapefruit juice:* increased drug blood level

Patient monitoring

- Monitor for drug efficacy.

Patient teaching

- Advise patient to take before anticipated sexual activity.

Caution patient never to take concurrently with nitrates.

Instruct patient to stop sexual activity and contact prescriber immediately if chest pain, dizziness, or nausea occurs.

- Instruct patient to contact prescriber if erection lasts more than 4 hours.
- Tell patient drug can cause serious interactions with many common drugs. Instruct him to tell all prescribers he's taking it.
- Caution patient to avoid driving and other hazardous activities until he knows how drug affects concentration and alertness.
- Inform patient that drug may cause temporary blood pressure drop, leading to light-headedness if he stands up suddenly. Advise him to rise slowly and carefully.
- As appropriate, review all other significant and life-threatening adverse reactions and interactions, especially those related to the drugs, tests, and foods mentioned above.

tamoxifen citrate

Nolvadex, Nolvadex-D✱, Novo-Tamoxifen✱, Tamofen✱

Pharmacologic class: Nonsteroidal antiestrogen

Therapeutic class: Antineoplastic

Pregnancy risk category D

Action

Competes with estrogen receptors in tumor cells for binding to target tissues (such as breast); reduces DNA synthesis and estrogen response

Availability

Tablets: 10 mg, 20 mg

Tablets (enteric-coated): 20 mg

Indications and dosages

➢ Adjunctive treatment of breast cancer

Adults: 20 to 40 mg P.O. daily for 5 years. Daily dosages of 20 mg may be taken as a single dose; daily dosages above 20 mg should be divided and taken b.i.d. (morning and evening).

➢ To reduce breast cancer incidence in high-risk women; treatment of ductal carcinoma in situ

Adults: 20 mg P.O. daily for 5 years

Off-label uses

- Mastalgia
- Ovulation stimulation

Contraindications

- Hypersensitivity to drug
- Concurrent warfarin use
- Women with a history of deep-vein thrombosis or pulmonary embolism
- Pregnancy or breastfeeding

Precautions

Use cautiously in:

- decreased bone marrow reserve, leu-

kopenia, thrombocytopenia, cataracts, hyperlipidemia
• females of childbearing age.

Administration
• Don't break or crush enteric-coated tablets.
• Know that drug is indicated for reducing breast cancer risk only in high-risk women, defined as those older than age 35 who have at least a 1.67% chance of developing breast cancer over 5 years.

Route	Onset	Peak	Duration
P.O.	Unknown	5 hr	Unknown

Adverse reactions
CNS: confusion, depression, headache, weakness, fatigue, light-headedness
CV: chest pain, **deep-vein thrombosis**
EENT: blurred vision, ocular lesion, retinopathy, corneal opacity
GI: nausea, vomiting, abdominal cramps, anorexia
GU: vaginal bleeding, discharge, or dryness; irregular menses; amenorrhea; oligomenorrhea; ovarian cyst; pruritus vulvae; **endometrial or uterine cancer**
Hematologic: leukopenia, thrombocytopenia
Metabolic: hypercalcemia, fluid retention
Musculoskeletal: bone pain
Respiratory: cough, **pulmonary embolism**
Skin: skin changes, hair thinning or partial hair loss
Other: altered taste, weight loss, tumor flare, tumor pain, hot flashes, edema

Interactions
Drug-drug. *Aminoglutethimide, estrogens:* decreased tamoxifen effects
Antineoplastics: increased risk of thromboembolic events
Bromocriptine: increased tamoxifen blood level
Warfarin: increased anticoagulant effect
Drug-diagnostic tests. *Aspartate aminotransferase, bilirubin, calcium, creatinine, hepatic enzymes:* increased levels
Platelets, white blood cells: decreased counts

Patient monitoring
• Monitor lipid panel, calcium level, mammography results, and gynecologic exam results.
🔈 Watch for signs and symptoms of thromboembolic events, including cerebrovascular accident and pulmonary embolism.
• Monitor menstrual cycle pattern for changes that may signal endometrial or uterine cancer.

Patient teaching
• Tell patient to swallow enteric-coated tablets whole without breaking or crushing.
🔈 Instruct patient to immediately report leg or calf pain, swelling, or tenderness; unexpected shortness of breath; sudden chest pain; coughing up blood; new breast lumps; vaginal bleeding; menstrual irregularities; changes in vaginal discharge; pelvic pain or pressure; and vision changes.
• Inform patient that increase in bone or tumor pain usually means drug will be effective. Advise her to discuss pain management with prescriber.
• Stress importance of undergoing regular blood tests, mammograms, and gynecologic exams to identify early signs of serious adverse reactions.
• As appropriate, review all other significant and life-threatening adverse reactions and interactions, especially those related to the drugs and tests mentioned above.

tamsulosin hydrochloride

Flomax

Pharmacologic class: Alpha-adrenergic blocker

Therapeutic class: Anti-adrenergic

Pregnancy risk category B

Action

Decreases smooth muscle contractions of prostate by binding to $alpha_1$-adrenergic receptors. This action increases urine flow and reduces symptoms of benign prostatic hyperplasia (BPH).

Availability

Capsules: 0.4 mg

Indications and dosages

➢ BPH

Adults: 0.4 mg/day P.O. after a meal. After 2 to 4 weeks, may increase to 0.8 mg/day.

Contraindications

- Hypersensitivity to drug or its components

Precautions

Use cautiously in:

- patients receiving other alpha-adrenergic blockers concurrently
- patients at increased risk for prostate cancer.

Administration

- Give 30 minutes after same meal each day.

Route	Onset	Peak	Duration
P.O.	Unknown	4-5 hr	9-15 hr

Adverse reactions

CNS: dizziness, headache, asthenia, insomnia, drowsiness, syncope, vertigo

CV: orthostatic hypotension, chest pain

EENT: rhinitis, amblyopia, pharyngitis, sinusitis

GU: retrograde or diminished ejaculation, decreased libido

Musculoskeletal: back pain

Respiratory: increased cough

Other: tooth disorder, infection

Interactions

Drug-drug. *Cimetidine:* increased tamsulosin blood level, greater risk of toxicity

Doxazosin, prazosin, terazosin: increased risk of hypotension

Drug-behaviors. *Alcohol use:* increased risk of hypotension

Patient monitoring

- Monitor blood pressure. Stay alert for orthostatic hypotension.

Patient teaching

- Tell patient to take 30 minutes after same meal each day.
- Instruct patient not to chew or open capsule. Advise him to swallow it whole.
- Tell patient to move slowly when sitting up or standing, to avoid dizziness or light-headedness from sudden blood pressure decrease.
- Caution patient to avoid hazardous activities on first day of therapy.
- Inform patient that drug may cause abnormal ejaculation. Advise him to discuss this issue with prescriber.
- As appropriate, review all other significant adverse reactions and interactions, especially those related to the drugs and behaviors mentioned above.

tegaserod maleate

Zelnorm

Pharmacologic class: Partial serotonin type 4 (5-HT_4) receptor agonist

Therapeutic class: Serotonin agonist

Pregnancy risk category B

Action

Unknown. Thought to activate 5-HT_4 receptors in GI tract, normalizing intestinal peristalsis reflex and relieving abdominal pain and discomfort.

Availability

Tablets: 2 mg, 6 mg

Indications and dosages

➢ Irritable bowel syndrome in women with constipation

Adults: 6 mg P.O. b.i.d. before meals for 4 to 6 weeks. Patients who respond may receive 4 to 6 more weeks of therapy.

➢ Chronic idiopathic constipation in patients younger than age 65

Adults: 6 mg P.O. b.i.d. before meals

Contraindications

- Hypersensitivity to drug or its components
- Severe renal disease
- Moderate to severe hepatic disease
- Gallbladder disease
- Abdominal adhesions
- Sphincter of Oddi dysfunction
- Diarrhea or history of frequent diarrhea
- History of bowel obstruction

Precautions

Use cautiously in:

- hypovolemia, hypotension, syncope, new or worsening abdominal pain
- pregnant patients
- breastfeeding (use not recommended).

Administration

- Give 1 hour before or 2 hours after meals.

Route	Onset	Peak	Duration
P.O.	1 hr	1-1.3 hr	Unknown

Adverse reactions

CNS: headache, dizziness, migraine, depression, syncope
CV: hypotension
GI: nausea, vomiting, diarrhea, abdominal pain, flatulence, **ischemic colitis**
Metabolic: hypovolemia
Musculoskeletal: joint, back, or leg pain
Other: facial edema, accidental trauma

Interactions

Drug-drug. *Digoxin, hormonal contraceptives:* decreased effects of these drugs

Drug-diagnostic tests. *Alanine aminotransferase, amylase, aspartate aminotransferase, blood and urine glucose, creatinine kinase, triglycerides:* increased levels

Drug-food. *Any food:* decreased drug absorption

Patient monitoring

- Assess for abdominal pain. Stop drug if patient develops new or sudden exacerbation of abdominal pain (especially with severe diarrhea), hypovolemia, hypotension, or syncope.
- Monitor patient for depression.

Patient teaching

- Instruct patient to take 1 hour before or 2 hours after meals.
- Advise patient to report severe diarrhea; diarrhea accompanied by severe abdominal pain, cramping, or dizziness; or sudden increase in abdominal pain.
- Tell patient to report depression.
- Caution female patient not to breastfeed during therapy.

• As appropriate, review all other significant and life-threatening adverse reactions and interactions, especially those related to the drugs, tests, and foods mentioned above.

telmisartan

Micardis

Pharmacologic class: Angiotensin II receptor antagonist

Therapeutic class: Antihypertensive

Pregnancy risk category C (first trimester), ***D*** (second and third trimesters)

Action

Inhibits vasoconstricting effects and blocks aldosterone-producing effects of angiotensin II at various receptor sites, including vascular smooth muscle and adrenal glands

Availability

Tablets: 20 mg, 40 mg, 80 mg

Indications and dosages

➢ Hypertension

Adults: 40 mg P.O. daily, titrated up or down within range of 20 to 80 mg daily based on response and tolerance

Contraindications

• Hypersensitivity to drug or its components

• Pregnancy (second and third trimesters), breastfeeding

Precautions

Use cautiously in:

• heart failure, impaired renal function secondary to primary renal disease or renal stenosis, obstructive biliary disorders, hepatic impairment, volume or sodium depletion

• patients receiving high-dose diuretics

• pregnant patients in first trimester

• females of childbearing age

• children younger than age 18 (safety not established).

Administration

• Don't remove tablet from blister pack until just before giving.

• Know that drug may be used alone or with other antihypertensives.

Route	Onset	Peak	Duration
P.O.	Unknown	0.5-1 hr	24 hr

Adverse reactions

CNS: dizziness, headache, fatigue

CV: chest pain, peripheral edema, hypertension

EENT: sinusitis, pharyngitis

GI: nausea, vomiting, diarrhea, dyspepsia, abdominal pain

GU: urinary tract infection

Musculoskeletal: myalgia, back and leg pain

Respiratory: cough, upper respiratory infection

Other: pain, flu or flulike symptoms

Interactions

Drug-drug. *Antihypertensives, diuretics:* increased risk of hypotension

Digoxin: increased digoxin blood level

Warfarin: decreased warfarin blood level

Drug-diagnostic tests. *Creatinine:* slight elevation

Drug-food. *Any food:* slightly reduced drug bioavailability

Patient monitoring

• Watch for signs and symptoms of hypotension.

• Correct volume deficits as appropriate before therapy starts. Monitor fluid intake and output and creatinine level during therapy.

Patient teaching

• Tell patient to take 1 hour before or 2 hours after meals.

t

• Caution patient not to remove tablet from blister pack until just before taking.
• Advise patient to report swelling or chest pain.
• Teach patient to measure blood pressure regularly and report significant changes.
• Tell patient to report suspected pregnancy to prescriber. Caution her not to breastfeed.
• As appropriate, review all other significant adverse reactions and interactions, especially those related to the drugs, tests, and foods mentioned above.

temazepam

Restoril

Pharmacologic class: Benzodiazepine
Therapeutic class: Sedative-hypnotic
Controlled substance schedule IV
Pregnancy risk category X

Action

Depresses CNS at limbic, thalamic, and hypothalamic levels. Enhances effects of gamma-aminobutyric acid, resulting in sedation, hypnosis, skeletal muscle relaxation, and anticonvulsant and anxiolytic activity.

Availability

Capsules: 7.5 mg, 15 mg, 30 mg

Indications and dosages

➢ Insomnia
Adults: 15 mg P.O. at bedtime p.r.n. Range is 7.5 to 30 mg.

Dosage adjustment

• Elderly or debilitated patients

Contraindications

• Hypersensitivity to drug or other benzodiazepines
• Pregnancy

Precautions

Use cautiously in:
• chronic pulmonary insufficiency, hepatic dysfunction, renal disease, psychoses, drug abuse
• history of suicide attempt or drug abuse
• elderly or debilitated patients
• breastfeeding patients
• children younger than age 15.

Administration

• Give at bedtime with or without food.

Route	Onset	Peak	Duration
P.O.	30 min	1.2-1.6 hr	Unknown

Adverse reactions

CNS: hangover, headache, dizziness, drowsiness, lethargy, fatigue, paradoxical stimulation, light-headedness, talkativeness, irritability, nervousness, confusion, euphoria, relaxed feeling, tremor, incoordination, impaired memory, nightmares, paresthesia
CV: chest pain, palpitations, tachycardia
EENT: eye irritation, pain, and swelling; photophobia; tinnitus
GI: nausea, vomiting, constipation, diarrhea, heartburn, abdominal pain, dry mouth, anorexia
Musculoskeletal: joint pain
Other: altered taste, body pain, physical or psychological drug dependence, drug tolerance

Interactions

Drug-drug. *Antidepressants, antihistamines, opioid analgesics, other sedative-hypnotics:* additive CNS depression
Digoxin: increased digoxin blood level, greater risk of toxicity

Probenecid: faster temazepam onset and prolonged effects
Theophylline: antagonism of temazepam's sedative effects
Drug-herbs. *Chamomile, hops, kava, skullcap, valerian:* increased CNS depression
Drug-behaviors. *Alcohol use:* additive CNS depression
Smoking: increased drug metabolism

Patient monitoring

- Monitor neurologic status carefully. Check for paradoxical reactions, especially in elderly patient.
- Watch for signs and symptoms of physical and psychological drug dependence. Stay alert for drug hoarding.

Patient teaching

- Advise patient to establish effective bedtime routine, to minimize insomnia.
- Inform patient (and significant other if appropriate) that drug may cause psychological and physical dependence and should be used only as prescribed and needed.
- Caution patient to avoid driving and other hazardous activities on day after taking drug, until he knows how it affects concentration and alertness.
- Instruct patient not to drink alcohol.
- Advise patient not to smoke or use herbs without consulting prescriber.
- Instruct patient to report suspected pregnancy.
- As appropriate, review all other significant adverse reactions and interactions, especially those related to the drugs, herbs, and behaviors mentioned above.

temozolomide

Temodal✱, Temodar

Pharmacologic class: Alkylating agent
Therapeutic class: Antineoplastic
Pregnancy risk category D

Action

Rapidly converts to monomethyl triazeno imidazole carboxamide, an active compound that prevents DNA transcription

Availability

Capsules: 5 mg, 20 mg, 100 mg, 250 mg

Indications and dosages

➢ Refractory anaplastic astrocytoma
Adults: 150 mg/m² P.O. daily for 5 consecutive days of each 28-day treatment cycle. Adjust dosage as appropriate based on absolute neutrophil count.

Contraindications

- Hypersensitivity to drug, its components, or dacarbazine
- Pregnancy or breastfeeding

Precautions

Use cautiously in:

- severe hepatic or renal impairment, active infection, decreased bone marrow reserve, other chronic debilitating illness
- elderly patients
- patients with childbearing potential
- children (safety not established).

Administration

- Follow facility policy for handling and disposing of chemotherapeutic drugs.
- Give daily with a full glass of water, consistently either with or without food.

• Be aware that dosages in 28-day cycle depend on nadir neutrophil and platelet counts.

Route	Onset	Peak	Duration
P.O.	Rapid	1 hr	Unknown

Adverse reactions

CNS: fatigue, headache, dysphasia, poor coordination, ataxia, anxiety, depression, dizziness, drowsiness, confusion, amnesia, insomnia, mental status changes, weakness, paresis, hemiparesis, paresthesias, **seizures**
CV: peripheral edema
EENT: abnormal vision, diplopia, pharyngitis, sinusitis
GI: nausea, vomiting, constipation, diarrhea, abdominal pain, anorexia
GU: urinary incontinence or frequency, urinary tract infection, breast pain (in women)
Hematologic: anemia, **leukopenia, thrombocytopenia**
Metabolic: adrenal hypercorticism
Musculoskeletal: abnormal gait, back pain, myalgia
Respiratory: cough, upper respiratory infection
Skin: pruritus, rash
Other: fever, viral infection, weight gain

Interactions

Drug-drug. *Antineoplastics:* additive bone marrow depression
Live-virus vaccines: decreased antibody response to vaccine, greater risk of adverse reactions
Valproic acid: decreased oral clearance of temozolomide
Drug-diagnostic tests. *Neutrophils, platelets:* decreased counts

Patient monitoring

🔈 Monitor CBC with white cell differential. Stay alert for evidence of bone marrow depression.
• Assess neurologic status carefully.
• Monitor fluid intake and output, and weigh patient regularly.

Patient teaching

• Tell patient to take consistently with or without food, and with a full glass of water.
• If drug causes nausea or vomiting, advise patient to take it 1 hour before or 2 hours after a meal.
• Inform patient that drug may cause abnormal gait and dizziness.
🔈 Instruct patient to immediately report unusual bleeding or bruising.
• Advise patient to avoid live-virus vaccines.
• Caution patient to avoid driving and other hazardous activities until he knows how drug affects concentration, alertness, and vision.
• Instruct patient to report suspected pregnancy. Caution her not to breastfeed.
• As appropriate, review all other significant and life-threatening adverse reactions and interactions, especially those related to the drugs and tests mentioned above.

tenecteplase

TNKase

Pharmacologic class: Tissue plasminogen activator
Therapeutic class: Thrombolytic enzyme
Pregnancy risk category C

Action

Binds to fibrin and converts plasminogen to plasmin, which breaks down fibrin clots and lyses thrombi and emboli. Causes systemic fibrinolysis.

Availability

Powder for injection: 50 mg/vial with 10-ml syringe and TwinPak Dual Cannula Device and 10-ml vial of sterile water for injection

Indications and dosages

➢ To reduce mortality associated with acute myocardial infarction

Adults weighing 90 kg (198 lb) or more: 50 mg I.V. bolus given over 5 seconds

Adults weighing 80 kg to 89 kg (176 to 197 lb): 45 mg I.V. bolus given over 5 seconds

Adults weighing 70 kg to 79 kg (154 to 175 lb): 40 mg I.V. bolus given over 5 seconds

Adults weighing 60 to 69 kg (132 to 153 lb): 35 mg I.V. bolus given over 5 seconds

Adults weighing less than 60 kg (132 lb): 30 mg I.V. bolus given over 5 seconds

Contraindications

- Hypersensitivity to drug or other tissue plasminogen activators
- Active internal bleeding
- Bleeding diathesis
- Recent intracranial or intraspinal surgery or trauma
- Severe uncontrolled hypertension
- Intracranial neoplasm
- Arteriovenous malformation or aneurysm
- History of cerebrovascular accident (CVA)

Precautions

Use cautiously in:

- previous puncture of noncompressible vessels, organ biopsy, hypertension, acute pericarditis, high risk of left ventricular thrombosis, subacute bacterial endocarditis, hemostatic defects, diabetic hemorrhagic retinopathy, septic thrombophlebitis, obstetric delivery
- patients taking warfarin concurrently
- patients older than age 75
- pregnant or breastfeeding patients.

Administration

- Reconstitute by mixing contents of prefilled syringe with 10 ml of sterile water for injection. Swirl gently; don't shake. Draw up prescribed dosage from vial, then discard remainder. Give I.V. over 5 seconds through designated line.
- Don't deliver in same I.V. line with dextrose solutions. Flush I.V. line with normal saline solution before giving drug if patient has been receiving dextrose.
- Give with heparin if ordered, but not through same I.V. line.

Route	Onset	Peak	Duration
I.V.	Immediate	Unknown	Unknown

Adverse reactions

CNS: intracranial hemorrhage, CVA

CV: hypotension, **arrhythmia, myocardial rupture, myocardial reinfarction, cardiogenic shock, atrioventricular block, cardiac arrest, cardiac tamponade, heart failure**, pericarditis, **pericardial effusion, mitral regurgitation, thrombosis, embolism, hemorrhage**

EENT: epistaxis, minor pharyngeal bleeding

GI: nausea, vomiting, **hemorrhage**

GU: hematuria

Hematologic: anemia, **bleeding tendency**

Respiratory: respiratory depression, pulmonary edema, apnea

Skin: bleeding at puncture sites, hematoma

Interactions

Drug-drug. *Anticoagulants, aspirin, dipyridamole, indomethacin, phenylbutazone:* increased bleeding risk

Drug-diagnostic tests. *Coagulation tests:* fibrinogen degradation in blood sample

Patient monitoring

Monitor ECG. Stay alert for reperfusion arrhythmias.

Monitor vital signs carefully. Watch for signs and symptoms of respiratory depression and reinfarction.
Evaluate all body systems closely for signs and symptoms of bleeding. If bleeding occurs, stop drug and give antiplatelet agents, as ordered.
- Monitor CBC and coagulation studies. However, know that drug may skew coagulation results.

Patient teaching

Inform patient that drug increases risk of bleeding. Advise him to immediately report signs and symptoms of bleeding.
- Teach patient safety measures to avoid bruising and bleeding.
- Tell patient he'll undergo regular blood tests during therapy.
- As appropriate, review all other significant and life-threatening adverse reactions and interactions, especially those related to the drugs and tests mentioned above.

tenofovir disoproxil fumarate

Viread

Pharmacologic class: Nucleoside analog reverse transcriptase inhibitor
Therapeutic class: Antiretroviral
Pregnancy risk category B

Action

Inhibits activity of human immunodeficiency virus (HIV) by competing with natural substrate deoxyadenosine 5'-triphosphate; disrupts cellular DNA by causing chain termination

Availability

Tablets: 300 mg

Indications and dosages

➢ HIV-1 infection
Adults: 300 mg P.O. daily

Dosage adjustment

- Renal impairment

Contraindications

- Hypersensitivity to drug
- Renal insufficiency
- Hepatotoxicity
- Lactic acidosis
- Breastfeeding

Precautions

Use cautiously in:
- elderly patients
- pregnant patients
- children.

Administration

- Give without regard to meals.
- Know that drug is usually given with other antiretrovirals. If patient is also receiving didanosine, give tenofovir at least 2 hours before or 1 hour after didanosine.

Route	Onset	Peak	Duration
P.O.	Rapid	45-75 min	Unknown

Adverse reactions

CNS: headache, asthenia
GI: nausea, vomiting, diarrhea, abdominal pain, flatulence, anorexia
GU: glycosuria
Hepatic: severe hepatomegaly with steatosis
Metabolic: hyperglycemia, **lactic acidosis**
Other: body fat redistribution

Interactions

Drug-drug. *Acyclovir, cidofovir, didanosine, ganciclovir, indinavir, iopinavir, probenecid, ritonavir, valacyclovir, valganciclovir, other drugs eliminated by active tubular secretion:* increased blood level of either drug

Drug-diagnostic tests. *Alanine aminotransferase, amylase, aspartate aminotransferase, blood and urine glucose, creatine kinase, triglycerides:* increased levels
Neutrophils: decreased count
Drug-food. *Any food:* decreased drug bioavailability and efficacy

Patient monitoring

🔈 Watch for and report signs and symptoms of lactic acidosis or hepatotoxicity.
- Monitor kidney and liver function tests.
- Assess nutritional status and hydration in light of adverse GI reactions and underlying disease.

Patient teaching

- Tell patient to take once daily with or without food.
- If patient is also receiving didanosine, instruct him to take tenofovir at least 2 hours before or 1 hour after didanosine.

🔈 Instruct patient to immediately report unusual tiredness or yellowing of skin or eyes.
- Tell patient drug may cause weakness and headache. Caution him to avoid driving and other hazardous activities until he knows how drug affects performance.
- Caution female patient not to breastfeed.
- As appropriate, review all other significant and life-threatening adverse reactions and interactions, especially those related to the drugs, tests, and foods mentioned above.

terazosin hydrochloride
Hytrin

Pharmacologic class: Anti-adrenergic (peripherally acting)
Therapeutic class: Antihypertensive
Pregnancy risk category C

Action

Blocks postsynaptic alpha$_1$-adrenergic receptors, causing vasodilation and decreasing smooth muscle contractions in bladder neck and prostate

Availability

Tablets: 1 mg, 2 mg, 5 mg, 10 mg

Indications and dosages

➤ Hypertension
Adults: Initially, 1 mg P.O., increased slowly as needed up to 5 mg/day. Usual range is 1 to 5 mg/day, not to exceed 20 mg/day.
➤ Benign prostatic hyperplasia
Adults: 1 mg P.O. at bedtime. To achieve desired response, may increase gradually to 2 mg/day, then to 5 mg/day, and then to a maximum of 10 mg/day.

Contraindications

- Hypersensitivity to drug or other quinazoline derivatives

Precautions

Use cautiously in:
- prostate cancer, hepatic disease, dehydration, volume or sodium depletion
- pregnant or breastfeeding patients
- children (safety not established).

Administration

🔈 Don't stop therapy suddenly. Dosage must be tapered.

t

• Know that drug may be given as a single dose at bedtime or in two divided doses.

Route	Onset	Peak	Duration
P.O.	15 min	2-3 hr	24 hr

Adverse reactions

CNS: dizziness, headache, weakness, drowsiness, nervousness, paresthesia, vertigo, fatigue, syncope
CV: orthostatic hypotension (with first dose), rebound hypertension, chest pain, palpitations, peripheral edema, tachycardia, **arrhythmias**
EENT: blurred vision, conjunctivitis, amblyopia, nasal congestion, sinusitis
GI: nausea, vomiting, diarrhea, abdominal pain, dry mouth
GU: urinary frequency or incontinence, erectile dysfunction, priapism
Musculoskeletal: joint, back, and extremity pain; arthritis
Respiratory: dyspnea
Skin: pruritus
Other: fever, weight gain, flulike symptoms

Interactions

Drug-drug. *Estrogens, nonsteroidal anti-inflammatory drugs (NSAIDs), sympathomimetics:* decreased antihypertensive effects
Midodrine: antagonism of terazosin's action
Nitrates, other antihypertensives: additive hypotension
Drug-herbs. *Ephedra (ma huang):* antagonism of terazosin's action
Drug-behaviors. *Alcohol use:* additive hypotension

Patient monitoring

• Monitor blood pressure. Stay alert for orthostatic hypotension (first-dose effect) when therapy begins.
• Assess cardiovascular status. Report chest pain, peripheral edema, palpitations, and other significant effects.

Patient teaching

• Instruct patient to take at same time every day, with or without food.
Caution patient not to stop therapy abruptly. Dosage must be tapered.
Advise patient to immediately report swelling, breathing difficulty, palpitations, chest pain, and other cardiovascular reactions.
• Tell patient drug may cause erectile dysfunction and other sexual problems.
• Caution patient not to use NSAIDs or drink alcohol.
• Instruct patient to move slowly when sitting up or standing, to avoid dizziness from sudden blood pressure decrease.
• As appropriate, review all other significant and life-threatening adverse reactions and interactions, especially those related to the drugs, herbs, and behaviors mentioned above.

terbinafine hydrochloride

Desenex Max, Lamisil, Lamisil AT

Pharmacologic class: Synthetic allylamine derivative
Therapeutic class: Antifungal
Pregnancy risk category B

Action

Unclear. Thought to interfere with sterol biosynthesis of fungal cell membrane permeability by inhibiting enzymes responsible for normal fungal growth and maturation, resulting in cell death.

Availability

Cream: 1%
Tablets: 250 mg

Indications and dosages

➤ Tinea cruris; tinea corporis; tinea pedis; tinea versicolor
Adults and children: Massage cream

into affected area and surrounding area once or twice daily for 7 to 14 days, not to exceed 4 weeks.

➢ Onychomycosis of fingernail or toenail

Adults: For fingernail infection, 250 mg P.O. daily for 6 weeks. For toenail infection, 250 mg P.O. daily for 12 weeks.

Contraindications

- Hypersensitivity to drug or its components
- Chronic active hepatic disease

Precautions

Use cautiously in:

- renal impairment (use not recommended)
- pregnant or breastfeeding patients (use not recommended)
- children (safety and efficacy not established).

Administration

- Give with or without food, but not with coffee, cola, or tea.
- Don't put occlusive dressing over affected area after cream application.

Route	Onset	Peak	Duration
P.O.	Unknown	≤ 2 hr	Unknown
Topical	Unknown	Unknown	Unknown

Adverse reactions

CNS: headache
EENT: visual disturbances
GI: nausea, diarrhea, dyspepsia, abdominal pain, flatulence
Hematologic: neutropenia
Hepatic: hepatic failure
Skin: burning, stinging, dryness, itching, and local irritation (with topical form); rash; pruritus; urticaria; **erythema multiforme; Stevens-Johnson syndrome**
Other: taste disturbances

Interactions

Drug-drug. *Cimetidine:* decreased terbinafine clearance
Cyclosporine: increased cyclosporine clearance
Dextromethorphan: increased dextromethorphan blood level
Rifampin: increased terbinafine clearance
Warfarin: altered warfarin efficacy
Drug-diagnostic tests. *Hepatic enzymes:* increased levels
Neutrophils: decreased count
Drug-food. *Caffeine-containing foods and beverages:* decreased caffeine clearance
Drug-herbs. *Chaparral, comfrey, germander, jin bu huan, kava, pennyroyal:* increased risk of hepatotoxicity
Cola nut, guarana, yerba maté: decreased clearance of these herbs

Patient monitoring

- Monitor CBC and liver function tests.

[Clinical alert] Watch for signs and symptoms of erythema multiforme. Report early indications before they progress to Stevens-Johnson syndrome.

Patient teaching

- Tell patient he may take with or without food.
- Instruct patient to avoid coffee, tea, and colas, which can worsen adverse drug reactions.
- Tell patient drug may take 4 weeks to be effective in fingernail infections and 10 weeks in toenail infections. Urge him to keep taking it even though symptoms don't improve right away.

[Clinical alert] Advise patient to immediately report rash, sore throat, cough, fever, or yellowing of skin or eyes.

- Instruct patient not to place occlusive dressing over affected area after applying cream.
- Caution patient not to let cream contact eyes, nose, or mouth.
- As appropriate, review all other significant and life-threatening adverse

t

reactions and interactions, especially those related to the drugs, tests, foods, and herbs mentioned above.

terbutaline sulfate

Brethair, Brethine, Bricanyl

Pharmacologic class: Selective $beta_2$-adrenergic receptor agonist

Therapeutic class: Bronchodilator

Pregnancy risk category B

Action

Relaxes bronchial smooth muscle by stimulating $beta_2$-adrenergic receptors; inhibits release of hypersensitivity mediators, especially from mast cells

Availability

Inhaler: 0.2 mg/inhalation
Injection: 1 mg/ml
Tablets: 2.5 mg, 5 mg

Indications and dosages

➢ Bronchospasm in reversible obstructive airway disease

Adults and children older than age 12: 0.25 mg subcutaneously, repeated in 15 to 30 minutes p.r.n., up to a maximum of 0.5 mg in 4 hours. Or 2.5 to 5 mg P.O. q 6 hours t.i.d. while awake, up to a maximum of 15 mg/day in adults; 2.5 mg P.O. q 6 hours t.i.d. while awake, up to a maximum of 7.5 mg/day in children. Or 0.2 to 0.5 mg by inhaler (one to two inhalations) q 4 to 6 hours.

Dosage adjustment

- Renal impairment

Off-label uses

- Tocolytic in preterm labor

Contraindications

- Hypersensitivity to drug, its components, or sympathomimetic amines

Precautions

Use cautiously in:

- cardiovascular disorders, hypertension, arrhythmias, hyperthyroidism, diabetes mellitus, seizure disorders, glaucoma
- concurrent use of MAO inhibitors, tricyclic antidepressants, or beta-adrenergic blockers
- elderly patients
- breastfeeding patients.

Administration

- Inject subcutaneously into lateral deltoid.

Route	Onset	Peak	Duration
P.O.	30 min	2-3 hr	4-8 hr
Subcut.	15 min	30 min	1.5-4 hr
Inhalation	Unknown	Unknown	Unknown

Adverse reactions

CNS: tremors, anxiety, nervousness, insomnia, headache, dizziness, drowsiness, stimulation
CV: palpitations, chest discomfort, tachycardia
GI: nausea, vomiting
Skin: diaphoresis, flushing

Interactions

Drug-drug. *Beta-adrenergic blockers:* blockage of bronchodilating effect
MAO inhibitors, tricyclic antidepressants: potentiation of terbutaline's adverse cardiovascular reactions
Other sympathomimetic amines: additive adverse cardiovascular reactions

Patient monitoring

- Monitor vital signs.
- Assess neurologic status.

Patient teaching

- Tell patient he may take with or without food.
- Advise patient or parents to establish effective bedtime routine to minimize insomnia.

• Instruct patient or parents to space doses evenly during waking hours, to avoid taking drug at bedtime.
• As appropriate, review all other significant adverse reactions and interactions, especially those related to the drugs mentioned above.

teriparatide (recombinant)

Forteo

Pharmacologic class: Biosynthetic fragment of human parathyroid hormone
Therapeutic class: Parathyroid hormone
Pregnancy risk category C

Action

Stimulates new bone growth by binding to specific high-affinity cell-surface receptors

Availability

Injection: 750 mcg/3 ml (controlled pen device)

Indications and dosages

➢ Osteoporosis in patients at high risk for bone fracture
Adults: 20 mcg/day subcutaneously for up to 2 years

Contraindications

• Hypersensitivity to drug
• Conditions that increase osteosarcoma risk (such as Paget's disease, unexplained alkaline phosphatase elevation, open epiphyses, skeletal radiation therapy)
• Bone cancer metastases or history of bone cancer
• Metabolic bone disease other than osteoporosis
• Hypercalcemia

Precautions

Use cautiously in:
• urolithiasis, hypotension
• concurrent use of cardiac glycosides
• pregnant or breastfeeding patients.

Administration

• Inject subcutaneously into thigh or abdominal wall, with patient lying down.
• Know that prefilled injection pen delivers 20 mcg of drug per actuation and may be reused for up to 28 days after first injection. Discard pen in protected container after 28 days, even if it's not empty.

Route	Onset	Peak	Duration
Subcut.	Rapid	Rapid	Unknown

Adverse reactions

CNS: dizziness, headache, insomnia, depression, vertigo, asthenia
CV: hypertension, angina, syncope
EENT: rhinitis, pharyngitis
GI: nausea, vomiting, diarrhea, dyspepsia, anorexia
Metabolic: hyperuricemia
Musculoskeletal: joint pain, cramps
Respiratory: cough, dyspnea, pneumonia
Skin: rash, sweating
Other: pain

Interactions

Drug-drug. *Digoxin:* increased digoxin toxicity
Drug-diagnostic tests. *Calcium:* increased level

Patient monitoring

• Monitor respiratory and neurologic status and assess patient's mood.
• Monitor bone mineral density tests and calcium level.

Patient teaching

• Instruct patient to promptly report such adverse reactions as cough and difficulty breathing.

• Tell patient that prefilled injection pen delivers 20 mcg of drug per actuation. Inform him that he may reuse it for up to 28 days after first injection, and should then discard it in appropriate receptacle, even if it's not empty.
• Advise patient to establish effective bedtime routine to minimize insomnia.
• Caution patient to avoid driving and other hazardous activities until he knows how drug affects strength and balance.
• As appropriate, review all other significant adverse reactions and interactions, especially those related to the drugs and tests mentioned above.

testosterone

Androderm, AndroGel, Striant, Testim, Testoderm, Testoderm TTS, Testopel Pellets

testosterone cypionate

Depo-Testosterone

testosterone enanthate

Delatestryl

Pharmacologic class: Hormone
Therapeutic class: Androgenic and anabolic steroid, antineoplastic
Controlled substance schedule III
Pregnancy risk category X

Action

Responsible for normal growth and development of male sex organs and maintenance and maturation of secondary sex characteristics. Also decreases estrogen activity, which aids treatment of some breast cancers.

Availability

testosterone
Buccal system: 30 mg
Gel: 1% (25 mg, 50 mg)
Injection (aqueous suspension): 100 mg/ml
Pellets (subcutaneous implant): 75 mg
Transdermal system: 2.5 mg/24 hours, 4 mg/24 hours, 5 mg/24 hours, 6 mg/24 hours
testosterone cypionate
Injection: 100 mg/ml, 200 mg/ml
testosterone enanthate
Injection (in oil): 200 mg/ ml

Indications and dosages

➢ Male hypogonadism
Adult males: 10 to 25 mg (testosterone) I.M. two to three times weekly or 50 to 400 mg (enanthate) I.M. q 2 to 4 weeks for 3 to 4 years. Or 150 to 450 mg (pellet) implanted subcutaneously q 3 to 6 months. Or 5 mg daily transdermal (nonscrotal) system (Androderm); may increase up to 7.5 mg daily or 5 mg daily (Testoderm TTS), adjusted after 3 to 4 weeks and possibly increased to 10 mg daily. Or 4 to 6 mg daily transdermal scrotal system (Testoderm), adjusted after 3 to 4 weeks. Or 50 mg testosterone gel (AndroGel 1%) daily applied topically, adjusted up to 75 mg daily within 14 days, with subsequent dosages up to 100 mg daily. Or 30 mg (buccal system) to gum region b.i.d. Or 50 to 400 mg I.M. (cypionate) q 2 to 4 weeks.
➢ Delayed puberty
Adult males: 50 to 200 mg I.M. (enanthate only) q 2 to 4 weeks for limited duration (4 to 6 months); or 150 to 450 mg subcutaneously (pellets) q 3 to 6 months
➢ Inoperable breast cancer in women 1 to 5 years after menopause
Adults: 200 to 400 mg I.M. (enanthate) q 2 to 4 weeks

Contraindications

• Hypersensitivity to drug, its components, or tartrazine
• Serious cardiac, hepatic, or renal disease

• Males with breast cancer or suspected prostate cancer
• Females (buccal or transdermal systems or gel)
• Pregnancy or breastfeeding

Precautions

Use cautiously in:
• diabetes mellitus, cardiovascular or hepatic disease, sleep apnea, or hypercalcemia.

Administration

• Inspect aqueous solution for injection. If crystals are visible, warm bottle and shake contents to dissolve crystals.
• Rotate I.M. injection sites within upper outer quadrant of gluteus maximus. Inject deeply into muscle.
• Apply gel once daily to clean, dry, intact skin on shoulder, upper arm, or abdomen.
• Place buccal system just above incisor tooth. Have patient hold it in place for 30 seconds to ensure adhesion. Rotate to other side of mouth with each application.

Route	Onset	Peak	Duration
Buccal	Slow	10-12 hr	Unknown
I.M.	Unknown	10-100 min	Unknown
Subcut.	Unknown	Unknown	3-4 mo
Topical gel	30 min	Unknown	Unknown
Transdermal	Unknown	2-4 hr	Unknown

Adverse reactions

CNS: headache, depression, emotional lability, nervousness, anxiety, asthenia, memory loss, dizziness, vertigo, **cerebrovascular accident**
CV: edema, peripheral edema, **deep-vein phlebitis, heart failure**
GI: bleeding
GU: hematuria, urinary tract infection, impaired urination, scrotal cellulitis, benign prostatic hyperplasia, scrotal papilloma (with transdermal use), prostatitis, libido changes, breast pain or tenderness, gynecomastia, virilization in females, excessive hormonal effects in males
Hematologic: polycythemia, leukopenia, suppressed clotting factors
Hepatic: hepatic adenoma (with long-term enanthate use)
Metabolic: hyperphosphatemia, hypernatremia, hypercalcemia, **hypoglycemia, hyperkalemia**
Musculoskeletal: myalgia
Respiratory: sleep apnea
Skin: acne; rash, itching, burning, discomfort, irritation, burn-like blister, erythema (with transdermal use); pain, local edema, and induration at injection site (with I.M. or subcutaneous use)
Other: accidental injury, flulike symptoms, hypersensitivity reaction

Interactions

Drug-drug. *Corticosteroids:* increased risk of edema
Hepatotoxic drugs: increased risk of hepatotoxicity
Insulin, oral hypoglycemics: decreased blood glucose level
Oral anticoagulants: increased anticoagulant effect
Oxyphenbutazone: increased oxyphenbutazone blood level
Propranolol: increased propranolol clearance
Drug-diagnostic tests. *Bilirubin, liver function tests:* abnormal results
Calcium, cholesterol, hematocrit, hemoglobin, phosphate, prostate-specific antigen (with topical use), sodium: increased levels
Clotting factors, creatine excretion, glucose, serum creatinine, thyroxine, thyroxine-binding globulin: decreased levels
Urine creatine and creatinine: decreased excretion
Urine 17-ketosteroids: increased excretion

t

Drug-herbs. *Chaparral, comfrey, germander, jin bu huan, kava, pennyroyal:* increased risk of hepatotoxicity

Patient monitoring

- Monitor electrolyte levels, liver function tests, blood and urine calcium levels, lipid panels, CBC with white cell differential, and semen studies.
- Assess diabetic patient carefully for hypoglycemia.
- Closely monitor neurologic status. Stay alert for sleep apnea.
- Assess for early signs of excessive hormonal effects in females (virilization). If these occur, drug withdrawal may be indicated.

Patient teaching

🔊 Instruct patient to immediately report signs and symptoms of liver problems, including nausea, vomiting, yellowing of skin or eyes, and ankle swelling.
- Teach prepubertal male about signs and symptoms of excessive hormonal effects, such as acne, priapism, increased body and facial hair, and penile enlargement.
- Teach postpubertal male about signs and symptoms of excessive adverse hormonal effects, such as erectile dysfunction, gynecomastia, epididymitis, testicular atrophy, and infertility.

🔊 Tell female patient to immediately report signs of masculinization, such as excessive body or facial hair, deepening of voice, clitoral enlargement, and menstrual irregularities.
- Advise female of childbearing age to use barrier contraceptives. Caution her not to breastfeed.
- Tell patient which transdermal patches can be applied to scrotum. Instruct him to apply patch daily to clean, dry skin after removing protective liner to expose drug-containing film. To prevent irritation, instruct him to apply each patch to a different site, waiting at least 1 week before reusing same site.
- Advise patient to apply topical gel once daily to clean, dry skin on shoulder, upper arm, or abdomen. Tell him that after opening packet, he should squeeze entire contents into palm and apply immediately. Instruct him to wait until gel dries before getting dressed.
- Teach patient to place buccal system in comfortable position just above incisor tooth and hold it in place for about 30 seconds to ensure adhesion. Tell him to use opposite side of mouth with each application. Caution him to not to dislodge buccal system, especially when eating, drinking, brushing teeth, or using mouthwash. If system doesn't properly adhere or falls out during 12-hour dosing interval, tell him to discard it and apply new system. If it falls out within 4 hours of next dose, tell him to apply new system and keep it in place until next regularly scheduled dose.
- Tell patient drug shouldn't be used to enhance athletic performance or physique.
- As appropriate, review all other significant and life-threatening adverse reactions and interactions, especially those related to the drugs, tests, and herbs mentioned above.

tetracycline hydrochloride

Actisite, Apo-Tetra✱, Bristacycline, Novotetra✱, Nu-Tetra✱, Sumycin, Sumycin Syrup

Pharmacologic class: Tetracycline
Therapeutic class: Anti-infective
Pregnancy risk category B (topical form), ***D*** (oral form)

Action

Unknown. Thought to inhibit bacterial protein synthesis at level of 30S and 50S bacterial ribosomes and to alter cytoplasmic membrane of susceptible organisms.

Availability

Capsules: 250 mg, 500 mg
Ointment: 3%
Oral suspension: 125 mg/5 ml

Indications and dosages

➢ Mild to moderate infections caused by susceptible organisms
Adults: 500 mg P.O. b.i.d. or 250 mg P.O. q.i.d.
➢ Severe infections caused by susceptible organisms
Adults: 500 mg P.O. q.i.d.
Children older than age 8: 25 to 50 mg/kg P.O. q.i.d.
➢ Syphilis in penicillin-allergic patients
Adults: 500 mg P.O. q.i.d. for 14 days
➢ Late syphilis (except neurosyphilis)
Adults: 500 mg P.O. q.i.d. for 28 days
➢ Leptospirosis when penicillin is contraindicated or ineffective
Adults: 1 to 2 g P.O. daily in two to four divided doses for 5 to 7 days
➢ Yaws
Adults: 1 to 2 g P.O. daily in two to four divided doses for 10 to 14 days
➢ Gonorrhea in penicillin-allergic patients
Adults: Initially, 1.5 g P.O., followed by 500 mg P.O. q 6 hours for 4 days, up to a total of 9 g
➢ Uncomplicated urethral, endocervical, or rectal infections caused by *Chlamydia trachomatis*
Adults: 500 mg P.O. q.i.d for 7 days
➢ Rickettsial and mycoplasmal infections
Adults: 1 to 2 g P.O. daily in two to four divided doses for 7 days
➢ *Helicobacter pylori* infection
Adults: In patients with active duodenal ulcer, 500 mg P.O. q.i.d. at meals and bedtime for 14 days, given with other drugs (such as metronidazole, bismuth subsalicylate, amoxicillin, or omeprazole)
➢ Brucellosis
Adults: 500 mg P.O. q.i.d. for 3 weeks, given with streptomycin I.M. b.i.d. during week 1 and streptomycin once daily during week 2
➢ Granuloma inguinale; chancroid
Adults: 1 to 2 g P.O. daily in two to four divided doses for 2 to 4 weeks
➢ Cholera
Adults: 500 mg P.O. q 6 hours for 48 to 72 hours
➢ Plague when streptomycin is contraindicated or ineffective
Adults: 2 to 4 g P.O. q.i.d. for 10 days
Children older than age 8: 30 to 40 mg/kg P.O. q.i.d. for 10 to 14 days
➢ Tularemia as an alternative to streptomycin
Adults: 1 to 2 g P.O. daily in two to four divided doses for 1 to 2 weeks
➢ *Campylobacter* infection
Adults: 1 to 2 g P.O. daily in two to four divided doses for 10 days
➢ Relapsing fever caused by *Borrelia recurrentis*
Adults: 1 to 2 g P.O. daily in two to four divided doses for 7 days or until patient is afebrile
➢ Adjunctive treatment of inflammatory acne
Adults and adolescents: 500 mg to 1 g P.O. q.i.d. for 1 to 2 weeks, decreased gradually to 125 to 500 mg P.O. daily
➢ Acne vulgaris
Adults and children older than age 11: 3% ointment applied to affected area b.i.d. (morning and evening) until skin is thoroughly wet

Dosage adjustment

- Renal impairment

Off-label uses

- Rosacea
- Anthrax
- Arthritis

• Lyme disease
• Sclerosing agent to control pleural effusions

Contraindications

• Hypersensitivity to drug, other tetracyclines, bisulfites, or alcohol (in some products)

Precautions

Use cautiously in:
• renal disease, hepatic impairment, nephrogenic diabetes insipidus
• cachectic or debilitated patients
• pregnant or breastfeeding patients (except in anthrax treatment or with topical form)
• children younger than age 11 (with topical form)
• children younger than age 8 (except in anthrax treatment).

Administration

• Give with 8 oz of water at least 1 hour before or 2 hours after a meal (especially if it includes milk or other dairy products), antacids, laxatives, or antidiarrheal drugs.

Route	Onset	Peak	Duration
P.O.	Rapid	2-3 hr	6-12 hr
Topical	Unknown	Unknown	Unknown

Adverse reactions

CNS: paresthesia, **benign intracranial hypertension**
CV: pericarditis
EENT: abnormal conjunctival pigmentation, hoarseness, pharyngitis
GI: nausea, vomiting, diarrhea, loose bulky stools, esophageal ulcers, epigastric distress, enterocolitis, oral and anogenital candidiasis, stomatitis, black hairy tongue, glossitis, anorexia, **pancreatitis**
GU: dark yellow or brown urine, vaginal candidiasis, anogenital lesions
Hematologic: eosinophilia, **hemolytic anemia, neutropenia, thrombocytopenia, thrombocytopenia purpura**
Hepatic: fatty liver
Musculoskeletal: retarded bone growth, polyarthralgia
Respiratory: pulmonary infiltrates
Skin: stinging and yellowing of skin (with topical form), photosensitivity, maculopapular or erythematous rash, increased pigmentation, urticaria, onycholysis
Other: permanent tooth discoloration (in children younger than age 8), tooth enamel defects, superinfection, hypersensitivity reactions including **anaphylaxis, serum sickness–like reaction, exacerbation of systemic lupus erythematosus**

Interactions

Drug-drug. *Adsorbent antidiarrheals, antacids, calcium, cholestyramine, cimetidine, colestipol, iron, magnesium, sodium bicarbonate:* decreased tetracycline absorption
Digoxin: increased digoxin blood level, greater risk of toxicity
Hormonal contraceptives: decreased contraceptive efficacy
Insulin: reduced insulin requirement
Lithium: increased or decreased lithium blood level
Methoxyflurane: increased risk of nephrotoxicity
Penicillin: decreased penicillin activity
Sucralfate: prevention of tetracycline absorption from GI tract
Warfarin: enhanced warfarin effects
Drug-diagnostic tests. *Alanine aminotransferase, alkaline phosphatase, amylase, aspartate aminotransferase, bilirubin, blood urea nitrogen:* increased levels
Hemoglobin, neutrophils, platelets, white blood cells: decreased levels
Urinary catecholamines: false elevation
Drug-food. *Dairy products, foods containing calcium:* decreased drug absorption
Drug-behaviors. *Alcohol use:* decreased drug efficacy

Sun exposure: increased risk of photosensitivity

Patient monitoring

- Monitor for signs and symptoms of superinfection and hypersensitivity reaction.
- With long-term use, monitor CBC, liver function tests, and (in prepubertal patients) bone growth.
- Assess neurologic status. Stay alert for benign intracranial hypertension (especially in children).

Patient teaching

- Tell patient to take oral form with 8 oz of water at least 1 hour before or 2 hours after eating a meal, consuming dairy products, or taking antacids, laxatives, or antidiarrheal drugs. Advise him to take last daily dose at least 1 hour before bedtime.
- Stress importance of completing entire course of therapy as ordered, even after symptoms improve.

Caution patient not to use outdated tetracycline, because it may cause serious kidney disease.

- Teach patient to recognize and report signs and symptoms of yeast infection and other infections.
- With long-long therapy, tell patient he'll undergo regular blood testing. Advise parents that prepubertal child should have periodic bone X-rays.
- Instruct patient using topical form not to let drug touch eyes, nose, or mouth. Tell him drug may turn skin yellow.
- Caution patient to avoid alcohol during therapy.
- Tell parents that tetracycline use during tooth development period (last half of pregnancy, infancy, and childhood to age 8) may cause permanent yellow, gray, or brownish tooth discoloration.
- As appropriate, review all other significant and life-threatening adverse reactions and interactions, especially those related to the drugs, tests, foods, and behaviors mentioned above.

thalidomide

Thalomid

Pharmacologic class: Synthetic glutamic acid derivative
Therapeutic class: Immunomodulator, angiogenesis inhibitor
Pregnancy risk category X

Action

Suppresses excess levels of tumor necrosis factor-alpha in patients with erythema nodosum leprosum (ENL). Alters leukocyte migration by changing cell surface characteristics.

Availability

Capsules: 50 mg, 100 mg, 200 mg

Indications and dosages

➢ Cutaneous manifestations of moderate to severe ENL; to prevent and suppress recurrent ENL

Adults weighing 50 kg (110 lb) or more: 100 to 300 mg P.O. daily, or up to 400 mg P.O. daily, depending on disease severity or previous response. Continue therapy until symptoms of active reactions subside (usually after 2 weeks); then may taper in 50-mg decrements q 2 to 4 weeks.

Adults weighing less than 50 kg (110 lb): Initially, 100 mg P.O. daily, or up to 400 mg P.O. daily, depending on disease severity or previous response. Continue therapy until symptoms of active reactions subside (usually after 2 weeks); then may taper in 50-mg decrements q 2 to 4 weeks.

Off-label uses

- Aphthous stomatitis
- Wasting syndrome associated with human immunodeficiency virus (HIV)

• Multiple myeloma
• Refractory Crohn's disease

Contraindications

• Hypersensitivity to drug or its components
• Pregnancy

Precautions

Use cautiously in:
• breastfeeding patients (use not recommended)
• children younger than age 12 (safety not established).

Administration

🔊 Follow all instructions provided by System for Thalidomide Education and Prescribing Safety (S.T.E.P.S.™) program, accessible at http://www.steps-info.com.
• Give with 8 oz of water just before bedtime, at least 1 hour after evening meal.
• Know that patients who need prolonged maintenance therapy to prevent cutaneous ENL recurrence and those who have flares during tapering should receive minimum effective dosage, with tapering attempted every 3 to 6 months. To taper, decrease dosage by 50 mg every 2 to 4 weeks.

Route	Onset	Peak	Duration
P.O.	48 hr	1-2 mo	Unknown

Adverse reactions

CNS: drowsiness, dizziness, vertigo, sedation, tremor, asthenia, peripheral neuropathy
CV: bradycardia, orthostatic hypotension, peripheral edema
EENT: rhinitis, sinusitis, pharyngitis
GI: nausea, constipation, diarrhea, abdominal pain, oral moniliasis
GU: erectile dysfunction
Hematologic: neutropenia
Musculoskeletal: back pain
Skin: exfoliative, purpuric, bullous, or maculopapular rash; pruritus; fungal dermatitis; nail disorder; photosensitivity; toxic epidermal necrolysis, **Stevens-Johnson syndrome**
Other: tooth pain, chills, accidental injury, hypersensitivity reactions, increased HIV viral load, **severe birth defects, fetal death**

Interactions

Drug-drug. *Barbiturates, chlorpromazine, reserpine, sedative-hypnotics, and other CNS depressants:* increased sedation
Drugs linked to peripheral neuropathy: increased risk of peripheral neuropathy
Drug-diagnostic tests. *Alanine aminotransferase, aspartate aminotransferase, lactate dehydrogenase, lipids, liver function tests:* increased values
Hemoglobin, neutrophils, white blood cells: decreased values
Drug-food. *High-fat meal:* interference with drug absorption
Drug-behaviors. *Alcohol use:* increased sedation

Patient monitoring

🔊 Monitor for signs and symptoms of hypersensitivity reaction. If rash occurs, discontinue drug and contact prescriber immediately. Don't restart drug if Stevens-Johnson syndrome, toxic epidermal necrolysis, or exfoliative, purpuric, or bullous rash occurs.
• Watch for and report signs and symptoms of peripheral neuropathy.
• Assess CBC with white cell differential.
• Carefully monitor patient's reproductive status.

Patient teaching

• Instruct patient to take with 8 oz of water just before bedtime, at least 1 hour after dinner.
🔊 Tell patient to immediately report signs and symptoms of hypersensitivity reaction, especially rash.

• Teach patient about risks of fetal exposure to drug. Carefully review relevant portions of S.T.E.P.S.™ program with patient.
• Instruct female of childbearing age to use two highly effective birth control methods simultaneously, from 1 month before first thalidomide dose until 1 month after last dose.
• Explain mandatory pregnancy testing schedule to female patient, and stress importance of compliance.
Clinical alert: Advise female patient to contact prescriber immediately if she suspects she's pregnant.
• Caution female patient not to breastfeed.
• Instruct male patient to use latex condoms during every sexual encounter.
• Tell patient to avoid alcohol during drug therapy.
• As appropriate, review all other significant and life-threatening adverse reactions and interactions, especially those related to the drugs, tests, foods, and behaviors mentioned above.

theophylline

Apo-Theo LA♣, Elixophyllin, Pulmophyllin ELX♣, Quibron-T, Theochron, Theolair, Theo-24, T-Phyl, Uniphyl

Pharmacologic class: Xanthine derivative

Therapeutic class: Bronchodilator, spasmolytic

Pregnancy risk category C

Action

Relaxes bronchial smooth muscles, suppressing airway response to stimuli. Also inhibits phosphodiesterase and release of slow-reacting substance of anaphylaxis and histamine.

Availability

Capsules (immediate-release): 100 mg, 200 mg
Capsules (timed-release, 8 to 12 hours): 50 mg, 60 mg, 65 mg, 75 mg, 100 mg, 125 mg, 130 mg
Capsules (timed-release, 12 hours): 50 mg, 125 mg, 130 mg, 250 mg, 260 mg
Capsules (timed-release, 24 hours): 100 mg, 200 mg, 300 mg
Elixir: 80 mg/15 ml
Injection (with dextrose): 0.4 mg/ml, 0.8 mg/ml, 1.6 mg/ml, 2 mg/ml, 3.2 mg/ml, 4 mg/ml
Solution: 80 mg/15 ml, 150 mg/15 ml
Syrup (cherry): 80 mg/15 mg, 150 mg/15 ml
Tablets (immediate-release): 100 mg, 125 mg, 200 mg, 250 mg, 300 mg
Tablets (timed-release, 8 to 12 hours): 100 mg, 200 mg, 250 mg, 300 mg, 500 mg
Tablets (timed-release, 8 to 24 hours): 100 mg, 200 mg, 300 mg, 450 mg
Tablets (timed-release, 12 to 24 hours): 100 mg, 200 mg, 300 mg, 450 mg
Tablets (timed-release, 24 hours): 200 mg, 250 mg, 260 mg, 400 mg, 600 mg

Indications and dosages

➢ Acute bronchospasm in patients not receiving theophylline

Adults (otherwise healthy nonsmokers): Initially, 6 mg/kg P.O., followed in next 12 to 16 hours by 3 mg/kg P.O. q 6 hours for two doses, then a maintenance dosage of 3 mg/kg P.O. q 8 hours

Children ages 9 to 16; young adult smokers: Initially, 6 mg/kg P.O., followed in next 12 to 16 hours by 3 mg/kg P.O. q 4 hours for three doses, then a maintenance dosage of 3 mg/kg P.O. q 6 hours

Children ages 1 to 9: Initially, 6 mg/kg P.O., followed in next 12 to 16 hours by 4 mg/kg P.O. q 4 hours for three doses, then a maintenance dosage of 4 mg/kg P.O. q 6 hours

t

➢ Acute bronchospasm in patients receiving theophylline

Adults and children: Loading dose based partly on time, amount, and administration route of last dose and on expectation that each 0.5 mg/kg will produce 1 mcg/ml rise in theophylline blood level. In significant respiratory distress, loading dose may be 2.5 mg/kg P.O. or I.V. to increase theophylline level by approximately 5 mcg/ml.

➢ Chronic bronchospasm

Adults and children: *Immediate-release forms*—16 mg/kg or 400 mg P.O. daily (whichever is lower) in three to four divided doses q 6 to 8 hours. *Timed-release forms*—12 mg/kg or 400 mg P.O. daily (whichever is lower) in three to four divided doses q 8 to 12 hours. May increase dosage of either immediate- or timed-release form at 2- to 3-day intervals, to a maximum of 13 mg/kg or 900 mg daily (whichever is lower) in patients older than age 16, 18 mg/kg daily in children ages 12 to 16, 20 mg/kg daily in children ages 9 to 12, or 24 mg/kg daily in children up to age 9.

Dosage adjustment

- Cor pulmonale or heart failure
- Elderly patients
- Young adults

Off-label uses

- Essential tremor
- Apnea and bradycardia in premature infants

Contraindications

- Hypersensitivity to drug or other xanthines (such as coffee, theobromine)
- Active peptic ulcer
- Seizure disorder

Precautions

Use cautiously in:

- alcoholism; heart failure or other cardiac or circulatory impairment; hypertension; renal or hepatic disease; COPD; hypoxemia; hyperthyroidism; diabetes mellitus; glaucoma; peptic ulcer disease
- elderly patients
- children younger than age 1.

Administration

- For I.V. delivery, use infusion solution designed for drug, or mix with dextrose 5% in water. Administer by controlled infusion pump.
- Know that for acute bronchospasm, theophylline preferably is given I.V. as 20 mg/ml of theophylline (or 25 mg/ml of aminophylline).
- Don't give timed-release form to patient with acute bronchospasm.

Route	Onset	Peak	Duration
P.O.	Rapid	1-2 hr	6 hr
P.O. (timed)	Delayed	4-8 hr	8-24 hr
I.V.	Rapid	End of infusion	6-8 hr

Adverse reactions

CNS: irritability, dizziness, nervousness, restlessness, headache, insomnia, reflex hyperexcitability, **seizures**

CV: palpitations, marked hypotension, sinus tachycardia, extrasystole, **circulatory failure, ventricular arrhythmias**

GI: nausea, vomiting, diarrhea, hematemesis, gastroesophageal reflux

GU: increased diuresis, proteinuria

Metabolic: hyperglycemia, **syndrome of inappropriate antidiuretic hormone secretion**

Musculoskeletal: muscle twitching

Respiratory: tachypnea, **respiratory arrest**

Skin: urticaria, rash, alopecia, flushing

Other: fever, hypersensitivity reaction

Interactions

Drug-drug. *Allopurinol, calcium channel blockers, cimetidine, corticosteroids, disulfiram, ephedrine, hormonal contraceptives, influenza virus vaccine, interferon, macrolides, mexiletine, nonselective*

beta-adrenergic blockers, quinolones, thiabendazole: increased theophylline blood level, greater risk of toxicity
Aminoglutethimide, barbiturates, ketoconazole, rifampin, sulfinpyrazone, sympathomimetics: decreased theophylline blood level and effects
Carbamazepine, isoniazid, loop diuretics: increased or decreased theophylline blood level
Halothane: increased risk of arrhythmias
Hydantoins: decreased hydantoin blood level
Lithium: decreased therapeutic effect of lithium
Nondepolarizing muscle relaxants: reversal of neuromuscular blockade
Propofol: antagonism of propofol's sedative effects
Tetracyclines: increased risk of adverse reactions to theophylline
Drug-diagnostic tests. *Glucose:* increased level
Drug-food. *Any food:* altered bioavailability and absorption of some timed-release theophylline forms, causing rapid release and possible toxicity
Caffeine- or xanthine-containing foods and beverages: increased theophylline blood level and greater risk of adverse CNS and cardiovascular reactions
Diet high in protein and charcoal-broiled beef and low in carbohydrates: increased theophylline elimination, decreased efficacy
High-carbohydrate, low-protein diet: decreased theophylline elimination, increased risk of adverse reactions
Drug-herbs. *Caffeine-containing herbs (such as cola nut, guarana, maté):* increased theophylline blood level, greater risk of adverse CNS and cardiovascular reactions
Ephedra (ma huang): increased stimulant effect
St. John's wort: decreased theophylline blood level and efficacy
Drug-behaviors. *Nicotine (in cigarettes, gum, transdermal patches):* increased theophylline metabolism, decreased efficacy

Patient monitoring

- Monitor for signs and symptoms of hypersensitivity reaction, including rash and fever.
- Assess respiratory status. Monitor pulmonary function tests to gauge drug efficacy and identify adverse effects.
- Monitor cardiovascular and neurologic status carefully.
- Assess glucose level in diabetic patient.

Patient teaching

- Advise patient to take oral form with 8 oz of water 1 hour before or 2 hours after meals.
- Tell patient not to crush or chew timed-release form.
- Caution patient not to use different drug brands interchangeably.
- Instruct patient to immediately report worsening dyspnea and other respiratory problems.
- Teach patient to recognize and report adverse neurologic reactions.
- Tell patient that all nicotine forms (including cigarettes, patches, and gum) decrease drug efficacy. Discourage nicotine use.
- Advise patient that a diet high in protein and charcoal-broiled beef and low in carbohydrates makes drug less effective.
- Tell patient that a high-carbohydrate, low-protein diet increases risk of adverse reactions, as do products containing caffeine.
- Caution patient to avoid herbs, especially ephedra and St. John's wort.
- Advise patient not to take over-the-counter drugs without prescriber's approval. Tell him to inform all prescribers he's taking drug, because it interacts with many other drugs.

t

• As appropriate, review all other significant and life-threatening adverse reactions and interactions, especially those related to the drugs, tests, foods, herbs, and behaviors mentioned above.

thioridazine hydrochloride

Apo-Thioridazine✱, Novo-Ridazine✱, PMS Thioridazine✱

Pharmacologic class: Phenothiazine
Therapeutic class: Antipsychotic
Pregnancy risk category C

Action

Blocks dopamine receptors in CNS. Exerts strong alpha-adrenergic and anticholinergic blocking activity; also depresses cerebral cortex, hypothalamus, and limbic system.

Availability

Oral solution (concentrated): 30 mg/ml, 100 mg/ml
Oral suspension: 10 mg/5 ml, 25 mg/5 ml, 100 mg/5 ml
Tablets: 10 mg, 15 mg, 25 mg, 50 mg, 100 mg, 150 mg, 200 mg

Indications and dosages

➢ Schizophrenia

Adults: Initially, 50 to 100 mg P.O. t.i.d.; may increase gradually as needed to a maintenance dosage of up to 800 mg/day

Severely disturbed, hospitalized children ages 2 to 12: Initially, 0.5 mg/kg/day P.O. in divided doses. May increase gradually as needed until optimal effects occur; maximum daily dosage is 3 mg/kg.

Dosage adjustment

• Renal or hepatic impairment
• Elderly patients

Contraindications

• Hypersensitivity to drug, its components, or other phenothiazines
• Severe CNS depression
• Severe hypertension or hypotension
• Bone marrow depression or blood dyscrasias
• Genetic defect that inhibits CYP450-2D6
• Congenital long-QT syndrome
• Prolonged QTc interval
• History of arrhythmias
• Concurrent use of other drugs that prolong the QTc interval (such as fluoxetine, paroxetine) or reduce phenothiazine clearance by other means (such as fluvoxamine, pindolol, propranolol)

Precautions

Use cautiously in:
• cardiovascular or respiratory disease, mitral insufficiency, hepatic or renal impairment, glaucoma, depression, seizure disorder, risk factors for electrolyte imbalance (such as dehydration or diuretic therapy)
• sulfite or tartrazine sensitivity (with some products)
• alcohol intolerance (with concentrate)
• elderly or debilitated patients
• pregnant or breastfeeding patients.

Administration

• Due to risk of potentially life-threatening proarrhythmic effects, know that drug is indicated only for schizophrenic patients who don't respond adequately to other antipsychotics.
• Keep liquid form away from skin to avoid contact dermatitis.
• Before starting therapy, correct hypokalemia as ordered.
• Discontinue at least 48 hours before myelography, because of seizure risk.

Route	Onset	Peak	Duration
P.O.	Unknown	Unknown	8-12 hr

Adverse reactions

CNS: sedation, extrapyramidal reactions, tardive dyskinesia, **neuroleptic malignant syndrome, seizures**
CV: orthostatic hypotension, tachycardia, **prolonged QTc interval, arrhythmias**
EENT: lens opacities, pigmentary retinopathy, dry eyes
GI: constipation, ileus, dry mouth, anorexia
GU: urinary retention, dark urine, galactorrhea, gynecomastia
Hepatic: jaundice
Hematologic: agranulocytosis, leukopenia
Skin: rash, photosensitivity reaction, pigmentation changes
Other: allergic reactions, hyperthermia

Interactions

Drug-drug. *Anticholinergic and anticholinergic-like drugs (such as antihistamines, antidepressants, atropine, disopyramide, haloperidol, other phenothiazines):* additive anticholinergic effects
Antihypertensives, nitrates: additive hypotension
CNS depressants (such as antihistamines, general anesthetics, opioid analgesics, sedative-hypnotics): additive CNS depression
Diuretics: increased risk of electrolyte imbalances and arrhythmias
Drugs that inhibit CYP450-2D6 (such as fluoxetine, paroxetine), prolong the QTc interval (such as arsenic trioxide, azole antifungals, floxin antibiotics, octreotide), or decrease phenothiazine clearance by other means (such as fluvoxamine, pindolol, propranolol): increased risk of life-threatening arrhythmias
Lithium: disorientation, loss of consciousness, increased risk of extrapyramidal reactions
Drug-diagnostic tests. *Alanine aminotransferase, alkaline phosphatase, aspartate aminotransferase, serum bilirubin:* increased levels
Granulocytes, hematocrit, hemoglobin, platelets, white blood cells: decreased levels
Pregnancy tests, urine bilirubin: false-positive results
Drug-herbs. *Kava:* increased risk of adverse drug reactions
Drug-behaviors. *Alcohol use:* additive hypotension

Patient monitoring

🔈 Monitor neurologic status closely. Stay alert for signs and symptoms of neuroleptic malignant syndrome.
- Watch for tardive dyskinesia and extrapyramidal symptoms.
- Assess for urinary retention, constipation, and blurred vision.
- Monitor bilirubin level, CBC, liver function tests, and vision exams. Be aware that signs and symptoms of agranulocytosis, leukopenia, or hepatic dysfunction may warrant withdrawal.

🔈 Closely monitor depressed patient for suicidal ideation.

Patient teaching

- Instruct patient to dilute concentrate with water or fruit juice and then take dose right away, with or without food.

🔈 Caution patient not to stop therapy suddenly. Dosage must be tapered.
🔈 Tell patient or caregiver to immediately report signs and symptoms of serious CNS reactions, including high fever, sweating, unstable blood pressure, stupor, muscle rigidity, tongue protrusion, cheek puffing, mouth puckering, chewing movements, and involuntary leg or arm movements.
- Caution patient to keep liquid form away from skin. If it contacts skin, advise him to wash it off thoroughly and immediately.
- Tell patient to report urinary retention, blurred vision, or constipation.
- Advise patient to avoid driving and other hazardous activities.

t

• Caution patient not to drink alcohol. Tell him that concentrate form contains alcohol.
• Teach patient effective ways to counteract photosensitivity.
• As appropriate, review all other significant and life-threatening adverse reactions and interactions, especially those related to the drugs, tests, herbs, and behaviors mentioned above.

thyroid, desiccated

Armour Thyroid, Thyrar, Thyroid Strong, Westhroid

Pharmacologic class: Hormone supplement
Therapeutic class: Thyroid hormone
Pregnancy risk category A

Action

Regulates cell growth and differentiation and increases metabolic rate of body tissues; effects mediated at cellular level

Availability

Tablets: 15 mg, 30 mg, 60 mg, 90 mg, 120 mg, 180 mg, 240 mg, 300 mg

Indications and dosages

➢ Mild hypothyroidism
Adults: Initially, 60 mg/day P.O.; may increase by 60 mg q 30 days to desired response. Usual maintenance dosage is 60 to 180 mg/day.
➢ Severe hypothyroidism
Adults: Initially, 15 mg/day P.O. daily; may increase to 30 mg/day after 2 weeks and then to 60 mg/day 2 weeks later. Assess after 1 month, and again 1 month later at 60 mg-dose. If necessary, dosage may then increase to 120 mg/day P.O. for 2 months, with assessment repeated. Subsequent assessments and dosage increases may occur up to a maximum of 180 mg/day.
➢ Congenital or severe hypothyroidism
Children: Initially, 15 mg P.O. daily; may increase to 30 mg/day after 2 weeks, with subsequent increases at 2-week intervals. Maintenance dosage may be higher in growing children than in hypothyroid adults.

Dosage adjustment

• Cardiovascular disease
• Elderly patients

Contraindications

• Hypersensitivity to drug or its components
• Adrenal insufficiency
• Thyrotoxicosis

Precautions

Use cautiously in:
• tartrazine sensitivity (some products)
• cardiovascular disease
• elderly patients
• breastfeeding patients.

Administration

• Give before breakfast each day.

Route	Onset	Peak	Duration
P.O.	Unknown	12-48 hr	Unknown

Adverse reactions

CNS: insomnia, tremors, headache
CV: palpitations, angina pectoris, hypertension, tachycardia, **arrhythmias, cardiac arrest**
GI: nausea, vomiting, diarrhea
GU: menstrual irregularities
Metabolic: heat intolerance, **thyroid storm**
Musculoskeletal: accelerated bone maturation (in children)
Skin: sweating
Other: weight loss, appetite changes, fever

Interactions

Drug-drug. *Anticoagulants, catecholamines, sympathomimetics:* increased effects of these drugs
Bile acid sequestrants: decreased thyroid hormone absorption
Digoxin, insulin, oral hypoglycemics: decreased effects of these drugs
Estrogen: decreased thyroid hormone effects
Oral anticoagulants: increased risk of bleeding
Drug-diagnostic tests. *Aspartate aminotransferase, creatine kinase, glucose, lactate dehydrogenase, protein-bound iodine:* increased levels
Thyroid function tests: decreased values
Drug-herbs. *Bugleweed, soy:* increased adverse drug reactions

Patient monitoring

Monitor for chest pain. If it occurs, withhold drug and contact prescriber.
• Assess vital signs and temperature frequently.
Monitor thyroid function tests closely. Immediately report evidence of thyroid storm.
• In diabetic patient, monitor blood glucose level closely.
• In children, monitor sleeping pulse rate and morning basal temperature.
• In female on long-term therapy, monitor bone density tests.

Patient teaching

• Tell patient to take each morning before breakfast.
Caution patient not to stop therapy abruptly. Dosage must be tapered.
Advise patient to immediately report chest pain or signs and symptoms of drug toxicity (fever, chest pain, rapid pulse, skipped heartbeats, heat intolerance, excessive sweating, nervousness, emotional instability).
• Instruct patient to tell all prescribers he's taking drug. Caution him not to use over-the-counter preparations without consulting prescriber.
• Tell diabetic patient that drug may alter blood glucose level. Encourage frequent glucose self-monitoring.
• As appropriate, review all other significant and life-threatening adverse reactions and interactions, especially those related to the drugs, tests, and herbs mentioned above.

tiagabine hydrochloride

Gabatril Filmtabs

Pharmacologic class: Nipecotic acid derivative
Therapeutic class: Anticonvulsant
Pregnancy risk category C

Action

Unknown. Thought to raise seizure threshold by enhancing activity of gamma-aminobutyric acid (a major inhibitory neurotransmitter in CNS).

Availability

Tablets: 2 mg, 4 mg, 12 mg, 16 mg, 20 mg

Indications and dosages

➢ Adjunctive treatment of partial seizures
Adults older than age 18: Initially, 4 mg P.O. once daily for 1 week; may increase as needed by 4 to 8 mg/day at weekly intervals, up to 56 mg/day in two to four divided doses
Adolescents ages 12 to 18: Initially, 4 mg P.O. once daily. May increase total daily dosage by 4 mg at start of week 2; thereafter, may increase by 4 to 8 mg q week until clinical response occurs or patient is receiving up to 32 mg/day. Give total daily dosage in two to four divided doses.

t

Dosage adjustment
• Hepatic impairment

Off-label uses
• Anxiety

Contraindications
• Hypersensitivity to drug or its components

Precautions
Use cautiously in:
• hepatic impairment
• pregnant or breastfeeding patients
• children younger than age 12 (safety not established).

Administration
◀ Don't stop drug suddenly. Dosage must be tapered.
• Be aware that concomitant anticonvulsant therapy need not be modified unless indicated.

Route	Onset	Peak	Duration
P.O.	Unknown	45 min	Unknown

Adverse reactions
CNS: dizziness, insomnia, drowsiness, nervousness, asthenia, confusion, poor concentration, impaired memory, depression, emotional lability, hostility, agitation, ataxia, abnormal gait, tremors, paresthesia, speech disorder, language problems
CV: vasodilation
EENT: nystagmus, epistaxis, pharyngitis
GI: nausea, vomiting, diarrhea, abdominal pain, mouth ulcers
Musculoskeletal: myasthenia
Respiratory: increased cough
Skin: rash, pruritus
Other: increased appetite, weight changes, pain, allergic reaction

Interactions
Drug-drug. *Carbamazepine, phenobarbital, phenytoin, primidone:* increased tiagabine clearance, decreased blood level

Patient monitoring
◀ Watch for signs or symptoms of depression and suicidal ideation.
• Assess vital signs and cardiovascular status.
• Monitor closely for severe generalized weakness. If present, consult prescriber regarding possible dosage reduction.

Patient teaching
• Tell patient to take on regular schedule with food.
◀ Caution patient not to stop therapy suddenly. Dosage must be tapered.
• Instruct patient to report signs or symptoms of depression.
◀ Advise patient to report neurologic reactions. Tell him to contact prescriber immediately if severe overall weakness or severe depression occurs.
• Advise female patient to tell prescriber if she suspects she's pregnant.
• As appropriate, review all other significant adverse reactions and interactions, especially those related to the drugs mentioned above.

ticarcillin disodium
Ticar

Pharmacologic class: Penicillin (extended-spectrum)
Therapeutic class: Anti-infective
Pregnancy risk category B

Action
Inhibits bacterial cell-wall synthesis and division during replication, causing osmotically unstable cells to lyse and die

Availability
Powder for injection: 1 g, 3 g, 6 g, 20 g, 30 g

Indications and dosages

➢ Complicated urinary tract infections (UTIs)

Adults and children: 150 to 200 mg/kg/day I.V. infusion in divided doses q 4 to 6 hours

➢ Uncomplicated UTIs

Adults and children weighing more than 40 kg (88 lb): 1 g I.M. or direct I.V. q 6 hours

Children older than 1 month who weigh less than 40 kg (88 lb): 50 to 100 mg/kg/day I.M. or direct I.V. in divided doses q 6 hours to 8 hours, not to exceed adult dosage

➢ Bacterial septicemia

Adults and children: 200 to 300 mg/kg/day by I.V. infusion in divided doses q 4 or 6 hours, depending on patient's weight and severity of infection

Dosage adjustment

- Hepatic or renal impairment

Contraindications

- Hypersensitivity to drug or other penicillins

Precautions

Use cautiously in:

- cystic fibrosis, renal or hepatic disease
- pregnant or breastfeeding patients.

Administration

- Ask patient about penicillin allergy before giving.
- For direct I.V. injection, dilute with sodium chloride solution, dextrose 5% in water, or lactated Ringer's solution as directed. Give by slow I.V. injection into vein or I.V. tubing, preferably no faster than 50 mg/ml to reduce vein irritation.
- For intermittent or continuous I.V. infusion, reconstitute and dilute with compatible I.V. solution to a concentration of 10 to 100 mg/ml. Give by slow or intermittent I.V. infusion over 30 minutes to 2 hours (in adults).
- Change I.V. site every 2 days.
- For I.M. use, reconstitute 1-g vial with 2 ml of sterile water for injection, sodium chloride injection, or 1% lidocaine solution without epinephrine. Solution will contain approximately 385 mg ticarcillin per ml. Inject I.M. deep into large muscle, such as gluteus maximus. Don't exceed 2 g per injection.
- Give at least 1 hour before aminoglycosides (such as amikacin, gentamicin, or tobramycin).

Route	Onset	Peak	Duration
I.V.	Rapid	End of infusion	Unknown
I.M.	Rapid	30-75 min	Unknown

Adverse reactions

CNS: headache, giddiness, dizziness, lethargy, fatigue, hyperreflexia, neuromuscular excitability, asterixis, hallucinations, stupor, **seizures**

GI: nausea, vomiting, diarrhea, flatulence, **pseudomembranous colitis**

Hematologic: eosinophilia, transient **neutropenia** and **leukopenia** (with high doses)

Skin: urticaria, rash

Other: unpleasant taste; pain, induration, and erythema at I.M. injection site; fever; overgrowth of nonsusceptible organisms; pain, vein irritation, erythema, phlebitis, and **thrombophlebitis** at I.V. site; hypersensitivity reactions including **anaphylaxis**

t

Interactions

Drug-drug. *Aminoglycosides:* physical incompatibility, causing aminoglycoside inactivation when mixed in same I.V. solution

Aminoglycosides, tetracyclines: additive activity against some bacteria

Lithium: altered lithium elimination

Probenecid: increased ticarcillin blood level

Drug-diagnostic tests. *Alanine aminotransferase, alkaline phosphatase, aspar-*

tate aminotransferase, eosinophils, lactate dehydrogenase, sodium: increased levels
Bleeding time: prolonged
Granulocytes, hemoglobin, platelets, white blood cells: decreased levels
Liver function tests: transient elevations
Urine glucose, urine protein: false-positive results

Patient monitoring

- Monitor liver function tests and CBC with white cell differential.
- Assess for superinfection and severe allergic reactions.
- Monitor neurologic status. Stay alert for seizures.

Patient teaching

Advise patient to promptly report skin reactions or severe diarrhea.
Tell patient drug may increase risk of other infections. Instruct him to report signs and symptoms of new infection right away.
- Advise patient to limit sodium intake (ticarcillin contains sodium).
- As appropriate, review all other significant and life-threatening adverse reactions and interactions, especially those related to the drugs and tests mentioned above.

ticarcillin disodium and clavulanate potassium

Timentin

Pharmacologic class: Penicillin (extended-spectrum)
Therapeutic class: Anti-infective
Pregnancy risk category B

Action

Ticarcillin disodium inhibits bacterial cell-wall synthesis during replication; clavulanic acid extends ticarcillin's antibiotic spectrum by inactivating beta-lactamase enzymes (which otherwise would degrade ticarcillin).

Availability

Injection: 3 g ticarcillin and 100 mg clavulanic acid in 3.1-g vials

Indications and dosages

➢ Systemic and urinary tract infections caused by susceptible organisms
Adults weighing more than 60 kg (132 lb): 3.1 g (30:1 fixed-ratio combination of 3 g ticarcillin and 100 mg clavulanic acid) by I.V. infusion q 4 to 6 hours
Adults weighing less than 60 kg (132 lb): 200 to 300 mg/kg/day (based on ticarcillin content) by I.V. infusion in divided doses q 4 to 6 hours
➢ Gynecologic infections caused by susceptible organisms
Adults weighing more than 60 kg (132 lb): For moderate infections, 200 mg/kg/day (based on ticarcillin content) by I.V. infusion in divided doses q 6 hours. For severe infections, 300 mg/kg/day (based on ticarcillin content) by I.V. infusion in divided doses q 4 hours.
Adults weighing less than 60 kg (132 lb): 200 to 300 mg/kg/day by I.V. infusion q 4 to 6 hours
➢ Mild to moderate or severe infections in children caused by susceptible organisms
Children weighing more than 60 kg (132 lb): For mild to moderate infections, 3.1 g (30:1 fixed-ratio combination of 3 g ticarcillin and 100 mg clavulanic acid) by I.V. infusion q 6 hours. For severe infections, 3.1 g (30:1 fixed-ratio combination of 3 g ticarcillin and 100 mg clavulanic acid) by I.V. infusion q 4 hours.
Children ages 3 months to 16 years weighing less than 60 kg (132 lb): For mild to moderate infections, 200 mg/kg/day (based on ticarcillin content) by I.V. infusion in divided doses q 6 hours. For severe infections, 300 mg/ kg/day

(based on ticarcillin content) by I.V. infusion in divided doses q 4 hours.

Dosage adjustment

- Renal impairment

Contraindications

- Hypersensitivity to drug or other penicillins

Precautions

Use cautiously in:

- cystic fibrosis, renal or hepatic disease
- pregnant or breastfeeding patients.

Administration

- Ask patient about penicillin allergy before giving.
- Add 13 ml of sterile water or normal saline solution to vial; shake gently. Dilute further to 10 to 100 mg/ml of ticarcillin; infuse I.V. over 30 minutes.
- Give at least 1 hour before I.V. aminoglycosides (such as amikacin or gentamicin).

Route	Onset	Peak	Duration
I.V.	Immediate	Immediate	Unknown

Adverse reactions

CNS: headache, giddiness, dizziness, lethargy, fatigue, hyperreflexia, neuromuscular excitability, asterixis, hallucinations, stupor, **seizures**
GI: nausea, vomiting, diarrhea, flatulence, **pseudomembranous colitis**
Hematologic: eosinophilia, transient **neutropenia** and **leukopenia** (with high doses)
Skin: urticaria, rash
Other: unpleasant taste; fever; overgrowth of nonsusceptible organisms; pain, vein irritation, erythema, phlebitis, and **thrombophlebitis** at I.V. site; hypersensitivity reactions including **anaphylaxis**

Interactions

Drug-drug. *Aminoglycosides:* physical incompatibility, causing aminoglycoside inactivation when mixed in same I.V. solution
Aminoglycosides, tetracyclines: additive activity against some bacteria
Lithium: altered lithium elimination
Probenecid: increased ticarcillin blood level
Drug-diagnostic tests. *Alanine aminotransferase, alkaline phosphatase, aspartate aminotransferase, eosinophils, lactate dehydrogenase, sodium:* increased levels
Bleeding time: prolonged
Granulocytes, hemoglobin, platelets, white blood cells: decreased levels
Liver function tests: transient increases
Urine glucose, urine protein: false-positive results

Patient monitoring

- Monitor liver function tests and CBC with white cell differential.
- Watch closely for signs and symptoms of superinfection and severe allergic reactions.
- Assess neurologic status, and stay alert for seizures.

Patient teaching

🔊 Advise patient to report skin reactions and severe diarrhea right away.
🔊 Tell patient drug may increase risk of other infections. Advise him to promptly report signs and symptoms of new infection.

- Instruct patient to limit sodium intake (drug contains sodium).
- As appropriate, review all other significant and life-threatening adverse reactions and interactions, especially those related to the drugs and tests mentioned above.

t

ticlopidine hydrochloride

Ticlid

Pharmacologic class: Platelet aggregation inhibitor

Therapeutic class: Antiplatelet agent

Pregnancy risk category B

Action

Inhibits release of first and second phases of adenosine diphosphate–induced effects on platelet aggregation, preventing thrombus formation

Availability

Tablets: 250 mg

Indications and dosages

➢ To reduce risk of thrombotic cerebrovascular accident when aspirin is ineffective or intolerable

Adults: 250 mg P.O. b.i.d. with meals

➢ Adjunctive therapy to prevent subacute stent thrombosis in patients with implanted coronary stents

Adults: 250 mg P.O. b.i.d. with meals, given with antiplatelet doses of aspirin for up to 30 days after successful stent implantation

Dosage adjustment

- Renal impairment

Off-label uses

- Chronic arterial occlusion
- Coronary artery bypass graft
- Open-heart surgery
- Intermittent claudication
- Primary glomerulonephritis
- Sickle cell disease
- Subarachnoid hemorrhage
- Uremic patients with atrioventricular shunts or fistulas

Contraindications

- Hypersensitivity to drug
- Hematopoietic disorders
- Hemostatic disorders or active bleeding
- Severe hepatic disease
- History of thrombotic thrombocytopenia purpura (TTP) or aplastic anemia

Precautions

Use cautiously in:

- renal or hepatic impairment
- high risk for bleeding
- elderly patients
- pregnant or breastfeeding patients
- children younger than age 18 (safety not established).

Administration

- Give with meals.
- Don't give within 2 hours of antacids.

Route	Onset	Peak	Duration
P.O.	Within 4 days	8-11 days	2 wk

Adverse reactions

CNS: dizziness, headache, weakness, **intracerebral bleeding**

EENT: conjunctival hemorrhage, tinnitus, epistaxis

GI: nausea, vomiting, diarrhea, full sensation, GI pain, dyspepsia, flatulence, anorexia, **GI bleeding**

GU: hematuria

Hematologic: ecchymosis, eosinophilia, purpura, **TTP, thrombocytosis, neutropenia, agranulocytosis, bone marrow depression**

Skin: rashes, bruising, pruritus, urticaria

Other: pain, posttraumatic or perioperative bleeding

Interactions

Drug-drug. *Antacids:* decreased ticlopidine blood level

Aspirin: potentiation of aspirin's effect on platelets

Cimetidine (long-term use): reduced ticlopidine clearance

Digoxin: slightly decreased digoxin blood level
Phenytoin: increased phenytoin blood level, greater risk of toxicity
Theophylline: decreased theophylline clearance, greater risk of toxicity
Vitamin A: altered anticoagulant effects
Drug-diagnostic tests. *Alanine aminotransferase, alkaline phosphatase, aspartate aminotransferase:* increased levels
Granulocytes, neutrophils, platelets, white blood cells: decreased counts
Liver function tests: abnormal results
Drug-food. *Any food:* increased ticlopidine absorption
Drug-herbs. *Alfalfa, anise, arnica, astragalus, bilberry, black current seed oil, bladderwrack, bogbean, boldo, borage oil, buchu, capsacin, cat's claw, celery, chapparal, cinchona bark, clove oil, coenzyme Q10, dandelion, dong quai, evening primrose oil, fenugreek, feverfew, garlic, ginger, gingko, guggal, papaya extract, red clover, rhubarb, safflower oil, skullcap, St. John's wort, tan shen:* altered anticoagulant effects

Patient monitoring

🔊 Closely monitor coagulation studies and CBC with white cell differential. Watch for evidence of bleeding tendency and blood dyscrasias.
🔊 Assess neurologic status carefully. Stay alert for signs and symptoms of intracranial bleeding.
- Monitor liver function tests.

Patient teaching

- Tell patient to take with meals, but not within 2 hours of antacids.

🔊 Instruct patient to immediately report easy bruising or bleeding.
- Advise patient to stop taking drug 10 to 14 days before elective surgery.
- Tell patient to inform all prescribers that he's taking drug.
- Inform patient that aspirin-containing products and many herbs increase risk of bleeding. Urge him to consult prescriber before taking over-the-counter drugs or herbs.
- Caution patient to avoid activities that can cause injury. Tell him to use soft toothbrush and electric razor to avoid gum and skin injury.
- As appropriate, review all other significant and life-threatening adverse reactions and interactions, especially those related to the drugs, tests, foods, and herbs mentioned above.

timolol maleate

Apo-Timol✤, Blocadren, Novo-Timol✤, Timoptic

Pharmacologic class: Beta-adrenergic blocker (nonselective)
Therapeutic class: Antihypertensive, vascular headache suppressant, antiglaucoma agent
Pregnancy risk category C

Action

Blocks stimulation of $beta_1$-adrenergic (myocardial) and $beta_2$-adrenergic (pulmonary, vascular, uterine) receptor sites. May reduce aqueous production, which decreases intraocular pressure (IOP).

Availability

Ophthalmic gel: 0.25%, 0.5%
Ophthalmic solution: 0.25%, 0.5%
Tablets: 5 mg, 10 mg, 20 mg

Indications and dosages

➢ Hypertension
Adults: Initially, 10 mg P.O. b.i.d., given alone or with a diuretic; may increase at 7-day intervals as needed. Usual maintenance dosage is 10 to 20 mg daily in two divided doses, up to 60 mg/day.

t

➢ Acute myocardial infarction (MI)
Adults: 10 mg P.O. b.i.d. starting 1 to 4 weeks after MI

➢ To prevent vascular headaches
Adults: Initially, 10 mg P.O. b.i.d. For maintenance, 20 mg may be given as a single daily dose. Total daily dosage may be increased to a maximum of 30 mg in divided doses or decreased to 10 mg/day, depending on response and tolerance. Withdraw drug if satisfactory response doesn't occur after 6 to 8 weeks at maximum dosage.

➢ Elevated IOP in patients with ocular hypertension or open-angle glaucoma
Adults: One drop of 0.25% to 0.5% ophthalmic solution in affected eye b.i.d., or 0.25% to 0.5% ophthalmic gel in affected eye once daily

Off-label uses

- Angina pectoris
- Supraventricular arrhythmias

Contraindications

- Hypersensitivity to drug or other beta-adrenergic blockers
- Uncompensated heart failure
- Bradycardia or heart block
- Cardiogenic shock
- Bronchial asthma (current or previous), severe chronic obstructive pulmonary disease

Precautions

Use cautiously in:
- renal or hepatic impairment, diabetes mellitus, thyrotoxicosis
- elderly patients
- pregnant or breastfeeding patients
- children (safety not established).

Administration

- Measure apical pulse before giving. If patient has significant bradycardia or tachycardia, withhold dose and consult prescriber.

Route	Onset	Peak	Duration
P.O.	Unknown	1-2 hr	12-24 hr
Ophthalmic	≤ 30 min	1-2 hr	≤ 24 hr

Adverse reactions

CNS: fatigue, dizziness, asthenia, insomnia, headache, vertigo, nervousness, depression, paresthesia, hallucinations, memory loss, disorientation, emotional lability, clouded sensorium
CV: hypotension, angina pectoris exacerbation, bradycardia, **atrioventricular or sinoatrial block, arrhythmias, heart failure**
EENT: visual disturbances, dry eyes, tinnitus, nasal congestion
GI: nausea, constipation, diarrhea, abdominal discomfort
GU: erectile dysfunction, decreased libido
Metabolic: hyperuricemia, **hypoglycemia, hyperkalemia**
Musculoskeletal: joint pain
Respiratory: dyspnea, crackles, **bronchospasm, pulmonary edema**
Skin: itching, rash

Interactions

Drug-drug. *Antihypertensives, nitrates:* additive hypotension
Insulin, oral hypoglycemics: altered efficacy of these drugs
Nonsteroidal anti-inflammatory drugs: decreased antihypertensive effect of timolol
Quinidine: inhibited timolol metabolism, leading to increased beta-adrenergic blockade and bradycardia
Reserpine: increased risk of hypotension and bradycardia
Theophylline: reduced effects of both drugs
Drug-diagnostic tests. *Antinuclear antibodies:* increased titer
Blood urea nitrogen, liver function tests, potassium, uric acid: increased values
Glucose, high-density lipoproteins, hematocrit, hemoglobin: decreased values

Drug-herbs. *Ephedra (ma huang), St. John's wort, yohimbine:* decreased timolol efficacy

Patient monitoring

- Closely monitor vital signs, blood pressure, cardiovascular status, and ECG.
- Assess respiratory status. Check breath sounds for wheezing and bronchospasm.
- Monitor blood glucose level in patient with diabetes mellitus.

Patient teaching

- Teach patient how to measure pulse before each dose. Instruct him to contact prescriber if pulse is outside established safe range.
- Caution patient not to stop taking drug abruptly. Dosage must be tapered.
- Teach patient how to administer eye drops. Instruct him to use drops only as prescribed, because they are absorbed systemically. Caution him not to touch dropper tip to eye or any other surface.
- Teach patient to recognize and immediately report significant adverse respiratory, cardiac, and neurologic reactions.
- Inform patient that many over-the-counter drugs and herbs may decrease the efficacy of timolol. Advise him to consult prescriber before using these products.
- Advise diabetic patient that drug may lower blood glucose level. Encourage regular blood glucose monitoring.
- As appropriate, review all other significant and life-threatening adverse reactions and interactions, especially those related to the drugs, tests, and herbs mentioned above.

tinzaparin sodium

Innohep

Pharmacologic class: Low-molecular-weight heparin
Therapeutic class: Anticoagulant
Pregnancy risk category B

Action

Enhances inhibition of factor Xa and thrombi by binding to and accelerating activity of antithrombin III; has only slight effect on thrombin and clotting time

Availability

Injection: 20,000 anti-Xa international units/ml in 2-ml vials

Indications and dosages

➢ Deep-vein thrombosis

Adults: 175 anti-Xa international units/kg subcutaneously daily for at least 6 days and until patient is adequately anticoagulated with warfarin for 2 consecutive days

Off-label uses

- Pulmonary embolism

Contraindications

- Hypersensitivity to drug, heparin, sulfites, benzyl alcohol, or pork products
- Active major bleeding
- History of heparin-induced thrombocytopenia

Precautions

Use cautiously in:

- renal impairment; bacterial endocarditis; uncontrolled hypertension; congenital or acquired bleeding disorders; hepatic failure and GI ulcers; recent brain, spinal, or ophthalmic surgery; diabetic retinopathy

t

- pregnant or breastfeeding patients
- elderly patients.

Administration

Be aware that tinzaparin sodium is a high-alert drug.
- Give by deep subcutaneous injection into abdominal wall while patient is sitting or lying down.
- Don't rub injection site after removing needle.
- Observe injection site closely for hematoma.
- Rotate injection sites among four quadrants of abdominal wall.

Don't give I.V. or I.M.
- Know that warfarin therapy usually starts within 1 to 3 days after tinzaparin therapy begins.

Route	Onset	Peak	Duration
Subcut.	2-3 hr	4-5 hr	18-24 hr

Adverse reactions

CNS: dizziness, insomnia, confusion, headache, **cerebral or intracranial bleeding**
CV: hypotension, hypertension, angina pectoris, chest pain, tachycardia, dependent edema, **thromboembolism, arrhythmias, myocardial infarction (MI)**
EENT: ocular hemorrhage, epistaxis
GI: nausea, vomiting, constipation, flatulence, dyspepsia, melena, **GI hemorrhage, retroperitoneal or intra-abdominal bleeding**
GU: urinary tract infection, hematuria, urinary retention, dysuria, **vaginal hemorrhage**
Hematologic: anemia, **thrombocytopenia, granulocytopenia, agranulocytosis, pancytopenia, hemorrhage**
Musculoskeletal: back pain, **intra-articular hemorrhage**
Respiratory: dyspnea, pneumonia, respiratory disorder, **pulmonary embolism**
Skin: pruritus, rash, bullous eruption, cellulitis, purpura, skin necrosis
Other: injection site hematoma and reactions, pain, fever, impaired healing, infection, hypersensitivity reaction, congenital anomaly, **fetal distress, fetal death**

Interactions

Drug-drug. *Oral anticoagulants, platelet inhibitors (such as dextran, dipyridamole, nonsteroidal anti-inflammatory drugs [NSAIDs], salicylate, sulfinpyrazone), thrombolytics:* increased risk of bleeding
Vitamin A: increased anticoagulant effect
Drug-diagnostic tests. *Alanine aminotransferase, aspartate aminotransferase:* reversible elevations
Granulocytes, hemoglobin, platelets, red blood cells, white blood cells: decreased values
Drug-herbs. *Alfalfa, anise, arnica, astragalus, bilberry, black currant seed oil, bladderwrack, bogbean, boldo (with fenugreek), borage oil, buchu, capsacin, cat's claw, celery, chaparral, chincona bark, clove oil, dandelion, dong quai, evening primrose oil, fenugreek, feverfew, garlic, ginger, ginkgo, guggul, papaya extract, red clover, rhubarb, safflower oil, skullcap, tan-shen:* increased anticoagulant effect

Patient monitoring

- Monitor vital signs and ECG closely.

Assess neurologic status. Stay alert for indications of intracranial or intracerebral bleeding.
- Evaluate closely for signs and symptoms of bleeding in all body systems.

Monitor respiratory status carefully to detect pneumonia, pulmonary embolism, and other serious adverse reactions.
- Monitor cardiovascular status closely. Watch for signs and symptoms of thrombophlebitis and edema.
- Monitor CBC, platelet count, and coagulation studies. Assess stools for occult blood.

Patient teaching

Tell patient to immediately report unusual bleeding or bruising. Inform him that drug can cause serious adverse reactions, especially bleeding. Instruct him to report new symptoms right away.
- Advise patient that aspirin products, NSAIDs, and many herbs increase the bleeding risk. Urge him to consult prescriber before using these products.
- Instruct patient to avoid activities that can cause injury. Tell him to use soft toothbrush and electric razor to avoid gum and skin injury.
- Tell patient he'll undergo regular blood tests during therapy.
- As appropriate, review all other significant and life-threatening adverse reactions and interactions, especially those related to the drugs, tests, and herbs mentioned above.

tirofiban hydrochloride

Aggrastat

Pharmacologic class: Glycoprotein (GP IIb/IIIa)-receptor inhibitor

Therapeutic class: Platelet aggregation inhibitor

Pregnancy risk category B

Action

Inhibits reversible platelet aggregation by binding to GP IIb/IIIa receptor on platelets

Availability

Injection: 25-ml and 50-ml vials (250 mcg/ml), 100-ml and 250-ml premixed vials (50 mcg/ml)

Indications and dosages

➢ Acute coronary syndrome (given with heparin); patients undergoing percutaneous transluminal coronary angioplasty (PTCA) or atherectomy

Adults: Loading dose of 0.4 mcg/kg/minute I.V. for 30 minutes, followed by continuous I.V. infusion of 0.1 mcg/kg/minute for 48 to 108 hours in patients being managed medically. Continue infusion for 12 to 24 hours after PTCA or atherectomy.

Dosage adjustment

- Renal insufficiency

Contraindications

- Hypersensitivity to drug or its components
- Active internal bleeding or history of bleeding diathesis within past 30 days
- Cerebrovascular accident (CVA) within past 30 days, or history of hemorrhagic CVA
- History of intracranial hemorrhage, intracranial neoplasm, arteriovenous malformation, aneurysm, or thrombocytopenia after previous tirofiban use
- History, symptoms, or findings that suggest aortic dissection
- Severe hypertension
- Acute pericarditis
- Major surgery or severe trauma within past 30 days
- Concurrent use of other parenteral GP IIb/IIIa inhibitors

Precautions

Use cautiously in:
- renal disease
- elderly patients
- pregnant or breastfeeding patients
- children younger than age 18 (safety not established).

Administration

Know that drug comes both in premixed vials of 50 mcg/ml and injection concentrate of 250 mcg/ml.
- Dilute injection concentrate to same concentration as premixed vial (50 mcg/ml) by withdrawing and discarding 50 ml of solution from 250-ml

t

plastic bag of normal saline solution or dextrose 5% in water, or by withdrawing and discarding 100 ml of solution from 500-ml plastic bag of same solution and replacing with equal volume of concentrated drug form.
• Mix I.V. solution well and inspect visually before administering.
• Squeeze plastic bag and check for leaks; discard if it has leaks.
• Don't use drug in series connections with other plastic bags. Don't add other drugs to bag containing tirofiban.

Route	Onset	Peak	Duration
I.V.	Immediate	Immediate	4-6 hr

Adverse reactions

CNS: headache, dizziness, **spinal-epidural hematoma, intracranial hemorrhage**
CV: vasovagal reaction, bradycardia, **hemopericardium, coronary artery dissection**
GI: nausea, vomiting, occult bleeding, hematemesis, **retroperitoneal hemorrhage**
GU: pelvic pain, hematuria
Hematologic: bleeding, **thrombocytopenia**
Musculoskeletal: leg pain
Respiratory: pulmonary hemorrhage
Skin: diaphoresis
Other: infusion site bleeding, chills, fever, edema, allergic reactions, **anaphylaxis**

Interactions

Drug-drug. *Clopidogrel, dipyridamole, nonsteroidal anti-inflammatory drugs, oral anticoagulants (such as thrombolytics, ticlopidine, warfarin), other drugs affecting hemostasis:* increased risk of bleeding
Levothyroxine, omeprazole: increased renal clearance of tirofiban
Vitamin A: increased risk of bleeding
Drug-diagnostic tests. *Hematocrit, hemoglobin, platelets:* decreased values
Drug-herbs. *Alfalfa, anise, arnica, astragalus, bilberry, black currant seed oil, bladderwrack, bogbean, boldo (with fenugreek), borage oil, buchu, capsaicin, cat's claw, celery, chaparral, chincona bark, clove oil, dandelion, dong quai, evening primrose oil, fenugreek, feverfew, garlic, ginger, ginkgo, guggul, papaya extract, red clover, rhubarb, safflower oil, skullcap, tan-shen:* increased risk of bleeding

Patient monitoring

Monitor CBC, platelet count, and coagulation studies. Assess stool for occult blood.
• Watch for bleeding at puncture sites, especially at cardiac catheterization access site. Immobilize access site to reduce bleeding risk.
Monitor for signs and symptoms of bleeding in cranium and other body systems (especially respiratory, GI, and GU).
• Monitor vital signs and ECG.
Assess cardiovascular status. Stay alert for signs and symptoms of coronary artery dissection or hemopericardium.

Patient teaching

Teach patient to recognize and immediately report serious adverse reactions.
• Tell patient he will be closely monitored and undergo regular blood testing during therapy.

tizanidine hydrochloride

Zanaflex

Pharmacologic class: Alpha-adrenergic agonist (centrally acting)
Therapeutic class: Skeletal muscle relaxant
Pregnancy risk category C

Action

Stimulates $alpha_2$-adrenergic agonist receptor sites and reduces spasticity by inhibiting presynaptic motor neurons

Availability

Tablets: 2 mg, 4 mg

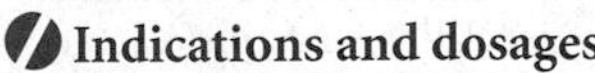

Indications and dosages

➢ Increased muscle tone associated with spasticity

Adults: Initially, 4 mg P.O. q 6 to 8 hours (no more than three doses in 24 hours). Increase in increments of 2 to 4 mg, up to 8 mg/dose or 24 mg/day (not to exceed 36 mg/day), as needed.

Contraindications

- Hypersensitivity to drug or its components

Precautions

Use cautiously in:
- renal or hepatic impairment
- elderly patients
- pregnant or breastfeeding patients
- children (safety not established).

Administration

- Give with or without food.

Route	Onset	Peak	Duration
P.O.	Unknown	1-2 hr	3-6 hr

Adverse reactions

CNS: drowsiness, asthenia, dizziness, speech disorder, dyskinesia, nervousness, anxiety, depression, hallucinations, sedation, paresthesia
CV: hypotension, bradycardia
EENT: blurred vision, pharyngitis, rhinitis
GI: vomiting, diarrhea, constipation, abdominal pain, dyspepsia, dry mouth
GU: urinary frequency, urinary tract infection
Hepatic: hepatitis
Musculoskeletal: back pain, myasthenia
Skin: rash, skin ulcers, sweating
Other: fever, infection, flulike symptoms

Interactions

Drug-drug. *Alpha$_2$-adrenergic agonist antihypertensives:* increased risk of hypotension
CNS depressants (such as antihistamines, opioids, sedative-hypnotics): additive CNS depression
Hormonal contraceptives: increased tizanidine blood level, greater risk of adverse reactions
Drug-diagnostic tests. *Alanine aminotransferase, alkaline phosphatase, aspartate aminotransferase, glucose:* increased levels
Drug-food. *Any food:* increased drug bioavailability, shorter time to peak concentration (with no effect on absorption)
Drug-behaviors. *Alcohol use:* additive CNS depression

Patient monitoring

- Monitor temperature and vital signs. Watch for orthostatic hypotension, bradycardia, and fever or other signs and symptoms of infection.
- Assess liver function tests.

Patient teaching

- Advise patient he may take with or without food.
- Tell patient to report signs or symptoms of infection or depression.
- Instruct patient to move slowly when sitting up or standing, to avoid dizziness from sudden blood pressure decrease.

Tell patient to immediately report unusual tiredness or yellowing of skin or eyes.
- Caution patient not to drink alcohol.
- Instruct patient to avoid driving and other hazardous activities until he knows how drug affects concentration and alertness.

• As appropriate, review all other significant and life-threatening adverse reactions and interactions, especially those related to the drugs, tests, foods, and behaviors mentioned above.

tobramycin
Aktob, TOBI, Tobrex

tobramycin sulfate
Nebcin

Pharmacologic class: Aminoglycoside
Therapeutic class: Anti-infective
Pregnancy risk category B (inhalation, ophthalmic), ***D*** (parenteral)

Action
Interferes with protein synthesis in bacterial cell by binding to 30S ribosomal subunit

Availability
Injection: 10 mg/ml, 40 mg/ml, 1.2-g vial
Nebulizer solution: 300 mg/5 ml in 5-ml ampule
Ophthalmic ointment: 0.3%
Ophthalmic solution: 0.3%
Pediatric solution for injection: 20 mg/2 ml

Indications and dosages
➢ Serious infections caused by susceptible organisms
Adults: 3 mg/kg/day I.V. or I.M. in evenly divided doses q 8 hours. For life-threatening infections, may increase up to 5 mg/kg/day I.V. or I.M. in three or four evenly divided doses, then reduce to 3 mg/kg/day as soon as possible.
Children older than 1 week: 6 to 7.5 mg/kg/day in three or four evenly divided doses, such as 2 to 2.5 mg/kg I.V. or I.M. q 8 hours or 1.5 to 1.9 mg/kg I.V. or I.M. q 6 hours
Neonates less than 1 week old: Up to 4 mg/kg/day I.V. or I.M. in evenly divided doses q 12 hours
➢ *Pseudomonas aeruginosa* in cystic fibrosis patients
Adults and children older than age 6: 300 mg inhalation b.i.d. (preferably q 12 hours but no less than 6 hours apart) for 28 days, then off for 28 days; then repeat cycle
➢ Ocular infections caused by susceptible organisms
Adults and children: For mild to moderate infections, apply a ribbon of ophthalmic ointment (approximately 1 cm) to infected eye two or three times daily, or instill one to two drops of ophthalmic solution into infected eye q 4 hours. For severe infections, apply ophthalmic ointment q 3 to 4 hours or instill two drops of ophthalmic solution into infected eye q 30 to 60 minutes; decrease dosing frequency when improvement occurs. Therapy should continue for at least 48 hours after infection is under control.

Dosage adjustment
• Renal impairment

Contraindications
• Hypersensitivity to drug, other aminoglycosides, bisulfites (with some products), or benzyl alcohol (in neonates, with some products)

Precautions
Use cautiously in:
• renal or hearing impairment, neuromuscular diseases, obesity
• elderly patients
• pregnant or breastfeeding patients
• neonates and premature infants.

Administration
• Dilute I.V. dose in 50 to 100 ml of normal saline solution or dextrose 5%

in water. For child, smaller volumes are needed.
• Infuse over at least 30 minutes. Flush line after administration.
• Give cephalosporins or penicillin, if ordered, 1 hour before or after tobramycin.
• Give inhalation doses by nebulizer over 10 to 15 minutes.

Route	Onset	Peak	Duration
I.V.	Rapid	15-30 min	Unknown
I.M.	Rapid	30-90 min	Unknown
Inhalation, ophthalmic	Unknown	Unknown	Unknown

Adverse reactions

CNS: confusion, lethargy, headache, delirium, dizziness, vertigo
EENT: eye stinging (with ophthalmic form), ototoxicity, hearing loss, roaring in ears, tinnitus
GI: nausea, vomiting, diarrhea, stomatitis
GU: proteinuria, **oliguria, nephrotoxicity**
Hematologic: anemia, eosinophilia, **leukocytosis, leukopenia, thrombocytopenia, granulocytopenia**
Metabolic: hypocalcemia, hyponatremia, hypokalemia, hypomagnesemia
Musculoskeletal: muscle weakness
Respiratory: apnea
Skin: rash, urticaria, itching
Other: superinfection, fever, pain and irritation at injection site

Interactions

Drug-drug. *Cephalosporins, vancomycin:* increased risk of nephrotoxicity
Dimenhydrinate: masking of ototoxicity symptoms
General anesthetics, neuromuscular blockers: increased neuromuscular blockade and respiratory depression
Indomethacin: increased tobramycin trough and peak levels
Loop diuretics: increased risk of ototoxicity
Penicillins: physical incompatibility, tobramycin inactivation when mixed in same I.V. solution
Polypeptide anti-infectives: increased risk of respiratory paralysis and renal dysfunction
Drug-diagnostic tests. *Alanine aminotransferase, aspartate aminotransferase, bilirubin, blood urea nitrogen, creatinine, lactate dehydrogenase, nonprotein nitrogen, urine protein:* increased levels
Calcium, granulocytes, hemoglobin, magnesium, platelets, potassium, sodium, white blood cells: decreased levels

Patient monitoring

• Draw sample for peak drug level 1 hour after I.M. or 30 minutes after I.V. administration. Draw sample for trough level just before next dose.
• Assess liver and kidney function tests.
• Monitor CBC with white cell differential.
• Closely monitor patient's hearing.

Patient teaching

Tell patient drug may cause hearing impairment and other serious adverse reactions, such as unusual bleeding or bruising. Instruct him to report these reactions at once.
• Advise patient to report new signs or symptoms of infection.
• With inhalation form, teach patient how to use nebulizer. Instruct him to administer dose over 10 to 15 minutes by breathing normally through mouthpiece while sitting or standing. Remind him to use only the hand-held nebulizer and compressor originally dispensed with drug. Advise him to use a nose clip to help him breathe through his mouth. If he uses other inhaled drugs, instruct him to take tobramycin last.
• Teach patient proper use of eye drops. Caution him not to touch dropper to eye or any other surface.
• As appropriate, review all other significant and life-threatening adverse

t

reactions and interactions, especially those related to the drugs and tests mentioned above.

tocainide hydrochloride

Tonocard

Pharmacologic class: Local anesthetic; class IB antiarrhythmic
Therapeutic class: Antiarrhythmic
Pregnancy risk category C

Action

Makes myocardial cells less excitable by reducing sodium and potassium conductance

Availability

Tablets: 400 mg, 600 mg

Indications and dosages

➢ Life-threatening ventricular arrhythmias

Adults: Dosage individualized based on antiarrhythmic response and tolerance. Recommended initial dosage is 400 mg P.O. q 8 hours. Usual dosage ranges from 1,200 to 1,800 mg daily in three divided doses.

Dosage adjustment

- Renal or hepatic impairment

Contraindications

- Hypersensitivity to drug or local amide anesthetics
- Second- or third-degree atrioventricular block (except in patients with artificial pacemakers)

Precautions

Use cautiously in:

- blood dyscrasias; heart failure or minimum cardiac reserve; increasing depression of cardiac conductivity; severe hepatic, renal, or pulmonary disease
- elderly patients
- pregnant or breastfeeding patients
- children (safety and efficacy not established).

Administration

- Know that initial doses should be given only in hospital setting.
- Before starting drug, correct hypokalemia (may make drug ineffective).
- Give with or without food.

Route	Onset	Peak	Duration
P.O.	Unknown	0.5-2 hr	Unknown

Adverse reactions

CNS: dizziness, tiredness, drowsiness, fatigue, lethargy, paresthesia, tremor, confusion, disorientation, hallucinations, headache, nervousness, altered mood or awareness, incoordination, unsteadiness, gait disturbance, anxiety, ataxia, vertigo
CV: hypotension, bradycardia, palpitations, chest pain, premature ventricular contractions, tachycardia, bradycardia, **heart failure (HF), HF progression, conduction disorders, left ventricular failure, increased ventricular arrhythmias**
EENT: blurred vision, visual disturbances, nystagmus, tinnitus, hearing loss
GI: nausea, vomiting, anorexia, diarrhea
Musculoskeletal: arthritis, arthralgia, myalgia
Skin: diaphoresis, rash, skin lesions, **lupus**
Other: hot or cold sensation

Interactions

Drug-drug. *Lidocaine:* increased CNS adverse reactions, including seizures
Metoprolol: additive effects on capillary wedge pressure and cardiac index
Drug-diagnostic tests. *Liver function tests:* altered results

Patient monitoring

🔊 Closely monitor cardiovascular status, including ECG. Watch for increasing arrhythmias and other serious problems.
🔊 Closely monitor respiratory and neurologic status and CBC with white cell differential. Stay alert for serious pulmonary problems, seizures, and blood dyscrasias (rare).
🔊 Watch for rash, skin lesions, and signs and symptoms of lupus.
- Monitor liver function tests and electrolyte levels, especially potassium.

Patient teaching

- Tell patient he may take with or without food.

🔊 Instruct patient to immediately report increasing cardiac problems, easy bruising or bleeding, respiratory problems, rash, or skin lesions.
- Caution patient to avoid driving and other hazardous activities until he knows how drug affects concentration and alertness.
- Tell patient he'll undergo regular blood testing during therapy.
- As appropriate, review all other significant and life-threatening adverse reactions and interactions, especially those related to the drugs and tests mentioned above.

tolbutamide sodium

Apo-Tolbutamide✤, Novo-Butamide✤

Pharmacologic class: Sulfonylurea (first-generation)
Therapeutic class: Hypoglycemic
Pregnancy risk category C

Action

Stimulates insulin release from pancreatic beta cells. Increases peripheral tissue sensitivity to insulin, either by increasing the number of insulin receptors or enhancing insulin binding to cellular receptors.

Availability

Powder for injection: 1 g
Tablets: 500 mg

Indications and dosages

➢ Adjunct in type 2 (non-insulin-dependent) diabetes mellitus not controlled by diet and exercise
Adults: Initially, 1 to 2 g P.O. daily. May adjust to maintenance dosage of 250 mg to 2 g P.O. daily; maximum dosage is 3 g daily.
➢ To aid diagnosis of pancreatic islet cell adenoma
Adults: 1g I.V.

Dosage adjustment

- Hepatic insufficiency

Contraindications

- Hypersensitivity to drug, its components, or other sulfonylureas
- Diabetic coma or ketoacidosis
- Sole therapy for type 1 (insulin-dependent) diabetes mellitus

Precautions

Use cautiously in:
- severe renal or hepatic disease
- stress caused by infection, fever, trauma, or surgery
- pregnant or breastfeeding patients (use not recommended)
- children (safety and efficacy not established).

Administration

- Give oral doses as prescribed, either as a single dose in morning or in divided doses after meals (based on GI tolerance).
- When giving I.V. to aid diagnosis of pancreatic islet cell adenoma, expect blood glucose level to fall rapidly for 30 to 45 minutes, followed by rise to

t

normal level in next 90 to 180 minutes. In patients with insulinomas, blood glucose decrease typically has greater magnitude and longer duration than in healthy persons.

Route	Onset	Peak	Duration
P.O.	1 hr	3-4 hr	6-12 hr
I.V.	Rapid	20 min	Unknown

Adverse reactions

CNS: malaise, paresthesia, vertigo, headache, fatigue, dizziness
CV: increased risk of cardiovascular mortality
GI: nausea, heartburn, epigastric fullness
Metabolic: syndrome of inappropriate antidiuretic hormone secretion, severe hypoglycemia
Skin: transient rash, pruritus, erythema, urticaria, photosensitivity
Other: taste alteration, weight gain

Interactions

Drug-drug. *Androgens, anticoagulants, azole antifungals, chloramphenicol, clofibrate, fenfluramine, fluconazole, gemfibrozil, histamine$_2$ antagonists, magnesium salts, methyldopa, MAO inhibitors, phenylbutazone, probenecid, salicylates, sulfonamides, tricyclic antidepressants, urinary acidifiers:* increased hypoglycemia
Beta-adrenergic blockers, calcium channel blockers, cholestyramine, corticosteroids, diazoxide, estrogens, hormonal contraceptives, hydantoins, isoniazid, nicotinic acid, phenothiazines, rifampin, sympathomimetics, thiazide diuretics, thyroid agents, urinary alkalizers: decreased hypoglycemic effect
Charcoal: decreased tolbutamide absorption
Digoxin: increased digoxin blood level and risk of toxicity
Drug-diagnostic tests. *Glucose:* decreased level
Radioactive iodine: decreased thyroid uptake
Urine albumin: false-positive reaction
Drug-herbs. *Aloe, bitter melon, fenugreek, St. John's wort:* increased risk of hypoglycemia
Drug-behaviors. *Alcohol use:* disulfiram-like effect

Patient monitoring

- Monitor blood glucose level frequently.
- Assess vital signs and cardiovascular and neurologic status.
- Monitor nutritional status; report significant problems.

Patient teaching

- Tell patient to take as prescribed, either as a single dose in morning or in divided doses after meals.
- Stress importance of adhering to prescribed diet and exercise.
- Advise patient to report significant adverse reactions.
- Instruct patient to monitor blood glucose level carefully.
- Caution patient not to drink alcohol.
- Tell patient some herbs affect blood glucose level. Advise him to consult prescriber before using.
- Teach patient effective ways to counteract photosensitivity.
- Tell patient he'll undergo regular blood testing during therapy.
- Advise female patient that drug isn't recommended during pregnancy or breastfeeding.
- As appropriate, review all other significant and life-threatening adverse reactions and interactions, especially those related to the drugs, tests, herbs, and behaviors mentioned above.

tolcapone

Tasmar

Pharmacologic class: Catecholamine inhibitor

Therapeutic class: Antiparkinsonian

Pregnancy risk category C

Action

Unknown. When given with levodopa-carbidopa, thought to reversibly inhibit catechol *O*-methyltranferase, leading to increased levodopa bioavailability and stimulation in brain.

Availability

Tablets: 100 mg, 200 mg

Indications and dosages

➢ Adjunct to levodopa-carbidopa in idiopathic Parkinson's disease

Adults: Initially, 100 mg P.O. t.i.d. given with levodopa-carbidopa. If beneficial, may increase dosage to 200 mg P.O. t.i.d.; maximum dosage is 600 mg daily. If response inadequate after 3 weeks, stop therapy.

Contraindications

- Hypersensitivity to drug
- Nontraumatic rhabdomyolysis
- Drug-related hyperpyrexia or confusion
- Hepatic disease, alanine aminotransferase or aspartate aminotransferase elevation
- History of tolcapone-induced hepatocellular injury

Precautions

Use cautiously in:

- renal or cardiac disease, hypertension, asthma
- concurrent use of nonselective MAO inhibitor (such as phenelzine, tranylcypromine)
- pregnant or breastfeeding patients.

Administration

Before giving first dose, obtain patient's written informed consent for drug therapy.

- Check liver function tests before starting drug.

Don't stop drug abruptly, because this may cause a syndrome similar to neuroleptic malignant syndrome.

- Know that levodopa-carbidopa dosage may be decreased to minimize dyskinesia.

Route	Onset	Peak	Duration
P.O.	Unknown	2 hr	Unknown

Adverse reactions

CNS: dizziness, asthenia, headache, fatigue, hypokinesia, mental deficiency, agitation, tremor, hyperactivity, paresthesia, irritability, syncope, depression, speech disorder, confusion, sleep disorder, excessive dreaming, hallucinations, drowsiness, hypertonia, imbalance, falling, hyperkinesias, dystonia, dyskinesia

CV: hypotension, chest discomfort or pain, orthostatic hypotension, palpitations

EENT: tinnitus, sinus congestion, pharyngitis

GI: nausea, vomiting, diarrhea, constipation, dyspepsia, abdominal pain, flatulence, dry mouth, anorexia

GU: hematuria, urinary tract infection (UTI), urinary incontinence, urine discoloration, urinary disorder, erectile dysfunction

Hepatic: jaundice, **severe hepatocellular injury (including fulminant hepatic failure, death)**

Musculoskeletal: neck pain, arthritis, muscle cramps, stiffness, **rhabdomyolysis**

Respiratory: upper respiratory infection, dyspnea, bronchitis

Skin: rash, dermal bleeding, diaphoresis

Other: fever, influenza

t

Interactions

Drug-drug. *Desipramine:* increased risk of adverse tolcapone reactions
Nonselective MAO inhibitors (such as phenelzine, tranylcypromine): inhibition of principal pathways of tolcapone metabolism
Warfarin: increased warfarin blood level
Drug-diagnostic tests. *Alanine aminotransferase, aspartate aminotransferase:* increased levels

Patient monitoring

- Monitor parkinsonian symptoms during first 3 weeks of therapy. Report improvement (or lack thereof) to help determine if therapy should continue.
- Assess neurologic status closely.

◀≡ Monitor liver function tests. Watch closely for signs and symptoms of hepatic impairment.

- Closely monitor temperature. Stay alert for fever and other indications of infection (particularly upper respiratory infection, influenza, and UTI).

Patient teaching

- Tell patient to take drug with first levodopa-carbidopa dose of day.

◀≡ Advise patient to immediately report signs or symptoms of liver problems (persistent nausea, fatigue, appetite loss, dark urine, itching, tenderness on right side of abdomen, and yellowing of skin or eyes).

- Instruct patient to promptly report signs and symptoms of infection.

◀≡ Advise female patient to immediately report suspected pregnancy. Caution her not to breastfeed.

- Tell patient drug may cause involuntary movements, hallucinations, lightheadedness, and other significant reactions. Urge him to use safety measures as needed.
- Caution patient to avoid driving and other hazardous activities until he knows how drug affects concentration and alertness.
- Advise patient to move slowly when sitting up or standing, to avoid dizziness from sudden blood pressure decrease.
- As appropriate, review all other significant and life-threatening adverse reactions and interactions, especially those related to the drugs and tests mentioned above.

tolterodine

Detrol, Detrol LA

Pharmacologic class: Anticholinergic
Therapeutic class: Urinary tract antispasmodic
Pregnancy risk category C

Action

Competitively antagonizes muscarinic receptors, inhibiting bladder contractions and reducing urinary frequency

Availability

Capsules (extended-release): 2 mg, 4 mg
Tablets: 1 mg, 2 mg

Indications and dosages

➢ Overactive bladder

Adults: 2 mg (immediate-release) P.O. b.i.d.; may decrease to 1 mg P.O. b.i.d. depending on response and tolerance. Or 4 mg (extended-release) P.O. daily; may decrease to 2 mg P.O. daily, depending on response.

Dosage adjustment

- Hepatic impairment or disease
- Renal impairment
- Concurrent use of potent CYP3A4 inhibitors

Contraindications

- Hypersensitivity to drug or its components
- Urinary or gastric retention
- Uncontrolled angle-closure glaucoma

Precautions

Use cautiously in
- GI obstruction, significant bladder outflow obstruction, controlled angle-closure glaucoma, significant hepatic impairment, renal impairment
- pregnant or breastfeeding patients
- children (safety not established).

Administration

- Give with food to increase bioavailability.

Route	Onset	Peak	Duration
P.O.	Unknown	Unknown	12 hr

Adverse reactions

CNS: headache, dizziness, vertigo, drowsiness, paresthesia, fatigue
CV: chest pain
EENT: vision abnormalities, xerophthalmia, pharyngitis
GI: diarrhea, constipation, abdominal pain, dyspepsia, dry mouth
GU: dysuria, urinary retention or frequency, urinary tract infection
Musculoskeletal: joint pain
Skin: dry skin
Other: weight gain, flulike symptoms, infection

Interactions

Drug-drug. *Clarithromycin, erythromycin, itraconazole, ketoconazole, miconazole:* inhibited metabolism and increased effects of tolterodine
Drug-food. *Any food:* increased drug bioavailability

Patient monitoring

- Monitor bladder function.
- Assess blood pressure and stay alert for chest pain.
- Monitor neurologic status. Report paresthesia or visual impairment.

Patient teaching

- Tell patient to take with food.
- If patient takes extended-release form, instruct him not to chew or crush it.
- Advise patient to use sugarless gum or hard candy to relieve dry mouth.
- As appropriate, review all other significant adverse reactions and interactions, especially those related to the drugs and foods mentioned above.

topiramate

Topamax

Pharmacologic class: Sulfamate-substituted monosaccharide derivative
Therapeutic class: Anticonvulsant
Pregnancy risk category C

Action

Blocks sodium channels, enhancing the action of gamma-amino butyrate (a neurotransmitter); also inhibits amino acid excitatory receptors

Availability

Sprinkle capsules: 15 mg, 25 mg
Tablets: 25 mg, 50 mg, 100 mg, 200 mg

Indications and dosages

➢ Adjunct in partial-onset seizures, primary generalized tonic-clonic seizures, and seizures associated with Lennox-Gastaut syndrome
Adults and children older than age 17: Initially, 25 to 50 mg P.O. daily. To achieve adequate response, may increase by 25 to 50 mg weekly, up to 200 mg b.i.d.
Children ages 2 to 16: Initially, less than 25 mg P.O. daily; increase at 1- or 2-week intervals in increments of 1 to 3 mg/kg/day given in two divided doses to achieve adequate response.
➢ Migraine prophylaxis
Adults: Dosage titrated to 100 mg P.O. daily as follows: 25 mg/day during week 1, 25 mg b.i.d. during week 2, 25

t

mg in morning and 50 mg in evening during week 3, and 50 mg b.i.d. during week 4

Dosage adjustment
- Renal impairment

Off-label uses
- Cluster headaches
- Infantile spasms
- Mood stabilization

Contraindications
- Hypersensitivity to drug or its components

Precautions
Use cautiously in:
- renal or hepatic impairment, dehydration, urolithiasis, glaucoma, myopia
- pregnant or breastfeeding patients.
- children younger than age 2 (safety and efficacy not established).

Administration
- Give without regard to meals.
- Don't break tablets, because of bitter taste.
- Administer capsules either whole or by opening capsule carefully and sprinkling entire contents into small amount of soft food. Instruct patient to swallow mixture immediately without chewing sprinkles.

🔊 Don't stop therapy suddenly. Dosage must be tapered.

Route	Onset	Peak	Duration
P.O.	Unknown	2 hr	12 hr

Adverse reactions
CNS: dizziness, drowsiness, fatigue, malaise, poor memory and concentration, nervousness, psychomotor slowing, speech and language problems, aggressive reaction, agitation, anxiety, confusion, depression, irritability, ataxia, paresthesia, hyperesthesia, tremor, **suicide attempt, increased seizures**
EENT: abnormal vision, diplopia, nystagmus, acute myopia, secondary angle-closure glaucoma, decreased hearing, rhinitis, sinusitis, epistaxis, pharyngitis
GI: nausea, constipation, abdominal pain, dry mouth, gastroenteritis, increased salivation (in children), anorexia
GU: renal calculi, urinary incontinence, leukorrhea
Hematologic: purpura, **leukopenia, thrombocytopenia**
Metabolic: hypocalcemia, hyperchloremia, hypernatremia, hyponatremia, hypophosphatemia, **hypoglycemia**
Musculoskeletal: myalgia, back pain, leg pain
Respiratory: pneumonia
Skin: rash, skin disorder, alopecia, dermatitis, hypertrichosis, eczema, seborrhea, skin discoloration
Other: altered taste, weight loss, thirst, fever, flulike symptoms, hot flashes, infection, edema, allergic reaction

Interactions
Drug-drug. *Carbamazepine:* decreased topiramate blood level and effects
Carbonic anhydrase inhibitors (such as acetazolamide): increased risk of renal calculi
CNS depressants: increased risk of CNS depression and other adverse cognitive or neuropsychiatric reactions
Hormonal contraceptives: decreased contraceptive efficacy
Phenytoin: increased phenytoin blood level and effects, decreased topiramate blood level and effects
Valproic acid: decreased effects of both drugs
Drug-diagnostic tests. *Alanine aminotransferase, alkaline phosphatase, aspartate aminotransferase, creatinine:* increased levels
Calcium, cholesterol, glucose, phosphate: decreased levels
Sodium: increased or decreased level

Drug-behaviors. *Alcohol use:* increased CNS depression

Patient monitoring

🔊 Monitor seizure type and pattern. Report new seizure types or worsening seizure pattern.
- Assess neurologic status closely. Report significant adverse reactions.

🔊 Watch for and immediately report signs and symptoms of depression or suicidal ideation.
- Monitor fluid intake and output. Report indications of urinary tract infection, urinary incontinence, or renal calculi.

🔊 Monitor vision. If patient becomes acutely nearsighted with symptoms of angle-closure glaucoma (cloudy vision, eye pain), stop drug and contact prescriber right away.

Patient teaching

- Tell patient he may take with or without food.
- Caution patient not to crush or break tablets.
- If patient takes capsules, tell him he may open them, sprinkle contents onto small amount of soft food, and consume immediately. Tell him not to store this mixture.

🔊 Caution patient not to stop drug suddenly. Dosage must be tapered.
- Instruct patient to drink plenty of fluids to reduce risk of kidney stones.

🔊 Tell patient drug may cause new seizure types or worsen seizure pattern. Instruct him to report these developments immediately.

🔊 Instruct patient (and significant other as appropriate) to immediately report signs or symptoms of depression or suicidal thoughts.

🔊 Advise patient to immediately report vision changes, especially nearsightedness, cloudy vision, or eye pain.
- Caution patient not to drive or perform other hazardous activities.
- Tell patient not to drink alcohol during drug therapy.
- Advise female patient to notify prescriber of suspected pregnancy.
- As appropriate, review all other significant and life-threatening adverse reactions and interactions, especially those related to the drugs, tests, and behaviors mentioned above.

topotecan hydrochloride

Hycamtin

Pharmacologic class: DNA topoisomerase inhibitor

Therapeutic class: Antineoplastic

Pregnancy risk category D

Action

Regulates DNA replication and repair of broken DNA strands, relieving torsional strain; exerts cytotoxic effects during DNA synthesis

Availability

Injection: 4 mg in single-dose vials

Indications and dosages

➢ Metastatic ovarian cancer or small-cell lung cancer after first-line chemotherapy fails

Adults: 1.5 mg/m^2 daily by I.V. infusion given over 30 minutes for 5 consecutive days, starting on day 1 of 21-day cycle

Dosage adjustment

- Renal impairment
- Neutropenia

Contraindications

- Hypersensitivity to drug or its components
- Severe bone marrow depression
- Pregnancy or breastfeeding

t

Precautions

Use cautiously in:

- children (safety and efficacy not established).

Administration

🔊 Before starting therapy, check blood counts. Patient must have baseline neutrophil count above 1,500 cells/mm^3 and platelet count above 100,000 cells/mm^3 to receive drug.

🔊 Prepare drug under vertical laminar-flow hood, wearing gloves and protective clothing. Follow facility policy for discarding used drug containers and I.V. equipment.

- If skin contacts drug, wash immediately with soap and water.
- To reconstitute, add 4 ml of sterile water to 4-mg vial. Dilute further in normal saline solution or dextrose 5% in water. Give immediately over 30 minutes using infusion pump.

Route	Onset	Peak	Duration
I.V.	Unknown	Unknown	Unknown

Adverse reactions

CNS: asthenia, headache, fatigue, paresthesia

GI: nausea, vomiting, diarrhea, constipation, abdominal pain, stomatitis, anorexia

Hematologic: anemia, **leukopenia, thrombocytopenia, neutropenia**

Musculoskeletal: back pain, skeletal pain

Respiratory: coughing, dyspnea

Skin: erythematous or maculopapular rash, pruritus, urticaria, dermatitis, bullous eruption, alopecia

Other: fever, body pain, **sepsis**

Interactions

Drug-drug. *Cisplatin:* severe bone marrow depression

Granulocyte colony-stimulating factor: prolonged neutropenia

Live-virus vaccines: increased risk of infection from vaccine

Drug-diagnostic tests. *Alanine aminotransferase, aspartate aminotransferase, bilirubin:* increased levels

Patient monitoring

- Closely monitor CBC with white cell differential.
- Assess for signs and symptoms of bleeding tendency.
- Monitor closely for sepsis, other infections, and increased hepatic enzyme levels.

Patient teaching

🔊 Advise patient to immediately report unusual bleeding or bruising, sore throat, fever, or chills.

- Teach patient safety measures to avoid bruising and bleeding.
- Tell patient to minimize GI upset by eating small, frequent servings of food and drinking plenty of fluids.

🔊 Advise female patient to notify prescriber of suspected pregnancy. Caution her not to breastfeed during therapy.

- Inform patient that drug may cause hair loss.
- Tell patient he'll undergo regular blood testing during therapy.
- As appropriate, review all other significant and life-threatening adverse reactions and interactions, especially those related to the drugs and tests mentioned above.

torsemide

Demadex

Pharmacologic class: Loop diuretic

Therapeutic class: Diuretic, antihypertensive

Pregnancy risk category B

Action

Inhibits sodium and chloride reabsorption from ascending loop of Henle and distal renal tubule; increases renal excretion of water, sodium, chloride, magnesium, calcium, and hydrogen. Also may exert renal and peripheral vasodilatory effects. Net effect is natriuretic diuresis.

Availability

Injection: 10 mg/ml
Tablets: 5 mg, 10 mg, 20 mg, 100 mg

Indications and dosages

➢ Heart failure
Adults: 10 to 20 mg P.O. or I.V. daily. If response inadequate, double dosage until desired response occurs. Don't exceed 200 mg as a single dose.
➢ Hypertension
Adults: 5 mg P.O. daily. May increase to 10 mg daily after 4 to 6 weeks; if drug still isn't effective, additional antihypertensives may be prescribed.
➢ Chronic renal failure
Adults: 20 mg P.O. or I.V. daily. If response inadequate, double dosage until desired response occurs. Don't exceed 200 mg as a single dose.
➢ Hepatic cirrhosis
Adults: 5 or 10 mg P.O. or I.V. daily, given with aldosterone antagonist or potassium-sparing diuretic. If response inadequate, double dosage. Don't exceed 40 mg as a single dose.

Contraindications

- Hypersensitivity to drug, thiazides, or sulfonylureas
- Anuria

Precautions

Use cautiously in:
- severe hepatic disease accompanied by cirrhosis or ascites, preexisting uncorrected electrolyte imbalances, diabetes mellitus, worsening azotemia
- elderly patients
- pregnant or breastfeeding patients
- children younger than age 18.

Administration

- Give I.V. by direct injection over at least 2 minutes or by continuous I.V. infusion.
- Flush I.V. line with normal saline solution before and after administering.

Route	Onset	Peak	Duration
P.O.	Within 1 hr	1-2 hr	6-8 hr
I.V.	Within 10 min	Within 1 hr	6-8 hr

Adverse reactions

CNS: dizziness, headache, asthenia, insomnia, nervousness, syncope
CV: hypotension, ECG changes, chest pain, volume depletion, **atrial fibrillation, ventricular tachycardia, shunt thrombosis**
EENT: rhinitis, sore throat
GI: nausea, diarrhea, vomiting, constipation, dyspepsia, anorexia, rectal bleeding, **GI hemorrhage**
GU: excessive urination
Metabolic: hyperglycemia, hyperuricemia, hypokalemia
Musculoskeletal: joint pain, myalgia
Respiratory: increased cough
Skin: rash
Other: edema

Interactions

Drug-drug. *Aminoglycosides, cisplatin:* increased risk of ototoxicity
Amphotericin B, corticosteroids, mezlocillin, piperacillin, potassium-wasting diuretics, stimulant laxatives: additive hypokalemia
Antihypertensives, nitrates: additive hypotension
Lithium: increased lithium blood level and toxicity
Neuromuscular blockers: prolonged neuromuscular blockade
Nonsteroidal anti-inflammatory drugs, probenecid: inhibited diuretic response
Sulfonylureas: decreased glucose tolerance, hyperglycemia in patients with previously well-controlled diabetes

Drug-diagnostic tests. *Glucose, uric acid:* increased levels
Potassium: decreased level
Drug-herbs. *Dandelion:* interference with diuresis
Ephedra (ma huang): reduced hypotensive effect of torsemide
Geranium, ginseng: increased risk of diuretic resistance
Licorice: rapid potassium loss
Drug-behaviors. *Acute alcohol ingestion:* additive hypotension

Patient monitoring

- Monitor vital signs, especially for hypotension.
- Assess ECG for arrhythmias and other changes.
- Monitor weight and fluid intake and output to assess drug efficacy.
- Monitor electrolyte levels, particularly potassium. Stay alert for signs and symptoms of hypokalemia.
- Assess hearing for signs and symptoms of ototoxicity.
- Monitor blood glucose level carefully in diabetic patient.

Patient teaching

- Advise patient to take in morning with or without food.
- Instruct patient to move slowly when sitting up or standing, to avoid dizziness from sudden blood pressure drop.
- Tell patient to monitor weight and report sudden increases.
- Instruct diabetic patient to monitor blood glucose level carefully.
- Caution patient to avoid alcohol during drug therapy.
- Advise patient to consult prescriber before using herbs.
- As appropriate, review all other significant and life-threatening adverse reactions and interactions, especially those related to the drugs, tests, herbs, and behaviors mentioned above.

tramadol hydrochloride

Ultram

Pharmacologic class: Opioid agonist
Therapeutic class: Analgesic
Pregnancy risk category C

Action

Inhibits reuptake of serotonin and norepinephrine in CNS

Availability

Tablets: 50 mg

Indications and dosages

➢ Moderate to moderately severe pain
Adults: In rapid titration, 50 to 100 mg P.O. q 4 to 6 hours p.r.n. (not to exceed 400 mg/day, or 300 mg/day in patients older than age 75). In gradual titration, initially 25 mg P.O. daily; increase by 25 mg/day q 3 days to 100 mg/day, then increase by 50 mg/day q 3 days, up to 200 mg/day p.r.n.

Dosage adjustment

- Renal or hepatic impairment

Contraindications

- Hypersensitivity to drug, its components, or opioids
- Acute intoxication with alcohol, sedative-hypnotics, centrally acting analgesics, opioid analgesics, or psychotropic agents
- Physical opioid dependence

Precautions

Use cautiously in:
- seizure disorder or risk factors for seizures, renal or hepatic impairment, increased intracranial pressure, head trauma, acute abdomen
- history of opioid dependence or recent use of large opioid doses

• elderly patients
• pregnant or breastfeeding patients
• children younger than age 16 (safety not established).

Administration

• Give as prescribed, preferably before pain becomes severe.

Route	Onset	Peak	Duration
P.O.	1 hr	2-3 hr	4-6 hr

Adverse reactions

CNS: dizziness, vertigo, headache, drowsiness, anxiety, stimulation, confusion, incoordination, euphoria, nervousness, sleep disorder, asthenia, hypertonia, **seizures**
CV: vasodilation
EENT: visual disturbances
GI: nausea, vomiting, diarrhea, constipation, abdominal pain, dyspepsia, flatulence, dry mouth, anorexia
GU: urinary retention and frequency, proteinuria, menopausal symptoms
Respiratory: respiratory depression (with large doses, concomitant anesthetic use, or alcohol ingestion)
Skin: pruritus, sweating
Other: physical or psychological drug dependence, drug tolerance

Interactions

Drug-drug. *Anesthetics, antihistamines, CNS depressants, other opioids, psychotropic agents, sedative-hypnotics:* increased risk of CNS depression
Carbamazepine: increased tramadol metabolism and decreased efficacy
MAO inhibitors: increased risk of serotonin syndrome and seizures
Drug-diagnostic tests. *Creatinine, hepatic enzymes:* increased levels
Hemoglobin: decreased level
Drug-herbs. *Chamomile, hops, kava, skullcap, valerian:* increased CNS depression
Drug-behaviors. *Alcohol use:* increased CNS depression

Patient monitoring

• Assess patient's response to drug 30 minutes after administration.
• Monitor respiratory status. Withhold drug and contact prescriber if respirations become shallow or slower than 12 breaths/minute.
• Monitor for physical and psychological drug dependence. Report signs to prescriber.

Patient teaching

• Tell patient drug works best when taken before pain becomes severe.
• Inform patient (and significant other as appropriate) that drug may cause respiratory depression if used with alcohol. Recommend abstinence.
Instruct patient to immediately report seizure.
• Tell patient drug interacts with many common over-the-counter drugs and herbal remedies. Instruct him to consult prescriber before taking these products.
• Inform patient that drug can cause physical and psychological dependence. Urge him to take it only as prescribed and needed.
• Caution patient to avoid driving and other hazardous activities until he knows how drug affects concentration and alertness.
• As appropriate, review all other significant and life-threatening adverse reactions and interactions, especially those related to the drugs, tests, herbs, and behaviors mentioned above.

t

trandolapril

Mavik

Pharmacologic class: Angiotensin-converting enzyme (ACE) inhibitor

Therapeutic class: Antihypertensive

Pregnancy risk category C *(first trimester),* ***D*** (second and third trimesters)

Action

Inhibits conversion of angiotensin I to the potent vasoconstrictor angiotensin II, promoting vasodilation. Also increases plasma renin and stimulates aldosterone secretion, inducing diuresis.

Availability

Tablets: 1 mg, 2 mg, 4 mg

Indications and dosages

➢ Hypertension

Adults: For patients not receiving diuretics, 1 mg/day P.O. in nonblack patients or 2 mg/day P.O. in black patients. If response inadequate, may increase at weekly intervals up to 4 mg/day. For patients receiving diuretics, start with 0.5 mg/day P.O.

➢ Heart failure or left ventricular dysfunction after myocardial infarction

Adults: Initially, 1 mg P.O. daily. Titrate up to 4 mg daily, if tolerated.

Dosage adjustment

- Renal or hepatic impairment

Contraindications

- Hypersensitivity to drug or other ACE inhibitors
- Angioedema with previous ACE inhibitor use
- Pregnancy (second and third trimesters)

Precautions

Use cautiously in:

- renal or hepatic impairment, hypovolemia, hyponatremia, aortic stenosis or hypertrophic cardiomyopathy, cerebrovascular or cardiac insufficiency, surgery and anesthesia
- family history of angioedema
- concurrent diuretic therapy
- black patients with hypertension
- elderly patients
- pregnant patients (first trimester) or breastfeeding patients
- children (safety not established).

Administration

- Give once or twice daily as prescribed, with or without food.

Route	Onset	Peak	Duration
P.O.	Within 1 hr	4-10 hr	Up to 24 hr

Adverse reactions

CNS: insomnia, paresthesia, dizziness, drowsiness, asthenia, syncope, **cerebrovascular accident**

CV: chest pain, hypotension, palpitations, intermittent claudication, bradycardia, **first-degree atrioventricular block, cardiogenic shock**

EENT: epistaxis, sinusitis, throat inflammation

GI: vomiting, diarrhea, constipation, abdominal pain or distention, gastritis, dyspepsia, **pancreatitis**

GU: urinary tract infection, erectile dysfunction, decreased libido

Hematologic: agranulocytosis, neutropenia

Metabolic: hypocalcemia, gout, **hyperkalemia**

Musculoskeletal: muscle cramps, myalgia, extremity pain

Respiratory: cough, dyspnea, upper respiratory infection

Skin: rash, flushing, pruritus, angioedema

Other: edema

Interactions

Drug-drug. *Antacids:* decreased trandolapril absorption
Digoxin: increased digoxin blood level, greater risk of toxicity
Diuretics, general anesthetics, nitrates, other antihypertensives: additive hypotension
Indomethacin: reduced hypotensive effect of trandolapril
Lithium: increased lithium blood level, greater risk of toxicity
Phenothiazines: increased trandolapril effects
Potassium-sparing diuretics, potassium supplements, salt substitutes containing potassium: additive hyperkalemia
Drug-diagnostic tests. *Neutrophils, platelets:* decreased counts
Potassium: increased level
Drug-food. *Salt substitutes containing potassium:* hyperkalemia
Drug-herbs. *Capsaicin:* increased incidence of cough
Ephedra (ma huang), yohimbine: antagonism of trandolapril effects
Drug-behaviors. *Acute alcohol ingestion:* additive hypotension

Patient monitoring

- Monitor vital signs, especially for hypotension and bradycardia when therapy begins.
- Assess CBC with white cell differential. Watch for signs and symptoms of bleeding and infection.
- Monitor electrolyte levels, especially potassium. Stay alert for hyperkalemia.
- Assess renal function tests and fluid intake and output.

Patient teaching

- Tell patient drug may cause bleeding tendency or increase his infection risk. Teach him which warning signs to report.
- Teach patient to recognize and report signs or symptoms of hyperkalemia.
- Instruct patient to move slowly when sitting up or standing, to avoid dizziness from sudden blood pressure drop.
- Caution patient not to exercise vigorously in hot environments.
- Advise patient not to use salt substitutes containing potassium. Tell him to avoid high-potassium foods.
- As appropriate, review all other significant and life-threatening adverse reactions and interactions, especially those related to the drugs, tests, foods, herbs, and behaviors mentioned above.

tranylcypromine sulfate

Parnate

Pharmacologic class: MAO inhibitor
Therapeutic class: Antidepressant
Pregnancy risk category C

Action

Unknown. Thought to increase concentrations of serotonin, epinephrine, and norepinephrine in CNS by inhibiting effects of MAO.

Availability

Tablets: 10 mg

Indications and dosages

➤ Depression
Adults: 10 mg P.O. t.i.d., increased if needed by 10 mg P.O. daily at intervals of 1 to 3 weeks. Maximum dosage is 60 mg daily.

Contraindications

- Hypersensitivity to drug or other MAO inhibitors
- Pheochromocytoma
- Heart failure or other cardiovascular disease
- Confirmed or suspected cerebrovascular disorder
- Severe renal impairment
- Hypertension

• History of hepatic disease or elevated liver function tests
• History of headache
• Upcoming elective surgery
• Concurrent use of other MAO inhibitors, dibenzazepine derivatives, CNS depressants, anesthetics, antihypertensives, bupropion, sympathomimetics, selective serotonin reuptake inhibitors (SSRIs), or dextromethorphan
• Consumption of caffeine, certain cheeses, and other foods with high tryptophan or tyramine content

Precautions

Use cautiously in:
• seizure disorders, diabetes mellitus, hyperactivity, schizophrenia, severe depression, suicidal attempt or ideation
• pregnant or breastfeeding patients
• children.

Administration

◀ Don't stop therapy suddenly. Dosage must be tapered.

Route	Onset	Peak	Duration
P.O.	Unknown	1-3.5 hr	10 days

Adverse reactions

CNS: dizziness, headache, hyperreflexia, tremor, mania, hypomania, confusion, impaired memory, hypersomnia or insomnia, weakness, fatigue, drowsiness, restlessness, increased anxiety, myoclonic movements, **suicidal behavior or ideation** (especially in child or adolescent)
CV: orthostatic hypotension, tachycardia, palpitations, syncope, paradoxical hypertension, **hypertensive crisis**
EENT: blurred vision
GI: nausea, diarrhea, constipation, GI disturbances, abdominal pain, dry mouth, anorexia
GU: urinary retention, impaired ejaculation, erectile dysfunction
Hematologic: anemia, **agranulocytosis, leukopenia, thrombocytopenia**
Musculoskeletal: muscle twitching
Other: weight gain, chills, edema

Interactions

Drug-drug. *Anesthetics, antihypertensives, bupropion, CNS depressants, dextromethorphan, dibenzazepine derivatives, other MAO inhibitors, SSRIs, sympathomimetics:* potentially fatal reactions
Beta-adrenergic blockers: bradycardia
Carbamazepine: hypertensive crisis, severe seizures, coma, circulatory collapse
Hypoglycemics: potentiation of hypoglycemic response
Levodopa: hypertensive reactions
Methylphenidate: increased risk of hypertensive crisis
Sulfonamides: sulfonamide or tranylcypromine toxicity
Thiazide diuretics: exaggerated hypotension
Drug-diagnostic tests. *Transaminases:* increased levels
Drug-food. *Foods containing high caffeine, tyramine, or tryptophan content:* hypertension
Drug-herbs. *Cacao:* vasopressor effects
Ephedra (ma huang): severe reactions, including hypertensive crisis
Ginseng: tremor, headache, mania
Licorice: increased tranylcypromine activity
L-tryptophan: serotonin syndrome (overreactive reflexes, high body temperature, jaw clenching, sweating, drowsiness, euphoria, and even death)
Drug-behaviors. *Alcohol use:* increased CNS effects

Patient monitoring

◀ Monitor vital signs and cardiovascular status carefully. Stay alert for indications of impending hypertensive crisis (palpitations, frequent headaches). Keep phentolamine at hand to lower blood pressure if needed.
• Monitor CBC and liver function tests.

Observe patient closely for suicidal ideation and drug hoarding.

Patient teaching

Instruct patient or caregiver to immediately report rapid heartbeat and frequent headaches (possible symptoms of hypertensive crisis).
- Advise patient to read food labels carefully and to avoid foods high in tyramine, tryptophan, and caffeine.
- Tell patient drug causes serious interactions with many common drugs. Instruct him to tell all prescribers he's taking it.

Teach patient or caregiver to recognize and immediately report increasing depression or suicidal ideation (especially in child or adolescent).
- Advise patient to avoid alcohol and herbal remedies, because serious reactions may occur.

Caution patient not to stop therapy suddenly. Dosage must be tapered.
- Instruct patient to move slowly when sitting up or standing, to avoid dizziness from sudden blood pressure drop.
- Caution patient to avoid driving and other hazardous activities until he knows how drug affects concentration, vision, and alertness.
- As appropriate, review all other significant and life-threatening adverse reactions and interactions, especially those related to the drugs, tests, foods, herbs, and behaviors mentioned above.

trastuzumab

Herceptin

Pharmacologic class: Recombinant DNA-derived monoclonal antibody
Therapeutic class: Antineoplastic
Pregnancy risk category B

Action

Selectively binds to human epidermal growth factor receptor 2 (HER2), inhibiting proliferation of human tumor cells that overexpress HER2

Availability

Lyophilized powder: 440-mg vial (each vial contains 20 ml bacteriostatic water for injection, 1.1% benzyl alcohol)

Indications and dosages

➢ Metastatic breast cancer in patients whose tumors overexpress HER2
Adults: As monotherapy, loading dose of 4 mg/kg I.V. infusion over 90 minutes, followed by weekly maintenance dose of 2 mg/kg I.V. infusion given over 30 minutes if loading dose was tolerated. Don't give by I.V. push.

Contraindications

- Hypersensitivity to drug

Precautions

Use cautiously in
- hypersensitivity to Chinese hamster ovary cell protein or to benzyl alcohol
- cardiac disease, anemia, leukopenia
- elderly patients
- pregnant or breastfeeding patients
- children younger than age 18 (safety and efficacy not established).

Administration

- Follow facility policy for handling, administering, and disposal of carcinogenic, mutagenic, and teratogenic agents.
- Give antiemetic, as prescribed, before administering trastuzumab.

Administer by I.V. infusion only. Don't give by I.V. push or bolus.
- To reconstitute, add 20 ml of bacteriostatic water for injection to vial, pointing diluent stream at lyophilized cake. Swirl vial gently; don't shake. Withdraw prescribed dose and add it to 250 ml of normal saline solution. (Don't use dextrose 5% in water.)

t

• Infuse loading dose I.V. over 90 minutes. Infuse weekly doses I.V. over 30 minutes.
• Immediately after reconstituting, write a date that is 28 days from reconstitution date in the space after "Do not use after" on vial label.
• If patient has benzyl alcohol hypersensitivity, reconstitute with sterile water for injection. Use immediately after reconstitution; discard unused portion.
🔊 Never administer intrathecally; doing so causes death.
• Know that for patient who hasn't previously received chemotherapy for metastatic disease, drug is given at same dosage but in combination with paclitaxel.

Route	Onset	Peak	Duration
I.V.	Unknown	Unknown	Unknown

Adverse reactions

CNS: dizziness, headache, depression, paresthesia, insomnia, ataxia, confusion, manic reaction, **seizures**
CV: peripheral edema, hypotension, tachycardia, syncope, **arrhythmias, shock, pericardial effusion, vascular thrombosis, heart failure, cardiotoxicity, cardiac arrest**
EENT: amblyopia, hearing loss
GI: nausea, vomiting, diarrhea, gastroenteritis, hematemesis, colitis, esophageal ulcer, stomatitis, ileus, anorexia, **intestinal obstruction, pancreatitis**
GU: urinary tract infection, hematuria, hemorrhagic cystitis, hydronephrosis, pyelonephritis, **renal failure**
Hematologic: coagulation disorder, pancytopenia, leukemia
Hepatic: ascites, **hepatitis, hepatic failure**
Metabolic: hypothyroidism, hypercalcemia, hyponatremia
Musculoskeletal: back, bone, or joint pain; myopathy; fractures; **bone necrosis**
Respiratory: upper respiratory infection, dyspnea, **acute respiratory distress syndrome**
Skin: cellulitis, rash, acne, herpes simplex, herpes zoster, skin ulcers
Other: weight loss, edema, infection, fever, chills, flulike syndrome, lymphangitis, hypersensitivity reactions including **anaphylaxis, infusion reaction**

Interactions

Drug-drug. *Anthracyclines, cyclophosphamide:* cardiotoxicity

Patient monitoring

🔊 Monitor closely for signs and symptoms of infusion reaction (including respiratory distress). Halt infusion if these occur.
• Monitor vital signs, especially for hypotension and bradycardia.
🔊 Use with extreme caution in patients with cardiac dysfunction. Assess cardiovascular status carefully; stay alert for heart failure and peripheral edema.
• Assess neurologic status for depression and paresthesia.
• Monitor respiratory status. Report increased dyspnea or flulike symptoms.
• Watch closely for signs and symptoms of infection, including herpes simplex.
• Monitor electrolyte levels and CBC with white cell differential.

Patient teaching

🔊 Instruct patient to immediately report difficulty breathing, flulike symptoms, and fever, chills, and other signs and symptoms of infection.
🔊 Advise patient to monitor weight. Tell him to report sudden weight gain as well as swelling and other signs and symptoms of heart failure.
🔊 Instruct patient to immediately report abdominal pain, change in bowel habits, yellowing of skin or eyes, and easy bruising or bleeding.
• Tell patient drug may cause depression. Advise him (or significant other

as appropriate) to contact prescriber if this occurs.
- As appropriate, review all other significant and life-threatening adverse reactions and interactions, especially those related to the drugs mentioned above.

trazodone hydrochloride
Desyrel, Trazorel✦

Pharmacologic class: Triazolopyridine derivative
Therapeutic class: Antidepressant
Pregnancy risk category C

Action
Unclear. Thought to selectively inhibit serotonin and norepinephrine uptake in brain.

Availability
Tablets: 50 mg, 100 mg, 150 mg, 300 mg

Indications and dosages
➢ Major depression
Adults: 150 mg/day P.O. in three divided doses; may increase by 50 mg/day q 3 to 4 days until desired response occurs. Don't exceed 400 mg/day in outpatient or 600 mg/day in hospitalized patient.

Dosage adjustment
- Elderly patients

Off-label uses
- Alcohol dependence
- Cocaine withdrawal
- Anxiety neurosis
- Insomnia

Contraindications
- Hypersensitivity to drug
- Recovery period after myocardial infarction

Precautions
Use cautiously in:
- cardiovascular disease, severe hepatic or renal disease, suicidal behavior or ideation
- elderly patients
- pregnant or breastfeeding patients
- children (safety not established).

Administration
- Give after meals or snacks.
- Know that drug is often used in conjunction with psychotherapy.

Route	Onset	Peak	Duration
P.O.	1-2 wk	2-4 wk	Wks

Adverse reactions
CNS: drowsiness, confusion, dizziness, fatigue, hallucinations, headache, insomnia, nightmares, slurred speech, syncope, weakness, tremor, **suicidal behavior or ideation** (especially in child or adolescent)
CV: chest pain, hypotension, hypertension, palpitations, tachycardia, **arrhythmias**
EENT: blurred vision, tinnitus
GI: nausea, vomiting, diarrhea, constipation, excessive salivation, flatulence, dry mouth
GU: urinary frequency, hematuria, erectile dysfunction, priapism
Hematologic: anemia, **leukopenia**
Musculoskeletal: myalgia
Skin: rash

Interactions
Drug-drug. *Antihypertensives, nitrates:* additive hypotension
Digoxin, phenytoin: increased blood levels of these drugs
Fluoxetine: increased trazodone blood level, greater risk of toxicity
Other CNS depressants (such as opioid analgesics, sedative-hypnotics): additive CNS depression
Drug-diagnostic tests. *Alkaline phosphatase, bilirubin, glucose:* increased levels

t

Urinary catecholamines: false increases
Urinary 5-hydroxyindole acetic acid, vanillylmandelic acid: decreased levels
Drug-herbs. *Chamomile, hops, kava, skullcap, valerian:* increased CNS depression
S-adenosylmethionine (SAM-e), St. John's wort, increased risk of serotonergic effects (including serotonin syndrome)
Drug-behaviors. *Alcohol use:* additive CNS depression and hypotension

Patient monitoring

- Monitor vital signs and ECG.
- Monitor neurologic status. Report significant adverse reactions.
- Assess patient's mood frequently. Stay alert for worsening depression and suicidal ideation.
- Watch for drug hoarding or overuse.

Patient teaching

- Tell patient to take with meals or snacks to improve drug absorption.
- Instruct patient to take only as prescribed. Caution him not to overuse or hoard drug.
- Advise patient (and significant other as appropriate) to monitor his mood. Explain that drug should ease depression.

Caution patient (and parent or significant other) to immediately report suicidal thoughts or behavior, especially in child or adolescent.

- Tell patient drug may cause significant adverse reactions. Instruct him to report priapism, hallucinations, fainting spells, and other serious problems.
- Instruct patient not to drink alcohol during drug therapy.
- Tell patient that many common herbs worsen drug's adverse reactions. Tell him to consult prescriber before taking these products.
- Caution patient to avoid driving and other hazardous activities until he knows how drug affects concentration, vision, and alertness. Reassure him that dizziness and drowsiness usually subside after first few weeks.
- As appropriate, review all other significant and life-threatening adverse reactions and interactions, especially those related to the drugs, tests, herbs, and behaviors mentioned above.

treprostinil sodium

Remodulin

Pharmacologic class: Synthetic prostacyclin analog

Therapeutic class: Antiplatelet agent, vasodilator

Pregnancy risk category B

Action

Dilates pulmonary and systemic arterial vascular beds, reducing right and left ventricular afterload and increasing cardiac output and stroke volume. Also inhibits platelet aggregation.

Availability

Injection: 1 mg/ml, 2.5 mg/ml, 5 mg/ml, 10 mg/ml

Indications and dosages

➢ To diminish exercise-induced symptoms of pulmonary artery hypertension (PAH) in patients with NYHA class II-IV symptoms
Adults: Initially, 1.25 ng/kg/minute by continuous subcutaneous infusion; if initial dose isn't tolerated, reduce infusion rate to 0.625 ng/kg/minute. For maintenance, may increase infusion rate in increments of no more than 1.25 ng/kg/minute q week for first 4 weeks, then in increments of no more than 2.5 ng/kg/minute q week, if needed. Maximum dosage is 40 ng/kg/minute.

Dosage adjustment
- Hepatic insufficiency

Contraindications
- Hypersensitivity to drug, its components, or structurally related compounds

Precautions
Use cautiously in:
- renal disease
- history of hepatic disease
- elderly patients
- pregnant or breastfeeding patients
- children.

Administration
🔊 Give first dose in setting where resuscitation equipment is available and other health care personnel can assist if an emergency arises.
- Administer by continuous subcutaneous infusion through subcutaneous catheter with infusion pump made specifically for subcutaneous infusions.
- Expect to adjust dosage for first 6 to 12 weeks as prescriber balances symptom improvement against adverse reactions.

🔊 Don't stop infusion abruptly (may worsen PAH).

Route	Onset	Peak	Duration
Subcut.	Unknown	Unknown	Unknown

Adverse reactions
CNS: dizziness, headache, anxiety, restlessness
CV: vasodilation, edema, hypotension
EENT: jaw pain
GI: nausea, vomiting, diarrhea
Skin: rash, pruritus
Other: infusion site pain or reaction (such as erythema, rash, induration)

Interactions
Drug-drug. *Anticoagulants:* increased risk of bleeding
Antihypertensives, diuretics, other vasodilators: increased risk of hypotension
Vitamin A: increased risk of bleeding
Drug-herbs. *Alfalfa, anise, arnica, astragalus, bilberry, black currant seed oil, bladderwrack, bogbean, boldo (with fenugreek), borage oil, buchu, capsaicin, cat's claw, celery, chaparral, chincona bark, clove oil, dandelion, dong quai, evening primrose oil, fenugreek, feverfew, garlic, ginger, ginkgo, guggul, papaya extract, red clover, rhubarb, safflower oil, skullcap, tan-shen:* increased risk of bleeding

Patient monitoring
🔊 Especially after first dose, watch closely for severe vasodilation leading to chest pain and hypotension. These signs and symptoms call for emergency measures.

🔊 Monitor vital signs. Assess carefully for indications of right ventricular failure.
- Assess neurologic status. Institute safety measures as needed to prevent injury.

🔊 Watch for infusion site reaction.

Patient teaching
- Tell patient drug is a long-term measure to control PAH and requires a commitment to maintain infusion system.

🔊 Instruct patient to immediately report signs and symptoms of infusion site reaction (such as redness, rash, and hardened tissue).
- Teach patient which symptoms reflect underlying disease and which may reflect adverse reactions that he should report.
- As appropriate, review all other significant adverse reactions and interactions, especially those related to the drugs and herbs mentioned above.

t

tretinoin

Avita, Renova, Retin-A, Retin-A Micro, Vesanoid

Pharmacologic class: Retinoid
Therapeutic class: Antineoplastic, dermatologic agent (topical)
Pregnancy risk category C (topical), *D* (oral)

Action

Unknown. Thought to cause differentiation of promyelocytic leukemic blast cells, leading to apoptosis (cell shrinkage and death) and cancer remission.

Availability

Capsules: 10 mg
Topical cream: 0.02%, 0.025%, 0.05%, 0.1%
Topical gel: 0.01%, 0.025%, 0.04%, 0.1%
Topical liquid: 0.05%

Indications and dosages

➢ Acute promyelocytic leukemia (APL) when anthracycline chemotherapy fails or is contraindicated
Adults and children ages 1 and older: 45 mg/m²/day P.O. in two evenly divided doses. Discontinue after 90 days of therapy or 30 days after complete remission occurs, whichever comes first.

➢ Acne vulgaris
Adults: Apply Avita cream, Retin-A cream, gel, or liquid, or Retin-A Micro gel daily before bedtime or in evening. Cover entire affected area lightly.

➢ Adjunct for mitigating fine wrinkles in patients who use comprehensive skin care and sun avoidance programs
Adults: Apply Renova 0.02% cream to face daily in evening for up to 52 weeks, using only enough to lightly cover entire affected area.

➢ Adjunct for mitigating fine wrinkles, mottled hyperpigmentation, and tactile roughness of facial skin when comprehensive skin care and sun avoidance programs alone fail
Adults ages 50 and younger: Apply Renova 0.05% cream to face daily in evening for up to 48 weeks, using only enough to lightly cover entire affected area.

Contraindications

- Hypersensitivity to drug or parabens
- Pregnancy or breastfeeding (oral use)

Precautions

Use cautiously in:
- eczema, sunburn, photosensitivity
- concurrent use of over-the-counter (OTC) acne products or abrasive soaps or cleansers with strong drying effects or high alcohol or lime content (with all topical forms)
- concurrent use of astringents, spices, permanent wave solutions, electrolysis, hair depilatories or waxes, or photosensitizing drugs (such as fluoroquinolones, phenothiazines, tetracyclines, thiazides)
- heavily pigmented, elderly, pregnant, or breastfeeding patients (safety and efficacy not established for topical use)
- children younger than age 1 for oral use or younger than age 18 for topical use (safety and efficacy not established).

Administration

- Verify that female patient has had required pregnancy test before P.O. therapy starts.
- Know that Renova topical cream isn't indicated for acne vulgaris, and that other topical forms are indicated only for acne vulgaris. Also know that some absorption of topical products occurs.

Route	Onset	Peak	Duration
P.O.	Unknown	1-2 hr	Unknown
Topical	Unknown	Unknown	Unknown

Adverse reactions

CNS: dizziness, headache, asthenia, paresthesia, confusion, agitation, hallucinations, anxiety, aphasia, depression, agnosia, insomnia, asterixis, cerebellar edema, hypotaxia, drowsiness, slow speech, facial paralysis, hemiplegia, hyporeflexia, hypotaxia, dementia, spinal cord disorder, tremors, dysarthria, **cerebrovascular accident (CVA), coma, seizures, intracranial hypertension, cerebral hemorrhage**
CV: heart murmur, chest discomfort, peripheral edema, hypertension, hypotension, phlebitis, edema, enlarged heart, ischemia, **arrhythmias, secondary cardiomyopathy, myocarditis, myocardial infarction (MI), heart failure, pericardial effusion, impaired myocardial contractility, progressive hypoxemia**
EENT: vision disturbances, visual acuity changes, visual field defect, absence of light reflex, hearing loss, earache, full sensation in ears
GI: nausea, vomiting, constipation, diarrhea, abdominal pain and distention, GI disorders, mucositis, dyspepsia, ulcer, anorexia, **GI hemorrhage**
GU: dysuria, urinary frequency, enlarged prostate, **renal insufficiency, renal tubular necrosis, acute renal failure**
Hematologic: leukocytosis, disseminated intravascular coagulation (DIC), hemorrhage
Hepatic: ascites, **hepatosplenomegaly, hepatitis**
Metabolic: fluid imbalance, **acidosis**
Musculoskeletal: bone pain or inflammation, myalgia, flank pain
Respiratory: respiratory tract disorders, dyspnea, expiratory wheezing, crackles, pneumonia, **laryngeal edema, pulmonary infiltrates, pleural effusion, bronchial asthma, pulmonary hypertension**
Skin: rash; pallor; flushing; diaphoresis; alopecia; dry skin and mucous membranes; skin changes; pruritus; cellulitis; burning, erythema, peeling, and stinging (with topical use)
Other: weight changes, fever, lymphatic disorder, hypothermia, infections, facial edema, pain, **retinoic acid-APL syndrome, multisystem failure, septicemia**

Interactions

Drug-drug. *Photosensitizing drugs (such as fluoroquinolones, phenothiazines, tetracyclines, thiazides):* increased risk of photosensitivity reaction (with topical forms)
Drug-diagnostic tests. *Cholesterol, triglycerides:* increased levels
Drug-food. *Any food:* enhanced tretinoin absorption
Drug-behaviors. *Sun exposure:* increased risk of photosensitivity

Patient monitoring

🔊 Watch closely for septicemia, multisystem failure, and retinoic acid-APL syndrome (which causes pulmonary and pericardial effusion, fever, weight gain, and dyspnea).
🔊 Monitor for significant adverse CNS reactions, including seizures, CVA, and cerebral hemorrhage.
🔊 Monitor cardiovascular status. Stay alert for signs and symptoms of arrhythmias, MI, and heart failure.
🔊 Closely monitor liver and kidney function tests. Watch for evidence of hepatitis and renal failure.
🔊 Monitor coagulation studies. Watch closely for DIC and hemorrhage.
• Evaluate respiratory status. Stay alert for indications of pulmonary hypertension and respiratory insufficiency.

t

• Frequently assess lipid panel and CBC with white cell differential.

Patient teaching

• Instruct patient to take oral doses with food.

Teach patient to recognize and immediately report serious adverse reactions.

• Tell patient he'll undergo regular blood testing during oral therapy.

• Instruct patient using topical form to gently wash face with mild soap, pat skin dry, and then wait 20 to 30 minutes before applying. Advise him to apply to face in evening, using only enough to cover entire affected area lightly and only for prescribed duration.

• Caution patient to avoid OTC acne drugs and extreme weather conditions (such as wind and cold). Urge him to adhere to prescribed skin care and sunlight avoidance programs when using topical form.

• Tell patient using topical form that transient burning, erythema, peeling, pruritus, and stinging may occur. Advise him to notify prescriber if these symptoms become severe.

• As appropriate, review all other significant and life-threatening adverse reactions and interactions, especially those related to the drugs, tests, foods, and behaviors mentioned above.

triamcinolone

Aristocort, Kenacort

triamcinolone acetonide

Aristocort, Aristocort A, Azmacort HFA, Azmacort Inhalation Aerosol, Kenalog, Kenalog-10, Kenalog-40, Nasacort AQ

triamcinolone diacetate

Kenacort

triamcinolone hexacetonide

Aristospan Intra-Articular, Aristospan Intralesional

Pharmacologic class: Synthetic corticosteroid

Therapeutic class: Anti-inflammatory (steroidal)

Pregnancy risk category C

Action

Unknown. Thought to decrease inflammation mainly by inhibiting activities of mast cells, macrophages, and other mediators of allergic reactions. Also suppresses immune system by depressing lymphatic activity.

Availability

triamcinolone

Tablets: 1 mg, 2 mg, 4 mg, 8 mg

triamcinolone acetonide

Cream: 0.025%, 0.1%, 0.5%

Inhalation aerosol (intranasal): 55 mcg/inhalation (metered spray) in 20-g canister (240 metered inhalations)

Inhalation aerosol (oral): 100 mcg/inhalation (metered spray)

Injectable suspension: 3 mg/ml, 10 mg/ml, 40 mg/ml

Lotion: 0.025%, 0.1%

Ointment: 0.025%, 0.1%, 0.5%
Solution: 50 mcg/metered spray
Suspension: 55 mcg/metered spray
triamcinolone diacetate
Injectable suspension: 25 mg/ml, 40 mg/ml
triamcinolone hexacetonide
Injectable suspension: 5 mg/ml, 20 mg/ml

Indications and dosages

➢ Allergic rhinitis

Adults and children older than age 12: 8 to 12 mg (tablets) P.O. daily. Or 110 mcg (two sprays of inhalation aerosol or acetonide suspension) in each nostril daily; may increase to 220 mcg (four sprays) in each nostril daily (110 mcg b.i.d. or 55 mcg q.i.d.). Or 100 mcg (two sprays of acetonide solution) in each nostril daily; may increase to 400 mcg (four sprays) in each nostril daily or two sprays in each nostril b.i.d.
Children ages 6 to 12: 55 mcg (one spray of inhalation aerosol or acetonide suspension) in each nostril daily

➢ Chronic asthma

Adults and children older than age 12: Two metered inhalations three to four times daily or four metered inhalations b.i.d. (100 mcg/metered inhalation), not to exceed 16 inhalations/day
Children ages 6 to 12: One to two metered inhalations three to four times daily or two to four metered inhalations b.i.d. (100 mcg/metered inhalation), not to exceed 12 inhalations/day

➢ Severe inflammation; immunosuppression

Adults and children older than age 12: 4 to 48 mg (tablets) P.O. daily in one to four divided doses. Or 60 mg (acetonide) I.M. at 6-week intervals. For intralesional or sublesional use, 1 mg at each injection site, repeated one or more times weekly; for intra-articular, intrasynovial, or soft-tissue injection, 2.5 to 40 mg, repeated when symptoms recur. Or 200 mcg (two sprays of acetonide inhalation aerosol) three to four times daily. Or 40 mg (diacetate) I.M. weekly. Or 5 to 48 mg (diacetate) by intralesional or sublesional injection, not to exceed 75 mg/week intralesionally. Or 2 to 40 mg (diacetate) by intra-articular, intrasynovial, or soft-tissue injection; may repeat at 1- to 8-week intervals. Or 0.5 mg/square inch of affected skin (hexacetonide) by intralesional or sublesional injection or 2 to 20 mg by intra-articular injection; may repeat at 3- to 4-week intervals.
Children ages 6 to 12: 100 or 200 mcg (one or two sprays of acetonide inhalation aerosol) three to four times daily, or 0.03 to 0.2 mg/kg or 1 to 6.25 mg/m^2 I.M. at intervals of 1 to 7 days

➢ Corticosteroid-responsive dermatoses

Adults and children older than age 12: Apply cream, ointment, or lotion sparingly to affected area two to four times daily.

➢ Adrenocortical insufficiency

Adults and children older than age 12: 4 to 12 mg (tablets) P.O. daily, used with mineralocorticoid therapy

➢ Rheumatic disorders; dermatologic disorders; severe psoriasis

Adults and children older than age 12: 8 to 16 mg (tablets) P.O. daily

➢ Systemic lupus erythematosus

Adults and children older than age 12: Initially, 20 to 32 mg (tablets) P.O. daily, continued until desired response occurs. Severe symptoms may warrant initial dosage of 48 mg.

➢ Acute rheumatic carditis

Adults and children older than age 12: Initially, 20 to 60 mg (tablets) P.O. daily (usually given with anti-infectives and salicylates) until desired clinical response occurs. Then dosage may be reduced to maintenance level and continued for 6 weeks or up to 3 months.

➢ Ophthalmic inflammatory diseases; sympathetic ophthalmia

Adults and children older than age 12: 12 to 40 mg (tablets) P.O. daily, depending on severity of condition and degree of ocular structure involvement. Response is usually rapid and length of therapy is usually brief.

➢ Respiratory diseases; tuberculous meningitis; nephrotic syndrome

Adults and children older than age 12: 16 to 48 mg (tablets) P.O. daily; or 32 to 48 (tablets) P.O. daily in divided doses in tuberculous meningitis. For tuberculosis, give with antitubercular therapy, as prescribed.

➢ Thrombocytopenia (in adults); autoimmune hemolytic anemia; erythroblastopenia; congenital hypoplastic anemia

Adults and children older than age 12: 16 to 60 mg (tablets) P.O. daily. Reduce dosage after adequate response.

➢ Palliative therapy in acute leukemia of childhood

Children: 1 to 2 mg/kg (tablets) P.O. daily, with expected initial response occurring in 6 to 21 days. Therapy usually continues for 4 to 6 weeks.

➢ Palliative therapy in acute leukemia or lymphoma in adults

Adults: 16 to 40 mg P.O. daily; may increase to 100 mg daily in leukemia

Contraindications

- Hypersensitivity to drug, tartrazine, chlorofluorocarbon propellants, alcohol, propylene glycol, or polyethylene glycol
- Acute asthma attacks, status asthmaticus (inhalation use only)
- Systemic fungal infections (oral and parenteral use)
- Idiopathic thrombocytopenic purpura (I.M. use)
- Administration of live-virus vaccines (with immunosuppressant doses of triamcinolone)

Precautions

Use cautiously in:

- active untreated infection, systemic infection, immunosuppression, hypertension, osteoporosis, diabetes mellitus, glaucoma, renal disease, hypothyroidism, cirrhosis, diverticulitis, nonspecific ulcerative colitis, recent intestinal anastomoses, thromboembolic disorders, seizures, myasthenia gravis, heart failure, ocular herpes simplex, emotional instability
- pregnant or breastfeeding patients
- children younger than age 6 (safety not established).

Administration

🔊 Don't withdraw systemic corticosteroids abruptly when patient begins inhalation steroid therapy.

🔊 Know that patient will need additional steroids during times of stress or trauma.

- Use hand-held nebulizer supplied with aerosol form.

🔊 Apply cream, lotion, or ointment sparingly. Know that triamcinolone is a high-potency steroid; it can be absorbed systemically and should not be withdrawn abruptly.

🔊 Avoid intralesional injection to face or head (may cause blindness).

- Don't apply topical form near eyes.
- Know that occlusive dressing may be used with topical form when treating psoriasis or other recalcitrant conditions, but should be removed if infection occurs.

Route	Onset	Peak	Duration
P.O.	Unknown	Unknown	2.25 days
I.M.	Unknown	Unknown	1-4 wk
Intralesional, sublesional, intra-articular	Slow	Unknown	Unknown
Inhalation	Immediate	Unknown	Unknown
Topical	Unknown	Unknown	Unknown

Adverse reactions

CNS: headache, vertigo, paresthesia, syncope, personality changes, **pseudotumor cerebri, seizures**

CV: hypertension, **thrombophlebitis, arrhythmias, thromboembolism, heart failure**
EENT: cataract, glaucoma, increased intraocular pressure, exophthalmos, otitis, nasal or sinus congestion, rhinitis, epistaxis, sneezing, dry mucous membranes, pharyngitis, throat discomfort
GI: nausea, vomiting, dyspepsia, abdominal distention or pain, peptic ulcer, ulcerative esophagitis, oral candidiasis, dry mouth, **pancreatitis**
GU: cystitis, urinary tract infection, glycosuria, menstrual irregularities, vaginal candidiasis
Metabolic: fluid retention, hypernatremia, hypokalemia, hyperglycemia, hypocalcemia, decreased growth (in children), carbohydrate intolerance, exacerbation of latent diabetes mellitus, cushingoid appearance (moon face, buffalo hump), **hypokalemic alkalosis, acute adrenal insufficiency** (with abrupt withdrawal or acute stress in long-term use)
Musculoskeletal: muscle weakness; steroid myopathy; loss of muscle mass; myalgia; bursitis; tenosynovitis; osteoporosis; fractures; aseptic necrosis; with intra-articular injection—osteonecrosis, tendon rupture, post-injection flare
Respiratory: cough, wheezing, chest congestion
Skin: delayed wound healing; thin and fragile skin; petechiae; bruising; with topical use—local eruptions, pruritus, hypopigmentation or hyperpigmentation, scarring, stinging, skin maceration, secondary infection, cutaneous or subcutaneous atrophy, diaphoresis, facial erythema
Other: toothache, weight gain, fever, pain, voice alteration, hypersensitivity reaction

Interactions

Drug-drug. *Erythromycin, indinavir, itraconazole, ketoconazole, ritonavir, saquinavir:* increased triamcinolone blood level and effects
Fluoroquinolones: increased risk of tendon rupture
Live-virus vaccines: decreased antibody response to vaccine
Nonsteroidal anti-inflammatory drugs (including aspirin): increased risk of adverse GI reactions
Potassium-wasting drugs (including amphotericin B, thiazide and loop diuretics, mezlocillin, piperacillin, ticarcillin): additive hypokalemia
Drug-diagnostic tests. *Cholesterol:* increased level
Skin tests: suppressed reaction

Patient monitoring

- Monitor respiratory status. Watch for worsening signs and symptoms.
- With long-term use, assess for adverse endocrine and musculoskeletal reactions.
- Monitor carefully for signs and symptoms of infection, which drug may mask.

Patient teaching

- Teach patient correct use of drug. Make sure he has received manufacturer's patient information sheet.

(Clinical alert) Advise patient to contact prescriber immediately if acute asthma attack occurs. Tell him inhalation aerosol isn't meant for rapid relief of bronchospasm.

- Inform patient that drug can affect many body systems. Urge him to report serious adverse effects promptly.
- Tell parents drug may make child more vulnerable to childhood infections, such as chicken pox and measles.
- As appropriate, review all other significant and life-threatening adverse reactions and interactions, especially those related to the drugs and tests mentioned above.

t

triamterene

Dyrenium

Pharmacologic class: Potassium-sparing diuretic
Therapeutic class: Diuretic
Pregnancy risk category B

Action

Depresses sodium resorption and potassium excretion in renal distal tubule

Availability

Capsules: 50 mg, 100 mg

Indications and dosages

➤ Edema

Adults: 100 mg P.O. b.i.d. Do not exceed 300 mg/day.

Dosage adjustment

- Concurrent antihypertensive drug therapy
- Elderly patients

Off-label uses

- Diabetes insipidus

Contraindications

- Hypersensitivity to drug
- Hyperkalemia
- Severe hepatic disease
- Anuria, severe renal dysfunction (except nephrosis)
- Concurrent use of other potassium-sparing diuretics or potassium supplements

Precautions

Use cautiously in:

- hepatic dysfunction, renal insufficiency, diabetes mellitus
- history of gout or renal calculi
- elderly or debilitated patients
- pregnant or breastfeeding patients
- children (safety not established).

Administration

- Give after meals.
- Know that drug may be used alone or as adjunct to thiazide or loop diuretics.
- Make sure patient stops taking potassium supplements before starting triamterene.

Route	Onset	Peak	Duration
P.O.	2-4 hr	Unknown	12-16 hr

Adverse reactions

CNS: headache, fatigue, asthenia, dizziness
GI: nausea, vomiting, diarrhea, dry mouth
GU: azotemia, renal calculi
Hematologic: megaloblastic anemia, thrombocytopenia
Hepatic: jaundice
Metabolic: hyperglycemia, **hyperkalemia, metabolic acidosis**
Skin: rash, photosensitivity
Other: anaphylaxis

Interactions

Drug-drug. *Amantadine:* increased amantadine blood level, greater risk of toxicity
Angiotensin-converting enzyme inhibitors, cyclosporine, indomethacin, potassium-sparing diuretics, potassium supplements, other potassium-containing preparations: increased risk of hyperkalemia
Antihypertensives, nondepolarizing muscle relaxants, other diuretics, preanesthetic and anesthetic agents: potentiated effects of these drugs
Chlorpropamide: increased risk of hyponatremia
Cimetidine: increased bioavailability and decreased renal clearance of triamterene

Indomethacin: increased risk of acute renal failure
Lithium: decreased lithium clearance, greater risk of lithium toxicity
Drug-diagnostic tests. *Alkali reserves, hemoglobin, platelets:* decreased values
Blood urea nitrogen (BUN), creatinine, glucose, hepatic enzymes, potassium: increased levels
Liver function tests: increased values
Quinidine blood level: interference with fluorescent measurement
Drug-food. *Salt substitutes containing potassium:* increased risk of hyperkalemia
Drug-herbs. *Gossypol, licorice:* increased risk of hypokalemia

Patient monitoring

- Monitor BUN, creatinine, and electrolyte levels. Stay alert for hyperkalemia.
- Assess CBC with white cell differential.

Patient teaching

- Advise patient to take after meals to reduce nausea.
- Instruct patient to take last daily dose in early evening to avoid nocturia.
- Teach patient to recognize and report signs and symptoms of electrolyte imbalances.
- Tell patient to avoid salt substitutes. Advise him not to use herbs without consulting prescriber.
- As appropriate, review all other significant and life-threatening adverse reactions and interactions, especially those related to the drugs, tests, foods, and herbs mentioned above.

triazolam

Apo-Triazo♣, Gen-Triazolam♣, Halcion, Novo-Triolam♣

Pharmacologic class: Benzodiazepine
Therapeutic class: Sedative-hypnotic
Controlled substance schedule IV
Pregnancy risk category X

Action

Inhibits gamma-aminobutyric acid, a neurotransmitter that activates receptors at limbic, thalamic, and hypothalamic levels of CNS

Availability

Tablets: 0.125 mg, 0.25 mg, 0.5 mg

Indications and dosages

➢ Insomnia
Adults: 0.125 to 0.5 mg P.O. at bedtime p.r.n. After 7 to 10 days, decrease dosage gradually and then discontinue.

Dosage adjustment

- Elderly or debilitated patients

Off-label uses

- Presurgical hypnotic

Contraindications

- Hypersensitivity to drug or other benzodiazepines
- Concurrent use of itraconazole, ketoconazole, or nefazodone
- Pregnancy

Precautions

Use cautiously in:
- hepatic or renal dysfunction, sleep apnea, respiratory compromise, psychosis
- history of suicide attempt or drug abuse
- elderly or debilitated patients
- breastfeeding patients

t

• children younger than age 18 (safety and efficacy not established).

Administration

• Don't give with grapefruit juice.

Route	Onset	Peak	Duration
P.O.	15-30 min	2 hr	Unknown

Adverse reactions

CNS: dizziness, excessive sedation, hangover, headache, anterograde or traveler's amnesia, confusion, incoordination, lethargy, depression, paradoxical excitation, light-headedness, psychological disturbance, euphoria
GI: nausea, vomiting
Other: physical or psychological drug dependence, drug tolerance, withdrawal symptoms (tremor, abdominal and muscle cramps, vomiting, diaphoresis, dysphoria, perceptual disturbances, insomnia)

Interactions

Drug-drug. *Antidepressants, antihistamines, chloral hydrate, opioid analgesics, other psychotropic drugs:* additive CNS depression
Cimetidine, disulfiram, fluconazole, hormonal contraceptives, isoniazid, itraconazole, ketoconazole, nefazodone, rifampin, and other drugs that inhibit CYP450-3A4–mediated metabolism: decreased oxidative metabolism and increased action of triazolam
Digoxin: increased digoxin blood level, greater risk of toxicity
Macrolide anti-infectives (such as azithromycin, clarithromycin, erythromycin): increased triazolam bioavailability
Probenecid: rapid onset and prolonged effects of triazolam
Ranitidine: increased triazolam blood level
Theophylline: decreased sedative effect of triazolam
Drug-food. *Grapefruit juice:* increased triazolam blood level and effects
Drug-herbs. *Chamomile, hops, kava, skullcap, valerian:* increased CNS depression
Drug-behaviors. *Alcohol use:* increased CNS depression
Smoking: increased triazolam clearance

Patient monitoring

• Monitor neurologic status. Watch for paradoxical or rebound drug effects.
• Observe for signs of drug hoarding and drug abuse.

Patient teaching

• Tell patient to take at bedtime with a liquid other than grapefruit juice.
• Explain that drug is meant only for short-term use (7 to 10 days).
• Tell patient rebound insomnia may occur for 1 to 2 nights after he discontinues drug.
• Instruct patient to avoid alcohol use and smoking.
• Caution patient to avoid driving and other hazardous activities while under drug's influence.
• As appropriate, review all other significant adverse reactions and interactions, especially those related to the drugs, foods, herbs, and behaviors mentioned above.

trifluoperazine hydrochloride

Apo-Trifluoperazine♣, Novo-Flurazine♣, PMS-Trifluoperazine♣, Solazine♣, Terfluzine♣

Pharmacologic class: Piperazine phenothiazine
Therapeutic class: Antipsychotic
Pregnancy risk category C

Action

Unknown. Thought to act on subcortical levels of hypothalamic and limbic systems by producing antidopaminergic effects. Also lowers seizure threshold and exhibits some adrenergic, muscarinic, and anticholinergic activity.

Availability

Injection: 2 mg/ml in 10-ml vials
Oral solution: 10 mg/ml in 60-ml bottles
Tablets: 1 mg, 2 mg, 5 mg, 10 mg, 20 mg

Indications and dosages

➢ Schizophrenia

Adults: 2 to 5 mg P.O. b.i.d.; may increase gradually to obtain adequate response. Usual maintenance dosage is 15 to 20 mg/day. For prompt control of severe symptoms, 1 to 2 mg I.M. q 4 to 6 hours; some patients may need more than 6 mg/day.
Children ages 6 to 12: Initially, 1 mg P.O. once or twice daily in hospitalized patients or those under close supervision; may increase gradually up to 15 mg/day P.O. until symptoms are controlled or adverse reactions are intolerable. For prompt control of severe symptoms, 1 mg I.M. once or twice daily.

➢ Nonpsychotic anxiety

Adults: 1 to 2 mg P.O. b.i.d. Do not exceed 6 mg/day or 12 weeks' duration.

Dosage adjustment

- Hepatic disease
- Elderly or debilitated patients

Contraindications

- Hypersensitivity to drug, other phenothiazines, or bisulfites
- Severe hepatic disease
- Bone marrow depression
- Blood dyscrasias
- Coma
- Concomitant use of other CNS depressants in high doses

Precautions

Use cautiously in:

- seizure disorders, cardiovascular disorders, GI obstruction, glaucoma, retinopathy
- elderly or debilitated patients
- pregnant or breastfeeding patients.

Administration

- Mix oral solution in at least 60 ml of liquid or semisolid food just before giving.
- Administer I.M. injection deep into muscle.
- Know that parenteral solution should be colorless to pale yellow; discard if it's markedly discolored.

Route	Onset	Peak	Duration
P.O.	Unknown	2-4 hr	12-24 hr
I.M.	Unknown	Unknown	4-6 hr

Adverse reactions

CNS: sedation, dizziness, drowsiness, insomnia, fatigue, extrapyramidal effects, **neuroleptic malignant syndrome**
CV: tachycardia, hypotension, orthostatic hypotension, peripheral edema, **prolonged QT interval, torsades de pointes**
EENT: dry eyes, blurred vision, miosis, mydriasis, epithelial keratopathy, pigmentary retinopathy
GI: constipation, biliary stasis, dry mouth, anorexia, **adynamic ileus**
GU: urinary retention, glycosuria, amenorrhea, ejaculatory disorders, galactorrhea, gynecomastia
Hematologic: leukopenia, agranulocytosis
Hepatic: cholestatic jaundice
Musculoskeletal: muscle weakness
Skin: photosensitivity, altered pigmentation, erythema, rash
Other: mild fever, weight gain, allergic reaction

Interactions

Drug-drug. *Alpha-adrenergic blockers:* additive effect

t

Antacids containing aluminum: decreased trifluoperazine absorption
Anticholinergics, anticholinergic-like drugs (including antidepressants, antihistamines, disopyramide, other phenothiazines, quinidine): additive anticholinergic effects
Anticonvulsants: decreased seizure threshold
Antihistamines, CNS depressants, general anesthetics, opioids, sedative-hypnotics: additive CNS depression
Barbiturates: decreased blood levels of both drugs
Guanethidine: decreased antihypertensive effect
Lithium: increased risk of extrapyramidal reactions, disorientation, and unconsciousness
Oral anticoagulants: decreased anticoagulant effect
Phenytoin: interference with phenytoin metabolism, causing phenytoin toxicity
Propranolol: increased blood levels of both drugs
Thiazide diuretics: additive orthostatic hypotension
Drug-diagnostic tests. *Hepatic enzymes:* increased levels
Phenylketonuria test: false-positive result
Prolactin: increased level, causing interference with gonadotropin tests
Urine bilirubin: false-positive result
Drug-herbs. *St. John's wort:* increased risk of photosensitivity
Drug-behaviors. *Alcohol use:* additive CNS depression and hypotension
Sun exposure: increased risk of photosensitivity

Patient monitoring

- Monitor ECG and blood pressure. Watch closely for hypotension.
- Assess CBC (including platelet count) and liver function tests. Stay alert for signs and symptoms of hepatic damage and blood dyscrasias.

🔈 Monitor neurologic status, especially for indications of neuroleptic malignant syndrome (unstable blood pressure, high fever, sweating, stupor, muscle rigidity, and autonomic dysfunction).

Patient teaching

- Instruct patient taking oral solution to add solution to 60 ml or more of liquid (tomato or fruit juice, milk, carbonated beverage, coffee, tea, or water) or semisolid food (such as soup or pudding) just before taking.
- Tell patient that drug's full effect usually occurs in 1 to 2 weeks.
- Instruct patient to move slowly when sitting up or standing, to avoid dizziness from sudden blood pressure drop.

🔈 Teach patient to recognize and immediately report signs and symptoms of neuroleptic malignant syndrome.

- Caution patient to avoid driving and other hazardous activities until he knows how drug affects him.
- Tell patient to avoid alcohol and certain herbs.
- Advise patient to avoid sun exposure and to wear sunscreen and protective clothing when going outdoors.
- As appropriate, review all other significant and life-threatening adverse reactions and interactions, especially those related to the drugs, tests, herbs, and behaviors mentioned above.

trihexyphenidyl hydrochloride

Apo-Trihex✤, Novo-Hexidyl✤, PMS-Trihexyphenidyl✤

Pharmacologic class: Anticholinergic
Therapeutic class: Antidyskinetic
Pregnancy risk category C

Action
Inhibits parasympathetic nervous system, relaxing smooth muscles and decreasing involuntary movements

Availability
Capsules (sustained-release): 5 mg
Elixir: 2 mg/5 ml
Tablets: 2 mg, 5 mg

Indications and dosages
➢ Adjunct in idiopathic, postencephalitic, or arteriosclerotic parkinsonism
Adults: 1 mg P.O. on first day; may increase in 2-mg increments q 3 to 5 days, up to a maximum of 6 to 10 mg/day. In postencephalitic parkinsonism, 12 to 15 mg P.O. daily. May give sustained-release form (Artane Sequels) in same dosage as conventional form, as a single dose or in two divided doses q 12 hours after daily dosage is determined using conventional tablets or liquid.
➢ Drug-induced extrapyramidal symptoms
Adults: Initially, 1 mg P.O. daily, increased progressively if extrapyramidal symptoms aren't controlled within several hours. Usual dosage range is 5 to 15 mg/day P.O. in divided doses.

Dosage adjustment
- Concurrent use of levodopa or other parasympathetic inhibitor
- Elderly patients

Off-label uses
- Dystonia

Contraindications
- Hypersensitivity to drug, its components, or alcohol (elixir only)
- Angle-closure glaucoma
- Pyloric or duodenal obstruction
- Stenosing peptic ulcer
- Megacolon
- Prostatic hypertrophy or bladder-neck obstruction
- Achalasia
- Myasthenia gravis

Precautions
Use cautiously in:
- chronic renal, hepatic, pulmonary, or cardiac disease; hypertension; tachycardia secondary to cardiac insufficiency; hyperthyroidism
- elderly patients
- pregnant or breastfeeding patients
- children (safety not established).

Administration
- Give with meals. However, if drug causes severe dry mouth, give before meals.
- Administer last dose at bedtime.
- Know that sustained-release capsules shouldn't be used for initial therapy because of their greater strength. Once patient is stabilized on conventional form, he may be switched to sustained-release capsules on basis of milligram-per-milligram of total daily dosage.

Route	Onset	Peak	Duration
P.O.	1 hr	2-3 hr	6-12 hr
P.O. (sustained)	Unknown	Unknown	12-24 hr

Adverse reactions
CNS: dizziness, nervousness, drowsiness, asthenia, headache
CV: orthostatic hypotension, tachycardia
EENT: blurred vision, mydriasis, increased intraocular pressure (IOP), angle-closure glaucoma (with long-term use)
GI: nausea, vomiting, constipation, dry mouth
GU: urinary hesitancy or retention

Interactions
Drug-drug. *Amantadine, other anticholinergics (including disopyramide, phenothiazines, quinidine, tricyclic antidepressants):* additive anticholinergic effects

Other CNS depressants (such as antihistamines, opioids, sedative-hypnotics): additive CNS depression
Phenothiazines: decreased phenothiazine effects
Drug-herbs. *Angel's trumpet, jimsonweed, scopolia:* increased anticholinergic effects
Drug-behaviors. *Alcohol use:* additive CNS depression

Patient monitoring

- With prolonged use, monitor vision and IOP regularly.
- Assess drug efficacy to help guide dosage titration.
- Monitor vital signs. Watch for orthostatic hypotension.
- Closely monitor fluid intake and output. Stay alert for urinary retention.

Patient teaching

- Instruct patient to take with meals or, if severe dry mouth occurs, before meals.
- Tell patient drug has a bitter taste, which may be followed by numbness and tingling in mouth.
- Stress importance of follow-up eye exams.
- Instruct patient to consult prescriber before taking over-the-counter preparations or herbs.
- Advise patient to avoid alcohol and hazardous activities during drug therapy.
- Tell patient to move slowly when sitting up or standing, to avoid dizziness from sudden blood pressure decrease.
- As appropriate, review all other significant adverse reactions and interactions, especially those related to the drugs, herbs, and behaviors mentioned above.

trimethobenzamide hydrochloride

Tigan

Pharmacologic class: Anticholinergic
Therapeutic class: Antiemetic
Pregnancy risk category C

Action

Unclear. Thought to block dopamine receptors and emetic impulses in chemoreceptor trigger zone, preventing nausea and vomiting.

Availability

Capsules: 100 mg, 250 mg, 300 mg
Injection: 100 mg/ml in 2-ml ampules and prefilled syringes and in 20-ml vials
Suppositories: 100 mg, 200 mg

Indications and dosages

➢ Nausea and vomiting
Adults: 250 mg P.O. three to four times daily or 200 mg I.M. or P.R. three to four times daily
Children weighing 13.6 to 40.8 kg (30 to 90 lb): 100 to 200 mg P.O. or P.R. three to four times daily
Children weighing less than 13.6 kg (30 lb): 100 mg P.R. three to four times daily. Don't use in infants.

Contraindications

- Hypersensitivity to drug, benzocaine, or similar local anesthetics (with suppositories)
- Parenteral form in children
- Suppositories in infants

Precautions

Use cautiously in:
- arrhythmias, encephalitis, gastroenteritis, dehydration, electrolyte imbalances
- elderly or debilitated patients

• pregnant or breastfeeding patients
• children with known or suspected viral illnesses.

Administration

• In I.M. use, inject deep into upper outer quadrant of gluteus maximus.
• Withhold drug in children with signs or symptoms of Reye's syndrome.

Route	Onset	Peak	Duration
P.O., P.R.	10-40 min	Unknown	3-4 hr
I.M.	15-35 min	Unknown	2-3 hr

Adverse reactions

CNS: drowsiness, dizziness, headache, depression, disorientation, parkinsonian symptoms, **coma, seizures**
CV: hypotension
EENT: blurred vision
GI: diarrhea, rectal irritation (with suppositories)
Hematologic: blood dyscrasias
Hepatic: jaundice
Musculoskeletal: muscle cramps, opisthotonos
Skin: rash, urticaria, flushing
Other: pain and stinging at I.M. injection site, hypersensitivity reaction

Interactions

Drug-drug. *Antidepressants, antihistamines, CNS depressants, opioids, sedative-hypnotics:* additive CNS depression
Drug-behaviors. *Alcohol use:* additive CNS depression

Patient monitoring

• Monitor neurologic status, especially for parkinsonian symptoms and other serious adverse reactions.
• Assess CBC and liver function tests. Watch for blood dyscrasias and jaundice.
• Evaluate injection site for pain and stinging.
• Closely monitor patient's nutritional and hydration status. Report continuing nausea.

Patient teaching

• Advise patient to take as needed for nausea and vomiting, but only as prescribed.
• Tell patient to contact prescriber promptly if nausea persists despite therapy.
• Instruct patient to minimize nausea and vomiting by eating small, frequent servings of healthy food and drinking plenty of fluids.
• Advise patient to avoid alcohol.
• Caution patient to avoid driving and other hazardous activities until drug effects are known.
• As appropriate, review all other significant and life-threatening adverse reactions and interactions, especially those related to the drugs and behaviors mentioned above.

trimethoprim

Primsol, Proloprim

Pharmacologic class: Folate antagonist, dihydrofolate reductase inhibitor
Therapeutic class: Anti-infective
Pregnancy risk category C

Action

Inhibits dihydrofolate reductase (an enzyme required for production of tetrahydrofolic acid), preventing bacterial synthesis

Availability

Oral solution: 50 mg/5 ml
Tablets: 100 mg, 200 mg

Indications and dosages

➢ Urinary tract infections
Adults: 100 mg P.O. q 12 hours or 200 mg P.O. daily for 10 days

Dosage adjustment

• Renal impairment

t

Off-label uses
- *Pneumocystis jiroveci* pneumonia

Contraindications
- Hypersensitivity to drug or its components
- Megaloblastic anemia caused by folate deficiency

Precautions
Use cautiously in:
- renal or hepatic disease, folate deficiency
- pregnant or breastfeeding patients.

Administration
- Administer with or without food.

Route	Onset	Peak	Duration
P.O.	Rapid	1-4 hr	Unknown

Adverse reactions
GI: nausea, vomiting, epigastric distress, glossitis
Hematologic: methemoglobinemia, thrombocytopenia, leukopenia, neutropenia, megaloblastic anemia
Skin: rash, pruritus, **exfoliative dermatitis**
Other: fever

Interactions
Drug-drug. *Phenytoin:* increased phenytoin effects
Drug-diagnostic tests. *Alanine aminotransferase, aspartate aminotransferase, bilirubin, blood urea nitrogen, creatinine:* increased levels
Creatinine (determined by Jaffe reaction): false elevation
Hemoglobin, platelets, white blood cells: decreased levels
Methotrexate assay: interference with test results

Patient monitoring
- With prolonged use, monitor CBC (including platelet count). Watch for evidence of bone marrow depression.
- Assess kidney and liver function tests.

Patient teaching
- Explain drug therapy to patient. Urge him to take entire amount prescribed, even if symptoms improve.
- Advise patient to drink at least 2 L of fluid daily (unless contraindicated).
- Instruct patient to promptly report adverse reactions or worsening signs and symptoms.
- As appropriate, review all other significant and life-threatening adverse reactions and interactions, especially those related to the drugs and tests mentioned above.

trimipramine maleate
Apo-Trimip♣, Novo-Tripramine♣, Rhotrimine♣, Surmontil

Pharmacologic class: Dibenzazepine derivative tricyclic

Therapeutic class: Tricyclic antidepressant

Pregnancy risk category C

Action
Unknown. Thought to inhibit presynaptic norepinephrine and serotonin reuptake at CNS and peripheral receptors, causing increased synaptic concentrations of these neurotransmitters.

Availability
Capsules: 25 mg, 50 mg, 100 mg

Indications and dosages
➢ Depression

Adults: In outpatients, 75 mg/day P.O. in divided doses, increased gradually p.r.n. to a maximum of 200 mg/day; maintenance dosage is 50 to 150 mg/day P.O. for approximately 3 months. In hospitalized patients, 100 mg/day P.O. in divided doses, increased over several days p.r.n. to 200 mg/day; if no improvement occurs in 2 to 3 weeks, may increase to a maximum of 300 mg/day.

Dosage adjustment
- Hepatic disease
- Elderly patients

Off-label uses
- Depression in adolescents

Contraindications
- Hypersensitivity to drug or other dibenzazepines
- Acute recovery phase after myocardial infarction (MI)
- MAO inhibitor use within past 14 days

Precautions
Use cautiously in:
- increased intraocular pressure, angle-closure glaucoma, urinary retention, cardiac or hepatic disease, hyperthyroidism, urethral or ureteral spasm, seizure disorders, severe depression, suicidal ideation or behavior
- elderly patients
- pregnant or breastfeeding patients.

Administration
Don't give within 14 days of MAO inhibitors.

Route	Onset	Peak	Duration
P.O.	Unknown	2 hr	Unknown

Adverse reactions
CNS: confusion, drowsiness, dizziness, asthenia, fatigue, headache, disorientation, hallucinations, delusions, restlessness, anxiety, agitation, insomnia, nightmares, hypomania, psychosis exacerbation, paresthesia, incoordination, ataxia, tremor, peripheral neuropathy, extrapyramidal symptoms, EEG changes, **seizures, cerebrovascular accident (CVA), suicide or suicidal ideation** (especially in child or adolescent)
CV: hypotension, hypertension, tachycardia, palpitations, **heart block, arrhythmias, MI**
EENT: blurred vision, mydriasis, abnormal accommodation, tinnitus
GI: nausea, vomiting, diarrhea, constipation, epigastric distress, abdominal cramps, stomatitis, black tongue, dry mouth, **paralytic ileus**
GU: urinary retention or frequency, delayed voiding, urinary tract dilation, gynecomastia, galactorrhea, increased or decreased libido, erectile dysfunction, testicular swelling
Hematologic: eosinophilia, purpura, **thrombocytopenia, agranulocytosis**
Hepatic: jaundice, **hepatic dysfunction**
Metabolic: hyperglycemia, **hypoglycemia, syndrome of inappropriate antidiuretic hormone secretion**
Skin: rash, petechiae, pruritus, urticaria, alopecia, diaphoresis, flushing, photosensitivity
Other: abnormal taste, swollen face and tongue, weight changes, parotid gland swelling

Interactions
Drug-drug. *Anticholinergics (such as some antidepressants, antihistamines, atropine, disopyramide, haloperidol, phenothiazines, quinidine):* additive anticholinergic effects
Antihistamines, CNS depressants, opioids, sedative-hypnotics: additive CNS depression
Antithyroid drugs: increased risk of cardiotoxicity
Barbiturates: decreased trimipramine blood level, increased depressant effect
Cimetidine, flecainide, fluoxetine, paroxetine, phenothiazines, quinidine, sertraline: increased trimipramine blood level, greater risk of toxicity
Clonidine: increased risk of hypertensive crisis
Guanethidine: blocked guanethidine effects

Local anesthetics containing epinephrine, local decongestants, sympathomimetic amines: increased effects of these drugs
MAO inhibitors: hypertension, hyperpyrexia, seizures, death
Drug-diagnostic tests. *Alanine aminotransferase, aspartate aminotransferase:* increased levels
Glucose: increased or decreased level
Drug-herbs. *Angel's trumpet, belladonna, henbane, jimsonweed, scopolia:* increased anticholinergic effects
Chamomile, hops, kava, scopolia, skullcap, valerian: increased CNS depression
St. John's wort: decreased trimipramine blood level and efficacy
Drug-behaviors. *Alcohol use:* increased CNS depression
Sun exposure: increased risk of photosensitivity

Patient monitoring

- Monitor neurologic status. Watch for improvement in depression, as well as signs and symptoms of CVA or seizures.

Assess for suicide risk and drug hoarding.

- Monitor CBC and liver function tests. Stay alert for blood dyscrasias and hepatic dysfunction.

Patient teaching

- Tell patient he may take with or without food.
- Instruct patient to use only as prescribed.
- Caution patient not to stop drug abruptly, because doing so may cause nausea, headache, and malaise.

Instruct patient (or parent, as appropriate) to promptly report loss of consciousness, worsening depression, bleeding, bruising, or suicidal thoughts or behavior (especially in child or adolescent).

- Advise patient to avoid alcohol and herbs.
- Tell patient to avoid exposure to sun and to wear sunscreen and protective clothing when going outdoors.
- Caution patient to avoid driving and other hazardous activities until drug effects are known.
- As appropriate, review all other significant and life-threatening adverse reactions and interactions, especially those related to the drugs, tests, herbs, and behaviors mentioned above.

triptorelin pamoate

Trelstar Depot, Trelstar LA

Pharmacologic class: Synthetic agonist analog of luteinizing hormone-releasing hormone (LHRH)
Therapeutic class: Antineoplastic
Pregnancy risk category X

Action

Initially causes surge in luteinizing hormone (LH), follicle-stimulating hormone (FSH), and testosterone levels. After several weeks of therapy, LH and FSH secretion decrease, causing sustained testosterone reduction equivalent to pharmacologic castration.

Availability

Microgranules for injection (lyophilized): 3.75 mg (depot), 11.25 mg (long-acting)

Indications and dosages

➤ Palliative treatment of advanced prostate cancer
Adults: 3.75 mg (depot) I.M. monthly as a single injection or 11.25 mg (long-acting) I.M. q 84 days as a single injection

Off-label uses

- Infertility
- Endometriosis

• Uterine fibroids
• Precocious puberty

Contraindications
• Hypersensitivity to drug, LHRH, or other LHRH agonists
• Pregnancy
• Women of childbearing potential

Precautions
Use cautiously in:
• renal insufficiency
• prostate cancer with impending spinal cord compression or severe urinary tract disorder
• breastfeeding patients (use not recommended).

Administration
• Reconstitute with 2 ml of sterile water for injection, using accompanying syringe (don't use other diluents). Add syringe contents to vial containing particles; shake well. Withdraw vial contents and inject I.M. immediately.
• Inject deep I.M. into either buttock. Rotate injection sites.
Keep epinephrine and emergency equipment at hand in case of anaphylactic reaction.

Route	Onset	Peak	Duration
I.M. (depot)	Slow	4 days	1 mo
I.M. (long-acting)	Slow	2-3 days	3 mo

Adverse reactions
CNS: insomnia, dizziness, headache, emotional lability, fatigue
CV: hypertension
GI: vomiting, diarrhea
GU: urinary retention, urinary tract infection, gynecomastia, erectile dysfunction
Hematologic: anemia
Musculoskeletal: skeletal or leg pain
Skin: pruritus
Other: temporary worsening of disease, edema, hot flashes, pain at injection site, hypersensitivity reactions including **anaphylaxis**

Interactions
Drug-drug. *Metoclopramide and other drugs that can cause hyperprolactinemia:* increased prolactin production and risk of severe hyperprolactinemia
Drug-diagnostic tests. *Hemoglobin:* decreased value
Pituitary-gonadal function tests: misleading results (with continuous or long-term use)

Patient monitoring
• Monitor serum testosterone and prostate-specific antigen levels periodically to assess drug efficacy.

Patient teaching
• Explain drug therapy to patient. Stress need for follow-up laboratory tests.
• Tell patient prostate cancer symptoms may worsen during first few weeks of therapy.
• Instruct patient to monitor weight and report sudden weight gain or leg swelling.
• Advise female patient to tell prescriber before starting therapy if she is or plans to become pregnant. Caution her not to breastfeed during therapy.
• As appropriate, review all other significant and life-threatening adverse reactions and interactions, especially those related to the drugs and tests mentioned above.

t

tromethamine
Tham

Pharmacologic class: Protein substrate
Therapeutic class: Systemic alkalizer
Pregnancy risk category C

Action

Combines with hydrogen ions to form bicarbonate and a buffer, correcting acidosis. Also shows some diuretic activity.

Availability

Injection: 18 g/500 ml

Indications and dosages

➢ Metabolic acidosis associated with cardiac bypass surgery

Adults: 9 ml/kg (0.32 g/kg) by slow I.V. infusion; 500 ml (18 g) is usually adequate. Maximum single dosage is 500 mg/kg infused over at least 1 hour.

➢ Metabolic acidosis associated with cardiac arrest

Adults: 3.6 to 10.8 g by I.V. injection into large peripheral vein if chest isn't open, or 2 to 6 g I.V. directly into ventricular cavity if chest is open. After reversal of cardiac arrest, patient may need additional amounts to control persistent acidosis.

➢ To correct acidity of acid-citrate-dextrose (ACD) blood in cardiac bypass surgery

Adults: 0.5 to 2.5 g added to each 500 ml of ACD blood used for priming pump-oxygenator. Usual dosage is 2 g.

Dosage adjustment

- Elderly patients

Contraindications

- Hypersensitivity to drug
- Anuria
- Uremia

Precautions

Use cautiously in:

- renal disease, severe respiratory disease, respiratory depression
- pregnant patients
- infants.

Administration

Keep intubation equipment nearby in case respiratory depression occurs.

- For metabolic acidosis associated with cardiac bypass surgery, give by slow I.V. infusion through large-bore I.V. catheter into large antecubital vein. Elevate arm after infusion.
- If extravasation occurs, discontinue drug and infiltrate affected area with 1% procaine hydrochloride (containing hyaluronidase).
- Be aware that in cardiac arrest, drug is used with standard resuscitative measures. When giving by direct I.V. injection into open chest, never inject into cardiac muscle.

Route	Onset	Peak	Duration
I.V.	Immediate	Immediate	Unknown

Adverse reactions

GU: oliguria

Hepatic: hemorrhagic hepatic necrosis

Metabolic: metabolic alkalosis, transient hypoglycemia, fluid-solute overload, hyperkalemia

Respiratory: respiratory depression

Other: fever; I.V. site infection; extravasation with venous thrombosis or phlebitis, inflammation, necrosis, and sloughing

Interactions

Drug-diagnostic tests. *Glucose:* decreased level

Potassium: increased level

Patient monitoring

- Maintain continuous cardiac monitoring.
- Monitor arterial blood gas levels. Watch for alkalosis and signs and symptoms of respiratory depression.
- Assess liver function tests. Stay alert for signs and symptoms of hepatic impairment.

• Monitor glucose and potassium levels. Watch for hypoglycemia and hyperkalemia.
• Closely monitor fluid intake and output. Check for fluid and electrolyte imbalances and oliguria related to hyperkalemia.

Patient teaching
• Explain drug therapy to patient. Assure him he'll be monitored continuously.
• As appropriate, review all significant and life-threatening adverse reactions and interactions, especially those related to the tests mentioned above.

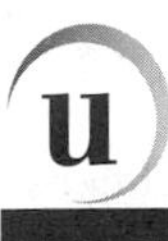

urea
Ureaphil

Pharmacologic class: Diamide salt of carbonic acid
Therapeutic class: Osmotic diuretic
Pregnancy risk category C

Action
Increases osmotic pressure of glomerular filtrate, inhibits tubular reabsorption of water and electrolytes, and elevates plasma osmolarity, increasing water influx into extracellular fluid

Availability
Powder for reconstitution: 40 g/150 ml

Indications and dosages
➤ Increased intracranial pressure (ICP) or intraocular pressure (IOP)
Adults: 1 to 1.5 g/kg as 30% solution I.V., infused slowly over 1 to 2½ hours at a rate no faster than 4 ml/minute. Maximum dosage is 120 g/day.

Off-label uses
• Abortifacient

Contraindications
• Hypersensitivity to drug
• Severe renal impairment
• Marked dehydration
• Active intracranial bleeding
• Hepatic failure
• Infusion into lower leg veins in elderly patients

Precautions
Use cautiously in:
• hepatic or renal disease, electrolyte imbalances, diabetes mellitus, sickle cell disease, membrane rupture, cervical stenosis, uterine fibroids
• pregnant or breastfeeding patients.

Administration
• Add dextrose 5% or 10% in water to container with 40 g of urea, to yield a final concentration of 300 mg/ml. Infuse I.V. no faster than 4 ml/minute.
• Infuse through large-bore catheter into large vein only.
🔊 Don't stop infusion abruptly.

Route	Onset	Peak	Duration
I.V.	30-45 min	1-2 hr	3-10 hr

Adverse reactions
CNS: headache, dizziness, agitation, confusion, disorientation, syncope, nervousness, drowsiness (with prolonged use in sickle cell patients), **subdural hemorrhage**
CV: hypotension, tachycardia, ECG changes, **capillary bleeding, cardiotoxicity**
GI: nausea, vomiting
GU: oliguria
Hematologic: hemolysis (with rapid administration)
Metabolic: hypervolemia, hyponatremia, hypokalemia, electrolyte imbalances
Skin: irritation or necrotic sloughing with extravasation

Other: pain, thrombosis, chemical phlebitis, or infection at injection site; fever; hyperthermia

Interactions

Drug-drug. *Lithium:* increased lithium clearance and decreased efficacy
Drug-diagnostic tests. *Potassium, sodium:* decreased levels

Patient monitoring

- Institute continuous cardiac monitoring.
- Closely monitor vital signs, ICP, and neurologic and cardiac status.
- Monitor electrolyte levels and kidney function tests.
- Assess fluid intake and output.
- When drug is used for IOP reduction, monitor IOP.

Patient teaching

- Explain drug therapy to patient.
- Tell patient drug may affect many body systems. Instruct him to immediately report such symptoms as headache or confusion.
- As appropriate, review all significant and life-threatening adverse reactions and interactions, especially those related to the drugs and tests mentioned above.

urokinase

Abbokinase, Abbokinase Open-Cath

Pharmacologic class: Plasminogen activator
Therapeutic class: Thrombolytic enzyme
Pregnancy risk category B

Action

Promotes thrombolysis by directly converting plasminogen to plasmin

Availability

Injection: 250,000 international units/vial

Indications and dosages

➤ Pulmonary emboli
Adults: Loading dose of 4,400 international units/kg I.V. given at a rate of 90 ml/hour over 10 minutes, followed by a continuous infusion of 4,400 international units/kg/hour at 15 ml/hour for 12 hours

Off-label uses

- Central venous catheter occlusion
- Myocardial infarction

Contraindications

- Hypersensitivity to drug
- Active bleeding
- Intraspinal surgery
- Severe uncontrolled arterial hypertension
- Cerebral embolism, thrombosis, or hemorrhage
- CNS or intracranial neoplasm, arteriovenous malformation, or aneurysm
- Bleeding diathesis
- History of cerebrovascular accident

Precautions

Use cautiously in:
- hypertension, known or suspected left-sided thrombus, acute pericarditis, subacute bacterial endocarditis, hemostatic defects, severe hepatic or renal dysfunction, diabetic hemorrhagic retinopathy or other hemorrhagic ophthalmic condition, septic thrombophlebitis, cerebrovascular disease
- recent GI or GU bleeding
- concurrent anticoagulant therapy
- elderly patients
- pregnant or breastfeeding patients
- children (safety and efficacy not established).

Administration

◀ Keep emergency equipment and epinephrine readily available in case anaphylaxis occurs.

- Before giving, check activated partial thromboplastin time (APTT), hematocrit, and platelet count. APPT must be less than twice the normal control value before drug can be given.
- Discontinue heparin as ordered before starting urokinase. (Heparin therapy may resume after urokinase therapy ends, if APPT is less than twice the normal control value.)
- Immediately before giving, reconstitute powder with preservative-free sterile water for injection; reconstituted solution should be clear or a light straw color. Solution may be filtered through 0.45-micron or smaller cellulose-membrane filter. Dilute further with normal saline solution or dextrose 5% in water, to yield a total volume not exceeding 195 ml.
- After infusion, make sure entire dose has been given by flushing (at a rate of 15 ml/hour) any urokinase still in I.V. tubing with a volume of compatible I.V. solution roughly equal to that of drug remaining in tubing.

◀ Keep blood products and aminocaproic acid at hand in case of serious spontaneous bleeding.

Route	Onset	Peak	Duration
I.V.	Immediate	20 min-4 hr	12-24 hr

Adverse reactions

CNS: intracranial bleeding
CV: hypotension, hypertension, **reperfusion arrhythmias**
GI: GI or retroperitoneal bleeding
GU: GU bleeding
Hematologic: hemorrhage
Respiratory: altered respiration, **bronchospasm**
Skin: rash, urticaria, pruritus, flushing, surface bleeding
Other: fever; phlebitis at I.V. injection site; bleeding at external excision, I.V. puncture, or I.M. site; **anaphylaxis**

Interactions

Drug-drug. *Abciximab, anticoagulants, aspirin, cephalosporins (selected), clopidogrel, dipyridamole, eptifibatide, indomethacin, nonsteroidal anti-inflammatory drugs, phenylbutazone, plicamycin, ticlopidine, tirofiban, valproic acid, other drugs that affect platelet activity:* increased risk of bleeding
Drug-diagnostic tests. *Hematocrit, hemoglobin:* decreased values
Drug-herbs. *Ginkgo:* increased risk of bleeding

Patient monitoring

◀ Monitor vital signs and watch for reperfusion arrhythmias. Check blood pressure manually.

◀ Stay alert for other reperfusion reactions, such as fever, chills, hypotension or hypertension, nausea, vomiting, hypoxia, cyanosis, dyspnea, acidosis, or back pain. If such a reaction occurs, discontinue drug immediately and give antihistamines, adrenergics, or corticosteroids, as prescribed.

◀ Monitor hemoglobin, hematocrit, prothrombin time, International Normalized Ratio, and APTT closely. Stay alert for signs and symptoms of bleeding in all body systems.

- Monitor puncture sites. After needle puncture, apply pressure dressing for at least 30 minutes.

◀ Evaluate respiratory status closely, especially for bronchospasm.

Patient teaching

- Explain drug therapy to patient.
- As appropriate, review all significant and life-threatening adverse reactions and interactions, especially those related to the drugs, tests, and herbs mentioned above.

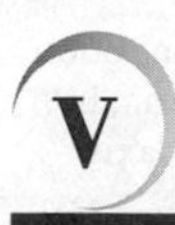

valacyclovir hydrochloride

Valtrex

Pharmacologic class: Acyclic purine nucleoside analog
Therapeutic class: Antiviral
Pregnancy risk category B

Action

Rapidly converts to acyclovir, which interferes with viral DNA synthesis and replication

Availability

Caplets: 500 mg, 1 g

Indications and dosages

➢ Herpes zoster (shingles)
Adults: 1 g P.O. t.i.d. for 7 days. Therapy should begin at first sign or symptom of herpes zoster, within 48 hours of onset of zoster rash.

➢ Genital herpes
Adults: For initial episode, 1 g P.O. b.i.d. for 10 days. For recurrent episodes, 500 mg P.O. b.i.d. for 3 days. For chronic suppression, 1 g P.O. daily for no more than 1 year; in patients with history of fewer than nine yearly recurrences, 500 mg P.O. daily for no more than 1 year.

➢ To reduce risk of genital herpes in immunocompetent patients
Adults: 500 mg P.O. daily for source partner, along with counseling regarding safe sex practices

➢ Herpes labialis
Adults: 2 g b.i.d. for 1 day taken 12 hours apart. Begin therapy at first symptom of lesion.

Dosage adjustment

- Renal impairment

Off-label uses

- Cytomegalovirus prophylaxis

Contraindications

- Hypersensitivity to drug, its components, or acyclovir

Precautions

Use cautiously in:
- renal impairment
- pregnant or breastfeeding patients
- children.

Administration

- Be aware that therapy may be ineffective if begun more than 72 hours after initial genital herpes outbreak, or more than 24 hours after symptom onset in herpes recurrence.

Route	Onset	Peak	Duration
P.O.	Unknown	1.5-2.5 hr	8-24 hr

Adverse reactions

CNS: headache, dizziness, depression
GI: nausea, vomiting, diarrhea, abdominal pain
GU: dysmenorrhea
Hematologic: anemia, **leukopenia, thrombocytopenia**
Musculoskeletal: joint pain
Other: hypersensitivity reaction

Interactions

Drug-drug. *Cimetidine, probenecid:* increased valacyclovir blood level
Drug-diagnostic tests. *Alanine aminotransferase, alkaline phosphatase, aspartate aminotransferase:* increased levels

Patient monitoring

- Monitor CBC. Stay alert for signs and symptoms of blood dyscrasias.
- Assess liver and kidney function tests.

Patient teaching

- Inform patient that herpes transmission can occur even when he's asymptomatic.

• Tell patient and significant other that no cure exists for herpes. Urge them to practice safe sex.
• Inform pregnant patient of risk of neonatal herpes infection.
• Instruct pregnant patient or female of childbearing age to tell health care provider that she has herpes. After delivery, tell her to inform neonatal care providers.
Instruct patient to promptly report unusual bleeding or bruising, urinary changes, or serious adverse CNS reactions.
• As appropriate, review all other significant and life-threatening adverse reactions and interactions, especially those related to the drugs and tests mentioned above.

valdecoxib

Bextra

Pharmacologic class: Nonsteroidal anti-inflammatory drug (NSAID), selective cyclooxygenase-2 (COX-2) inhibitor

Therapeutic class: Anti-inflammatory

Pregnancy risk category C (first and second trimesters), ***D*** (third trimester)

Action

Inhibits prostaglandin synthesis by inhibiting COX-2, reducing inflammation

Availability

Tablets: 10 mg, 20 mg

Indications and dosages

➢ Osteoarthritis; adult rheumatoid arthritis
Adults: 10 mg P.O. daily
➢ Primary dysmenorrhea
Adults: 20 mg P.O. b.i.d. p.r.n.

Off-label uses

• Postoperative pain

Contraindications

• Hypersensitivity to drug, its components, other NSAIDs (including aspirin), iodides, or sulfonamides
• Third trimester of pregnancy

Precautions

Use cautiously in:
• hypertension, bleeding, severe dehydration, heart failure, asthma, anemia
• history of hepatic or renal dysfunction, coagulation defects or GI ulcers, bleeding, or perforation
• pregnant women in first or second trimester, breastfeeding patients
• children younger than age 18.

Administration

• Give with or without food.

Route	Onset	Peak	Duration
P.O.	Variable	2-3 hr	Unknown

Adverse reactions

CNS: headache, dizziness, asthenia, fatigue, depression, drowsiness, insomnia, tremor, confusion, vertigo, paresthesia, anxiety, migraine, hypertonia
CV: palpitations, hypotension, hypertension, tachycardia, peripheral edema, angina pectoris, **arrhythmias, myocardial infarction (MI), heart failure**
EENT: blurred vision, conjunctivitis, tinnitus, rhinitis, epistaxis, pharyngitis, sinusitis
GI: nausea, vomiting, diarrhea, constipation, abdominal pain or cramps, bloating, eructation, flatulence, dyspepsia, gastritis, gastroenteritis, melena, peptic ulcer, hematemesis, stomatitis, dry mouth
GU: urinary frequency, polyuria, urinary tract infection, hematuria, albuminuria, cystitis, menstrual disorder, vaginal bleeding, erectile dysfunction
Hematologic: anemia, eosinophilia, **leukopenia, thrombocytopenia**

V

Hepatic: hepatitis
Metabolic: hyperglycemia, hypokalemia, **hyperkalemia**
Musculoskeletal: joint pain, myalgia, back pain
Respiratory: dyspnea, upper respiratory tract infection, bronchitis, cough, pneumonia, **bronchospasm**
Skin: diaphoresis, rash, pruritus, alopecia, eczema, bruising, photosensitivity
Other: altered taste, appetite changes, weight changes, excessive thirst, chills, fever, edema, facial edema, lymphadenopathy, accidental injury, flulike symptoms, pain, allergic reaction

Interactions

Drug-drug. *Angiotensin-converting enzyme inhibitors, furosemide, thiazide diuretics:* decreased effects of these drugs
Antineoplastics, lithium: increased blood levels and risk of toxicity of these drugs
Dextromethorphan: increased dextromethorphan blood level
Fluconazole, ketoconazole: increased valdecoxib blood level
Glucocorticoids, NSAIDs: increased GI reactions, greater risk of bleeding
Oral anticoagulants: increased anticoagulant effect
Drug-diagnostic tests. *Alanine aminotransferase, alkaline phosphatase, aspartate aminotransferase, blood urea nitrogen, creatinine, eosinophils, glucose, potassium:* increased levels
Hematocrit, hemoglobin, platelets, potassium, white blood cells: decreased levels

Patient monitoring

- Monitor kidney and liver function tests, CBC, and electrolyte levels. Stay alert for signs and symptoms of organ dysfunction and blood dyscrasias.

Patient teaching

- Tell patient he may take with or without food.
- Explain risks and benefits of drug therapy. Emphasize need for periodic laboratory tests.

🔊 Instruct patient to immediately report signs or symptoms of GI bleeding or ulcers, heart failure, or liver problems (such as fatigue, nausea, or yellowing of skin or eyes).

- Tell female of childbearing age to inform prescriber if she is pregnant or breastfeeding or plans to become pregnant or to breastfeed.

🔊 Advise patient to stop taking drug and contact prescriber immediately if rash or other signs or symptoms of hypersensitivity reaction occur.

- As appropriate, review all other significant and life-threatening adverse reactions and interactions, especially those related to the drugs and tests mentioned above.

valganciclovir hydrochloride

Valcyte

Pharmacologic class: Synthetic guanine derivative
Therapeutic class: Antiviral
Pregnancy risk category C

Action

Converts to its active form, inhibiting activity of cytomegalovirus (CMV)

Availability

Tablets: 450 mg

Indications and dosages

➢ Active CMV retinitis in AIDS patients
Adults: For induction therapy, 900 mg P.O. b.i.d. for 21 days. For maintenance, 900 mg P.O. daily.

➢ CMV prevention in high-risk kidney, heart, and kidney-pancreas transplant patients
Adults: 900 mg P.O. daily with food, starting within 10 days of transplantation and continuing until 100 days after transplantation

Dosage adjustment
- Renal impairment

Contraindications
- Hypersensitivity to drug, its components, or ganciclovir
- Absolute neutrophil count below 500 cells/mm^3, platelet count below 25,000 cells/mm^3, or hemoglobin below 8 g/dl

Precautions
Use cautiously in:
- cytopenia, impaired renal function
- patients receiving myelosuppressive drug therapy or radiation therapy
- elderly patients
- pregnant or breastfeeding patients.

Administration
- Avoid direct contact with broken or crushed tablet. If skin contact occurs, wash thoroughly with soap and water; if eye contact occurs, rinse eyes thoroughly with plain water.

Route	Onset	Peak	Duration
P.O.	Unknown	1-3 hr	Unknown

Adverse reactions
CNS: headache, insomnia, sedation, dizziness, peripheral neuropathy, paresthesia, hallucinations, confusion, agitation, psychosis, ataxia, **seizures**
EENT: retinal detachment
GI: nausea, vomiting, diarrhea, abdominal pain
Hematologic: anemia, **bone marrow depression, aplastic anemia, pancytopenia, thrombocytopenia, neutropenia**
Other: fever, catheter-related infection, local or systemic infection, hypersensitivity reaction, **sepsis**

Interactions
Drug-drug. *Cytotoxic drugs (such as adriamycin, amphotericin B, co-trimoxazole, dapsone, doxorubicin, flucytosine, pentamidine, vinblastine, vincristine):* additive toxicity
Cilastatin, imipenem: seizures
Didanosine: decreased valganciclovir blood level, increased didanosine blood level
Nephrotoxic drugs (such as amphotericin B, cyclosporine): increased creatinine level
Probenecid: decreased renal clearance of valganciclovir
Zidovudine: increased risk of granulocytopenia and anemia
Drug-diagnostic tests. *Alanine aminotransferase, alkaline phosphatase, aspartate aminotransferase, creatinine:* increased levels
Creatinine clearance: decreased value
Granulocytes, hemoglobin, neutrophils, platelets, white blood cells: decreased levels
Drug-food. *Any food:* increased drug absorption

Patient monitoring
- Monitor CBC with white cell differential and platelet count. Watch for signs and symptoms of blood dyscrasias.

◀ Stay alert for hypersensitivity reaction and signs and symptoms of infection.

- Closely monitor neurologic status. Observe for signs and symptoms of impending seizure.
- Periodically assess creatinine level and creatinine clearance.

Patient teaching
- Instruct patient to take with food.

V

• Explain drug therapy to patient. Stress importance of taking drug exactly as prescribed to prevent overdose.
Clinical alert: Tell patient drug can cause serious adverse reactions. Teach him which ones to report immediately.
• Active patient to avoid driving and other hazardous activities.
• Caution female of childbearing age to avoid pregnancy and breastfeeding.
• Urge male patient to use barrier contraception during and for 90 days after therapy.
• Instruct patient to have follow-up eye exams every 4 to 6 weeks, as well as periodic laboratory tests.
• As appropriate, review all other significant and life-threatening adverse reactions and interactions, especially those related to the drugs, tests, and foods mentioned above.

valproate sodium
Depacon

valproic acid
Depakene

divalproex sodium
Depakote, Depakote ER, Depakote Sprinkle

Pharmacologic class: Carboxylic acid derivative

Therapeutic class: Anticonvulsant, mood stabilizer, antimigraine agent

Pregnancy risk category D

Action
Increases level of gamma-aminobutyric acid in brain, reducing seizure activity

Availability
valproate sodium
Injection: 100 mg/ml in 5-ml vial
Syrup: 250 mg/5 ml
valproic acid
Capsules (liquid-filled): 250 mg
divalproex sodium
Capsules (containing coated particles or sprinkles): 125 mg
Tablets (enteric-coated, delayed-release): 125 mg, 250 mg, 500 mg
Tablets (extended-release): 250 mg, 500 mg

Indications and dosages
➢ Complex partial seizures
Adults and children older than age 10: Initially, 10 to 15 mg/kg/day P.O. May increase by 5 to 10 mg/kg/day q week until blood drug level is 50 to 100 mcg/ml or adverse reactions occur; don't exceed 60 mg/kg/day. If daily dosage exceeds 250 mg, give in two divided doses.
➢ Simple or complex absence seizures
Adults and children older than age 10: Initially, 15 mg/kg/day P.O. May increase by 5 to 10 mg/kg/day at weekly intervals until therapeutic blood drug level is reached or adverse reactions occur; don't exceed 60 mg/kg/day. If daily dosage exceeds 250 mg, give in two divided doses.
➢ Mania
Adults: Initially, 750 mg (divalproex delayed-release) P.O. daily in divided doses. Titrate rapidly to desired effect or trough level of 50 to 125 mcg/ml. Don't exceed 60 mg/kg/day.
➢ To prevent migraine
Adults: 250 mg (divalproex delayed-release) P.O. b.i.d. Or 500 mg (divalproex extended-release) P.O. daily for 1 week (up to 1 g/day). Maximum dosage is 1 g/day.

Off-label uses
• Chorea
• Photosensitivity-related seizures
• Sedative-hypnotic withdrawal

Contraindications

- Hypersensitivity to drug or tartrazine (some products)
- Hepatic impairment
- Urea cycle disorders
- Pregnancy

Precautions

Use cautiously in:
- bleeding disorders, organic brain disease, bone marrow depression, renal impairment
- posttraumatic seizures caused by head injury (use not recommended)
- history of hepatic disease
- breastfeeding patients
- children.

Administration

- Give I.V. only when oral therapy isn't feasible.
- For I.V. use, dilute valproate sodium in at least 50 ml of dextrose 5% in water, lactated Ringer's solution, or normal saline solution. Infuse over 1 hour at a rate slower than 20 mg/minute.
- Know that I.V. and P.O. dosages and dosing frequencies are identical. However, patient should be switched to oral therapy as soon as possible.
- Give oral forms with food.
- Be aware that divalproex extended-release and delayed-release forms are not bioequivalent.
- Make sure patient swallows divalproex extended-release tablets whole without chewing or crushing.
- If patient can't swallow capsule containing coated particles, sprinkle entire contents of capsule onto about 5 ml of semisolid food, such as pudding or applesauce, immediately before giving.
- Don't give syrup in carbonated beverages (may cause mouth and throat irritation).

Route	Onset	Peak	Duration
P.O. (capsules)	Rapid	1-4 hr	6-24 hr
P.O. (delayed, extended)	Unknown	Unknown	Unknown
P.O. (syrup)	Rapid	15-120 min	6-24 hr
I.V.	Rapid	End of 1-hr infusion	Unknown

Adverse reactions

CNS: confusion, dizziness, headache, sedation, ataxia, paresthesia, asthenia, tremor, drowsiness, emotional lability, abnormal thinking, amnesia
EENT: amblyopia, blurred vision, nystagmus, tinnitus, pharyngitis
GI: nausea, vomiting, diarrhea, abdominal pain, dyspepsia, anorexia, **pancreatitis**
Hematologic: leukopenia, thrombocytopenia
Hepatic: hepatotoxicity
Musculoskeletal: back pain
Respiratory: dyspnea
Skin: rash, alopecia, bruising
Other: abnormal taste, increased appetite, weight gain, flulike symptoms, infection, infusion site pain and reaction

Interactions

Drug-drug. *Activated charcoal, cholestyramine:* decreased valproate absorption
Antiplatelet agents (including abciximab, aspirin and other nonsteroidal anti-inflammatory drugs, eptifibatide, tirofiban), cefamandole, cefoperazone, cefotetan, heparin, thrombolytics, warfarin: increased risk of bleeding
Barbiturates, primidone: decreased metabolism and greater risk of toxicity of these drugs, decreased valproate efficacy
Carbamazepine: increased carbamazepine blood level, decreased valproate blood level, poor seizure control

V

Chlorpromazine: decreased valproate clearance and increased trough level
Cimetidine: decreased valproate clearance
Clonazepam: absence seizures in patients with history of these seizures
CNS depressants (such as antihistamines and antidepressants, MAO inhibitors, opioid analgesics, sedative-hypnotics): additive CNS depression
Diazepam: displacement of diazepam from binding site, inhibited diazepam metabolism
Erythromycin, felbamate: increased valproate blood level, greater risk of toxicity
Ethosuximide: inhibited ethosuximide metabolism
Lamotrigine: decreased valproate blood level, increased lamotrigine blood level
Phenytoin: increased phenytoin effects and risk of toxicity, decreased valproate effects
Salicylates (large doses in children): increased valproate effects
Tricyclic antidepressants: increased blood levels of these drugs, greater risk of adverse reactions
Zidovudine: decreased zidovudine clearance in patients with human immunodeficiency virus
Drug-diagnostic tests. *Alanine aminotransferase, alkaline phosphatase, aspartate aminotransferase, bilirubin:* increased levels
Bleeding time: prolonged
Ketone bodies: false-positive results
Platelets, white blood cells: decreased counts
Thyroid function tests: interference with results
Drug-behaviors. *Alcohol use:* additive CNS depression

Patient monitoring

- 🔊 Closely monitor neurologic status. Watch for seizures.
- 🔊 Evaluate GI status. Stay alert for signs and symptoms of pancreatitis.
- Monitor I.V. infusion site for local reactions.
- Assess CBC (including platelet count), prothrombin time, International Normalized Ratio, and liver function tests.
- Monitor valproate blood level; therapeutic range is 50 to 100 mcg/ml.

Patient teaching

- Instruct patient to take with food to minimize GI upset.
- Tell patient taking extended-release tablets to swallow them whole without chewing or breaking.
- Inform patient taking capsules that he may swallow them whole or open them and sprinkle contents onto a teaspoon of semisolid food, such as pudding or applesauce.
- Tell patient (or parents) that valproate syrup shouldn't be taken with carbonated beverages.
- 🔊 Advise patient to immediately report malaise, weakness, lethargy, appetite loss, vomiting, or yellowing of skin or eyes.
- If patient's taking drug for seizure control, tell him to avoid driving and other hazardous activities.
- 🔊 Caution patient not to stop therapy abruptly.
- Instruct patient to avoid alcohol.
- Stress importance of follow-up laboratory tests.
- As appropriate, review all other significant and life-threatening adverse reactions and interactions, especially those related to the drugs, tests, and behaviors mentioned above.

valsartan
Diovan

Pharmacologic class: Angiotensin II receptor antagonist
Therapeutic class: Antihypertensive
Pregnancy risk category C (first trimester), *D* (second and third trimesters)

Action
Blocks the vasoconstrictive and aldosterone-producing effects of angiotensin II at various receptor sites, including vascular smooth muscle and adrenal glands

Availability
Tablets: 40 mg, 80 mg, 160 mg, 320 mg

Indications and dosages
➢ Hypertension
Adults: Initially, 80 to 160 mg P.O. daily. May increase as needed to a maximum of 320 mg P.O. daily, or a diuretic may be added.
➢ Heart failure in patients intolerant of angiotensin-converting enzyme inhibitors
Adults: Initially, 40 mg P.O. b.i.d.; may increase to 160 mg P.O. b.i.d. as needed. May be given alone or with other drugs, up to a maximum of 320 mg/day.

Off-label uses
- Left ventricular hypertrophy
- Diabetic nephropathy

Contraindications
- Hypersensitivity to drug or its components
- Second or third trimester of pregnancy

Precautions
Use cautiously in:
- severe heart failure; volume or sodium depletion; hepatic or renal impairment; obstructive biliary disorders; angioedema; aortic, mitral valve, or renal artery stenosis; hyperkalemia
- concurrent use of high-dose diuretics
- black patients
- females of childbearing age
- pregnant patients in first trimester
- children younger than age 18 (safety not established).

Administration
- Give with or without food.

Route	Onset	Peak	Duration
P.O.	Within 2 hr	4-6 hr	24 hr

Adverse reactions
CNS: dizziness, fatigue, headache
CV: hypotension, palpitations
EENT: sinus disorders
GI: nausea, diarrhea, constipation, abdominal pain, dry mouth
GU: albuminuria, **renal impairment**
Hematologic: neutropenia
Metabolic: hyperkalemia
Musculoskeletal: back pain, joint pain, muscle cramps
Skin: alopecia, angioedema
Other: dental pain, fever, viral infection

Interactions
Drug-drug. *Other antihypertensives:* increased risk of hypotension
Potassium-sparing diuretics, potassium supplements: increased risk of hyperkalemia
Drug-diagnostic tests. *Urine albumin, urine potassium:* increased levels
Drug-food. *Salt substitutes containing potassium:* increased risk of hyperkalemia
Drug-herbs. *Ephedra (ma huang):* reduced hypotensive effect of valsartan
Drug-behaviors. *Alcohol use:* increased CNS depression

Patient monitoring

- Monitor blood pressure closely, especially during initial therapy and dosage adjustments.
- Assess potassium level. Stay alert for hyperkalemia.
- Be aware that in black patients, drug may be ineffective when used alone. Additional agents may be required.

Patient teaching

- Tell patient he may take with or without food.

Instruct female of childbearing age to report pregnancy immediately.

- Advise patient to avoid potassium-containing salt substitutes.
- Caution patient to avoid alcohol.
- As appropriate, review all other significant and life-threatening adverse reactions and interactions, especially those related to the drugs, tests, foods, herbs, and behaviors mentioned above.

vancomycin hydrochloride

Vancocin

Pharmacologic class: Tricyclic glycopeptide
Therapeutic class: Anti-infective
Pregnancy risk category C

Action

Binds to bacterial cell wall, inhibiting cell-wall synthesis and causing secondary damage to bacterial membrane

Availability

Capsules: 125 mg, 250 mg
Powder for injection: 500-mg vial, 1-g vial, 5-g vial, 10 g-vial
Powder for oral solution: 1-g and 10-g bottles

Indications and dosages

➢ Severe, life-threatening infections caused by susceptible strains of methicillin-resistant staphylococci, *Staphylococcus epidermidis, Streptococcus viridans* or *Streptococcus bovis* (alone or combined with an aminoglycoside), or *Enterococcus faecalis* (combined with an aminoglycoside)

Adults: 500 mg I.V. q 6 hours or 1 g I.V. q 12 hours
Children: 10 mg/kg I.V. q 6 hours
Infants and neonates: Initially, 15 mg/kg I.V., followed by 10 mg/kg I.V. q 8 hours in infants 8 days to 1 month old, or 10 mg/kg I.V. q 12 hours in infants less than 8 days old

➢ Endocarditis prophylaxis in penicillin-allergic patients at moderate risk who are scheduled for dental and other invasive procedures

Adults: 1 g I.V. slowly over 1 to 2 hours, with infusion completed 30 minutes before invasive procedure begins
Children: 20 mg/kg I.V. over 1 to 2 hours, with infusion completed 30 minutes before invasive procedure begins

➢ Enterocolitis caused by *Streptococcus aureus;* antibiotic-related pseudomembranous diarrhea caused by *Clostridium difficile*

Adults: 500 mg to 2 g P.O. daily in three or four divided doses for 7 to 10 days
Children: 40 mg/kg P.O. daily in three or four divided doses for 7 to 10 days, up to a maximum of 2 g/day

Dosage adjustment

- Renal impairment
- Elderly patients

Off-label uses

- Peritonitis
- Meningitis
- Intraocular infections
- Febrile neutropenia

Contraindications

- Hypersensitivity to drug

Precautions

Use cautiously in:

- renal impairment, preexisting hearing loss
- concurrent use of anesthetics, immunosuppressants, or nephrotoxic or ototoxic drugs
- elderly patients
- pregnant or breastfeeding patients
- neonates.

Administration

🔈 Know that I.V. therapy is ineffective against enterocolitis and pseudomembranous diarrhea.

- For intermittent I.V. infusion, dilute by adding 10 or 20 ml of sterile water for injection to vial containing 500 mg or 1 g of drug, respectively, to yield a concentration of 50 mg/ml. Dilute further by adding at least 100 ml or 200 ml, respectively, of dextrose 5% in water or normal saline solution; infuse over at least 1 hour.
- Don't give by I.M. route.

🔈 Keep emergency equipment and epinephrine on hand in case of anaphylaxis.

Route	Onset	Peak	Duration
P.O.	Unknown	Unknown	Unknown
I.V.	Immediate	Immediate	Unknown

Adverse reactions

CV: hypotension, **cardiac arrest, vascular collapse**
EENT: permanent hearing loss, ototoxicity, tinnitus
GI: nausea, vomiting, **pseudomembranous colitis**
GU: nephrotoxicity, severe uremia
Hematologic: eosinophilia, **leukopenia, neutropenia**
Respiratory: wheezing, dyspnea
Skin: "red man" syndrome (nonallergic histamine reaction with rapid I.V. infusion), rash, urticaria, pruritus, necrosis
Other: chills, fever, thrombophlebitis at injection site, **anaphylaxis**

Interactions

Drug-drug. *Aminoglycosides, amphotericin B, bacitracin, cephalosporins, cisplatin, colistin, nondepolarizing neuromuscular blockers, pentamidine:* increased risk of nephrotoxicity and ototoxicity
Warfarin: increased risk of bleeding
Drug-diagnostic tests. *Albumin, blood urea nitrogen (BUN), creatinine:* increased levels
Eosinophils, neutrophils: decreased counts

Patient monitoring

🔈 Monitor closely for signs and symptoms of hypersensitivity reactions, including anaphylaxis.

- Check drug blood level weekly. Therapeutic peak ranges from 30 to 40 g/L; therapeutic trough, 5 to 10 mg/L.
- Assess BUN and creatinine levels every 2 days, or daily in patients with unstable renal function.
- Monitor urine output daily. Weigh patient at least weekly.
- Assess hearing before and during therapy; stay alert for hearing loss. Patient may require baseline and weekly audiograms.
- Check I.V. site often for phlebitis.
- Watch for "red-man" syndrome, which can result from rapid infusion. Signs and symptoms include hypotension, pruritus, and maculopapular rash on face, neck, trunk, and limbs.
- Monitor CBC. Watch for signs and symptoms of blood dyscrasias.
- Closely monitor respiratory status. Stay alert for wheezing and dyspnea.

🔈 Monitor vital signs and cardiovascular status, especially for vascular collapse and other signs of impending cardiac arrest.

V

Patient teaching

- Tell patient he may take with or without food.
- Instruct patient to take oral drug exactly as prescribed for as long as prescribed, even if symptoms improve.
- Explain importance of prophylactic I.V. therapy to patients at risk for endocarditis who are scheduled for invasive procedures.

Advise patient to promptly report rash, hearing loss, breathing problems, and signs and symptoms of "red-man" syndrome, nephrotoxicity, and blood dyscrasias.

- As appropriate, review all other significant and life-threatening adverse reactions and interactions, especially those related to the drugs and tests mentioned above.

vardenafil hydrochloride

Levitra

Pharmacologic class: Phosphodiesterase-5 (PDE5) inhibitor

Therapeutic class: Erectile dysfunction agent

Pregnancy risk category B

Action

Selectively blocks PDE5, which neutralizes cyclic guanosine monophosphate, resulting in enhanced erectile function

Availability

Tablets: 2.5 mg, 5 mg, 10 mg, 20 mg

Indications and dosages

➢ Erectile dysfunction

Adult males: 10 or 20 mg P.O. approximately 1 hour before anticipated sexual activity. Maximum dosing frequency is once daily.

Dosage adjustment

- Patients older than age 65
- Concurrent use of CYP450-3A4 inhibitors
- Concurrent HIV therapy (except highly active antiretroviral therapy)

Contraindications

- Hypersensitivity to drug
- Concurrent use of nitrates or nitrate patches to treat angina
- Concurrent use of alpha-adrenergic blockers

Precautions

Use cautiously in:

- cardiovascular disease, retinitis pigmentosa, hepatic or renal impairment, reduced hepatic blood flow
- patients at increased risk for priapism (as from sickle-cell disease, leukemia, multiple myeloma, polycythemia, or history of priapism).

Administration

- Advise patient not to take more than one tablet daily.

Route	Onset	Peak	Duration
P.O.	Unknown	1 hr	4 hr

Adverse reactions

CNS: headache
CV: hypotension
EENT: blurred vision, altered color perception, light sensitivity, rhinitis
GI: dyspepsia
Skin: flushing
Other: flulike symptoms

Interactions

Drug-drug. *Alpha-adrenergic blockers, nitrates:* hypotension
Erythromycin, itraconazole, ketoconazole, protease inhibitors: increased vardenafil blood level
Drug-diagnostic tests. *Creatine kinase:* increased level

Patient monitoring
- Monitor blood pressure and heart rate, particularly if patient has cardiovascular disease.

Patient teaching
- Tell patient he may take with or without food.
- Instruct patient to take one tablet about 1 hour before anticipated sexual activity. Caution him not to take more than one tablet daily.
- Instruct patient to promptly contact prescriber if erection lasts more than 4 hours, because irreversible damage to penis may occur.
- Caution patient not to take nitrates. Tell him to inform prescriber of other drugs he's taking.
- As appropriate, review all other significant adverse reactions and interactions, especially those related to the drugs and tests mentioned above.

venlafaxine hydrochloride
Effexor, Effexor XR

Pharmacologic class: Phenethylamine derivative

Therapeutic class: Antidepressant, anxiolytic

Pregnancy risk category C

Action
Inhibits neuronal serotonin and norepinephrine reuptake and slightly inhibits dopamine reuptake

Availability
Capsules (extended-release): 37.5 mg, 75 mg, 150 mg
Tablets: 25 mg, 37.5 mg, 50 mg, 75 mg, 100 mg

Indications and dosages
➢ Depression

Adults: In outpatients, 75 mg P.O. daily in two or three divided doses; may increase in increments of 75 mg/day q 4 or more days to a maximum of 225 mg/day; extended-release form can be given as a single daily dose. In hospitalized patients, 75 mg P.O. daily in two or three divided doses; may increase in increments of 75 mg/day q 4 days to a maximum of 375 mg/day given in three divided doses.

➢ Generalized anxiety disorder

Adults: Single dose of 37.5 to 75 mg (extended-release) P.O. daily; may increase in increments of 75 mg/day q 4 days to a maximum of 225 mg/day

Dosage adjustment
- Hepatic or renal impairment

Off-label uses
- Premenstrual dysphoric disorder

Contraindications
- Hypersensitivity to drug
- MAO inhibitor use within past 14 days

Precautions
Use cautiously in:
- cardiovascular disease; hypertension; heart failure, recent myocardial infarction, and other conditions in which increased heart rate poses a danger; hepatic or renal impairment; glaucoma; hyperthyroidism; hyponatremia; syndrome of inappropriate antidiuretic hormone secretion (SIADH)
- history of seizures, neurologic impairment, or drug abuse
- pregnant or breastfeeding patients
- children younger than age 18.

V

Administration
Don't give within 14 days of MAO inhibitors.

Route	Onset	Peak	Duration
P.O.	Within 2 wk	2-4 wk	Unknown

Adverse reactions

CNS: abnormal dreams, anxiety, dizziness, headache, insomnia, nervousness, abnormal thinking, agitation, confusion, depersonalization, drowsiness, emotional lability, worsening depression, twitching, tremor, asthenia, paresthesia, mania, hypomania, **suicidal ideation or behavior** (especially in child or adolescent)
CV: chest pain, hypertension, palpitations, tachycardia, vasodilation
EENT: visual disturbances, blurred vision, mydriasis, tinnitus, rhinitis
GI: nausea, vomiting, diarrhea, constipation, abdominal pain, dyspepsia, flatulence, dry mouth, anorexia
GU: urinary frequency or retention, sexual dysfunction, abnormal ejaculation, anorgasmia, erectile dysfunction
Metabolic: hyponatremia, **SIADH**
Skin: bruising, pruritus, rash, diaphoresis, photosensitivity
Other: altered taste, weight loss, chills, yawning

Interactions

Drug-drug. *Cimetidine:* increased venlafaxine effects
MAO inhibitors: potentially fatal reactions
Sumatriptan, trazodone: serotonin syndrome (including altered level of consciousness)
Drug-diagnostic tests. *Sodium:* decreased level
Drug-herbs. *Chamomile, hops, kava, skullcap, valerian:* increased CNS depression
S-adenosylmethionine (SAM-e), St. John's wort: increased risk of sedative or hypnotic effects

Patient monitoring

🔊 Monitor neurologic status, particularly for seizures, worsening depression, and suicidal ideation.
• Closely monitor vital signs and cardiovascular status. Stay alert for hypertension and tachycardia.
• Monitor nutritional status, hydration, and weight.

Patient teaching

• Tell patient taking extended-release capsules to swallow them whole without chewing, breaking, dividing, or dissolving.
🔊 Caution patient not to stop therapy abruptly.
🔊 Advise patient to promptly report seizures, worsening depression, or suicidal thoughts (especially in child or adolescent).
• Caution patient to avoid driving and other dangerous activities until drug effects are known.
• As appropriate, review all other significant and life-threatening adverse reactions and interactions, especially those related to the drugs, tests, and herbs mentioned above.

verapamil hydrochloride

Apo-Verap✤, Calan, Calan SR, Covera-HS, Isoptin, Isoptin SR, Novo-Veramil✤, Nu-Verap✤, Verelan, Verelan PM

Pharmacologic class: Calcium channel blocker
Therapeutic class: Antianginal, antiarrhythmic (class IV), antihypertensive
Pregnancy risk category C

Action

Decreases conduction of sinoatrial and atrioventricular (AV) nodes by inhibiting calcium influx into cardiac and vascular smooth muscle cells, inhibiting excitatory contraction. These effects prolong AV node refractoriness and decrease myocardial oxygen consumption.

Availability

Capsules (extended-release): 100 mg, 120 mg, 180 mg, 200 mg, 240 mg, 300 mg, 360 mg
Capsules (sustained-release): 120 mg, 180 mg, 240 mg, 360 mg
Injection: 2.5 mg/ml in 2- and 4-ml vials, ampules, and syringes
Tablets (extended-release): 120 mg, 180 mg, 240 mg
Tablets (immediate-release): 40 mg, 80 mg, 120 mg

Indications and dosages

➢ Angina
Adults: Initially, 80 mg (immediate-release) P.O. t.i.d.; may titrate at daily or weekly intervals to 360 mg/day. Or initially, 180 mg (extended-release) P.O. once daily at bedtime, titrated up to 480 mg/day at bedtime.

➢ Supraventricular tachyarrhythmias (SVTs)
Adults: 5 to 10 mg (0.075 to 0.15 mg/kg) I.V. bolus over 2 minutes; may give additional 10 mg after 30 minutes if response inadequate. Or 240 to 480 mg (immediate-release) P.O. daily in three or four divided doses.

➢ To control ventricular rate in chronic atrial flutter or atrial fibrillation in patients receiving digoxin
Adults: 240 to 320 mg P.O. daily in three or four divided doses

➢ Hypertension
Adults: Initially, 180 mg (extended-release tablet) or 200 mg (extended-release capsule) P.O. daily at bedtime. For maintenance, may titrate up to 480 mg (extended-release tablet) or 400 mg (extended-release capsule) P.O. daily at bedtime. Or initially, 80 mg (immediate-release tablet) P.O. t.i.d.; may titrate at daily or weekly intervals up to 360 to 480 mg/day. Or initially, 240 mg (sustained-release capsule) P.O. q day in morning; for maintenance, may titrate up to 240 mg P.O. b.i.d. or 480 mg P.O. once daily in morning. Titrate based on response.

Dosage adjustment

- Renal or hepatic impairment
- Concurrent digoxin therapy

Off-label uses

- Ventricular tachycardia
- Migraine headache prophylaxis
- Neurogenic bladder
- Premature labor

Contraindications

- Hypersensitivity to drug or other calcium channel blockers
- Sick sinus syndrome
- Second- or third-degree AV block (except in patients with artificial pacemakers)
- Hypotension
- Heart failure, severe ventricular dysfunction, or cardiogenic shock (except when associated with SVTs)
- Atrial flutter or atrial fibrillation associated with accessory bypass tracts (such as Wolff-Parkinson-White or Lown-Ganong-Levine syndrome)

Precautions

Use cautiously in:
- renal or severe hepatic impairment; first-degree AV block; idiopathic hypertrophic cardiomyopathy; neuromuscular transmission defects (such as Duchenne's muscular dystrophy); respiratory depression; digital ulcers, ischemia, or gangrene
- elderly patients
- pregnant or breastfeeding patients.

Administration

- Give I.V. over at least 2 minutes.

• Discontinue disopyramide 48 hours before starting verapamil. Don't restart disopyramide for at least 24 hours after verapamil therapy ends.

Route	Onset	Peak	Duration
P.O. (immediate)	30 min	1-2 hr	3-7 hr
P.O. (extended)	Unknown	5-7 hr	24 hr
P.O. (sustained)	Unknown	Unknown	Unknown
I.V.	Immediate	3-5 min	2 hr

Adverse reactions

CNS: anxiety, confusion, dizziness, syncope, drowsiness, headache, jitteriness, abnormal dreams, disturbed equilibrium, psychiatric disturbances, asthenia, paresthesia, tremor, fatigue
CV: chest pain, hypotension, palpitations, peripheral edema, tachycardia, **arrhythmias, heart failure, bradycardia, AV block**
EENT: blurred vision, epistaxis, tinnitus
GI: nausea, vomiting, diarrhea, constipation, dyspepsia, dry mouth, anorexia
GU: dysuria, urinary frequency, nocturia, polyuria, sexual dysfunction, gynecomastia
Hematologic: anemia, **leukopenia, thrombocytopenia**
Metabolic: hyperglycemia
Musculoskeletal: joint stiffness, muscle cramps
Respiratory: cough, dyspnea, shortness of breath, **pulmonary edema**
Skin: dermatitis, flushing, diaphoresis, photosensitivity, pruritus, urticaria, rash, **erythema multiforme, Stevens-Johnson syndrome**
Other: gingival hyperplasia, edema, weight gain

Interactions

Drug-drug. *Antihypertensives:* additive hypotension
Aspirin: increased risk of bleeding
Beta-adrenergic blockers, other antiarrhythmics: additive adverse cardiovascular reactions
Carbamazepine, cyclosporine: increased blood levels of these drugs
CYP450-3A4 inducers (such as rifampin): decreased verapamil blood level
CYP450-3A4 inhibitors (such as erythromycin, ritonavir): increased verapamil blood level
Digoxin: increased digoxin blood level, greater risk of toxicity
Lithium: increased or decreased lithium blood level
Neuromuscular blockers (succinylcholine, tubocurarine, vecuronium): prolonged neuromuscular blockade
Theophylline: decreased verapamil clearance, increased blood level, and possible toxicity
Drug-diagnostic tests. *Alanine aminotransferase, alkaline phosphatase, aspartate aminotransferase, blood urea nitrogen, glucose, lactate dehydrogenase:* increased levels
Granulocytes: decreased count
Drug-food. *Coffee, tea:* increased caffeine blood level
Grapefruit juice: increased verapamil blood level and effects
Drug-herbs. *Black catechu:* increased drug effects
Cola nut, guarana: increased caffeine blood level
Ephedra (ma huang), St. John's wort: reduced hypotensive effect of verapamil
Yerba maté: decreased clearance of this herb
Drug-behaviors. *Alcohol use:* additive hypotension

Patient monitoring

• With I.V. use, monitor vital signs and ECG continuously.
• Assess blood pressure when therapy begins and when dosage is adjusted.
• Watch closely for signs and symptoms of heart failure.
[Clinical alert] Monitor for signs and symptoms of erythema multiforme (fever, rash,

sore throat, mouth sores, cough, iris lesions). Report early indications immediately, before condition can progress to Stevens-Johnson syndrome.
- Assess CBC. Watch for blood dyscrasias.
- Monitor blood glucose level. Stay alert for hyperglycemia in diabetic patients.

Patient teaching
- Instruct patient to avoid chewing, breaking, or crushing extended-release form.

Advise patient to immediately report rash, unusual bleeding or bruising, fainting, and (in long-term use) fatigue, nausea, or yellowing of skin or eyes.
- Caution patient not to take with grapefruit juice.
- Instruct patient to limit caffeine intake and avoid alcohol.
- Advise patient to seek medical advice before using over-the-counter medications or herbs.
- Tell patient to avoid sun exposure and to wear sunscreen and protective clothing when going outdoors.
- As appropriate, review all other significant and life-threatening adverse reactions and interactions, especially those related to the drugs, tests, foods, herbs, and behaviors mentioned above.

vinblastine sulfate (VLB)

Pharmacologic class: Vinca alkaloid
Therapeutic class: Antineoplastic
Pregnancy risk category D

Action
Arrests mitosis and blocks cell division, interfering with nucleic acid synthesis. Cell-cycle-phase specific.

Availability
Lyophilized powder for injection: 10-mg vial

Indications and dosages
➤ Hodgkin's disease; advanced testicular cancer; lymphoma; AIDS-related Kaposi's sarcoma; bladder cancer; renal cancer; non-small-cell lung cancer; melanoma; breast cancer; choriocarcinoma; histiocytosis X; mycosis fungoides

Adults: 3.7 mg/m^2 I.V. weekly; may increase to a maximum of 18.5 mg/m^2 I.V. weekly, based on response. Withhold weekly dose if white blood cell (WBC) count is less than 4,000 cells/mm^3. May increase dosage in increments of 1.8 mg/m^2 if needed, but not after WBC count drops to approximately 3,000 cells/mm^3.

Dosage adjustment
- Hepatic impairment

Contraindications
- Hypersensitivity to drug
- Significant granulocytopenia from causes other than disease being treated
- Uncontrolled bacterial infections
- Intrathecal use
- Elderly patients with cachexia or skin ulcers

Precautions
Use cautiously in:
- hepatic or pulmonary dysfunction, renal disease with hypertension, malignant-cell infiltration of bone marrow, neuromuscular disease
- females of childbearing age
- pregnant or breastfeeding patients (use not recommended).

Administration
Follow facility protocol for handling and preparing chemotherapeutic drugs. Take special care to avoid eye contamination.

V

• Know that patient is usually premedicated with antiemetic.

🔊 Give by I.V. route only. (Intrathecal injection is fatal.)

• Reconstitute powder in 10-mg vial with 10 ml of normal saline solution for injection, to a concentration of 1 mg/ml. Refrigerate solution and protect from light; discard after 28 days.

• Inject I.V. dose into tubing of running I.V. line, or inject directly into vein over about 1 minute.

• Avoid extravasation, which may cause tissue necrosis. If extravasation occurs, stop injection, inject hyaluronidase locally, and apply moderate heat.

Route	Onset	Peak	Duration
I.V.	Unknown	Unknown	Unknown

Adverse reactions

CNS: headache, malaise, depression, paresthesia, loss of deep tendon reflexes, peripheral neuropathy and neuritis, **cerebrovascular accident, seizures**
CV: hypertension, tachycardia, **myocardial infarction**
EENT: pharyngitis
GI: nausea, vomiting, diarrhea, constipation, bleeding ulcer, abdominal pain, stomatitis, anorexia, **paralytic ileus**
GU: aspermia
Hematologic: anemia, **thrombocytopenia, leukopenia**
Metabolic: hyperuricemia, **syndrome of inappropriate antidiuretic hormone secretion**
Musculoskeletal: bone pain, muscle pain and weakness
Respiratory: shortness of breath, **acute bronchospasm, pulmonary infiltrates**
Skin: alopecia, skin irritation
Other: weight loss; jaw pain; tumor site pain; sloughing, cellulitis, and phlebitis at I.V. site; tissue necrosis (with extravasation)

Interactions

Drug-drug. *Erythromycin, other CYP450 inhibitors:* increased vinblastine toxicity
Mitomycin: increased risk of bronchospasm and shortness of breath
Phenytoin: decreased phenytoin blood level

Patient monitoring

🔊 Assess respiratory status closely. Drug may cause acute shortness of breath and bronchospasm, especially in patients who previously received mitomycin.

• Check injection site for extravasation.

• Monitor blood pressure.

• Assess CBC. Stay alert for signs and symptoms of infection.

• Monitor closely for numbness and tingling of hands or feet and other adverse reactions.

Patient teaching

• Explain drug therapy to patient. Emphasize importance of follow-up laboratory tests.

• Tell patient to promptly report signs and symptoms of infection and to take his temperature daily.

• Inform patient that drug may cause pain over tumor site.

• Instruct female of childbearing age to avoid pregnancy. Caution her not to breastfeed during therapy.

• Encourage patient to practice good oral hygiene to help prevent infected mouth sores.

• Inform patient that hair loss is a common side effect but typically reverses after treatment ends.

• As appropriate, review all other significant and life-threatening adverse reactions and interactions, especially those related to the drugs mentioned above.

vincristine sulfate (VCR)
Vincasar PFS

Pharmacologic class: Vinca alkaloid
Therapeutic class: Antineoplastic
Pregnancy risk category D

Action
Unknown. Thought to block cell division and interfere with synthesis of nucleic acid. Cell-cycle-phase specific.

Availability
Solution for injection: 1 mg/ml in 1-, 2-, and 5-ml vials

Indications and dosages
➢ Acute leukemia
Adults: 0.4 to 1.4 mg/m² I.V. weekly, not to exceed 2 mg/dose. (Dosages higher than 2 mg may be used depending on patient, physician, protocol, and facility.)
Children weighing more than 10 kg (22 lb): 2 mg/m² I.V. weekly
Children weighing 10 kg (22 lb) or less: 0.05 mg/kg I.V. weekly

Dosage adjustment
- Hepatic impairment

Off-label uses
- Brain, hepatic, ovarian, testicular, and other cancers
- Neuroblastoma
- Kaposi's sarcoma
- Idiopathic thrombocytopenic purpura

Contraindications
- Hypersensitivity to drug
- Demyelinating form of Charcot-Marie-Tooth disease
- Intrathecal use

Precautions
Use cautiously in:
- infections, decreased bone marrow reserve, hepatic impairment, acute uric acid nephropathy, neuromuscular disease, pulmonary dysfunction, other chronic debilitating illnesses
- females of childbearing age
- pregnant or breastfeeding patients (use not recommended).

Administration
Follow facility protocol for handling and preparing chemotherapeutic drugs. Be especially careful to avoid eye contamination.
- Be aware that patient is usually premedicated with antiemetic.

Give by I.V. route only. (Intrathecal injection is fatal.)
- Inject into tubing of running I.V. line, or inject directly into vein over 1 minute.
- Avoid extravasation (may cause tissue necrosis). If extravasation occurs, stop injection, inject hyaluronidase locally, and apply moderate heat.
- Know that drug may be used with other antineoplastics in some diseases.

Route	Onset	Peak	Duration
I.V.	Unknown	4 days	7 days

Adverse reactions
CNS: agitation, insomnia, depression, mental status changes, ascending peripheral neuropathy, transient cortical blindness, **seizures, coma**
EENT: diplopia
GI: nausea, vomiting, constipation, abdominal cramps, stomatitis, anorexia, **paralytic ileus**
GU: nocturia, urinary retention, gonadal suppression, **oliguria**
Hematologic: anemia, **leukopenia, thrombocytopenia** (mild and brief)
Metabolic: hyperuricemia, **syndrome of inappropriate antidiuretic hormone secretion**

V

Respiratory: bronchospasm
Skin: alopecia
Other: tissue necrosis (with extravasation), phlebitis at I.V. site

Interactions

Drug-drug. *Asparaginase:* decreased hepatic metabolism of vincristine
Live-virus vaccines: decreased antibody response to vaccine, increased risk of adverse reactions
Mitomycin: increased risk of bronchospasm and shortness of breath
Drug-diagnostic tests. *Platelets:* increased or decreased count
Uric acid: increased level
White blood cells: decreased count (slight leukopenia) 4 days after therapy, resolving within 7 days

Patient monitoring

Assess respiratory status. Drug may cause bronchospasm, especially in patients who previously received mitomycin.
- Monitor blood pressure.
- Evaluate neurologic status. Know that neurotoxicity is a dose-limiting adverse reaction.
- Monitor CBC with platelet count. Watch for signs and symptoms of blood dyscrasias.
- Stay alert for signs and symptoms of infection.

Patient teaching

- Explain drug therapy to patient. Emphasize importance of follow-up laboratory tests.
- Advise patient to promptly report signs and symptoms of infection and to take his temperature daily.
- Urge patient to practice good oral hygiene, to help prevent infected mouth sores.
- Instruct female of childbearing age to avoid pregnancy. Caution her not to breastfeed during therapy.
- Tell patient that hair loss is a common side effect but typically reverses once treatment ends.
- As appropriate, review all other significant and life-threatening adverse reactions and interactions, especially those related to the drugs and tests mentioned above.

vinorelbine tartrate

Navelbine

Pharmacologic class: Vinca alkaloid
Therapeutic class: Antineoplastic
Pregnancy risk category D

Action

Blocks cell division and interferes with nucleic acid synthesis. Cell-cycle-phase specific.

Availability

Injection: 10 mg/ml in 1-ml and 5-ml vials

Indications and dosages

➢ Inoperable non-small-cell lung cancer
Adults: As monotherapy, 30 mg/m^2 I.V. weekly given over 6 to 10 minutes. In combination therapy, 25 mg/m^2 weekly given with cisplatin q 4 weeks. Alternatively, in combination therapy, 30 mg/m^2 I.V. given with cisplatin on days 1 and 29, then q 6 weeks.

Dosage adjustment

- Hepatic impairment
- Neurotoxicity

Off-label uses

- Cervical, breast, or ovarian cancer

Contraindications

- Hypersensitivity to drug
- Pretreatment granulocyte count below 1,000 cells/mm^3

Precautions

Use cautiously in:
- hepatic impairment, decreased bone marrow reserve, past or present neuropathy
- history of radiation therapy
- females of childbearing age
- pregnant or breastfeeding patients (use not recommended)
- children (safety not established).

Administration

🔊 Follow facility protocols for handling and preparing chemotherapeutic drugs. Be especially careful to avoid eye contamination.
- Know that patient is usually premedicated with antiemetic.

🔊 Give by I.V. route only. (Intrathecal injection is fatal.)
- Before use, dilute drug in syringe with dextrose 5% in water or normal saline solution to yield a concentration of 1.5 to 3 mg/ml. Or dilute in I.V. bag of compatible solution to yield a concentration of 0.5 to 2 mg/ml.
- Administer into tubing of running I.V. line or directly into vein over 6 to 10 minutes. Immediately after injection, flush line with 75 to 125 ml of compatible I.V. solution.

Route	Onset	Peak	Duration
I.V.	Unknown	7-10 days	7-15 days

Adverse reactions

CNS: fatigue, **neurotoxicity**
CV: chest pain, phlebitis
GI: nausea, vomiting, diarrhea, constipation, abdominal pain, anorexia, **pancreatitis, intestinal obstruction, paralytic ileus**
Hematologic: anemia, **bone marrow depression, severe granulocytopenia, neutropenia, thrombocytopenia**
Metabolic: hyponatremia
Musculoskeletal: joint, back, or jaw pain; myalgia
Respiratory: acute respiratory distress syndrome, acute shortness of breath, bronchospasm, interstitial pulmonary changes
Skin: alopecia, rash, skin reactions
Other: tumor site pain; irritation, pain, and phlebitis at I.V. site; **sepsis**

Interactions

Drug-drug. *Cisplatin, other antineoplastics:* increased risk and severity of bone marrow depression
Mitomycin: increased risk of acute pulmonary reaction
Drug-diagnostic tests. *Bilirubin, hepatic enzymes, liver function tests:* increased values
Granulocytes, hemoglobin, platelets, white blood cells: decreased levels

Patient monitoring

- Monitor vital signs closely.
- Assess liver function tests and CBC with platelet count.
- Watch for signs and symptoms of infection.
- Observe injection site closely for reactions and extravasation.

🔊 Closely monitor neurologic and respiratory status. Drug may lead to acute pulmonary changes, especially in patients who previously received mitomycin.

Patient teaching

- Explain drug therapy to patient. Emphasize importance of follow-up laboratory tests.
- Advise patient to promptly report signs and symptoms of infection and to take his temperature daily.
- Tell patient that hair loss is a common side effect but typically reverses once treatment ends.
- Instruct female of childbearing age to avoid pregnancy. Caution her not to breastfeed during therapy.
- Urge patient to practice good oral hygiene, to help prevent infected mouth sores.
- As appropriate, review all other significant and life-threatening adverse

V

reactions and interactions, especially those related to the drugs and tests mentioned above.

voriconazole

Vfend

Pharmacologic class: Triazole
Therapeutic class: Antifungal
Pregnancy risk category D

Action

Inhibits fungal cytochrome P450–mediated 14-alpha-lanosterol demethylation, preventing fungal biosynthesis and inactivating fungal cell

Availability

Lyophilized powder for injection: 200 mg
Powder for oral suspension: 45 g in 100-ml bottle
Tablets: 50 mg, 200 mg

Indications and dosages

➢ Invasive aspergillosis; serious fungal infections caused by *Scedosporium apiospermum* and *Fusarium* species
Adults and children older than age 12: Initially, 6 mg/kg I.V. q 12 hours for two doses (each dose infused over 1 to 2 hours), followed by a maintenance dose of 4 mg/kg I.V. q 12 hours given no faster than 3 mg/kg/hour. Change to oral dosing as described below when patient can tolerate it.
Adults and children older than age 12 weighing more than 40 kg (88 lb): 200 mg P.O. q 12 hours 1 hour before or after a meal; may increase to 300 mg P.O. q 12 hours p.r.n.
Adults and children older than age 12 weighing less than 40 kg (88 lb): 100 mg P.O. q 12 hours at least 1 hour before or after a meal; may increase to 150 mg P.O. q 12 hours p.r.n.

➢ Esophageal candidiasis
Adults and children older than age 12 weighing 40 kg (88 lb) or more: 200 mg P.O. q 12 hours for at least 14 days, and for at least 7 days after symptoms resolve
Adults and children older than age 12 weighing less than 40 kg (88 lb): 100 mg P.O. q 12 hours for at least 14 days, and for at least 7 days after symptoms resolve

Dosage adjustment

- Hepatic cirrhosis
- Renal impairment

Off-label uses

- Febrile neutropenia (as empiric therapy)

Contraindications

- Hypersensitivity to drug or its components
- Concurrent use of long-acting barbiturates, ergot alkaloids, rifabutin, rifampin, CYP450-3A4 substrates (such as astemizole, cisapride, pimozide, quinidine, terfenadine), sirolimus, ritonavir, efavirenz, or carbamazepine

Precautions

Use cautiously in:
- hypersensitivity to other azoles
- renal disease, mild to moderate hepatic cirrhosis, lactose or galactose intolerance
- pregnant or breastfeeding patients.

Administration

- Correct electrolyte disturbances before therapy starts.

🔊 Don't give concurrently with astemizole, cisapride, or terfenadine (no longer available in U.S.); carbamazepine; efavirenz; ergot alkaloids; long-acting barbiturates; pimozide; quinidine; rifabutin; rifampin; ritonavir; or sirolimus.

- Reconstitute powder with 19 ml of water for injection, to yield a volume of 20 ml. Shake vial until powder dissolves. Withdraw prescribed dose, then dilute further in compatible I.V. solution to a final concentration of 0.5 to 5 mg/ml. Give I.V. over 1 to 2 hours at a rate not exceeding 3 mg/kg/hour.

- Don't give through same I.V. line with other drugs, blood products, or electrolytes.
- To reconstitute powder for oral suspension, tap bottle to release powder. Add 46 ml of water, and shake vigorously for about 1 minute. Remove cap, push bottle adapter into neck of bottle, and replace cap. After reconstitution, suspension volume is 75 ml, providing usable volume of 70 ml (40 mg/ml). Shake bottle before each use. Use only 5-ml oral dispenser supplied. Don't mix with other drugs, and don't dilute further.
- Give oral suspension 1 hour before or after a meal.

Route	Onset	Peak	Duration
P.O.	1-2 hr	Unknown	Unknown
I.V.	Start of infusion	Unknown	Unknown

Adverse reactions

CNS: dizziness, headache, hallucinations
CV: hypotension, hypertension, tachycardia, chest pain, vasodilation, peripheral edema
EENT: photophobia, blurred vision, visual disturbances, eye hemorrhage, chromatopsia
GI: nausea, vomiting, diarrhea, abdominal pain, dry mouth
GU: renal dysfunction, acute renal failure
Hematologic: anemia, **pancytopenia, leukopenia, thrombocytopenia**
Hepatic: cholestatic jaundice, **hepatic failure**
Metabolic: hypomagnesemia, hypokalemia
Respiratory: respiratory disorders
Skin: pruritus, maculopapular rash, **erythema multiforme, toxic epidermal necrolysis, Stevens-Johnson syndrome**
Other: chills, fever, **sepsis, anaphylaxis**

Interactions

Drug-drug. *Barbiturates (long-acting), carbamazepine, phenytoin, rifampin:* decreased voriconazole blood level
Benzodiazepines: sedation
Calcium channel blockers, HMG-CoA reductase inhibitors: increased blood levels of these drugs
Cyclosporine, sirolimus, tacrolimus: increased blood levels of these drugs, greater risk of nephrotoxicity
CYP450-3A4 substrates: increased blood levels of these drugs, causing prolonged QT interval and risk of torsades de pointes
Ergot alkaloids: increased blood levels of these drugs, resulting in ergotism
Non-nucleoside reverse transcriptase inhibitors, protease inhibitors: inhibited voriconazole metabolism
Rifabutin: decreased voriconazole blood level, increased rifabutin blood level
Sulfonylureas: increased sulfonylurea blood level, greater risk of hypoglycemia
Vinca alkaloids: increased risk of neurotoxicity
Warfarin, other coumarin derivatives: increased partial thromboplastin time
Drug-diagnostic tests. *Alanine aminotransferase, alkaline phosphatase, aspartate aminotransferase, bilirubin, creatinine:* increased levels
Drug-herbs. *Gossypol:* increased risk of nephrotoxicity

V

Patient monitoring

- Monitor kidney and liver function tests. Watch for signs and symptoms of organ toxicity.
- Assess electrolyte levels and CBC, including platelet count.

Monitor ECG. Stay alert for prolonged QT interval.

• Check for vision problems in therapy exceeding 28 days.

Patient teaching

• Explain therapy to patient. Stress importance of follow-up laboratory tests.
• Tell patient using oral form to take doses 1 hour before or after a meal.
• Emphasize importance of taking drug exactly as directed for entire duration prescribed.
• Instruct patient to promptly report adverse reactions.
• Tell female of childbearing age to immediately report pregnancy.
• Caution patient to avoid driving and other hazardous activities, because drug may cause visual disturbances.
• Advise patient to minimize GI upset by eating small, frequent servings of food and drinking plenty of fluids.
• As appropriate, review all other significant and life-threatening adverse reactions and interactions, especially those related to the drugs, tests, and herbs mentioned above.

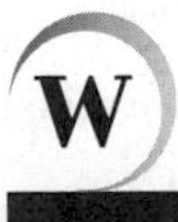

warfarin sodium

Coumadin, Warfilone*

Pharmacologic class: Coumarin derivative

Therapeutic class: Anticoagulant

Pregnancy risk category X

Action

Interferes with synthesis of vitamin K–dependent clotting factors (II, VII, IX, and X) and anticoagulant proteins C and S in liver

Availability

Injection: 5.4 mg/vial (2 mg/ml when reconstituted)

Tablets: 1 mg, 2 mg, 2.5 mg, 3 mg, 4 mg, 5 mg, 6 mg, 7.5 mg, 10 mg

Indications and dosages

➢ Venous thrombosis; pulmonary embolism; atrial fibrillation; myocardial infarction (MI); thromboembolic complications of cardiac valve placement

Adults: Initially, 2.5 to 10 mg P.O. or I.V. daily for 2 to 4 days, then adjusted based on prothrombin time (PT) or International Normalized Ratio (INR). Usual maintenance dosage is 2 to 10 mg P.O. daily.

Dosage adjustment

• Elderly or debilitated patients

Off-label uses

• Acute coronary syndrome
• Intracoronary stent placement
• Prevention of catheter thrombosis

Contraindications

• Hypersensitivity to drug
• Uncontrolled bleeding
• Open wounds
• Severe hepatic disease
• Hemorrhagic or bleeding tendency
• Cerebrovascular hemorrhage
• Cerebral aneurysm or dissecting aorta
• Blood dyscrasias
• Pericarditis or pericardial effusion
• Bacterial endocarditis
• Malignant hypertension
• Recent brain, eye, or spinal cord injury or surgery
• Lumbar puncture and other procedures that may cause uncontrollable bleeding
• Major regional or lumbar block anesthesia
• Threatened abortion, eclampsia, preeclampsia

• Unsupervised senile, alcoholic, or psychotic patients
• Pregnancy, females of childbearing potential

Precautions

Use cautiously in:
• cancer, heparin-induced thrombocytopenia, moderate to severe renal impairment, moderate to severe hypertension, infectious GI disease, known or suspected deficiency in protein C–mediated anticoagulant response, polycythemia vera, vasculitis, severe diabetes mellitus
• indwelling catheter use
• history of poor compliance
• elderly or debilitated patients
• breastfeeding patients
• children younger than age 18 (safety and efficacy not established).

Administration

Be aware that warfarin is a high-alert drug.
• Know that I.V. form is reserved for patients who can't tolerate oral form. I.V. and oral dosages are identical.
• For I.V. use, reconstitute vial with 2.7 ml of sterile water for injection; administer over 1 to 2 minutes. After reconstitution, drug is stable for 4 hours at room temperature.
• Be aware that vitamin K reverses warfarin effects. If major bleeding occurs, fresh frozen plasma may be given.
• When converting to warfarin from heparin, give both drugs concomitantly for 4 to 5 days until therapeutic effect of warfarin occurs.

Route	Onset	Peak	Duration
P.O.	Several hr	0.5-3 days	2-5 days
I.V.	Unknown	Unknown	Unknown

Adverse reactions

GI: nausea, vomiting, diarrhea, abdominal cramps, stomatitis, anorexia
GU: hematuria
Hematologic: eosinophilia, **bleeding, hemorrhage, agranulocytosis, leukopenia**
Hepatic: hepatitis
Skin: rash, dermatitis, urticaria, pruritus, alopecia, dermal necrosis
Other: fever, "purple toes" syndrome (bilateral painful, purple lesions on toes and sides of feet), hypersensitivity reaction

Interactions

Drug-drug. *Abciximab, acetaminophen (chronic use), androgens, aspirin, capecitabine, cefamandole, cefoperazone, cefotetan, chloral hydrate, chloramphenicol, clopidogrel, disulfiram, eptifibatide, fluconazole, fluoroquinolones, itraconazole, metronidazole (including vaginal use), nonsteroidal anti-inflammatory drugs, plicamycin, quinidine, quinine, sulfonamides, thrombolytics, ticlopidine, tirofiban, valproic acid, zafirlukast:* increased response to warfarin, greater risk of bleeding
Barbiturates, hormonal contraceptives containing estrogen: decreased anticoagulant effect
Drug-diagnostic tests. *Alanine aminotransferase, aspartate aminotransferase, INR:* increased values
Partial thromboplastin time, PT: prolonged
Drug-food. *Vitamin K–rich foods (large amounts):* antagonism of anticoagulant effect
Drug-herbs. *Angelica:* prolonged PT
Anise, arnica, asafetida, bromelain, chamomile, clove, danshen, devil's claw, dong quai, fenugreek, feverfew, garlic, ginger, ginkgo, ginseng, horse chestnut, licorice, meadowsweet, motherwort, onion, papain, parsley, passionflower, quassia, red clover, Reishi mushroom, rue, sweet clover, turmeric, white willow, others: increased risk of bleeding
Coenzyme Q10, green tea, St. John's wort: decreased anticoagulant effect

W

Drug-behaviors. *Alcohol use:* enhanced warfarin activity

Patient monitoring

- Monitor PT, INR, and liver function tests.
- Watch for signs and symptoms of bleeding and hepatitis.

Patient teaching

Clinical alert: Explain therapy to patient. Stress importance of adhering to schedule for laboratory tests.

Clinical alert: Instruct patient to promptly report unusual bleeding or bruising.

- Caution patient to consult prescriber before taking over-the-counter preparations or herbs.
- Advise patient to inform all other health care providers (including dentist) that he's taking warfarin.
- Tell patient not to vary his intake of foods high in vitamin K (such as leafy green vegetables, fish, pork, green tea, and tomatoes), to avoid alterations in drug's anticoagulant effect.

Clinical alert: Instruct females of childbearing age to report pregnancy immediately.

- Stress importance of avoiding contact sports and other activities that could cause injury and bleeding.
- Caution patient to avoid alcohol during therapy.
- As appropriate, review all other significant and life-threatening adverse reactions and interactions, especially those related to the drugs, tests, foods, herbs, and behaviors mentioned above.

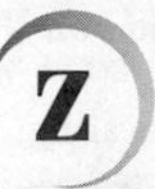

zafirlukast

Accolate

Pharmacologic class: Leukotriene receptor antagonist

Therapeutic class: Antiasthmatic, bronchodilator

Pregnancy risk category B

Action

Antagonizes activity of three leukotrienes at specific receptor sites in airway smooth muscle, inhibiting inflammation

Availability

Tablets (coated): 10 mg, 20 mg

Indications and dosages

➢ Prophylaxis and long-term treatment of asthma

Adults and children ages 12 and older: 20 mg P.O. b.i.d.

Children ages 5 to 11: 10 mg P.O. b.i.d.

Dosage adjustment

- Hepatic impairment

Off-label uses

- Exercise-induced bronchospasm
- Chronic urticaria

Contraindications

- Hypersensitivity to drug or its components

Precautions

Use cautiously in:

- hepatic disease, acute asthma attacks
- patients older than age 55
- pregnant patients
- breastfeeding patients (use not recommended)

• children younger than age 7 (safety not established).

Administration

• Give at least 1 hour before or 2 hours after a meal.

Route	Onset	Peak	Duration
P.O.	30 min	3.5 hr	12 hr

Adverse reactions

CNS: headache, dizziness, asthenia
GI: nausea, vomiting, diarrhea, abdominal pain, dyspepsia
Musculoskeletal: joint or back pain, myalgia
Other: fever, infection, pain

Interactions

Drug-drug. *Aspirin:* increased zafirlukast blood level
Erythromycin, theophylline: decreased zafirlukast blood level
Warfarin: increased warfarin effects, greater risk of bleeding
Drug-food. *Any food:* decreased rate and extent of zafirlukast absorption

Patient monitoring

• Assess patient's respiratory status to help evaluate drug efficacy.

Patient teaching

• Tell patient to take at least 1 hour before or 2 hours after a meal.
• Advise patient to take exactly as prescribed, even if he's symptom-free.
Tell patient to immediately report asthma attack. Advise him not to use drug for rapid relief of bronchospasm.
• Instruct patient to continue taking other asthma drugs unless prescriber directs otherwise.
• Instruct female patient to consult prescriber if she plans to breastfeed.
• As appropriate, review all other significant adverse reactions and interactions, especially those related to the drugs and foods mentioned above.

zalcitabine (dideoxycytidine, ddC)

Hivid

Pharmacologic class: Nucleoside reverse transcriptase inhibitor
Therapeutic class: Antiretroviral
Pregnancy risk category C

Action

After conversion to active metabolite dideoxycytidine-5′-triphosphate, blocks activity of reverse transcriptase, inhibiting replication of human immunodeficiency virus (HIV)

Availability

Tablets: 0.375 mg, 0.75 mg

Indications and dosages

➢ Advanced HIV infection (CD4+ cell count of 300/mm^3 or lower)
Adults and children older than age 13: 0.75 mg P.O. q 8 hours, given with other antiretrovirals

Dosage adjustment

• Renal impairment

Contraindications

• Hypersensitivity to drug or its components

Precautions

Use cautiously in:
• HIV complications, lymphoma, renal or hepatic disease, peripheral neuropathy, heart failure, decreased CD4+ cell count
• known risk factors for, or history of, pancreatitis
• pregnant or breastfeeding patients.
• children younger than age 13 (safety and efficacy not established).

Z

Administration

- Give at least 1 hour before or 2 hours after a meal.

Route	Onset	Peak	Duration
P.O.	Unknown	1-2 hr	Unknown

Adverse reactions

CNS: headache, fatigue, dizziness, insomnia, depression, peripheral neuropathy, confusion, poor concentration, amnesia, tremor, hypertonia, anxiety, **seizures**
CV: chest pain, **cardiomyopathy, heart failure**
EENT: abnormal vision, eye pain, ototoxicity, nasal discharge, pharyngitis
GI: nausea, vomiting, diarrhea, constipation, abdominal pain, esophageal ulcer, glossitis, stomatitis, anorexia, **pancreatitis**
Hematologic: anemia, **leukopenia, thrombocytopenia, neutropenia**
Hepatic: severe hepatomegaly with steatosis
Metabolic: hypoglycemia, lactic acidosis
Musculoskeletal: myalgia, joint pain
Respiratory: cough
Skin: pruritus; urticaria; erythematous, maculopapular, or follicular rash
Other: night sweats, fever

Interactions

Drug-drug. *Aminoglycosides, amphotericin B, foscarnet, other drugs that can impair renal function:* increased risk of nephrotoxicity
Antacids containing aluminum or magnesium: decreased zalcitabine bioavailability
Chloramphenicol, cisplatin, dapsone, didanosine, disulfiram, ethionamide, glutethimide, gold salts, hydralazine, iodoquinol, isoniazid, metronidazole, phenytoin, other drugs that can cause peripheral neuropathy (such as ribavirin, stavudine, vincristine): increased risk of peripheral neuropathy
Cimetidine, probenecid: increased zalcitabine blood level
Pentamidine: increased risk of pancreatitis
Drug-diagnostic tests. *Alanine aminotransferase, alkaline phosphatase, aspartate aminotransferase:* increased levels
Hemoglobin, platelets, white blood cells: decreased levels
Liver function tests: abnormal results
Drug-food. *Any food:* decreased drug absorption

Patient monitoring

- Monitor CD4+ cell count, CBC, and electrolyte levels before and periodically during therapy.
- Assess kidney function tests.
- Watch closely for signs and symptoms of peripheral neuropathy and worsening HIV infection.
- Monitor for signs and symptoms of pancreatitis.

Assess for hepatic dysfunction and lactic acidosis, which can be fatal.

Patient teaching

- Instruct patient to take at least 1 hour before or 2 hours after a meal.
- Explain therapy to patient. Tell him that drug doesn't cure HIV infection. Stress importance of practicing safe sex.
- Advise female of childbearing age to use effective contraception.
- Caution female patient not to breastfeed, because of risk of transmitting HIV to infant.

Teach patient to recognize and immediately report signs and symptoms of pancreatitis, lactic acidosis, and liver impairment.

- Emphasize importance of follow-up laboratory tests.
- As appropriate, review all other significant and life-threatening adverse reactions and interactions, especially those related to the drugs, tests, and foods mentioned above.

zaleplon

Sonata

Pharmacologic class: Pyrazolopyrimidine, nonbenzodiazepine hypnotic

Therapeutic class: Sedative-hypnotic

Controlled substance schedule IV

Pregnancy risk category C

Action

Binds to omega-1 receptor of gamma-aminobutyric acid receptor complex, relaxing smooth muscles, reducing anxiety, and producing sedation. Also has anticonvulsant effect.

Availability

Capsules: 5 mg, 10 mg

Indications and dosages

➢ Insomnia

Adults younger than age 65: 10 mg P.O. at bedtime. Dosage above 20 mg is not recommended.

Dosage adjustment

- Mild to moderate hepatic impairment
- Elderly or debilitated patients

Contraindications

- Hypersensitivity to drug or its components

Precautions

Use cautiously in:

- tartrazine sensitivity
- severe renal impairment (use not recommended), mild to moderate hepatic impairment, respiratory impairment, depression
- history of suicide attempt
- patients weighing less than 50 kg (110 lb)
- patients older than age 65
- pregnant or breastfeeding patients (use not recommended)
- children younger than age 18 (safety not established).

Administration

- Give at bedtime.
- Don't administer with high-fat meal.

Route	Onset	Peak	Duration
P.O.	Rapid	1 hr	3-4 hr

Adverse reactions

CNS: headache, amnesia, anxiety, hallucinations, light-headedness, dizziness, drowsiness, depersonalization, transient memory or psychomotor impairment, incoordination, malaise, vertigo, asthenia, hyperesthesia, paresthesia, tremor

CV: peripheral edema

EENT: abnormal vision, eye pain, ear pain, hearing sensitivity, epistaxis

GI: nausea, abdominal pain, colitis, dyspepsia, anorexia

GU: dysmenorrhea

Musculoskeletal: myalgia

Skin: photosensitivity

Other: altered sense of smell, fever

Interactions

Drug-drug. *Cimetidine:* decreased metabolism and increased effects of zaleplon

CNS depressants (including antihistamines, opioids, other sedative-hypnotics, phenothiazines, tricyclic antidepressants): additive CNS depression

CYP450-3A4 inducers (such as carbamazepine, phenobarbital, phenytoin, rifampin): decreased blood level and reduced efficacy of zaleplon

CYP450-3A4 inhibitors (such as erythromycin, ketoconazole): increased zaleplon blood level

Drug-food. *High-fat meal:* delayed drug absorption

Drug-herbs. *Chamomile, hops, kava, skullcap, valerian:* increased CNS depression

Z

Drug-behaviors. *Alcohol use:* increased CNS depression

Patient monitoring

- Monitor drug efficacy. Insomnia persisting after 7 to 10 days warrants reevaluation for underlying psychological or physical illness.
- Stay alert for adverse drug reactions.

Patient teaching

- Explain therapy to patient. Emphasize importance of taking drug just before bedtime or after trying to sleep—but only if he'll be able to get at least 4 hours of sleep.
- Inform patient that high-fat meal slows drug absorption and delays drug effects.
- Caution patient to avoid driving and other hazardous activities while under drug's influence.
- Instruct patient to avoid alcohol during therapy.
- Tell patient rebound insomnia may occur for 1 or 2 nights after he stops taking drug.
- Advise female of childbearing age to notify prescriber if she is or plans to become pregnant or if she's breastfeeding.
- As appropriate, review all other significant adverse reactions and interactions, especially those related to the drugs, foods, herbs, and behaviors mentioned above.

zanamivir

Relenza

Pharmacologic class: Neuraminidase inhibitor

Therapeutic class: Antiviral

Pregnancy risk category C

Action

Inhibits influenza virus neuraminidase, an enzyme essential for viral replication

Availability

Powder for inhalation: 5 mg/blister

Indications and dosages

➢ Influenza virus A or B

Adults and children ages 7 and older: Two oral inhalations (5 mg/inhalation) b.i.d. for 5 days

Contraindications

- Hypersensitivity to drug or its components

Precautions

Use cautiously in:

- chronic obstructive pulmonary disease, asthma, lactose intolerance
- pregnant or breastfeeding patients
- children younger than age 7 (safety not established).

Administration

- Give two doses on day 1, spaced at least 2 hours apart. On subsequent days, space doses 12 hours apart, and give at approximately same time each day.

Route	Onset	Peak	Duration
Inhalation	Rapid	1-2 hr	12 hr

Adverse reactions

CNS: headache, dizziness
EENT: sinusitis, EENT infections
GI: nausea, vomiting, diarrhea
Respiratory: bronchitis, cough
Other: allergic reaction

Interactions

None significant

Patient monitoring

- Assess respiratory status. Watch closely for signs and symptoms of declining respiratory function.

Patient teaching

- Explain therapy to patient. Demonstrate how to use Diskhaler device.
- Tell patient to take drug exactly as prescribed for as long as directed, even if symptoms improve.
- If patient's also taking an inhaled bronchodilator, advise him to take bronchodilator before zanamivir.
- Emphasize that drug doesn't prevent spread of influenza to others.
- Instruct patient to immediately report worsening respiratory symptoms.
- As appropriate, review other significant adverse reactions.

zidovudine

Apo-Zidovudine✦, Novo-AZT✦, Retrovir

Pharmacologic class: Nucleoside reverse transcriptase inhibitor

Therapeutic class: Antiretroviral

Pregnancy risk category C

Action

After conversion to its active metabolite, inhibits activity of human immunodeficiency virus (HIV) reverse transcriptase and terminates viral DNA growth

Availability

Capsules: 300 mg
Injection: 10 mg/ml in 20-ml vial
Syrup: 50 mg/5 ml
Tablets: 100 mg

Indications and dosages

➢ HIV infection

Adults and children older than age 12: 200 mg P.O. t.i.d. or 300 mg P.O. b.i.d. for a total daily dosage of 600 mg/day, or 1 mg/kg I.V. five to six times daily; usually given with other antiretrovirals

Children ages 6 weeks to 12 years: 160 mg/m^2 P.O. q 8 hours (480 mg/m^2/day, to a maximum of 200 mg q 8 hours), given with other antiretrovirals

➢ To prevent maternal-fetal HIV transmission

Pregnant women: 500 mg P.O. daily in divided doses (usually as five 100-mg doses) until labor begins; then 2 mg/kg I.V. over 1 hour followed by a continuous infusion of 1 mg/kg/hour until umbilical cord is clamped

Neonates: 2 mg/kg P.O. q 6 hours starting within 12 hours of delivery and continuing for 6 weeks

Dosage adjustment

- Hepatic or renal impairment

Off-label uses

- Occupational exposure to HIV

Contraindications

- Hypersensitivity to drug or its components
- Concomitant use of Combivir or Trizivir (zidovudine-containing products)

Precautions

Use cautiously in:

- renal or hepatic impairment, decreased bone marrow reserve, hemoglobin less than 9.5 g/dl, granulocyte count less than 1,000 cells/mm^3
- pregnant or breastfeeding patients.

Administration

- For I.V. use, remove dose from vial and add to I.V. solution containing dextrose 5% in water, to yield a final concentration no higher than 4 mg/ml. Infuse over 1 hour.
- In adults, give by I.V. route only until patient can tolerate oral dose.

Route	Onset	Peak	Duration
P.O.	Variable	30-90 min	4 hr
I.V.	Rapid	End of infusion	4 hr

Adverse reactions

CNS: headache, paresthesia, malaise, insomnia, dizziness, drowsiness, asthenia, **seizures**
GI: nausea, vomiting, constipation, abdominal pain, dyspepsia, anorexia, **pancreatitis**
Hematologic: severe anemia (necessitating transfusions), **agranulocytopenia, severe bone marrow depression**
Musculoskeletal: myalgia, back pain, myopathy
Respiratory: dyspnea
Skin: diaphoresis, rash, altered nail pigmentation
Other: abnormal taste, fever

Interactions

Drug-drug. *Acetaminophen, aspirin, indomethacin:* increased risk of zidovudine toxicity
Amphotericin B, dapsone, flucytosine, pentamidine: increased risk of nephrotoxicity and bone marrow depression
Cyclosporine: extreme drowsiness, lethargy
Cytotoxic drugs, myelosuppressants, nephrotoxic drugs (such as ganciclovir, interferon alfa): increased risk of hematologic toxicity
Fluconazole, methadone, probenecid, valproic acid: increased zidovudine blood level, greater risk of toxicity
Ribavirin: antagonism of zidovudine's antiviral activity
Drug-diagnostic tests. *Granulocytes, hemoglobin, platelets:* decreased levels
Drug-herbs. *St. John's wort:* decreased zidovudine efficacy

Patient monitoring

- Monitor neurologic status, especially for signs and symptoms of impending seizure.
- [Clinical alert] Periodically assess CBC and kidney and liver function tests. Be aware that drug can cause hepatotoxicity.
- Watch for signs and symptoms of pancreatitis.

Patient teaching

- Tell patient he may take with or without food.
- Instruct patient to take capsules with at least 4 oz of fluid and to stay upright after taking.
- Explain therapy to patient. Emphasize that drug doesn't cure HIV infection.
- Urge patient to take drug exactly as prescribed.
- [Clinical alert] Teach patient to recognize and immediately report signs and symptoms of serious side effects, such as seizures.
- Stress importance of follow-up laboratory testing.
- Advise female of childbearing age to use effective contraception.
- Inform pregnant patient that drug reduces risk of, but may not prevent, HIV transmission to neonate.
- As appropriate, review all other significant and life-threatening adverse reactions and interactions, especially those related to the drugs, tests, and herbs mentioned above.

ziprasidone hydrochloride

Geodon

Pharmacologic class: Benzisoxazole derivative

Therapeutic class: Antipsychotic

Pregnancy risk category C

Action

Unknown. Thought to antagonize dopamine$_2$ and serotonin$_2$ receptors.

Availability

Capsules: 20 mg, 40 mg, 60 mg, 80 mg
Injection: 20 mg/ml

Indications and dosages

➢ Schizophrenia
Adults: Initially, 20 mg P.O. b.i.d. with food; may increase q 2 days up to 80

mg b.i.d. Usual maintenance dosage is 20 to 80 mg P.O. b.i.d.; maximum recommended dosage is 80 mg b.i.d. For prompt control of acute agitation, 10 to 20 mg I.M. as a single dose; depending on patient's response, may repeat 10-mg I.M. dose q 2 hours or 20-mg I.M. dose q 4 hours to a maximum daily dosage of 40 mg.

Contraindications

- Hypersensitivity to drug
- History of arrhythmias, prolonged QT interval
- Recent myocardial infarction
- Uncompensated heart failure
- Concomitant use of arsenic trioxide, chlorpromazine, class IA or III antiarrhythmics, or other drugs that prolong the QT interval

Precautions

Use cautiously in:
- cardiovascular disorders, dysphagia, hyperprolactinemia, bradycardia, hypokalemia, hypomagnesemia
- adverse reactions with previous use of atypical antipsychotics (such as risperidone or clozapine)
- pregnant patients.

Administration

- Give with food.
- Know that P.O. therapy should replace I.M. therapy as soon as possible.
- Don't give with drugs that prolong the QT interval.

Route	Onset	Peak	Duration
P.O.	Several hr	1-3 days	Unknown
I.M.	Unknown	1 hr	Unknown

Adverse reactions

CNS: dizziness, drowsiness, dystonia, hypertonia, asthenia, akathisia, extrapyramidal reactions, agitation, headache, insomnia, personality disorder, paresthesia, speech disorder, **neuroleptic malignant syndrome, seizures, suicide attempt**
CV: orthostatic hypotension, hypertension, tachycardia, **arrhythmias** (from prolonged QT interval)
EENT: abnormal vision, rhinitis
GI: nausea, vomiting, diarrhea, constipation, dyspepsia, dry mouth, anorexia
GU: dysmenorrhea, priapism
Musculoskeletal: myalgia
Respiratory: cough, cold symptoms
Skin: urticaria, rash, fungal dermatitis, diaphoresis, photosensitivity
Other: accidental injury, pain at I.M. injection site

Interactions

Drug-drug. *Antihypertensives:* additive hypotension
Carbamazepine: decreased ziprasidone blood level
Centrally acting drugs: additive CNS effects
Dopamine agonists, levodopa: antagonism of these drugs' effects
Drugs that decrease potassium or magnesium level (such as diuretics) or prolong QT interval (such as dofetilide, moxifloxacin, pimozide, quinidine, sotalol, sparfloxacin, thioridazine): increased risk of arrhythmias
Ketoconazole: increased ziprasidone blood level
Drug-herbs. *Chamomile, hops, kava, skullcap, valerian:* increased CNS depression

Patient monitoring

- Monitor ECG before and during therapy. Stay alert for prolonged QT interval.
- Assess blood pressure for hypertension and orthostatic hypotension.
- 🔊 Monitor neurologic status, especially for and neuroleptic malignant syndrome.
- 🔊 Watch for adverse reactions. Know that dizziness, syncope, or palpitations may signify life-threatening arrhythmias caused by prolonged QT interval.
- 🔊 Be aware that patient with bradycardia, hypokalemia, or hypomagne-

Z

semia is at greater risk for torsades de pointes and sudden death.

Patient teaching

- Tell patient to take with food.
- Explain therapy and need for follow-up laboratory testing.

Advise patient to promptly report fainting, seizures, high fever, sweating, unstable blood pressure, stupor, muscle rigidity, or suspected infection.

- Instruct patient to consult prescriber before taking over-the-counter preparations.
- Caution patient to avoid driving and other hazardous activities until drug effects are known.
- Instruct patient to move slowly when sitting up or standing, to avoid dizziness from sudden blood pressure drop.
- Advise patient to avoid sun exposure and to wear sunscreen and protective clothing when going outdoors.
- As appropriate, review all other significant and life-threatening adverse reactions and interactions, especially those related to the drugs and herbs mentioned above.

zoledronic acid

Zometa

Pharmacologic class: Third-generation bisphosphonate

Therapeutic class: Calcium regulator

Pregnancy risk category D

Action

Inhibits osteoclast-mediated bone by blocking resorption of mineralized bone and cartilage, eventually causing cell death and limiting tumor growth. Also limits calcium release produced by tumor.

Availability

Lyophilized powder for injection: 4 mg/vial

Indications and dosages

➢ Hypercalcemia caused by cancer

Adults: 4 mg I.V. as a single dose infused over 15 minutes. If albumin-corrected calcium level doesn't return to normal or stay normal, retreatment with 4 mg I.V. begins no sooner than 7 days after initial treatment. For single dose, maximum recommended dosage is 4 mg.

➢ Multiple myeloma; bone metastasis from solid tumors

Adults: 4 mg I.V. as a single dose infused over 15 minutes q 3 to 4 weeks. Treatment may continue for 9 to 15 months, depending on clinical condition.

Dosage adjustment

- Renal impairment

Off-label uses

- Paget's disease

Contraindications

- Hypersensitivity to drug, its components, or other bisphosphonates
- Bone metastasis with severe renal impairment
- Pregnancy

Precautions

Use cautiously in:

- asthma, renal dysfunction, hepatic insufficiency, history of hypoparathyroidism
- breastfeeding patients.

Administration

- Before starting therapy, make sure patient is adequately hydrated.
- Reconstitute by adding 5 ml of sterile water for injection to 4-mg vial. Dilute further by adding reconstituted drug to 100 ml of normal saline solution or dextrose 5% in water.

◀ Give by I.V. infusion over no less than 15 minutes. (Faster infusion may cause renal failure.)
• Be aware that patient usually receives daily oral calcium supplement of 500 mg and multivitamin containing 400 international units of vitamin D.

Route	Onset	Peak	Duration
I.V.	Unknown	Unknown	7-28 days

Adverse reactions

CNS: headache, agitation, confusion, insomnia, anxiety, drowsiness, fatigue, paresthesia
CV: hypotension
EENT: conjunctivitis
GI: nausea, vomiting, diarrhea, constipation, dysphagia, anorexia
GU: urinary tract infection, **renal toxicity**
Hematologic: anemia, **neutropenia**
Metabolic: dehydration, hypomagnesemia, hypercalcemia, hypophosphatemia
Musculoskeletal: myalgia, joint or bone pain
Respiratory: dyspnea, cough, **pleural effusion**
Other: infection, fever, chills, infusion site reactions

Interactions

Drug-drug. *Aminoglycosides, loop diuretics, thalidomide:* increased risk of renal toxicity
Drug-diagnostic tests. *Calcium, hemoglobin, magnesium, phosphorus, platelets, potassium, red blood cells, white blood cells:* decreased levels
Creatinine: increased or decreased level

Patient monitoring

• Monitor electrolyte levels (especially calcium). Watch for signs and symptoms of electrolyte imbalance.
• Assess vital signs. Stay alert for hypotension, dyspnea, and pleural effusion.
◀ Closely monitor fluid intake and output and creatinine level. Check for signs and symptoms of renal toxicity.
• Monitor CBC with platelet count.

Patient teaching

• Explain therapy to patient, including associated risk of renal failure and need for follow-up laboratory tests.
• Tell patient to report shortness of breath, unusual bleeding or bruising, decreased urine output, or other significant problems.
• Instruct patient to take daily 500-mg oral calcium supplement and multivitamin containing 400 international units of vitamin D (unless prescriber directs otherwise).
• Advise female of childbearing age to avoid pregnancy and breastfeeding.
• As appropriate, review all other significant and life-threatening adverse reactions and interactions, especially those related to the drugs and tests mentioned above.

zolmitriptan

Zomig, Zomig-ZMT

Pharmacologic class: Selective 5-hydroxytryptamine receptor agonist
Therapeutic class: Antimigraine agent
Pregnancy risk category C

Action

Blocks serotonin release, constricting inflamed and dilated cerebral and cranial blood vessels and reducing nerve transmission in trigeminal pain pathways

Availability

Nasal spray: 5-mg single-use spray device
Tablets (immediate-release): 2.5 mg, 5 mg
Tablets (orally disintegrating): 2.5 mg

Indications and dosages

➢ Acute migraine

Adults: 1.25 to 2.5 mg (immediate-release) P.O., repeated if migraine returns in 2 hours or less; maximum dosage is 10 mg in any 24-hour period. Or 2.5 mg (orally disintegrating tablet) P.O., repeated if migraine returns in 2 hours or less; maximum dosage is 10 mg in any 24-hour period. Alternatively, one dose of nasal spray (5 mg); if migraine returns, may repeat dose after 2 hours; don't exceed maximum daily dosage of 10 mg in any 24-hour period.

Dosage adjustment

- Hepatic impairment

Contraindications

- Hypersensitivity to drug
- Hemiplegic or basilar migraine
- Ischemic cardiac disease or other significant cardiac disease
- Uncontrolled hypertension
- Cerebrovascular accident or transient ischemic attack
- Peripheral vascular disease, including ischemic bowel disease
- Use of ergot-type or ergot-containing drugs or other 5-HT_1 agonists within past 24 hours
- MAO inhibitor use within past 14 days

Precautions

Use cautiously in:

- hepatic or renal impairment
- risk factors for coronary artery disease (such as strong family history of this disease, diabetes mellitus, obesity, cigarette smoking, high cholesterol level, men older than age 40, postmenopausal women)
- elderly patients
- pregnant or breastfeeding patients
- children.

Administration

- Place orally disintegrating tablet on patient's tongue, where it should dissolve.
- Don't break orally disintegrating tablet in half.
- Know that each nasal spray unit is intended for one use only.

Route	Onset	Peak	Duration
P.O.	Unknown	2 hr	Unknown
Nasal	15 min	2-5 hr	24 hr

Adverse reactions

CNS: paresthesia, asthenia, dizziness, insomnia, hyperesthesia, drowsiness, syncope, vertigo, agitation, depression, anxiety, emotional lability, fatigue, malaise
CV: chest pain, heaviness, or tightness; hypertension; palpitations; angina; **arrhythmias**
EENT: dry eyes, ear pain, tinnitus, epistaxis, altered sense of smell, laryngitis
GI: nausea, vomiting, dyspepsia, dysphagia, gastroenteritis, esophagitis, dry mouth
GU: urinary frequency, hematuria, polyuria, cystitis
Hepatic: hepatic dysfunction
Metabolic: hyperglycemia
Musculoskeletal: leg cramps, neck pain, tenosynovitis, myasthenia, myalgia, back pain
Respiratory: bronchitis, hiccups
Skin: pruritus, rash, diaphoresis, bruising, urticaria, photosensitivity
Other: unusual taste, flushing, sweating or redness in face (with nasal spray); fever; chills; excessive thirst; facial or tongue edema; pressure or tightness in throat or jaw; yawning; warm or cold sensation

Interactions

Drug-drug. *Cimetidine:* doubling of zolmitriptan's half-life
Ergot-containing drugs: vasospasm

Fluoxetine, fluvoxamine, paroxetine, sertraline: weakness, incoordination, hyperreflexia
MAO inhibitors: increased zolmitriptan effects
Drug-diagnostic tests. *Blood glucose:* increased level
Drug-herbs. *S-adenosylmethionine (SAM-e), St. John's wort:* serotonin syndrome
Drug-behaviors. *Smoking:* increased risk of adverse cardiovascular effects

Patient monitoring
- Assess therapeutic response to help gauge drug efficacy.
- Watch for adverse cardiovascular and respiratory reactions, particularly dyspnea and chest pain or tightness.
- Assess blood glucose level in diabetic patient.

Patient teaching
- Tell patient to immediately report shortness of breath or pain or tightness in chest or throat.
- Explain that drug is intended to treat migraine, not prevent it.
- Tell patient to remove orally disintegrating tablet from blister pack just before taking it, and then place it on his tongue and let it dissolve. Instruct him not to break it.
- Teach patient proper use of nasal spray. Tell him each unit is intended for one use only.
- Caution patient to avoid driving and other hazardous activities during severe migraine or if drug causes adverse CNS effects.
- Inform patient that smoking may increase drug's cardiovascular risks.
- Advise female of childbearing age not to take drug if she is, might be, or plans to become pregnant.
- Advise patient to avoid sun exposure and to wear sunscreen and protective clothing when going outdoors.
- As appropriate, review all other significant and life-threatening adverse reactions and interactions, especially those related to the drugs, tests, herbs, and behaviors mentioned above.

zolpidem tartrate
Ambien

Pharmacologic class: Imidazopyridine
Therapeutic class: Sedative-hypnotic
Controlled substance schedule IV
Pregnancy risk category B

Action
Depresses CNS by binding to gamma-aminobutyric acid receptors

Availability
Tablets: 5 mg, 10 mg

Indications and dosages
➢ Insomnia
Adults: 10 mg P.O. at bedtime

Dosage adjustment
- Hepatic impairment
- Elderly or debilitated patients

Off-label uses
- Long-term treatment of insomnia
- Insomnia related to selective serotonin reuptake inhibitors
- Postoperative sedation

Contraindications
- Hypersensitivity to drug

Precautions
Use cautiously in:
- pulmonary disease, hepatic or severe renal impairment
- history of psychiatric illness, suicide attempt, or substance abuse
- elderly or debilitated patients
- pregnant or breastfeeding patients
- children (safety not established).

Administration

• Don't give with or immediately after a meal.
• Know that dosage may need to be decreased if patient's receiving other CNS depressants.

Route	Onset	Peak	Duration
P.O.	Rapid	30 min-2 hr	6-8 hr

Adverse reactions

CNS: amnesia, ataxia, confusion, euphoria, vertigo, daytime drowsiness, dizziness, drugged feeling
EENT: diplopia, abnormal vision
GI: nausea, vomiting, diarrhea, dry mouth
Other: hypersensitivity reaction, physical or psychological drug dependence, drug tolerance

Interactions

Drug-drug. *Antihistamines, opioid analgesics, phenothiazines, sedative-hypnotics, tricyclic antidepressants:* increased CNS depression
Ketoconazole, ritonavir: increased blood level and enhanced effects of zolpidem
Rifampin: decreased zolpidem efficacy
Drug-herbs. *Chamomile, hops, kava, skullcap, valerian:* increased CNS depression
Drug-behaviors. *Alcohol use:* increased CNS depression

Patient monitoring

• Monitor for physical and psychological drug dependence. Watch for drug hoarding.
• Assess for adverse reactions, including confusion, ataxia, and amnesia.

Patient teaching

• Tell patient to take immediately before bedtime (and not after a meal), because it works quickly.
• Advise patient to take only when he's able to get a full night's sleep (7 to 8 hours) before he needs to be active again.
• Stress that drug is meant only for short-term use (7 to 10 days).
• Tell patient rebound insomnia may occur for 1 to 2 nights after he discontinues drug.
• Inform patient that drug may cause amnesia, drowsiness, and a drugged feeling the next day.
• Caution patient to avoid driving and other hazardous activities while under drug's influence.
• As appropriate, review all other significant adverse reactions and interactions, especially those related to the drugs, herbs, and behaviors mentioned above.

zonisamide

Zonegran

Pharmacologic class: Sulfonamide
Therapeutic class: Anticonvulsant
Pregnancy risk category C

Action

Raises seizure threshold and reduces seizure duration, probably by stabilizing neuronal membranes through action on sodium and calcium channels

Availability

Capsules: 25 mg, 50 mg, 100 mg

Indications and dosages

➢ Adjunctive treatment of partial seizures
Adults and children older than age 16: Initially, 100 mg P.O. daily for 2 weeks, then, if required, increased to 200 mg P.O. daily for at least 2 weeks. May increase in 100-mg increments at 2-week intervals to 300 to 400 mg daily as required. Daily dosage ranges from 100 to 600 mg.

Dosage adjustment
- Hepatic or renal impairment
- Elderly patients

Off-label uses
- Infantile spasms
- Progressive myoclonic epilepsy
- Weight loss

Contraindications
- Hypersensitivity to drug or other sulfonamides

Precautions
Use cautiously in:
- hepatic or renal disease
- pregnant or breastfeeding patients
- children younger than age 16 (safety not established).

Administration
- Give with or without food.

Route	Onset	Peak	Duration
P.O.	Unknown	2-6 hr	24 hr

Adverse reactions
CNS: drowsiness, fatigue, agitation, irritability, depression, dizziness, psychomotor slowing, psychosis, asthenia, abnormal gait, incoordination, tremor, ataxia, headache, confusion, impaired memory, hyperesthesia, paresthesia, **seizures**
EENT: diplopia, amblyopia, nystagmus, tinnitus, rhinitis, pharyngitis
GI: nausea, vomiting, diarrhea, dyspepsia, dry mouth, anorexia
GU: renal calculi
Hematologic: anemia, **leukopenia**
Respiratory: cough
Skin: rash, pruritus, bruising, **Stevens-Johnson syndrome**
Other: abnormal taste, weight loss, allergic reactions, oligohidrosis and hyperthermia (in children), flulike symptoms, accidental injury

Interactions
Drug-drug. *Carbamazepine, phenobarbital, phenytoin, valproic acid:* decreased zonisamide blood level and effects
CYP450-3A4 inducers: decreased zonisamide half-life
CYP450-3A4 inhibitors: increased zonisamide blood level
Drug-diagnostic tests. *Blood urea nitrogen, creatinine:* increased levels
Platelets, white blood cells: decreased counts

Patient monitoring
- Monitor CBC with white cell differential.
- Assess neurologic status; report significant adverse reactions.
- Monitor renal function tests. Watch for signs and symptoms of renal calculi.

[Clinical alert] Monitor for rash, which may be first sign of Stevens-Johnson syndrome. If rash occurs, discontinue drug and notify prescriber immediately.

Patient teaching
- Explain therapy to patient. Instruct him to keep seizure diary and show it to prescriber.
- Instruct patient to swallow capsules whole. Advise him to drink 6 to 8 glasses of water daily to help prevent kidney stones.

[Clinical alert] Warn patient that stopping drug abruptly may cause status epilepticus.

- Caution patient to avoid driving and other hazardous activities until he knows how drug affects him and until seizures are well controlled.

[Clinical alert] Tell patient to immediately report rash, fever, sore throat, sudden back pain, depression, speech or language problems, or painful urination.

- As appropriate, review all other significant and life-threatening adverse reactions and interactions, especially those related to the drugs and tests mentioned above.

Z

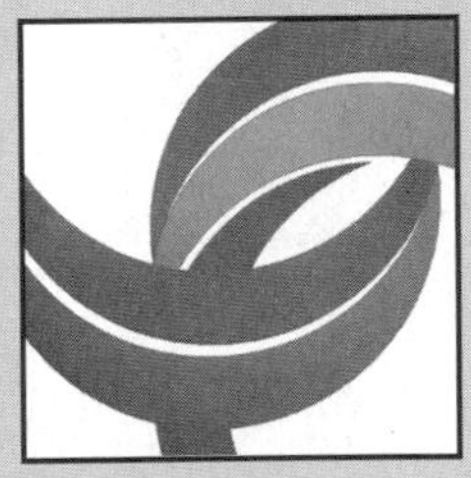

Part 2

Drug classes

Vitamins and minerals

Herbs and supplements

Drug classes

The collective monographs below cover the most common drug classes, and provide general information for the most commonly used generic drugs in each class. The drugs listed in each class are those covered in individual monographs in this book; the list is not intended to be comprehensive.

Keep in mind that drugs in the same class may vary as to contraindications, precautions, adverse reactions, interactions, and patient monitoring. For specific information on a particular drug, see the individual monograph. Also, because pregnancy risk category and interactions may differ for the drugs in a given class, this information is not included in the monographs below.

alpha$_1$-adrenergic agents

Alpha$_1$-adrenergic blockers: alfuzosin hydrochloride, doxazosin mesylate, prazocin hydrochloride, tamsulosin hydrochloride, terazosin hydrochloride

Centrally acting alpha-adrenergic agonists: clonidine hydrochloride, methyldopa

Peripherally acting alpha-adrenergic agonists: midodrine hydrochloride

Action

Alpha$_1$-adrenergic blockers selectively block postsynaptic alpha$_1$-adrenergic receptors, causing dilation of arterioles and veins, in turn lowering supine and standing blood pressure. *Centrally acting alpha-adrenergic agonists* reduce sympathetic outflow from CNS and decrease peripheral resistance, renal vascular resistance, heart rate, and blood pressure. *Peripherally acting alpha-adrenergic agonists* activate alpha-adrenergic receptors of the arteriolar and venous vasculature, increasing vascular tone and blood pressure.

Indications

Hypertension, refractory heart failure, peripheral vascular disorders, benign prostatic hypertrophy, orthostatic hypotension (midodrine only), severe pain in cancer patients (injectable clonidine only)

Contraindications and precautions

• Contraindicated in hypersensitivity to drug
• Use cautiously in renal insufficiency, angina pectoris, overt heart failure, when adding diuretics to drug regimen, in pregnant or breastfeeding patients, and in children (safety not established).

Adverse reactions

CNS: dizziness, headache, asthenia, drowsiness, nervousness, paresthesia, vertigo, fatigue
CV: orthostatic hypotension (with first dose of alpha$_1$-adrenergic blocker), rebound hypertension, chest pain, palpitations, peripheral edema, tachycardia, **arrhythmias**
EENT: blurred vision, conjunctivitis, nasal congestion, sinusitis
GI: nausea, vomiting, diarrhea, abdominal pain, dry mouth
GU: urinary frequency or incontinence, priapism, erectile dysfunction, gynecomastia (with centrally acting agonists)
Musculoskeletal: joint, back, or extremity pain
Respiratory: dyspnea

Skin: pruritus, angioedema, urticaria, alopecia (with centrally acting agonists)
Other: fever, weight gain

Patient monitoring

• Monitor electrolyte levels, ECG, and vital signs.

antacids

aluminum hydroxide, calcium carbonate, magaldrate, magnesium hydroxide, magnesium oxide, sodium bicarbonate

Action

Neutralize gastric acidity, which increases pH of stomach and duodenal bulb. Aluminum-containing antacids bind with phosphate ions in intestine to form insoluble aluminum phosphate, which is excreted in feces.

Indications

Peptic ulcer, gastric hyperacidity, upset stomach associated with hyperacidity. Magnesium oxide is indicated for magnesium deficiency or depletion caused by malnutrition, restricted diet, alcoholism, or magnesium-depleting drugs.

Contraindications and precautions

• Contraindicated in hypersensitivity to drug, renal calculi, hypercalcemia, and hypophosphatemia
• Use cautiously in renal impairment, chronic pain syndrome, recent massive GI hemorrhage, and pregnant patients.

Adverse reactions

CNS: aluminum toxicity, encephalopathy (aluminum-containing antacids)
GI: diarrhea (magnesium-containing antacids); constipation, possibly leading to intestinal obstruction (aluminum-containing antacids)
Metabolic: dose-dependent rebound hyperacidity; milk-alkali syndrome; hypermagnesemia in renal failure patients (magnesium-containing antacids); hypophosphatemia, aluminum accumulation in blood (aluminum-containing antacids)
Musculoskeletal: osteomalacia, aluminum accumulation in bone (aluminum-containing antacids)

Patient monitoring

• Assess for constipation.
• Monitor serum electrolyte levels as appropriate.

anti-Alzheimer's agents

donepezil hydrochloride, galantamine hydrobromide, memantine, rivastigmine tartrate, tacrine hydrochloride

Action

Reversibly inhibit acetylcholinesterase hydrolysis in CNS, which increases acetylcholine level and promotes nerve impulse transmission. Unlike donepezil, galantamine, and rivastigmine, memantine binds preferentially to cation channels operated by *N*-methyl-D-aspartate and doesn't affect reversible acetylcholinesterase inhibition.

Indications

Mild to moderate Alzheimer's disease, moderate to severe Alzheimer's disease (memantine only)

Contraindications and precautions

• Contraindicated in hypersensitivity to drug, piperidine derivatives, or acridines; angle-closure glaucoma; undiagnosed skin lesions; and jaundice with previous use of these drugs

• Use cautiously in moderate to severe renal or hepatic dysfunction, GI bleeding, seizures, cardiovascular disease, sick sinus syndrome, asthma or chronic obstructive pulmonary disease, impaired urinary outflow, diabetes mellitus, obesity, history of ulcer, postmenopausal patients, elderly patients, pregnant or breastfeeding patients, and children.

Adverse reactions

CNS: tremor, confusion, insomnia, psychosis, hallucinations, depression, dizziness, headache, anxiety, nervousness, drowsiness, fatigue, abnormal dreams, irritability, paresthesia, aggression, vertigo, ataxia, restlessness, abnormal crying, syncope, aphasia, **seizures**
CV: chest pain, hypotension, hypertension, peripheral edema, vasodilation, **atrial fibrillation**
EENT: cataract, blurred vision, eye irritation, rhinitis, pharyngitis, sore throat
GI: nausea, vomiting, diarrhea, constipation, abdominal pain, flatulence, eructation, anorexia
GU: urinary tract infection, urinary frequency or incontinence, increased libido
Metabolic: dehydration, hot flashes
Musculoskeletal: back and joint pain, bone fracture, muscle cramps, arthritis
Respiratory: upper respiratory infection, cough, bronchitis, dyspnea, influenza
Skin: rash, pruritus, urticaria, diaphoresis, flushing
Other: toothache, weight loss, pain, accidental trauma, flulike symptoms

Patient monitoring

• Assess for severe nausea, vomiting, and diarrhea (which may lead to dehydration and weight loss).
Watch closely for adverse reactions in patients with a history of GI bleeding, arrhythmias, seizures, pulmonary conditions, or use of nonsteroidal anti-inflammatory drugs.
• Monitor alanine aminotransferase level weekly during first 18 weeks of therapy.

antiarrhythmics

acebutolol hydrochloride, adenosine, amiodarone hydrochloride, bretylium tosylate, digoxin, disopyramide phosphate, dofetilide, esmolol, flecainide acetate, ibutilide fumarate, lidocaine hydrochloride, mexiletine, moricizine hydrochloride, phenytoin, phenytoin sodium, procainamide hydrochloride, propafenone hydrochloride, propranolol hydrochloride, quinidine gluconate, quinidine sulfate, sotalol hydrochloride, tocainide hydrochloride, verapamil hydrochloride

Action

Varies with classification and subdivision (which are based on drug's action on cardiac muscle). *Class I* antiarrhythmics decrease rate of sodium entry during depolarization, reduce rate of action potential, and lengthen effective refractory period of fast-response fibers. Class I antiarrhythmics fall into three subdivisions. *Class IA* drugs (such as disopyramide, procainamide, and quinidine) depress phase 0 and lengthen the action potential. *Class IB* drugs (such as lidocaine, phenytoin, and tocainide) somewhat depress phase 0 and shorten the action potential. *Class IC* drugs (such as flecainide and propafenone) greatly depress phase 0 and slow conduction. Moricizine shares properties of class IA, IB, and IC antiarrhythmics.

Class II antiarrhythmics (such as propranolol) competitively block beta-adrenergic receptors and depress phase 4 depolarization.

Class III antiarrhythmics (such as amiodarone, bretylium, dofetilide, ibutilide, and sotalol) prolong duration of the action potential but don't affect polarization phase or resting membrane potential.

Class IV antiarrhythmics (calcium channel blockers such as verapamil) slow conduction velocity and increase atrioventricular (AV) node refractoriness.

Indications

Arrhythmias, premature ventricular tachycardia, atrial flutter, atrial fibrillation, AV heart block

Contraindications and precautions

• Contraindicated in hypersensitivity to drug, congenital or acquired long-QT syndrome, baseline QT or QTc interval greater than 440 msec, sick sinus syndrome, second- or third-degree AV block (unless patient has an artificial pacemaker), systolic pressure below 90 mm Hg, recent myocardial infarction or pulmonary congestion, pulmonary hypertension, aortic stenosis, severe renal impairment, digoxin toxicity, pregnancy, breastfeeding, and neonates

• Use cautiously in mild to moderate renal or hepatic impairment, enlarged prostate, myasthenia gravis, glaucoma, diabetes mellitus, potassium imbalance, conduction abnormalities, ventricular tachycardia, ventricular arrhythmias, history of serious ventricular arrhythmias or heart failure, elderly patients, and children (safety not established).

Adverse reactions

CNS: dizziness, light-headedness, agitation, jitteriness, anxiety, depression, fatigue, drowsiness, headache, syncope, malaise, involuntary movements, ataxia, paresthesia, peripheral neuropathy, incoordination, tremor, abnormal dreams, insomnia, confusion, acute psychosis, psychiatric disturbances
CV: chest pain, palpitations, peripheral edema, bradycardia, tachycardia, **hypotension,** development or worsening of **arrhythmias, heart failure, heart block**
EENT: blurred vision, angle-closure glaucoma, corneal microdeposits, optic neuritis or neuropathy, photophobia, dry eyes, tinnitus, disturbed equilibrium, epistaxis, dry nose, altered smell perception
GI: nausea, vomiting, diarrhea, constipation, abdominal pain, bloating, flatulence, dry mouth, anorexia
GU: dysuria, nocturia, polyuria, urinary hesitancy, urinary retention, erectile or other sexual dysfunction, decreased libido, epididymitis
Hematologic: anemia, **leukopenia, thrombocytopenia, agranulocytosis**
Hepatic: jaundice, **hepatic dysfunction**
Metabolic: hypokalemia, hypothyroidism, hyperthyroidism, **hypoglycemia**
Musculoskeletal: muscle weakness, aches, or cramps; joint stiffness
Respiratory: cough, dyspnea, pneumonia, **pulmonary fibrosis, adult respiratory distress syndrome**
Skin: bluish skin discoloration, rash, dermatosis, pruritus, alopecia, flushing, photosensitivity, toxic epidermal necrolysis, **Stevens-Johnson syndrome**
Other: gingival hyperplasia, edema, weight gain

Patient monitoring

• Monitor antiarrhythmic blood level.
• Assess blood pressure and pulse. Report heart rate below 50 or above 120 beats/minute.
• Monitor blood glucose and electrolyte levels and liver and kidney function tests.

Closely monitor extent of palpitations. Stay alert for fluttering or missed heartbeats, chest pain, and fainting episodes. Obtain ECG to document arrhythmias.

anticholinergics

atropine sulfate, benztropine mesylate, biperiden, dicyclomine hydrochloride, dimenhydrinate, glycopyrrolate, hyoscyamine, hyoscyamine sulfate, ipratropium bromide, meclizine hydrochloride, oxybutynin chloride, propantheline bromide, scopolamine hydrobromide, trihexyphenidyl hydrochloride, trimethobenzamide hydrochloride, tolterodine tartrate

Action

Block acetylcholine action in CNS and on autonomic effectors; also block vagal effects on sinoatrial and atrioventricular nodes, causing heart rate to increase. Small doses decrease salivary and bronchial secretions and reduce sweating; intermediate doses dilate pupils, inhibit accommodation, and increase heart rate; large doses decrease GI and GU motility; even higher doses reduce gastric acid secretion.

Indications

Bradyarrhythmias, symptomatic bradycardia, heart block caused by vagal activity, peptic ulcer disease, pylorospasm, small-intestine hypertoxicity, colonic hypermotility, mild dysentery, diverticulitis, bronchospasm, spastic or overactive bladder, cystitis, infant colic, biliary or renal colic, pancreatitis, acute iritis, acute rhinitis, sialorrhea, hyperhidrosis, anticholinesterase poisoning, nausea, vomiting, dizziness, motion sickness, drug-induced extrapyramidal disorders, parkinsonism, adjunct for Parkinson's disease. Also used for cycloplegic refraction, to control gastric secretions and block cardiac vagal reflexes preoperatively, to promote diagnostic hypotonic duodenography, and to increase radiologic visibility of kidney.

Contraindications and precautions

- Contraindicated in hypersensitivity to drug, GI or GU tract obstruction, reflux esophagitis, severe ulcerative colitis, glaucoma, myasthenia gravis, intestinal atony, unstable cardiovascular status in acute hemorrhage, arrhythmias, tachycardia caused by cardiac insufficiency or thyrotoxicosis, toxic megacolon, GI infection, severe prostatic hypertrophy, bladder neck obstruction, bronchial asthma, chronic obstructive pulmonary disease, breastfeeding, and infants less than 6 months old
- Use cautiously in alcohol, sulfite, or tartrazine intolerance; high environmental temperatures; hepatic or renal impairment; autonomic neuropathy; mild to moderate prostatic hypertrophy; hyperthyroidism; coronary disease; heart failure; hypertension; hiatal hernia; ulcerative colitis; brain damage; Down syndrome; spasticity; phenylketonuria; elderly patients; pregnant patients (safety not established); neonates; and immature infants.

Adverse reactions

CNS: asthenia, nervousness, stimulation, insomnia, drowsiness, dizziness, headache, confusion
CV: palpitations, tachycardia
EENT: increased intraocular pressure, dilated pupils, blurred vision, photophobia
GI: nausea, vomiting, constipation, abdominal distention, epigastric distress, heartburn, gastroesophageal reflux, dry mouth, **paralytic ileus**

GU: urinary hesitancy or retention, erectile dysfunction, lactation suppression
Skin: urticaria, decreased diaphoresis
Other: taste loss, fever, irritation at I.M. injection site, allergic reaction, **anaphylaxis**

Patient monitoring

- Closely monitor vital signs and urine output.

anticoagulants

argatroban, bivalirudin, dalteparin sodium, danaparoid sodium, enoxaparin sodium, fondaparinux sodium, heparin calcium, heparin sodium, lepirudin, tinzaparin sodium, warfarin sodium

Action

Interfere with one or more parts of the pathways that lead to stable fibrin clot formation. May inhibit coagulation factors, bind to antithrombin, cause release of tissue factor pathway inhibitors, and prevent conversion of fibrinogen to fibrin.

Indications

Treatment or prophylaxis of venous thrombosis, pulmonary embolism, atrial fibrillation with embolization, myocardial infarction, or thromboembolic events (including deep-vein thrombosis); during cardiovascular surgery; prevention of thrombus formation and embolization after prosthetic valve placement; after abdominal surgery or total hip or knee replacement surgery

Contraindications and precautions

- Contraindicated in hypersensitivity to drug, uncontrolled or active major bleeding, or thrombocytopenia caused by antiplatelet antibodies associated with low-molecular-weight heparins
- Use cautiously in severe hepatic or renal disease; hypertensive or diabetic retinopathy; untreated or severe uncontrolled hypertension; hemorrhagic stroke; severe thrombocytopenia; active GI bleeding or ulcers or recent history of ulcer disease; cancer; bacterial endocarditis; history of congenital or acquired bleeding disorder; recent brain, spinal, or ophthalmic surgery; spinal or epidural anesthesia; patients weighing less than 45 kg (99 lb); elderly patients; pregnant or breastfeeding patients; and children (safety not established).

Adverse reactions

CNS: headache, dizziness, insomnia, confusion, **spinal hematoma, cerebral or intracranial bleeding**
CV: hypotension, hypertension, angina pectoris, tachycardia, **arrhythmias, pulmonary embolism, thromboembolism, myocardial infarction**
EENT: ocular hemorrhage, rhinitis, epistaxis
GI: nausea, vomiting, constipation, dyspepsia, hematemesis, anorectal bleeding, melena, flatulence, **retroperitoneal or intra-abdominal bleeding, GI hemorrhage**
GU: dysuria, hematuria, urinary tract infection, urinary retention, **vaginal hemorrhage**
Hematologic: purpura, anemia, **granulocytopenia, thrombocytopenia, agranulocytosis, pancytopenia, hemorrhage**
Hepatic: hepatitis
Musculoskeletal: back pain
Respiratory: dyspnea, pneumonia, respiratory disorder
Skin: rash, pruritus, bullous eruption, skin necrosis, urticaria, cellulitis, injection site or wound hematoma, alopecia
Other: fever, pain, infection, dependent edema, impaired healing, hyper-

sensitivity reaction, **congenital anomalies, fetal distress, fetal death**

Patient monitoring

🔊 Watch for tarry stools and unusual bleeding or bruising.

- Assess baseline coagulation tests and CBC with white cell differential.
- Monitor venipuncture sites for bleeding, hematoma, and inflammation.

anticonvulsants

carbamazepine, clonazepam, clorazepate dipotassium, diazepam, divalproex sodium, fosphenytoin sodium, gabapentin, lamotrigine, levetiracetam, magnesium sulfate, oxcarbazepine, pentobarbital, phenobarbital sodium, phenytoin, phenytoin sodium, primidone, tiagabine hydrochloride, topiramate, valproate sodium, valproic acid, zonisamide

Action

Selectively depress hyperactive brain areas responsible for seizures

Indications

Prophylaxis and treatment of status epilepticus and generalized tonic-clonic, mixed, petit mal, petit mal variant, akinetic, complex-partial, and myoclonic seizures; management of panic disorder, trigeminal neuralgia, migraine, anxiety, psychoneurotic reactions, and alcohol withdrawal; skeletal muscle relaxation for endoscopy or cardioversion

Contraindications and precautions

- Contraindicated in hypersensitivity to drug or intolerance of alcohol, propylene glycol, tartrazine, or tricyclic antidepressants; bone marrow depression; severe hepatic disease; and MAO inhibitor use within past 14 days
- Use cautiously in mild to moderate hepatic or renal disease, severe cardiac or respiratory disease, acute or chronic pain, fever, hyperthyroidism, diabetes mellitus, severe anemia, uremia, angle-closure glaucoma, coma, CNS depression, sinus bradycardia, sinoatrial block, second- or third-degree heart block, Stokes-Adams syndrome, obesity, history of suicide attempt or drug abuse, elderly or debilitated patients, and pregnant or breastfeeding patients.

Adverse reactions

CNS: dizziness, light-headedness, syncope, drowsiness, lethargy, sedation, depression, apathy, fatigue, disorientation, anger, hostility, mania or hypomania, restlessness, confusion, crying, delirium, headache, slurred speech, dysarthria, stupor, rigidity, tremor, dystonia, vertigo, euphoria, nervousness, poor concentration, vivid dreams, psychomotor retardation, paresthesia, extrapyramidal symptoms, mild paradoxical stimulation (first 2 weeks of therapy)
CV: hypertension, hypotension, palpitations, bradycardia, tachycardia, aggravation of coronary artery disease, **cardiovascular collapse, heart failure, arrhythmias**
EENT: blurred vision, diplopia, corneal opacities, nystagmus and other abnormal eye movements, conjunctivitis
GI: nausea, vomiting, diarrhea, constipation, abdominal pain, dysphagia, gastric disorders, stomatitis, glossitis, dry mouth, increased salivation, pharyngeal dryness, anorexia
GU: urinary hesitancy, retention, frequency, or incontinence; albuminuria; glycosuria; dysuria; nocturia; menstrual irregularities; libido changes; erectile dysfunction; gynecomastia
Hematologic: eosinophilia, **leukopenia, agranulocytosis, aplastic anemia, thrombocytopenia**

Hepatic: hepatitis
Metabolic: syndrome of inappropriate antidiuretic hormone secretion
Musculoskeletal: muscle rigidity
Respiratory: pneumonitis
Skin: photosensitivity, rash, urticaria, diaphoresis, **erythema multiforme, Stevens-Johnson syndrome**
Other: chills, fever, hiccups, weight changes, edema, lymphadenopathy, physical and psychological drug dependence, drug tolerance

Patient monitoring

- Monitor CBC, glucose and uric acid levels, urinalysis, and kidney and liver function tests.

[Clinical alert] With I.V. use, watch closely for respiratory depression and cardiovascular collapse.

- Monitor for sore throat, easy bruising and bleeding, and epistaxis.
- Stay alert for oversedation.

antidepressants

amitriptyline hydrochloride, amoxapine, bupropion hydrochloride, citalopram hydrobromide, clomipramine hydrochloride, desipramine hydrochloride, doxepin hydrochloride, duloxetine hydrochloride, escitalopram oxalate, fluoxetine hydrochloride, fluvoxamine maleate, imipramine pamoate, mirtazapine, nefazodone hydrochloride, nortriptyline hydrochloride, paroxetine hydrochloride, phenelzine, sertraline hydrochloride, tranylcypromine sulfate, trazodone hydrochloride, trimipramine maleate, venlafaxine hydrochloride

Action

Produce changes in serotonin or norepinephrine receptor systems; inhibit neuronal serotonin, norepinephrine, or dopamine reuptake

Indications

Endogenous or reactive depression, including depression associated with anxiety and sleep disturbances

Contraindications and precautions

- Contraindicated in hypersensitivity to drug
- Use cautiously in cardiovascular disease; hypertension; hepatic or renal impairment; severe depression; increased intraocular pressure; angle-closure glaucoma; hyperthyroidism; prostatic hypertrophy; acute recovery phase after myocardial infarction (MI); electroshock therapy; elective surgery; suicidal tendency; history of seizures, neurologic impairment, mania, or drug abuse; pregnant or breastfeeding patients; and children younger than age 18.

Adverse reactions

CNS: lethargy, sedation, hallucinations, delusions, disorientation, anxiety, nervousness, EEG changes, fatigue, peripheral neuropathy, insomnia, restlessness, drowsiness, dizziness, syncope, extrapyramidal effects, **neuroleptic malignant syndrome, seizures, coma, cerebrovascular accident** (CVA)
CV: hypotension, hypertension, ECG changes, tachycardia, palpitations, chest pain, **arrhythmias, MI**
EENT: visual disturbances, blurred vision, mydriasis, increased intraocular pressure, dry eyes, tinnitus, rhinitis
GI: nausea, vomiting, diarrhea, constipation, epigastric or abdominal pain, dyspepsia, dry mouth, anorexia, **paralytic ileus**
GU: urinary frequency or retention, gynecomastia, sexual dysfunction
Hematologic: leukopenia, agranulocytosis, thrombocytopenia
Hepatic: hepatitis

Metabolic: blood glucose changes
Skin: rash, urticaria, diaphoresis, bruising, pruritus, photosensitivity
Other: altered taste, increased appetite, weight changes, edema, chills, yawning, hypersensitivity reaction

Patient monitoring

- Monitor CBC, blood glucose level, and kidney and liver function tests.

🔊 Assess ECG and heart sounds. Watch for tachycardia and more frequent angina attacks (which may precede MI or CVA).

- Evaluate neurologic function.
- Watch for sleep disturbances, lethargy, apathy, impaired thought processes, and poor therapeutic response.
- Check results of periodic eye exams. Report vision changes, perception of halos, eye pain, dilated pupils, headache, and nausea.

antidiabetic drugs (hypoglycemics)

acarbose, chlorpropamide, diazoxide, glimepiride, glipizide, glyburide, insulins, metformin hydrochloride, miglitol, nateglinide, pioglitazone hydrochloride, repaglinide, rosiglitazone maleate, tolazamide, tolbutamide sodium

Action

Bind to plasma membrane of functional pancreatic beta cells, decreasing potassium permeability and membrane depolarization. These effects increase intracellular calcium transport and enhance release of secretory granules containing insulin.

Insulins promote glucose transport and stimulate carbohydrate metabolism, which inhibits the release of free fatty acids and stimulates protein metabolism and synthesis.

Indications

Type 1 (insulin-dependent) or type 2 (non-insulin-dependent) diabetes mellitus

Contraindications and precautions

- Contraindicated in hypersensitivity to drug and in diabetes mellitus complicated by ketoacidosis
- Use cautiously in severe cardiovascular, hepatic, or renal disease; heart failure; intestinal disorders; thyroid, pituitary, or adrenal dysfunction; malnutrition; high fever; prolonged nausea or vomiting; dehydration; hypoxemia; excessive alcohol ingestion (acute or chronic); elderly patients; and pregnant or breastfeeding patients.

Adverse reactions

CNS: lethargy, sedation, hallucinations, delusions, disorientation, peripheral neuropathy, EEG changes, nervousness, restlessness, anxiety, fatigue, insomnia, drowsiness, dizziness, syncope, asthenia, extrapyramidal effects, **neuroleptic malignant syndrome, seizures, coma, cerebrovascular accident**
CV: hypotension, hypertension, ECG changes, tachycardia, palpitations, chest pain, **arrhythmias, myocardial infarction**
EENT: blurred vision, visual disturbances, mydriasis, dry eyes, increased intraocular pressure, tinnitus, rhinitis
GI: nausea, vomiting, diarrhea, constipation, epigastric or abdominal pain, dyspepsia, dry mouth, anorexia, **paralytic ileus**
GU: urinary frequency or retention, gynecomastia, sexual dysfunction
Hematologic: leukopenia, agranulocytosis, thrombocytopenia
Hepatic: hepatitis
Metabolic: hypokalemia, sodium retention, blood glucose changes, **hypoglycemia**

Skin: rash, urticaria, pruritus, diaphoresis, bruising, photosensitivity
Other: altered taste, increased appetite, weight changes, edema, chills, yawning, hypersensitivity reaction, injection site reaction

Patient monitoring
- Monitor blood glucose level, especially during times of increased stress (such as infection, fever, surgery, and trauma).
- Assess weight and nutritional status.
- Evaluate liver and kidney function tests.

antiemetics

5-HT_3 receptor antagonists: dolasetron mesylate, granisetron hydrochloride, ondansetron hydrochloride, palonosetron hydrochloride

Anticholinergics: dimenhydrinate, diphenhydramine hydrochloride, meclizine hydrochloride, trimethobenzamide hydrochloride

Antidopaminergics: chlorpromazine hydrochloride, metoclopramide hydrochloride, perphenazine, prochlorperazine, promethazine hydrochloride

Other: aprepitant, dronabinol

Action
Block activity of central neurotransmitters, dopamine in chemoreceptor trigger zone, acetylcholine in vomiting center, or 5-HT_3 receptors on vagal neurons in GI tract

Indications
Prevention of nausea and vomiting caused by chemotherapy or radiation therapy, prevention or treatment of postoperative nausea or vomiting

Contraindications and precautions
- 5-HT_3 receptor antagonists are contraindicated in hypersensitivity to drug. Antidopaminergics are contraindicated in coma and drug- or alcohol-induced CNS depression.
- Use cautiously in hepatic disease; premature infants (if drug contains benzyl alcohol); or sulfite or tartrazine sensitivity (if drug contains sulfite or tartrazine). Also use cautiously in patients who have or may develop prolonged conduction intervals, especially marked QTc prolongation.

Adverse reactions
CNS: anxiety, agitation, confusion, asthenia, dizziness, drowsiness, sedation, headache, malaise, fatigue, weakness, pain, vertigo, paresthesia, tremor, sleep disorder, depersonalization, ataxia, twitching, extrapyramidal syndrome
CV: hypertension, hypotension, angina, syncope, bradycardia, tachycardia, **arrhythmias, Mobitz I heart block**
EENT: epistaxis
GI: nausea, vomiting, diarrhea, constipation, dyspepsia, abdominal pain, dry mouth, anorexia
GU: hematuria, dysuria, polyuria, urinary retention, **oliguria**
Hematologic: anemia, purpura, hematoma, **leukopenia, thrombocytopenia**
Respiratory: hypoxia
Skin: rash, flushing, increased diaphoresis, pruritus
Other: altered taste, fever, chills, cold sensation, edema, facial or peripheral edema, injection site reaction, **anaphylaxis**

Patient monitoring
- Monitor CBC, liver function tests, and ECG changes.

🔊 Stay alert for prolonged PR interval and widened QRS complexes, especially in patients receiving concurrent antiarrhythmics.

• Watch for excessive diuresis.
• When giving antidopaminergics, monitor for signs and symptoms of neuroleptic malignant syndrome.

antifungals

amphotericin B, caspofungin acetate, fluconazole, flucytosine, griseofulvin, itraconazole, ketoconazole, miconazole, nystatin, terbinafine hydrochloride, voriconazole

Action

Varies with specific drug. See individual monographs.

Indications

Meningitis, visceral leishmaniasis in immunocompetent patients, invasive fungal infections, systemic fungal infections (histoplasmosis, coccidioidomycosis, blastomycosis, cryptococcosis, phycomycosis, disseminated candidiasis, zygomycosis), oral and perioral candidal infections, GI tract infections caused by *Candida albicans*

Contraindications and precautions

• Contraindicated in hypersensitivity to antifungals and concurrent use of cisapride or pimozide
• Use cautiously in renal, hepatic, or cardiac disease; achlorhydria; pregnant or breastfeeding patients; and children younger than age 2.

Adverse reactions

CNS: anxiety, confusion, headache, insomnia, asthenia, abnormal thinking, agitation, depression, dizziness, hallucinations, hypertonia, vertigo, psychosis, drowsiness, speech disorder, malaise, **stupor, seizures**
CV: chest pain, vasodilation, hypotension, orthostatic hypotension, hypertension, phlebitis, tachycardia, bradycardia, **supraventricular tachycardia, cardiac arrest, asystole, atrial fibrillation, shock**
EENT: diplopia, amblyopia, blurred vision, eye hemorrhage, hearing loss, tinnitus, epistaxis, rhinitis, sinusitis, pharyngitis
GI: nausea, vomiting, diarrhea, abdominal pain, abdominal distention, melena, stomatitis, dry mouth, oral candidiasis, anorexia, **GI hemorrhage**
GU: dysuria, hematuria, albuminuria, glycosuria, urinary retention or incontinence, **oliguria, renal failure, abnormal renal function with hypokalemia**
Hematologic: anemia, eosinophilia, **leukocytosis, thrombocytopenia, leukopenia, agranulocytosis**
Hepatic: jaundice, **acute hepatic failure, hepatitis**
Metabolic: dehydration, hypomagnesemia, hypokalemia, hypocalcemia, hypernatremia, hyperglycemia, hypoproteinemia, hyperlipidemia, **acidosis**
Musculoskeletal: myalgia; joint, neck, or back pain
Respiratory: increased cough, wheezing, dyspnea, tachypnea, hypoxia, hyperventilation, hemoptysis, asthma, **pulmonary edema, pleural effusion, bronchospasm, respiratory failure**
Skin: pruritus, acne, alopecia, diaphoresis, skin discoloration, nodules, ulcers, urticaria, maculopapular rash
Other: gingivitis, weight changes, chills, fever, infection, peripheral or facial edema, pain or reaction at injection site, tissue damage (with extravasation), allergic reactions including **anaphylaxis, sepsis, multisystem failure**

Patient monitoring

• Monitor vital signs and fluid intake and output.
• Assess electrolyte levels, CBC, and kidney and liver function tests.

antigout agents (antihyperuricemia agents)

allopurinol, colchicine, probenecid, rasburicase

Action

Decrease uric acid levels by inhibiting uric acid production or tubular reabsorption of urate or by catalyzing enzymatic oxidation of uric acid into allantoin (an inactive and soluble metabolite)

Indications

Primary or secondary gout, calcium oxalate calculi, management of uric acid levels during chemotherapy

Contraindications and precautions

- Contraindicated in hypersensitivity to drug, blood dyscrasias, or methemoglobinemia and G6PD deficiency
- Use cautiously in acute gout attack during initiation of therapy, bone marrow depression, renal or hepatic disease, cardiac disease, idiopathic hemochromatosis, seizure disorders, peptic ulcer, and children (except those with cancer-related hyperuricemia).

Adverse reactions

CNS: headache, somnolence, peripheral neuropathy, neuritis, paresthesia
CV: vasculitis, **necrotizing angiitis**
EENT: epistaxis
GI: nausea, vomiting, diarrhea, abdominal pain, gastritis, dyspepsia
GU: uremia, **renal failure**
Hematologic: ecchymosis, purpura, eosinophilia, **leukopenia, leukocytosis, thrombocytopenia**
Hepatic: cholestatic jaundice, **hepatomegaly, granulomatous hepatitis, hepatic necrosis**
Metabolic: acute gout attack
Musculoskeletal: arthralgia, myopathy
Skin: rash, vesicular bullous dermatitis, eczematoid dermatitis, pruritus, urticaria, onycholysis, lichen planus, alopecia, purpura, toxic epidermal necrolysis, **Stevens-Johnson syndrome**
Other: taste loss or perversion, fever, hypersensitivity reaction

Patient monitoring

- Assess fluid intake and output. Intake should be sufficient to yield daily output of at least 2 liters of slightly alkaline urine.
- Monitor uric acid level.

antihistamines

brompheniramine, cetirizine hydrochloride, chlorpheniramine maleate, cyproheptadine hydrochloride, desloratadine, diphenhydramine hydrochloride, fexofenadine hydrochloride, hydroxyzine hydrochloride, hydroxyzine pamoate, loratadine, promethazine

Action

Bind either nonselectively to central and peripheral histamine$_1$ (H_1) receptors or selectively to peripheral H_1 receptors, causing either CNS stimulation or depression

Indications

Sedation, nausea and vomiting, cough, parkinsonian symptoms, motion sickness, allergy symptoms, adjunct to pre- or postoperative analgesia

Contraindications and precautions

- Contraindicated in hypersensitivity to specific or structurally related antihistamines, angle-closure glaucoma, stenosing peptic ulcer, symptomatic prostatic hypertrophy, bladder neck

obstruction, pyloroduodenal obstruction, MAO inhibitor use within past 14 days, elderly or debilitated patients (cyproheptadine), premature infants, and neonates
• Use cautiously in respiratory or cardiovascular disease, seizure disorders, ulcer disease, sleep apnea, renal or hepatic impairment, elderly patients, pregnant or breastfeeding patients, and children.

Adverse reactions

CNS: drowsiness, sedation, weakness, dizziness, syncope, incoordination, fatigue, lassitude, confusion, restlessness, excitation, euphoria, tremor, headache, insomnia, nightmares, paresthesia, catatonic-like state, hallucinations, disorientation, pseudoschizophrenia, vertigo, hysteria, tongue protrusion, neuritis, **seizures**
CV: orthostatic hypotension, hypotension, hypertension, palpitations, bradycardia, tachycardia, reflex tachycardia, extrasystoles, ECG changes, venous thrombosis at injection site (with I.V. promethazine), **cardiac arrest**
EENT: blurred vision; diplopia; oculogyric crisis; tinnitus; labyrinthitis; nasal stuffiness; dry mouth, nose, and throat; sore throat; **laryngeal edema**
GI: nausea, vomiting, diarrhea, constipation, epigastric distress, stomatitis, anorexia
GU: dysuria, glycosuria, urinary frequency, urinary retention, lactation, early menses, gynecomastia, inhibited ejaculation
Hematologic: thrombocytopenic purpura; hemolytic, hypoplastic, or aplastic anemia; thrombocytopenia; leukopenia; agranulocytosis; pancytopenia
Musculoskeletal: torticollis; tingling, heaviness, and weakness of hands
Respiratory: thickened bronchial secretions, chest tightness, wheezing, asthma, **respiratory depression**
Skin: rash, dermatitis, erythema, urticaria, excessive perspiration, angioedema, photosensitivity
Other: appetite increase, weight gain, peripheral edema, chills, **lupus erythematosus–like syndrome, anaphylaxis**

Patient monitoring

• Monitor cardiovascular status, especially in patients with cardiovascular disease.
• Use side rails as needed. Supervise patient during ambulation.

antihyperlipidemics

Bile acid suppressants: cholestyramine, colesevelam hydrochloride, colestipol hydrochloride

Fibric acid derivatives: fenofibrate, gemfibrozil

HMG-CoA reductase inhibitors: atorvastatin calcium, fluvastatin sodium, lovastatin, pravastatin sodium, rosuvastatin, simvastatin

Other: ezetimibe, niacin

Action

Bile acid suppressants bind bile acids in intestine to form an insoluble complex that's excreted in feces; increased fecal loss of bile acids enhances cholesterol oxidation to bile acids, which lowers low-density lipoprotein (LDL) and cholesterol levels. *Fibric acid derivatives* inhibit peripheral lipolysis and decrease hepatic extraction of free fatty acids, reducing hepatic triglyceride production. They also inhibit synthesis and increase clearance of apolipoprotein B (which carries very-low-density lipoproteins [VLDLs]), thus lowering VLDL production. *HMG-CoA reductase inhibitors* competitively inhibit HMG-CoA reductase (an enzyme that catalyzes the first step in cholesterol synthesis pathway); this inhibition decreases total cholesterol, LDL, VLDL, triglyceride, and apolipoprotein B levels while increasing high-density lipoprotein levels.

Indications

Elevated LDL, total cholesterol, triglyceride, or apolipoprotein B levels in primary hypercholesterolemia or mixed dyslipidemia (Fredrickson types IIa and IIb); primary dysbetalipoproteinemia (Fredrickson type III); adjunct to diet in hypertriglyceridemia (Fredrickson type IV)

Contraindications and precautions

- Contraindicated in hypersensitivity to drug; active hepatic disease; complete biliary obstruction; persistent, unexplained elevations in liver function tests; pregnancy; and breastfeeding
- Use cautiously in severe metabolic, endocrine, or electrolyte disorders; visual disturbances; uncontrolled seizures; myopathy; cerebral arteriosclerosis; coronary artery disease; severe hypotension or hypertension; history of hepatic disease, alcoholism, renal impairment, severe acute infection, major surgery, or trauma; females of childbearing age; and children younger than age 18 (safety not established).

Adverse reactions

CNS: amnesia, abnormal dreams, malaise, asthenia, emotional lability, facial paralysis, headache, hyperkinesia, incoordination, paresthesia, drowsiness, syncope, peripheral neuropathy
CV: orthostatic hypotension, palpitations, vasodilation, phlebitis, **arrhythmias**
EENT: eye hemorrhage, amblyopia, glaucoma, altered refraction, dry eyes, hearing loss, tinnitus, epistaxis, sinusitis, pharyngitis
GI: nausea, vomiting, diarrhea, constipation, abdominal cramps, abdominal or biliary pain, dyspepsia, gastroenteritis, colitis, flatulence, melena, tenesmus, dysphagia, esophagitis, pancreatitis, dry mouth, stomatitis, glossitis, anorexia, **GI ulcers, rectal hemorrhage**
GU: dysuria, nocturia, hematuria, urinary frequency or urgency, urinary retention, cystitis, renal calculi, nephritis, abnormal ejaculation, decreased libido, epididymitis, erectile dysfunction
Hematologic: anemia, **thrombocytopenia**
Hepatic: jaundice, **hepatic failure, hepatitis**
Metabolic: gout, hyperglycemia, **hypoglycemia**
Musculoskeletal: joint or back pain, bursitis, leg cramps, neck rigidity, torticollis, myalgia, myositis, myasthenia gravis
Respiratory: dyspnea, pneumonia, bronchitis
Skin: diaphoresis, acne, pruritus, rash, urticaria, alopecia, contact dermatitis, eczema, dry skin, skin ulcers, seborrhea, photosensitivity
Other: gingival hemorrhage, taste loss, increased appetite, weight gain, flulike symptoms, infection, fever, allergic reaction

Patient monitoring

- Monitor liver function tests and blood lipid panel.

anti-infectives

Aminoglycosides: amikacin sulfate, gentamicin sulfate, kanamycin, neomycin sulfate, streptomycin sulfate, tobramycin sulfate

Carbapenems: ertapenem sodium, imipenem cilastatin, meropenem

Cephalosporins, first generation: cefadroxil, cefazolin sodium, cephalexin hydrochloride, cephradine

Cephalosporins, second generation: cefaclor, cefamandole, cefmetazole sodium, cefonicid sodium, cefotetan disodium, cefoxitin sodium, cefprozil, cefuroxime axetil, loracarbef

Cephalosporins, third generation: cefdinir, cefditoren pivoxil, cefepime hydrochloride, cefixime, cefoperazone sodium, cefotaxime sodium, cefpodoxime proxetil, ceftazidime, ceftibuten, ceftizoxime sodium, ceftriaxone sodium

Fluoroquinolones: ciprofloxacin, enoxacin, gatifloxacin, levofloxacin, lomefloxacin hydrochloride, moxifloxacin hydrochloride, nalidixic acid, norfloxacin, ofloxacin

Lincosamides: clindamycin hydrochloride, clindamycin palmitate hydrochloride, clindamycin phosphate

Macrolides: azithromycin, clarithromycin, dirithromycin, erythromycin

Monobactams: aztreonam

Penicillins: amoxicillin, amoxicillin trihydrate, amoxicillin and clavulanate potassium, ampicillin sodium, ampicillin sodium and sulbactam sodium, dicloxacillin sodium, nafcillin sodium, oxacillin sodium, penicillin G benzathine, penicillin G potassium, penicillin G procaine, penicillin V potassium, piperacillin sodium, piperacillin sodium and tazobactam sodium, ticarcillin disodium, ticarcillin disodium and clavulanate potassium

Streptogramins: quinupristin

Sulfonamides: sulfadiazine, sulfisoxazole, sulfasalazine, sulfinpyrazone, sulfisoxazole acetyl

Tetracyclines: demeclocyline hydrochloride, doxycycline, minocycline hydrochloride, tetracycline hydrochloride

Other: chloramphenicol, dapsone, linezolid, metronidazole, nitrofurantoin, pentamidine, vancomycin

Action

Bactericidal anti-infectives (aminoglycosides, cephalosporins, carbapenems, dapsone, fluoroquinolones, lincosamides, linezolid, macrolides and nitrofurantoin at high concentrations, metronidazole, monobactams, penicillins, quinupristin, and vancomycin) kill bacterial cells by inhibiting cell-wall synthesis of actively dividing bacterial cells via binding to one or more penicillin-bound proteins or 30S ribosomal subunits or via inhibition of DNA gyrase and topoisomerase IV.

Bacteriostatic anti-infectives (chloramphenicol, dapsone, linezolid [against enterococci and staphylococci only], macrolides and nitrofurantoin at low concentrations, quinupristin/dalfopristin [bacteriostatic against *Enterococcus faecium*], sulfonamides, telithromycin, and tetracyclines) inhibit bacterial cell growth or multiplication by giving the host immune system adequate time to mount a lethal response.

Indications

Vary with drug. See individual monographs.

Contraindications and precautions

- Contraindicated in hypersensitivity to drug. (For additional contraindications, see individual monographs.)
- Use cautiously in renal impairment, cirrhosis or other hepatic disease, neuromuscular disease, CNS disease, bradycardia, acute myocardial ischemia, parkinsonism, hearing impairment, dialysis patients, obese patients, elderly patients, pregnant or breastfeeding patients, neonates, and premature infants.

Adverse reactions

CNS: dizziness, vertigo, tremor, numbness, depression, confusion, lethargy, nystagmus, headache, paresthesia, **neuromuscular blockade, seizures, neurotoxicity**
CV: hypotension, hypertension, palpitations, phlebitis, **thrombophlebitis**
EENT: visual disturbances; eye stinging, redness, itching, or dryness; photophobia; tinnitus; hearing loss; ototoxicity; increased salivation; hoarseness (with tetracyclines)
GI: nausea, vomiting, diarrhea, abdominal cramps, stomatitis, oral candidiasis, black "hairy" tongue, anorexia, splenomegaly, **pseudomembranous colitis**
GU: polyuria, dysuria, azotemia, increased urinary cast excretion, erectile dysfunction, vaginal candidiasis, **nephrotoxicity, renal failure**
Hematologic: purpura, eosinophilia, lymphocytosis, **leukemoid reaction, hemolytic or aplastic anemia, neutropenia, agranulocytosis, leukopenia, thrombocytopenia, pancytopenia, hypoprothrombinemia, bone marrow depression**
Hepatic: hepatomegaly, hepatic necrosis
Metabolic: blood glucose changes
Musculoskeletal: joint pain, tendinitis, tendon rupture
Respiratory: dyspnea, apnea
Skin: rash, urticaria, pruritus, exfoliative dermatitis, alopecia, sterile abscess, **Stevens-Johnson syndrome**
Other: permanent tooth discoloration, tooth enamel defects, weight loss, superinfection, pain, irritation at I.M. injection site, induration, chills, fever, edema, **serum sickness, anaphylaxis**

Patient monitoring

- Monitor vital signs and fluid intake and output. Push fluids to help prevent renal tubular irritation.
- Monitor drug blood level.
- Watch for signs and symptoms of overgrowth of resistant organisms.
- Assess CBC and kidney function tests.
- Monitor International Normalized Ratio in prolonged therapy and in patients with malnutrition or high risk of renal or hepatic impairment.
- Assess for ototoxicity by comparing current and baseline audiograms.

antimalarials

chloroquine hydrochloride, chloroquine phosphate, dapsone, doxycycline, hydroxychloroquine sulfate, mefloquine hydrochloride, primaquine hydrochloride, pyrimethamine, quinine sulfate

Action

Varies. See individual monographs.

Indications

Prophylaxis or treatment of malaria

Contraindications and precautions

• Contraindicated for prophylactic use in severe renal insufficiency, marked hepatic parenchymal damage, or blood dyscrasias. Also contraindicated in hypersensitivity to drug, megaloblastic anemia caused by folate deficiency, depression (current or previous), generalized anxiety disorder, psychosis, schizophrenia or other major psychiatric disorder, history of seizures, pregnancy at term, breastfeeding, and infants younger than 2 months old.
• Use cautiously in hepatic dysfunction, cardiac disease, and ocular lesions.

Adverse reactions

CNS: headache, psychic stimulation, psychotic episodes, **seizures**
CV: hypotension, ECG changes, **cardiomyopathy**
EENT: irreversible retinal damage; visual disturbances; night blindness; scotomatous vision with field defects of paracentral and pericentral ring types and typically temporal scotomas
GI: vomiting, abdominal cramps, atrophic glossitis, anorexia
GU: hematuria
Hematologic: hemolytic or megaloblastic anemia, leukopenia, thrombocytopenia, pancytopenia, methemoglobinemia, agranulocytosis
Skin: pruritus, lichen planus–like eruptions, skin and mucosal pigment changes, pleomorphic skin eruptions, alopecia, toxic epidermal necrolysis, **erythema multiforme, Stevens-Johnson syndrome**
Other: hypersensitivity reactions including **anaphylaxis**

Patient monitoring

• Monitor liver function tests, CBC, and G6PD levels in susceptible patients before and periodically during therapy.

antimigraine drugs

Ergotamine derivatives: dihydroergotamine mesylate, ergotamine tartrate

Serotonin (5-hydroxytryptamine [5-HT$_1$]) receptor agonists: almotriptan malate, eletriptan, frovatriptan, naratriptan hydrochloride, rizatriptan hydrochloride, sumatriptan, topiramate, zolmitriptan

Action

Ergotamine derivatives exert partial agonist or antagonist activity against tryptaminergic, dopaminergic, and alpha-adrenergic receptors (depending on their site), causing peripheral and cranial vasoconstriction and depression of central vasomotor centers.

5-HT$_1$ receptor agonists activate serotonin 5-HT$_1$B/1D receptors, causing cranial vasoconstriction, inhibition of neuropeptide release, and reduced impulse transmission in trigeminal pain pathways.

Indications

Migraine

Contraindications and precautions

• Contraindicated in hypersensitivity to drug; hemiplegic or basilar migraine; ischemic heart or bowel disease; severe renal or hepatic impairment; Prinzmetal's angina or other significant underlying cardiovascular disease; uncontrolled hypertension; use of ergotamine-containing preparations, ergot-type drugs, or other 5-HT$_1$ agonists within past 24 hours; MAO inhibitor use within past 14 days; and I.V. use
• Use cautiously in hypertension, hypercholesterolemia, diabetes mellitus, cardiovascular disease, smoking, obesi-

ty, men older than age 40, menopausal women, pregnant or breastfeeding patients, and children younger than age 18.

Adverse reactions

CNS: dizziness, paresthesia, hypoesthesia, asthenia, drowsiness, somnolence, fatigue, headache, myasthenia, vertigo
CV: chest tightness, pressure, or heaviness
EENT: rhinitis, sinusitis, pharyngitis
GI: nausea; vomiting; diarrhea; abdominal pain or discomfort; stomach pain, cramps, or pressure; dyspepsia; dysphagia; dry mouth
Musculoskeletal: neck, throat, or jaw pain; stiffness
Other: altered taste, hot or cold sensations, hot flushes, application site reaction

Patient monitoring

- Monitor ECG for changes.

antineoplastics

Alkylating agents: busulfan, carboplatin, carmustine, chlorambucil, cisplatin, cyclophosphamide, dacarbazine, ifosfamide, lomustine, mechlorethamine hydrochloride, melphalan hydrochloride, oxaliplatin, procarbazine hydrochloride, streptozocin, temozolomide, thiotepa

Antibiotic antineoplastics: bleomycin, dactinomycin, daunorubicin hydrochloride, doxorubicin hydrochloride, epirubicin, idarubicin, mitomycin, mitoxantrone, plicamycin

Antimetabolites: capecitabine, cytarabine, floxuridine, fludarabine phosphate, fluorouracil, gemcitabine, mercaptopurine, methotrexate sodium, pentostatin

Antimitotics: docetaxel, paclitaxel, vinblastine, vincristine, vinorelbine

Biological antineoplastics: aldesleukin, alemtuzumab, denileukin diftitox, ibritumomab tiuxetan, interferon alfa-2a, interferon alfa-2b, rituximab, trastuzumab

Cytoprotective agents: amifostine, mesna

DNA topoisomerase inhibitors: irinotecan, topotecan

Enzyme antineoplastics: asparaginase, pegasparaginase

Epipodophyllotoxins: etoposide, teniposide

Hormonal antineoplastics: anastrozole, bicalutamide, exemestane, flutamide, fulvestrant, goserelin, letrozole, leuprolide, medroxyprogesterone acetate, megestrol, nilutamide, raloxifene, tamoxifen citrate, triptorelin pamoate

Other: arsenic trioxide, bexarotene, bortezomib, gefitinib, hydroxyurea, imatinib, porfimer, tretinoin

Action

Varies with specific drug. Generally, antineoplastics inhibit normal substrate use in tumor cells, forming dysfunctional macromolecules by inserting themselves into abnormal cells; also intercalate between DNA strands and interfere with DNA templates. Some antineoplastics modify growth of hormone-dependent tumors.

Indications

Hodgkin's or non-Hodgkin's lymphoma, testicular teratomas, mycosis fungoides, breast cancer, ovarian cancer, prostate cancer, lung cancer, head and neck cancer, colorectal cancer, pancreatic cancer, bronchogenic carcinoma, malignant melanoma, chronic lymphatic or chronic myeloid leukemia, other cancers

Contraindications and precautions

• Contraindicated in hypersensitivity to drug or its components
• Use cautiously in heart disease, renal or hepatic impairment, decreased bone marrow reserve, active infections, severe myocardial insufficiency, coagulation and bleeding disorders, active thrombophlebitis or thromboembolic disorders, shock, trauma, major surgery within previous month, elderly or debilitated patients, patients with childbearing potential, and pregnant or breastfeeding patients.

Adverse reactions

CNS: dizziness, fatigue, lethargy, asthenia, drowsiness, malaise, headache, sensory or motor dysfunction, impaired memory, confusion, agitation, depression, emotional lability, sleep disturbances, hallucinations, rigors, peripheral neuropathy, paresthesia, tremor, ataxia, flaccid paresis, abnormal gait, vertigo, syncope, cranial nerve dysfunction, hemiparesis, mental status changes, acute cerebellar dysfunction, **demyelinization, seizures, leukoencephalopathy, cerebrovascular accident, suicidal ideation**
CV: hypotension, hypertension, chest pain, peripheral edema, tachycardia, **cardiomegaly, prolonged QT interval, thromboembolic events, arrhythmias, cardiac tamponade, torsades de pointes, cardiac arrest, capillary leak syndrome, myocardial infarction, left-sided heart failure, pericardial effusion**
EENT: retinal thrombosis, corneal opacity, photophobia, diplopia, visual changes, nystagmus, lacrimation, lacrimal duct stenosis, stye, epistaxis, pharyngitis
GI: nausea, vomiting, diarrhea, constipation, fecal incontinence, abdominal pain, dyspepsia, GI ulcer, ascites, dry mouth, mucositis, oral candidiasis, dysphagia, anorexia, **intestinal perforation, paralytic ileus, GI bleeding**
GU: proteinuria, hematuria, dysuria, urinary hesitancy or retention, urinary obstruction, cystitis, bladder fibrosis, vaginitis, vaginal hemorrhage, breast swelling and tenderness, menstrual abnormalities, abortion, gynecomastia, sterility, libido loss, erectile dysfunction, decreased testes size, reduced sperm count, **progressive azotemia, hemolytic uremic syndrome, nephrotoxicity, oliguria or anuria, renal failure**
Hematologic: anemia, eosinophilia, **neutropenia, thrombocytopenia, leukopenia, leukocytosis, bone marrow depression, agranulocytosis, pancytopenia, coagulation disorders, hemorrhage**
Hepatic: jaundice, **hepatitis, hepatotoxicity**
Metabolic: hyperglycemia, fluid retention, **hyperkalemia**
Musculoskeletal: muscle twitching, joint or bone pain, decreased bone density, carpal tunnel syndrome
Respiratory: tachypnea, dyspnea, wheezing, pulmonary congestion, cough, chronic obstructive pulmonary disease, upper respiratory tract infection, **tracheoesophageal fistula, pleural effusion, interstitial pneumonitis, bronchospasm, pulmonary toxicity, pulmonary edema, respiratory failure, apnea, development or worsening of pulmonary fibrosis**
Skin: erythema, pruritus, rash, diaphoresis, night sweats, dry skin, urticaria, alopecia, phlebitis at I.V. site, palmar-plantar erythrodysesthesia, nail loss, bruising, petechiae, exacerbation of

postradiation erythema, painful plaque erosions, epidermal necrolysis, exfoliative dermatitis, **Stevens-Johnson syndrome**
Other: increased appetite, weight gain, fever, chills, pain, flulike symptoms, herpes simplex or other infection, tumor flare, hypersensitivity reaction, **risk of second malignancy, anaphylaxis, sepsis, tumor lysis syndrome**

Patient monitoring

Watch for bleeding. If platelet count is low, avoid giving I.M. injections and taking rectal temperature.
- Stay alert for bone marrow depression, neutropenia, and anemia.
- Monitor fluid intake and output.
- Monitor for GI upset. Give antiemetics as needed and prescribed.

antiparkinsonian drugs

Anticholinergics: benztropine, biperiden, trihexyphenidyl hydrochloride

Antivirals: amantadine hydrochloride

Dopaminergics: bromocriptine mesylate, carbidopa-levodopa, carbidopa-levodopa-entacapone, entacapone, levodopa, pergolide mesylate, pramipexole, ropinirole hydrochloride, tolcapone

MAO inhibitor: selegiline

Action

Block central cholinergic receptors or inhibit prolactin secretion; also may act as dopamine receptor agonists by activating postsynaptic dopamine receptors

Indications

Parkinson's disease

Contraindications and precautions

- Contraindicated in hypersensitivity to drug, angle-closure glaucoma, tardive dyskinesia, stenosing peptic ulcer, achalasia, pyloric or duodenal obstruction, prostatic hypertrophy, bladder neck obstruction, myasthenia gravis, and children younger than age 3
- Use cautiously in seizure disorders, arrhythmias, tachycardia, hypertension, hypotension, hepatic or renal dysfunction, alcoholism, exposure to hot environments, elderly patients, and pregnant or breastfeeding patients (safety not established).

Adverse reactions

CNS: confusion, headache, dizziness, fatigue, light-headedness, drowsiness, nervousness, insomnia, nightmares, mania, delusions, **seizures, cerebrovascular accident**
CV: hypotension, palpitations, extrasystole, bradycardia, **arrhythmias, acute myocardial infarction**
EENT: diplopia, blurred vision, burning sensation of eyes, nasal congestion
GI: nausea, vomiting, diarrhea, constipation, abdominal cramps, dry mouth, anorexia, **GI hemorrhage**
GU: urinary incontinence, frequency, or retention; diuresis; erectile dysfunction
Hepatic: hepatic failure
Musculoskeletal: leg cramps, numb fingers
Skin: urticaria; pale, cool fingers and toes; facial and arm rash; alopecia
Other: hyperthermia, **heat stroke**

Patient monitoring

- Monitor fluid intake and output and assess vital signs (especially blood pressure).

antiplatelet drugs

abciximab, anagrelide hydrochloride, cilostazol, clopidogrel bisulfate, dipyridamole, eptifibatide, ticlopidine hydrochloride, treprostinil sodium

Action

Inhibit platelet aggregation by reversibly preventing fibrinogen, von Willebrand's factor, and other adhesion ligands from binding to glycoprotein (GP) IIb/IIIa receptor or by inhibiting platelet fibrinogen induced by adenosine diphosphate

Indications

Acute coronary syndrome, cerebrovascular accident (CVA)

Contraindications and precautions

- Contraindicated in hypersensitivity to drug, CVA or abnormal bleeding within past 30 days, history of bleeding diathesis, history of hemorrhagic CVA, major surgery within past 6 weeks, concurrent or planned use of other parenteral GP IIb/IIIa inhibitors, dependence on renal dialysis, severe uncontrolled hypertension (systolic pressure above 200 mm Hg or diastolic pressure above 110 mm Hg), platelet count below 100,000/mm^3, or serum creatinine of 4 mg/dl or more
- Use cautiously in hemorrhagic retinopathy; severe renal insufficiency; chronic hemodialysis; hepatic failure; platelet count below 150,000/mm^3; hypotension, pulmonary edema, or pulmonary veno-occlusive disease (treprostinil); or concurrent use of thrombolytics or other drugs that affect hemostasis.

Adverse reactions

CNS: depression, somnolence, confusion, insomnia, nervousness, amnesia, migraine, dizziness, headache, **intracranial hemorrhage**
CV: chest pain, angina pectoris, orthostatic hypotension, hypertension, vasodilation, syncope, bradycardia, cardiovascular disease, **arrhythmias, thrombosis, aortic dissection, heart failure**
EENT: amblyopia, abnormal vision, visual field abnormality, diplopia, tinnitus, epistaxis, rhinitis, sinusitis
GI: nausea, diarrhea, constipation, gastritis, abdominal pain, dyspepsia, melena, eructation, aphthous stomatitis, **GI hemorrhage**
GU: dysuria, hematuria, urinary tract infection
Hematologic: anemia, ecchymosis, **bleeding, thrombocytopenia**
Hepatic: hemorrhage
Metabolic: dehydration
Musculoskeletal: arthralgia, myalgia, leg cramps or pain, pelvic pain
Respiratory: respiratory disease, pneumonia, bronchitis, asthma
Skin: skin disease, diaphoresis, alopecia, photosensitivity
Other: lymphadenopathy, fever, chills, edema, flulike symptoms, accidental injury

Patient monitoring

- Monitor CBC, platelet count, and coagulation studies.
- Watch for unusual bleeding or bruising.
- Assess vital signs and cardiovascular status.

antipsychotics

aripiprazole, atomoxetine hydrochloride, chlorpromazine hydrochloride, clozapine, fluphenazine, haloperidol, lithium carbonate, lithium citrate, loxapine, olanzapine, perphenazine, pimozide, prochlorperazine, quetiapine fumarate, risperidone, thioridazine hydrochloride, trifluoperazine hydrochloride, ziprasidone

Action

Block postsynaptic mesolimbic and mesocortical dopamine receptors in brain, relieving hallucinations, delusions, and psychoses. Also thought to relieve anxiety by filtering internal arousal stimuli to reticular system in brain stem.

Indications

Acute or chronic psychosis, acute intermittent porphyria, nausea and vomiting, intractable hiccups, preoperative sedation

Contraindications and precautions

• Contraindicated in hypersensitivity to drug, phenothiazines, sulfites (when injected), or benzyl alcohol (sustained-release forms); angle-closure glaucoma; bone marrow depression; blood dyscrasias; myeloproliferative disorders; subcortical brain damage; cerebral arteriosclerosis; hepatic damage; coronary artery disease; severe hypotension or hypertension; coma; and severe depression
• Use cautiously in diabetes mellitus; respiratory disease; prostatic hypertrophy; CNS tumors; seizure disorders; intestinal obstruction; elderly or debilitated patients; pregnant or breastfeeding patients (safety not established); and children with acute illness, infection, gastroenteritis, or dehydration.

Adverse reactions

CNS: drowsiness, sedation, extrapyramidal reactions, tardive dyskinesia, pseudoparkinsonism, **seizures, neuroleptic malignant syndrome**
CV: hypotension (increased with I.M. or I.V. use), tachycardia
EENT: blurred vision, lens opacities, dry eyes, nasal congestion
GI: constipation, anorexia, dry mouth, **paralytic ileus**
GU: urinary retention, menstrual irregularities, inhibited ejaculation, priapism, galactorrhea
Hematologic: eosinophilia, **hemolytic anemia, agranulocytosis, leukopenia, aplastic anemia, thrombocytopenia**
Hepatic: jaundice, **hepatitis**
Skin: photosensitivity, pigmentation changes, rash, sterile abscess
Other: allergic reactions, hyperthermia, pain at injection site

Patient monitoring

• Monitor vital signs (especially blood pressure), ECG, CBC, urinalysis, liver and kidney function tests, and periodic eye exams.

antirheumatic drugs

Biological response modifiers: adalimumab, anakinra, etanercept, infliximab

Disease-modifying agents: auranofin, aurothioglucose, azathioprine, cyclosporine, hydroxychloroquine sulfate, leflunomide, methotrexate, methotrexate sodium

Action

Biological response modifiers bind specifically to tumor necrosis factor

(TNF) alpha or competitively inhibit binding of interleukin-1 (IL-1) to IL-1 type I receptors, thereby blocking biologic activity of TNF alpha or IL-1.

Disease-modifying agents suppress the immune system and decrease inflammation.

Indications

Rheumatoid arthritis

Contraindications and precautions

- Contraindicated in hypersensitivity to drug, moderate to severe heart failure, demyelinating CNS disorder, hematologic abnormalities, poorly controlled or advanced diabetes mellitus, and significant exposure to varicella virus
- Use cautiously in severe myocardial, hepatic, or renal disease; decreased bone marrow reserve; active infection; hypotension; coma; history of or exposure to tuberculosis; elderly patients; pregnant or breastfeeding patients; and children.

Adverse reactions

CNS: confusion, hallucinations, headache, fatigue, insomnia, depression, EEG abnormalities, peripheral neuropathy, sensorimotor effects, **encephalitis, seizures**
CV: hypertension
EENT: iritis, corneal ulcers, gold deposits in ocular tissues, rhinitis, pharyngitis, sinusitis
GI: nausea, vomiting, diarrhea, constipation, abdominal cramps, flatulence, dyspepsia, dysphagia, ulcerative enterocolitis, melena, occult blood in stool, anorexia, **GI bleeding**
GU: hematuria, proteinuria, urinary tract infection, **nephrotic syndrome or glomerulitis, acute renal failure, acute tubular necrosis, acute nephritis, degeneration of proximal tubular epithelium**
Hematologic: eosinophilia, anemia, **thrombocytopenia, leukopenia, neutropenia, agranulocytosis, pancytopenia, hypoplastic anemia, aplastic anemia, pure red-cell aplasia, granulocytopenia, panmyelopathy, hemorrhagic diathesis**
Hepatic: jaundice, intrahepatic cholestasis, **hepatitis with jaundice, toxic hepatitis**
Musculoskeletal: arthralgia, back pain, myalgia, synovial destruction
Respiratory: upper respiratory infection, cough, dyspnea, **tuberculosis**
Skin: rash; urticaria; pruritus; erythema; papular, vesicular, or exfoliative dermatitis; abscess; alopecia; nail shedding; angioedema; photosensitivity
Other: bad taste, fever, chest pain, candidiasis, infection, chrysiasis, lupus-like syndrome, lymphoproliferative disease, hypersensitivity reaction, **cancer**

Patient monitoring

- Monitor for signs and symptoms of hypersensitivity reaction and infection.
- Monitor CBC with white cell differential and platelet count; assess liver and kidney function tests.
- Assess for heart failure in patients with history of cardiac disease.

antituberculars

dapsone, ethambutol hydrochloride, isoniazid, pyrazinamide, rifabutin, rifampin, rifapentine, streptomycin sulfate

Action

Unknown. May interfere with synthesis of one or more bacterial metabolites, altering RNA synthesis during cell division.

Indications
Tuberculosis and atypical mycobacterial infections caused by *Mycobacterium tuberculosis*

Contraindications and precautions
• Contraindicated in hypersensitivity to drug (including drug-induced hepatitis)
• Use cautiously in severe renal impairment, malnutrition, diabetes mellitus, chronic alcoholism, diabetic retinopathy, cataracts, optic neuritis and other ocular defects, history of hepatic damage or chronic alcohol ingestion, patients older than age 50, Black or Hispanic females, postpartal patients, pregnant or breastfeeding patients, and children younger than age 13.

Adverse reactions
CNS: confusion, dizziness, hallucinations, headache, malaise, peripheral neuritis
EENT: optic neuritis, blurred vision, decreased visual acuity, eye pain, red-green color blindness
GI: nausea, vomiting, abdominal pain, anorexia
Hematologic: thrombocytopenia
Hepatic: hepatitis
Metabolic: hyperuricemia
Musculoskeletal: joint pain, gouty arthritis
Respiratory: bloody sputum
Skin: rash, toxic epidermal necrolysis
Other: fever, **anaphylaxis**

Patient monitoring
• Monitor vital signs (especially blood pressure), ECG, CBC, urinalysis, liver and kidney function tests, and periodic eye exams.

antiulcer drugs
Histamine$_2$ (H_2)-receptor antagonists: cimetidine hydrochloride, famotidine, nizatidine, ranitidine hydrochloride

Proton pump inhibitors: esomeprazole magnesium, lansoprazole, omeprazole, pantoprazole sodium, rabeprazole sodium

Other: bismuth subsalicylate, misoprostol, sucralfate

Action
Reduce gastric acid level either by blocking H_2 receptors or by inhibiting the proton pump

Indications
Short-term treatment of active duodenal ulcer or benign gastric ulcer; prophylaxis of duodenal ulcer (at lower doses); treatment of gastroesophageal reflux disease, heartburn, acid indigestion, and gastric hypersecretory states (such as Zollinger-Ellison syndrome); prevention and treatment of stress-induced upper GI bleeding in critically ill patients

Contraindications and precautions
• Contraindicated in hypersensitivity to any antiulcer drug and in alcohol intolerance
• Use cautiously in renal impairment, elderly patients, and pregnant or breastfeeding patients.

Adverse reactions
CNS: confusion, dizziness, drowsiness, hallucinations, headache, peripheral neuropathy, **brain stem dysfunction**
CV: hypotension, **arrhythmias, cardiac arrest**

GI: nausea, diarrhea, constipation
GU: decreased sperm count, erectile dysfunction, gynecomastia
Hematologic: anemia, **neutropenia, thrombocytopenia, agranulocytosis, aplastic anemia**
Hepatic: hepatitis
Other: altered taste, pain at I.M. injection site, hypersensitivity reaction

Patient monitoring
- Monitor for resolution of GI symptoms.
- Assess CBC and liver function tests.

antivirals and antiretrovirals
Antivirals: acyclovir sodium, amantadine hydrochloride, famciclovir, foscarnet sodium, ganciclovir, oseltamivir phosphate, ribavirin, rimantadine hydrochloride, valacyclovir hydrochloride, valganciclovir hydrochloride, zanamivir

Antiretrovirals: abacavir sulfate, adefovir dipivoxil, amprenavir, cidofovir, delavirdine mesylate, didanosine, emtricitabine, efavirenz, enfurvitide, indinavir sulfate, lamivudine, nelfinavir mesylate, nevirapine, ritonavir, saquinavir, stavudine, tenofovir disoproxil fumarate, zalcitabine, zidovudine

Action
Antivirals kill viral cells by inhibiting release of enzymes required for DNA synthesis; inhibiting viral nucleic acid, DNA, or protein synthesis; inhibiting viral replication; or inhibiting protease reaction.

Antiretrovirals inhibit activity of human immunodeficiency virus (HIV) protease or HIV-1 reverse transcriptase, or bind directly to reverse transcriptase and block RNA- and DNA-dependent DNA polymerase activities. These actions inhibit HIV replication.

Indications
Genital herpes, herpes simplex, varicella zoster, herpes zoster (shingles), influenza type A virus, hepatitis, cytomegalovirus, HIV

Contraindications and precautions
- Contraindicated in hypersensitivity to drug or its components
- Use cautiously in renal or hepatic impairment; peripheral neuropathy; phenylketonuria; hyperuricemia; hypercholesterolemia; amylase elevation; history of mental illness, substance abuse, or hepatic impairment (including hepatitis B or C infection); sodium-restricted diet; elderly or debilitated patients; pregnant or breastfeeding patients; and children.

Adverse reactions
CNS: dizziness, asthenia, anxiety, abnormal thinking, hypoesthesia, agitation, confusion, hypertonia, **seizures, coma**
CV: hypotension, palpitations, bradycardia, weak pulse, pseudoaneurysm, **embolism, thrombophlebitis, nodal arrhythmias, atrioventricular block, ventricular tachycardia**
EENT: ocular hypotony, iritis, retinal detachment, diplopia
GI: nausea, vomiting, diarrhea, abdominal distention, dyspepsia, gastroesophageal reflux, hematemesis, dysphagia, dry mouth, **paralytic ileus**
GU: urinary retention, frequency, or incontinence; dysuria; prostatitis; **nephrotoxicity**
Hematologic: anemia, petechiae, **leukocytosis, thrombocytopenia, neutropenia, bleeding**
Hepatic: hepatomegaly

Metabolic: diabetes mellitus, **hyperkalemia**
Musculoskeletal: muscle contractions
Respiratory: bronchitis, dyspnea, wheezing, pneumonia, pleurisy, **pleural effusion, pulmonary edema, bronchospasm, pulmonary embolism**
Skin: rash, diaphoresis, urticaria, pruritus, bullous eruptions, pallor
Other: pain, peripheral coldness, edema, drug toxicity

Patient monitoring

- Monitor CBC and liver and kidney function tests.
- As indicated, monitor viral load and T-cell levels.

anxiolytics

Benzodiazepines: alprazolam, chlordiazepoxide hydrochloride, clorazepate, clonazepam, diazepam, lorazepam, oxazepam

Other: buspirone hydrochloride, doxepin, hydroxyzine hydrochloride, hydroxyzine pamoate

Action

Benzodiazepines potentiate effects of gamma-aminobutyric acid (GABA) and other inhibitory transmitters by binding to specific benzodiazepine receptor sites.

Other anxiolytics have unknown actions. They are thought to act on brain by inhibiting neuronal firing and reducing serotonin transmission.

Indications

Anxiety disorders

Contraindications and precautions

- Contraindicated in hypersensitivity to drug, psychosis, acute angle-closure glaucoma, significant hepatic disease, intra-arterial use (lorazepam injection), concurrent use of ketoconazole or itraconazole, breastfeeding (diazepam), and children younger than 6 months
- Use cautiously in hepatic disease, asthma, severe pulmonary disease, open-angle glaucoma, obesity, or concurrent use of CNS depressants.

Adverse reactions

CNS: sedation, somnolence, depression, lethargy, apathy, fatigue, hypoactivity, light-headedness, dizziness, memory impairment, disorientation, anterograde amnesia, restlessness, confusion, crying, sobbing, delirium, agitation, headache, slurred speech, aphonia, dysarthria, stupor, syncope, vertigo, euphoria, nervousness, irritability, poor concentration, inability to perform complex mental functions, rigidity, tremor, dystonia, akathisia, hemiparesis, paresthesia, hypotonia, unsteadiness, ataxia, incoordination, weakness, vivid dreams, psychomotor retardation, extrapyramidal symptoms, paradoxical reactions, behavior problems, hysteria, psychosis, **seizures, coma, suicidal tendency**
CV: bradycardia, tachycardia, hypertension, hypotension, palpitations, decreased systolic pressure, **cardiovascular collapse**
EENT: visual disturbances, diplopia, nystagmus, decreased hearing, auditory disturbances, nasal congestion
GI: nausea, vomiting, diarrhea, constipation, gastritis, coated tongue, difficulty swallowing, increased salivation, dry mouth, anorexia
GU: urinary incontinence or retention, menstrual irregularities, gynecomastia, galactorrhea, libido changes
Hematologic: anemia, eosinophilia, **leukopenia, agranulocytosis, thrombocytopenia**
Hepatic: hepatic dysfunction
Metabolic: dehydration

Musculoskeletal: muscle disturbances, joint pain
Respiratory: respiratory disturbances, partial airway obstruction
Skin: urticaria; pruritus; morbilliform, urticarial, or maculopapular rash; dermatitis; alopecia; hirsutism; ankle or facial edema; diaphoresis
Other: sore gums; appetite and weight changes; glassy-eyed appearance; fever; hiccups; edema; lymphadenopathy; pain, burning, and redness at I.M. injection site; phlebitis and thrombosis at I.V. site

Patient monitoring

- Monitor CBC and kidney and liver function tests.
- Taper dosage gradually to termination; do not withdraw quickly.

beta-adrenergic blockers

Alpha/beta-adrenergic blockers: carvedilol, labetalol

Beta-adrenergic blockers: acebutolol hydrochloride, atenolol, bisoprolol fumarate, carteolol hydrochloride, esmolol hydrochloride, metoprolol, nadolol, pindolol, propranolol hydrochloride, sotalol hydrochloride, timolol maleate

Action

Alpha/beta-adrenergic blockers combine selective competitive postsynaptic alpha$_1$-adrenergic blockade with nonselective, competitive beta-adrenergic blockade, causing blood pressure to decrease.

Beta-adrenergic blockers combine reversibly with beta-adrenergic receptors, blocking responses to sympathetic nerve impulses, catecholamines, or adrenergic drugs. Beta$_1$ blockade decreases heart rate, myocardial contractility, and cardiac output while slowing atrioventricular conduction. Beta$_2$ blockade increases bronchiolar airway resistance and enhances the inhibitory effect of catecholamines on peripheral vessels.

Indications

Hypertension; angina pectoris; myocardial infarction (MI); stable, symptomatic (class II or III) heart failure of ischemic, hypertensive, or cardiomyopathic origin; ventricular arrhythmias or tachycardia; tremors; chronic intraocular glaucoma; aggressive behavior; drug-induced akathisia; anxiety; migraine prophylaxis

Contraindications and precautions

- Contraindicated in hypersensitivity to drug, heart failure (unless secondary to tachyarrhythmia treatable with specific beta-adrenergic blocker), shock, sinus bradycardia, and heart block greater than first degree. Alpha/beta-adrenergic blockers are contraindicated in bronchial asthma and symptomatic hepatic impairment.
- Use cautiously in renal or hepatic impairment, pulmonary disease (especially asthma), pulmonary edema, diabetes mellitus, thyrotoxicosis, history of severe allergic reactions, elderly patients, pregnant or breastfeeding patients, and children (safety not established).

Adverse reactions

CNS: insomnia, headache, hyperactivity, malaise, CNS stimulation, dizziness, drowsiness, syncope, tremor, restlessness, nervousness, apprehension, anxiety, hyperkinesia, asthenia, vertigo, paresthesia
CV: hypertension, hypotension, tachycardia, angina, chest pain, palpitations, **arrhythmias**
EENT: abnormal vision, dry eyes, epistaxis, nasal congestion, sore throat (in-

haled drug form), nasal dryness and irritation, hoarseness
GI: nausea, vomiting, heartburn, cholestasis, anorexia
GU: acute urinary bladder retention, difficulty voiding, ejaculation failure, erectile dysfunction, priapism, Peyronie's disease
Metabolic: hypokalemia, **hypoglycemia**
Musculoskeletal: muscle cramps
Respiratory: cough, wheezing, dyspnea, bronchitis, increased sputum, paradoxical airway resistance (with repeated, excessive use of inhaled form), **pulmonary edema, bronchospasm**
Skin: pallor; flushing; diaphoresis; generalized maculopapular, lichenoid, urticarial, or psoriaform rash; bullous lichen planus; facial erythema; reversible alopecia
Other: bad or unusual taste, increased appetite, edema, fever, antimitochondrial antibodies, hypersensitivity reaction, **systemic lupus erythematosus**

Patient monitoring

- Monitor CBC, ECG, blood glucose and electrolyte levels, and liver and kidney function tests.
- Assess vital signs, fluid intake and output, and weight.

bisphosphonates

alendronate sodium, etidronate disodium, pamidronate disodium, risendronate, zoledronic acid

Action

Inhibit normal and abnormal bone resorption

Indications

Osteoporosis in postmenopausal women and men, glucocorticoid-induced osteoporosis, Paget's disease, heterotopic ossification, hypercalcemia of malignancy, breast cancer, multiple myeloma, bone metastases of solid tumors

Contraindications and precautions

- Contraindicated in hypersensitivity to drug, hypocalcemia, esophageal abnormalities, clinically overt osteomalacia, renal impairment (class Dc and higher), inability to stand or sit upright for at least 30 minutes after dosing, and pregnancy
- Use cautiously in renal impairment less than class Dc; history of hypoparathyroidism or aspirin-sensitive asthma; or concurrent use of loop diuretics, aminoglycosides, or other nephrotoxic drugs.

Adverse reactions

CNS: agitation, anxiety, confusion, asthenia, depression, dizziness, headache, hypertonia, hypoesthesia, insomnia, neuralgia, fatigue, paresthesia, psychosis, somnolence, vertigo, **seizures**
CV: angina pectoris, cardiovascular disorder, chest pain, hypertension, hypotension, syncope, vasodilation, tachycardia, **atrial flutter or fibrillation, heart failure**
EENT: amblyopia, cataract, conjunctivitis, dry eyes, tinnitus, rhinitis, sinusitis, pharyngitis
GI: nausea, vomiting, diarrhea, constipation, abdominal pain, abdominal distention, acid reflux, belching, colitis, dyspepsia, gastritis, gastroenteritis, dysphagia, flatulence, esophageal ulcer, dry mouth, anorexia, **GI hemorrhage**
Hematologic: anemia, ecchymosis, **granulocytopenia, leukopenia, neutropenia, thrombocytopenia**
Metabolic: dehydration, **fluid overload**
Musculoskeletal: arthralgia, arthritis, arthrosis, back or neck pain, bone disorder, bone fracture, bone or skeletal pain, bursitis, joint disorder, leg or other muscle cramps, myalgia

Respiratory: bronchitis, cough, dyspnea, pneumonia, crackles, upper respiratory infection, **pleural effusion**
Skin: alopecia, dermatitis, pruritus, rash
Other: taste perversion, weight loss, pain, edema, fever, flulike symptoms, infection, infusion-site reaction, allergic reaction

Patient monitoring

- Watch for signs and symptoms of GI irritation, including ulcers.
- Monitor blood pressure and calcium, potassium, phosphate and creatinine levels.

bronchodilators

albuterol, aminophylline, dyphylline, ephedrine, epinephrine, ipratropium bromide, isoproterenol, levalbuterol hydrochloride, metaproterenol sulfate, pirbuterol acetate, salmeterol, terbutaline sulfate, theophylline

Action

Inhibit phosphodiesterase, an enzyme that degrades cyclic adenosine monophosphate (cAMP) by stimulating cAMP release and inhibiting release of slow-reacting substance of anaphylaxis and histamine. These actions cause bronchodilation, produce CNS and cardiac stimulation, promote diuresis, and increase gastric acid secretion.

Indications

Prevention of exercise-induced bronchospasm, prevention and treatment of bronchospasm in reversible obstructive airway disease

Contraindications and precautions

- Contraindicated in hypersensitivity to drug, angina, arrhythmias associated with tachycardia, ventricular arrhythmias that warrant inotropic therapy, cardiac dilatation or insufficiency, cerebral arteriosclerosis, organic brain damage, angle-closure glaucoma, local anesthesia of certain areas (such as toes or fingers), and labor
- Use cautiously in heart failure or other cardiac or circulatory impairment, hypertension, chronic obstructive pulmonary disease, renal or hepatic disease, hyperthyroidism, peptic ulcer, severe hypoxemia, diabetes mellitus, seizure disorders, glaucoma, elderly patients, pregnant or breastfeeding patients, young children, and infants.

Adverse reactions

CNS: insomnia, headache, hyperactivity, asthenia, malaise, dizziness, apprehension, anxiety, restlessness, CNS stimulation, nervousness, hyperkinesia, vertigo, drowsiness, tremor
CV: hypertension, hypotension, tachycardia, angina, chest pain, palpitations, **arrhythmias**
EENT: nasal congestion, nasal dryness and irritation, epistaxis, sore throat (with inhaled drug), hoarseness
GI: nausea, vomiting, heartburn, anorexia
Metabolic: hypokalemia, **hypoglycemia**
Musculoskeletal: muscle cramps
Respiratory: cough, wheezing, dyspnea, bronchitis, paradoxical airway resistance (with repeated, excessive use of inhaled drug), increased sputum, **bronchospasm, pulmonary edema**
Skin: pallor, flushing, diaphoresis
Other: unusual or bad taste, increased appetite, hypersensitivity reaction

Patient monitoring

- Monitor vital signs, ECG, and fluid intake and output.

calcium channel blockers

amlodipine, diltiazem hydrochloride, felodipine, isradipine, nicardipine hydrochloride, nifedipine, nimodipine, nisoldipine, verapamil hydrochloride

Action

Inhibit calcium influx through membranes of cardiac and smooth-muscle cells; this action depresses automaticity and conduction velocity in cardiac muscle, reducing myocardial contractility. Also decrease depolarization rate, atrial conduction, and total peripheral resistance.

Indications

Hypertension, angina pectoris, vasospastic (Prinzmetal's) angina, supraventricular tachyarrhythmias, rapid ventricular rate in atrial flutter or fibrillation

Contraindications and precautions

• Contraindicated in hypersensitivity to drug, sick sinus syndrome, second- or third-degree atrioventricular block (unless patient has artificial pacemaker in place), and systolic pressure below 90 mm Hg

• Use cautiously in severe renal or hepatic impairment, advanced aortic stenosis, cardiogenic shock (unless associated with supraventricular tachyarrhythmias), history of serious ventricular arrhythmias or heart failure, concurrent use of I.V. beta-adrenergic blockers, elderly patients, pregnant or breastfeeding patients, and children (safety not established).

Adverse reactions

CNS: headache, abnormal dreams, anxiety, confusion, dizziness, syncope, drowsiness, nervousness, paresthesia, tremor, asthenia, psychiatric disturbances
CV: peripheral edema, chest pain, hypotension, palpitations, bradycardia, tachycardia, **arrhythmias, heart failure**
EENT: blurred vision, disturbed equilibrium, tinnitus, epistaxis
GI: nausea, vomiting, diarrhea, constipation, dyspepsia, dry mouth, anorexia
GU: dysuria, nocturia, polyuria, sexual dysfunction, gynecomastia
Hematologic: anemia, **leukopenia, thrombocytopenia**
Metabolic: hyperglycemia
Musculoskeletal: joint stiffness, muscle cramps
Respiratory: cough, dyspnea
Skin: rash, dermatitis, pruritus, urticaria, flushing, diaphoresis, photosensitivity reaction, **erythema multiforme, Stevens-Johnson syndrome**
Other: gingival hyperplasia, altered taste, weight gain

Patient monitoring

• Monitor blood glucose and electrolyte levels, fluid intake and output, and liver and kidney function tests.

• Assess vital signs, ECG, weight, and blood pressure in both arms (with patient lying down, sitting, and standing).

cholinergics

bethanechol chloride, cevimeline hydrochloride, edrophonium chloride, neostigmine, pyridostigmine bromide

Action

Stimulate cholinergic receptors, causing urinary bladder contraction, decreased bladder capacity, more frequent ureteral peristaltic waves, increased GI tone and peristalsis, increased lower esophageal sphincter pressure, and increased gastric secretions

Indications

Postpartum or postoperative nonobstructive urinary retention, urinary retention caused by neurogenic bladder, diagnosis of myasthenia gravis (Tensilon test), antidote for curare (to reverse nondepolarizing neuromuscular blockade)

Contraindications and precautions

- Contraindicated in hypersensitivity to drug or sulfites, hyperthyroidism, peptic ulcer, latent or active bronchial asthma, pronounced bradycardia or atrioventricular (AV) conduction defects, vasomotor instability, coronary artery disease, coronary occlusion, hypotension, hypertension, seizure disorders, parkinsonism, GI or GU tract obstruction, impaired GI or GU wall integrity, spastic GI disturbances, acute inflammatory GI tract lesions, peritonitis, marked vagotonia, and when GI tract or urinary bladder activity is undesirable (for instance, postoperatively)
- Use cautiously in arrhythmias, toxic megacolon, poor GI motility, and pregnant patients.

Adverse reactions

CNS: asthenia, dysarthria, dysphonia, dizziness, drowsiness, headache, syncope, **loss of consciousness, seizures**
CV: hypotension, AV block, bradycardia, **cardiac arrest, thrombophlebitis** (with I.V. use)
EENT: diplopia, miosis, conjunctival hyperemia, excessive lacrimation and salivation
GI: nausea, vomiting, diarrhea, abdominal cramps, dysphagia
GU: urinary frequency or incontinence
Musculoskeletal: muscle cramps, fasciculations
Respiratory: dyspnea, **respiratory muscle paralysis, central respiratory paralysis, laryngospasm, bronchospasm, respiratory arrest**
Skin: rash, diaphoresis, flushing
Other: anaphylaxis

Patient monitoring

- Monitor ECG, glucose and electrolyte levels, urinalysis, and liver and kidney function tests.

(Clinical alert) Assess platelet count in long-term use. Report unusual bleeding or bruising, petechiae, skin disorders, and signs and symptoms of diabetes mellitus.

CNS stimulants

amphetamine, dexmethylphenidate hydrochloride, dextroamphetamine sulfate, doxapram, methylphenidate hydrochloride, modafinil, pemoline

Action

Cause norepinephrine release from central adrenergic neurons and increase central stimulation, which enhances motor activity and mental alertness, lifts mood, and suppresses appetite

Indications

Attention deficit hyperactivity disorder, narcolepsy

Contraindications and precautions

- Contraindicated in hypersensitivity to drug or tartrazine, advanced arteriosclerosis, cardiovascular disease, moderate to severe hypertension, agitation, hyperexcitable states (including hyperthyroidism), glaucoma, history of Tourette's syndrome or drug abuse, suicidal or homicidal tendency, concurrent MAO inhibitor use, breastfeeding, and children younger than age 6

• Use cautiously in mild hypertension, diabetes mellitus, depression, seizures, psychosis, long-term amphetamine use, elderly or debilitated patients, and pregnant patients.

Adverse reactions

CNS: nervousness, insomnia, dizziness, headache, dyskinesia, chorea, drowsiness, hyperactivity, restlessness, tremor, depression, Tourette's syndrome, **toxic psychosis**
CV: angina, palpitations, hypertension, hypotension, tachycardia, **arrhythmias**
EENT: blurred vision, poor accommodation
GI: nausea, vomiting, diarrhea, constipation, abdominal pain and cramps, anorexia, dry mouth
GU: erectile dysfunction, increased libido
Hematologic: anemia, **leukopenia, thrombocytopenia**
Hepatic: hepatic dysfunction, hepatic coma
Skin: rash, alopecia, exfoliative dermatitis
Other: metallic taste, weight loss, fever, psychological or physical drug dependence, drug tolerance, abnormal behavior (with abuse)

Patient monitoring

• Watch for and report fever, excitation, delirium, tremors, and twitching.
🔊 Monitor vital signs. Stay alert for arrhythmias, tachycardia, hypertension, and cardiovascular changes with psychotic syndrome.
• Watch for and report signs of drug abuse.

corticosteroids

beclomethasone dipropionate, betamethasone, budesonide, cortisone acetate, dexamethasone, fludrocortisone, hydrocortisone, methylprednisolone, mometasone, prednisolone, prednisone, triamcinolone

Action

Reduce the immune response by inhibiting prostaglandin synthesis, macrophage and leukocyte accumulation at inflammation site, phagocytosis, and lysosomal enzyme release. Also reduce numbers of T lymphocytes, monocytes, and eosinophils and interfere with immunoglobulin binding to cell-surface receptors. Some corticosteroids regulate metabolic pathways involving protein, carbohydrate, and fat; others regulate electrolyte and water balance.

Indications

Adrenocortical insufficiency; adrenal, inflammatory, allergic, hematologic, neoplastic, and autoimmune disorders; asthma; cerebral edema; Crohn's disease; hypercalcemia; acute spinal cord injury; nausea and vomiting caused by chemotherapy; prevention of organ rejection in transplant patients; prevention of neonatal respiratory distress in high-risk pregnancies

Contraindications and precautions

• Contraindicated in hypersensitivity to drug or intolerance of alcohol, bisulfites, or tartrazine and in active untreated infections
• Use cautiously in hypertension, osteoporosis, diabetes mellitus, glaucoma, immunosuppression, seizure disorders, renal disease, hypothyroidism, cirrhosis, diverticulitis, active or latent

peptic ulcer, inflammatory bowel disease, ulcerative colitis, thromboembolic disorder or tendency, myasthenia gravis, heart failure, metastatic cancer, emotional instability, recent GI surgery, pregnant or breastfeeding patients, and children younger than age 6 (safety not established).

Adverse reactions

CNS: headache, nervousness, restlessness, depression, euphoria, personality changes, psychosis, vertigo, paresthesia, insomnia, **increased intracranial pressure, seizures**
CV: hypotension, hypertension, Churg-Strauss syndrome, **heart failure, thrombophlebitis, thromboembolism, fat embolism, arrhythmias, shock**
EENT: glaucoma (with long-term use), increased intraocular pressure, cataract, nasal congestion and irritation, perforated nasal septum, epistaxis, nasopharyngeal or oropharyngeal fungal infection, sneezing, dysphonia, hoarseness, throat irritation
GI: nausea, vomiting, abdominal distention, peptic ulcer, esophageal candidiasis or ulcer, pancreatitis, dry mouth, anorexia
GU: amenorrhea, irregular menses
Metabolic: decreased growth (in children), diabetes mellitus, cushingoid state, sodium and fluid retention, hyperglycemia, hypokalemia, hypocalcemia, hypercholesterolemia, **adrenal suppression, hypothalamic-pituitary-adrenal suppression** (with systemic use for more than 5 days)
Musculoskeletal: muscle wasting, muscle pain and weakness, myopathy, spontaneous fractures, aseptic joint necrosis, tendon rupture, osteoporosis, osteonecrosis
Respiratory: cough, wheezing, **bronchospasm**
Skin: rash, pruritus, contact dermatitis, acne, decreased wound healing, bruising, hirsutism, thin and fragile skin, petechiae, purpura, striae, subcutaneous fat atrophy, injection site atrophy, angioedema
Other: bad taste, increased appetite (with long-term use), weight gain, facial edema, increased susceptibility to infection, aggravation or masking of infection, immunosuppression, hypersensitivity reaction

Patient monitoring

- Monitor ECG, blood glucose and electrolyte levels, urinalysis, and kidney and liver function tests.

🔊 Assess platelet count in long-term therapy. Report unusual bleeding or bruising, petechiae, skin disorders, and signs and symptom of diabetes mellitus.

- Monitor appearance for changes that suggest Cushing's syndrome.

diuretics

Carbonic anhydrase inhibitor: acetazolamide

Loop diuretics: bumetanide, furosemide, torsemide

Osmotic diuretics: mannitol, urea

Potassium-sparing diuretics: amiloride hydrochloride, spironolactone, triamterene

Thiazide and thiazide-like diuretics: chlorothiazide, chlorthalidone, hydrochlorothiazide, indapamide, metolazone

Action

Carbonic anhydrase inhibitors inhibit carbonic anhydrase in kidneys, decreasing reabsorption of water, sodium, potassium, and bicarbonate. *Loop* diuretics inhibit reabsorption of sodium and chloride (and therefore water)

in proximal and distal tubules and loop of Henle. *Osmotic* diuretics increase plasma osmolality, drawing water from body tissues into extracellular fluid and then out through the kidney. *Potassium-sparing* diuretics inhibit sodium reabsorption in distal renal tubule, causing sodium and water loss. *Thiazide and thiazide-like* diuretics decrease rate of sodium and chloride reabsorption by distal renal tubule and increase water excretion.

Indications

Hypertension or edema secondary to heart failure or other causes, cerebral edema, hemolytic transfusion reaction, drug toxicity, prevention of oliguria or acute renal failure

Contraindications and precautions

• Contraindicated in hypersensitivity to drug, alcohol intolerance (some liquid furosemide forms), anuria, renal decompensation, hepatic coma or precoma, severe electrolyte depletion, severe pulmonary congestion or edema, severe dehydration, and active intracranial bleeding (except during craniotomy)
• Use cautiously in severe hepatic disease accompanied by cirrhosis or ascites, electrolyte depletion, worsening azotemia, renal insufficiency (blood urea nitrogen above 30 mg/dl or creatinine clearance below 30 ml/minute), diabetes mellitus, elderly or debilitated patients, pregnant or breastfeeding patients, and children younger than age 18.

Adverse reactions

CNS: dizziness, headache, insomnia, nervousness, vertigo, asthenia, paresthesia, confusion, fatigue, drowsiness, **encephalopathy**
CV: hypotension, chest pain, volume depletion, **thrombophlebitis, arrhythmias**
EENT: blurred vision, nystagmus, hearing loss, tinnitus
GI: nausea, vomiting, diarrhea, constipation, dyspepsia, gastric irritation, dry mouth, anorexia, **acute pancreatitis**
GU: polyuria, nocturia, glycosuria, premature ejaculation, erectile dysfunction, nipple tenderness, **renal failure, oliguria**
Hematologic: leukopenia, other blood dyscrasias
Hepatic: jaundice
Metabolic: dehydration, hyperglycemia, hyperuricemia, hypokalemia, hypomagnesemia, **hypochloremic alkalosis**
Musculoskeletal: joint pain, muscle cramps, myalgia
Skin: rash, pruritus, urticaria, diaphoresis, photosensitivity
Other: weight gain

Patient monitoring

• Monitor fluid intake and output and weight.
• Monitor CBC and blood glucose, blood urea nitrogen, creatinine, carbon dioxide, and electrolyte levels (especially potassium).
• Assess vital signs during rapid diuresis.

erectile dysfunction agents

Phosphodiesterase type 5 (PDE5) inhibitors: sildenafil citrate, tadalafil, vardenafil hydrochloride

Other: alprostadil

Action

PDE5 inhibitors cause degradation of cyclic guanylic acid in smooth-muscle cells of corpus cavernosum, enhancing effects of nitric oxide released during sexual stimulation. These actions increase blood flow to penis and induce erection.

Alprostadil relaxes the trabecular smooth muscle and dilates cavernosal arteries, causing expansion of lacunar spaces and blood entrapment from compression of venules against the tunica albuginea. These effects induce erection.

Indications
Erectile dysfunction

Contraindications and precautions
- Contraindicated in hypersensitivity to drug or its components and in concurrent use of nitrates (regularly or intermittently), nitric oxide donors, or alpha-adrenergic blockers
- Use cautiously in anatomic penile deformation, conditions that predispose to priapism (such as sickle cell anemia, multiple myeloma, leukemia), bleeding disorders, active peptic ulcer, retinitis pigmentosa or other retinal abnormality, coronary ischemia, heart failure, multidrug antihypertensive regimen, or concurrent use of erythromycin, cimetidine, or other drugs that could prolong the half-life of erectile dysfunction agent.

Adverse reactions
CNS: dizziness, headache, fainting, hypoesthesia
CV: abnormal ECG, hypertension, hypotension, vasodilation, vasovagal reaction, peripheral vascular disorder, supraventricular extrasystoles
EENT: abnormal vision, mydriasis, nasal congestion, rhinitis, sinusitis
GI: nausea, diarrhea, dyspepsia, dry mouth
GU: urinary frequency and urgency, impaired urination, hematuria, urinary tract infection, inguinal hernia, prostate disorder, scrotal disorder or edema, testicular pain
Metabolic: hyperglycemia
Musculoskeletal: back or limb pain, leg cramps, myalgia
Respiratory: cough
Skin: rash, nonapplication site pruritus, diaphoresis, flushing, skin disorder or neoplasm
Other: accidental injury, flulike symptoms, infection, localized pain

Patient monitoring
- Monitor cardiovascular status and vision.
- Assess for drug efficacy. Watch for priapism or erections lasting beyond 4 hours, which may permanently damage penile tissue.

hematopoietic agents
Colony-stimulating factors: filgrastim, pegfilgrastim, sargramostim

Human erythropoietins: darbepoetin alfa, epoetin alfa

Action
Varies with specific drug. See individual monographs.

Indications
Colony-stimulating factors—to reduce incidence of infection in myelosuppressive chemotherapy; to reduce time to neutrophil recovery and fever duration in patients with acute myelogenous leukemia and nonmyeloid cancer who are undergoing myeloablative chemotherapy followed by bone marrow transplant; mobilization of peripheral blood progenitor cell collection; severe chronic neutropenia
Human erythropoietins—anemia associated with chronic renal failure, zidovudine therapy in patients with human immunodeficiency virus, cancer patients on chemotherapy, reduction of allogeneic blood transfusions in surgery patients

Contraindications and precautions

• Contraindicated in hypersensitivity to drug or human albumin and in uncontrolled hypertension
• Use cautiously in cardiac disease, hypertension, seizures, and porphyria.

Adverse reactions

CNS: fatigue, headache, generalized weakness
CV: chest pain, hypertension, tachycardia
GI: nausea, vomiting, diarrhea, constipation, mucositis, stomatitis, anorexia
Metabolic: hyperkalemia
Musculoskeletal: skeletal pain, arthralgia, myalgia
Hematologic: neutropenic fever
Respiratory: dyspnea, cough, sore throat
Skin: alopecia, rash, urticaria
Other: fever, stinging at injection site, flulike symptoms, hypersensitivity reaction

Patient monitoring

• Monitor CBC before and frequently throughout therapy. Also monitor liver function tests and uric acid levels.
• Assess for signs and symptoms of splenic rupture, such as left upper quadrant abdominal pain, shoulder pain, and splenic enlargement.
• Watch for signs and symptoms of infection, sepsis, adult respiratory distress syndrome, and neutropenic fever.

immunosuppressants

azathioprine, basiliximab, cyclosporine, daclizumab, glatiramer acetate, methotrexate sodium, muromonab-CD3, mycophenolate mofetil, sirolimus, tacrolimus, thalidomide

Action

Inhibit binding of interleukin (IL)-1 to IL-1 receptors; prevent proliferation and differentiation of activated B and T cells; inhibit lymphokine production and IL-2 release; react with T-lymphocyte membranes, depleting blood of CD3+ T cells; and bind to intracellular proteins to prevent T-cell activation

Indications

Moderate to severely active rheumatoid arthritis, prevention of organ transplant rejection

Contraindications and precautions

• Contraindicated in hypersensitivity to drug or its components, fluid overload, uncompensated heart failure, seizure disorders, and pregnant patients with rheumatoid arthritis
• Use cautiously in renal or hepatic disease, cancer, diabetes mellitus, hyperkalemia, hyperuricemia, infection, hypertension, pregnant patients (except those with rheumatoid arthritis), breastfeeding patients, and children younger than age 13.

Adverse reactions

CNS: headache, insomnia, paresthesia, dizziness, tremor, drowsiness, anxiety, confusion, agitation, rigors, asthenia, **coma, seizures**
CV: hypotension, hypertension, tachycardia, palpitations, chest pain, ECG

abnormalities, **torsades de pointes, prolonged QT interval**
EENT: blurred vision, painful red eye, dry and irritated eyes, eyelid edema, earache, tinnitus, nasopharyngitis, epistaxis, postnasal drip, sinusitis, sore throat
GI: nausea, vomiting, diarrhea, constipation, fecal incontinence, dyspepsia, abdominal pain, dry mouth, oral blisters, oral candidiasis, anorexia, **GI hemorrhage**
GU: urinary incontinence, breakthrough bleeding, **vaginal hemorrhage, renal impairment, oliguria, renal failure**
Hematologic: anemia, **thrombocytopenia, neutropenia, hemorrhage, disseminated intravascular coagulation**
Metabolic: hypomagnesemia, hyperglycemia, hypokalemia, **hyperkalemia, hypoglycemia, acidosis**
Musculoskeletal: myalgia; joint, bone, back, neck, or limb pain
Respiratory: dyspnea, cough, hypoxia, wheezing, tachypnea, decreased or abnormal breath sounds, hemoptysis, upper respiratory infection, **pleural effusion**
Skin: pruritus, dermatitis, bruising, dry skin, diaphoresis, night sweats, flushing, erythema, petechiae, hyperpigmentation, urticaria, skin lesions, pallor, local exfoliation
Other: weight changes, fever, lymphadenopathy, edema, facial edema, bacterial infection, herpes simplex infection, pain, hypersensitivity reaction, **sepsis**

Patient monitoring

- Assess for signs and symptoms of infection and injection site reaction.
- Monitor vital signs, CBC with platelet count, fluid intake and output, electrolyte and blood glucose levels, and liver and kidney function tests.

inotropics

digoxin, inamrinone lactate, milrinone lactate

Action

Inhibit sodium- and potassium-activated adenosine triphosphatase phosphodiesterase, which raises intracellular and extracellular calcium levels. These effects increase myocardial contractility, prolong atrioventricular (AV) node refractory period, decrease conduction through sinoatrial and AV nodes, and relax and dilate vascular smooth muscle to reduce preload and afterload.

Indications

Heart failure, tachyarrhythmias, atrial fibrillation or flutter, paroxysmal atrial tachycardia

Contraindications and precautions

- Contraindicated in hypersensitivity to drug, known alcohol intolerance (elixir only), and ventricular fibrillation
- Use cautiously in electrolyte abnormalities (such as hypokalemia, hypercalcemia, hypomagnesemia), myocardial infarction, AV block, idiopathic hypertrophic subaortic stenosis, constrictive pericarditis, renal impairment, obesity, elderly patients, pregnant or breastfeeding patients, and children.

Adverse reactions

CNS: fatigue, headache, asthenia
CV: bradycardia, ECG changes, **arrhythmias**
EENT: blurred or yellow vision
GI: nausea, vomiting, diarrhea, anorexia
GU: gynecomastia
Hematologic: thrombocytopenia

Patient monitoring
• Monitor vital signs, weight, electrolyte levels, fluid intake and output, drug blood level, and kidney function tests.

laxatives
bisacodyl, calcium polycarbophil, castor oil, docusate, glycerin, lactulose, magnesium salts, methylcellulose, psyllium, senna, sodium phosphate

Action
Stimulate smooth muscle of bowel, increasing intestinal contractions; increase stool bulk by causing water retention and inhibiting digestion in stomach. Also soften hard feces, promoting their passage through lower intestine.

Indications
Treatment of constipation, prevention of constipation in patients who should not strain during defecation (for example, after anorectal surgery or myocardial infarction), colonic evacuation for rectal and bowel examination

Contraindications and precautions
• Contraindicated in hypersensitivity to drug or its components, intestinal obstruction, undiagnosed abdominal pain, suspected appendicitis, and fecal impaction
• Use cautiously in severe cardiovascular disease, anal or rectal fissures, enteritis, ulcerative colitis, diverticulitis, pregnant or breastfeeding patients, and children younger than age 2.

Adverse reactions
GI: nausea; vomiting; diarrhea; esophageal, gastric, small-intestine, or rectal obstruction (with dry form of drug); abdominal cramps in severe constipation; anorexia
GU: reddish-pink discoloration of alkaline urine, yellow-brown discoloration of acidic urine
Metabolic: alkalosis, fluid and electrolyte imbalances
Musculoskeletal: tetany
Other: laxative dependence (with excessive long-term use)

Patient monitoring
• Monitor fluid and electrolyte balance.

neuromuscular blockers
Depolarizing blocker: succinylcholine chloride

Nondepolarizing blockers: atracurium besylate, botulinum toxin type A, cisatracurium besylate, doxacurium chloride, mivacurium chloride, pancuronium bromide, rocuronium bromide, tubocurarine chloride, vecuronium bromide

Action
Depolarizing neuromuscular blockers initially excite skeletal muscle, then prevent muscle contraction by prolonging the refractory period. *Nondepolarizing* (competitive) neuromuscular blockers bind competitively to cholinergic receptors on motor end plates, preventing muscle contraction.

Indications
Adjunct to anesthesia to facilitate endotracheal intubation; skeletal and smooth muscle relaxation; to facilitate orthopedic manipulation; reduction of muscle contractions during pharmacologically or electrically induced seizures; myasthenia gravis diagnosis

Contraindications and precautions

• Contraindicated in hypersensitivity to drug, low plasma pseudocholinesterase level, angle-closure glaucoma, myopathy with elevated creatine kinase level, penetrating eye injury, and personal or family history of malignant hyperthermia

• Use cautiously in heart disease; electrolyte imbalance; dehydration; neuromuscular, respiratory, or hepatic disease; pregnant or breastfeeding patients, and children younger than age 2.

Adverse reactions

CV: hypotension, bradycardia, **arrhythmias, cardiac arrest**
Musculoskeletal: profound and prolonged muscle relaxation, residual muscle weakness
Respiratory: cyanosis, **prolonged apnea, bronchospasm, respiratory depression**
Skin: rash, flushing, pruritus, urticaria
Other: hypersensitivity reaction

Patient monitoring

🔊 Monitor vital signs, pulmonary status, and temperature continuously.

nonopioid analgesics

acetaminophen, acetylsalicylic acid, celecoxib, diclofenac, diflunisal, etodolac, ibuprofen, indomethacin, ketoprofen, ketorolac tromethamine, meloxicam, nabumetone, naproxen, naproxen sodium, oxaprozin, piroxicam, salsalate, valdecoxib

Action

Inhibit cyclooxygenase, an enzyme needed for prostaglandin synthesis. This inhibition stimulates the anti-inflammatory response and blocks pain impulses.

Indications

Inflammatory conditions (such as osteoarthritis, rheumatoid arthritis, and ankylosing spondylitis), dysmenorrhea, actinic keratoses, fever

Contraindications and precautions

• Contraindicated in hypersensitivity to drug or sulfonamides and in history of asthma, urticaria, or allergic reaction to aspirin or other nonsteroidal anti-inflammatory drugs

• Use cautiously in severe cardiovascular, renal, or hepatic disease; GI disorders; cardiac decompensation; active GI bleeding or ulcer; asthma; history of ulcer disease; and chronic alcohol use or abuse.

Adverse reactions

CNS: dizziness, headache, insomnia, fatigue, paresthesia, tremor, vertigo, syncope, anxiety, confusion, depression, nervousness, drowsiness, malaise, **seizures**
CV: palpitations, tachycardia, angina pectoris, hypertension, hypotension, **arrhythmias, heart failure, myocardial infarction**
EENT: abnormal vision, conjunctivitis, hearing loss, tinnitus, pharyngitis
GI: nausea, vomiting, diarrhea, constipation, abdominal pain, dyspepsia, flatulence, colitis, duodenal or gastric ulcer, gastritis, gastroesophageal reflux, esophagitis, dry mouth, **GI hemorrhage, pancreatitis**
GU: albuminuria, hematuria, urinary frequency, urinary tract infection, **renal failure**
Hematologic: anemia, purpura, **leukopenia, thrombocytopenia, other blood dyscrasias**
Hepatic: hepatitis
Metabolic: dehydration
Musculoskeletal: myalgia, joint or back pain

Respiratory: dyspnea, cough, asthma, upper respiratory infection, **bronchospasm**
Skin: rash, urticaria, diaphoresis, pruritus, alopecia, bullous eruption, angioedema, photosensitivity
Other: altered taste, increased appetite, weight changes, flulike symptoms, edema, accidental injury, fever, allergic reaction

Patient monitoring

• Monitor CBC and liver and kidney function tests.

opioid analgesics

alfentanil, buprenorphine hydrochloride, butorphanol tartrate, codeine, fentanyl, hydrocodone, hydromorphone, levorphanol tartrate, meperidine hydrochloride, methadone hydrochloride, morphine sulfate, nalbuphine hydrochloride, oxycodone, oxymorphone hydrochloride, pentazocine, propoxyphene, remifentanil hydrochloride, sufentanil, tramadol

Action

Attach to specific CNS receptors, decreasing cell membrane permeability, slowing pain impulse transmission, and altering response to pain

Indications

Moderate to severe pain, intraoperative anesthesia, labor, cough, diarrhea

Contraindications and precautions

• Contraindicated in hypersensitivity to drug, diarrhea caused by poisoning, acute bronchial asthma, and upper airway obstruction
• Use cautiously in severe cardiovascular, renal, or hepatic disease; cardiac decompensation; GI disorders; history of ulcer disease; chronic alcohol use or abuse; elderly patients; pregnant or breastfeeding patients; and children younger than age 13.

Adverse reactions

CNS: drowsiness, sedation, dizziness, tremor, irritability, syncope, stimulation (in children)
CV: hypertension, hypotension, palpitations, bradycardia, tachycardia, extrasystole, **arrhythmias**
EENT: blurred vision, nasal dryness and congestion, dry or sore throat
GI: nausea, vomiting, constipation, epigastric distress, dry mouth, anorexia, **intestinal obstruction**
GU: urinary retention or hesitancy, dysuria, early menses, decreased libido, erectile dysfunction
Hematologic: hemolytic anemia, hypoplastic anemia, thrombocytopenia, agranulocytosis, leukopenia, pancytopenia
Respiratory: thickened bronchial secretions, chest tightness, wheezing
Skin: urticaria, rash, diaphoresis
Other: hypersensitivity reaction (with I.V. use), **anaphylactic shock**

Patient monitoring

• Assess vital signs and respiratory status.
• Monitor CBC, electrolyte levels, and liver and kidney function tests.

plasma expanders

albumin (human normal serum), dextran, hetastarch, plasma protein fraction

Action

Maintain plasma colloid osmotic pressure and carry intermediate metabolites in transport and exchange of tissue products; crucial to regulation of circulating blood volume

Indications
Shock, burns, hypoproteinemia, adult respiratory distress syndrome, cardiopulmonary bypass, acute hepatic failure, acute nephrosis, hyperbilirubinemia and erythroblastosis fetalis, sequestration of protein-rich fluids, leukapheresis, erythrocyte resuspension, renal dialysis

Contraindications and precautions
- Contraindicated in hypersensitivity to drug, severe anemia, heart failure, severe bleeding disorders, and renal failure with oliguria or anuria
- Use cautiously in normal or increased intravascular volume, cardiopulmonary bypass, chronic nephrosis, hepatic or renal failure caused by increased protein load, sodium restriction, and critically ill patients.

Adverse reactions
CNS: headache
CV: hypotension, tachycardia, pulse and blood pressure changes, **vascular overload**
EENT: blurred vision, throat tightness
GI: nausea, vomiting, increased salivation, submaxillary and parotid gland enlargement
Musculoskeletal: back pain, muscle pain
Respiratory: dyspnea, respiratory changes, **pulmonary edema**
Skin: flushing, urticaria, rash, pruritus
Other: allergic or pyrogenic reactions, chills, flulike symptoms

Patient monitoring
- Monitor for hemorrhagic shock after injury or surgery. (Rapid postinfusion blood pressure rise may cause bleeding from severed vessels.)
- Check vital signs frequently.
- Watch for signs and symptoms of heart failure and pulmonary edema.
- Evaluate fluid intake and output.
- Monitor hemoglobin, hematocrit, urine protein, and electrolyte levels.

renin-angiotensin system antagonists

Angiotensin-converting enzyme (ACE) inhibitors: benazepril hydrochloride, captopril, enalapril maleate, enalaprilat, fosinopril sodium, lisinopril, moexipril, perindopril erbumine, quinapril hydrochloride, ramipril, trandolapril

Angiotensin II receptor antagonists: candesartan cilexetil, eprosartan mesylate, irbesartan, losartan potassium, olmesartan medoxomil, telmisartan, valsartan

Selective aldosterone receptor antagonist: eplerenone

Action
ACE inhibitors lower blood pressure by preventing conversion of angiotensin I to angiotensin II, a potent vasoconstrictor that decreases peripheral resistance and aldosterone secretion.

Angiotensin II receptor antagonists block vasoconstrictive and aldosterone-secreting effects of angiotensin II by selectively blocking binding of angiotensin II to angiotensin I receptors in vascular smooth muscle, adrenal, and other tissues.

Selective aldosterone receptor antagonists bind to mineralocorticoid receptors and block binding of aldosterone, a component of the renin-angiotensin-aldosterone system. This effect decreases blood pressure.

Indications

Hypertension, heart failure, left ventricular dysfunction, multiple sclerosis, diabetic neuropathy

Contraindications and precautions

• Contraindicated in hypersensitivity to drug
• Use cautiously in renal or hepatic impairment, hypovolemia, hyponatremia, aortic stenosis and hypertrophic cardiomyopathy, cerebrovascular or cardiac insufficiency, surgery and anesthesia, concurrent diuretic therapy, family history of angioedema, Black patients with hypertension, elderly patients, pregnant or breastfeeding patients, and children (safety not established for most ACE inhibitors).

Adverse reactions

CNS: dizziness, fatigue, headache, insomnia, asthenia, drowsiness, vertigo
CV: hypotension, angina pectoris, tachycardia, **myocardial infarction**
EENT: sinusitis
GI: nausea, diarrhea, anorexia
GU: proteinuria, erectile dysfunction, decreased libido, **renal failure**
Hematologic: bone marrow depression, agranulocytosis
Hepatic: cholestatic jaundice progressing to **hepatic necrosis and death**
Metabolic: hyperkalemia
Respiratory: cough, bronchitis, dyspnea, asthma, **eosinophilic pneumonitis**
Skin: rash, angioedema
Other: taste disturbances, fever, **anaphylaxis**

Patient monitoring

• Monitor vital signs, including blood pressure in both arms with patient lying down, standing, and sitting.
• Assess fluid intake and output, electrolyte levels, CBC, and kidney and liver function tests.
• Evaluate urine for protein.
• Watch for microalbuminuria, especially in diabetic patients.

sedative-hypnotics

Barbiturates: pentobarbital, phenobarbital

Nonbarbiturates: chloral hydrate, dexmedetomidine hydrochloride, flurazepam hydrochloride, temazepam, triazolam, zaleplon, zolpidem tartrate

Action

Barbiturates cause drowsiness, sedation, and hypnosis by depressing the sensory cortex, decreasing motor activity, and altering cerebellar function.

Nonbarbiturates produce sedative, anxiolytic, muscle relaxant, and anticonvulsant effects by interacting with the gamma-aminobutyric acid–benzodiazepine receptor complex.

Indications

Short-term treatment of insomnia, sedation, preanesthesia

Contraindications and precautions

• Contraindicated in hypersensitivity to drug, barbiturate sensitivity, manifest or latent porphyria, marked hepatic dysfunction, severe respiratory disease, and nephritis
• Use cautiously in depression, respiratory compromise, pulmonary insufficiency, seizure disorders, hepatic or severe renal impairment, anxiety, elderly or debilitated patients, or history of drug abuse.

Adverse reactions

CNS: headache, nervousness, talkativeness, slurred speech, apprehension, ir-

ritability, anxiety, light-headedness, dizziness, euphoria, relaxed feeling, weakness, poor concentration, incoordination, confusion, memory impairment, depression, abnormal dreams, nightmares, insomnia, paresthesia, restlessness, fatigue, dysesthesia, drowsiness, somnolence, staggering, falling, ataxia, agitation, hyperkinesia, psychiatric disturbances, hallucinations, abnormal thinking, vertigo, lethargy, hangover effect
CV: palpitations, chest pain, tachycardia, hypotension, bradycardia, **circulatory collapse**, **thrombophlebitis** (with I.V. use)
EENT: blurred vision, burning eyes, difficulty focusing, visual disturbances, tinnitus
GI: nausea, vomiting, diarrhea, constipation, dyspepsia, GI pain, dry mouth, excessive salivation, glossitis, stomatitis, anorexia
Hepatic: jaundice, **hepatic failure** (in patients also receiving diuretics)
Hematologic: leukopenia, granulocytopenia
Musculoskeletal: joint pain
Respiratory: shortness of breath, hypoventilation, **respiratory depression**
Skin: dermatitis, diaphoresis, flushing, pruritus, rash, angioedema, exfoliative dermatitis
Other: altered taste, body pain, pain at I.M. injection site, fever (especially with long-term phenobarbital use)

Patient monitoring

- Monitor vital signs, respiratory status, CBC with white cell differential, liver function tests, and blood urea nitrogen, creatinine, and electrolyte levels. Stay alert for hyperkalemia.
- Assess neurologic status. Watch for signs and symptoms of drug dependence.

sex hormones

5-alpha reductase inhibitors: dutasteride, finasteride

Androgens: danazol, fluoxymesterone, nandrolone, oxandrolone, testosterone

Estrogens: conjugated estrogens, esterified estrogens, estradiol, estrogens, etonogestrel and ethinyl estradiol vaginal ring, norelgestromin/ethinyl estradiol, norethindrone acetate, norgestrel

Progestins: medroxyprogesterone, megestrol acetate, progesterone

Selective estrogen receptor modulator: raloxifene

Action

Varies with specific drug. See individual monographs.

Indications

Vary with specific drug. See individual monographs.

Contraindications and precautions

- Contraindicated in hypersensitivity to drug or its components; known or suspected breast cancer or estrogen-dependent neoplasia; undiagnosed abnormal genital bleeding; porphyria; active deep-vein thrombosis, pulmonary embolism, or history of these conditions; active or recent arterial thromboembolic disease; active thrombophlebitis or thromboembolic disorders; history of thrombophlebitis, thrombosis, or thromboembolic disorders associated with previous estrogen use; and pregnancy

• Use cautiously in endometrial or ovarian cancer, endometriosis, gallbladder disease, vision disturbances, hypertension, familial hyperlipoproteinemia, hypothyroidism, conditions that predispose to fluid retention, hypocalcemia, asthma, diabetes mellitus, seizure disorders, migraine, hepatic or renal disease, and elderly patients.

Adverse reactions

CNS: headache, migraine, syncope, depression, insomnia, vertigo, neuralgia, hypoesthesia
CV: chest pain, varicose veins
EENT: conjunctivitis, neuro-ocular lesions (such as retinal thrombosis, optic neuritis), steepened corneal curvature, contact lens intolerance, sinusitis, rhinitis, laryngitis, pharyngitis
GI: nausea, vomiting, diarrhea, dyspepsia, flatulence, abdominal pain, GI disorder, gastroenteritis
GU: urinary tract infection, cystitis, leukorrhea, uterine or endometrial disorder, urinary tract disorder, breast tenderness or pain, breast enlargement, decreased lactation, amenorrhea, vaginal candidiasis, vaginitis, **vaginal hemorrhage, invasive cervical cancer**
Musculoskeletal: arthralgia, myalgia, leg cramps, arthritis, tendon disorder
Respiratory: cough, bronchitis, pneumonia
Skin: rash, diaphoresis, hot flashes
Other: fever, infection, flulike symptoms

Patient monitoring

• Monitor liver function tests, fluid intake and output, and phosphatase, calcium glucose, and folic acid levels.
• Assess abdomen for liver enlargement.
• Monitor for breast tenderness and swelling.
• Assess bone density annually.

skeletal muscle relaxants

baclofen, carisoprodol, chlorzoxazone, cyclobenzaprine hydrochloride, dantrolene sodium, diazepam, methocarbamol, tizanidine hydrochloride

Action

Unknown. Thought to cause muscle relaxation through sedative properties and by inhibiting activity in descending reticular formation and spine. Also decrease muscle tone and involuntary movements.

Indications

Muscle spasms (as from trauma or inflammation), hyperreflexia and hypertonia (as in parkinsonism), tetanus, cerebral palsy, multiple sclerosis, tension headache

Contraindications and precautions

• Contraindicated in hypersensitivity to drug or polyethylene glycol (parenteral forms), renal impairment (parenteral forms), active hepatic disease, upper motor neuron disorder, and patients who use spasticity to maintain posture or balance
• Use cautiously in cardiac, hepatic, or renal dysfunction; history of allergies; seizure disorders (parenteral forms); pregnant or breastfeeding patients; and children (safety not established).

Adverse reactions

CNS: dizziness, anxiety, abnormal thinking, hyperesthesia, agitation, confusion, hypertonia, **seizures, coma**
CV: palpitations, hypotension, bradycardia, weak pulse, fistula, pseudoaneurysm, **thrombophlebitis, complete or incomplete atrioventricular block, pulmonary embolism, nodal**

arrhythmias, ventricular tachycardia
EENT: diplopia
GI: nausea, vomiting, diarrhea, dyspepsia, gastroesophageal reflux, hematemesis, dysphagia, **paralytic ileus, GI bleeding**
GU: urinary frequency or incontinence, dysuria, cystalgia, prostatitis, **renal dysfunction**
Hepatic: hepatitis
Musculoskeletal: muscle rigidity
Respiratory: abnormal breath sounds, dyspnea, wheezing, bronchitis, pneumonia, pleurisy, **pleural effusion, pulmonary edema, pulmonary embolism, bronchospasm**
Skin: rash, urticaria, pruritus, edema
Other: chills, fever

Patient monitoring

- Monitor vital signs and liver function tests.

thrombolytics

alteplase, anistreplase, drotrecogin alfa, reteplase, streptokinase, tenecteplase, urokinase

Action

Convert plasminogen to plasmin, an enzyme that degrades fibrin clots and lyses thrombi and emboli

Indications

Acute massive pulmonary embolism, acute ischemic cerebrovascular accident (CVA), thrombotic coronary arterial obstruction in acute myocardial infarction, deep-vein thrombosis, arterial emboli or thromboses, occlusion of venous access device

Contraindications and precautions

- Contraindicated in hypersensitivity to drug or other thrombolytics, active internal bleeding, bleeding diathesis, severe uncontrolled hypertension, intracranial neoplasm, arteriovenous malformation or aneurysm, recent CVA, or recent intracranial or intraspinal surgery or trauma
- Use cautiously in GI or GU bleeding, hypertension, left-sided cardiac thrombus (including mitral stenosis), acute pericarditis, subacute bacterial endocarditis, hemostatic defects, diabetic hemorrhagic retinopathy, septic thrombophlebitis, previous puncture of noncompressible vessels, trauma, obstetric delivery, organ biopsy, major surgery, patients older than age 75, and pregnant or breastfeeding patients.

Adverse reactions

CNS: intracranial hemorrhage
CV: hypotension, **arrhythmias, cholesterol embolization, venous thrombosis**
GI: nausea, vomiting, **GI or retroperitoneal bleeding**
GU: hematuria
Hematologic: anemia, **bone marrow depression, hemorrhage, bleeding tendency**
Respiratory: respiratory depression, apnea
Skin: bruising, urticaria
Other: fever, edema, phlebitis or hemorrhage at I.V. site, hypersensitivity reactions including **anaphylaxis, sepsis**

Patient monitoring

- Monitor vital signs and neurologic status closely.
- (Clinical alert) Assess for unusual bleeding or bruising.
- Monitor International Normalized Ratio, prothrombin time, and partial thromboplastin time.

thyroid hormones

levothyroxine sodium; liothyronine sodium; liotrix; thyroid, desiccated

Action

Regulate growth and development by controlling protein synthesis; stimulate normal metabolism by oxygenating body tissues

Indications

Hypothyroidism, euthyroid or multinodal goiter, subacute or chronic lymphocytic thyroiditis

Contraindications and precautions

- Contraindicated in hypersensitivity to drug, recent myocardial infarction, adrenal insufficiency, and thyrotoxicosis
- Use cautiously in cardiovascular disease, severe renal insufficiency, uncorrected adrenocortical disorders, angina pectoris, ischemia, diabetes mellitus, myxedema, elderly patients, and pregnant or breastfeeding patients.

Adverse reactions

CNS: insomnia, irritability, nervousness, tremor, headache
CV: tachycardia, angina pectoris, hypotension, hypertension, increased cardiac output, palpitations, **arrhythmias, cardiovascular collapse**
GI: vomiting, diarrhea, abdominal cramps
GU: menstrual irregularities
Metabolic: hyperthyroidism
Musculoskeletal: accelerated bone maturation in children
Skin: alopecia (in children), diaphoresis
Other: weight loss, appetite changes, heat intolerance

Patient monitoring

- Monitor vital signs, weight, ECG, and thyroid function tests.

thyroid hormone antagonists

methimazole, potassium iodide, propylthiouracil, sodium iodide ^{131}I

Action

Rapidly inhibit iodine release and synthesis in thyroid gland, decreasing thyroid vascularity and preventing iodine uptake

Indications

Hyperthyroidism, thyroid cancer, thyrotoxicosis, to control hyperthyroidism before thyroidectomy or radioactive iodine therapy

Contraindications and precautions

- Contraindicated in hypersensitivity to thyroid hormone antagonists and in breastfeeding
- Use cautiously in bone marrow depression, tuberculosis, bronchitis, hyperkalemia, renal impairment, recent myocardial infarction, large nodular goiter, vomiting and diarrhea, patients younger than age 30, and pregnant patients.

Adverse reactions

CNS: headache, vertigo, paresthesia, neuritis, neuropathy, CNS stimulation, depression, drowsiness
CV: chest pain, tachycardia
EENT: pain on swallowing, sore throat
GI: nausea, vomiting, diarrhea, constipation, epigastric distress, GI irritation, dry mouth, salivary gland enlargement, anorexia, **paralytic ileus**
GU: nephritis

Hematologic: anemia, eosinophilia, **bone marrow depression, leukopenia, thrombocytopenia, leukemia, agranulocytosis**
Hepatic: jaundice, **hepatic dysfunction, hepatitis**
Metabolic: hypothyroidism, thyroid hyperplasia, **hyperkalemia**
Musculoskeletal: joint pain, myalgia
Respiratory: cough
Skin: rash, urticaria, skin discoloration, pruritus, erythema nodosum, exfoliative dermatitis, alopecia, acneiform eruption
Other: taste loss, fullness in neck, fever, lupuslike syndrome, lymphadenopathy, lymphedema, **radiation sickness** (with sodium iodide ^{131}I)

Patient monitoring

- Monitor CBC and thyroid function tests.

vasodilators

bosentan, hydralazine hydrochloride, isosorbide dinitrate, isosorbide mononitrate, minoxidil, nesiritide, nitroglycerin, nitroprusside sodium

Action

Relax vascular smooth muscle by stimulating intracellular production of cyclic guanosine monophosphate

Indications

Acute angina, prophylaxis and long-term management of recurrent angina, heart failure associated with acute myocardial infarction (MI), to control blood pressure in perioperative hypertension associated with surgery

Contraindications and precautions

- Contraindicated in hypersensitivity to drug, severe anemia, angle-closure glaucoma, orthostatic hypotension, early MI, head trauma, cerebral hemorrhage, and as primary therapy in cardiogenic shock or systolic pressure below 90 mm Hg
- Use cautiously in acute MI (associated with hypertension, tachycardia, or congestive heart failure), cerebral hemorrhage, gastric hypermotility or malabsorption syndrome (with sustained-release forms), head trauma, hyperthyroidism, hypertrophic cardiomyopathy, increased intraocular pressure, orthostatic hypotension, volume depletion, and alcohol use.

Adverse reactions

CNS: headache, apprehension, malaise, rigors, restlessness, weakness, asthenia, vertigo, dizziness, agitation, anxiety, confusion, insomnia, nervousness, nightmares, incoordination, hypoesthesia, hypokinesia
CV: tachycardia, retrosternal discomfort, palpitations, orthostatic hypotension, rebound hypertension, hypotension, syncope, crescendo angina, premature ventricular contractions, **arrhythmias, atrial fibrillation**
EENT: blurred vision, diplopia
GI: nausea, vomiting, diarrhea, dyspepsia, abdominal pain, tenesmus, fecal incontinence
GU: dysuria, urinary frequency, urinary incontinence, erectile dysfunction
Hematologic: methemoglobinemia, hemolytic anemia
Musculoskeletal: arthralgia, muscle twitching, stiff neck
Respiratory: bronchitis, pneumonia, upper respiratory infection
Skin: pallor; cold sweats; increased perspiration; rash; contact or exfoliative dermatitis; cutaneous vasodilation with flushing; crusty skin lesions; pruritus; topical allergic reaction; erythematous, vesicular, or pruritic lesions; local burning or tingling sensation in oral cavity (with sublingual forms);

anaphylactoid reactions with oral mucosal and conjunctival edema
Other: tooth disorder, increased appetite, edema

Patient monitoring

- Closely monitor ECG and vital signs (especially blood pressure).
- In suspected overdose, assess for signs and symptoms of increased intracranial pressure.
- Check arterial blood gas values and methemoglobin levels.

Vitamins and minerals

ascorbic acid (vitamin C)

Cecon, Cevi-Bid, Dull-C, Vita-C

Action

Water-soluble vitamin with antioxidant properties; stimulates collagen formation and enhances tissue repair

Availability

Capsules: 500 mg
Crystals: 1,000 mg/½ tsp
Injection: 250 mg/ml, 500 mg/ml
Liquid: 50 mg/ml, 500 mg/5 ml
Powder: 60 mg/½ tsp, 1,060 mg/½ tsp
Solution: 100 mg/ml
Tablets: 25 mg, 50 mg, 100 mg, 125 mg, 250 mg, 500 mg, 1,000 mg, 1,500 mg
Tablets (chewable): 60 mg, 100 mg, 250 mg, 500 mg, 1,000 mg
Tablets (timed-release): 500 mg, 1,000 mg, 1,500 mg

Indications and dosages

➢ Recommended dietary allowance
Adults: 60 mg daily
➢ Scurvy
Adults: 300 mg to 1 g P.O., subcutaneously, I.M., or I.V. daily
Children: 100 to 300 mg P.O., subcutaneously, I.M., or I.V. daily depending on severity

Contraindications and precautions

• Prolonged use of excessive doses contraindicated in diabetes mellitus, sodium-restricted diet, concurrent anticoagulant use, and history of recurrent renal calculi
• Use cautiously in hypersensitivity to tartrazine or sulfites (if product contains these compounds), before tests for occult blood in stool, and in breast-feeding patients. Don't exceed recommended amount in pregnant patients.
• Avoid rapid I.V. infusion.

Adverse reactions

Transient mild soreness at I.M. or subcutaneous injection site; transient light-headedness or dizziness (with rapid I.V. administration)

cholecalciferol (vitamin D_3)

Delta-D

Action

Biologically active vitamin D metabolite; controls intestinal absorption of dietary calcium, tubular reabsorption of calcium by kidney, and (in conjunction with parathyroid hormone [PTH]), calcium mobilization from skeleton. Acts directly on bone cells to stimulate skeletal growth and on parathyroid glands to suppress PTH synthesis and secretion.

Availability

Tablets: 400 international units, 1,000 international units

Indications and dosages

➢ Recommended dietary allowance (RDA)
Adults: 400 to 1,000 international units/day
Children: 400 international units/day

Contraindications and precautions

• Contraindicated in hypercalcemia, vitamin D toxicity, malabsorption syn-

drome, and abnormal sensitivity to vitamin D effects
• Don't exceed RDA during normal pregnancy. Use cautiously in breast-feeding patients. Safety and efficacy of dosages exceeding RDA have not been established for children.

Adverse reactions

Nausea, vomiting, constipation, pancreatitis, weakness, headache, irritability, drowsiness, overt psychosis, dry mouth, metallic taste, muscle or bone pain, hypertension, hypotension, polyuria, polydipsia, anorexia, weight loss, hypercalciuria, reversible azotemia, nephrocalcinosis, conjunctivitis, photophobia, pruritus, albuminuria, elevated liver function tests results, **arrhythmias**

chromium (chromic chloride)

Chroma-Pak

Action

Serves as a component of glucose tolerance factor, which activates insulin-mediated reactions; helps maintain normal glucose metabolism and peripheral nerve function

Availability

Injection: 4 mcg/ml (as 20.5 mcg chromic chloride hexahydrate), 20 mcg/ml (as 102.5 mcg chromic chloride hexahydrate)

Indications and dosages

➢ Supplement to I.V. solutions used in total parenteral nutrition
Adults: 10 to 15 mcg/day. For metabolically stable adults with intestinal fluid loss, 20 mcg/day.
Children: 0.14 to 0.2 mcg/kg/day

Contraindications and precautions

• Preparations containing benzyl alcohol contraindicated in premature infants (may cause fatal gasping syndrome)
• Avoid use or adjust dosage in patients with renal or GI dysfunction.
• Use cautiously in pregnant patients.
• Multiple trace element solutions may cause overdose if patient's requirement for one element in formulation exceeds that for others. Chromium may need to be given separately.

Adverse reactions

Toxicity is rare at recommended dosages; hypersensitivity reaction to iodide may occur.

copper

Cupric Sulfate

Action

Serves as cofactor for ceruloplasmin, an oxidase needed for proper formation of transferrin (an iron carrier protein); helps maintain normal rate of red and white blood cell formation

Availability

Injection: 0.4 mg/ml, 2 mg/ml

Indications and dosages

➢ Supplement to I.V. solutions used in total parenteral nutrition
Adults: 0.5 to 1.5 mg/day to prevent deficiency; 3 mg/day to treat deficiency
Children: 20 mcg/kg/day to prevent deficiency; 20 to 30 mcg/kg/day to treat deficiency

Contraindications and precautions

• Multidose preparations contraindicated in patients with sensitivity to benzyl alcohol (such as premature in-

fants, who may experience fatal gasping syndrome)
• Use cautiously in renal or GI dysfunction, Wilson's disease, and pregnant patients.
• Be aware that giving copper without zinc (or vice versa) may decrease blood level of the other mineral. Monitor levels before giving subsequent doses.
• Multiple trace element solutions may cause overdose if patient's requirement for one element in formulation exceeds that for others. Copper may need to be given separately.

Adverse reactions
None known

cyanocobalamin (vitamin B_{12})
Big Shot B-12, Cyanoject, Rubramin

hydroxocobalamin, crystalline (vitamin B_{12})
Hydro-Crysti-12, LA-12

Action
Essential to growth, cell reproduction, hematopoiesis, and nucleoprotein and myelin synthesis; also participates in nucleic acid synthesis. Plays a role in red blood cell formation through activation of folic acid coenzymes.

Availability
cyanocobalamin
Injection: 100 mcg/ml, 1,000 mcg/ml
Intranasal gel: 500 mcg/0.1 ml
Tablets: 25 mcg, 50 mcg, 100 mcg, 200 mcg, 250 mcg, 500 mcg, 1,000 mcg, 1,500 mcg
Tablets (extended-release): 100 mcg, 200 mcg, 500 mcg, 1,000 mcg
hydroxocobalamin
Injection: 1,000 mcg/ml

Indications and dosages
➢ Recommended dietary allowance
Adults and children older than age 11: 2 mcg cyanocobalamin daily
Children ages 9 to 11: 1.8 mcg daily
Children ages 4 to 8: 1.2 mcg daily
Children ages 1 to 3: 0.9 mcg daily
➢ Vitamin B_{12} deficiency
Adults: 30 mcg hydroxocobalamin I.M. daily for 5 to 10 days, depending on cause and severity; for maintenance, 100 to 200 mcg I.M. monthly
Children: Total dosage of 1 to 5 mg hydroxocobalamin I.M. given over 2 or more weeks in divided doses of 100 mcg; then a maintenance dosage of 30 to 50 mcg I.M. q 4 weeks
➢ Pernicious anemia
Adults: 100 mcg cyanocobalamin subcutaneously or I.M. daily for 7 days; then 100 mcg subcutaneously or I.M. every other day for 14 days; then 100 mcg subcutaneously or I.M. q 3 to 4 days for 2 to 3 weeks or until remission; then 100 mcg I.M. monthly or 1,000 to 2,000 mcg P.O. daily
➢ Vitamin B_{12} deficiency and malabsorption in patients in remission
Adults: 500 mcg nasal gel intranasally once weekly

Contraindications and precautions
• Contraindicated in hypersensitivity to vitamin B_{12}, cobalt, or product components

Adverse reactions
Mild transient diarrhea, nausea, vomiting, dyspepsia, headache, anxiety, dizziness, nervousness, hypoesthesia, sore throat, severe and rapid optic nerve atrophy, back pain, myalgia, arthritis, paresthesia, abnormal gait, dyspnea, rhinitis, itching, rash, polycythemia vera; with parenteral forms—injection site pain, **pulmonary edema, heart failure, peripheral vascular thrombosis, anaphylactic shock**

doxercalciferol
Hectorol

Action
Synthetic vitamin D analogue; acts directly on parathyroid gland to stimulate and suppress parathyroid hormone (PTH) synthesis and secretion

Availability
Capsules: 0.5 mcg, 2.5 mcg
Injection: 2 mcg/vial

Indications and dosages
➢ Elevated intact PTH levels (iPTH) in secondary hyperparathyroidism caused by chronic renal dialysis
Adults: Dosage individualized. Recommended initial dosage is 10 mcg P.O. three times weekly at dialysis (approximately every other day). Adjust as needed to lower blood iPTH level to 150 to 300 pg/ml. Maximum dosage is 20 mcg P.O. three times weekly.

Contraindications and precautions
• Contraindicated in hypersensitivity to product components, hypercalcemia, and evidence of vitamin D toxicity
• Use cautiously in elderly patients with coronary disease, renal impairment, or arteriosclerosis.

Adverse reactions
Nausea, vomiting, constipation, dyspepsia, headache, malaise, dizziness, sleep disorder, weight gain, anorexia, edema, arthralgia, abscess, dyspnea, pruritus, bradycardia

folic acid
Folvite

Action
Stimulates production of red and white blood cells and platelets in some megaloblastic anemias

Availability
Injection: 5 mg/ml
Tablets: 0.4 mg, 0.8 mg, 1 mg

Indications and dosages
➢ Recommended dietary allowance
Adults and children older than age 11: 150 to 400 mcg
Children younger than age 11: 25 to 100 mcg
➢ Megaloblastic anemia related to folic acid deficiency in sprue, nutritional deficiency, pregnancy, childhood, or infancy
Adults: Up to 1 mg/day P.O., I.M., I.V., or subcutaneously (given P.O. except in severe disease or severely impaired GI absorption). Higher dosages may be needed in severe cases, with a maintenance dosage of 0.4 mg/day. In pregnant or breastfeeding patients, 0.8 mg/day.
Children older than age 4: Maintenance dosage of 0.4 mg/day P.O., I.M., or subcutaneously (given P.O. except in severe disease or severely impaired GI absorption)
Children younger than age 4: Maintenance dosage of up to 0.3 mg/day P.O., I.M., or subcutaneously (given P.O. except in severe disease or severely impaired GI absorption)

Contraindications and precautions
• Contraindicated in pernicious, aplastic, or normocytic anemia
• Use cautiously in breastfeeding patients.

Adverse reactions
Altered sleep pattern, malaise, poor concentration, impaired judgment, hyperactivity, anorexia, nausea, flatulence, bitter taste, allergic reaction (including rash, pruritus, erythema), **bronchospasm**

manganese, chelated

manganese chloride

Action
Serves as a cofactor in various enzyme systems; stimulates hepatic cholesterol and fatty acid synthesis and influences mucopolysaccharide synthesis

Availability
Injection: 0.1 mg/ml (as 0.36 mg manganese chloride)
Tablets: 20 mg and 50 mg of chelated manganese

Indications and dosages
➢ Recommended dietary allowance
Adults: 1.9 to 2.3 mg/day in males; 1.6 to 1.8 mg/day in females
➢ Supplement to I.V. solutions used for total parenteral nutrition
Adults: 0.15 to 0.8 mg/day
Children: 2 to 10 mcg/kg/day

Contraindications and precautions
- Use cautiously in pregnant patients and premature infants (may reach toxic levels in kidney).
- Reduce dosage in renal or GI dysfunction.
- Multiple trace element solutions may cause overdose if patient's requirement for one element in formulation exceeds that for others. Manganese may need to be given separately.

Adverse reactions
None known

niacin (nicotinic acid, vitamin B_3)
Slo-Niacin

niacinamide (nicotinamide)

Action
Serves as a component of two coenzymes essential to oxidation-reduction reactions

Availability
Capsules (extended-release): 100 mg, 250 mg, 400 mg, 500 mg
Capsules (sustained-release): 125 mg, 500 mg
Capsules (timed-release): 250 mg, 500 mg
Tablets: 25 mg, 50 mg, 100 mg, 125 mg, 250 mg, 400 mg, 500 mg
Tablets (extended-release): 250 mg, 500 mg, 750 mg, 1,000 mg
Tablets (sustained-release): 500 mg
Tablets (timed-release): 250 mg, 500 mg

Indications and dosages
➢ Recommended dietary allowance (RDA)
Adults: 15 to 20 mg P.O. daily in males; 13 to 15 mg P.O. daily in females
➢ Pellagra
Adults: Up to 500 mg daily P.O. given in divided doses
➢ Niacin deficiency
Adults: Up to 100 mg P.O. daily
➢ Hyperlipidemia
Adults: Initially, 250 mg P.O. daily; increase up to 1 or 2 g/day (given in divided doses) at 4- to 7-day intervals. Don't exceed 6 g/day.

Contraindications and precautions

- Contraindicated in hypersensitivity to niacin, hepatic dysfunction, active peptic ulcer, severe hypotension, and arterial bleeding
- Use cautiously in heart disease (give only under doctor's supervision), gout, regular consumption of large amounts of alcohol, history of hepatic disease, and pregnant or breastfeeding patients. Don't exceed RDA in children (safety and efficacy not established).

Adverse reactions

Flushing, pruritus, urticaria, rash, dry skin, tingling, acanthosis nigricans, hyperpigmentation, diaphoresis, nausea, vomiting, diarrhea, dyspepsia, GI distress, abdominal pain, peptic ulcer, hyperuricemia, gout, decreased glucose tolerance, chills, dizziness, insomnia, migraine, transient headache, toxic amblyopia, cystoid macular edema, orthostasis, edema, hypotension, palpitations, syncope, dyspnea, abnormal liver function tests, **fulminant hepatic necrosis, hepatotoxicity, atrial fibrillation, other arrhythmias**

paricalcitol

Zemplar

Action

Synthetic vitamin D analog; suppresses parathyroid hormone in patients with chronic renal failure

Availability

Injection: 2 mcg/ml, 5 mcg/ml

Indications and dosages

➢ Hyperparathyroidism associated with chronic renal failure

Adults: 0.04 to 0.1 mcg/kg (2.8 to 7 mcg) as a single I.V. bolus dose given no more often than every other day during dialysis. Dosage may be increased by 2 to 4 mcg at 2- to 4-week intervals.

Contraindications and precautions

- Contraindicated in hypersensitivity to components of formulation, hypercalcemia, and vitamin D toxicity
- Use cautiously in breastfeeding patients.

Adverse reactions

Nausea, vomiting, dry mouth, pruritus, allergic reaction, rash, urticaria, edema, light-headedness, chills, fever, flulike symptoms, malaise, palpitations, pneumonia, **GI bleeding, sepsis**

phytonadione (vitamin K_1)

AquaMEPHYTON, Mephyton

Action

Promotes hepatic synthesis of active prothrombin, proconvertin, plasma thromboplastin component, and Stuart factor

Availability

Aqueous colloidal solution for injection: 2 mg/ml

Tablets: 5 mg

Indications and dosages

➢ Hypoprothrombinemia caused by anticoagulant therapy

Adults: Initially, 2.5 to 10 mg P.O., I.M., subcutaneously, or I.V. (at doses not exceeding 1 mg/minute); repeat if needed within 12 to 48 hours after P.O. dose or within 6 to 8 hours of I.M., subcutaneous, or I.V. dose. Subsequent dosages determined by prothrombin time or clinical condition.

➢ Hypoprothrombinemia secondary to other causes

Adults: 2.5 to 25 mg (rarely, up to 50

mg); dosage and administration route depend on severity and response.
Children: 5 to 10 mg; dosage and administration route depend on severity and response.

➢ Prevention and treatment of hemorrhagic disease of newborn
Neonates: For prevention, 0.5 to 1 mg I.M. as a single dose within 1 hour of birth. For treatment, 1 mg I.M. or subcutaneously if mother received oral anticoagulants.

Contraindications and precautions

- Contraindicated in hypersensitivity to drug or its components. (Life-threatening reactions resembling hypersensitivity or anaphylaxis have occurred during and immediately after I.V. injection.)
- Use cautiously in pregnant or breast-feeding patients, children, and neonates (if product contains benzyl alcohol).
- Avoid P.O. use in disorders that may prevent adequate absorption.

Adverse reactions

Hyperbilirubinemia (in infants); with parenteral administration—pain, swelling, tenderness at injection site; itchy rash after repeated injections; transient flushing sensations; peculiar taste; **anaphylactoid reactions**

pyridoxine hydrochloride (vitamin B_6)

Beesix, Doxine, Nestrex, Rodex

Action

Converts to physiologically active forms of vitamin B_6 (pyridoxal phosphate and pyridoxamine phosphate), which promote metabolic functions affecting carbohydrate, protein, and lipid use

Availability

Capsules (extended-release): 150 mg
Injection: 100 mg/ml
Tablets: 10 mg, 25 mg, 50 mg, 100 mg, 200 mg, 250 mg, 500 mg
Tablets (enteric-coated): 20 mg
*Tablets (extended-release):*100 mg, 200 mg, 500 mg

Indications and dosages

➢ Recommended dietary allowance (RDA)
Adults: 1.7 to 2 mg daily in males; 1.4 to 1.6 mg daily in females

➢ Prophylaxis or treatment of pyridoxine deficiency, including drug-induced deficiency (as from isoniazid, hydralazine, or hormonal contraceptives)
Adults: For prophylaxis, 25 to 100 mg daily P.O., I.V., or I.M. For established neuropathy, 200 mg daily.

Contraindications and precautions

- Contraindicated in hypersensitivity to pyridoxine or components of formulation
- Don't exceed RDA in children (safety and efficacy not established).
- Use cautiously in breastfeeding patients.
- Be aware that drug abuse and dependence have occurred after withdrawal from dosage of 200 mg/day.

Adverse reactions

Sensory neuropathic syndrome (including unstable gait, ataxia, clumsiness of hands, pedal and perioral numbness, paresthesia, and decreased sensation to touch, temperature, and vibration), photoallergic reaction, nausea, headache, decreased folic acid level, aspartate aminotransferase elevation, **seizures**

retinol (vitamin A)

Aquasol A, Palmitate-A 5000

Action

Stimulates and supports retinal function, reproduction, bone growth, epithelial tissue differentiation, and embryonic development

Availability

Capsules: 10,000 international units, 15,000 international units, 25,000 international units
Injection: 50,000 international units/ml
Tablets: 5,000 international units

Indications and dosages

➢ Recommended dietary allowance (RDA)
Adults: 1,000 mcg retinol equivalents (RE) daily in males; 800 mcg RE daily in females
➢ Severe vitamin A deficiency with corneal changes
Adults and children older than age 8: 100,000 international units I.M. daily for first 3 days, followed by 50,000 international units I.M. daily for 2 weeks. Or 500,000 international units P.O. for 3 days, followed by 50,000 international units P.O. daily for 14 days, then 10,000 to 20,000 international units P.O. daily for 60 days. Or 50,000 to 100,000 international units P.O. daily for 1 to 7 days, followed by 5,000 to 75,000 international units daily for several weeks.
➢ Vitamin A deficiency with xerophthalmia
Children: 5,000 to 15,000 international units (1,500 to 4,500 RE) I.M. for 10 days or 5,000 international units/kg P.O. for 5 days or until recovery

Contraindications and precautions

- Hypersensitivity to vitamin A or components of formulation, hypervitaminosis A
- Don't exceed RDA during normal pregnancy.
- Use cautiously in patients with renal failure and in I.V. use.

Adverse reactions

Headache, irritability, vertigo, lethargy, malaise, fever, headache, hypercalcemia, weight loss, vision changes, anorexia, sticky skin, hypervitaminosis A, **increased intracranial pressure, anaphylactic shock and death** (with I.V. use)

riboflavin (lactoflavin, vitamin B_2)

Action

Serves as two coenzymes that catalyze oxidation-reduction reactions, such as glucose oxidation, amino acid deamination, and fatty acid breakdown

Availability

Tablets: 10 mg, 25 mg, 50 mg, 100 mg, 250 mg

Indications and dosages

➢ Recommended dietary allowance (RDA)
Adults: 1.4 to 1.8 mg in males; 1.2 to 1.3 mg in females
➢ Riboflavin deficiency
Adults: 5 to 30 mg P.O. daily in divided doses

Contraindications and precautions

- Use cautiously when giving more than RDA to pregnant or breastfeeding women.

Adverse reactions

None known

selenium

Sele-Pak, Selepen

Action

Guards cell components against oxidative damage caused by peroxides generated during cellular metabolism

Availability

Injection: 40 mcg/ml

Indications and dosages

➢ Recommended dietary allowance

Adults: 40 to 70 mcg in males; 45 to 55 mcg in females

➢ Supplement to I.V. solutions used in total parenteral nutrition for prophylaxis and treatment of selenium deficiency

Adults and adolescents: 20 to 40 mcg daily for prophylaxis; 100 mcg daily for 24 to 31 days for treatment

Children: 3 mcg/kg daily (for prophylaxis or treatment)

Contraindications and precautions

- Use cautiously in renal or GI dysfunction, pregnant patients, or premature infants (if product contains benzyl alcohol, which is associated with fatal gasping syndrome). May need to decrease dosage in renal or GI dysfunction.
- Multiple trace element solutions may cause overdose if patient's requirement for one element in formulation exceeds that for others. Selenium may need to be given separately.

Adverse reactions

Lethargy, alopecia, hair discoloration, vomiting, abdominal pain, garlic breath, tremor, diaphoresis

thiamine (vitamin B_1)

Biamine, Thiamilate, Thiamine Hydrochloride

Action

Water-soluble vitamin; combines with adenosine triphosphate and thiamine diphosphokinase to form thiamine pyrophosphate, a coenzyme essential for normal growth and aerobic metabolism, nerve impulse transmission, and acetylcholine synthesis

Availability

Injection: 100 mg/ml

Tablets: 5 mg, 10 mg, 25 mg, 50 mg, 100 mg, 250 mg, 500 mg

Tablets (enteric-coated): 20 mg

Indications and dosages

➢ Recommended dietary allowance

Adults: 1.2 to 1.5 mg/day in males; 1 to 1.1 mg/day in females

➢ Thiamine deficiency (beriberi)

Adults: 10 to 20 mg I.M. t.i.d. for 2 weeks, then 5 to 30 mg P.O. daily for 1 month

➢ Wernicke's encephalopathy

Adults: Initially, 100 mg I.V., followed by 50 to 100 mg daily I.M. until patient can consume a regular balanced diet

Contraindications and precautions

- Contraindicated in thiamine hypersensitivity
- Use cautiously in pregnant or breast-feeding patients.

Adverse reactions

Warm sensation, pruritus, urticaria, weakness, diaphoresis, tenderness and induration (with I.M. use), hypersensitivity reaction, **cyanosis, pulmonary edema, GI tract hemorrhage, cardiovascular collapse, angioedema, anaphylactic shock, death**

tocopherols (alpha tocopherols, vitamin E)

Aquavit E, d'Apha E, Nutr-E-Sol, Vita-Plus E

Action

Protects cellular components from oxidation, prevents formation of toxic oxidation products, maintains integrity of red blood cell (RBC) wall, protects RBCs against hemolysis, stimulates steroid metabolism, suppresses prostaglandin production, and inhibits platelet aggregation

Availability

Capsules: 100, 200, 400, 600, and 1,000 international units
Drops: 15 international units/0.3 ml
Liquid: 15 international units/30 ml
Solution (water-miscible): 50 international units/ml
Tablets: 100, 200, 400, 500, 600, 800, and 1,000 international units

Indications and dosages

➢ Recommended dietary allowance
Adults: 15 international units in males; 12 international units in females
➢ To prevent or treat vitamin E deficiency
Adults: 60 to 75 international units P.O. daily, to a maximum of 1,000 international units daily

Contraindications and precautions

None

Adverse reactions

Hypervitaminosis E, nausea, vomiting, diarrhea, fatigue, weakness, blurred vision, headache, rash, gonadal dysfunction, **bleeding, necrotizing enterocolitis** (in infants)

zinc chloride

zinc gluconate

zinc sulfate

Zinca-Pak

Action

Serves as cofactor for more than 70 enzymes; promotes wound healing and helps maintain normal growth rate, normal skin hydration, and taste and smell sensations

Availability

Capsules: 220 mg
Injection: 1 mg/ml (as 2.09 mg chloride)
Tablets (gluconate): 10 mg, 15 mg, 50 mg
Tablets (sulfate): 66 mg, 110 mg

Indications and dosages

➢ Recommended dietary allowance
Adults: 12 to 15 mg
➢ Dietary supplement
Adults: 25 to 50 mg P.O. daily
➢ Supplement to I.V. solution used in total parenteral nutrition (TPN)
Metabolically stable adults: 2.5 to 4 mg/day; may give additional 2 mg/day in acute catabolic states. In patients with fluid loss from small bowel, give additional 12.2 mg/L of TPN solution.

Contraindications and precautions

- Use cautiously in renal or GI dysfunction, pregnant patients, and premature infants (if product contains benzyl alcohol, which is associated with fatal gasping syndrome).
- Dosage may need to be decreased in renal or GI dysfunction.

• Multiple trace element solutions may cause overdose if patient's requirement one element in formulation exceeds that for others. Zinc may need to be given separately.

Adverse reactions

Restlessness, dizziness, nausea, vomiting, diarrhea, gastric ulcer

Herbs and supplements

The information provided in these monographs reflects commonly held beliefs about the actions and uses of common herbs and nutritional supplements. However, not all of these beliefs have been confirmed by clinical trials. Although herbal remedies have been used for thousands of years, few have undergone well-designed scientific studies to determine how they work, if they're safe, and whether they're effective in treating the medical conditions for which they're commonly used. Advise patients to consult a health care practitioner before using herbs or supplements to help determine if such use may be safe.

aloe

Purported action
With topical use, exerts a moisturizing effect on burns and wounds, which prevents air from drying the wound and increases blood flow to stimulate healing. With internal use, may exert a laxative effect by stimulating the large intestine and increasing peristalsis.

Reported uses
Used topically (as a gel) to inhibit infection and promote healing of minor burns, abrasions, wounds, and frostbite and to treat certain skin diseases (such as psoriasis and seborrheic dermatitis). Used internally (as liquid extract concentrate, capsules, or dried aloe latex) as a strong laxative.

Contraindications and precautions
Internal use is contraindicated in inflammatory bowel disease, elderly patients with suspected intestinal obstruction, pregnant or breastfeeding patients, and children younger than age 12.

Adverse reactions
- With topical use: redness, itching, and burning sensation in dermabraded skin
- With P.O. use: edema, cramps, diarrhea, weight loss, electrolyte abnormalities, **arrhythmias**

Interactions
Antiarrhythmics, corticosteroids, licorice, stimulant laxatives, thiazide diuretics: hypokalemia
Cardiac glycosides: increased effects of these drugs

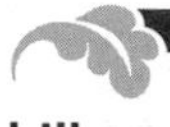

bilberry

Purported action
Relieves mild GI tract inflammation, easing diarrhea; reduces oral mucous membrane irritation; increases microcirculation by redistributing new capillary formation; strengthens capillary walls; promotes overall health of circulatory system; and exerts a protective effect on stomach and liver (possibly through increased prostaglandin production)

Reported uses
Nonspecific diarrhea, mouth and throat irritation, to improve visual acuity and accommodation. Further studies are needed to confirm that bil-

berry promotes circulatory, GI, or hepatic health.

Contraindications and precautions
Contraindicated in bleeding disorders, pregnancy, and breastfeeding

Adverse reactions
- At typical dosages: GI distress, rash, drowsiness
- At higher dosages: unknown

Interactions
Anticoagulants, antiplatelet drugs, salicylates: potentiated effects, causing increased prothrombin time
Hypoglycemics: reduced blood glucose level

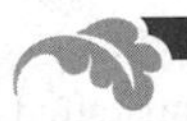

black cohosh

Purported action
Binds to estrogen receptors, directly or indirectly influencing luteinizing hormone release. Studies show black cohosh increases bone mineral density in rats but not in humans.

Reported uses
Menopause symptoms (as alternative to hormone replacement therapy), premenstrual syndrome, dysmenorrhea, arthritis, renal problems, malaria, sore throat

Contraindications and precautions
Contraindicated in pregnancy (may cause premature birth or miscarriage)

Adverse reactions
Headache, dizziness, CNS and visual disturbances, GI distress, nausea, vomiting, reduced heart rate, increased perspiration, weight gain

Interactions
Antihypertensives: additive hypotension
Docetaxel: increased docetaxel blood level
Hepatotoxic drugs: increased risk of hepatotoxicity

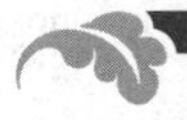

cat's claw

Purported action
Stimulates the immune system, enhances phagocytosis, dilates peripheral vessels, inhibits sympathetic nervous system activity, slows heart rate, decreases cholesterol levels, promotes diuresis, inhibits urinary bladder contraction, relaxes smooth muscle, and exerts local anesthetic effects. Studies show cat's claw has some anticancer and immunostimulant properties.

Reported uses
AIDS; inflammation; GI disorders (including colitis, inflammatory bowel disease, Crohn's disease); as an astringent, antiviral, anti-infective, and general tonic

Contraindications and precautions
Contraindicated in multiple sclerosis, tuberculosis, autoimmune disease, pregnancy, and breastfeeding. Use cautiously in GI disease (increases stomach acid secretion).

Adverse reactions
- Hypotension
- With decoction: few known risks

Interactions
Anticoagulants, antiplatelets: inhibited platelet aggregation, prolonged bleeding time
Antihypertensives: potentiated antihypertensive effects

Benzodiazepines: increased CNS depression
CYP450-3A4 substrates (such as amiodarone, amlodipine, fentanyl, flutamide, imipramine): increased levels of these drugs
Food: enhanced cat's claw absorption
Immunosuppressants: negated immunosuppressant effects

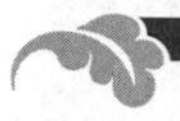

chamomile

Purported action
Reduces inflammation and fever, promotes healing of burns, and prevents ulcer formation. May also exert antispasmodic, anxiolytic, and sedative effects through action on CNS receptors.

Reported uses
Vomiting, flatulence, colic, fever, cystitis, parasitic worm infections, spasms, inflammation, anxiety; as an antibacterial, astringent, deodorant, or skin wash (to increase sloughing of necrotic tissue and promote granulation and epithelialization)

Contraindications and precautions
Contraindicated in ragweed allergy, hepatic or renal disease, pregnancy, and breastfeeding. Use cautiously in patients receiving anticoagulants.

Adverse reactions
Contact dermatitis in patients allergic to ragweed, asters, chrysanthemums, or other members of the Compositae family (such as arnica, feverfew, tansy, and yarrow), **anaphylaxis, other severe hypersensitivity reactions**

Interactions
Anticoagulants: increased anticoagulant effect
Concurrently administered drugs: delayed drug absorption
Sedatives (such as benzodiazepines): enhanced sedative effects

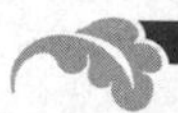

chondroitin

Purported action
A glycosaminoglycan (complex polysaccharide) found in extracellular matrix of connective tissue, including cornea and cartilage; thought to have protective properties (as for corneal endothelial cells and other ocular structures) without interfering with epithelialization and healing

Reported uses
Osteoarthritis, hyperlipidemia, ischemic heart disease, dry eyes, surgical aid in cataract extraction or lens implantation

Contraindications and precautions
Contraindicated in clotting disorders, prostate cancer, risk factors for prostate cancer, and patients receiving anticoagulants. Use cautiously in asthma.

Adverse reactions
Allergic reactions, alopecia, nausea, diarrhea, constipation, epigastric pain, extrasystoles, edema

Interactions
Warfarin: increased warfarin effects (with high chondroitin doses)

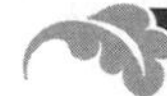

coenzyme Q10

Purported action
Fat-soluble, vitamin-like compound present in cells (especially concentrated

in heart, liver, kidney, and pancreas). Exerts antioxidant activity, stabilizes membranes, and serves as cofactor in many metabolic pathways, especially adenosine triphosphate production in oxidative respiration.

Reported uses

Mitochondrial cytopathies (FDA-approved claim), cardiac risk reduction, heart failure, hypertension, prophylaxis of doxorubicin-induced cardiotoxicity, diabetes mellitus, immunostimulation, muscular dystrophy, statin-induced myopathy, chronic fatigue syndrome, breast cancer, Huntington's disease, Parkinson's disease, periodontal disease

Contraindications and precautions

Use cautiously in biliary obstruction, hepatic insufficiency, hypertension, diabetes mellitus, patients receiving antihypertensives, and patients undergoing chemotherapy or radiation therapy.

Adverse reactions

Anxiety, nausea, vomiting, diarrhea, flatulence, headache, mania or hypomania

Interactions

Antihypertensives: additive blood pressure reduction
Chemotherapy: possible cancer-cell protection
Warfarin: reduced warfarin effects

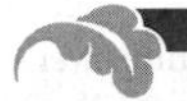

dong quai

Purported action

Exerts antispasmodic effect on smooth muscles, including those of airway and uterus. Forms containing coumarin have anticoagulant effects.

Reported uses

Asthma, allergies, menstrual disorders, menopausal symptoms, rheumatic pain, anemia, constipation, hypertension, psoriasis, skin depigmentation, ulcers; as an antispasmodic, anti-inflammatory, and anticoagulant

Contraindications and precautions

Contraindicated in patients receiving warfarin concurrently and in pregnant or breastfeeding patients (may influence uterine contractions or cause unknown effects in fetus)

Adverse reactions

- With authentic dong quai: no known reactions
- With other dong quai forms: increased risk of phototoxicity, abortion, uterine stimulation, and altered menstrual cycle

Interactions

Anticoagulants: increased anticoagulant effect

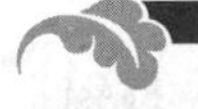

echinacea

Purported action

Stimulates immune system; with topical use, may have mild antibacterial and antiviral properties

Reported uses

Urinary tract and yeast infections, promotion of wound healing, prevention and treatment of upper respiratory infections (including colds and flu), allergic rhinitis, psoriasis, herpes simplex infection (topical form)

Contraindications and precautions
Contraindicated in patients receiving immunosuppressant therapy (because of immune-stimulating properties)

Adverse reactions
Nausea, mild GI upset, allergic reactions, **anaphylaxis**

Note: Adverse reactions may be more common in patients with allergies to daisy-type plants.

Interactions
Corticosteroids: interference with chemotherapeutic effects of these drugs
CYP450-3A4 substrates (such as amiodarone, amlodipine, fentanyl, flutamide, imipramine): increased levels of these drugs
Immunosuppressants: interference with immunosuppressant effects

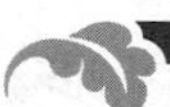

evening primrose oil

Purported action
Contains essential fatty acids (EFAs) that may improve cellular structural elements and serve as precursors to prostaglandins, which help regulate metabolic functions (including cervical ripening)

Reported uses
Disorders thought to stem from EFA deficiency or disturbed EFA metabolism, including cardiovascular disease, premenstrual syndrome, mastalgia and other breast disorders, rheumatoid arthritis, multiple sclerosis, atopic dermatitis and other dermatologic disorders, Raynaud's disease, Sjögren's syndrome, Alzheimer's disease, schizophrenia, and attention deficit hyperactivity disorder

Contraindications and precautions
Contraindicated in pregnancy, breastfeeding, and history of seizures or allergy to evening primrose oil

Adverse reactions
Headache, nausea, vomiting, diarrhea, abdominal pain, indigestion, flatulence, allergic reaction

Interactions
Anesthetics, phenothiazines: lowered seizure threshold
Anticoagulants: bleeding, bruising
Anticonvulsants: lowered seizure threshold, decreased anticonvulsant efficacy

feverfew

Purported action
Inhibits prostaglandin synthesis and serotonin release from platelets and polymorphonuclear leukocyte granules; extract may inhibit phagocytosis and platelet deposition on collagen surfaces. Exhibits antithrombotic potential and in vitro antibacterial activity, inhibits mast cell release of histamine, exerts cytotoxic activity, and suppresses enzyme release from white blood cells in inflamed joints and skin. May promote contraction and relaxation of vascular smooth muscle.

Reported uses
Menstrual pain, allergies, tinnitus, vertigo, asthma, dermatitis, psoriasis, arthritis, fever, migraine prophylaxis

Contraindications and precautions
Contraindicated in pregnancy, breastfeeding, and children younger than age 2

Adverse reactions

- Hypersensitivity reaction, increased heart rate, oral mucosa and tongue inflammation
- After withdrawal: cluster of CNS reactions (rebound migraine, anxiety, disturbed sleep pattern), muscle and joint stiffness

Interactions

Anticoagulants, aspirin: increased antithrombotic effect of these drugs

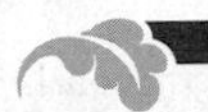

fish oils

Purported action

Contain omega-3 fatty acids, which exert anti-inflammatory and antithrombotic effects by competing with arachidonic acid in cyclooxygenase and lipoxygenase pathways and which also may suppress cyclooxygenase-2, interleukin-1 alpha, and tumor necrosis factor-alpha. Also inhibit arachidonic acid synthesis of thromboxane A_2, which causes platelet aggregation and vasoconstriction; and increase production of prostacyclin, a prostaglandin that causes vasoconstriction and reduces platelet aggregation.

Reported uses

Coronary heart disease, cardiovascular disease, cerebrovascular accident, hypertension, asthma, Crohn's disease, type 2 (non-insulin-dependent) diabetes mellitus, dysmenorrhea, fatigue, headache, herpes simplex virus type 2, hypercholesterolemia, hypertriglyceridemia, multiple sclerosis, rheumatoid arthritis, acne, rosacea, eczema, psoriasis, scleroderma, immune support; to improve circulation; to enhance cognitive performance and memory

Contraindications and precautions

Avoid large doses (more than 3 g/day) in diabetes mellitus and immunodeficiency. Use cautiously in aspirin sensitivity, bleeding disorders, cirrhosis, familial adenomatous polyposis, major depressive disorders, bipolar disorder, and concurrent antihypertensive use.

Adverse reactions

- Belching, halitosis, heartburn, increased low-density lipoprotein level, weight gain
- With large doses: bleeding, hemorrhagic stroke, immunosuppression, loose stools, nausea, hyperglycemia

Interactions

Anticoagulants, antiplatelet drugs, salicylates: increased risk of bleeding
Antihypertensives: additive hypotension
Hormonal contraceptives: interference with triglyceride-lowering effects of fish oils

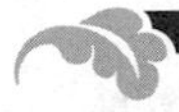

flaxseed oil

Purported action

Contains linolenic, linoleic, and alpha-linolenic acid. Linoleic acid and alpha-linolenic acid are required for structural integrity of cell membranes. Alpha-linolenic acid increases blood levels of omega-3 polyunsaturated fatty acids, including eicosapentaenoic acid and docosahexaenoic acid.

Reported uses

Atherosclerosis, hyperlipidemia, benign prostatic hypertrophy, constipation, diverticulitis, enteritis, gastritis, irritable bowel syndrome, menopausal symptoms, skin inflammation, systemic lupus erythematosus, nephritis, cancer prevention

Contraindications and precautions
Contraindicated in bowel obstruction, breast cancer, endometriosis, esophageal stricture, intestinal inflammation, ovarian cancer, uterine cancer, and uterine fibroids. Avoid medicinal doses in pregnant patients. Use cautiously in bleeding disorders or diabetes mellitus.

Adverse reactions
Diarrhea, allergic reactions, **anaphylactoid reactions, intestinal obstruction**

Interactions
Anticoagulants, antiplatelet drugs, salicylates: increased risk of bleeding
Hypoglycemics, insulins: increased risk of hypoglycemia

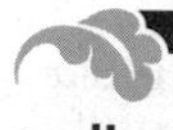

garlic

Purported action
Inactivates thiol enzymes (such as coenzyme A and HMG-CoA reductase) and oxidizes glutamate synthase complex, both of which are required for lipid synthesis. Also may exert mild antibacterial, antifungal, and hypotensive activity.

Reported uses
To reduce blood lipid levels (transient effect); as an antibacterial, antiseptic, or antithrombotic. Insufficient data exist regarding effects of garlic on clinical cardiovascular conditions, such as claudication and myocardial infarction.

Contraindications and precautions
Pregnant and breastfeeding patients should avoid large amounts. Use cautiously in severe renal or hepatic disease and in children.

Adverse reactions
Headache, insomnia, fatigue, vertigo, GI distress, shortness of breath, facial flushing, contact dermatitis, allergic reaction

Interactions
Anticoagulants, antiplatelet drugs, nonsteroidal anti-inflammatory drugs, other drugs and herbs with anticoagulant effects: increased prothrombin time, bleeding time, and International Normalized Ratio
Cyclosporine: decreased cyclosporine efficacy
Hormonal contraceptives: decreased contraceptive efficacy
Nonnucleoside reverse-transcriptase inhibitors, protease inhibitors: decreased efficacy of these drugs

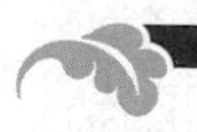

ginger

Purported action
Inhibits prostaglandin and thromboxane biosynthesis and promotes platelet aggregation. Also possesses antiemetic, antithrombotic, antibacterial, antioxidant, antihepatotoxic, anti-inflammatory, antimutagenic, stimulant, cardiotonic, immunostimulant, diuretic, and spasmolytic properties.

Reported uses
Dyspepsia, colic, anorexia, bronchitis, and rheumatism; to stimulate digestion, increase intestinal peristalsis, promote gastric secretions, reduce cholesterol level, raise blood glucose level, and stimulate peripheral circulation; to treat nausea and vomiting associated with motion sickness, hyperemesis gravidarum, and migraine

Contraindications and precautions
Large amounts are controversial in pregnant patients. Avoid use in gallstones, bleeding disorders, hypertension, hypotension, and diabetes mellitus.

Adverse reactions
CNS depression, interference with cardiac function or anticoagulant activity

Interactions
Anticoagulants: increased bleeding time
Antacids, histamine$_2$ blockers, hypoglycemics, insulin, proton pump inhibitors: interference with actions of these drugs
Barbiturates: enhanced barbiturate effects

ginkgo

Purported action
Exerts antioxidant and neuroprotective activity, including arteriolar vasodilation, increased tissue perfusion and cerebral blood flow, decreased arterial spasms, and reduced platelet aggregation

Reported uses
Raynaud's disease, cerebral insufficiency, anxiety, stress, tinnitus, dementia, circulatory disorders, asthma, memory impairment, headache, depression, impotence; as an adjunct in schizophrenia treatment

Contraindications and precautions
Pregnant or breastfeeding patients should avoid ginkgo. Use cautiously in diabetes mellitus, hypertension, and in patients receiving antiplatelet drugs or anticoagulants.

Adverse reactions
- Headache, dizziness, palpitations, GI and skin disorders
- With excessive use: **seizures, subdural hematoma**
- Ginkgo pollen can be strongly allergenic; contact with fleshy fruit pulp causes allergic dermatitis similar to that from poison ivy.

Interactions
Anticonvulsants: decreased efficacy of these drugs, increased risk of seizures
Buspirone, fluoxetine: hypomania
Drugs that lower seizure threshold: increased risk of seizures
Insulin: altered insulin metabolism and excretion
Thiazide diuretics: increased blood pressure
Trazodone: possible coma

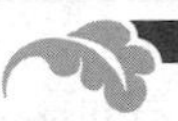

ginseng

Purported action
Increases natural "killer" cell activity, stimulates interferon production, accelerates nuclear RNA synthesis, decreases blood glucose level, and increases high-density lipoprotein level; also possesses depressant, anticonvulsant, and analgesic properties

Reported uses
Fatigue, poor concentration, nervousness, hypertension or hypotension, erectile dysfunction, gastritis, cancer, some CNS and endocrine conditions

Contraindications and precautions
Contraindicated in pregnant or breastfeeding patients. Patients taking MAO inhibitors should avoid ginseng. Use cautiously in hypertension or diabetes mellitus.

Adverse reactions
Nervousness, stimulation, hypoglycemia, diffuse mammary nodules, vaginal bleeding, ginseng abuse

Interactions
Alcohol: increased alcohol clearance
Antipsychotics, MAO inhibitors: inhibition of antipsychotic effect
Caffeine-containing preparations, stimulants: stimulant potentiation
Hypoglycemics, insulin: increased hypoglycemic effect
Immunosuppressants: decreased immunosuppressant activity
Loop diuretics: poor diuretic response
Warfarin: decreased warfarin efficacy

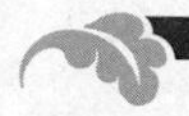

glucosamine

Purported action
Serves as a building block for cartilage glycosaminoglycans (GAG), aiding treatment of osteoarthritis (marked by progressive GAG degeneration). Also may possess chondroprotective, antireactive, and antiarthritic properties.

Reported uses
Osteoarthritis, joint pain and inflammation, temporomandibular joint syndrome, glaucoma; to aid weight loss

Contraindications and precautions
Diabetic patients should consult health care professional before using glucosamine because it may increase blood glucose level.

Adverse reactions
Gastric discomfort (such as nausea, vomiting, diarrhea, heartburn), headache, drowsiness, insomnia, tachycardia, pruritus

Interactions
Acetaminophen: interference with glucosamine activity
Antimitotic therapy: resistance to chemotherapeutic effects of these drugs
Diuretics: decreased glucosamine effects

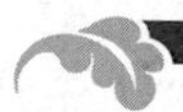

goldenseal

Purported action
Contains alkaloids (hydrastine and berberine) that exert modest antimicrobial activity. May have cardiostimulatory, anti-inflammatory, peripheral vasoconstrictive, antihemorraghic, and muscle relaxant effects.

Reported uses
Topical infections (such as wounds and herpes labialis lesions), conjunctivitis, inflamed mucous membranes (as an ingredient in cold and flu preparations), postpartum hemorrhage; as a diuretic or laxative

Contraindications and precautions
Contraindicated in hypertension, heart disease (especially arrhythmias), heart failure, and pregnancy

Adverse reactions
Rash, headache, insomnia, nausea, vomiting, abdominal pain, tachycardia, bradycardia, **seizures, respiratory depression** (with high doses)

Interactions
Antacids, histamine$_2$ antagonists, proton pump inhibitors: decreased effects of these drugs
Antihypertensives: decreased antihypertensive effect
CNS depressants: additive sedation

grapeseed

Purported action
Exerts antioxidant, anticarcinogenic, cytoprotective, and vascular activity; also inhibits proteolytic enzymes, causing collagen stabilization

Reported uses
Prevention of cancer, cardiovascular disease, and dental caries; treatment of venous insufficiency, edema, and allergic rhinitis

Contraindications and precautions
Contraindicated in known hypersensitivity to grapeseed. Use cautiously in hepatic disease. Safety during pregnancy has not been established.

Adverse reactions
Hepatotoxicity

Interactions
Warfarin: increased risk of bleeding

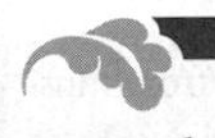

green tea

Purported action
Maintains significant blood levels of catechin, which may exert antioxidant activity against lipoproteins. Delays lipid peroxidation, exerts antimicrobial effects against oral bacteria and diarrhea-causing bacteria, and contributes antimutagenic potential against dietary carcinogens.

Reported uses
Atherosclerosis, headache, diarrhea, stomach disorders, cancer, elevated lipid levels, wounds, dental caries prophylaxis

Contraindications and precautions
Because of caffeine content, green tea should be avoided by pregnant or breastfeeding patients and by females who may become pregnant. Use cautiously in cardiac disease, renal disease, and hyperthyroidism.

Adverse reactions
Nervousness, insomnia, tachycardia, constipation, diarrhea, increased blood glucose and cholesterol levels, impaired iron metabolism, **asthma, esophageal cancer** (with heavy use)

Interactions
Hypoglycemics, insulin: interference with blood glucose control
Stimulants: increased stimulant effect
Warfarin: increased risk of bleeding

hawthorn

Purported action
Increases coronary blood flow and heart rate; exerts antiarrhythmic and positive inotropic effects

Reported uses
Atherosclerosis, angina pectoris; to regulate blood pressure and heart rhythm; as an antispasmodic or sedative

Contraindications and precautions
Contraindicated in severe renal or hepatic disease and in pregnancy and breastfeeding

Adverse reactions
Agitation, dizziness, hypotension, sedation, nausea, sweating, **toxicity** (with high doses)

Interactions
Antiarrhythmics: enhanced antiarrhythmic action
Antihypertensives, nitrates: increased effects of these drugs
Cardiac glycosides: increased risk of cardiac glycoside toxicity
CNS depressants: increased CNS effects

kava

Purported action
Produces mild anxiolytic and anticonvulsant effects; also may exert antithrombotic effect on platelets

Reported uses
Anxiety, stress, restlessness, seizure disorders, headache, infection, local anesthesia

Contraindications and precautions
Contraindicated in history of hepatic problems. Pregnant or breastfeeding patients should avoid kava. Use cautiously in neutropenia, renal disease, and thrombocytopenia.

Adverse reactions
Morning fatigue, headache, drowsiness, mydriasis, mild GI disturbances, diarrhea, hematuria, hypertension, shortness of breath, visual disturbances, scaly rash (with heavy use)

Interactions
CNS depressants: potentiation of CNS effects
Hepatotoxic drugs: increased hepatotoxicity
Levodopa: reduced levodopa efficacy

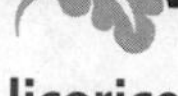

licorice

Purported action
Licorice root derivative (carbenoxolone) soothes inflamed mucous membranes, increases life span of gastric epithelial cells by stimulating secretin release, and inhibits peptic and prostaglandin activity

Reported uses
GI complaints, cough, asthma, gastric and duodenal ulcers; used investigationally in lupus and inflammation

Contraindications and precautions
Contraindicated in renal, hepatic, and cardiovascular disease. Pregnant or breastfeeding patients should avoid licorice.

Adverse reactions
- Headache, lethargy, water retention, hypokalemia, hypernatremia, visual disturbances, hypertension, **pulmonary edema**
- With prolonged, daily use of large amounts: reactions ranging from muscle weakness to quadriplegia

Interactions
Antihypertensives, corticosteroids, diuretics: increased blood pressure
Corticosteroids, furosemide, thiazide diuretics: increased potassium loss
Digoxin: increased risk of digoxin toxicity
Estrogen: interference with estrogen therapy
Ethacrynic acid: increased mineralocorticoid activity
Insulin: hypokalemia, sodium retention

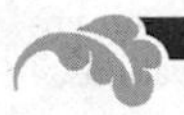

lutein

Purported action
Serves as antioxidant and blue light filter, protecting underlying ocular tissues from photodamage. Evidence links high dietary lutein intake with reduced risk of age-related macular degeneration and cataracts. Also, serum lutein level may be inversely related to breast cancer risk.

Reported uses
Cataracts, macular degeneration, colorectal cancer

Contraindications and precautions
Use with caution in bleeding disorders and diabetes mellitus.

Adverse reactions
None reported

Interactions
Beta carotene: interference with lutein availability

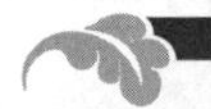

melatonin

Purported action
Endogenous melatonin plays a role in circadian rhythms: light inhibits melatonin synthesis and darkness stimulates it. Exogenous melatonin increases melatonin blood levels without affecting endogenous melatonin production; also affects body temperature regulation, cardiovascular function, and reproduction.

Reported uses
Short-term sleep pattern regulation, jet lag, tinnitus, depression, cluster headaches, cancer, thrombocytopenia caused by chemotherapy

Contraindications and precautions
Contraindicated in hepatic insufficiency, cerebrovascular disease, depression, and neurologic disorders

Adverse reactions
Headache, depression, confusion, tachycardia, pruritus

Interactions
Anticoagulants, antiplatelet drugs: increased risk of bleeding
Benzodiazepines: decreased endogenous melatonin
CNS depressants: additive sedation
Flumazenil: inhibition of melatonin effects
Fluvoxamine: increased melatonin blood level and effects
Hormonal contraceptives: increased melatonin effects
Hypoglycemics, insulin: increased insulin resistance, impaired glucose use
Immunosuppressants: interference with immunosuppressant effects
Nifedipine: interference with antihypertensive effect, increased heart rate
Verapamil: increased melatonin excretion

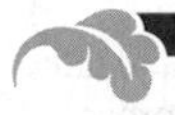

milk thistle

Purported action
Exerts a hepatoprotective effect, possibly by stimulating RNA and DNA synthesis. Thought to scavenge prooxidant free radicals and increase intracellular concentrations of glutathione (a substance needed to detoxify hepatic cell reactions). Also alters the outer membrane of hepatic cells and may produce an anti-inflammatory effect on platelets.

Reported uses
Hepatic dysfunction (including damage caused by acute viral hepatitis and long-term phenothiazine or butyrophenone use), dyspepsia, gallbladder and spleen disorders; antidote for Amanita mushroom poisoning; to reduce increased total cholesterol and low-density lipoprotein levels

Contraindications and precautions
Contraindicated in pregnancy and breastfeeding

Adverse reactions
Brief GI disturbances, diarrhea, cramping, mild allergic reactions, urticaria

Interactions
Estrogens, glucuronidated drugs: increased clearance of these drugs

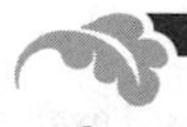

red yeast rice

Purported action
Contains mevinic acids (including lovastatin), which competitively inhibit HMG-CoA reductase, thereby blocking cholesterol biosynthesis

Reported uses
Diarrhea, indigestion, hyperlipidemia, poor blood circulation; to improve spleen and stomach health

Contraindications and precautions
Contraindicated in pregnancy and breastfeeding. Use cautiously in hepatic dysfunction, abnormal liver function tests, concurrent use of hepatotoxic drugs, and in persons who consume more than two alcoholic drinks daily.

Adverse reactions
Gastritis, abdominal discomfort, heartburn, flatulence, dizziness, hepatic enzyme and creatine kinase elevations, **anaphylaxis**

Interactions
Cyclosporine: increased risk of myopathy
CYP450-3A4 inhibitors: increased red yeast blood level, increased adverse reactions
Gemfibrozil, niacin: increased risk of myopathy
Grapefruit juice, HMG-CoA inhibitors (statins): increased risk of adverse reactions
Levothyroxine: abnormal thyroid function

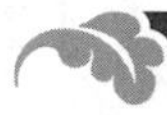

S-adenosylmethionine (SAM-e)

Purported action
Naturally occurring molecule; plays an essential role in biochemical reactions involving enzymatic transmethylation. Contributes to synthesis, activation, and metabolism of hormones, neurotransmitters, nucleic acids, proteins, phospholipids, and some drugs.

Reported uses
Cardiovascular disease, fibromyalgia, headache, insomnia, hepatic disease, osteoarthritis, rheumatoid arthritis, depression

Contraindications and precautions
Contraindicated in concurrent use of MAO inhibitors. Use cautiously in bleeding disorders and diabetes mellitus.

Adverse reactions
Anxiety, nausea, vomiting, diarrhea, flatulence, headache, mania or hypomania

Interactions
Antidepressants: additive effects (including additive serotonergic effects)

saw palmetto

Purported action
Reduces enlarged prostate by inhibiting testosterone 5-alpha reductase (an enzyme that converts testosterone to 5-alpha-testosterone in prostate). Inhibits cell proliferation induced by prolactin and growth factor; also may exert anti-inflammatory, immunostimulant, antiandrogenic, antiestrogenic, and astringent activity.

Reported uses
Symptomatic treatment of benign prostatic hypertrophy, including urinary frequency, reduced urinary flow, and nocturia; bronchitis; asthma

Contraindications and precautions
Contraindicated in pregnancy and in patients receiving concurrent hormone therapy (including hormonal contraceptives and hormone replacement therapy). Use cautiously in patients receiving drugs that may alter immunostimulant or anti-inflammatory activity.

Adverse reactions
Headache, hypertension, nausea, diarrhea, constipation, abdominal pain, GI upset, urinary retention

Interactions
Anticoagulants, antiplatelet drugs: increased risk of bleeding
Estrogens: interference with estrogen activity
Hormonal contraceptives: interference with contraceptive activity

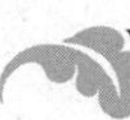

shark cartilage

Purported action
Helps control cancer by inhibiting new blood vessel formation (angiogenesis) in tumors; also may have anti-inflammatory effects

Reported uses
Prostate cancer, AIDS-associated Kaposi's sarcoma, arthritis, eczema

Contraindications and precautions
Contraindicated in pregnancy or breastfeeding and in children. Use cautiously in hepatic disease.

Adverse reactions
Hepatitis

Interactions
None known

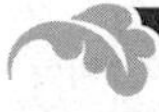

soy

Purported action
Isoflavones (phytoestrogens found in soybean) produce effects similar to those of estradiol (a female hormone). They also limit cholesterol absorption in intestine by binding to cholesterol and may enhance immune function, produce antioxidant effects, and exert beneficial effects on GI function.

Reported uses
Menopausal symptoms, osteoporosis, minor GI problems; to reduce total cholesterol and low-density lipoprotein levels. Also serves as source of fiber, protein, and minerals.

Contraindications and precautions
Contraindicated in estrogen-dependent tumors and peanut allergy (cross-sensitivity may occur)

Adverse reactions
Some experts are concerned that phytoestrogens in soy-based infant formulas may influence CNS and psychomotor development.

Interactions
Antibiotics: decreased action of isoflavones
Estrogens: interference with hormone replacement therapy
Tamoxifen: antagonism of tamoxifen
Warfarin: decreased International Normalized Ratio, inhibited platelet aggregation

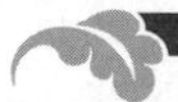

St. John's wort

Purported action
Inhibits postsynaptic serotonin reuptake or antagonizes MAO

Reported uses
Depression, wounds, muscle pain, burns; used investigationally to treat human immunodeficiency virus and certain other viruses

Contraindications and precautions
Contraindicated in concurrent use of antidepressants, in pregnant patients, and in patients planning pregnancy

Adverse reactions
Abdominal pain, constipation, other GI symptoms, dry mouth, dizziness, confusion, fatigue, mania, photosensitivity

Interactions
Bexarotene: decreased effects of St. John's wort and bexarotene
Cyclosporine, digoxin, paclitaxel, protease inhibitors, telithromycin, theophylline, tricyclic antidepressants, vinca alkaloids, warfarin: decreased efficacy of these drugs
Hormonal contraceptives: breakthrough bleeding
MAO inhibitors, selective serotonin reuptake inhibitors, serotonin agonists: increased risk of serotonin syndrome

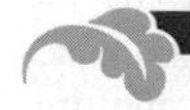

valerian

Purported action
Binds to gamma-aminobutyric acid (GABA) and benzodiazepine receptors, stimulating release of these substances. Glutamine, a free amino acid in valerian extract, can cross the blood-brain barrier and may be metabolized to GABA, causing sedation.

Reported uses
Anxiety, nervousness, attention deficit hyperactivity disorder, depression, seizures, menopausal symptoms, menstrual cramps, tremors, restlessness, sleep disorders; as an antispasmodic

Contraindications and precautions
Avoid use in hepatic dysfunction and in pregnant or breastfeeding patients.

Adverse reactions
With overdose or prolonged use: excitability, headache, insomnia, nausea, blurred vision, **cardiac dysfunction, hepatotoxicity**

Interactions
Alcohol, antihistamines, CNS depressants: additive sedation

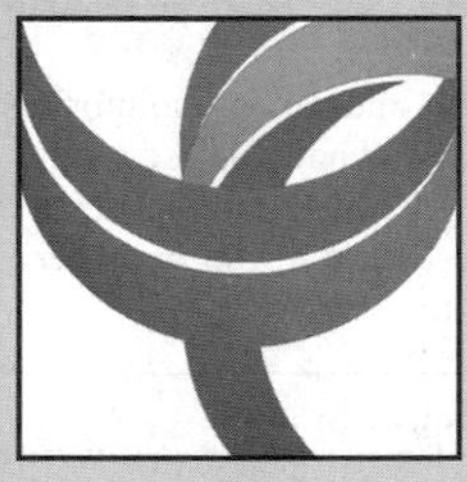

Part 3

Appendices
Selected references
Index

Common anesthetic drugs

This chart describes the indications, dosages, administration, and patient monitoring for commonly used anesthetic drugs. Although these potent and potentially dangerous drugs usually are given by specially trained personnel (such as anesthesiologists or anesthetists), the nurse is responsible for monitoring the patient during and after administration.

Drug	Indications and dosages
atracurium besylate Tracrium	➢ Adjunct to general anesthesia to promote endotracheal intubation and relax skeletal muscles during surgery **Adults and children ages 2 and older:** Initially, 0.4 to 0.5 mg/kg by I.V. bolus. For prolonged surgery, give maintenance dosage of 0.08 to 0.1 mg/kg within 20 to 45 minutes of initial dose; may repeat q 15 to 25 minutes p.r.n. During prolonged procedures, may give a continuous infusion of 5 to 9 mcg/kg/minute. **Children ages 1 month to 2 years:** 0.3 to 0.4 mg/kg I.V. Repeat if needed.
doxacurium chloride Nuromax	➢ To sustain neuromuscular blockade during prolonged procedures **Adults:** Initially, 0.05 mg/kg I.V.; for maintenance, 0.005 to 0.01 mg/kg (prolongs blockade for 30 to 45 minutes on average) ➢ Adjunct to general anesthesia to relax skeletal muscles during surgery **Adults:** 0.05 mg/kg rapid I.V.; produces adequate blockade for endotracheal intubation in 5 minutes when used as part of thiopental-narcotic induction. At this dosage, adequate blockade lasts 100 minutes on average. **Children older than age 2:** Initially, 0.03 mg/kg I.V. given with halothane anesthesia; produces adequate blockade in 7 minutes, with a duration of 30 minutes. Or 0.05 mg/kg, which produces adequate blockade in 4 minutes, with a duration of 45 minutes.

Administration and patient monitoring

- Before giving, make sure emergency respiratory equipment is at hand and that patient receives a sedative or general anesthetic.
- Give by I.V. route only (bolus, intermittent infusion, or continuous infusion). Never give I.M.
- Know that patient can hear while drug is in effect. Explain events as they occur and provide ongoing reassurance.
- Be ready to reverse drug's effects with anticholinesterase drug once spontaneous recovery begins.
- Watch for anaphylaxis and injection site reaction.
- Check vital signs and airway patency until patient recovers completely from drug effects.
- Assess for pain; give analgesics p.r.n. Be aware that patient may be unable to verbalize pain while drug is in effect.
- Evaluate patient's recovery with muscle strength tests, nerve stimulation, and train-of-four monitoring.

- Be aware that drug contains benzyl alcohol, linked to fatal complications in neonates.
- Keep lifesaving equipment in immediate area. Drug may cause profound, prolonged paralysis leading to respiratory insufficiency, apnea, fatal bronchospasm, ventricular fibrillation, or acute myocardial infarction.
- Know that children need higher dosages than adults (on mg/kg basis) to achieve same level of blockade.
- Dilute each 1 mg with 10 ml of dextrose 5% in water, normal saline solution, lactated Ringer's solution, or dextrose 5% in lactated Ringer's solution, to yield a concentration of 0.1 mg/ml.
- Give by I.V. push over 5 to 10 seconds.
- Always give concurrently with a sedative, amnesiac, or analgesic, as prescribed.
- Evaluate patient for adequate neuromuscular blockade.
- Assess vital signs. Monitor closely for hypoxia and hypercapnia.
- Watch for respiratory depression, which may occur up to 48 hours after doxacurium administration.
- Support ventilation until patient recovers fully from neuromuscular blockade.

(continued)

Common anesthetic drugs (continued)

Drug	Indications and dosages
fentanyl citrate Sublimaze **fentanyl transdermal system** Duragesic, Duragesic 25, Duragesic 50, Duragesic 75, Duragesic 100 **fentanyl transmucosal** Actiq, Fentanyl Oralet	➢ Short-term analgesia during anesthesia and immediate preoperative and postoperative periods **Adults:** 0.05 to 0.1 mg I.M. 30 to 60 minutes before surgery and as adjunct to general anesthesia; total dosage is 0.002 mg/kg. Maintenance dosage during surgery is 0.025 to 0.1 mg I.V. or I.M. Postoperatively, 0.05 to 0.1 mg I.M. to control pain, tachypnea, or emergence delirium; repeat in 1 to 2 hours if needed. **Children ages 2 to 12:** 2 to 3 mcg/kg I.V., depending on vital signs; or 5 to 15 mcg/kg transmucosally ➢ General anesthesia (given only with oxygen) **Adults:** 0.05 to 0.1 mg/kg I.V. for high-dose therapy. Up to 0.12 mg/kg may be necessary. ➢ Adjunct to regional anesthesia **Adults:** 0.05 to 0.1 mg I.M. or slow I.V. over 1 to 2 minutes
midazolam hydrochloride Apo-Midazolam*, Versed	➢ To induce general anesthesia **Adults younger than age 55:** 0.3 to 0.35 mg/kg I.V. over 20 to 30 seconds if patient is not premedicated, or 0.15 to 0.35 mg/kg (usual dosage of 0.25 mg/kg) I.V. over 20 to 30 seconds if patient is premedicated. Wait 2 minutes to evaluate effect. Additional increments of 25% of initial dosage may be needed to complete induction. ➢ Continuous infusion to initiate sedation **Adults:** For rapid sedation, loading dose of 0.01 to 0.05 mg/kg by slow I.V.; repeat dose q 10 to 15 minutes until adequate sedation occurs. To maintain sedation, infuse at initial rate of 0.02 to 0.10 mg/kg/hour (1 to 7 mg/hour); adjust rate as needed.
mivacurium chloride Mivacron	➢ Adjunct to general anesthesia; skeletal muscle relaxation for endotracheal intubation **Adults:** 0.15 mg/kg I.V. bolus administered over 5 to 15 seconds. To maintain neuromuscular blockade after spontaneous recovery from initial dose, 9 to 10 mcg/kg/minute by I.V. infusion. **Children ages 7 months to 12 years:** 0.2 mg/kg I.V. over 5 to 15 seconds. To maintain neuromuscular blockade after spontaneous recovery from initial dose, 11 to 14 mcg/kg/minute. **Children ages 2 to 6 months:** 0.15 mg/kg I.V. over 5 to 15 seconds. To maintain neuromuscular blockade after spontaneous recovery from initial dose, 11 to 14 mcg/kg/minute.

Administration and patient monitoring

- Know that I.V. dose is given slowly over 1 to 2 minutes.
- Keep narcotic antagonist (naloxone) and emergency equipment at hand when giving I.V.
- Know that drug is not recommended for control of mild or intermittent pain.
- Assess for muscle rigidity in patients receiving high doses. Discuss need for neuromuscular blocker with prescriber. If blocker is given, patient will require ventilator.
- Monitor respiratory and cardiovascular functions and urinary output.
- If patient develops fever, assess for signs and symptoms of opioid toxicity, because more drug is absorbed at higher body temperatures.
- Carefully monitor hematologic studies and hepatic enzyme levels.

- Keep oxygen and resuscitation equipment at hand in case severe respiratory depression occurs.
- Inject I.M. deep into large muscle mass.
- Know that drug may be mixed in same syringe as atropine, meperidine, morphine, or scopolamine.
- Dilute concentrate for I.V. infusion to 0.5 mg/ml using dextrose 5% in water or normal saline solution. Infuse over at least 2 minutes; wait at least 2 minutes before giving second dose. Be aware that excessive dose or rapid I.V. delivery may cause severe respiratory depression.
- Monitor vital signs, ECG, respiratory status, and oxygen saturation.
- Assess neurologic status closely, especially in children.
- Monitor for nausea and vomiting.

- Before giving, make sure emergency resuscitation equipment is at hand and patient is being monitored.
- Assess electrolyte levels before drug is administered; correct imbalances.
- Dilute to 0.5 mg/ml using dextrose 5% in water (D_5W), normal saline solution, D_5W in normal saline solution, lactated Ringer's solution, or dextrose 5% in lactated Ringer's solution.
- Infuse at prescribed rate. In adults, if continuous infusion begins with dosage of 0.15 mg/kg, use slower rate of 4 mcg/kg/minute.
- Be aware that muscle relaxation for endotracheal intubation usually is adequate within 2 to 3 minutes of I.V. bolus dose and lasts 15 to 20 minutes.
- Know that when drug is used with isoflurane or enflurane, dosage is reduced 35% to 40%.
- Know that children may receive higher dosages (on mg/kg basis) and faster continuous infusion rates than adults.
- During recovery and residual phase, watch for residual weakness and respiratory distress.
- Monitor recovery by checking hand grip, head lift, and ability to cough voluntarily.

(continued)

Common anesthetic drugs (continued)

Drug	Indications and dosages
nalbuphine hydrochloride Nubain	➢ Adjunct to balanced anesthesia **Adults:** 0.3 mg to 3 mg/kg I.V. over 10 to 15 minutes, followed by a maintenance dosage of 0.25 mg to 0.50 mg/kg I.V. in single doses p.r.n.
pancuronium bromide Pavulon	➢ Adjunct to balanced anesthesia to relax skeletal muscles for intubation **Adults and children ages 1 month and older:** Initially, 0.04 to 0.1 mg/kg I.V.; may follow with 0.01 mg/kg q 25 to 60 minutes if needed. (Dosage and infusion rates are based on type of anesthesia used and patient needs and response. Dosages listed here are typical.)
pentazocine hydrochloride Talwin **pentazocine hydrochloride and acetaminophen** Talacen **pentazocine hydrochloride and naloxone hydrochloride** Talwin NX	➢ Preoperative or preanesthetic medication; adjunct to surgical anesthesia **Adults:** 30 mg subcutaneously, I.M., or I.V. q 3 to 4 hours (not to exceed 30 mg I.V. or 60 mg I.M. or subcutaneously) ➢ Labor **Adults:** 20 mg I.V. for two or three doses at 2- to 3-hour intervals, or 30 mg I.M. as a single dose
procaine hydrochloride Novocain	➢ Infiltration anesthesia **Adults:** 350 to 600 mg of 0.25% to 0.5% of diluted solution injected as a single dose into area to be anesthetized ➢ Peripheral nerve block **Adults:** 100 ml of 1% diluted solution or 50 ml of 2% solution injected into area where peripheral nerve block is needed, or up to 200 ml of 0.5% diluted solution ➢ Spinal anesthesia **Adults:** 0.5, 1, or 2 ml of 10% solution injected into spinal area to be anesthetized, diluted in 0.5, 1, or 2 ml (respectively) of normal saline solution, sterile distilled water, or spinal fluid. Administer at 1 ml/5 seconds.

Administration and patient monitoring

- Make sure emergency resuscitation equipment and naloxone (antidote) are at hand before administration begins.
- Monitor vital signs. Watch for respiratory depression and heart rate changes.
- Evaluate patient for CNS changes. Institute safety measures as needed to prevent injury.
- Watch for hypersensitivity reactions, such as anaphylaxis.

- Know that drug should be given only by specially trained personnel in settings where respiratory support is available.
- Administer through established I.V. line containing normal saline solution, lactated Ringer's solution, or dextrose 5% in water.
- Know that neostigmine can reverse drug's effects.
- Make sure patient's analgesic and sedative needs are met; drug doesn't relieve pain or provide sedation.
- Monitor heart rhythm, vital signs, and pulse oximetry during and after administration.
- Evaluate fluid intake and output and potassium level.
- Assess muscle recovery using peripheral nerve stimulator and train-of-four monitoring.

- Inject each 5-mg dose over 1 minute by slow, direct I.V. infusion, with patient lying supine.
- Use subcutaneous route only when necessary (may cause tissue damage).
- Monitor vital signs. Stay alert for shock, dyspnea, and circulatory or respiratory depression.
- Monitor drug efficacy.

- Know that drug should be given only by specially trained personnel with expertise in avoiding intravascular injections and in assessing and managing dose-related toxicities and other acute emergencies that may arise.
- Make sure emergency resuscitation equipment is at hand before drug is given.
- Follow label directions to reconstitute drug for selected route.
- Be aware that if necessary, epinephrine may be added to slow procaine absorption, prolong its action, or maintain hemostasis.
- Monitor vital signs and ECG closely, especially when drug is used for spinal anesthesia. Stay alert for evidence of impending cardiac arrest.
- Watch for signs and symptoms of status asthmaticus and anaphylaxis.
- Monitor patient's position carefully, especially after spinal anesthesia, to help prevent damage to nerves and other body tissues.
- Inspect infusion site for extravasation.

(continued)

Common anesthetic drugs (continued)

Drug	Indications and dosages
propofol Diprivan	➢ General anesthesia induction **Healthy adults younger than age 55:** 40 mg or 2 to 2.5 mg/kg I.V. q 10 seconds until induction onset. In neurosurgical patients, 20 mg or 1 to 2 mg/kg q 10 seconds until induction onset. In cardiac anesthesia, 20 mg or 0.5 to 1.5 mg/kg q 10 seconds until induction onset. **Healthy children ages 3 to 16:** 2.5 to 3.5 mg/kg I.V. given over 20 to 30 seconds ➢ General anesthesia maintenance **Healthy adults younger than age 55:** 100 to 200 mcg/kg/minute by I.V. infusion, given with nitrous oxide and oxygen; or 25 to 50 mg (2.5 to 5 ml) by intermittent I.V. bolus, given with nitrous oxide **Healthy children ages 2 months to 16 years:** 7.5 to 18 mg/kg/hour I.V.
remifentanil hydrochloride Ultiva	➢ To induce anesthesia through intubation **Adults:** 0.5 to 1 mcg/kg/minute I.V., given with a hypnotic or volatile drug. May administer 1 mcg/kg I.V. over 30 to 60 seconds if endotracheal intubation will occur less than 8 minutes after drug infusion starts. ➢ To maintain anesthesia **Adults:** 0.25 to 0.4 mcg/kg/minute. Increase dosage by 25% to 100% or decrease by 25% to 50% q 2 to 5 minutes p.r.n. If rate exceeds 1 mcg/kg/minute, dosage may be increased. Supplemental I.V. bolus of 1 mcg/kg may be given ➢ To continue analgesic effect during immediate postoperative period **Adults:** Initially, 0.1 mcg/kg/minute I.V. Adjust in increments of 0.025 mcg/kg/minute q 5 minutes p.r.n. ➢ Analgesic component of monitored anesthesia care **Adults:** 0.5 to 1 mcg/kg I.V. over 30 to 60 seconds, given 90 seconds before anesthetic. As a continuous infusion, 0.05 to 0.1 mcg/kg/minute I.V. 5 minutes before anesthetic. After anesthetic is given, titrate rate to 0.025 to 0.05 mcg/kg/minute, then adjust by 0.025 mcg/kg/minute q 5 minutes p.r.n.

Administration and patient monitoring

- Before giving, ask patient about allergies to eggs, soybean oil, or glycerol.
- Know that drug usually doesn't require dilution. However, if dilution is ordered, use only dextrose 5% in water and dilute to a concentration of no less than 2 mg/ml; infuse at prescribed rate.
- Don't use drug if emulsion phases have separated.
- Don't use filter with pores smaller than 5 microns.
- Don't mix with other drugs before infusing.
- Don't deliver through same I.V. line as blood or plasma.
- After 12 hours, discard unused portion and tubing.
- Don't stop drug administration suddenly; dosage must be tapered.
- Monitor vital signs and ECG continuously.
- Monitor arterial blood gas findings and respiratory status.
- When giving drug in ICU, evaluate patient's neurologic status frequently to help determine minimal dosage required.
- Assess blood lipid levels.

- Keep emergency resuscitation equipment and naloxone at hand in case of respiratory arrest.
- Add 1 ml of diluent/mg of drug. Shake well to produce a clear, colorless solution of 1 mg/ml.
- Dilute drug further in normal or half-normal saline solution, dextrose 5% in water, dextrose 5% in normal saline solution, or dextrose 5% in lactated Ringer's solution.
- Use infusion control pump for continuous infusion. Choose site close to venous cannula. After administering, flush I.V. tubing to clear.
- Know that delivery rates above 0.2 mcg/kg/minute may cause respiratory depression.
- When giving high doses, assess for muscle rigidity. Be prepared to stop therapy.
- Continuously monitor respiratory and cardiovascular function, oxygenation, and vital signs.
- Assess fluid intake and output. Watch for urinary retention.

(continued)

Common anesthetic drugs (continued)

Drug	Indications and dosages
rocuronium bromide Zemuron (P/F)	➢ Adjunct to general anesthesia to allow endotracheal intubation and relax skeletal muscles during mechanical ventilation or surgery **Adults:** Initially, I.V. bolus of 0.6 to 1.2 mg/kg (usually allows endotracheal intubation within 2 minutes and paralyzes muscles for 30 minutes). Boluses of 0.1 to 0.2 mg/kg may be given at 25% recovery for maintenance. For continuous I.V. infusion, 0.01 to 0.012 mg/kg/minute only after early evidence of recovery from intubating dose.
ropivacaine hydrochloride Naropin	➢ Lumbar epidural block **Adults:** 15 to 30 ml (75 to 150 mg) I.V. of 0.5% solution, or 15 to 25 ml (113 to 188 mg) I.V. of 0.75% solution ➢ Lumbar epidural block during labor **Adults:** 10 to 20 ml (20 to 40 mg) of 0.2% solution, then 6 to 14 ml/hour (12 to 28 mg/hour) as a continuous I.V. infusion; or 10 to 15 ml/hour (20 to 30 mg/hour) of 0.2% solution as an incremental "top-up" injection ➢ Lumbar epidural block for cesarean section **Adults:** 20 to 30 ml (100 to 150 mg) I.V. of 0.5% solution, or 15 to 20 ml (113 to 150 mg) of 0.75% solution
succinylcholine chloride Anectine, Quelicin	➢ Adjunct to anesthesia to relax skeletal muscles during short surgical procedures; endotracheal intubation with mechanical ventilation; electrically induced convulsive therapy **Adults:** 0.6 mg/kg I.V. over 10 to 30 seconds, or a continuous I.V. infusion at 0.5 to 10 mg/minute, or 0.04 to 0.07 mg/kg I.V. intermittently p.r.n. **Older children and adolescents:** 1 mg/kg I.V. over 10 to 30 seconds **Infants and young children:** 2 mg/kg I.V. over 10 to 30 seconds

Administration and patient monitoring

- Keep emergency resuscitation equipment at hand when giving.
- Be aware that drug should be given only by personnel who are specially trained in administering anesthesia and neuromuscular blockers.
- Verify that patient has received a sedative or general anesthetic before therapy begins.
- Give by rapid I.V. injection or continuous I.V. infusion in compatible solution (dextrose 5% in water or normal saline solution, normal saline solution, sterile water for injection, or lactated Ringer's solution).
- Know that maintenance dose of 0.1 mg/kg provides an extra 12 minutes of muscle relaxation; 0.15 mg/kg, an extra 17 minutes; and 0.2 mg/kg, an extra 24 minutes.
- Assess respiratory status frequently.
- Monitor vital signs and ECG continuously until patient recovers fully from neuromuscular blockade. Closely monitor recovery with nerve stimulator and train-of-four monitoring.

- Know that drug should be given only by personnel specially trained in use of epidural blocks.
- Be aware that test dose (containing epinephrine) should be given.
- Use small, incremental doses for titration. Avoid rapid I.V. infusion.
- Monitor vital signs, ECG, and cardiovascular status continuously.
- Assess neurologic status. Stay alert for signs and symptoms of impending seizure.
- Watch carefully for warning signs of allergic reaction and respiratory distress.

- Make sure patient has received a sedative or general anesthetic before administering.
- Verify that emergency resuscitation equipment is at hand before giving.
- As ordered, give test dose of 5 to 10 mg I.V. after anesthesia administration. Drug may be given if test dose does not cause respiratory depression or if such depression lasts no longer than 5 minutes.
- For I.V. use, reconstitute with dextrose 5% in water or normal saline solution; administer via intermittent or continuous I.V. infusion. Don't mix with alkaline solution, such as sodium bicarbonate, barbiturates, or thiopental sodium.
- Be aware that continuous I.V. infusion isn't recommended for children or adolescents.
- Watch for life-threatening adverse reactions, including anaphylaxis, malignant hyperthermia, and hypersensitivity reaction.
- Monitor ECG and vital signs (especially respirations) until patient recovers fully.
- Assess recovery by checking hand grip, head lift, and voluntary cough response.

(continued)

Common anesthetic drugs (continued)

Drug	Indications and dosages
sufentanil Sufenta	➢ As a primary anesthetic to induce and maintain anesthesia **Adults:** Initially, 8 to 30 mcg/kg I.V., given with oxygen and a muscle relaxant. Maintenance dosage is 0.5 to 10 mcg/kg p.r.n.; maximum dosage is 30 mcg/kg **Children younger than age 12:** 10 to 25 mcg/kg I.V., given with oxygen. Maintenance dosage is 25 to 50 mcg. ➢ Analgesic adjunct to maintain balanced general anesthesia **Adults:** 1 to 8 mcg/kg I.V., with 75% of dose given immediately before intubation. Remainder can be given as 10- to 50-mcg bolus doses to maintain analgesia. ➢ Epidural analgesia during labor and delivery **Adults:** 10 to 15 mcg epidurally given with bupivacaine, with or without epinephrine. May repeat twice at intervals of more than 1 hour, for a total of three doses.
thiopental sodium Pentothal	➢ Slow anesthesia induction and maintenance **Adults:** 50 to 75 mg I.V. given slowly at 20- to 40-second intervals, based on response. May give additional doses of 25 to 50 mg I.V. p.r.n. ➢ Rapid anesthesia induction and maintenance before other general anesthetics are given **Adults:** 210 to 280 mg (3 to 4 mg/kg) I.V. in two to four divided doses ➢ Anesthesia maintenance without other general anesthetics for short procedures **Adults:** 0.2% or 0.4% solution intermittently by I.V. injection or continuous I.V. infusion ➢ Seizures associated with anesthesia or other causes in mechanically ventilated patients **Adults:** 75 to 125 mg I.V. infusion as soon as possible after seizure onset ➢ Increased intracranial pressure **Adults:** 1.5 to 3.5 mg/kg intermittent I.V. infusion

Administration and patient monitoring

- Know that drug should be given only by personnel who are specially trained in using I.V. and epidural anesthetics and in managing respiratory effects of potent opioids.
- Keep oxygen and resuscitation and intubation equipment at hand.
- Be aware that dosage is based on mean body weight.
- Monitor ECG and vital signs. Stay alert for signs and symptoms of shock and impending cardiac arrest.
- Assess airway patency closely. Watch for respiratory depression and airway spasms.
- Monitor neurologic status during and after administration. Institute safety measures as needed to prevent injury.
- Monitor fluid intake and output. Check for oliguria or urinary retention.

- Know that drug should be given only by personnel qualified in using I.V. anesthetics.
- Keep resuscitation equipment on hand.
- Reconstitute drug according to manufacturer's directions.
- Give test dose of 25 to 75 mg I.V., as ordered. Assess tolerance and monitor for hypersensitivity reaction for 1 minute.
- Administer I.V. injection over 20 to 30 seconds or by continuous I.V. infusion using infusion pump.
- Avoid extravasation to prevent severe tissue reaction (necrosis, sloughing). If extravasation occurs, stop infusion immediately, contact prescriber, apply moist heat, and inject 1% procaine hydrochloride, as prescribed.
- Monitor vital signs and ECG carefully.
- Closely monitor respiratory status, particularly for respiratory depression.
- Assess patient closely to detect early signs and symptoms of shock. Stop drug and contact prescriber immediately if these occur.
- Monitor neurologic status. Institute safety measures if seizures, agitation, or anxiety occurs.
- Assess injection site closely and frequently to prevent extravasation and detect thrombophlebitis.

(continued)

Common anesthetic drugs (continued)

Drug	Indications and dosages
tubocurarine chloride Tubocurarine	➢Adjunct to anesthesia to relax skeletal muscles **Adults:** 40 to 60 units (6 to 9 mg) I.V. when first incision is made, followed by 20 to 30 units in 3 to 5 minutes, if needed. Supplemental doses of 20 units may be required.
vecuronium bromide Norcuron	➢Adjunct to anesthesia to facilitate endotracheal intubation and relax skeletal muscles during surgery or mechanical ventilation **Adults and children older than age 9:** Initially, 0.08 to 0.1 mg/kg by I.V. bolus. During prolonged surgery, maintenance dose of 0.01 to 0.015 mg/kg is given by continuous I.V. infusion within 25 to 40 minutes of initial dose. In patients receiving balanced anesthesia, maintenance dose may be given q 12 to 15 minutes.

Administration and patient monitoring

- Assess renal function and electrolyte balance before giving.
- Keep oxygen, airway management equipment, atropine, and neostigmine or edrophonium at hand.
- Administer by I.V. route over at least 1 minute.
- Be aware that if suitable vein isn't accessible, drug may be given I.M. at same dosage as I.V. dosage.
- Monitor heart rhythm, blood pressure, and respiratory status.
- Assess muscle recovery using peripheral nerve stimulator and train-of-four monitoring.
- Monitor patient's need for sedative or analgesic. (Drug doesn't alter consciousness or relieve pain.)

- Know that drug should be given by specially trained personnel and only when respiratory support is available.
- When giving by I.V. bolus, administer over 1 to 2 minutes.
- When giving by continuous I.V. infusion, reconstitute by adding bacteriostatic water for injection to yield a concentration of 1 mg/ml. Dilute further with dextrose 5% in water, normal saline solution, or lactated Ringer's solution. Administer with infusion-control device.
- Monitor heart rhythm, blood pressure, and pulse oximetry during and after administration.
- Monitor fluid intake and output and measure temperature.
- Assess muscle recovery using peripheral nerve stimulator and train-of-four monitoring.
- Make sure patient's analgesic and sedative needs are met. (Drug doesn't relieve pain or provide sedation.)

Adult immunization schedule by age group

This 2005 schedule shows the recommended age groups for routine administration of vaccines for adults ages 19 and older. A person may receive a combination vaccine if any components of the combination are indicated (unless the vaccine's other components are contraindicated). Consult the package insert for detailed recommendations.

For more information about recommended vaccines and contraindications for immunization, visit www.cdc.gov/nip or call the National Immunization Hotline at 800-232-2522 (English) or 800-232-0233 (Spanish).

Vaccine	Ages 19-49	Ages 50-64	Ages 65 and older
Tetanus, diphtheria (Td)	1 dose booster every 10 years		
Influenza	1 dose annually		1 dose annually
Pneumococcal (polysaccharide)	1 dose		1 dose
Hepatitis B	3 doses (0, 1 to 2 months, and 4 to 6 months)		
Hepatitis A	2 doses (0, and 6 to 12 months)		
Measles, Mumps, Rubella (MMR)	1 dose if measles, mumps, or rubella vaccination history is unreliable 2 doses for persons with occupational or other indications		
Varicella	2 doses (0, 4 to 8 weeks) for susceptible persons		
Meningococcal (polysaccharide)	1 dose		

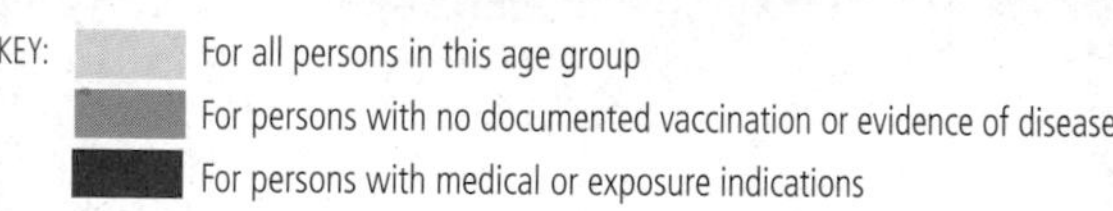

KEY:
- For all persons in this age group
- For persons with no documented vaccination or evidence of disease
- For persons with medical or exposure indications

Approved by Advisory Committee on Immunization Practices, American College of Obstetricians and Gynecologists, and American Academy of Family Physicians. Published by Advisory Committee on Immunization Practices, Department of Health and Human Services, Centers for Disease Control and Prevention.

Childhood and adolescent immunization schedule

This 2005 schedule shows recommended ages for routine administration of childhood vaccines for children through age 18. A child who doesn't receive a given dose at the recommended age should receive it at a subsequent visit. "Catch-up immunization" indicates ages at which children should receive the vaccine if they haven't previously received it. Consult the package insert for detailed recommendations.

For more information about vaccines (including precautions and contraindications for immunization and vaccine shortages), visit www.cdc.gov/nip or call the National Immunization Information Hotline at 800-232-2522 (English) or 800-232-0233 (Spanish).

Vaccine	Birth	1 mo	2 mo	4 mo	6 mo	12 mo	15 mo	18 mo	24 mo	4-6 yrs	11-12 yrs	13-18 yrs
Hepatitis B	HepB #1	only if mother HBsAg(-)									HepB series	
			HepB #2			HepB #3						
Diphtheria, Tetanus, Pertussis			DTaP	DTaP	DTaP		DTaP			DTaP	Td	Td
Haemophilus influenzae Type b			Hib	Hib	Hib	Hib						
Inactivated poliovirus			IPV	IPV		IPV				IPV		
Measles, Mumps, Rubella						MMR #1				MMR #2	MMR #2	
Varicella							Varicella				Varicella	
Pneumococcal			PCV	PCV	PCV	PCV			PCV		PPV	
Influenza						Influenza (yearly)					Influenza (yearly)	
Vaccines below this line are for selected populations.												
Hepatitis A											Hepatitis A series	

KEY:

- Range of recommended ages
- Catch-up immunization
- Preadolescent assessment

DTaP: Diphtheria, Tetanus, Pertussis
HBsAg(-): Hepatitis B surface antigen negative
HepB: Hepatitis B vaccine
HiB: *Haemophilus influenzae* type b
IPV: Inactivated poliovirus
MMR: Measles, Mumps, Rubella
PCV: Pneumococcal vaccine
PPV: Pneumococcal polysaccharide vaccine
Td: Tetanus and diphtheria toxoids

Approved by Advisory Committee on Immunization Practices, American Academy of Pediatrics, and American Academy of Family Physicians. Published by Advisory Committee on Immunization Practices, Department of Health and Human Services, Centers for Disease Control and Prevention.

Common combination drug products

Many drugs (especially over-the-counter preparations) are combination products that contain several active ingredients and are sold under a discrete trade name. The combination products below are listed by trade name, followed by active ingredients and therapeutic class.

Accuretic
hydrochlorothiazide, quinapril hydrochloride
Therapeutic class: Antihypertensive

Aceta with Codeine
acetaminophen
Therapeutic class: Opioid analgesic

Actifed
codeine phosphate, pseudoephedrine hydrochloride, triprolidine hydrochloride
Therapeutic class: Adrenergic, antihistamine, antitussive

Activella Tablets
estradiol, norethindrone acetate
Therapeutic class: Estrogen, progestin

Adderall
amphetamine aspartate, amphetamine sulfate, dextroamphetamine saccharate, dextroamphetamine sulfate
Therapeutic class: CNS stimulant

Advair Diskus
fluticasone propionate, salmeterol xinafoate
Therapeutic class: Corticosteroid, bronchodilator

Advicor
lovastatin, niacin
Therapeutic class: Antihyperlipidemic

Aggrenox
aspirin, dipyridamole
Therapeutic class: Antiplatelet drug

Aldactazide
hydrochlorothiazide, spironolactone
Therapeutic class: Diuretic

Aldoclor
chlorothiazide, methyldopa
Therapeutic class: Antihypertensive

Aldoril
hydrochlorothiazide, methyldopa
Therapeutic class: Antihypertensive

Allegra-D
fexofenadine hydrochloride, pseudoephedrine hydrochloride
Therapeutic class: Antihistamine, adrenergic

Apresazide
hydralazine hydrochloride, hydrochlorothiazide
Therapeutic class: Antihypertensive

Apri
desogrestrel, ethinyl estradiol
Therapeutic class: Estrogen, progestin

Arthrotec
diclofenac sodium, misoprostol
Therapeutic class: Anti-inflammatory, gastric protectant

Atacand HCT
candesartan cilexetil, hydrochlorothiazide
Therapeutic class: Antihypertensive

Atamet
carbidopa, levodopa
Therapeutic class: Antiparkinsonian

Augmentin
amoxicillin, clavulanate potassium
Therapeutic class: Anti-infective

Bactrim
sulfamethoxazole, trimethoprim
Therapeutic class: Anti-infective

Bancap HC
acetaminophen, hydrocodone bitartrate
Therapeutic class: Opioid analgesic

Caduet
amlodipine besylate, atorvastatin calcium
Therapeutic class: Antihypertensive, antihyperlipidemic

Capozide
captopril, hydrochlorothiazide
Therapeutic class: Antihypertensive

Ciprodex
ciprofloxacin, dexamethasone
Therapeutic class: Anti-infective, anti-inflammatory drug

Claritin-D
loratadine, pseudoephedrine sulfate
Therapeutic class: Antihistamine, adrenergic

CombiPatch
estradiol, norethindrone acetate
Therapeutic class: Estrogen, progestin

Combipres
chlorthalidone, clonidine hydrochloride
Therapeutic class: Antihypertensive

Combivent
albuterol sulfate, ipratropium bromide
Therapeutic class: Bronchodilator

Combivir
lamivudine, zidovudine
Therapeutic class: Antiviral

Combunox
ibuprofen, oxycodone hydrochloride
Therapeutic class: Opioid analgesic

Corzide
bendroflumethiazide, nadolol
Therapeutic class: Antihypertensive

Cosopt
dorzolamide, timolol maleate
Therapeutic class: Antihypertensive, carbonic anhydrase inhibitor

Darvocet N-100
acetaminophen, propoxyphene
Therapeutic class: Opioid analgesic

Demi-Regroton
chlorthalidone, reserpine
Therapeutic class: Antihypertensive

Dyazide
hydrochlorothiazide, triamterene
Therapeutic class: Diuretic

EMLA Cream
lidocaine, prilocaine
Therapeutic class: Anesthetic

Endocet
acetaminophen, oxycodone hydrochloride
Therapeutic class: Opioid analgesic

Epzicom
abacavir sulfate, lamivudine
Therapeutic class: Antiviral

Etrafon
amitriptyline hydrochloride, perphenazine
Therapeutic class: Antipsychotic, antidepressant

Fansidar
pyrimethamine, sulfadoxine
Therapeutic class: Antimalarial drug

femhrt
ethinyl estradiol, norethindrone acetate
Therapeutic class: Estrogen, progestin

Fioricet
acetaminophen, butalbital, caffeine
Therapeutic class: Barbiturate analgesic

Fiorinal
aspirin, butalbital, caffeine
Therapeutic class: Barbiturate analgesic

Glucovance
glyburide, metformin hydrochloride
Therapeutic class: Hypoglycemic

Helidac
bismuth subsalicylate, metronidazole, tetracycline hydrochloride
Therapeutic class: Anti-infective

Humulin 70/30
insulin suspension, isophane; insulin, recombinant human
Therapeutic class: Hypoglycemic

Hycodan
homatropine methylbromide, hydrocodone bitartrate
Therapeutic class: Opioid analgesic

Hydrocet
acetaminophen, hydrocodone bitartrate
Therapeutic class: Opioid analgesic

(continued)

Common combination drug products (continued)

Hyzaar
hydrochlorothiazide, losartan potassium
Therapeutic class: Antihypertensive

Inderide
hydrochlorothiazide, propranolol hydrochloride
Therapeutic class: Antihypertensive

Kaletra
lopinavir, ritonavir
Therapeutic class: Antiviral

Lexxel
enalapril maleate, felodipine
Therapeutic class: Antihypertensive

Librax
chlordiazepoxide hydrochloride, clidinium bromide
Therapeutic class: Anxiolytic

Lomotil
atropine sulfate, diphenoxylate hydrochloride
Therapeutic class: Antidiarrheal, anticholinergic

Lopressor HCT
hydrochlorothiazide, metoprolol tartrate
Therapeutic class: Antihypertensive

Lortab
acetaminophen, hydrocodone bitartrate
Therapeutic class: Opioid analgesic

Lotensin HCT
benazepril hydrochloride, hydrochlorothiazide
Therapeutic class: Antihypertensive

Lotrel
amlodipine besylate, benazepril hydrochloride
Therapeutic class: Antihypertensive

Maxzide
hydrochlorothiazide, triamterene
Therapeutic class: Antihypertensive, diuretic

Midrin
acetaminophen, dichloraiphenazone, isometheptene mucate
Therapeutic class: Vascular and tension headache suppressant

Minizide
polythiazide, prazosin hydrochloride
Therapeutic class: Antihypertensive

Moduretic
amiloride hydrochloride, hydrochlorothiazide
Therapeutic class: Diuretic

NovoLog Mix 70/30
insulin aspart (recombinant), insulin aspart protamine
Therapeutic class: Hypoglycemic

NuLYTELY
polyethylene glycol, potassium chloride, sodium bicarbonate, sodium chloride
Therapeutic class: Laxative

Ortho-Cyclen
ethinyl estradiol, norgestimate
Therapeutic class: Contraceptive

Pediazole
erythromycin ethylsuccinate, sulfisoxazole acetyl
Therapeutic class: Anti-infective

Percocet
acetaminophen, oxycodone hydrochloride
Therapeutic class: Opioid analgesic

Percodan
aspirin, oxycodone hydrochloride, oxycodone terephthalate
Therapeutic class: Opioid analgesic

Premphase
conjugated estrogens, medroxyprogesterone acetate
Therapeutic class: Contraceptive

Primaxin
cilastatin sodium, imipenem
Therapeutic class: Anti-infective

Quibron
guaifenesin, theophylline
Therapeutic class: Bronchodilator, expectorant

Rifamate
isoniazid, rifampin
Therapeutic class: Antitubercular

Rifater
isoniazid, pyrazinamide, rifampin
Therapeutic class: Antitubercular

Roxicet
acetaminophen, oxycodone hydrochloride
Therapeutic class: Opioid analgesic

Seasonale
ethinyl estradiol, levonorgestrel
Therapeutic class: Estrogen, progestin

Septra
sulfamethoxazole, trimethoprim
Therapeutic class: Anti-infective

Sinemet
carbidopa, levodopa
Therapeutic class: Antiparkinsonian

Solage
mequinol, tretinoin
Therapeutic class: Antineoplastic

Stalevo
carbidopa, entacapone, levodopa
Therapeutic class: Antiparkinsonian

Symbyax
fluoxetine hydrochloride, olanzapine
Therapeutic class: Mood stabilizer

Tarka
trandolapril, verapamil hydrochloride
Therapeutic class: Antihypertensive

Teczem
diltiazem malate, enalapril maleate
Therapeutic class: Antihypertensive

Tenoretic
atenolol, chlorthalidone
Therapeutic class: Antihypertensive

Truvada
emtricitabine, tenofovir disoproxil fumarate
Therapeutic class: Antiviral

Tussionex
chlorpheniramine polistirex, hydrocodone polistirex
Therapeutic class: Antitussive, antihistamine

Tylox
acetaminophen, oxycodone hydrochloride
Therapeutic class: Opioid analgesic

Ultracet
acetaminophen, tramadol hydrochloride
Therapeutic class: Nonopioid analgesic

Ultrase
amylase, lipase, protease
Therapeutic class: Digestive enzyme

Unasyn
ampicillin sodium, sulbactam sodium
Therapeutic class: Anti-infective

Vaseretic
enalapril maleate, hydrochlorothiazide
Therapeutic class: Antihypertensive, diuretic

Vicodin
acetaminophen, hydrocodone bitartate
Therapeutic class: Opioid analgesic

Vytorin
ezetimibe, simvastatin
Therapeutic class: Antihyperlipidemic

Zestoretic
hydrochlorothiazide, lisinopril
Therapeutic class: Antihypertensive

Ziac
bisoprolol fumarate, hydrochlorothiazide
Therapeutic class: Antihypertensive

Zyrtec-D
cetirizine hydrochloride, pseudoephedrine hydrochloride
Therapeutic class: Antihistamine/decongestant

Normal laboratory values for blood tests

The table below shows normal laboratory values for commonly ordered blood tests. Results may vary slightly among laboratories. Many of these values are monitored regularly to assess patient response and drug efficacy.

Hematology

White blood cell count
4,100 to 10,900/mm^3

Red blood cell count
Men: 4.5 to 6.2 million/mm^3
Women: 4.2 to 5.4 million/mm^3

Hemoglobin
Men: 14 to 18 g/dl
Women: 12 to 16 g/dl

Hematocrit
Men: 42% to 54%
Women: 38% to 46%

Platelet count
140,000 to 400,000/mm^3

Red blood cell indices
MCH: 26 to 32 pg
MCHC: 32 to 36 g/dl
MCV: 80 to 95 μm^3

Reticulocyte count
0.5% to 2% of total red blood cell count

White blood cell differential
Basophils: 0.3% to 2%
Eosinophils: 0.3% to 7%
Lymphocytes: 16.2% to 43%
Monocytes: 4% to 10%
Neutrophils: 47.6% to 76.8%

Coagulation studies

Partial thromboplastin time
60 to 70 seconds

Prothrombin time
10 to 14 seconds

International Normalized Ratio
2.0 to 3.0 in patients receiving warfarin

Bleeding time
3 to 6 minutes (template and Ivy methods)
1 to 3 minutes (Duke method)

D-Dimer
< 250 μg/L

Fibrinogen
215 to 519 mg/dl

Chemistry

Glucose
70 to 100 mg/dl

Blood urea nitrogen
8 to 20 mg/dl

Creatinine
Men: 0.8 to 1.2 mg/dl
Women: 0.6 to 1.1 mg/dl

Sodium
135 to 145 mEq/L

Potassium
3.5 to 5.0 mEq/L

Chemistry (continued)

Anion gap
8 to 16 mEq/L

Chloride
100 to 108 mEq/L

Carbon dioxide
22 to 34 mEq/L

Albumin
3.3 to 4.5 g/dl

Calcium
9 to 10.5 mg/dl

Magnesium
1.5 to 2.5 mEq/L

Phosphorus
2.5 to 4.5 mg/dl

Amylase
60 to 180 units/L

Lipase
0 to 110 units/L

Lactate dehydrogenase
48 to 115 IU/L

Lactic acid
3 to 12 mg/dl

Protein
6.0 to 8.5 g/dl

Uric acid
Men: 4.0 to 8.5 mg/dl
Women: 2.5 to 7.5 mg/dl

Erythrocyte sedimentation rate
Men: 0 to 15 mm/hour
Women: 0 to 20 mm/hour

KEY MCH: Mean corpuscular hemoglobin
MCHC: Mean corpuscular hemoglobin concentration
MCV: Mean corpuscular volume

Chemistry (continued)

Glucose-6-phosphate dehydrogenase
5 to 13 units/g hemoglobin

Hemoglobin A1c
< 6.0% of total hemoglobin

B-Type natriuretic peptide
< 100 pg/ml

Zinc
60 to 130 mcg/dl

Serotonin
Men: 21 to 321 ng/ml
Women: 0 to 420 ng/ml

Arterial blood gases

pH
7.35 to 7.45 mmHg

$Paco_2$
35 to 45 mmHg

Pao_2
75 to 100 mmHg

HCO_3^-
22 to 26 mEq/L

Sao_2
94% to 100%

Lipid studies

Low-density lipoproteins
Optimal: < 100 mg/dl
Near optimal: 100 to 129 mg/dl

High-density lipoproteins
Desirable: ≥ 60 mg/dl

Total cholesterol
Desirable: < 200 mg/dl

Triglycerides
Desirable: < 200 mg/dl

Liver function studies

Alanine aminotransferase
Men: 10 to 35 units/L
Women: 9 to 24 units/L

Alkaline phosphatase
39 to 117 units/L

Aspartate aminotransferase
Men: 8 to 20 units/L
Women: 5 to 40 units/L

Serum bilirubin
Direct: ≤ 0.4 mg/dl
Indirect: ≤ 1.3 mg/dl
Total: ≤ 1.3 mg/dl

Cardiac studies

Cardiac troponin I
< 1.0 μg/ml

Creatine kinase (CK)
Total CK—
- Men: 54 to 186 IU/L
- Women: 41 to 117 IU/L

Isoenzymes—
- CK-MM: 96% to 100% of total
- CK-MB: 0% to 4% of total
- CK-BB: 0% of total

High sensitivity C-reactive protein
Low cardiovascular risk: < 1.0 mg/L
Average cardiovascular risk: 1.0 to 3.0 mg/L

Prostate studies

Prostate-specific antigen
≤ 4 ng/ml

Prostatic acid phosphatase
< 0 to 2.7 ng/ml

Thyroid studies

Triiodothyronine (T_3)
60 to 181 ng/dl

Thyroxine (T_4)
4.5 to 12.5 mcg/dl

Thyroid-stimulating hormone
0.5 to 4.70 microIU/ml

Parathyroid hormone, intact
Ages 2 to 20 years: 9 to 52 pg/ml
Older than age 20: 8 to 97 pg/ml

Lymphocyte surface markers

CD3
Absolute: 840 to 3,060 cells/μL
Percentage: 57% to 85%

CD4
Absolute: 490 to 1,740 cells/μL
Percentage: 30% to 61%

CD8
Absolute: 180 to 1,170 cells/μL
Percentage: 12% to 42%

Helper: suppressor (CD4: CD8) ratio
0.86 to 5

(continued)

Normal laboratory values for blood tests (continued)

Iron studies

Serum iron
40 to 180 mcg/dl

Ferritin
Men: 18 to 270 μg/ml
Women: 18 to 160 μg/ml

Iron-binding capacity
200 to 450 mcg/dl

Transferrin
88 to 341 mg/dl

Transferrin saturation
12% to 57%

Hormone studies

Growth hormone
Age 1 day: 5 to 53 ng/ml
Age 1 week: 5 to 27 ng/ml
Age 1 to 12 months: 2 to 10 ng/ml
Age 1 year and older: < 5 ng/ml

Estradiol
Men: < 50 pg/ml
Women: Menstruating (day of cycle relative to LH peak) —
- Follicular (-12): 19 to 83 pg/ml
- Follicular (-4): 64 to 183 pg/ml
- Midcycle (-1): 150 to 528 pg/ml
- Luteal (+2): 58 to 157 pg/ml
- Luteal (+6): 60 to 211 pg/ml
- Luteal (+12): 55 to 150 pg/ml

Postmenopausal (no treatment): 0 to 31 pg/ml

Testosterone
Males > age 18: 241 to 827 ng/dl
Females > age 18: 14 to 76 ng/dl

Body surface area in adults

To estimate an adult's body surface area (BSA) with the nomogram below, use a straightedge to connect the patient's weight in the right column with height in the left column. The point of intersection in the middle column is the BSA. For example, a patient who weighs 120 lb and is 62" tall has a BSA of 1.60 m².

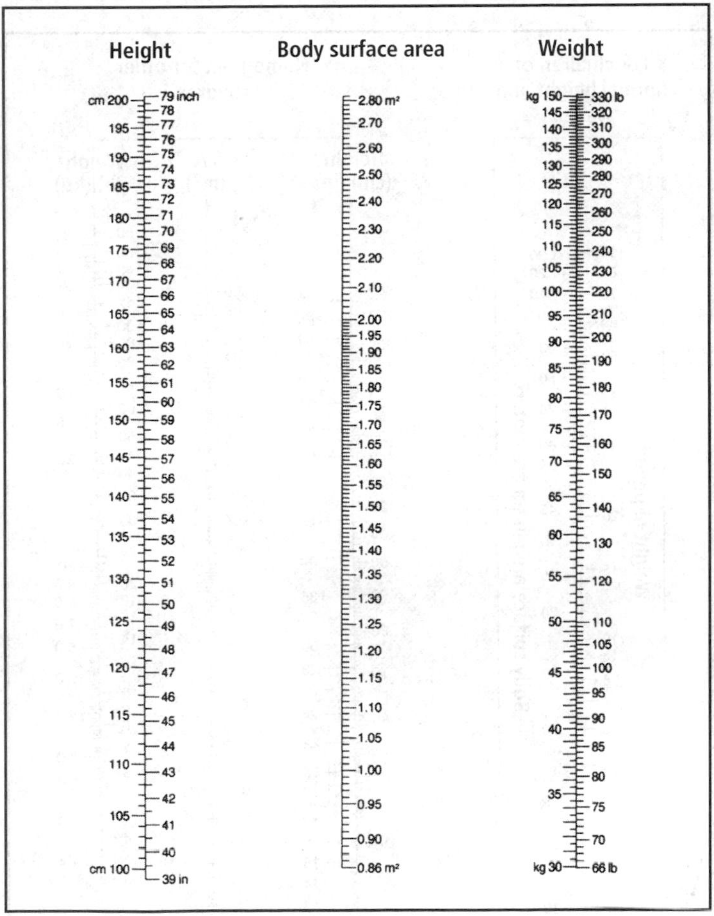

Height

cm 200 – 79 inch, 78, 77, 195, 76, 75, 190, 74, 73, 185, 72, 71, 180, 70, 69, 175, 68, 67, 170, 66, 65, 165, 64, 63, 160, 62, 61, 155, 60, 59, 150, 58, 57, 145, 56, 55, 140, 54, 53, 135, 52, 51, 130, 50, 49, 125, 48, 47, 120, 46, 45, 115, 44, 43, 110, 42, 41, 105, 40, cm 100 – 39 in

Body surface area

2.80 m², 2.70, 2.60, 2.50, 2.40, 2.30, 2.20, 2.10, 2.00, 1.95, 1.90, 1.85, 1.80, 1.75, 1.70, 1.65, 1.60, 1.55, 1.50, 1.45, 1.40, 1.35, 1.30, 1.25, 1.20, 1.15, 1.10, 1.05, 1.00, 0.95, 0.90, 0.86 m²

Weight

kg 150 – 330 lb, 145, 320, 140, 310, 135, 300, 290, 130, 280, 125, 270, 120, 260, 115, 250, 110, 240, 105, 230, 100, 220, 95, 210, 90, 200, 85, 190, 180, 80, 170, 75, 160, 70, 150, 65, 140, 60, 130, 55, 120, 50, 110, 105, 45, 100, 95, 90, 40, 85, 80, 35, 75, 70, kg 30 – 66 lb

From Lentner, C. (1981). *Geigy Scientific Tables: Units of Measurement, Body Fluid, Composition of Body, and Nutrition* (8th ed.). Basel, Switzerland: Novartis Medical Education. Used with permission from Icon Learning Systems, a division of MediMedia USA, Inc.

Body surface area in children

For children of average size, you can estimate body surface area (BSA) by using the nomogram on the left. Simply find the child's weight in pounds and then read across to the corresponding BSA on the right. For other children, use the nomogram on the right. With a straightedge, connect the patient's weight in the right column with height in the left column; the point of intersection in the middle column is the BSA.

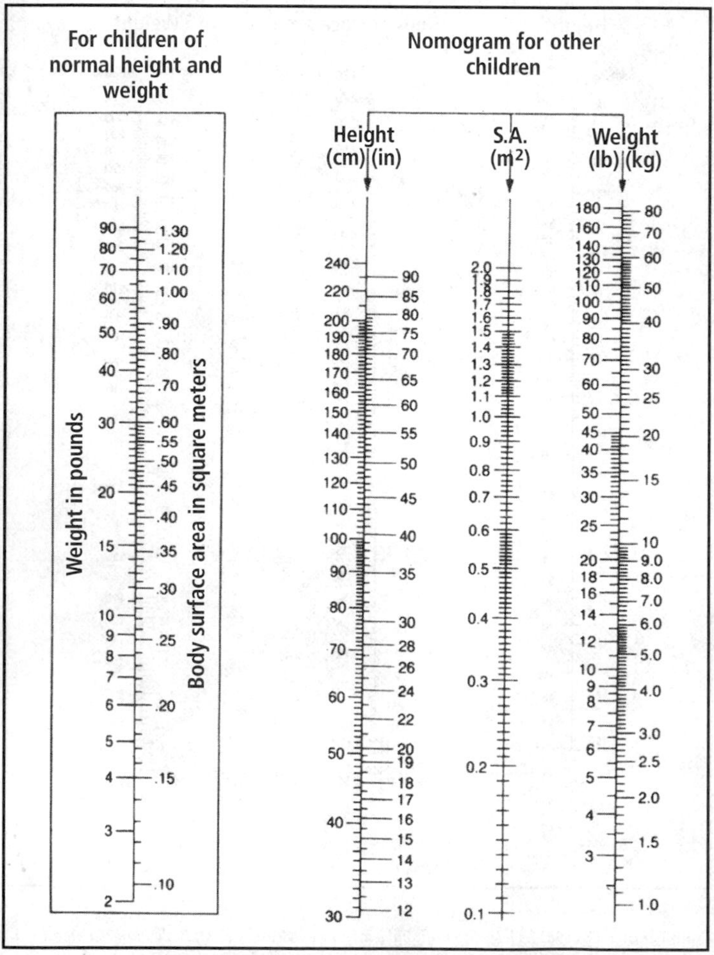

For children of normal height and weight

Weight in pounds	Body surface area in square meters
90	1.30
80	1.20
70	1.10
60	1.00
50	.90
	.80
40	.70
30	.60
	.55
	.50
20	.45
	.40
15	.35
	.30
10	
9	.25
8	
7	
6	.20
5	
4	.15
3	
	.10
2	

Nomogram for other children

Height (cm) (in): 240, 220, 200, 190, 180, 170, 160, 150, 140, 130, 120, 110, 100, 90, 80, 70, 60, 50, 40, 30 cm; 90, 85, 80, 75, 70, 65, 60, 55, 50, 45, 40, 35, 30, 28, 26, 24, 22, 20, 19, 18, 17, 16, 15, 14, 13, 12 in

S.A. (m^2): 2.0, 1.9, 1.8, 1.7, 1.6, 1.5, 1.4, 1.3, 1.2, 1.1, 1.0, 0.9, 0.8, 0.7, 0.6, 0.5, 0.4, 0.3, 0.2, 0.1

Weight (lb) (kg): 180, 160, 140, 130, 120, 110, 100, 90, 80, 70, 60, 50, 45, 40, 35, 30, 25, 20, 18, 16, 14, 12, 10, 9, 8, 7, 6, 5, 4, 3 lb; 80, 70, 60, 50, 40, 30, 25, 20, 15, 10, 9.0, 8.0, 7.0, 6.0, 5.0, 4.0, 3.0, 2.5, 2.0, 1.5, 1.0 kg

Reprinted from Behrman, R.E., Kliegman, R.M., and Jenson, H.B., eds. *Nelson Textbook of Pediatrics* (17th ed.), 2003, with permission from Elsevier.

Drug infusion rates

The tables below show infusion rates for common drug infusions. Before using these tables as your administration guide, make sure the concentration of the prescribed infusion matches the concentration shown in the table.

Dobutamine infusion rates

Using this table, you can determine the infusion rate for an infusion containing dobutamine 250 mg mixed in 250 ml of dextrose 5% in water (1,000 mcg/ml).

Dosage (mcg/kg/ minute)	Patient's weight (kg) 40	45	50	55	60	65	70	75	80	85	90	95	100	105	110
	Infusion rate (ml/hour)														
0.5	1	1	2	2	2	2	2	2	2	3	3	3	3	3	3
1.5	4	4	5	5	5	6	6	7	7	8	8	9	9	9	10
2.5	6	7	8	8	9	10	11	11	12	13	14	14	15	16	17
5.0	12	14	15	17	18	20	21	23	24	26	27	29	30	32	33
7.5	18	20	23	25	27	29	32	34	36	38	41	43	45	47	50
10.0	24	27	30	33	36	39	42	45	48	51	54	57	60	63	66
12.5	30	34	38	41	45	49	53	56	60	64	68	71	75	79	83
15.0	36	41	45	50	54	59	63	68	72	77	81	86	90	95	99
20.0	48	54	60	66	72	78	84	90	96	102	108	114	120	126	132
25.0	60	68	75	83	90	98	105	113	120	128	135	143	150	158	165
30.0	72	81	90	99	108	117	126	135	144	153	162	171	180	189	198
35.0	84	95	105	116	126	137	147	158	168	179	189	200	210	221	231
40.0	96	108	120	132	144	156	168	180	192	204	216	228	240	252	264

Nitroprusside infusion rates

Using this table, you can determine the infusion rate for an infusion containing nitroprusside 50 mg in 250 ml of dextrose 5% in water (200 mcg/ml).

Dosage (mcg/kg/ minute)	Patient's weight (kg) 40	45	50	55	60	65	70	75	80	85	90	95	100	105	110
	Infusion rate (ml/hour)														
0.3	4	4	5	5	5	6	6	7	7	8	8	9	9	9	10
0.5	6	7	8	8	9	10	11	11	12	13	14	14	15	16	17
1.0	12	14	15	17	18	20	21	23	24	26	27	29	30	32	33
1.5	18	20	23	25	27	29	32	34	36	38	41	43	45	47	50
2.0	24	27	30	33	36	39	42	45	48	51	54	57	60	63	66
3.0	36	41	45	50	54	59	63	68	72	77	81	86	90	95	99
4.0	48	54	60	66	72	78	84	90	96	102	108	114	120	126	132
5.0	60	68	75	83	90	98	105	113	120	128	135	143	150	158	165
6.0	72	81	90	99	108	117	126	135	144	153	162	171	180	189	198
7.0	84	95	105	116	126	137	147	158	168	179	189	200	210	221	231
8.0	96	108	120	132	144	156	168	180	192	204	216	228	240	252	264
9.0	108	122	135	149	162	176	189	203	216	230	243	257	270	284	297
10.0	120	135	150	165	180	195	210	225	240	255	270	285	300	315	330

(continued)

Drug infusion rates (continued)

Dopamine infusion rates

Using this table, you can determine the infusion rate for an infusion containing dopamine 400 mg in 250 ml of dextrose 5% in water (1,600 mcg/ml).

Dosage (mcg/kg/ minute)	Patient's weight (kg)													
	40	45	50	55	60	65	70	75	80	85	90	95	100	105
	Infusion rate (ml/hour)													
0.5	1	1	1	1	1	1	1	1	2	2	2	2	2	2
1.5	2	3	3	3	3	4	4	4	5	5	5	6	6	6
2.5	4	4	5	5	6	6	7	7	8	8	8	9	9	10
5.0	8	8	9	10	11	12	13	14	15	16	17	18	19	20
7.5	11	13	14	15	17	18	20	21	23	24	25	27	28	30
10.0	15	17	19	21	23	24	26	28	30	32	34	36	38	39
12.5	19	21	23	26	28	30	33	35	38	40	42	45	47	49
15.0	23	25	28	31	34	37	39	42	45	48	51	53	56	59
20.0	30	34	38	41	45	49	53	56	60	64	68	71	75	79
25.0	38	42	47	52	56	61	66	70	75	80	84	89	94	98
30.0	45	51	56	62	67	73	79	84	90	96	101	107	113	118
35.0	53	59	66	72	79	85	92	98	105	112	118	125	131	138
40.0	60	68	75	83	90	98	105	113	120	128	135	143	150	158
45.0	68	76	84	93	101	110	118	127	135	143	152	160	169	177
50.0	75	84	94	103	113	122	131	141	150	159	169	178	188	197

Nitroglycerin infusion rates

When infusing nitroglycerin, first find the prescribed concentration and then determine the infusion rate in ml/hour.

Dosage (mcg/minute)	Nitroglycerin 25 mg/250 ml D_5W (100 mcg/ml) Infusion rate (ml/hour)	Nitroglycerin 50 mg/250 ml D_5W (200 mcg/ml) Infusion rate (ml/hour)
5	3	2
10	6	3
15	9	5
20	12	6
25	15	8
30	18	9
40	24	12
50	30	15
60	36	18
70	42	21
80	48	24
90	54	27
100	60	30

KEY D_5W: dextrose 5% in water

Epinephrine infusion rates

Use this table to determine the rate at which to infuse epinephrine 1 mg in 250 ml of dextrose 5% in water (4 mcg/ml).

Dosage (mcg/minute)	Infusion rate (ml/hour)
1	15
2	30
3	45
4	60
5	75
6	90
7	105
8	120
9	135
10	150
15	225

Phenylephrine infusion rates

Using this table, you can determine the infusion rate for an infusion containing phenylephrine 20 mg in 250 ml of dextrose 5% in water or normal saline solution (80 mcg/ml).

Dosage (mcg/minute)	Rate (ml/hour)
9	7
11	8
12	9
13	10
15	11
16	12
17	13
19	14
20	15
21	16
23	17
24	18
25	19
27	20
29	22
32	24
35	26
37	28
40	30
43	32
45	34
48	36
51	38
53	40

Identifying life-threatening adverse reactions

Early recognition of a life-threatening adverse drug reaction is a crucial aspect of patient care and safety. This appendix helps you identify life-threatening adverse reactions that are relatively rare or cause symptoms you may not be readily familiar with. Some reactions are potentially lethal from the onset; others can become lethal if they progress.

Acute pancreatitis

Inflammation of the pancreas
Signs and symptoms: sudden onset of epigastric pain, nausea, and vomiting

Acute respiratory distress syndrome (ARDS)

Respiratory insufficiency in which abnormal permeability of the alveolar-capillary membrane causes fluid to fill the alveoli, disrupting gas exchange
Signs and symptoms: dyspnea, tachypnea, and progressive hypoxemia despite oxygen therapy; pulmonary edema

Adrenal suppression

Condition marked by inhibition of one or more of the enzymes essential to adrenocortical hormone production
Signs and symptoms: weakness, fatigue, abdominal pain, appetite and weight loss, dizziness, orthostatic hypotension, increased skin pigmentation

Adynamic ileus

Intestinal obstruction caused by a reduction in intestinal motility
Signs and symptoms: nausea, vomiting, decreased or absent bowel sounds, abdominal distention

Agranulocytopenia

Acute condition caused by deficiencies of neutrophils, basophils, and eosinophils in the blood
Signs and symptoms: chills, fever, headache, malaise, weakness, fatigue

Alkalosis

Increase in blood alkalinity caused by buildup of alkalis or reduction of acids
Signs and symptoms: in metabolic alkalosis—apathy, confusion, stupor (when severe); in respiratory alkalosis—air hunger, muscle twitching, numbness or tingling of extremities or circumoral area

Amyloidosis

Metabolic disorder caused by deposition of protein-containing fibrils in tissues, which may attack the heart and blood vessels, brain, kidneys, liver, spleen, intestines, or endocrine glands
Signs and symptoms: vary with area of invasion

Anaphylactoid shock

Hypersensitivity reaction marked by acute airway obstruction and vascular collapse within minutes of exposure to an antigen
Signs and symptoms: edema, rash, tachycardia, hypotension, respiratory distress, seizures, unconsciousness

Anaphylaxis

Hypersensitivity reaction to an antigen to which the patient has been previously sensitized, causing sudden release of immunologic mediators either locally or throughout the body
Signs and symptoms: urticaria, angioedema, flushing, wheezing, dyspnea, increased mucus production, nausea, vomiting

Angioedema
Vascular reaction involving deep dermal, submucosal, or subcutaneous tissues in which capillaries become dilated and more permeable; also called angioneurotic edema
Signs and symptoms: edema of skin, mucous membranes, and internal organs; urticaria; giant wheals; respiratory distress

Autoimmune phenomena
Immunologic responses, such as serum sickness, lupus, vasculitis, and hepatitis, associated with development of antibodies (as to a particular drug)
Signs and symptoms: possibly none; or signs and symptoms specific to the particular autoimmune condition

Bone marrow depression
Disruption of healthy blood cell development in the bone marrow (including red and white blood cells and platelets), which impairs or weakens the body's defense against pathogenic organisms, toxins, and irritants
Signs and symptoms: increased susceptibility to infection, fever, weakness

Cardiac tamponade
Condition marked by increased cardiac pressure, which inhibits filling of the heart chambers during diastole
Signs and symptoms: chest pain, weak peripheral pulses, distended neck veins, dyspnea, orthopnea, diaphoresis, anxiety, restlessness, pallor

Cardiomyopathy
Any disease or disorder of the heart that impairs normal cardiac performance
Signs and symptoms: shortness of breath, orthopnea, fatigue, chest pain, syncope

Cardiotoxicity
The quality of being poisonous or harmful to the heart (as with certain drugs)
Signs and symptoms: variable cardiac-related symptoms

Cardiovascular collapse
Sudden loss of effective blood flow to body tissues
Signs and symptoms: hypotension, vasovagal syncope, cardiogenic shock, cardiac arrest

Cerebral ischemia
Temporary lack of arterial or circulatory blood flow to the brain, possibly causing localized tissue death
Signs and symptoms: persistent focal neurologic deficit in the area of distribution of the involved cerebral artery

Chemical arachnoiditis
Inflammation of the arachnoid (middle) layer of the meninges of the brain and spinal cord in response to exposure to a toxic substance
Signs and symptoms: mild nausea or vomiting, headache, fever, neck or back pain and stiffness

Cholesterol embolism
Sudden obstruction of a blood vessel by cholesterol-containing plaques
Signs and symptoms: hypotension, sudden shortness of breath, weak pulse, cyanosis, chest pain, decreased level of consciousness

Disseminated intravascular coagulation
Disorder marked by abnormal activation of coagulation factors in the blood, causing hemostasis, thrombosis, and possibly, organ damage
Signs and symptoms: bleeding (possibly from multiple sites), hematomas, thrombosis, petechiae, ecchymosis, cutaneous oozing

Disulfiram-like reaction
Acute, unpleasant reaction to alcohol ingestion in a patient taking disulfiram (Antabuse) for alcohol aversion therapy
Signs and symptoms: flushing, dyspnea, headache, nausea, copious vomiting, blood pressure fluctuations

(continued)

Identifying life-threatening adverse reactions (continued)

Encephalopathy

Generalized dysfunction of the brain
Signs and symptoms: impaired speech, orientation, or cognition; sluggish reaction to stimuli

Eosinophilic pneumonitis

Infiltration of pulmonary alveoli by large numbers of eosinophils and mononuclear cells, causing inflammation
Signs and symptoms: dyspnea, cough, fever, night sweats, pulmonary edema, weight loss

Epileptiform seizures

Sudden, uncontrolled electrical discharge from the cerebral cortex caused by epilepsy
Signs and symptoms: variable; may include a cry, a fall, unconsciousness, overt seizure, amnesia, or incontinence

Erythema multiforme

Hypersensitivity reaction of the skin and mucous membranes; may take a severe multisystemic form
Signs and symptoms: rash, macules, papules, or blisters on the face, palms, and extremities

Fanconi syndrome

Congenital form of anemia caused by excessive amino acids in the blood secondary to renal tubular failure
Signs and symptoms: polyuria; growth impairment; soft, flexible, brittle bones

Granulocytopenia

Abnormal reduction in the number of granulocytes in the blood
Signs and symptoms: increased susceptibility to infection

Heart block

Interference with the normal electrical impulses of the heart, classified by the level of impairment that results (first-, second-, or-third-degree block)
Signs and symptoms: prolonged PR interval, widened QRS interval, and delayed or dropped beats on ECG; other symptoms vary with the degree of heart block and may include dizziness, syncope, shortness of breath, fatigue, and orthostatic hypotension

Hepatomegaly

Liver enlargement
Signs and symptoms: possibly none; or abdominal distention, abdominal pain, and constipation

Hepatotoxicity

Liver inflammation caused by exposure to a toxin or a toxic amount of a substance in the body
Signs and symptoms: jaundice, fatigue, weakness, altered mental status

Hyperkalemia

A condition marked by an excessive amount of potassium in the blood
Signs and symptoms: possibly none; with severe hyperkalemia—muscle weakness, arrhythmias

Hypertensive crisis

Severe blood pressure elevation, usually defined as diastolic pressure higher than 130 mmHg
Signs and symptoms: severe headache, dizziness, light-headedness

Hypertonia

Excessive tension or pressure within a muscle or an artery
Signs and symptoms: muscle pain and spasms

Impaired myocardial contractility

Decreased contractile ability of the middle layer of the heart muscle wall
Signs and symptoms: shortness of breath, chest pain, edema

Increased intracranial pressure
Increased pressure within the brain, as from increased cerebrospinal fluid pressure or a brain lesion or swelling; also called intracranial hypertension
Signs and symptoms: in infants—bulging fontanel, separated sutures, lethargy, vomiting; in older children and adults—lethargy, vomiting, headache, behavior changes, seizures, neurologic deficits, progressive decrease in level of consciousness

Interstitial pneumonia
Chronic, noninfectious inflammation of the pulmonary alveolar walls
Signs and symptoms: shortness of breath, either with activity or at rest

Ischemic colitis
Inflammation of the colon caused by lack of blood supply to mesenteric arteries of the small intestine
Signs and symptoms: abdominal pain, weight loss

Lactic acidosis
Accumulation of lactic acid in the blood caused by reduced oxygenation and perfusion to tissues, muscles, and major organs
Signs and symptoms: muscle pain, fatigue, hyperventilation, nausea, vomiting, dizziness, light-headedness

Leukocytosis
Abnormal increase in the number of white blood cells (leukocytes) in the blood
Signs and symptoms: fever, hemorrhage

Leukopenia
Abnormal reduction (below 5,000 cells/mm^3) in circulating white blood cells, as from drug-induced impairment of blood cell production
Signs and symptoms: infection, fever, stomatitis, sinusitis

Lupuslike syndrome
A syndrome similar to systemic lupus erythematosus that occurs in response to drug therapy and resolves when the drug is withdrawn
Signs and symptoms: fever; red, scaly, macular skin rash; joint inflammation

Lupus nephritis
Kidney inflammation associated with systemic lupus erythematosus (SLE), marked by deposition of antigen-antibody complexes in the mesangium and basement membrane
Signs and symptoms: hypertension, peripheral edema, proteinuria, renal failure, cardiac decompensation, other symptoms of active SLE (such as fatigue, fever, rash, arthritis, CNS disease)

Megaloblastic anemia
Anemia marked by production and proliferation of megaloblasts (large immature red blood cells) in the bone marrow or circulation
Signs and symptoms: weakness, fatigue, light-headedness, headache, rapid pulse, breathlessness

Metabolic acidosis
Increase in blood acidity caused by buildup of acids or loss of bicarbonate
Signs and symptoms: lethargy, drowsiness, headache, diminished muscle tone and reflexes, hyperventilation, arrhythmias, nausea, vomiting, diarrhea, abdominal pain

Methemoglobinemia
Condition in which a portion of the iron component of hemoglobin has been oxidized to the ferric state, making it incapable of transporting oxygen
Signs and symptoms: cyanosis, dizziness, drowsiness, headache

Neoplasm
Abnormal growth of new tissue, such as a tumor
Signs and symptoms: vary with tumor site

(continued)

Identifying life-threatening adverse reactions (continued)

Nephrotoxicity
The quality of causing damage to the kidney (as from a drug); usually leads to increased permeability to proteins, which results in edema and hypoalbuminemia
Signs and symptoms: proteinuria, hematuria, fluid retention

Neuroleptic malignant syndrome
Reaction to a drug that alters the brain's dopamine level or to withdrawal of a drug that increases the dopamine level
Signs and symptoms: sweating, altered mental status, seizures, renal failure

Neutropenia
Abnormal decrease in the level of neutrophils in the blood (usually below 1,500 per μL)
Signs and symptoms: infection, fever, mouth and throat sores

Osmotic nephrosis
Disruption of osmotic pressure in the kidney's renal tubule
Signs and symptoms: fluid retention, edema

Pancytopenia
Deficiency of all cellular elements of the blood, including red blood cells, white blood cells, and platelets
Signs and symptoms: bleeding from the nose and gums, easy bruising, fatigue, shortness of breath

Papilledema
Swelling and inflammation of the optic nerve
Signs and symptoms: severe headache, visual disturbances, blindness

Pericardial effusion
Escape of fluid from blood vessels into the pericardium
Signs and symptoms: hypotension, tachycardia, muffled heart sounds, decreased breath sounds, distended jugular vein, pulsus paradoxus, widened pulse pressure, weak peripheral pulses, pericardial friction rub, tachypnea, edema, cyanosis

Pseudomembranous colitis
Condition in which an inflammatory exudate forms on epithelial tissues of the colon
Signs and symptoms: diarrhea with blood and mucus, abdominal cramps

Pseudotumor cerebri
Benign intracranial hypertension without evidence of a brain tumor
Signs and symptoms: headache, papilledema, elevated cerebrospinal fluid pressure

Pulmonary toxicity
The quality of causing damage to the lungs and alveoli (as from certain drugs)
Signs and symptoms: any respiratory sign or symptom

Renal acidosis
Acidosis caused by accumulation of phosphoric and sulfuric acids in the body, which the kidneys fail to excrete
Signs and symptoms: appetite loss, altered level of consciousness, altered respiratory rate or effort

Renal failure
Condition marked by a serum creatinine increase of 25% or more, which impairs the kidney's ability to excrete wastes, concentrate urine, and conserve electrolytes
Signs and symptoms: dehydration, fluid overload, altered neurologic status, appetite loss, weight gain, bleeding

Respiratory acidosis
Acidosis resulting from accumulation and retention of carbon dioxide in the lungs
Signs and symptoms: dyspnea, diaphoresis, tremors, decreased reflexes, decreased level of consciousness

Rhabdomyolysis
Acute disorder in which byproducts of skeletal muscle destruction accumulate in the renal tubules, causing renal failure
Signs and symptoms: See "Hyperkalemia" and "Metabolic acidosis."

Salicylate toxicity
Toxic condition caused by overdose of a salicylate, such as aspirin or an aspirin derivative
Signs and symptoms: rapid breathing, irritability, headache, vomiting, and (if extreme) seizures and respiratory failure

Sarcoidosis
Multisystemic disease that causes granulomatous lesions of organs or tissues throughout the body
Signs and symptoms: fatigue, weight loss, shortness of breath, anorexia, skin lesions, cough, skeletal changes (in later stages)

Sepsis
Systemic inflammatory response caused by pathogenic microorganisms or their toxins
Signs and symptoms: tachycardia, fever, rapid breathing, hypothermia, evidence of reduced blood flow to major organs

Serotonin syndrome
Syndrome marked by changes in autonomic, neuromotor, and cognitive-behavioral function, resulting from increased serotonergic stimulation (as from certain drugs)
Signs and symptoms: fever, tremors, myoclonus, diaphoresis, agitation, muscle rigidity, chills, hyperreflexia

Serum sickness
Hypersensitivity reaction to administration of a nonprotein drug
Signs and symptoms: fever, rash, joint pain, edema, lymphadenopathy

Steatosis
Fatty liver degeneration
Signs and symptoms: possibly none; or right upper abdominal quadrant pain, abdominal discomfort, fatigue, malaise

Stevens-Johnson syndrome
Severe allergic reaction marked by severe skin and mucous membrane lesions, most often in response to a drug
Signs and symptoms: respiratory tract infection, fever, sore throat, chills, headache, malaise, vomiting, diarrhea, tachycardia, hypotension, corneal ulcers, conjunctivitis, epistaxis, dysuria, erosive vulvovaginitis, balanitis, seizures, altered level of consciousness, coma

Suicidal ideation
Thoughts of intentionally ending one's life
Signs and symptoms: depressed mood, giving away of possessions, statements indicating a wish to die, risk-taking behavior, alcohol or drug abuse

Sulfone syndrome
Syndrome resulting from sensitivity to the drug dapsone
Signs and symptoms: fever, rash, jaundice, anemia, mucocutaneous pemphigus lesions

Syndrome of inappropriate antidiuretic hormone secretion
Metabolic disturbance marked by an increase in antidiuretic hormone, which causes a decrease in serum sodium concentration
Signs and symptoms: weakness, fatigue, malaise, headache, altered mental status, lethargy, irritability, delirium, psychosis, personality changes, anorexia, nausea, vomiting, thirst, abdominal and muscle cramps

(continued)

Identifying life-threatening adverse reactions (continued)

Tardive dyskinesia

Disorder marked by slow, rhythmic involuntary movements of the face, limbs, and torso in patients who have received long-term dopaminergic antagonist therapy
Signs and symptoms: involuntary, repetitive facial grimacing and twisting; tongue protrusion; lip puckering and smacking; chewing or sucking motions; involuntary, snakelike writhing movements (such as wiggling or twisting); excessive blinking; involuntary flexion and extension movements of the fingers and hands

Tetany

Hyperexcitability of nerves and muscles caused by a decrease in extracellular calcium
Signs and symptoms: muscle twitching, cramps, sharp flexion of wrist and ankle joints, seizures

Thrombocytopenia

Abnormal decrease in the number of platelets caused by destruction of erythroid tissue in the bone marrow
Signs and symptoms: purpura, ecchymosis, petechiae, internal hemorrhage, hematuria, abdominal distention, melena

Torsade de pointes

Rapid form of ventricular tachycardia that appears as twisting or shifting QRS complexes on the ECG
Signs and symptoms: pallor, diaphoresis, rapid pulse, low or normal blood pressure, transient or prolonged loss of consciousness

Toxic epidermal necrolysis

Exfoliative skin condition that represents a severe cutaneous reaction (as to a drug, infection, or chemical exposure)
Signs and symptoms: scalded appearance of the skin, skin erosion and redness

Vascular leak syndrome

Leakage of blood from arteries, veins, and capillaries
Signs and symptoms: hypotension, bleeding, petechiae

Vascular thrombosis

Formation or presence of a blood clot in the vascular system
Signs and symptoms: vary with site of clot

Withdrawal phenomena

Physiologic changes caused by discontinuation of a drug or alcohol after prolonged use
Signs and symptoms: vary with type of substance used. In opioid withdrawal—rapid pulse and breathing, runny nose, yawning, restlessness, insomnia, fatigue, pupil dilation, nausea, vomiting, diarrhea, abdominal cramps, weakness, muscle aches, joint pain, hot and cold flushes. In benzodiazepine withdrawal—headache; aches and pains; anxiety; sleep disturbances; feelings of unreality; impaired memory; palpitations; hypersensitivity to noise, light, and touch.

Average wholesale price* per year of the top 30 brand-name drugs used by the elderly

The table below shows the annual average wholesale price per year of therapy in 2004 of the 30 most commonly prescribed brand-name drugs for the elderly. The drugs are ranked by the number of claims per year.

Brand-name drug	Dosage strength and form	Annual cost (2004)
1. Lipitor	10-mg tablet	$ 943
2. Plavix	75-mg tablet	$1,661
3. Fosamax	70-mg tablet	$ 953
4. Norvasc	5-mg tablet	$ 603
5. Celebrex	200-mg capsule	$2,273
6. Zocor	20-mg tablet	$1,747
7. Prevacid	30-mg capsule (CR)	$1,740
8. Protonix	40-mg tablet	$1,396
9. Lipitor	20-mg tablet	$1,369
10. Norvasc	10-mg tablet	$ 827
11. Toprol XL	50-mg tablet (CR)	$ 286
12. Nexium	40-mg capsule	$1,710
13. Xalatan	0.005% solution	$ 701
14. Vioxx	25-mg tablet	$1,100
15. Zocor	40-mg tablet	$1,747
16. Zoloft	50-mg tablet	$1,049
17. Evista	60-mg tablet	$1,033
18. Cozaar	50-mg tablet	$ 607
19. Combivent	1-mg aerosol	$ 957
20. Toprol XL	100-mg tablet (CR)	$ 429
21. Zocor	10-mg tablet	$1,001
22. Actonel	35-mg tablet	$ 916
23. Diovan	80-mg tablet	$ 640
24. Detrol LA	4-mg tablet	$1,220
25. Miacalcin	200 IU/actuation spray	$ 938
26. Pravachol	20-mg tablet	$1,203
27. Alphagan P	0.15% solution/5 ml	$ 535
28. Aricept	10-mg tablet	$1,893
29. Pravachol	40-mg tablet	$1,765
30. Celexa	20-mg tablet	$ 952

* = Cost per year based on average wholesale price as of 1/15/04 and calculated using the usual therapy dosage. This is not necessarily the retail price that seniors pay at the drugstore. However, it is the best measure available to examine base prices and the rate of price increases over time.

CR = Controlled-release

Source: "Annual Average Wholesale Price of the Top 30 Brand-Name Drugs Used by the Elderly" (Table A). Families USA Foundation, 2004. *Sticker Shock: Rising Prescription Drug Prices for Seniors.* Adapted and reprinted with permission.

Most commonly used drugs in nursing specialties

Nurses are often required to float to units in which they're not accustomed to working, where they might have to administer unfamiliar drugs. If you know ahead of time which drugs are most commonly used in the various nursing specialties, you'll be able to increase your confidence—and reduce the chance of making a drug error. The table below shows the 10 most commonly used drugs in nine nursing specialties.

Specialty	Top 10 drugs
Critical care nursing	amiodarone hydrochloride diltiazem hydrochloride dopamine hydrochloride epinephrine hydrochloride furosemide insulin lorazepam morphine sulfate nitroglycerin propofol
Emergency care nursing	acetaminophen aspirin diltiazem hydrochloride diphtheria and tetanus toxoids famotidine ibuprofen ketorolac levofloxacin metoclopramide nitroglycerin
Home care nursing	acetaminophen acetaminophen/oxycodone acetaminophen/propoxyphene napsylate digoxin diltiazem hydrochloride docusate sodium furosemide metformin hydrochloride potassium chloride warfarin
Long-term care nursing	carbidopa/levodopa digoxin docusate sodium donepezil hydrochloride enalapril maleate furosemide metoprolol tartrate mirtazapine pantoprazole sodium potassium chloride

Specialty	Top 10 drugs
Medical-surgical nursing	acetaminophen diltiazem hydrochloride enalapril maleate furosemide heparin sodium insulin levofloxacin metoprolol tartrate morphine sulfate potassium chloride
Obstetric nursing	acetaminophen/codeine acetaminophen/oxycodone dinoprostone ibuprofen magnesium sulfate nalbuphine hydrochloride oxytocin penicillin promethazine hydrochloride terbutaline sulfate
Pediatric nursing	albuterol amoxicillin/clavulanate potassium amoxicillin trihydrate cetirizine hydrochloride co-trimoxazole fluticasone propionate gentamicin sulfate hydrocortisone (topical) methylphenidate hydrochloride montelukast sodium
Post-anesthesia care nursing	bupivacaine hydrochloride fentanyl citrate hydromorphone hydrochloride lidocaine hydrochloride lorazepam meperidine hydrochloride metoclopramide hydrochloride midazolam hydrochloride morphine sulfate ondansetron hydrochloride
Psychiatric nursing	carbamazepine clonazepam divalproex sodium escitalopram oxalate lithium carbonate olanzapine paroxetine hydrochloride risperidone sertraline hydrochloride venlafaxine hydrochloride

Top 200 most commonly prescribed drugs

The table below lists the top 200 most commonly prescribed drugs in the United States in 2003, based on more than three billion prescriptions written. Drugs are listed by either generic name or brand name (capitalized).

1. hydrocodone/APAP
2. Lipitor
3. Synthroid
4. atenolol
5. Zithromax
6. amoxicillin
7. furosemide
8. hydrochlorothiazide
9. Norvasc
10. lisinopril
11. alprazolam
12. Zoloft
13. Albuterol Aerosol
14. Toprol-XL
15. Zocor
16. Premarin
17. Prevacid
18. Zyrtec
19. ibuprofen
20. Levoxyl
21. propoxyphene N/APAP
22. triamterene/HCTZ
23. Celebrex
24. Ambien
25. Allegra
26. cephalexin
27. Nexium
28. Fosamax
29. Vioxx
30. Singulair
31. Ortho Tri-Cyclen
32. prednisone
33. metoprolol tartrate
34. fluoxetine
35. Effexor XR
36. Neurontin
37. lorazepam
38. clonazepam
39. Celexa
40. Viagra
41. Wellbutrin SR
42. Paxil
43. Pravachol
44. Plavix
45. Trimox
46. potassium chloride
47. Protonix
48. Advair Diskus
49. Flonase
50. metformin
51. amoxicillin/clavulanate
52. amitriptyline
53. ranitidine hydrochloride
54. acetaminophen/codeine
55. Lexapro
56. Accupril
57. Levaquin
58. Altace
59. Diovan
60. Lotrel
61. warfarin
62. omeprazole
63. cyclobenzaprine
64. Glucotrol XL
65. Diflucan
66. verapamil
67. Bextra
68. penicillin VK
69. Cozaar
70. Actos

71. trazodone
72. glyburide
73. naproxen
74. Diovan HCT
75. Coumadin
76. Ortho Evra
77. Avandia
78. Paxil CR
79. Risperdal
80. Flomax
81. Aciphex
82. Digitek
83. Cipro
84. Nasonex
85. oxycodone/APAP
86. Glucophage XR
87. Lotensin
88. Evista
89. Zyprexa
90. diltiazem hydrochloride
91. Allegra-D
92. clonidine
93. Lanoxin
94. Hyzaar
95. Amoxil
96. Actonel
97. Oxycontin
98. Cotrim
99. Xalatan
100. Tricor
101. Amaryl
102. Concerta
103. Flovent
104. Glucovance
105. Combivent
106. Adderall XR
107. Prilosec
108. Seroquel
109. Yasmin 28
110. Valtrex
111. Depakote
112. Prempro
113. carisoprodol
114. isosorbide mononitrate
115. Levothroid
116. Avapro
117. diazepam
118. Detrol LA
119. Humulin N
120. Lantus
121. Coreg
122. enalapril
123. Ultracet
124. promethazine
125. Endocet
126. gemfibrozil
127. Topamax
128. Skelaxin
129. Biaxin XL
130. Cartia XT
131. monopril
132. Zetia
133. folic acid
134. Rhinocort Aqua
135. Omnicef
136. meclizine
137. Nasacort AQ
138. Augmentin ES-600
139. Macrobid
140. temazepam
141. doxycycline hyclate
142. Imitrex
143. Necon
144. Klor-Con
145. Klor-Con M20
146. allopurinol
147. Dilantin
148. sulfamethoxazole/trimethoprim
149. Microgestin Fe
150. Humalog
151. Cefzil
152. Duragesic
153. Bactroban
154. Patanol

(continued)

Top 200 most commonly prescribed drugs (continued)

155. Humulin 70/30
156. Aricept
157. MiraLax
158. Aviane
159. Zyrtec-D
160. Ditropan XL
161. Biaxin
162. ciprofloxacin
163. Niaspan
164. Strattera
165. Inderal LA
166. Elidel
167. Pulmicort
168. Trivora-28
169. albuterol
170. nifedipine ER
171. methylprednisolone
172. Tussionex
173. Mobic
174. timolol
175. Atacand
176. phenytoin
177. Alphagan P
178. Avelox
179. clotrimazole/betamethasone
180. trimcinolone
181. Lescol XL
182. Miacalcin
183. Ortho-Novum
184. Plendil
185. promethazine/codeine
186. NitroQuick
187. spironolactone
188. terazosin
189. Proscar
190. Avalide
191. Kariva
192. Low-Ogestrel
193. Tobradex
194. Remeron
195. Roxicet
196. Percocet
197. Atrovent
198. propranolol
199. Nifediac CC
200. Apri

Adapted with permission from NDCHealth, NDC Pharmaceutical Audit Suite, 2004

Selected references

Publications

American Heart Association. *ACLS Provider Manual.* Dallas: American Heart Association, 2003.

American Heart Association. *Handbook of Emergency Cardiovascular Care for Healthcare Providers.* Dallas: American Heart Association, 2000. (Summary of 2004 revisions available at www.americanheart.org/presenter.jhtml?identifier=3023110.)

American Heart Association and American Academy of Pediatrics. *PALS Provider Manual.* Dallas: American Heart Association, 2002.

Blumenthal, M., ed. *The ABC Clinical Guide to Herbs.* New York: Thieme Medical Publishers, 2003.

Blumenthal, M., et al, eds. *The Complete German Commission E Monographs: Therapeutic Guide to Herbal Medicines.* Newton, Mass.: Integrative Medicine Communication, 1998.

Blumenthal, M., et al, eds. *Herbal Medicine: Expanded Commission E Monographs.* Newton, Mass.: Integrative Medicine Communication, 2000.

Drug Facts and Comparisons 2005, 59th ed. St. Louis: Facts and Comparisons, 2005.

Drug Information for the Health Care Professional (USP DI), vol. 1. Greenwood Village, Colo.: Micromedex Thomson Healthcare, 2004.

Hansten, P.D., and Horn, J.R. *Hansten and Horn's Drug Interactions Analysis and Management.* St Louis: Facts and Comparisons, 1999 (plus quarterly updates).

Hansten, P.D., and Horn, J.R. *The Top 100 Drug Interactions: A Guide to Patient Management,* 2005 ed. Edmonds, Wash.: H & H Publications, 2005.

Hardman, J.G., et al, eds. *Goodman & Gilman's The Pharmacological Basis of Therapeutics,* 10th ed. New York: The McGraw Hill Companies, Inc., 2001.

King Guide to Parenteral Admixtures, 2005 ed. Napa, Calif.: King Guide Publications, Inc., 2005.

Lehne, R.A. *Pharmacology for Nursing Care,* 5th ed. Philadelphia: W.B. Saunders Co., 2003.

McEvoy, G. K., et al, eds. *AHFS Drug Information 2004.* Bethesda, Md.: American Society of Health-System Pharmacists, American Hospital Formulary Service, 2004.

Mosby's Drug Consult 2005, 15th ed. St Louis: Mosby, Inc., 2005.

PDR for Herbal Medicines, 3rd ed. Montvale, N.J.: Thomson Healthcare, 2004.

Physicians' Desk Reference 2004, 58th ed. Montvale, N.J.: Thomson Healthcare, 2003.

Physicians' Desk Reference Companion Guide 2004, 58th ed. Montvale, N.J.: Thomson Healthcare, 2003.

Pickar, G.D. *Dosage Calculations*, 7th ed. Clifton Park, N.Y.: Thomson Delmar Learning, 2004.

Polovich, M., ed. *Safe Handling of Hazardous Drugs*, 3rd ed. Pittsburgh: Oncology Nursing Society, 2003.

RxFACTS: Natural Products. St. Louis: Facts and Comparisons, 2002.

Sweetman, S.C. *Martindale: The Complete Drug Reference*, 34th ed. London: Pharmaceutical Press, 2004.

Shargel, L., Wu-Pong, S., and Yu, A.B. *Applied Biopharmaceutics & Pharmacokinetics*, 5th ed. New York: McGraw-Hill Medical, 2004.

Tatro, D.S. *Drug Interaction Facts 2005 Edition.* Philadelphia: Lippincott Williams & Wilkins, 2004.

2004 Dialysis of Drugs. Ann Arbor: Mich.: Nephrology Pharmacy Associates, 2005.

Walsh C.T., and Schwartz-Bloom, R.D. *Levine's Pharmacology: Drug Actions and Reactions*, 7th ed. New York: Taylor & Francis Group, 2004.

Websites

Drugs.com (drug information): www.drugs.com

Drugs@FDA (catalog of FDA-approved drugs): www.accessdata.fda.gov/scripts/cder/drugsatfda/

Druginfonet.com (drug information): www.druginfonet.com/index.php?pageID=official.htm

Health Canada (Canadian drug product database): www.hc-sc.gc.ca/hpb/drugs-dpd

Institute for Safe Medication Practices: www.ismp.org

National Library of Medicine and National Institutes of Health (drug information): www.nlm.nih.gov/medlineplus/druginformation.html

RxList: www.rxlist.com

United States Pharmacopeia: www.usp.org

U.S. Food and Drug Administration: www.fda.gov/cder/index.html

Index

B

E

F

G

H

I

M

N

O

Q

R

S

T

V

W

XYZ

Nurses Drug Handbook.com

We as

Home

SEARCH

HOME
SAFE DRUG ADMINISTRATION
IDENTIFYING DRUGS
MOST COMMONLY USED DRUGS
DRUG APPROVALS & UPDATES
FEDERAL GUIDELINES
PATIENT TEACHING AIDS
REPORTING INCIDENTS
CONTINUING EDUCATION
ORDER DRUG HANDBOOK
MORE...

NEWS

Medication Safety for Travelers

New Warnings for Infliximab

New Public Health Advisory for Viramune

Menactra – New Vaccine for Meningococcal Disease Protection

Lunesta — New Insomnia Treatment Option

More News...

Welcome to the compar
2006 Nursing Spectrum

Here you'll find a wide assortment of the l
downloadable patient teaching aids to cus
education modules, color guidelines and c

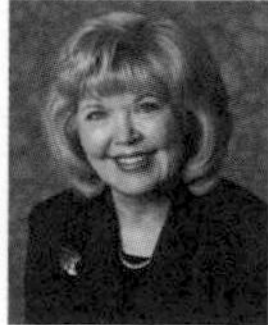

A note from th

I am happy to introduce t
2006 Nursing Spectrum
of practicing nurses, nurs
Many busy professional
Nursing Spectrum, thank
website is user-friendly, easy to navigate,
teaching materials and safety guidelines.

DRUG ALERT

New warnings for infliximab

Numerous serious adverse events have o
antibody used as a treatment for rheumat
The FDA is now requiring the manufacture
issue warnings to prescribing professiona

Nurses must be sure that patients who ta
of hepatic toxicity, including flulike sympto
and right upper quandrant pain. More...

From the Publishers of Nursing Spectrum NurseWeek

Home | Safe Drug Admin | Identifying Drugs
Federal Guidelines | Patient Teaching Aids |

WARNING: Every effort has been made to ensure that the
no guarantee is made to that effect and nursesdrughandbo